CASTLE CONNOLLY
AMERICA'S
TOP DOCTORS®
FOR CANCER

5th Edition

America's Trusted Source
For Identifying Top Doctors

Text by **DISCARDED**

John J. Connolly, Ed.D.

&

Jean Morgan, M.D.

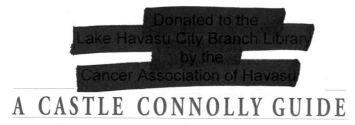

A CASTLE CONNOLLY GUIDE

The selection of medical providers for inclusion in this book was based in part on opinions solicited from physicians, and other healthcare professionals. The author and publishers cannot assure the accuracy of information provided to them by third parties, since such opinions are necessarily subjective and may be incomplete. The omission from this book of particular healthcare providers does not mean that such providers are not competent or reputable.

The purpose of this book is educational and informational. It is not intended to replace the advice of your physician or to assist the layman in diagnosing or treating illness, disease, or injury. Following the advice or recommendations set forth in this book is entirely at the reader's own risk. The author and publishers cannot ensure accuracy of, or assume responsibility for, the information in the book as such information is affected by constant change. Liability to any person or organization for any loss or damage caused by errors or omissions in this book is hereby disclaimed. Whenever possible, readers should consult their own primary care physician when selecting healthcare providers, including any selection based upon information contained in this book. In order to protect patient privacy the names of patients cited in anecdotes throughout the book have been omitted.

Reproduction in whole or part, or storage in any data retrieval system and reproduction therefrom, is strictly prohibited and violates Federal copyright and trademark laws. The contents of this book are intended for the personal use of the buyer. Use for any commercial purpose is strictly prohibited and will be pursued vigorously.

The confidence of our readers in our editorial integrity is crucial to the success of the Castle Connolly Guides. Any use of the Castle Connolly name, or of any list or listing (or portion of either) from any Castle Connolly Guide, for advertising or for any commercial purpose, without prior written consent, is strictly prohibited and may result in legal action.

For more information, please contact:

Castle Connolly Medical Ltd., 42 West 24th St, New York, New York 10010
212-367-8400x10
E-mail: info@castleconnolly.com
Web site: http://www.castleconnolly.com.
Library of Congress Catalog Card Number 2009934818
ISBN   1-883769-08-6;   978-1-883769-08-6   (paperback)
ISBN   1-883769-94-9;   978-1-883769-94-9   (hardcover)
Printed in the United States of America

Table of Contents

Table of Contents

Section III: Physician Listings by Medical Specialty

Table of Contents

America's Top Doctors® for Cancer 5th Edition

Table of Contents

America's Top Doctors® for Cancer 5th Edition

Table of Contents

Table of Contents

Table of Contents

Section IV: Appendices

Section V: Indices

America's Top Doctors® for Cancer 5th Edition

About the Publishers

John K. Castle, the Chairman of Castle Connolly Medical Ltd., has spent much of the last three decades involved with healthcare institutions and issues. Mr. Castle served as Chairman of the Board of New York Medical College for eleven years, an institution where he served on the Board of Trustees for twenty-two years.

Mr. Castle has been extensively involved in other healthcare and voluntary activities as well. He served for five years as a commissioner and officer of the Joint Commission formerly known as (JCAHO), the body which accredits most public and private hospitals throughout the United States. Mr. Castle has also served as a trustee of five different hospitals in the metropolitan New York region, including New York Presbyterian Hospital, where he continues to serve.

Mr. Castle has also served as the Chairman of the Columbia Presbyterian Science Advisory Council and as a Director of the Whitehead Institute for Biomedical Research. He is a Fellow of New York Academy of Medicine and has served as a Trustee of the Academy. He was Chairman of the United Hospital Fund of New York's Capital Campaign and continues as Director Emeritus of the United Hospital Fund. He is a Life Member of the MIT Corporation, the governing body of the Massachusetts Institute of Technology.

Mr. Castle's goal, as is the goal of Dr. John Connolly and all the Castle Connolly team, is to publish *America's Top Doctors®, America's Top Doctors® for Cancer, Top Doctors: New York Metro Area*, and other materials as well as build websites to help the public identify the very best in healthcare resources.

Mr. Castle received his bachelors degree from the Massachusetts Institute of Technology, his MBA as a Baker Scholar with High Distinction from Harvard, and two Honorary Doctorate degrees.

John J. Connolly, Ed.D. is the President & CEO of Castle Connolly Medical Ltd., and is the nation's foremost authority on identifying top physicians. Dr. Connolly's experience in healthcare is extensive.

For over a decade he served as President of New York Medical College, the nation's second largest private medical college. He is a Fellow of the New York Academy of Medicine, a Fellow of the New York Academy of Sciences, a Director of the New York Business Group on Health, a member of the President's Council of the United Hospital Fund, and a member of the Board of Advisors of Funding First, a Lasker Foundation initiative. Dr. Connolly has served as a trustee of two hospitals and as Chairman of the Board of one. He is extensively involved in healthcare and community activities and has served on a number of voluntary and corporate boards including the Board of the American Lyme Disease Foundation, of which he is a founder and past chairman, and the Board of Advisors of the Whitehead Institute for Biomedical Research. He is also a Director and Chairman of the Professional Examination Service. He holds a Bachelor of Science degree from Worcester State College, a Master's degree from the University of Connecticut, and a Doctor of Education degree in College and University Administration from Teacher's College, Columbia University.

Dr. Connolly has authored or edited nine books and has been interviewed by more than 100 television and radio stations nationwide including *Today Show*, *Good Morning America*, *20/20*, *48 Hours*, Fox Cable News, CNN, and *Weekend Today in New York*, and he and Castle Connolly have been featured in major newspapers and magazines including *The New York Times*, the *Chicago Tribune*, the *Daily News* and the *Boston Herald*, *Redbook*, *Town & Country*, *Good Housekeeping*, *Ladies Home Journal*, and regional magazines including *New York*, *Chicago*, *Philadelphia*, *Memphis*, *Palm Springs Life*, *Oklahoma*, *Pittsburgh* and *Atlanta* magazines.

Castle Connolly Medical Advisory Board

Castle Connolly Medical Ltd. is pleased to have associated with a distinguished group of medical leaders who offer invaluable advice and wisdom in our efforts to assist consumers in making good healthcare choices. We thank each member of the Medical Advisory Board for their valuable contributions.

Jeremiah A. Barondess, M.D.
President Emeritus
New York Academy of Medicine
Professor of Clinical Medicine Emeritus
Weill-Cornell Medical College

Roger Bulger, M.D.
National Institutes of Health

Menard M. Gertler, M.D., D.Sc.
Clinical Professor. of Medicine
Cornell University Med School

Arthur Hull Hayes, M.D.
Former President, E.M. Pharmaceuticals
Former Commissioner, U.S. Food & Drug Administration

Leo Henikoff, M.D.
President and CEO (retired)
Rush Presbyterian-St. Luke's Medical Center

Yutaka Kikkawa, M.D.
Professor and Chairman Emeritus
Department of Pathology, University of California,
Irvine College of Health Sciences

David Paige, M.D.
Professor
Bloomberg School of Public Health,
Johns Hopkins University

Ronald Pion, M.D.
Chairman and CEO
Medical Telecommunications Associates

Richard L. Reece, M.D.
Editor
Physician Practice Options

Leon G. Smith, M.D.
Chairman of Medicine
St. Michael's Medical Center, N.J.

Helen Smits, M.D.
Former Deputy Director
Health Care Financing Administration (HCFA)

Ralph Snyderman, M.D.
Chairman Emeritus
Duke University Health System

Foreword

Vincent T. DeVita, Jr., MD

Director, National Cancer Institute

(1980-1988)

As a physician, I've spent my professional career valuing the ability to find the right information and resources I need - quickly, efficiently and with the confidence that my sources are reliable. Similarly, healthcare consumers need to be able to find reliable information about the very best medical and healthcare services is critical, especially when confronting a diagnosis of cancer. That's why I like Castle Connolly's consumer guide, *America's Top Doctors® for Cancer*.

In creating this guide to more than 2,000 of the nation's leading medical specialists involved in the prevention, diagnosis and treatment of various cancer in both adults and children, Castle Connolly has invested a tremendous amount of time, energy and money in its research, screening and evaluation processes. To illustrate some of the complexity of doing this kind work, let me share a story with you. In my capacity as Director of the NCI from 1980 to 1988, I was often deluged with phone call requests, frequently from members of Congress or other well-placed individuals, to help them with their own personal problem with cancer or that of a friend or relative - and "pretty damn quick". They were not satisfied with just going to any doctor when their life, or the life of a friend or loved one was at stake - they wanted to know "who was doing what and where" and they wanted suggestions about the top doctors for their particular type of cancer. I often felt guilty that only a privileged few had access to this type of information. (This lack of fundamental information for the average patient is exactly what motivated Castle Connolly to start their "Top Doctors" series in 1991.)

Foreword

The National Cancer Act had been established in 1971 by an Act of the U.S. Congress as part of a national "War on Cancer." Among its mandates for National Cancer Institute (NCI) was the creation of a cancer information service to get relevant information rapidly to cancer patients. Two unique individuals deserve credit and recognition for the role that they played in creating this information service. This part of the Cancer Act mandate was actually the brainchild of the philanthropist Mary Lasker, who was also one of the main architects of the passage of the Cancer Act itself. She had her finger on the pulse of the American public and was concerned, and correctly so in my view, that researchers and organizations that supported them, like the NIH, had a tendency to ignore the practical applications of their work for the public, despite the fact that their research was paid for by tax dollars. From the time of the passage of the act, Mary Lasker pursued each subsequent National Cancer Institute Director to build this information service. In 1981, Mr. Richard Bloch, of H&R Block, then a member of the National Cancer Advisory Board, and himself a successfully treated lung cancer patient, approached the NCI Director about his dream that a patient could use computerized information services to enter their personal information and get, in return, the most up-to-date management recommendations, and names of doctors using them. He was motivated by his own experience. He had had to fight his way through the system, being told by several doctors that he was incurable before he found where to go, and the physicians to provide the treatment that ultimately cured him. It was his goal, a goal to which he dedicated the rest of his life; to see that cancer patients like him got the information they needed.

With the strong advocacy of Mary Lasker and Richard Bloch, in 1984 NCI launched the PDQ system at the National Library of Medicine. It was the first computerized database in the world, aimed at the general public, devoted to a single disease, cancer. PDQ included lists of institutions, treatment protocols, and physicians devoted to managing cancer patients, all geographically matrixed, to allow patients, regardless of their status, to find the most appropriate doctor, treatment, and or clinical trial for them anywhere in the country and in their locale as well. Ironically, this aspect of PDQ - a list of specialists that seemed so logical and necessary - was controversial. From cancer specialists themselves, we heard that since not all cancer specialists (for example Cancer Surgeons) are "certified" by boards that test their qualifications for the cancer part of their work, the PDQ lists did not include " board certification" as a selection criteria. The PDQ physician list was also constructed primarily by using input and lists from specialty organizations. By building our list with assistance from specialty organizations, we were told, we had abrogated peer review and would be including doctors who might be only marginally qualified as specialists. To identify all doctors who were capable of providing modern care for cancer patients, on an individual basis, was not within the capability of the NCI or any government or private institution at the time. And to identify who were among the most qualified to diagnosis and treat specific types of cancers was simply not within our purview. And yet we knew that finding the right doctor at the right time could be a matter of life and death.

Fast-forward to 2005 - PDQ and the Cancer Information Service have played a big part in the decline in national mortality rates from cancer in the US that began in 1990 and has continued since then. PDQ has now become a more complex information system about cancer and NCI cancer programs. But regrettably, the one thing that patients appreciated the most - the list of cancer doctors - is no longer a part of the PDQ system.

Castle Connolly's *America's Top Doctors® for Cancer* represents the much-needed and long-overdue answer for consumers – and physicians - seeking the top cancer specialists. Their physician-led Research Team has tackled some of the tough issues and developed criteria for selection, built on the foundation of Castle Connolly's well-respected national survey process that has enabled them to identify the leading physicians in more than twenty medical specialties associated with the prevention, diagnosis and treatment of cancers. The breadth and depth of the information they offer on each profiled physician will enable readers to be empowered consumers, to make informed decisions about the right doctor for their particular type of cancer. The guide also includes valuable information on some of the nation's most outstanding medical centers and specialty hospitals that are involved in the treatment of cancers.

America's Top Doctors® for Cancer will be an invaluable resource – a user-friendly, trusted source of information from an independent nationally renowned healthcare research and information company. I believe that using Castle Connolly's *America's Top Doctors® for Cancer* as a key source of information will help cancer patients and their loved ones navigate the complexities of the American healthcare system to find – and receive – the highest quality medical care.

Vincent T. DeVita, Jr., MD
Amy and Joseph Perella Professor of Medicine
Yale Cancer Center, Yale School of Medicine
(New Haven, Connecticut)
Director, National Cancer Institute (1980-1988)

Section I
Introduction

• 1 •

Cancer in the U.S. Today

If you or someone you love has been diagnosed with cancer, this book is for you. Although one in four Americans will be told they have cancer at some point during their lives, it is important to emphasize this no longer automatically carries a grim prognosis. Due to advances in treatment and, more importantly, early detection, people with cancer are living longer as well as healthier and more productive lives. While the overall quality of medical care throughout the United States is generally of very high quality, and in many places is superb, there are still those rare, complex or extremely difficult problems that demand resources beyond the ordinary or that require talents that are exceptional.

There is no denying fear is the most common reaction to the word "cancer," at least initially. Cancer has recently emerged as the leading cause of death of Americans under age 85. Bernadine Healy, M.D., former Director of the National Institutes of Health, wrote in U.S. News and World Report (Feb 14, 2005) that cancer is both "sneaky and inexplicably virulent in many of its forms." These characteristics go a long way toward making cancer even more formidable than heart disease, another major killer.

However, Dr. Healy also described how advances in identification and prevention have restrained cancer from "galloping" through our population. We are all familiar with PAP smears which can identify early forms of cervical cancer in women, or the Prostate-Specific Antigen (PSA) test for prostate cancer in men, as well as colonoscopies that permit doctors to remove potentially cancerous polyps from the colon.

Many cancers are potentially curable, provided they are detected in the early stages. Growing awareness of early warning signs and symptoms, together with advances in screening, have resulted in major improvements in cancer survival.

Many cancers are potentially curable, provided they are detected in the early stages.

Prevention is even more important. Jane E. Brody, one of the nation's leading health columnists, wrote in *The New York Times* about life-enhancing changes involving diet and exercise we can make that may enable us to live cancer-free beyond the age of 85.

At the same time that methods of diagnosis and prevention have advanced, so too has our ability to treat cancer. In fact, today, many people are completely cured or are able to cope with their cancer as a chronic disease. There are nearly 10 million cancer survivors in the U.S. alone.

Americans' risk of getting cancer and dying from cancer continues to decline and survival rates for many cancers continue to improve. The Annual Report to the Nation on the Status of Cancer, 1975-2002, which is a collaboration among the American Cancer Society (ACS), the Centers for Disease Control and Prevention (CDC), the National Cancer Institute (NCI), and the North American Association of Central Cancer Registries (NAACCR), provides updated information on cancer rates and trends in the United States, found that overall observed cancer incidence rates increased by 0.3 percent per year from 1987 to 2002, while death rates from all types of cancer combined dropped 1.1 percent per year from 1993 to 2002.

In keeping with the current hopeful climate for cancer patients, the purpose of this book is to help you approach your diagnosis and treatment in the most effective way possible.

Cancer can occur in any cell in the body when the mechanisms that regulate normal cell growth fail. As a result, the cell experiences uncontrolled and excessive growth. These rapidly multiplying cells may go on to invade local tissues or spread (metastasize) to other parts of the body.

The field of cancer research is growing in leaps and bounds. Research is essential, not only to improve current methods of treatment, but also to develop new ways of treating what had previously been considered intractable types of cancer. As medical research and technology advances, more treatments and drugs are being introduced to combat cancer. In fact, every day we can read of new developments which may give renewed hope to many cancer patients.

The huge amount of information now available about all aspects of cancer can be quite daunting. New tests, new drugs, new technology, all may present a bewildering choice for many patients. You need guidance, and also psychological support, as you navigate through this strange new world. That's why it's vital for you to consult and be treated by a physician highly experienced in and knowledgeable about your particular type of cancer.

In certain types of cancer, different specialists may combine their efforts to work together as a team. For example, in successful skull base tumor surgery, the otolaryngologist and neurological surgeon operate together.

Different major medical centers may concentrate on different types of cancer treatments, their physicians working together to provide the "team approach" as needed. In other words, you're not just selecting a single doctor, but an entire hospital for your treatment.

Research is essential, not only to improve on current methods of treatment, but also to develop new ways of treating what had previously been considered intractable types of cancer.

• 2 •

Why Top Doctors and Top Hospitals

Finding the best physicians and best hospitals for your care is a major factor in achieving the best possible outcome. The average person may not be familiar with the various medical specialties, or know what constitutes medical education and the specifics of doctor "training," that period of residencies and fellowships that follows medical school. As a result, it is difficult for most Americans to choose physicians or hospitals in a well-informed fashion. Most people still find a doctor by asking a friend for a recommendation, or picking a name from a health plan directory or even a phone book.

In addition to listing excellent physicians identified by the Castle Connolly research team through our surveys, this book will describe the process you can use to find a "top doctor" for any medical problem or need. It will also provide up-to-date information on leading hospitals, and list valuable resources for cancer patients and their families. These resources are found in the appendices.

At times, our healthcare system, while good, may seem less than consumer friendly. The United States (and Canada) has many thousands of exceptionally well-trained and dedicated professionals involved in providing the best healthcare possible. Managed care, despite its shortcomings, has brought some much-needed structure to the healthcare delivery system. Most plans require that you have a primary care physician as well as specify referrals to selected specialists and hospitals. The health plans have the ability to monitor and assess the care delivered to you at all times, regardless of provider or location, because the plan has all your medical records in order to affect appropriate payment.

Unfortunately, the advantages offered by managed care plans have too frequently been directed toward controlling costs rather than enhancing quality. The hospitals and doctors to which patients are referred for more services or complex care are often selected on the basis of cost rather than other, more medically relevant, criteria. Therefore, even though a health plan directory may list a number of "centers of excellence" and several specialists for a given problem, they may not be the best for your particular needs.

Asking your primary care physician for a referral to a specialist can be a good place to start. However, too many of us don't have a close relationship with that all important "quarterback" of our healthcare, and this type of referral also has its limitations. Is the recommendation being made on the basis of a personal or professional relationship? Is the specialist to whom you are being referred truly the best, or is he or she simply in your primary care physician's group or in the network of your health plan? Even if your primary care physician is making a referral free from outside considerations, how broad is his or her knowledge of this particular specialty? Most primary care physicians have a limited number of referral channels. They are busy caring for their own patients and rarely have the time to devote hours of research to identifying top doctors for referrals. Typically, their referral network is local rather than regional or national

If you are already under the care of an excellent specialist, and he or she refers you to another specialist or sub-specialist for a particular problem, you can be confident of a more "meaningful" referral. When physicians are continually dealing with a specific disease, such as cancer, they are usually more aware of advances in the field, as well as the names of the top practitioners.

As the patient, finding the best physicians and best hospitals for your care is your responsibility. "Get a second opinion" is a common refrain. Everyone has heard stories of patients who were told by one physician (even at a top hospital) that their case was hopeless and yet, when they continued their search, they found another doctor or hospital that provided a different plan of treatment and perhaps even a cure.

Even the best doctors and the best hospitals are not perfect. Cancer treatment, like other medical care, is a combination of art and science. Frequently, opinions on diagnosis and treatment may differ - even among top doctors. That's why it's so important for you to seek second or even third opinions when a diagnosis, even one not involving cancer, is serious or may necessitate major surgery.

Even the best doctors and the best hospitals are not perfect.
Cancer treatment is a combination of
art and science.

One of the best known and inspirational stories of a patient undertaking this kind of search is that of Lance Armstrong, the seven time Tour de France champion cyclist. When Armstrong was first diagnosed with testicular cancer he received a grim prognosis from a number of excellent physicians at some of the nation's leading cancer centers. The recommended courses of treatment would have destroyed his ability to continue competing professionally. Refusing to accept that limitation, he continued his search until he found a physician and institution that offered different treatment options. As most people know, the treatment was successful. Seven of Armstrong's cycling championships (1999-2005) have come since his recovery from cancer.

Of course, there is a difference between seeking additional medical opinions and simply bouncing around from doctor to doctor until you find one that tells you what you want to hear. You need to find a doctor, hospital and treatment plan in which you have confidence, and which you honestly believe, based on extensive research, will work for you. Depending on the circumstances, it may be possible to find another physician or hospital that can offer a superior plan, or it may be that no better treatment options currently exist.

"Hope springs eternal" is not just a trite saying. It is something that should drive every patient and every doctor, simply because there are always unexpected and sometimes unexplainable remissions or cures occurring with cancer, and new breakthroughs in treatment could be just around the corner.

There is a significant amount of evidence that patients who are optimistic and fight, rather than surrender to their disease, have generally better outcomes. A positive attitude and the support of family and friends, as well as physicians and nurses, can be an important factor in your recovery. Knowing as much as possible about your diagnosis and your treatment options is another.

Reaching an initial diagnosis usually involves a number of medical tests including x-rays, MRIs and analysis of tissue samples obtained by a biopsy. It may be necessary to repeat these tests, or perform more specialized ones, in order to gain more thorough information or firmly establish a questionable diagnosis.

In the case of breast cancer, the disease is first likely to be identified either through a mammogram or else the discovery of a lump during a routine self or physician exam. Any breast lumps need to be biopsied for confirmation of cancer. Once that occurs, you will be referred to a surgeon who has special expertise in this field. He or she will recommend one or more possible treatments, including a total mastectomy, a lumpectomy, radiation therapy and chemotherapy.

As the patient, finding the best physicians and best hospitals for your care is your responsibility.

A suspicion of prostate cancer usually occurs following evidence of an enlarged prostate or an elevated PSA test. A urologist will make a definitive diagnosis based on a biopsy and examination of that tissue by a pathologist. Once cancer is found, the urologist can treat it by removing the prostate or by radiation.

Both the breast cancer and prostate cancer patient face the same basic questions: Is the surgeon treating you the most qualified and, more importantly, is surgery the only or best solution to deal with your disease?

Just like a number of additional options exist for breast cancer, surgery is not the only way to deal with prostate cancer, and may have unwanted side effects. Other alternative treatments include radiation therapy. In addition, since prostate cancer usually develops very slowly, some patients, especially older ones, may choose "watchful waiting." However, because most patients initially see a surgeon at the time of their diagnosis, they may end up having surgery without fully exploring the other alternatives.

Knowledge is not just power; in some instances it can make all the difference in not only your long-term survival, but also the quality of your life. This is why it is essential for you to be an informed consumer and find the best possible healthcare for yourself. This book will help you find the very best doctors and hospitals to treat cancer.

Factors to Consider When Identifying a Top Doctor

1. Medical Education

2. Residency & Fellowships

3. Board Certification

4. Hospital Appointment

5. Academic and Other Professional titles

6. Insurance Accepted

7. Personality

• 3 •

How Castle Connolly Identified the Top Doctors for Cancer

Castle Connolly is best known for its series of consumer guides including *America's Top Doctors*®, and *Top Doctors: New York Metro Area*. These books list "top doctors" in their respective regions. The New York edition profiles primary care physicians as well as other specialists and sub-specialists. *America's Top Doctors*® does not include any primary care physicians, but it lists the nation's top referral specialists. The Castle Connolly Guides are trusted by consumers and physicians alike. In fact, over 50% of the physicians listed in the Guides use them to make referrals.

Doctors do not and cannot pay to be listed in any Castle Connolly Guides. They are selected based on their nomination by peers solicited through mail and phone surveys, and on an extensive review of their credentials by the Castle Connolly physician-led research team.

For *America's Top Doctors*® *for Cancer* 5th Edition, Castle Connolly sent nomination forms to all physicians listed in *America's Top Doctors*® (8th edition) and *America's Top Doctors*® *for Cancer* (4th edition). In addition, nominations were solicited from the presidents and vice presidents of over 300 of the nation's leading medical centers and specialty hospitals.

The physcians we have identified and listed are clearly among the best as nominated by their peers and screened by our research team.

Thousands of different physicians were nominated by their peers for inclusion in this guide. Of course, most of them received multiple nominations. In addition to the thousands of mail surveys, the Castle Connolly research team made hundreds of phone calls to leading specialists and sought additional nominations as well as using these conversations to reinforce the nominations received through the mail nomination process.

The Castle Connolly physician-led research team reviewed and analyzed the nominations and narrowed the field to those being considered for inclusion in *America's Top Doctors® for Cancer*. They contacted these physicians and asked them to complete an extensive biographical form describing their medical education, residencies, fellowships, hospital appointments and more. Particularly, we were interested in the physicians' area of special expertise; that is, the particular type of cancer (e.g. lung, breast, brain tumors, etc.,) or procedures (e.g. radical prostatectomy) in which the physician had particular experience, interest and expertise.

Finally, the research team checked on the disciplinary histories of the physicians by screening those that may have been disciplined by a medical board or state agency. After this intensive review, the final list was created.

The goal in creating this list was to select physicians viewed by their peers as the best in preventing, diagnosing and treating cancer and its related ramifications. Castle Connolly does not claim these are the only excellent doctors treating cancer in this country. Our nation is fortunate in having a generally excellent cadre of well-trained, dedicated physicians. The physicians we have identified and listed, however, are clearly among the very best as nominated by their peers and screened by our research team. In addition, they practice, for the most part, at major medical centers and leading specialty hospitals where they, and their patients, can receive the support of other highly skilled doctors, nurses and technicians as well as having access to the sophisticated and expensive equipment, laboratories and other resources that advance the level of cancer treatment and care from good to excellent. Furthermore, many of these physicians are engaged in teaching or research, or both. While the academic nature of their practice can limit the amount of time available to see patients, it keeps them, their colleagues and their institutions on the "cutting edge" of cancer treatment.

One important factor in our selection was geographic coverage. Some patients may be unable to travel long distances to a major medical center or specialty hospital due to financial resources, overall health status or some other reason. For them, a hospital in the immediate region is the only possible alternative. Since this is a guide for consumers and as many physicians use our guide to make referrals, we felt it was important to have broad geographic coverage and attempted to identify the top doctors for cancer in every state.

How Castle Connolly Identified the Top Doctors for Cancer

The reality is that the critical resources, the very best doctors and hospitals, are not dispersed evenly throughout the nation. For good reason they are clustered in large metropolitan areas or at academic medical centers that are part of major universities. It is only in these settings where it is possible to gather the combination of resources necessary to mount and maintain a superior medical program. The laboratories, technicians, intensive care beds, research fellows, scientists, specially trained nursing staff, equipment and, especially, the volume of patients and research subjects so necessary to enable these professional teams to continually develop and hone their skills, typically exist only in metropolitan areas or at university-based medical centers.

Therefore, it may be necessary for many Americans, if they are motivated to seek out the very best doctors and hospitals, to travel many miles, if possible, to obtain their care. It is also this reality that has motivated many outstanding medical centers and specialty hospitals to reach out and establish relationships with community hospitals throughout the nation. While it is not always possible to bring the labs, scientists, equipment and leading physicians to these communities, it is possible to raise the overall level of cancer care through these relationships.

Information on outcomes, procedure volume and malpractice is becoming increasingly available, but the public disclosure varies from state to state. Castle Connolly uses its best efforts to gather the information that is available and use it effectively. Ultimately, however, it is the professional judgment of the Castle Connolly editors, the Chief Medical and Research Officer and the research staff, which determines Castle Connolly Top Doctor™ selection.

Physicians may also be removed from the Castle Connolly lists if, in the judgment of the selection team, that is warranted. Some of the reasons physicians are removed include retirement, change in practice (taking a full time administrative post, for example), unavailability to patients, malpractice or disciplinary issues, negative physician or patient feedback, professional demeanor or a change in the "mix" of specialists Castle Connolly will present for a given community. Being removed from a Castle Connolly list does not necessarily indicate something negative about the physician. At the same time, Castle Connolly does not claim to identify every excellent physician in the nation or a region. The physicians identified through the Castle Connolly research process are clearly among the very best, but there are always other very good physicians not identified by Castle Connolly and that is why our guides, websites and other distribution channels for this critical information describe a process whereby consumers can identify excellent physicians using their own efforts.

• 4 •

Judging the Qualifications of a Physician

The National Cancer Institute (NCI) has declared its intention to eliminate suffering and death due to cancer by the year 2015. While that is clearly an ambitious goal, and one many may feel is unrealistic, it nonetheless demonstrates the optimism physicians and scientists are beginning to feel about the battle against cancer. As Ellen V. Sigal, Ph.D, founder and chairperson of Friends of Cancer Research in Washington, D.C. and a member of the National Cancer Institute's Board of Scientific Advisors, stated: "The consensus among the science community is that for the first time we understand the genetic underpinnings of this disease."

"How do you identify a top doctor?" is an important question for all Americans, not just those diagnosed with cancer. As we mentioned earlier, too many Americans are incredibly casual in selecting physicians and hospitals. They may pick a name from their health plan directory, or even from a phone book, with the location of the doctor's office being the primary factor in their selection. Others may simply ask a friend or relative and the recommendation they receive may be based on how well the person "likes" the doctor rather than on any particular medical expertise or skill.

The specialists listed in *America's Top Doctors® for Cancer* are clearly among the best in the nation and have been identified through a rigorous research process and thorough screening by the Castle Connolly physician-led research team. Through our extensive surveys and research we have done much of the work in finding a top referral specialist, but they are not the only excellent physicians in the nation.

The goal in creating this guide was to select physicians viewed by their peers as the best in preventing, diagnosing and treating cancer and its consequences.

So, how does one judge the qualifications of a physician who may not be listed in this Guide? If someone was trying to find a specialist on their own, how should they go about it? How can someone tell when a physician has the appropriate training in a specialty and how does one distinguish what is meaningful and what is not from among all those plaques and certificates on a doctor's wall?

The reality is that few of us see only one doctor in our lifetime. Each of us may be cared for by a primary care physician, an ophthalmologist, an orthopaedist, a dermatologist, a surgeon or a number of other specialists. The choices can be many and they can be among the most important choices we make.

The following pages will outline the process for selecting a well-qualified physician. In fact, what is written here reflects much of the logic that underlies the selection of physicians for this book. This section will help not only in finding a top specialist in this Guide, but it also should be helpful in choosing among the many specialists, primary care doctors and other physicians, that a person will need to consult throughout his/her life.

Education

The review of a prospective doctor's education and training should begin with medical school. While some may feel that the institution at which a physician earned a bachelor's degree could be an indication of the doctor's quality, most people in the medical field do not believe it plays a major role. A degree from a highly selective undergraduate college or university will help an aspiring doctor gain admission to a medical school, but once there, all students are peers. Furthermore, where a doctor trains (i.e. completes residency) is more important than medical school in judging quality. American medical schools are highly standardized, at least in terms of basic quality standards.

A group known as the Liaison Committee for Medical Education (LCME) accredits all U.S. medical schools that grant medical degrees (MDs) and osteopathic degrees (DOs). Most also are accredited by the appropriate state agency, if one exists, and by regional agencies that accredit colleges and universities of all kinds.

Fortunately, U.S. medical schools have universally high standards for admission, including success on the undergraduate level and on the Medical College Admissions Tests (MCATs). Although frequently criticized for being slow to change and for training too many specialists, the system of medical education in the United States has assured consistent high quality in medical practice. One recent positive change is a strong effort in most medical schools to diversify the composition of the student body. While these schools have been less successful in enrolling racial minorities, the number of women in U.S. medical schools has increased to the point that women now make up about 50 percent of most classes. In certain specialties preferred by women medical graduates (pediatrics, for example), it is possible that in coming years the majority of specialists will be female.

Most doctors practicing in the United States are graduates of U.S. medical schools, but there are two other groups of doctors who make up a significant portion (30+%) of the total physician population. They are (1) foreign nationals who graduated from foreign schools and (2) U.S. nationals who graduated from foreign schools. (Canadian medical schools are not considered foreign.)

Foreign Medical Graduates

Foreign medical schools vary greatly in quality. Even some of the oldest and finest European schools have become virtually "open door," with huge numbers of unscreened students making teaching and learning difficult. Others are excellent and provided the model for our system of medical education.

The fact that someone graduated from a foreign school does not mean that he or she is a poor doctor. Foreign schools, like those in the U.S., produce both good and poor doctors. Foreign medical graduates who wish to practice here must pass the same exam taken by U.S. graduates for licensure. It is true the failure rate for foreign graduates is significantly higher. In the first year of using the new United States Medical Licensing Exam (USMLE), 93 percent of U.S. medical school graduates passed Step II, the clinical exam, as compared with only 39 percent of the foreign graduates. It is clear that the quality of many foreign schools, if not individual doctors, is not the same as U.S. medical schools, at least as measured by our standards. Nonetheless, many communities and patients have been well served by foreign medical graduates practicing in this country—often in areas where it has been difficult to attract graduates of American schools. About 25% of practicing physicians in the U.S. today are graduates of foreign medical schools.

In addition, many foreign medical schools and their teaching hospitals are world renowned for their leadership in medical care, research and teaching, and many of the technologies and techniques we utilize in the U.S. today have been developed and perfected in foreign countries.

"How do you identify a top doctor?" is an important question for all Americans, not just those diagnosed with cancer.

Residency

Most doctors practicing today have at least three years of postgraduate training (following the MD or DO) in an approved residency program. This not only is an important step in the process of becoming a competent doctor, but it is also a requirement for board (specialty) certification. Most people assume that a prospective doctor needs to complete a three-year residency program to obtain a medical license. That is not an accurate assumption! New York State, for example, requires only one postgraduate year. However, since all approved residencies last at least three years and some, such as those in neurosurgery, general surgery, orthopaedic surgery and urology, may extend for five or more years, it is important to know the details of a doctor's training. Licensure alone is not enough of a basis on which to choose a physician.

Without undertaking extensive and detailed research on every residency program, the best assessment you can make of a doctor's residency program is to see if it took place in a large medical center whose name you recognize. The more prestigious institutions tend to attract the best medical students, sometimes regardless of the quality of the individual residency program. If in doubt about a doctor's training, ask the doctor if the residency he or she completed was in the specialty of the practice; if not, ask why not.

It is also important to be certain that a doctor completed a residency that has been approved by the appropriate governing board of the specialty, such as the American Board of Surgery, the American Board of Radiology, or the American Osteopathic Board of Pediatrics. These board groups are listed in Appendix A. If you are really concerned about a doctor's training, you should call the hospital that offered the residency and ask if the residency program was approved by the appropriate specialty group. If still in doubt, consult the publication Directory of Graduate Medical Education Programs, often called the "green book," found in medical school or hospital libraries, which lists all approved residencies.

If in doubt about a doctor's training, ask the doctor if the residency program he or she completed was in the specialty of the practice; if not, ask why not.

Board Certification

With an MD or DO degree and a license, an individual may practice in any medical specialty with or without additional specialized training. For example, doctors with a license, but no special training, may call themselves a surgeon, oncologist or radiologist. This is why board certification is such an important factor. It assures the physician has had specific training in that specialty and has passed the board exam. The American Board of Medical Specialties (ABMS) recognizes 25 specialties and more than 90 subspecialties. Visit www.abms.org or call 866-275-2267 for more information. Eighteen boards certify in 20 specialties under the aegis of the American Osteopathic Association (AOA). Visit www.osteopathic.org or call 800-621-1773 for more information. Doctors who have qualified for such specialization are called board certified; they have completed an approved residency and passed the board's exam.

(See Appendix A for an approved ABMS and AOA lists). While many doctors who are not board certified call themselves "specialists," board certification is the best standard by which to measure competence and training.

You can be confident that doctors who are board certified have, at a minimum, the proper training in their specialty and have demonstrated their proficiency through supervision and testing. While there are many non-board certified doctors who are highly competent, it is more difficult to assess the level of their training. While board certification alone does not guarantee competence, it is a standard that reflects successful completion of an appropriate training program. If it is impossible to find a doctor in your area who is board certified in a particular subspecialty, for example, Medical Oncology or Radiation Oncology, at least be certain the physician is board certified in a related specialty such as Internal Medicine or Radiology.

Board certified doctors are referred to as Diplomates of the Board. Some of the colleges of medical specialties (e.g., the American College of Radiology, the American College of Surgeons) have multiple levels of recognition. The first is basic membership and the second, more prestigious and difficult to obtain, is status as a Fellow. Fellowship status in the colleges is meaningful and is based on experience, professional achievement and recognition by one's peers, including extensive experience in patient care. It should be viewed as a significant professional qualification.

It is important to know the details of a doctor's training. Licensure alone is not enough of a basis on which to choose a physician.

Board Eligibility

Many doctors who have been more recently trained are waiting to take the boards. They are sometimes described as "board eligible," a common term that the ABMS advocates abandoning because of its ambiguity. Board eligible means that the doctor has completed an approved residency and is qualified to sit for the related board's exam. Another term that is used is "board qualified." Once again, the term has no official standing, but could mean the doctor has completed residency and is awaiting the board exam. It could also mean the doctor took and failed to pass the exam to become board certified.

Each member board of the ABMS has its own policy regarding the use and recognition of the board eligible term. Therefore, the description "board eligible" should not be viewed as a genuine qualification, especially if a doctor has been out of medical school long enough to have taken the certification exam. To the boards, a doctor is either board certified or not. Furthermore, most of the specialty boards permit unlimited attempts to pass the exam and, in some cases, doctors who have failed the exam twice or even ten times, continue to call themselves board eligible. In Osteopathic Medicine, the board eligible status is recognized only for the first six years after completion of a residency.

In addition to the approved lists of specialties and subspecialties of the ABMS and AOA, there are a wide variety of other doctors and groups of doctors who call themselves specialists. At present there are at least 100 such groups called "self-designated medical specialties." They range from doctors who are working to create a recognized body of knowledge and subspecialty training to less formal groups interested in a particular approach to the practice of medicine. These groups may or may not have standards for membership. It may be difficult to determine the true extent of their members' training, and neither the ABMS or the AOA recognizes them. While you should be cautious of doctors who claim they are specialists in these areas, many do have advanced training and the groups at least offer a listing of people interested in a particular approach to medical care. Rely on board certification to assure yourself of basic competence, and use membership in one of these groups to indicate strong interest and possible additional training in a particular aspect of medicine.

You can be confident that doctors who are board certified have, at a minimum, the proper training in their specialty and have demonstrated their proficiency through supervision and testing.

Recertification

A relatively new focus of the specialty boards is the area of recertification. Until recently, board certification lasted for an unlimited time. Now, almost all the boards have put time limits on the certification period. For example, in Internal Medicine and Radiology, the time limit is ten years. These more stringent standards reflect an increasing emphasis on recertification by both the medical boards and state agencies responsible for licensing doctors.

Since the policies of the boards vary widely, it is a good procedure to check a doctor's background to see when certification was awarded. If the date was seven to ten years ago, see if he or she has been recertified. Unfortunately, many boards permit "grandfathering," whereby already certified doctors do not have to be recertified, and recertification requirements apply only to newly certified doctors. Even if recertification is not required, it is good professional practice for doctors to undertake the process. It assures you, the patient, that they are attempting to stay current.

Many states have a continuing medical education requirement for doctors. These states typically require a minimum number of continuing medical education (CME) credits for a doctor to maintain a medical license. Seven states require 150 CME credits over a three-year period. Osteopathic doctors are required to take 120 hours of CME credits within three years to maintain certification.

Fellowships

The purpose of a fellowship is to provide advanced training in the clinical techniques and research of a particular specialty. Fellowships usually, but not always, are designed to lead to board certification in a subspecialty such as medical oncology which is a subspecialty of internal medicine. Many physicians listed in this Guide have had fellowship training. In the U.S. there are a variety of fellowship programs available to doctors, which fall into two broad categories: approved and unapproved. Approved fellowships are those that are approved by the appropriate medical specialty board (e.g., the American Board of Radiology) and lead to subspecialty certificates. Fellowship programs that are unapproved are often in the same areas of training as those that are approved, but they do not lead to subspecialty certificates.

Unfortunately, all too often, unapproved fellowships exist only to provide relatively inexpensive labor for the research and/or patient care activities of a clinical department in a medical school or hospital. In such cases, the learning that takes place is secondary and may be a good deal less than in an approved fellowship. On the other hand, any fellowship is better than none at all and some unapproved fellowships have status for a valid reason that should not reflect negatively on the program. For example, the fellowship may have been recently created, with approval being sought. There are also some areas of medicine not yet recognized for sub-specialty certification, such as Transplant Surgery.

Some physicians may have completed more than one fellowship and may be boarded in two or more subspecialties. In addition, some physicians may pursue fellowship training and subspecialty certification but then choose to practice in their primary field of certification. For example, a doctor who is board certified in internal medicine also may have obtained board certification in oncology, but may choose to practice primarily internal medicine. For the most part, the physicians in this guide practice in their sub-specialties.

Professional Reputation

There are practitioners who meet every professional standard on paper, but who are simply not good doctors. In all probability, the medical community has ascertained this and, while the individual may still practice medicine, his or her reputation will reflect that collective assessment. There are also doctors who are outstanding leaders in their fields because of research or professional activities but who are not particularly strong, or perhaps even active, in patient care. It is important to distinguish that kind of professional reputation from a reputation as a competent, caring doctor in delivering patient care or, in the case of this guide, as an outstanding practitioner in a given specialty.

Hospital Appointment

Most doctors are on the medical staff of one or more hospitals and are known as "attendings;" some, however, are not. If a doctor does not have admitting privileges or is not on the attending staff of a hospital, you may wish to consider choosing a different doctor. It can be very difficult to ascertain whether or not the lack of hospital appointment is for a good reason. For example, it is understandable that some doctors who are raising families or heading toward retirement choose not to meet the demands (meetings, committees, etc.) of being an attending. However, if you need care in a hospital, the lack of such an appointment means that another doctor will have to oversee that care. In some specialties, such as dermatology and psychiatry, doctors may conduct their entire practice in the office and a hospital appointment is not as essential, or as good a criterion for assessment, as in other specialties.

If a doctor does not have admitting privileges or is not on the attending staff of a hospital, you may wish to consider choosing a different doctor.

While mistakes are made, most hospitals are quite careful about admissions to their medical staffs. The best hospitals are highly selective, so a degree of screening (or "credentialing") has been done for you. In other words, the best doctors usually practice at the best hospitals. Since caring for a patient in a hospital is often a team effort involving a number of specialists, the reputation of the hospital to which the doctor admits patients carries special weight. Hospital medical staffs review their colleagues' credentials and authorize performance of specific procedures. In addition, they typically review and reappoint their medical staff every two or three years. In effect, this is an additional screening to protect patients. It is especially true of hospitals that have what are known as closed staffs, where it is impossible to obtain admitting privileges unless there is a vacancy that the administration and medical staff deem necessary to fill. If you are having a surgical procedure and are concerned about the doctor's skill or experience, it may be worthwhile to call the Medical Affairs Office at the doctor's hospital to see if he or she is authorized to perform that procedure in that hospital.

The reasons for a hospital's selectivity are easy to understand: no hospital wishes to expose itself to liability and every hospital wants to have the best reputation possible in order to attract patients. Obviously, the quality of the medical staff is immensely important in creating that reputation.

Physicians listed in this guide are primarily on the staffs of major medical centers, university teaching hospitals and leading specialty hospitals. Occasionally, some may be on staff at a community hospital for one or two days a week and spend the majority of their time at the teaching hospital. There are many excellent physicians on the staffs of community hospitals that call themselves "medical centers," but they are typically not physicians who attract complex cases and referrals regionally, nationally and even internationally.

To learn about a hospital, visit its website. It is also useful to review a hospital's accreditation status under the Joint Commission on the Accreditation of Healthcare Organizations at www.JCAHO.com. Also www.selectqualitycare.com offers data on hospital procedure numbers and outcome for an number of specific procedures.

A last and very important reason why a hospital appointment is an essential requirement in your choice of doctor is that some states permit doctors to practice without malpractice insurance. If you are injured as a result of a doctor's poor care, you could be without recourse. However, few hospitals permit doctors to practice in them unless they carry malpractice insurance. This not only protects the hospital, but the patient as well.

The best doctors usually practice at the best hospitals.

Medical School Faculty Appointment

Many doctors have appointments on the faculties of medical schools. There is a range of categories from "straight" appointments, meaning full-time appointment as professor, associate professor, assistant professor or instructor, to clinical ranks that may reflect lesser degrees of involvement in teaching or research. If someone carries what is known as a straight academic rank (e.g. "professor of surgery," without "clinical" in the title), this usually means that the individual is engaged full-time in medical school research, teaching activities and patient care. The title "clinical professor of surgery" usually identifies a part-time or adjunct appointment and less direct involvement in medical school activities such as teaching and research.

Doctors who are full-time academicians are more likely to be in the forefront of new techniques and research, especially when it comes to a disease like cancer. They also have the advantage of the support of other faculty, residents and medical students.

When you are seeking a subspecialist, a doctor's relationship to a medical school becomes more meaningful since medical school faculties tend to be made up of sub-specialists. You are less likely to find large numbers of general or primary care practitioners engaged full-time on a medical school faculty. The newest approaches and techniques in medicine, for the most part, are explored and developed by medical school faculties in their laboratories and clinical practice settings. This is where they practice their sub-specialties, as well as teach and conduct research.

Medical Society Membership

Most medical society memberships sound very prestigious and some are; however, there are many societies that are not selective and virtually any doctor can join. In addition, membership in many of the more prestigious societies is based on research and publication or on leadership in the field and may have little to do with direct patient care. While it is clearly an honor to be invited to join these groups, membership may be less than helpful in discerning whether a doctor can meet your needs.

Physicians listed in this guide are primarily on the staffs of major medical centers, university teaching hospitals and leading specialty hospitals.

Experience

Experience is difficult to assess. Obviously, in most cases, an older doctor has more experience; on the other hand, a younger doctor has been more recently immersed in the challenge of medical school, residency, or even a fellowship, and may be the more up-to-date. If a doctor is board certified, you may assume that assures at least a minimal amount of experience, but since it could be as little as a year, check the date of graduation from medical school or completion of residency to know precisely how long a doctor has been in practice.

There is a good deal of evidence that there is a positive relationship between quantity of experience and quality of care. That is, the more a doctor performs a procedure, the better he or she becomes at it. That is why it is important to ask a doctor about his or her experience with the procedure that you need. Does the doctor see and treat similar cases every day, every week or only rarely? Of course, with some rare diseases, "rarely" is the only possible answer, but it is the relative frequency that is critical. In some states, data is available on volume or numbers of certain procedures performed at hospitals. For volume and outcome information in other states, visit the web site of Healthcare Choices at www.healthcarechoices.org. There is a good deal of controversy, however, on the validity and usefulness of such data. Opponents cite the fact that some of the data is produced from Medicare patient records only and, therefore, is based solely on an elderly population that does not represent the total activity of a hospital or doctor. Proponents of the use of such volume data agree that it is not perfect, but suggest it can be one useful criterion in selecting the best places to receive care for these specific problems. While recognizing the limitations of such data, the healthcare consumer may, nonetheless, find it of interest and use.

The one type of experience you should specifically want to know about is that dealing with any special procedure, particularly a surgical one, that has recently been developed and introduced into practice. For example, in the 1980's many doctors using laparoscopic cholecystectomy, a then new, minimally invasive surgical technique for removing gallbladders, experienced a high percentage of problems because they were not properly trained. This prompted the American Board of Surgery to promulgate new standards for the training of surgeons using this technique. Do not hesitate to ask about your doctor's training in a procedure and how frequently and with what degree of success he or she has performed it. Practice may not lead to perfection, but it does improve skills and enhance the probability of success.

Doctors who are full-time academicians are more likely to be in the forefront of new techniques and research, especially when it comes to a disease like cancer.

In some cases, relatively young doctors have recently completed residency or fellowship training under recognized leaders who have developed new approaches or techniques for dealing with a particular problem. They may have learned the new techniques from their mentors and may be far ahead of the field (and ahead of more senior and distinguished colleagues) in using those approaches. So age and experience must be considered and weighed along with other factors when choosing a physician.

Most doctors will be supportive if you request a second opinion and many will recommend it. In many cases, insurance companies will pay for second opinions, but check ahead of time to make sure your insurance plan does cover them. In an HMO you may have to be more assertive because one way HMOs control costs is by limiting second opinions. Often, the opinion of a second doctor will confirm the opinion of the first, but the reassurance may be worth the time and extra cost. On the other hand, if the second opinion differs from the first, you have two alternatives: seek the opinion of a third doctor, or educate yourself as much as possible by talking to both doctors, reading up on the problem, and trusting your instincts about which diagnosis is correct. Sometimes obtaining a second opinion can be a major challenge. Occasionally, a physician may be offended. Nonetheless, you should not be dissuaded.

The simple logistics of getting a second opinion can be an obstacle. Tara Parker-Pope related in her column, *Health Journal* in *The Wall Street Journal*, the difficulty gathering her mother's records from five doctors, two radiology offices and the pathology lab. She also cited, in the same piece, a Northwestern University review of 340 breast cancer patients who sought second opinions. They reported that 20% of second opinions had no change in pathology or prognosis, but in the remaining 80% of patients some change did occur.

Office and Practice Arrangements

Some specialists will only see new patients who are referred to them by another doctor. Therefore, you may need to have your treating physician contact the specialist's office to arrange for your initial visit. Your health plan may also require that your primary care doctor provide a referral.

If English is not your first language, it may be advisable to determine whether someone in the specialist's office speaks your primary language or if a translator can be present during appointments or, perhaps take a bilingual person with you. This will ease communication and assure that all questions, responses and instructions are understood.

Research suggests that there is a positive relationship between quantity of experience and quality of care.

Accessibility of a physician's office may be a concern if you are wheelchair-bound, are elderly or cannot climb stairs or negotiate narrow corridors. Convenient parking may also be important to you.

When you are choosing a top specialist, these issues may be of lesser or greater importance, depending on the problem and type of care warranted. If you are traveling a great distance to have a specific procedure performed by a top specialist at a major medical center, continuing long-term monitoring or follow-up care by that physician may not be required or may not be feasible and such things as office practice arrangements are of less importance. On the other hand, if your disease needs to be monitored with follow-up care provided by the same top specialist, then such issues as accessibility of the doctor's office, appointment hours, waiting times and courtesy and professionalism of the staff become more significant.

Often, the opinion of a second doctor will confirm the opinion of the first, but the reassurance may be worth the time and extra cost.

Second Opinions

Second opinions are a valuable medical tool, too infrequently used in many instances and overused in others. Clearly, you do not want to seek another doctor's opinion on every ailment or problem that you face, but a second opinion should be pursued in the following situations:

- Before major surgery

- If a rare disease is diagnosed

- If a diagnosis is uncertain

- If the number of tests or procedures recommended might seem excessive

- If a test result has serious implications (e.g., a positive Pap smear)

- If the treatment suggested is risky or expensive

- If you are uncomfortable with the diagnosis and/or treatment

- If a course of treatment is not successful

- If you question your doctor's competence

- If your insurance company requires it

Personal Chemistry

One element of the doctor-patient relationship that we stress in our Guides is chemistry between doctor and patient, a part of which is often referred to as a doctor's "bedside manner." While this factor is of major importance in a long-term relationship such as you would have with your primary care physician, it is of less importance when you see a specialist only once or twice.

It is vital that there is a sense of mutual trust and respect between patient and doctor; this is a judgment that individuals must make for themselves. Among the many talented doctors listed in this Guide, there are very likely some to whom you would relate well and others with whom you may not feel as comfortable.

Patients prefer doctors who listen, demonstrate concern, are responsive to patient needs and spend sufficient time with them. The qualities of physicians in this regard, even the excellent ones in this Guide, vary widely.

You, the patient, are the only one who can assess these qualities because individuals react differently to various personalities. It is important for you to carefully judge your feelings towards a physician, especially if you are embarking on a long-term relationship. You should feel you can be open, trusting and responsive to your physician and that your relationship will be a positive one. Otherwise, find another doctor, since not doing so could adversely affect your care.

Once you have used this guide to identify the top specialist(s) best suited to treat your condition, there is much you can do to maximize the value of your first visit.

Patients prefer doctors who listen, demonstrate concern, are responsive to patient needs and spend sufficient time with them.

• 5 •

Maximizing Your First Appointment With a Top Doctor

After your research is done and you've secured an appointment for an initial consultation with a top doctor, known for his or her expertise in the diagnosis or treatment of your particular medical condition, what should you do?

Questions Concerning Payment

Other arrangements that may need to be made in advance of your first visit or discussed with the specialist's office staff concern payment. You may wish to ask the following:

- Is the specialist within your plan's network and will you need to make a co-payment? Or, is the specialist out-of-network and will you have to pay for your care out-of-pocket, meet a deductible or submit a form for reimbursement?

- Are credit cards an acceptable mode of payment?

- Does the specialist accept Medicare or Medicaid?

A specialist becoming newly involved in your care needs to learn as much as possible about the state of your health in a very limited time. Since top doctors are extremely busy people with many demands on their time, you should make certain that all relevant records and case summaries are obtained and sent to the specialist well in advance of your appointment.

Lastly, it may be advisable to take a relative or close friend with you for support.

Obtaining Your Records

All healthcare providers, including hospitals, doctors and their staffs, are under legal obligation to maintain the privacy of your medical records. In order to obtain release of those records, you must make a request in writing. If you need to obtain records from a number of providers, you should write one clear and concise letter authorizing release of your records and including your name, address, telephone number, date of birth, and hospital patient I.D. number. You then can make photocopies of this letter, but be sure to sign and date each copy as if it were an original. You also may want to specifically name those test results (e.g., pathology slides) or X-ray films (not just written reports or summaries) that must be included in addition to making a general request for your records. It's also a good idea to indicate the date of your appointment so the office staff can respond in a timely manner.

Although state laws require the timely release of medical records, hospital medical records departments and doctors' offices often take several weeks to pull and review patient charts and get them in the mail either to you or to another doctor. In addition to written authorization, you may be asked to pay the costs involved in copying your records, test results and X-ray films because many doctors' offices will not release the originals. Consider placing a call in advance to determine the procedure for releasing your records, how long you can expect it to take, and the costs involved so that you can save time by including payment with your release authorization letter. Be sure to allow sufficient time in advance of your consultation appointment for your request to be processed. Since you often must wait several weeks for an appointment with a specialist, allow at least that amount of time to obtain your records.

Even after making your written requests, you should follow up each letter with a telephone call to be sure that your records actually are sent. You should not assume that your request for records will be promptly fulfilled by an often overburdened, although well-intentioned, office staff.

It is vital that there is a sense of mutual trust and respect between patient and doctor; this is a judgment that individuals must make for themselves.

Remember, the more information the specialist has about your condition, the fewer repeat or additional tests or procedures you will need to undergo. This will lower the costs of your consultation and enable the specialist to more easily assess your condition.

The Facts and Only the Facts

Be thorough and organized in documenting your personal and familial medical histories, the medications you take and in relaying information about your condition. Even seemingly minor bits of information may provide subtle clues to the nature of your medical problem and the optimal way in which to treat it. It's also advisable to bring a list with you of names, addresses and telephone numbers of all physicians who have cared for you, especially those you have seen regarding your current medical problem.

Even though thoroughness is essential to presenting a clear picture of your medical condition, bear in mind that the specialist needs to get to your core health concerns as quickly as possible. Therefore, if you have a complex medical history, you may want to ask your current doctors to provide treatment summaries in addition to copies of your medical records. Hospital records should include your admission history and physical exam, dictated consultation and operation notes and discharge summaries for all hospitalizations. You may also be able to get a cumulative lab and X-ray summary for your hospital stays.

Unlike X-rays, which can be copied at reasonable cost, original pathology slides must be transported by mail or hand-carried. Your specialist may wish to have the pathologist with whom he or she works speak directly with the pathologist who initially interpreted your slides as part of the process of evaluating your case.

Being Prepared

To avoid leaving out important details of your condition or past treatment, prepare a concise, chronological summary before your consultation takes place. You may wish to type it and provide a copy to the specialist for inclusion in your chart. Highlight major medical results or significant events in the course of an illness or treatment if these will enlighten the doctor about your condition. Your personal perspective on the state of your health is vital to a full understanding of your medical problem.

You should make certain that all relevant records and case summaries are obtained and sent to the specialist well in advance of your appointment.

It is possible that the specialist will use terminology that you do not understand or may speak quickly assuming certain knowledge on your part about your condition or its treatment. Don't hesitate to ask for clarification as often or repeatedly as you may need to in order to fully comprehend what you are being told. If you are concerned that you may forget what the doctor tells you, ask the doctor's permission to take notes or ask if you might bring along a tape recorder so you can later replay what was said, especially any instructions you are given. You may prefer to bring along a relative or close friend to serve as a "second set of ears," but, again, seek the doctor's permission to do so in advance of your appointment.

Following this process will assure that you and the specialist you are consulting get the most from your appointment. After all, you both have the same goal: restoring you to optimal health and well being.

What To Do If You Can't Get an Appointment

At times it may be difficult, perhaps even impossible, to secure an appointment with the specific specialist you have identified. There are a number of reasons why this may occur. For example, the specialist may not be taking any new patients or may have such a busy schedule that it takes several weeks or months to get an appointment. He or she may only see patients during very limited hours because of teaching, research or other responsibilities or currently may have other limitations related to the acceptance of new patients.

However, bear in mind that the doctors in this guide are the leaders in their fields and therefore they work with and train the very best and brightest in their specialties. So, if you are unable to consult with a particular doctor, consider making an appointment with one of his or her outstanding colleagues. You can do this by asking a member of the doctor's office staff to refer you to an associate who is a member of the practice group or to another excellent physician who is specially trained to address your particular medical issue.

You can be comfortable knowing that you will receive high quality care from another specialist who practices in the same top setting.

Remember, the more information the specialist has about your condition, the fewer repeat or additional tests or procedures you will need to undergo.

Gathering The Facts

Have you done everything you can to prepare yourself and the specialist for the consultation? The following checklist will help you maximize the value of your visit to the specialist and will go a long way toward focusing you on the task at hand—getting the best advice or treatment for your health problem from one of the top doctors in the medical specialty related to your condition.

- Does the specialist have all the information needed to make a diagnosis of or treatment plan for your condition?

- Have your medical records, test results, and X-rays and MRIs been sent ahead of time to allow for their review by the specialist in advance of your first appointment?

- Have you written out your medical history, including that of your siblings, parents and grandparents, emphasizing the particular problem for which you are visiting this specialist?

- Are you prepared with a written list of questions?

- When you ask your questions, have you understood the answers?

• 6 •

Clinical Trials

The following information on special resources has been included to meet the needs of cancer patients and their families. These patients and their physicians may need to search for very new, cutting-edge, perhaps even experimental and not yet approved therapies. In such cases the search may lead to clinical trials, tests of new drugs and new medical devices, or innovative therapeutic approaches. Fortunately, these situations are rare, but when they do occur they are critical.

In addition to the outstanding private and public hospitals recognized in this guide, the U.S. government maintains its own unique, expert source of patient care and clinical research at the National Institutes of Health (NIH). In fact, the NIH operates its own hospital at which the care provided is usually related to clinical studies its researchers are undertaking.

In addition to those at the NIH, clinical trials also are conducted at leading medical centers and other organizations throughout the country. These facilities may be testing a new drug therapy, a new use for an existing medication or a medical device to deal with a problem that is not being resolved through the use of more traditional approaches.

This section will guide you in utilizing these special resources. These is also a listing of selected cancer resources in Appendix C.

If you are unable to consult with a particular doctor, consider making an appointment with one of his or her outstanding colleagues.

The Clinical Trial as a Treatment Option

For some patients the best medical treatment may only be available through clinical trials (also called treatment studies), which are designed to develop improved ways to use current medical treatments or to find new medical treatments by studying their effects on humans. Treatments are studied to determine if they are safe, effective and better treatments than conventional or standard therapies. Only if they meet all three of these criteria are they made available to the general public.

Many people are frightened by the term "clinical trial" because it conveys the notion of being a "guinea pig" in an experiment. Contrary to popular belief, however, new treatments are extensively studied by scientists in the laboratory before they are ever tested by physicians in clinical settings. Among the factors that keep patients from participating in clinical trials are: lack of awareness about clinical trials as a treatment option; fear of side effects or adverse reactions to treatment; refusal of insurance companies to pay for experimental treatments; failure of a physician to inform the patient about clinical trials; difficulty finding suitable clinical trials; unavailability of clinical trials for certain medical problems; distance of the patient from major medical centers conducting clinical trials; disruption of personal and family life; and the decision to stop medical treatment altogether.

Despite these and other obstacles, many people do seek out clinical trials. New medical treatments can offer participants hope for a cure, an extended lifespan, or an improvement in how they feel. Some participants also take comfort in knowing that others may benefit from their contribution to medical knowledge.

Deciding if a clinical trial is the right treatment option for you is no simple matter. Certainly, you will want to talk about it with your doctor(s) and other professionals involved in your care, as well as with family members and friends. But in order to fully benefit from what others have to say — based on either their professional knowledge or personal experience — you need to understand exactly what a clinical trial is and what your role as a volunteer will be.

Understanding Clinical Trials

Clinical trials are conducted for just about every medical condition, including life-threatening diseases such as AIDS or cancer; chronic illnesses such as diabetes and asthma; psychiatric disorders such as depression or anxiety; behavioral problems such as smoking and substance abuse; and even common ailments such as hair loss and acne. Chances are there is at least one trial (and probably more) that may be appropriate for you.

With more than 100 different types of cancer, it is understandable that a large number of clinical trials are cancer-related. Extensive information about clinical trials for cancer can be found on www.cancer.gov, the Web site of the National Cancer Institute (NCI). NCI is part of the NIH. CenterWatch, an online clinical trials listing service, identifies over 14,000 clinical trials that are actively recruiting patients. Veritas Medicine, another useful online organization, allows individuals to perform personalized searches of its clinical trials database. See "Selected Cancer Resources" in Appendix C for more information on clinical trials.

Most clinical trials study new medical treatments, combinations of treatments, or improvements in conventional treatments using drugs, surgery and other medical procedures, medical devices, radiation or other therapies. Newer types of clinical trials, called screening or prevention trials, study how to prevent the incidence or recurrence of disease through the use of medicines, vitamins, minerals or other supplements; and how to screen for disease, especially in its early stages. Another type of trial studies how to improve the quality of life for patients, including both their physical and emotional well-being.

Clinical trials are sponsored both by the federal government (through the National Institutes of Health, the National Cancer Institute and many others) and by private industry through pharmaceutical and biotechnology companies, and through healthcare institutions (hospitals or health maintenance organizations) and community-based physician-investigators. The National Cancer Institute sponsors clinical trials at more than 1,000 sites in the United States. Trials are carried out in major medical research centers such as teaching hospitals as well as in community hospitals, specialized medical clinics and in doctors' offices.

Though clinical trials often involve hospitalized patients, a fair number of trials are conducted on an outpatient basis. Many trials are part of a cooperative network which may include as few as one or two sites or hundreds of locations, although one center generally assumes responsibility for overall coordination of the research. More than 45 research-oriented institutions, recognized for their scientific excellence, have been designated by the NCI as comprehensive or clinical cancer centers. See "Selected Cancer Resources" in Appendix C to find out how to locate these centers.

Clinical research is based on a protocol (established rules or procedures) describing who will be studied, how and when medications, procedures and/or treatments will be administered and how long the study will last. Trials that are conducted simultaneously at different sites use the same protocol to ensure that all patients are treated identically and all data are collected uniformly so that study findings can be compared.

The National Cancer Institute sponsors clinical trials at more than 1,000 sites in the United States.

Clinical trials generally are conducted in three phases, as outlined in the study protocol. The first phase begins testing of the treatment on a small group of human subjects after rigorous and successful animal testing has been concluded. Phases 2 and 3, usually involve a broader test group and are designed to further evaluate the treatment's safety and more accurately determine appropriate dosage, application methods and side effects. In some trials there may be a fourth phase, conducted after the treatment is in widespread use, to monitor the results of long-term use and the occurrence of any serious side effects.

Some clinical trials test one treatment on one group of subjects, while others compare two or more groups of subjects. In such comparison studies participants are divided into two groups: the control group that receives the standard treatment and the experimental or treatment group which receives the new treatment. For example, the control group may undergo a surgical procedure while the experimental or treatment group undergoes a surgical procedure plus radiation to determine which treatment modality is more effective.

To ensure that patient characteristics do not unduly influence the study findings, patients may be randomly assigned to either the control or the experimental group, meaning that each patient's assignment is based purely on chance. In cases in which a standard treatment does not exist for a particular disease, the experimental group of patients receives the new treatment and the control group receives no treatment at all, or receives a placebo, an inactive medicine or procedure that has no treatment value. It is important to keep in mind that patients are never put into a control group without any treatment if there is a known treatment that could help them. Also, whether a patient is receiving an investigational drug or a placebo, he/she receives the same level and quality of medical care as those receiving the investigational treatment.

One of the most pressing reasons to participate in clinical trials is the opportunity to obtain treatment that might not be available otherwise.

Protecting the Rights of Participants

The safety of those who participate in clinical trials is a serious matter and is the number one priority of medical investigators. All clinical research, regardless of type of sponsorship results of long-term use and the occurrence of any serious side effect is guided by the same ethical and legal codes that govern the medical profession and the practice of medicine. Most clinical research is federally funded or federally regulated (at least in part) with built-in safeguards for patients. According to federal government regulations (and some state laws), every clinical trial in the United States must be approved and monitored by an Institutional Review Board (IRB), which is an independent committee of physicians, statisticians, community advocates and others (representing at least five distinct disciplines) to ensure that the protocol is being followed. Government regulations require researchers to fully inform participants about all aspects of a clinical trial before they agree to participate through a process called informed consent. To be sure that you understand your role in a clinical trial, you should jot down any questions beforehand so as not to forget them. You should also consider bringing along a friend or family member for support and additional input, and perhaps even tape recording the conversation (after asking permission to do so) to make sure you do not forget or misunderstand anything. Each participant in a clinical trial must be given a written consent form, which should be available in English and other languages. The consent form explains the issues listed in the box on page 46. Patients also are informed that they may leave the trial, or exclude themselves from any part of it, at any time. Informed consent means exactly what the term implies: you agree to join a clinical trial only after you completely understand exactly what your participation will involve for the duration of the study. By law, each patient must be provided with a copy of the signed consent form, which also must include the name and telephone number of a contact person for questions or additional information. Informed consent is a continuous process, so do not hesitate to ask questions before, during or after the trial.

The investigators must protect the privacy of each participant in a clinical trial by ensuring that all medical records are kept confidential except for inspection by the sponsoring agency, the Food and Drug Administration and other agencies involved in regulating the drug or treatment, and all data are collected anonymously by assigning a numeric code or initials to each individual.

During the course of the trial, participants are regularly seen by members of the research team to monitor their health and well-being. Participants also should be responsible for their own health by following the treatment plan (such as taking the proper dosage of medications on time), keeping all scheduled visits and informing members of the healthcare team about any symptoms that occur. If, during the course of the trial, the treatment proves to be ineffective or harmful, the patient is free to leave the study and still obtain conventional care. Conversely, as soon as there is evidence that one treatment modality is better than another, all patients in the trial are given the benefit of the new information.

Questions to Ask Your Doctor and the Trial's Research Team if You are Considering Participating in a clinical Trial:

- Who is sponsoring the trial?

- How many patients will be involved?

- Will the trial be testing a single treatment or a combination of treatments?

- Will there be one treatment group or more than one treatment group?

- If more than one treatment group, how are patients assigned to each group?

- Has this treatment been studied in previous clinical trials? What were the findings?

- What are the requirements for patient eligibility?

Enrolling in Clinical Trials

Each clinical trial has its own guidelines, called eligibility criteria, for determining who can participate. Treatment studies recruit participants who have a disease or other medical condition, while screening and prevention studies generally recruit healthy volunteers. Inclusion criteria (those that allow you to participate in a study) and exclusion criteria (those that keep you from participating in a study) ensure that the study will answer the research questions posed in the research protocol while maintaining the safety of participants. The disease being studied is a primary factor in selecting suitable patients, but other factors such as the patient's gender, age, treatment history and other diagnosed medical conditions may also be important. Unfortunately, eligibility also may depend upon ability to pay. Many health plans do not cover all of the costs associated with clinical trials because they define these trials as experimental procedures. However, trials sometimes pay volunteers for their time and/or reimburse them for travel, childcare, meals and lodging.

To prevent people who qualify from being excluded from clinical trials for financial reasons, agencies such as the National Cancer Institute are working with health plans to find solutions and a growing number of states require insurance companies to pay for all routine patient care costs in cancer trials. To encourage more senior citizens to participate in cancer trials, Medicare plans to revise its payment policy to cover those trials.

When choosing a clinical trial you should determine the factors that are most important to you. For instance, patients generally prefer to participate in trials near their homes so that they can maintain their usual day-to-day activities, be surrounded by family and friends and avoid travel and lodging costs. If travel or temporary relocation becomes necessary, try to find a trial site that is near to some family member or friend or one that is in a locale similar to your own city or town. Many organizations, such as the National Cancer Institute, will work with patients and their families to identify support networks for them wherever they participate.

Participating in a Clinical Trial

Clinical trials are conducted by a research team led by a principal investigator (usually a physician) and are comprised of physicians, nurses and other health professionals such as social workers, psychologists and nutritionists. As a participant you may be required to commit a fair amount of time to a clinical trial, often within more than one geographic region or state.

Some participants also take comfort in knowing that others may benefit from their contribution to medical knowledge.

Participants in clinical trials should remain under the care of their regular physician(s) since clinical trials tend to provide short-term treatment for a specific medical condition and do not generally provide comprehensive primary care. In fact, some trials require that a patient's regular physician sign a consent form before the patient is enrolled. In addition, your regular physician can collaborate with the research team to make sure there are no adverse reactions between your other medications or treatments and the investigational treatment.

Weighing the Benefits and Risks of a Clinical Trial

If you are considering participation in a clinical trial, you need to consider the medical, emotional and financial ramifications of participation. Of course, the obvious benefit of a clinical trial is the chance that a new treatment may improve your health and prognosis. You will have access to drugs and other medical interventions before they are widely available to the public and you will obtain expert and specialized medical care at leading healthcare facilities. Many patients receive an added psychological benefit by taking an active role in their treatment.

It is important to bear in mind that some medical interventions used in clinical trials may carry potential risks depending upon the type of treatment and the patient's condition. While many side effects or adverse reactions are temporary (such as hair loss and nausea caused by some anti-cancer drugs), other more serious reactions can be permanent and even life-threatening (for example, heart, liver or kidney damage).

Deciding whether or not to participate in a clinical trial is often a matter of determining if the trial's potential benefits outweigh its possible risks. This is a highly personal decision that may be difficult to make in situations involving experimental treatment in which limited medical information may be available.

Getting Information on Clinical Trials

The more information you have about a clinical trial, the easier it will be to make a decision about whether or not it is right for you, and the more confident you will be that you made an appropriate decision. In addition to the "Selected Cancer Resources," Appendix C in this guide, the staff at your local public library, community hospital, or major medical center can assist you in locating the information you need from books, consumer organizations and on the Internet.

It is important to keep in mind that patients are never put into a control group without any treatment if there is a known treatment that could help them.

Questions to Ask the Sponsors About Your Rights as a Participant in a Clinical Trial:

- Who is responsible for approving and monitoring this research? Is there an IRB?

- Who informs me about the trial process? Do I sign a consent form? Will I receive a copy?

- May I leave the trial at any time? Have previous patients dropped out?

- Whom do I contact if I am experiencing any difficulty with this trial?

Learning about the National Instututes of Health (NIH)

The National Institutes of Health (NIH) comprise one the world's leading medical research centers and the Federal government's principal agency for biomedical research. An agency of the United States Department of Health, United States Public Health Service, NIH encompasses 25 separate institutions and centers with its main campus located in Bethesda, Maryland. Research is also conducted at several field units across the country and abroad.

Paitent Care at the NIH

The Warren Grant Magnuson Clinical Center, NIH's principal medical research center and hospital located in Bethesda, Maryland, provides medical care only to patients participating in clinical research programs. Two categories of patients participate in the Clinical Center studies: children and adults who wish to improve their own health, such as those with newly diagnosed medical problems, ongoing medical problems or family history of disease; and healthy volunteers wishing to advance knowledge about the causes, progress and treatment of disease. The patient's case must fit into an ongoing NIH research project for which the patient has the precise kind or stage of illness under investigation. General diagnostic and treatment services common to community hospitals are not available.

The Magnuson Clinical Center is the world's largest biomedical research hospital and ambulatory care facility, housing 1,600 laboratories conducting basic and clinical research. There are 1,200 tenured physicians, dentists and researchers on staff along with 660 nurses and 570 allied healthcare professionals (dieticians, imaging technologists, medical technologists, medical records and clerical staff, pharmacists and therapists).

The Center's hospital is specially designed for medical research and accommodates 540 carefully selected patients who are participating in clinical research programs. Its 350-bed facility has 24 inpatient care units to which 7,000 patients are admitted annually. The Center also has an Ambulatory Care Research Facility (ACRF) that serves 68,000 outpatient visits each year. A new facility, called the Mark O. Hatfield Clinical Research Center, which began accepting patients in early 2005, has 242 beds for inpatient care and 90 day-hospital stations for outpatient care. The Mark O. Hatfield Center carries out the latest biomedical research that results in new forms of disease diagnosis, prevention and treatment, which is then incorporated into improved methods of patient care.

The Consent Form Should Explain the Following:

- Why the research is being done.

- What the researchers hope to accomplish.

- What types of treatment interventions (and other test or procedures) will be performed?

- How long the study will continue.

- What the expected benefits and the possible risks are.

- What other treatments are available.

- What costs will be covered by the study, by the patient or by third-party payers such as Medicare, Medicaid or private insurance.

This is a fine example of Translational Medicine where excellent research discoveries are translated into new and improved methods of clinical treatment. In other words, the laboratory discoveries are brought to the bedside.

The Clinical Center also maintains a Children's Inn for pediatric outpatients and their families. This family-centered residence operates 24 hours a day, 7 days a week, 365 days a year.

In an effort to bring clinical research to the community, NIH supports approximately 80 General Clinical Research Centers (GCRCs) around the country, located within hospitals of major academic medical centers.

It is important to note that, as part of the federal government, the Warren Grant Magnuson Clinical Center provides treatment in clinical trials at no cost to its patients. In some cases, patients receive a stipend to help cover the costs of traveling to Bethesda for treatment and follow-up care. Travel costs for the initial screening visit, however, are not covered.

Areas of Clinical Study at the NIH

At the Magnuson Clinical Center alone, NIH physician-scientists conduct nearly 1,000 studies each year. Among the areas of study are cancer and related diseases.

Not all of these clinical areas are under investigation at any given time, however. The Patient Recruitment and Public Liaison Office (PRPL) at the NIH Clinical Center assists patients, their families and their physicians in obtaining information about participation in NIH clinical trials. Trained nurses are available to answer questions about the research programs and admission procedures.

Cancer Care at the Warren Grant Magnuson Clinical Center

The National Cancer Institute (NCI) is the largest of the biomedical research institutes and centers at NIH. There, clinical studies are designed to evaluate new and promising ways to prevent, detect, diagnose and treat cancer. The Warren Grant Magnuson Clinical Center provides a separate outpatient division for cancer patients and also has several designated inpatient units.

The investigators must protect the privacy of each participant in a clinical trial by ensuring that all medical records are kept confidential.

Questions to ask the trial's sponsor about eligibility criteria:

- What are the inclusion and exclusion criteria for the clinical trial(s) I am considering?

- How can I improve my chances of being accepted? Pre-existing conditions? Problems?

- If I am not eligible for one trial, what other trials being conducted for my condition?

- Will I be paid for my time or reimbursed for my out-of-pocket expenses?

If you are interested in entering a cancer study at the Magnuson Clinical Center (or at the General Clinical Research Centers), you should first discuss treatment options with a physician. As a general rule, patients interested in participating in clinical studies must be referred by a physician. However, in some instances, self-referral may be permitted.

Patients with medical problems other than cancer or healthy volunteers who wish to participate in a clinical study should contact the particular NIH institute responsible for the clinical area involved.

Cancer Care at the NCI Clinical Centers and Comprehensive Cancer Centers

You may also obtain clinical oncology services (education, screening, diagnosis or treatment) or participate in clinical trials at one of the 21 Cancer Centers or 39 Comprehensive Cancer Centers designated by the NCI for their scientific excellence and extensive resources devoted to cancer and cancer-related problems. Centers are located in 32 states, with the majority of sites in California, New York and Pennsylvania. You can find out about clinical trials at the NCI-designated centers by contacting NCI's Clinical Studies Support Center (CSSC) or by calling each center directly (See Appendix C for contact information). Information about other cancer-related services at these centers also may be obtained from the center itself. For more information, you can visit the National Cancer Institute's website at www.cancer.gov.

Questions to Ask the Research Team or Your Physician About Your Role in a Clinical Trial:

- Who are the members of the health team? Who will be in charge of my care?

- How long will the trial last?

- How does treatment in the trial compare with or differ from the standard treatment?

- Will I be hospitalized? How often? For how long a period of time?

- What will occur during each visit? What treatments or procedures will I be given?

- Will I still be able to see my regular physician(s)?

- Will my doctor and the research team collaborate?

- Can I be put in touch with other patients who have participated in this trial?

To encourage more senior citizens to participate in cancer trials, Medicare plans to revise its payment policy to cover those trials.

If Your Physician Concurs that a Clinical Study might be Appropriate for you, the NIH Recommends that the Following Steps be Taken:

- Contact NCI's Clinical Studies Support Center (CSSC), which is staffed by trained oncology (cancer) nurses who can identify appropriate clinical studies for you. Summaries of these trials and other pertinent information about the type of treatment being offered and the type of patients eligible for inclusion can be mailed or faxed to you and/or your physician.

- Review the clinical trials summaries and other information with your physician to decide which study or studies you should consider. Your physician also can contact the CSSC to communicate directly with the investigator in charge of the study.

- In cases in which you meet the initial eligibility requirements, it may be necessary for you to schedule a screening visit at the Clinical Center to learn more about the trial and possibly undergo some medical tests.

- If accepted for a clinical trial, make sure that you understand the details about the treatment and any possible risks and benefits.

Section II
Using this Guide
to Find a
Top Doctor

• 7 •

How to Use This Book

We assume most people who purchase this book have either received a diagnosis of cancer, or know someone who has. Although it would have been possible to arrange the listings by type of cancer, e.g. lung, breast, prostate, etc., that would not have been practical. For any particular type of cancer, a patient may be seeking one or more of a variety of different specialists. For example, any of the cancers mentioned could require, among other specialists, the involvement of pathologists, medical oncologists, surgeons, urologists, radiation oncologists and, possibly, psychiatrists.

Therefore, this guide and its list of physicians is organized first by specialty. Then, because many patients may prefer care as close to home as possible, we organized the lists by region. (See map on page 56)

The Special Expertise Index we include in the book, may also be of great help in locating the specialists a patient needs. We asked physicians making nominations to recommend individuals who were nationally recognized as leaders in the prevention, diagnosis and treatment of particular types of cancer, as well as leaders in various treatment modalities. When physicians selected for inclusion in America's Top Doctors® for Cancer completed and submitted their professional biographies, we also asked them to list their areas of special expertise. As a result, the Special Expertise Index lists hundreds of these areas.

The physicians are listed alphabetically within their specialties and then within their regions. A sample biography is presented and explained on the next page.

SAMPLE PHYSICIAN LISTING

Smith, John MD [Ped] - **Spec Exp:** Asthma Allergy; **Hospital:** Children's Hosp (page 120);

Name [Specialty]   Special Expertise(s)   Admitting Hospital & Hospital Information Page

Address: 300 Ridge Road Boston, MA 12345; **Phone:** (617) 555-2343; **Board Cert:** Ped 75;

Office Address   Office Phone   Board Certification(s)

Med School: Harvard Med Sch 70; **Resid:** Ped, Children's Hosp 73;

Medical School   Residency(ies)

Fellow: AM, Children's Hosp 74; **Fac Appt:** Assoc Prof Ped, The Med Sch

Fellowship(s)   Faculty Appointment

Step-by-Step Directions for Finding the Specialist you Need

1. Look for a doctor first by specialty. Turn to the Special Cancer Expertise Index on p. 577. Review the list which is organized alphabetically, and find the particular disease, organ, procedure or treatment of interest to you. Write down the page numbers of physicians with that expertise and turn to those pages.

2. Look in the area of the country closest to you. Each specialty lists doctors alphabetically within their geographical region. These regions start in New England (northeast) and go around the country in a consistent order to finish the West Coast and Pacific. Each state is grouped into one of these seven geographical regions. See map of the United States and the regions on page 56. If you don't find a doctor in that particular specialty in your first geographic preference, expand your search to other regions.

3. Check further in the special expertise index. If you don't find a doctor to meet your needs, the last chapter contains those specialties which include a small number of doctors. The Special Cancer Expertise index may include some diseases which are not related to cancer because a physician who treats cancer patients also may treat patients with these diseases.

Locating A Specialist

This guide is organized to make finding the right specialists for you or your loved ones as simple as possible. Physicians' biographies are presented by specialty and are organized by geographic region within each specialty or subspecialty. Thus, you may search for a particular type of specialist or subspecialist in one or more regions or throughout the nation.

A second way to locate the right specialist is to use the **Special Expertise Index** beginning on page 577. This index is organized according to diseases, conditions and procedures or techniques. If you already know a specialist's name, you can find his/her listing by using the **Alphabetical Listing of Doctors** beginning on page 563.

The information reported in each doctor's listing is, for the most part, provided by the doctor or his/her office staff. Castle Connolly attempts to verify the data through other sources but cannot guarantee that in all cases all data has been so verified or accurate. All such information is subject to change from time to time due to changes in physician practices.

Geographic Regions & States

To assist you in using America's Top Doctors for Cancer in the most efficient and effective manner, the Guide is divided into seven geographic regions. This will help you to locate a specialist in your local or neighboring region. For example, if you live in Mississippi in the Southeast region and you are willing and able to travel to Louisiana in the Southwest region to consult with a specialist in medical oncology, you can review just those two regions, under the section headed "Medical Oncology." However, if you prefer to review the information on medical oncologists throughout the country, you can search the entire medical oncology section. Or, you can consult the "SPECIAL EXPERTISE INDEX" in the back of this Guide and choose a medical oncologist who has specific expertise to meet your particular needs.

The geographic regions are as follows:

New England   Great Plains and Mountains
Mid Atlantic   Southwest
Southeast   West Coast and Pacific
Midwest

The states that are included in each region are listed on the following page and a map of the regions is also provided. Please note that not all regions are represented in all specialties. For example, in "Interventional Radiology" there are no listings in the Southwest region.

Geographic Regions and States

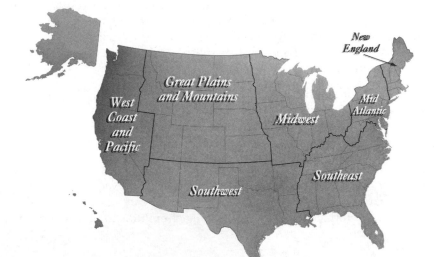

West Coast and Pacific:
Alaska
California
Hawaii
Nevada
Oregon
Washington

Great Plains and Mountains:
Colorado
Idaho
Kansas
Montana
Nebraska
North Dakota
South Dakota
Utah
Wyoming

Southwest:
Arizona
Arkansas
Louisiana
New Mexico
Oklahoma
Texas

Midwest:
Illinois
Indiana
Iowa
Michigan
Minnesota
Missouri
Ohio
Wisconsin

New England:
Connecticut
Maine
Massachusetts
New Hampshire
Rhode Island
Vermont

Mid Atlantic:
Delaware
Maryland
New Jersey
New York
Pennsylvania
Washington, DC
West Virginia

Southeast:
Alabama
Florida
Georgia
Kentucky
Mississippi
North Carolina
South Carolina
Tennessee
Virginia

• 8 •

Medical Specialties

In the pages that follow, each list of doctors in a medical specialty or subspecialty is preceded by a brief description of that specialty (or subspecialty) and the training required for board certification.

Critical Care Medicine has been excluded because in emergency situations there is neither time nor opportunity for choice. A number of other specialities not relevant to most patients (e.g., Forensic Psychiatry) have not been included as well.

The following descriptions of medical specialties and subspecialties were provided by the American Board of Medical Specialties (ABMS), an organization comprised of the 24 medical specialty boards that provide certification in 25 medical specialties. A complete listing of all specialists certified by the ABMS can be found in The Official ABMS Directory of Board Certified Medical Specialists, and is published by Marquis Who's Who. It is available (either in a multi-volume directory or on CD-ROM) in most public libraries, hospital libraries, university libraries and medical libraries. The ABMS also operates a toll-free phone line at 1-866-275-2267 and a website at www.abms.org to verify the certification status of individual doctors.

The following important policy statement, approved by the ABMS Assembly on March 19, 1987, remains valid.

The Purpose Of Certification
The intent of the certification process, as defined by the member boards of the American Board of Medical Specialties, is to provide assurance to the public that a certified medical specialist has successfully completed an approved educational program and an evaluation, including an examination process designed to assess the knowledge, experience and skills requisite to the provision of high quality patient care in that specialty.

Medical Specialty and Subspecialty Descriptions and Abbreviations

The following medical specialties and subspecialties are indicated in the doctors' listings by their abbreviations. Specialties are indicated in bold, subspecialties in italics, and the four primary care specialties in bold capitals. To review the official American Board of Medical Specialties (ABMS) organization of specialties, refer to Appendix A.

Addiction Psychiatry　　　　　　　　　　　　　　　　　　　　　　AdP
Deals with habitual psychological and physiological dependence on a substance or practice which is beyond voluntary control.

Adolescent Medicine　　　　　　　　　　　　　　　　　　　　　　AM
Involves the primary care treatment of adolescents and young adults.

Allergy & Immunology　　　　　　　　　　　　　　　　　　　　**A&I**
Diagnosis and treatment of allergies, asthma, and skin problems such as hives and contact dermatitis.

Anesthesiology　　　　　　　　　　　　　　　　　　　　　　　**Anes**
Provides pain relief in maintenance or restoration of a stable condition during and following an operation. Anesthesiologists also diagnose and treat acute and long standing pain problems.

Cardiac Electrophysiology (Clinical)　　　　　　　　　　　　　　　CE
Involves complicated technical procedures to evaluate heart rhythms and determine appropriate treatment for them.

Cardiovascular Disease　　　　　　　　　　　　　　　　　　　　　Cv
Involves the diagnosis and treatment of disorders of the heart, lungs, and blood vessels.

Child & Adolescent Psychiatry　　　　　　　　　　　　　　　　　ChAP
Deals with the diagnosis and treatment of mental diseases in children and adolescents.

Child Neurology　　　　　　　　　　　　　　　　　　　　　　　ChiN
Diagnosis and medical treatment of disorders of the brain, spinal cord, and nervous system in children.

Clinical Genetics　　　　　　　　　　　　　　　　　　　　　　**CG**
Deals with identifying the genetic causes of inherited diseases and ailments and preventing, when possible, their occurrence.

Colon and Rectal Surgery　　　　　　　　　　　　　　　　　　**CRS**
Surgical treatment of diseases of the intestinal tract, colon and rectum, anal canal, and perianal area.

Critical Care Medicine　　　　　　　　　　　　　　　　　　　　　CCM
Involves diagnosing and taking immediate action to prevent death or further injury of a patient. Examples of critical injuries include shock, heart attack, drug overdose, and massive bleeding.

Dermatology D

Diagnosis and treatment of benign and malignant disorders of the skin, mouth, external genitalia, hair and nails, as well as a number of sexually transmitted diseases.

Diagnostic Radiology DR

Involves the study of all modalities of radiant energy in medical diagnoses and therapeutic procedures utilizing radiologic guidance.

Endocrinology, Diabetes & Metabolism EDM

Involves the study and treatment of patients suffering from hormonal and chemical disorders.

FAMILY MEDICINE FP

Deals with and oversees the total healthcare of individual patients and their family members. Family practitioners are more common in rural areas and may perform procedures more commonly performed by specialists (e.g., minor surgery).

Forensic Psychiatry FPsy

Concerns the evaluation of certain diagnostic groups of patients that include those with sexual disorders, antisocial personality disorders, paranoid disorders, and addictive disorders.

Gastroenterology Ge

The study, diagnosis and treatment of diseases of the digestive organs including the stomach, bowels, liver, and gallbladder.

Geriatric Medicine Ger

Deals with diseases of the elderly and the problems associated with aging.

Geriatric Psychiatry GerPsy

Involves the diagnosis, prevention, and treatment of mental illness in the elderly.

Gynecologic Oncology GO

Deals with cancers of the female genital tract and reproductive systems.

Hand Surgery HS

Involves the treatment of injury to the hand through surgical techniques.

Hematology Hem

Involves the diagnosis and treatment of diseases and disorders of the blood, bone marrow, spleen, and lymph glands.

Infectious Disease Inf

The study and treatment of diseases caused by a bacterium, virus, fungus, or animal parasite.

INTERNAL MEDICINE IM

Diagnosis and nonsurgical treatment of diseases, especially those of adults. Internists may act as primary care specialists, highly trained family doctors, or they may subspecialize in specialties such as cardiology or nephrology.

Maternal & Fetal Medicine MF

Involves the care of women with high-risk pregnancies and their unborn fetuses.

Medical Oncology   Onc

Refers to the study and treatment of tumors and other cancers.

Neonatal-Perinatal Medicine   NP

Involves the diagnosis and treatments of infants prior to, during, and one month beyond birth.

Nephrology   Nep

Concerned with disorders of the kidneys, high blood pressure, fluid and mineral balance, dialysis of body wastes when the kidneys do not function, and consultation with surgeons about kidney transplantation.

Neurological Surgery   **NS**

Involves surgery of the brain, spinal cord, and nervous system.

Neurology   **N**

Diagnosis and medical treatment of disorders of the brain, spinal cord, and nervous system.

Neuroradiology   NRad

Involves the utilization of imaging procedures during diagnosis as they relate to the brain, spine and spinal cord, head, neck, and organs of special sense in adults and children.

Nuclear Medicine   **NuM**

Evaluation of the functions of all the organs in the body and treatment of thyroid disease, benign and malignant tumors, and radiation exposure through the use of radioactive substances.

Nuclear Radiology   NR

Involves the use of radioactive substances to diagnose and treat certain functions and diseases of the body.

OBSTETRICS & GYNECOLOGY   **ObG**

Deals with the medical aspects of and intervention in pregnancy and labor and the overall health of the female reproductive system.

Occupational Medicine   OM

Concentrates on the effect of the work environment on the health of employees.

Ophthalmology   **Oph**

Diagnosis and treatment of diseases of and injuries to the eye.

Orthopaedic Surgery   **OrS**

Involves operations to correct injuries which interfere with the form and function of the extremities, spine, and associated structures.

Otolaryngology   **Oto**

Explores and treats diseases in the interrelated areas of the ears, nose and throat.

Otology/Neurotology   ON

Concentrates on the management, prevention, cure and care of patients with diseases of the ear and temporal bone, including disorders of hearing and balance.

Pain Medicine
PM

Involves providing a high level of care for patients experiencing problems with acute or chronic pain in both hospital and ambulatory settings.

Pediatric Cardiology
PCd

Involves the diagnosis and treatment of heart disease in children.

Pediatric Critical Care Medicine
PCCM

Involves the care of children who are victims of life threatening disorders such as severe accidents, shock, and diabetes acidosis.

Pediatric Dermatology
PD

Diagnosis and treatment of benign and malignant disorders of the skin, mouth, external genitalia, hair and nails in children.

Pediatric Endocrinology
PEn

Involves the study and treatment of children with hormonal and chemical disorders.

Pediatric Gastroenterology
PGe

The study, diagnosis, and treatment of diseases of the digestive tract in children.

Pediatric Hematology-Oncology
PHO

The study and treatment of cancers of the blood and blood-forming parts of the body in children.

Pediatric Infectious Disease
PInf

The study and treatment of diseases caused by a virus, bacterium, fungus, or animal parasite in children.

Pediatric Nephrology
PNep

Deals with the diagnosis and treatment of disorders of the kidneys in children.

Pediatric Otolaryngology
POto

Involves the diagnosis and treatment of disorders of the ear, nose, and throat which affect children.

Pediatric Pulmonology
PPul

Involves the diagnosis and treatment of diseases of the chest, lungs, and chest tissue in children.

Pediatric Radiology
PR

Involves diagnostic imaging as it pertains to the newborn, infant, child, and adolescent.

Pediatric Rheumatology
PRhu

Involves the treatment of diseases of the joints and connective tissues in children.

Pediatric Surgery
PS

Treatment of disease, injury, or deformity in children through surgical techniques.

PEDIATRICS
Ped

Diagnosis and treatment of diseases of childhood and monitoring of the growth, development, and well-being of preadolescents.

Physical Medicine & Rehabilitation   **PMR**

The use of physical therapy and physical agents such as water, heat, light electricity, and mechanical manipulations in the diagnosis, treatment, and prevention of disease and body disorders.

Plastic Surgery   **PlS**

Involves reconstructive and cosmetic surgery of the face and other body parts.

Preventive Medicine   **PrM**

A specialty focusing on the prevention of illness and on the health of groups rather than individuals.

Psychiatry   **Psyc**

Examination, treatment, and prevention of mental illness through the use of psychoanalysis and/or drugs.

Public Health & General Preventive Medicine   PHGPM

Involves the investigation of the causes of epidemic disease and the prevention of a wide variety of acute and chronic illness.

Pulmonary Disease   Pul

Involves the diagnosis and treatment of diseases of the chest, lungs, and airways.

Radiation Oncology   RadRo

Involves the use of radiant energy and isotopes in the study and treatment of disease, especially malignant cancer.

Reproductive Endocrinology   RE

Deals with the endocrine system (including the pituitary, thyroid, parathyroid, adrenal glands, placenta, ovaries, and testes) and how its failure relates to infertility.

Rheumatology   Rhu

Involves the treatment of diseases of the joints, muscles, bones and associated structures.

Sleep Medicine   Sleep Med

Involves the investigation and treatment of patients with sleep disorders.

Spinal Cord Injury Medicine   SpCdInj

Involves the prevention, diagnosis, treatment and management of traumatic spinal cord injuries.

Sports Medicine   SM

Refers to the practice of an orthopaedist or other physician who specializes in injuries to the bone or other soft tissues (muscles, tendons, ligaments) caused by participation in Athletic activity.

Surgery   **S**

Treatment of disease, injury, and deformity by surgical procedures.

Surgery of the Hand   SHd

Involves providing appropriate care for all structures in the upper extremity directly affecting the hand and wrist function.

Surgical Critical Care   SCC

Involves specialized care in the management of the critically ill patient, particularly the trauma victim and postoperative patient in the emergency department, intensive care unit, trauma unit, burn unit, and other similar settings.

Thoracic Surgery (includes open heart surgery)   **TS**

Involves surgery on the heart, lungs, and chest area.

Urology   **U**

Diagnosis and treatment of diseases of the genitals in men and disorders of the urinary tract and bladder in both men and women.

Vascular & Interventional Radiology   VIR

Involves diagnosing and treating diseases by percutaneous methods guided by various radiologic imaging modalities.

Vascular Surgery   VascS

Involves the operative treatment of disorders of the blood vessels excluding those to the heart, lungs, or brain.

The Training of a Specialist

Excerpted from "Which Medical Specialist For You?," American Board of Medical Specialties, Evanston, IL, Revised 2000

Everyone knows that a "medical doctor" is a physician who has had years of training to understand the diagnosis, treatment and prevention of disease. The basic training for a physician specialist includes four years of premedical education in a college or university, four years of medical school, and after receiving the M.D. degree, at least three years of specialty training under supervision (called a "residency"). Training in subspecialties can take an additional one to three years.

Some specialists are primary care doctors such as family physicians, general internists and general pediatricians. Other specialists concentrate on certain body systems, specific age groups, or complex scientific techniques developed to diagnose or treat certain types of disorders. Specialties in medicine developed because of the rapidly expanding body of knowledge about health and illness and the constantly evolving new treatment techniques for disease.

A subspecialist is a physician who has completed training in a general medical specialty and then takes additional training in a more specific area of that specialty called a subspecialty. This training increases the depth of knowledge and expertise of the specialist in that particular field. For example, cardiology is a subspecialty of internal medicine and pediatrics, pediatric surgery is a subspecialty of surgery and child and adolescent psychiatry is a subspecialty of psychiatry. The training of a subspecialist within a specialty requires an additional one or more years of full-time education.

The training, or residency, of a specialist begins after the doctor has received the M.D. degree from a medical school. Resident physicians dedicate themselves for three to seven years to full-time experience in hospital and/or ambulatory care settings, caring for patients under the supervision of experienced specialists. Educational conferences and research experience are often part of that training. In years past, the first year of post-medical school training was called an internship, but is now called residency.

Licensure

The legal privilege to practice medicine is governed by state law and is not designed to recognize the knowledge and skills of a trained specialist. A physician is licensed to practice general medicine and surgery by a state board of medical examiners after passing a state or national licensure examination. Each state or territory has its own procedures to license physicians and sets the general standards for all physicians in that state or territory.

Who Credentials a Specialist and/or Subspecialist?

Specialty boards certify physicians as having met certain published standards. There are 24 specialty boards that are recognized by the American Board of Medical Specialties (ABMS) and the American Medical Association (AMA). All of the specialties and subspecialties recognized by the ABMS and the AMA are listed in the brief descriptions that follow. Remember, a subspecialist first must be trained and certified as a specialist.

In order to be certified as a medical specialist by one of these recognized boards a physician must complete certain requirements. See box on the next page.

All of the ABMS Member Boards now, or will soon, issue only time-limited certificates which are valid for six to ten years. In order to retain certification, diplomates must become "recertified," and must periodically go through an additional process involving continuing education in the specialty, review of credentials and further examination. Boards that may not yet require recertification have provided voluntary recertification with similar requirements.

How to Determine If a Physician is a Certified Specialist

Certified specialists are listed in The Official ABMS Directory of Board Certified Medical Specialists published by Marquis Who's Who. The ABMS Directory can be found in most public libraries, hospital libraries, university libraries and medical libraries, and is also available on CD-ROM. Alternatively, you could ask for that information from your county medical society, the American Board of Medical Specialties, or one of the specialty boards.

The ABMS operates a toll free number (1-866-275-2267) to verify the certification status of individual physicians. Additionally, information about the ABMS organization and links to an electronic directory of certified specialists can be accessed through the ABMS Web site at www.abms.org.

Almost all board certified specialists also are members of their medical specialty societies. These societies are dedicated to furthering standards, practice and professional and public education within individual medical specialties. Some, such as the American College of Surgeons and the American College of Obstetricians and Gynecologists, require board certification for full membership. A physician who has attained full membership is called a "Fellow" of the society and is entitled to use this designation in all formal communications such as certificates, publications, business cards, stationery and signage. Thus, "John Doe, M.D., F.A.C.S. (Fellow of the American College of Surgeons) is a board certified surgeon. Similarly, F.A.A.D. (Fellow of the American Academy of Dermatology) following the M.D. or D.O. in a physician's title would likely indicate board certification in that specialty.

To be Certified as a Medical Specialist by a Recognized Board, a Physician Must Complete Certain Requirements, these Include:

1 Completion of a course of study leading to the M.D. or D.O. (Doctor of Osteopathy) degree from a recognized school of medicine.

2 Completion of three to seven years of full-time training in an accredited residency program designed to train specialists in the field.

3 Many specialty boards require assessments and documentation of individual performance from the residency training director, or from the chief of service in the hospital where the specialist has practiced.

4 All of the ABMS Member Boards require that a person seeking certification have an unrestricted license to practice medicine in order to take the certification examination.

5 Finally, each candidate for certification must pass a written examination given by the specialty board. Fifteen of the 24 specialty boards also require an oral examination conducted by senior specialists in that field. Candidates who have passed the exams and other requirements are then given the status of "Diplomate" and are certified as specialists.

• 9 •

The Partnership for Excellence Program

Among the more than 6,000 acute care and specialty hospitals in the United States, many have extraordinary capabilities for superior patient care. These hospitals, renowned for their use of state-of-the-art equipment and up-to-the-minute technology, also attract outstanding physicians and other healthcare professionals. Many of their physicians are among those in the listings in this Guide.

To assist you in your search for top specialists and to supplement the information contained in the physician listings that follow, we invited a select group of these fine institutions to profile their services, special programs and centers of excellence in the Partnership for Excellence program. This special section contains pages sponsored by the included hospitals. This paid sponsorship program is totally separate from the physician selection process, which is based upon a completely independent review.

The Partnership for Excellence program provides an overview of the programs and services offered by the included hospitals with information related to their accreditation and sponsorship. Most also provide their physician referral numbers, should you wish to ask the hospitals for recommendations of doctors not listed in *America's Top Doctors® for Cancer* 4th edition.

In addition to the Partnership for Excellence program, profiled hospitals were also invited to highlight their special programs or services that focus on a particular disease or medical condition. These can be found in the "Centers of Excellence" sections that are interspersed throughout this book following the medical specialties and/or subspecialties to which they relate. Sponsored pages in the centers of excellence sections reflect the depth of commitment of these hospitals, which provide the staff, resources and financial support necessary to develop these special programs.

By visiting our website **www.CastleConnolly.com**, you may also link to the websites of these outstanding hospitals for even more detailed information on their cancer programs.

Participating Hospitals

- **City of Hope**

- **Cleveland Clinic Foundation**

- **Continuum Health Partners**

- **Fox Chase Cancer Center**

- **Hackensack University Medical Center**

- **IU Simon Cancer Center/Clarian Health**

- **Maimonides Medical Center**

- **Memorial Sloan-Kettering Cancer Center**

- **Mount Sinai Medical Center**

- **New York Eye & Ear Infirmary**

- **NewYork-Presbyterian Hospital**

- **NYU Langone Medical Center**

- **Penn Medicine**

- **Sylvester Comprehensive Cancer Center**

- **Thomas Jefferson University Hospital**

- **Wake Forest University Baptist Medical Center**

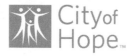

City of Hope

1500 East Duarte Road
Duarte, CA 91010
800-826-HOPE cityofhope.org

Sponsorship: Non-profit treatment and research center
Beds: 162 in-patient beds
Accreditation: The Joint Commission

City of Hope is a recognized worldwide leader for its compassionate patient care, innovative science and translational research, which rapidly turn laboratory breakthroughs into promising new therapies. One of only 40 National Cancer Institute-designated Comprehensive Cancer Centers nationwide and a founding member of the National Comprehensive Cancer Network, City of Hope is ranked as one of "America's Best Hospitals" in cancer and urology by *U.S.News & World Report*.

ACADEMIC AND CLINICAL AFFILIATIONS

As an independent academic institution, City of Hope enables its researchers to pursue all avenues of scientific inquiry while encouraging collaboration with other researchers and institutions around the world. This helps to speed the development of novel cancer therapies. City of Hope's Graduate School of Biological Sciences also provides a fertile academic environment to prepare future scientists for careers in academia, medical and industrial fields.

MEDICAL STAFF

Guided by a humanistic approach to medicine, nationally recognized physicians and nurses lead collaborative treatment teams that address the whole patient, not just the disease, including emotional, psychological, spiritual and nutritional needs.

PIONEERING, COMPREHENSIVE MEDICAL CARE

City of Hope's Helford Clinical Research Hospital integrates the best of science and human caring in one state-of-the-art facility. There, lifesaving research and superior clinical care join forces as multidisciplinary teams of medical professionals pool their knowledge to bring promising new therapies to patients quickly, safely and effectively.

PHYSICIAN REFERRAL

City of Hope welcomes patient referrals from physicians throughout the world. Referring physicians are encouraged to contact our specialists directly or call 800-826-HOPE.

Cleveland Clinic

Innovative Research and Outstanding Outcomes

At Cleveland Clinic Taussig Cancer Institute, more than 250 cancer specialists, researchers, nurses and technicians are dedicated to developing and applying the latest and most effective medical techniques to achieve the long-term survival and improve the quality of life for 7,500 new cancer patients every year. Because of our patient-centered care, leading-edge treatments, innovative research, 350 clinical trials and state-of-the-art medical technologies, *U.S.News & World Report* has rankedCleveland Clinic's cancer program one of the top cancer centers in the nation.

The Taussig Cancer Institute has more than 200,000 annual cancer patient visits at its main campus in Cleveland and at 10 locations throughout Northeast Ohio. Our areas of expertise include prostate and other urologic cancers, melanoma, blood and bone marrow cancers, multiple myeloma, colorectal cancer, lung cancer, breast cancer and brain and spinal cord tumors. **To schedule an appointment or get a second opinion, call 866.223.8100 today or visit clevelandclinic.org/cancerTCD.**

> ### Clinical Trials Now Online
>
> Cleveland Clinic offers a new online tool for patients, caregivers and physicians to search for open clinical trials at clevelandclinic.org/cancertrials. The site lists more than 100 trials being managed by oncologists in the Taussig Cancer Institute that are accepting patients at all Cleveland Clinic campuses, including main campus and our regional hospitals.
>
> Patients, family members and physicians who have questions about a specific trial or who are interested in enrolling in an open study can call the Cancer Answer Line at 866.223.8100 for more information.

Because of Taussig Cancer Institute's extensive cancer care system, the Leukemia & Lymphoma Society forged a groundbreaking partnership with Taussig Cancer Institute to make blood cancer clinical trials available to patients in their communities. This enables patients to stay with their primary doctors and participate in clinical trials near their hometown.

Outstanding Outcomes: Our Bone Marrow Transplant outcomes are unsurpassed by any program in the world. We have one of the most experienced teams in the nation, having performed more than 3,000 bone marrow transplant procedures since 1977.

Innovative Research: Taussig Cancer Institute is at the forefront of cancer research. Our world-renowned scientists are dedicated to developing novel, effective therapeutic options for cancer patients. Through understanding cellular abnormalities that lead to cancer, our researchers target specific genes with drugs or combinations of drugs to improve outcomes.

Cancer Genetics at the Center for Personalized Genetic Healthcare

Because some families are prone to developing cancer, advances in genetic research help us identify some of the risk factors. Cleveland Clinic's Center for Personalized Genetic Healthcare aims to prevent cancer by identifying high risk individuals and offers personalized medical management to them and their family members. For more information or to schedule an appointment, call 800.998.4785.

In our multidisciplinary clinics, medical, radiation and surgical oncologists work closely with pathologists, radiologists, oncology nurses and social workers to optimize the options for individual patients with complex problems.

To schedule an appointment or for more information about the Cleveland Clinic Taussig Cancer Institute, call 866.223.8100 or visit clevelandclinic.org/cancerTCD. Ask about our complimentary Medical Concierge service for patients who travel to Cleveland Clinic from outside Ohio.

Cleveland Clinic Taussig Cancer Institute | Cleveland, OH

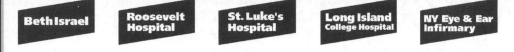

Sponsorship: Voluntary Not-for-profit **Beds:** 2,727 certified beds
Accreditation: Joint Commission of Accreditation of Healthcare Organizations (JCAHO), Accreditation Council for Graduate Medical Education, Medical Society of New York, in conjunction with the Accreditation Council for Continuing Medical Education

A STRONG PARTNERSHIP WITH A PROUD HERITAGE

Continuum Health Partners is a partnership of six venerable health care providers: Beth Israel Medical Center-Milton and Carroll Petrie Division, Beth Israel Medical Center-Kings Highway Division, St. Luke's Hospital, Roosevelt Hospital, Long Island College Hospital of Brooklyn, and The New York Eye and Ear Infirmary. Each of the six partner institutions was established more than a century ago by individuals committed to improving health and health care in their communities. Today, the system represents over 4,000 physicians and dentists and is superbly equipped to respond to the health care needs of the populations we serve. Our providers also see patients in group and private practice settings and in ambulatory centers in New York City and Westchester County.

LOCATIONS

Continuum Health Partners has campuses throughout Manhattan and Brooklyn. Beth Israel Medical Center has two divisions: the Milton and Caroll Petrie Division on the East Side, and the Kings Highway Division in Brooklyn. The Phillips Ambulatory Care Center, a state-of-art outpatient center, is located at Union Square. St. Luke's Hospital is in Morningside Heights and Roosevelt Hospital is in the Columbus Circle and Lincoln Center neighborhoods on the West Side. Long Island College Hospital of Brooklyn is located in the Brooklyn Heights/Cobble Hill section of Brooklyn. The New York Eye and Ear Infirmary is located on Second Avenue and 14th street.

ACADEMIC AFFILIATIONS

Beth Israel Medical Center is the University Hospital and Manhattan Campus for the Albert Einstein College of Medicine. St. Luke's-Roosevelt Hospital Center is an Academic Affiliate of Columbia University College of Physicians and Surgeons. Long Island College Hospital of Brooklyn is the primary teaching affiliate of the SUNY-Health Science Center in Brooklyn. The New York Eye and Ear Infirmary is the primary teaching center of the New York Medical College and affiliated teaching hospitals in the areas of ophthalmology and otolaryngology.

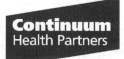

For a referral to a great doctor in your neighborhood, call (800) 420-4004.
Our Physician Referral Service can help you find a primary care
physician or specialist affiliated with Beth Israel, St. Luke's, Roosevelt,
Long Island College Hospital, or The New York Eye and Ear Infirmary.
Visit our Website at www.chpnyc.org

FOX CHASE
CANCER CENTER

333 Cottman Avenue
Philadelphia, PA 19111-2497
Phone: 1-888-FOX CHASE
www.fccc.edu

Sponsorship	Independent Nonprofit
Beds	100 licensed beds
Accreditation	The Joint Commission; American Hospital Association; American College of Surgeons Commission on Cancer; College of American Pathology; American College of Radiology

U.S. News & World Report consistently ranks Fox Chase Cancer Center among the nation's best. Fox Chase is also the first hospital in Pennsylvania and the nation's first cancer hospital to earn the Magnet Award for Nursing Excellence from the American Nurses Credentialing Center.

Overview

Fox Chase Cancer Center is one of the leading cancer research and treatments centers in the United States. Founded in 1904 in Philadelphia as one of the nation's first cancer hospitals, Fox Chase was also among the first institutions to be designated a National Cancer Institute Comprehensive Cancer Center in 1974. Fox Chase researchers have won the highest awards in their fields, including two Nobel Prizes. Fox Chase physicians are also routinely recognized in national rankings, and the Center's nursing program has received the Magnet status for excellence three consecutive times. Today, Fox Chase conducts a broad array of nationally competitive basic, translational, and clinical research, with special programs in cancer prevention, detection, survivorship, and community outreach.

- Fox Chase's 100-bed hospital is one of the few in the country devoted entirely to adult cancer care.
- Annual hospital admissions exceed 4,500 and outpatient visits to physicians total more than 75,000 a year.
- Fox Chase's board-certified specialists are recognized nationally and internationally in medical, radiation and surgical oncology, diagnostic imaging, diagnostic pathology, pain management, oncology nursing and oncology social work.
- The staff provides a coordinated approach to meet the treatment needs of each patient. Special multidisciplinary centers provide consultations and treatment recommendations for specific types of cancer.
- The nursing staff of specially trained oncology nurses provides one of the best nurse-to-patient ratios in the area.
- Fox Chase investigators have received numerous awards and honors, including Nobel Prizes in medicine and chemistry; a Kyoto Prize, a Lasker Clinical Research Award, memberships in the National Academy of Sciences and General Motors Cancer Research Foundation Prizes.
- Fox Chase is a founding member of the National Comprehensive Cancer Network, an alliance of the nation's leading academic cancer centers, and the hub of Fox Chase Cancer Center Partners, a select group of more than 22 community hospitals with Fox Chase-affiliated cancer programs.

**For more about Fox Chase physicians and services,
visit our web site, www.fccc.edu, or call 1-888-FOX CHASE.**

HACKENSACK UNIVERSITY MEDICAL CENTER

30 Prospect Avenue
Hackensack, New Jersey 07601
phone 201-996-3760
fax 201-996-3452

www.humc.com

Sponsorship	A not-for-profit, teaching and research hospital affiliated with the University of Medicine and Dentistry of New Jersey – New Jersey Medical School.
Beds	A 775-bed, Level II Trauma Center, providing tertiary and regional services for the New York/New Jersey metropolitan area.
Accreditation	Joint Commission on the Accreditation of Healthcare Organizations.

BACKGROUND

Founded in 1888 as Bergen County's first hospital, Hackensack University Medical Center (HUMC) has demonstrated more than a century of growth and progress in response to the needs of the communities it serves. The medical center continues to be the largest provider of inpatient and outpatient services in New Jersey and has been ranked as the fourth largest healthcare facility in the nation by number of inpatient admissions. Hackensack University Medical Center is Bergen County's largest employer with a work force of more than 7,200 employees and an annual budget of more than $1 billion.

MEDICAL AND DENTAL STAFF

There are nearly 1,500 members on the medical and dental staff. These physicians and dentists represent a full spectrum of medical and dental specialties and subspecialties.

ACCOMPLISHMENTS

One of America's 50 Best Hospitals – Hackensack University Medical Center has been recognized as one of America's 50 Best Hospitals by HealthGrades, the nation's leading independent healthcare ratings company. The designation recognizes hospitals that have demonstrated superior clinical quality over a seven-year time period, based upon an analysis of more than 75 million Medicare patient records from 1999-2005. These hospitals have achieved better survival rates and lower complication rates across dozens of medical procedures and diagnoses, from cardiac care to orthopedic surgery, consistently ranking among the top five percent in the nation for overall clinical outcomes. Hackensack University Medical Center is the only healthcare facility in New Jersey, New York, and New England to be named one of America's 50 Best Hospitals and has received this recognition for three years in a row.

Nursing Excellence – Honored since 1995 as the first hospital in New Jersey to receive the Magnet Award for Nursing Excellence from the American Nurses Credentialing Center. The medical center became the second hospital in the country to receive redesignation of this prestigious award and continues to have this highly honored recognition.

PREMIER AWARD FOR QUALITY

The Premier healthcare alliance has recognized Hackensack University Medical Center with its 2009 Premier Award for Quality. The medical center is the only one in New Jersey and one of oly 23 out of 3,796 eligible hospitals nationwide to be so honored.

Premier comprises 2,100 United States hospitals and 50,000+ other healthcare sites that work together to improve healthcare quality and affordability. The Award for Quality recognizes healthcare organizations that efficiently provide outstanding patient care and consistently set the standard in clinical excellence nationwide. The Award for Quality uses performance-based criteria – including clinical outcomes, resource utilization, and clinical process indicators – to measure top performing healthcare institutions. All acute inpatient facilities in the United States that submitted data to the Centers for Medicare & Medicaid Services (CMS) and the CMS Hospital Compare project were considered for the Award of Quality.

U.S. NEW AND WORLD REPORT

Hackensack University Medical Center has been ranked in **four specialties** including **geriatrics, heart and heart surgery, kidney disorders, and orthopedics** in *U.S. News and World Report's 200-10 publication of "America's Best Hospitals."*

IU SIMON CANCER CENTER
An IU School of Medicine & Clarian Health Partnership

The Indiana University Melvin and Bren Simon Cancer Center reflects the statewide nationally recognized health care delivery system of Clarian Health, supported by the scientific resources of Indiana University School of Medicine (IUSM), the second largest medical school in the United States.

SCIENTIFIC EXCELLENCE

The Indiana University Melvin and Bren Simon Cancer Center, a partnership between Clarian Health and IUSM, is the only National Cancer Institute (NCI)-designated cancer center in Indiana that provides patient care. This designation recognizes IU Simon Cancer Center's scientific excellence and helps fund life-saving research that ultimately benefits patients.

Nearly 40,000 patients turn to IU Simon Cancer Center for cancer care each year, seeking the multidisciplinary team approach pioneered in Indiana by each of our disease-specific clinical care programs. Our team approach combines treatment, research and supportive care expertise for each patient. With both standards of care and clinical trial options, IU Simon Cancer Center offers diagnostic, treatment and prevention regimens that meet the unique needs of each individual patient.

PATIENT/FAMILY FOCUS

Located in the heart of Indianapolis, the IU Simon Cancer Center offers the most advanced care in modern and comfortable facilities. Our CompleteLife program addresses the full spectrum of patient and family needs, including emotional, psychological and spiritual concerns. The benefits to patients are clear — a wide range of innovative treatment options, expert teams of diverse professionals focused on their specific cancer type and attention to all cancer care needs in one setting.

RESEARCH EXPERTISE

The IU Simon Cancer Center's research expertise is known around the world, offering renewed hope for patients and families and new options in cancer care. Researchers and physicians with IU Simon Cancer Center have improved the cure rate of testicular cancer from 10 percent to nearly 95 percent today. Our physicians have gained international recognition for treatment of the following conditions:

- Breast cancer
- Gastrointestinal cancers
- Genitourinary cancer
- Hematologic cancer
- Bone marrow and stem cell transplantation at Riley Hospital for Children and Indiana University Hospital
- Thoracic cancer

To schedule an appointment or for more information, call 888-600-4822 or visit cancer.iu.edu.

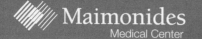

Memorial Sloan-Kettering Cancer Center

The Best Cancer Care. Anywhere.

1275 York Avenue
New York, NY 10065
Phone: (212) 639-2000
Physician Referral: (800) 525-2225
www.mskcc.org

Beds: 434
Sponsorship/Network Affiliation: Private, Non-Profit
Physician Referral: (800) 525-2225

THE MEMORIAL SLOAN-KETTERING ADVANTAGE: CANCER IS OUR ONLY FOCUS

At Memorial Sloan-Kettering Cancer Center (MSKCC), our only focus is cancer. Internationally recognized as one of the world's premier facilities for cancer care, we are consistently ranked as one of the nation's top cancer centers by *U.S. News & World Report*. We are proud to be a National Cancer Institute (NCI) Comprehensive Cancer Center and a member of the National Comprehensive Cancer Network.

A TEAM APPROACH TO CANCER CARE

Patients at MSKCC benefit from individualized treatment plans developed by a team of specialists with an unsurpassed depth and breadth of experience. The teams include surgeons, medical and radiation oncologists, radiologists, pathologists, nurses, and others who are specialists in treating patients with a specific type of cancer. They develop treatment plans that reflect their combined expertise, so that patients who need several different types of therapy will receive the best combination for them.

GREATER PRECISION IN DIAGNOSIS

Getting the correct diagnosis right from the start is crucial. At MSKCC, we use the most advanced imaging technologies, such as combined PET/CT and nuclear medicine scans, to accurately detect and precisely locate cancer. Our highly specialized pathologists analyze some 40,000 tumor samples annually to determine an exact diagnosis and the extent of disease. Increasingly, they use new technology to identify the molecular differences among tumors, allowing even greater precision in diagnosis.

UNPARALLELED SURGICAL EXPERTISE

Recent studies have shown that, for many cancers, patients have fewer complications and better outcomes if they have surgery at a hospital where high volumes of these operations are performed by surgeons with much experience in the procedure. MSKCC surgeons are among the most experienced cancer surgeons in the world. They use the latest surgical technology, including robotic and minimally invasive techniques, as well as interventional radiology for embolization, thermal ablation, and chemical ablation of tumors. In their quest to spare or reconstruct organs and preserve function, they are renowned for not only saving lives, but preserving the quality of life.

ADVANCES IN CHEMOTHERAPY

Our medical oncologists are leaders in developing new chemotherapy drugs that are safer and more effective than standard therapies. They also help manage any side effects of chemotherapy, such as nausea and fatigue, so patients can continue their usual activities wherever possible. Increasingly, our medical oncologists use advanced technologies, such as immunotherapies or vaccines, often in combination with chemotherapy.

LEADERS IN RADIATION THERAPY

MSKCC's radiation oncologists are highly skilled in complex treatment planning and sophisticated delivery techniques. For example, they have furthered intensity-modulated radiation therapy with image guidance (IGRT). IGRT enables them to image a tumor just before or even during a radiation treatment so they can adjust the radiation beams to pinpoint tumors with extreme accuracy. In some cases, our doctors may use radiation therapy combined with chemotherapy to make tumors more sensitive to the radiation, thus enhancing the chances of success.

RESEARCH EXPANDS TREATMENT OPTIONS

Through close collaboration between clinicians and research scientists, new therapies developed in the laboratory can be quickly translated into improved treatment options for patients.

INSURANCE

Memorial Sloan-Kettering Cancer Center is in-network with most New York–area insurance plans.

Physician Referral: (800) 525-2225

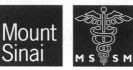

MOUNT SINAI
SCHOOL OF
MEDICINE

THE TISCH CANCER INSTITUTE
AT THE MOUNT SINAI MEDICAL CENTER
One Gustave L. Levy Place
Fifth Avenue and 100th Street
New York, NY 10029-6574
Physician Referral: 1-800-MD-SINAI (637-4624)
www.tischcancerinstitute.org

OVERVIEW
The Tisch Cancer Institute, part of The Mount Sinai Medical Center, is located on the Upper East Side of Manhattan. The Mount Sinai Medical Center was founded in 1852 and encompasses one of the oldest teaching hospitals in the country. In an atmosphere of learning, cutting-edge basic and clinical research, and superb patient care, The Tisch Cancer Institute coordinates a full-service diagnostic and treatment program for cancer patients. Because new treatments are developed at the Institute, patients often have access to these therapies before they are available anywhere else in the world.

A HERITAGE OF BREAKTHROUGHS
Teams of physicians and scientists at The Tisch Cancer Institute at Mount Sinai work together to rapidly translate laboratory research into new patient treatments. Among the advances pioneered at Mount Sinai are the first successful treatment of tumors of the bladder by transurethral electrocoagulation, the first demonstration of how asbestos can cause cancerous changes in the DNA of cells, and the first development of an ultrasound-guided technique to insert radioactive seeds into the prostate to treat prostate cancer.

THE TISCH CANCER INSTITUTE
The Tisch Cancer Institute employs a multidisciplinary treatment approach, providing access to clinical breakthroughs, innovative techniques, leading-edge technologies, and a wide range of diagnostic, therapeutic, and support services for all types of cancer. The Institute treats: head and neck cancer; thoracic cancer (including lung and esophagus); gynecologic cancer; hematological malignancies (including myelodysplastic syndrome and myeloproliferative disorders); brain tumors; and prostate, bladder, kidney, and liver cancer. In addition to surgical treatment, the Institute provides radiation and medical oncology therapies as well as bone marrow transplantation.

The Institute's multidisciplinary treatment approach involves collaboration with colleagues across the Medical Center, drawing upon the knowledge of a vast network of specialists who are outstanding in their fields. These experts consist of award-winning physicians and surgeons specializing in cardiac care, neurology, urology, pediatrics, digestive diseases, obstetrics and gynecology, and other therapeutic areas. Furthermore, Mount Sinai's nursing staff is an important part of the Medical Center's focus on delivering exceptional patient care, and it has received the prestigious Magnet Award for nursing excellence.

Mount Sinai is renowned for its palliative care program, which provides the highest level of care, focusing on the relief of pain, symptoms, and stress in cancer patients in both an inpatient and outpatient setting.

THE RUTTENBERG TREATMENT CENTER
The mission of the Ruttenberg Treatment Center at The Mount Sinai Medical Center is to reduce the burden of human cancer through its outstanding interdisciplinary programs in patient care and research, including cancer prevention, treatment, early detection, and education. Oncologists, surgeons, and specialists from across the medical spectrum work together to provide the highest quality care to all cancer patients. The members of the Center—scientists and physicians—are developing cancer therapies and prevention strategies to improve cancer care, and patients at the Center are the first to benefit from these treatments.

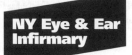
Sponsored Page

NewYork-Presbyterian
The University Hospital of Columbia and Cornell

Affiliated with Columbia University College of Physicians and Surgeons and Weill Medical College of Cornell University

NewYork-Presbyterian Hospital
Weill Cornell Medical Center
525 East 68th Street
New York, NY 10021

NewYork-Presbyterian Hospital
Columbia University Medical Center
622 West 168th Street
New York, NY 10032

Sponsorship: Voluntary Not-for-Profit
Beds: 2,369
Accreditation: Joint Commission on Accreditation of Healthcare Organizations (JCAHO), Commission on Accreditation of Rehabilitation Facilities (CARF) and College of American Pathologists (CAP)

The *U.S. News & World Report* has ranked NewYork-Presbyterian Hospital higher in more specialties than any other hospital in the New York area. NewYork-Presbyterian Hospital was named to the *Honor Roll of America's Best Hospitals.*

OVERVIEW:

NewYork-Presbyterian Hospital is the largest hospital in New York and one of the most comprehensive healthcare institutions in the world with 5,500 physicians, approximately 96,000 discharges and nearly 1 million outpatient visits annually, and with its affiliated medical schools, more than $330 million in research support.

AMONG ITS RENOWNED CENTERS OF EXCELLENCE ARE:

Morgan Stanley Children's Hospital and the Komansky Center for Children's Health – One of the largest, most comprehensive children's hospitals in the world providing highly sophisticated pediatric medical, surgical and intensive care, including a pediatric cardiovascular center, in a compassionate environment.

NewYork-Presbyterian Cancer Centers – Coordinated, multidisciplinary care and the latest therapeutic options and clinical trials available for all types of cancer.

NewYork-Presbyterian Heart – Expert diagnostic capabilities and medical and surgical innovations for simple to complex heart conditions.

NewYork-Presbyterian Neuroscience Centers – Latest research, diagnosis and treatment capabilities in Alzheimer's disease, Multiple Sclerosis, Parkinson's disease, aneurysms, epilepsy, brain tumors, stokes and other neurological disorders.

NewYork-Presbyterian Psychiatry – World-renowned center of excellence in psychiatric treatment, research and education.

NewYork-Presbyterian Transplant Institute – Adult and pediatric heart, liver, and kidney and adult pancreas and lung transplantation and cutting-edge research.

NewYork-Presbyterian Vascular Care Center – Comprehensive and integrated preventive, diagnostic and treatment program for diverse problems related to arteries and veins throughout the body.

NewYork-Presbyterian Digestive Disease Services – Expert capabilities in the broad range of conditions that affect the organs as well as other components of the digestive system.

William Randolph Hearst Burn Center – Largest and busiest burn center in the nation which also conducts research to improve survival and enhance quality of life for burn victims.

In addition, the Hospital offers extraordinary expertise, comprehensive programs and specialized resources in the fields of AIDS, Complementary Medicine, Gene Therapy, Reproductive Medicine and Infertility, Trauma Center and Women's Health Care.

ACADEMIC AFFILIATIONS:

NewYork-Presbyterian is the only hospital in the world affiliated with two Ivy League medical schools; The Joan and Sanford I Weill Medical College of Cornell University and the Columbia University College of Physicians and Surgeons.

Physician Referral: To find a NewYork-Presbyterian Hospital affiliated physician to meet your needs, call toll free 1-877-NYP-WELL (1-877-697-9355) or visit our website at www.nyp.org

Langone Medical Center

NYU Langone Medical Center
550 First Avenue (at 31st Street)
New York, New York 10016
www.nyumc.org
1-888-769-8633

NYU Langone Medical Center is one of the nation's premier centers of excellence in healthcare, biomedical research, and medical education. For over 168 years, NYU physicians and researchers have made countless contributions to the art and science of medicine.

Today the Medical Center consists of the three hospitals of NYU Hospitals Center—Tisch Hospital, a 705-bed acute-care general hospital; Rusk Institute of Rehabilitation Medicine, the first and largest facility of its kind; and the Hospital for Joint Diseases, a leader in musculoskeletal care—and NYU School of Medicine, including the Smilow Research Center, the Skirball Institute of Biomolecular Medicine, and the Sackler Institute of Graduate Biomedical Sciences.

With its specialized hospitals, NYU Langone Medical Center is internationally renowned for its services in orthopaedics and rehabilitation medicine. The medical center is also known for its excellence in areas such as cardiovascular disease, pediatrics, skin care, neurosurgery, urology, cancer care, bariatric surgery, plastic surgery, minimally invasive surgery, transplant surgery, infertility, women's health and day surgery. Many of these services are delivered through its major centers and institutes, including the NYU Cancer Institute, NYU Cardiac & Vascular Institute, Charles C. Harris Skin & Cancer Unit, Stephen D. Hassenfeld Children's Center for Cancer and Blood Disorders and the NYU Child Study Center.

As an integral part of an academic medical center, NYU Langone Medical Center's clinical services are continuously informed and enhanced by hundreds of ongoing basic and clinical research projects, as well as by major initiatives in translational research that promise to speed the transfer of laboratory discoveries to the patient's bedside. With this goal in mind, NYU Langone Medical Center recently established six Centers of Excellence that bring together some of its most distinguished scientists—researchers and clinicians—who share a deep passion and a common cause to improve and extend the lives of patients who suffer from Alzheimer's disease and other dementias; addiction; multiple sclerosis; skin cancer; urological diseases; and musculoskeletal diseases.

Additionally, the strengths of NYU Langone Medical Center include the talents of affiliates and partners, such as Bellevue Hospital Center and the Manhattan Veterans Affairs Medical Center.

Looking for information on our expert physicians?
1-888-769-8633

Sponsorship: Private; Not-for-Profit
Accreditations: The Joint Commission; Commission for Accreditation of Rehabilitation Facilities (CARF); NCI - designated Cancer Center and Magnet Status

Penn Medicine

OVERVIEW

For more than two centuries, Penn physicians and scientists have been committed to the highest standards of patient care, education and research. Our commitment has been recognized by our peers and by others throughout the greater Philadelphia region and across the nation.

Penn Medicine ranks second nationally in special grant funding from the National Institutes of Health, with several departments ranking first nationally. Overall, Penn has more individual departments ranked in the top five than any other academic medical center. *U.S.News* also consistently ranks the University of Pennsylvania Schools of Medicine and Nursing among the nation's best.

Our physicians and scientists are united in the health system's mission to expand the frontiers of medicine through new discoveries in the detection, treatment and prevention of human disease. Because we develop and test new treatments through clinical trials, our patients gain access to the very latest advances and future generations will benefit from the work we do today.

Penn continues to lead the way in discovering new treatment methods for diseases once considered incurable, including groundbreaking research in cancer, cardiac, neurosciences, orthopaedics, genetics and imaging.

Over the past 30 years, Penn physicians and scientists have participated in many important discoveries, including:

- The first general vaccine against pneumonia.

- The introduction of total intravenous feeding.

- The development of cognitive therapy.

- The development of magnetic resonance imaging and other imaging technologies.

- The discovery of the Philadelphia chromosome, which revolutionized cancer research by making the connection between genetic abnormalities and cancer.

- The development of a cure for atrial fibrillation.

- Pioneering new procedures in robotic-assisted surgery.

Locations

Patients are seen at:

- Hospital of the University of Pennsylvania
- Penn Presbyterian Medical Center
- Pennsylvania Hospital
- Penn Medicine at Cherry Hill
- Penn Medicine at Radnor
- Penn Medicine at Rittenhouse
- PennCare®, our primary care physician network, provides services in the local communities in Bucks, Chester, Delaware, Montgomery and Philadelphia counties in Pennsylvania and in Southern New Jersey.
- Hospice and home care services are provided by Penn Home Care and Hospice Services.

On the Web

Visit PennMedicine.org for the latest patient education with explanation of surgical procedures and follow-up care, screening tools, drug interactions and descriptions as well as an encyclopedia of health information.

To learn more about Penn physicians or services, call 800.789.PENN or visit PennMedicine.org

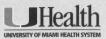
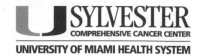
Sponsored Page

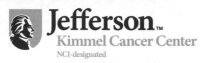

111 S. 11th Street, Philadelphia, PA 19107-5098, 215-955-6000, *www.JeffersonHospital.org*

Designated Center of Excellence

Thomas Jefferson University Hospitals is an academic medical center comprised of Thomas Jefferson University Hospital, Jefferson Hospital for Neuroscience (JHN), Methodist Hospital and multiple outpatient sites. It is home to the Kimmel Cancer Center at Jefferson, a National Cancer Institute-designated Center for Excellence in cancer research and treatment, where world-famous cancer specialists provide breakthrough treatment delivered with compassion, support and state-of-the-art technology. Jefferson doctors are ranked among the nation's best for cancer treatment on many prestigious lists, such as *Best Doctors in America*® database of experts. They also contribute to leading scientific and medical journals and hold leadership positions in many national and local cancer organizations.

At the Forefront of Cancer Care

Jefferson's Kimmel Cancer Center offers innovative therapies and clinical trial participation opportunities for brain, breast, colon and rectal, head and neck, lung, pancreatic, prostate, and complex and rare cancers. For example:

- Working together, Jefferson neurological surgeons and radiation oncologists have established radiosurgery as the standard for **brain cancer**. JHN introduced the region to Shaped Beam™ Stereotactic Radiosurgery, which precisely treats brain tumors while sparing healthy tissue.

- Jefferson patients with **breast cancer** may receive precisely targeted radiation therapy and intensity modulated radiation therapy technology to spare healthy breast tissue. Those patients with breast cancer on the left side may benefit from Active Breathing Coordination, a leading-edge treatment not widely available elsewhere. At the Jefferson-Honickman Breast Imaging Center, women have access to digital mammography, ultrasound and mammogram-guided core and stereotactic biopsies. PET-CT with MRI is also available.

- Utilizing the expertise of surgeons, medical oncologists, surgical pathologists, radiation oncologists, geneticists, nurses and ultrasound specialists, Jefferson's **colorectal cancer** program incorporates high-dose preoperative radiation and special sphincter-preservation surgical techniques. Jefferson's hereditary cancer testing program is among the Delaware Valley's most comprehensive. For screening, Jefferson offers colonoscopy, flexible sigmoidoscopy and fecal occult blood test, as well as virtual colonoscopy to eligible patients.

- **Head and neck cancer** experts in Jefferson's Department of Otolaryngology take a multidisciplinary approach to treatment of the esophagus, nose, mouth, voice box and thyroid. Otolaryngologists collaborate with neurological surgeons in offering minimally invasive cranial base surgery and endoscopic neurosurgery to remove skull-based tumors through the nose and nasal sinuses as an alternative to traditional open surgery.

- Jefferson medical oncologists and hematologists treat **hematologic malignancies** affecting the **bone marrow**, including leukemia, lymphoma and multiple myeloma. Jefferson offers autologous and allogeneic bone marrow transplantation for selected forms of cancer. Our phase I-II clinical trial in allogeneic stem cell transplant has resulted in several successful transplants of patients from half-match donors.

- Jefferson's multidisciplinary thoracic oncology team includes radiation and medical oncology specialists with expertise in treating **lung cancer**, as well as thoracic surgeons, pulmonary disease specialists, radiologists, nurses and social workers. Jefferson offers patients entry into national trials of new treatment regimens against lung cancers. Jefferson also offers minimally invasive video-assisted thoracic surgery (VATS), resulting in less pain, shorter hospital stays and faster recoveries for patients than traditional, open thoracotomy does.

- The Melanoma Hope Network has designated Jefferson's Kimmel Cancer Center as a Melanoma Center of Excellence. This designation recognizes Jefferson's exceptional care, knowledge and compassion to patients with melanoma, which is the most dangerous form of **skin cancer**.

- When possible, Jefferson surgeons treat **pancreatic cancer** by performing a "mini-Whipple" procedure that preserves the entire stomach, the pylorus and several centimeters of the upper duodenum. Jefferson's pancreatic cancer program is number one by surgical volume in the Delaware Valley; studies show that outcomes are better for patients who undergo procedures at high-volume centers.

- Jefferson's partnership of urologists and radiologists is at the national forefront for **prostate cancer** diagnosis. Jefferson urologists use robot-assisted laparoscopic prostatectomy, among other methods, to treat prostate cancer.

- Healthcare insurer Independence Blue Cross, a member of the Blue Cross and Blue Shield Association, has selected Thomas Jefferson University Hospital/Kimmel Cancer Center as a Blue Distinction Center for Complex and Rare Cancers such as **esophageal cancer**, **bladder cancer**, **liver cancer** and **thyroid cancer**.

Physician Referral: Outpatient healthcare services are available throughout the Delaware Valley at the offices of 205 primary care physicians and 572 specialists affiliated with Thomas Jefferson University Hospitals. For an appointment with a Jefferson doctor, call **1-800-JEFF-NOW** or visit *www.JeffersonHospital.org*

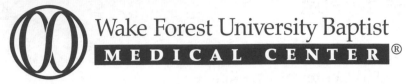

Medical Center Boulevard • Winston-Salem, NC 27157
PAL® (Physician-to-physician calls) 1-800-277-7654
Health On-Call® (Patient access) 1-800-446-2255
www.wfubmc.edu • www.brennerchildrens.org • www.besthealth.com

OVERVIEW

Wake Forest University Baptist Medical Center encompasses **Wake Forest University School of Medicine**, whose reputation attracts some of the nation's top doctors to its Wake Forest University Physicians faculty practice, and **North Carolina Baptist Hospital**, a nationally ranked, academic tertiary care facility. Internationally known for state-of-the-art treatment and technology, research leadership and teaching excellence, Wake Forest University Baptist Medical Center is ranked a top hospital by *U.S.News & World Report* (since 1993). More than 550 physicians offer preventive and highly specialized care.

COMPREHENSIVE SPECIALTY CENTERS AND SERVICES

Brenner Children's Hospital . . . the highest levels of neonatal and pediatric care in a state-of-the-art setting; **Heart Center** . . . groundbreaking research, technology and treatment, region's only transplant service; **Comprehensive Cancer Center of WFU** . . . NCI-designated for research, advanced technologies, treatments such as Gamma Knife, Intensity Modulated Radiation Therapy; **Neurosciences** . . . Stroke, ALS, Epilepsy, and Brain Tumor Centers, expertise in deep brain stimulation for Parkinson's; the region's most comprehensive, advanced service in **Digestive Health, Orthopaedics, Otolaryngology, Urology.**

RESEARCH EXCELLENCE

Wake Forest Baptist has more than 1,000 research and clinical trials under way, and a new Translational Science Institute is accelerating discovery that will benefit patients. At the **Wake Forest Institute for Regenerative Medicine**, doctors are applying tissue engineering to build more than 20 organs and tissues and have successfully implanted human, laboratory-grown bladders. The **Center for Human Genomics** is advancing knowledge of gene-based therapies for cardiovascular and pulmonary diseases, prostate cancer and diabetes. The **Brain Tumor Center** is at the forefront of molecular medicine therapies and radiation-induced brain injury research. The **Center for Biomolecular Imaging** is creating new ways to view the brain, heart and cancers.

TECHNOLOGY LEADERSHIP

Committed to serving our patients with "tomorrow's medicine" today, Wake Forest Baptist is home to one of North America's first **Integrated Brachytherapy Units**, a faster, extremely precise cancer treatment using radioactive seed implants . . . one of the nation's first **Bioanatomic Imaging and Treatment Programs**, allowing for new levels of accuracy in tumor identification and treatment . . . North Carolina's only **MEG** (magnetoencephalography), brain-function imaging that enables highly precise neurosurgical planning . . . N.C.'s first **Gamma Knife**, the gold standard for non-invasive brain surgeries.

OUTSTANDING CARE

WFUBMC is the **top consumer choice** in its area for health care, according to National Research Corp. surveys. **Patient satisfaction** scores are among the highest in the nation as compared to its peer group, according to Press Ganey. **Outstanding nursing** earned Wake Forest Baptist one of the nation's first 15 Magnet Awards for nursing excellence, awarded by the American Nurses Credentialing Center.

To make an appointment or find a specialist at Wake Forest University Baptist Medical Center, call Health On-Call® at **1-800-446-2255.**

KNOWLEDGE MAKES ALL THE DIFFERENCE.

Section III
Physician Listings by Medical Specialty

Colon & Rectal Surgery

A colon and rectal surgeon is trained to diagnose and treat various diseases of the intestinal tract, colon, rectum, anal canal and perianal area by medical and surgical means. This specialist also deals with other organs and tissues (such as the liver, urinary and female reproductive system) involved with primary intestinal disease.

Colon and rectal surgeons have the expertise to diagnose and often manage anorectal conditions such as hemorrhoids, fissures (painful tears in the anal lining), abscesses and fistulae (infections located around the anus and rectum) in the office setting. They also treat problems of the intestine and colon and perform endoscopic procedures to evaluate and treat problems such as cancer, polyps (pre-cancerous growths) and inflammatory conditions.

Training Required: Five Years of General Surgery followed by one year in Colon & Rectal Surgery.

COLON & RECTAL SURGERY

New England

Bleday, Ronald MD [CRS] - **Spec Exp:** Colon & Rectal Cancer; **Hospital:** Brigham & Women's Hosp, Dana-Farber Cancer Inst; **Address:** Brigham & Women's Hosp, Dept Genl Surg, 75 Francis St, ASB II, Boston, MA 02115; **Phone:** 617-732-8460; **Board Cert:** Surgery 1999; Colon & Rectal Surgery 2003; **Med School:** McGill Univ 1982; **Resid:** Surgery, Rhode Island Hosp 1989; Surgical Oncology, Brigham & Womens Hosp 1986; **Fellow:** Endoscopy, Mass Genl Hosp 1990; Colon & Rectal Surgery, Univ Minn 1991; **Fac Appt:** Assoc Prof S, Harvard Med Sch

Harnsberger, Jeffrey R MD [CRS] - **Spec Exp:** Colon & Rectal Cancer; **Hospital:** Dartmouth - Hitchcock Med Ctr, Elliot Hosp; **Address:** Dartmouth-Hitchcock Manchester, 100 Hitchcock Way, Manchester, NH 03104; **Phone:** 603-695-2840; **Board Cert:** Surgery 2001; Colon & Rectal Surgery 2005; **Med School:** Med Coll OH 1987; **Resid:** Surgery, Dartamouth-Hitchkock Med Ctr 1992; **Fellow:** Colon & Rectal Surgery, St Louis Univ Med Ctr 1993; **Fac Appt:** Asst Prof S, Dartmouth Med Sch

Hyman, Neil H MD [CRS] - **Spec Exp:** Colon & Rectal Cancer; **Hospital:** Fletcher Allen Health Care- Med Ctr Campus; **Address:** FAHC 111 Colchester Ave, 111 Colchester Ave, Burlington, VT 05401; **Phone:** 802-847-3339; **Board Cert:** Surgery 1998; Colon & Rectal Surgery 2003; **Med School:** Univ VT Coll Med 1984; **Resid:** Surgery, Mt Sinai Med Ctr 1989; **Fellow:** Colon & Rectal Surgery, Cleveland Clinic 1990; **Fac Appt:** Prof S, Univ VT Coll Med

Longo, Walter E MD [CRS] - **Spec Exp:** Colon & Rectal Cancer; Gastrointestinal Surgery; **Hospital:** Yale-New Haven Hosp; **Address:** Yale Univ School Medicine, Dept Surgery/Gastroenterology, Box 208062, New Haven, CT 06520-8062; **Phone:** 203-785-2616; **Board Cert:** Surgery 2001; Colon & Rectal Surgery 2006; **Med School:** NY Med Coll 1984; **Resid:** Surgery, Yale-New Haven Hosp 1990; **Fellow:** Research, Yale-New Haven Hosp 1988; Colon & Rectal Surgery, Cleveland Clinic 1991; **Fac Appt:** Prof S, Yale Univ

Nagle, Deborah A MD [CRS] - **Spec Exp:** Colon & Rectal Cancer; Anal Cancer; Laparoscopic Surgery; **Hospital:** Beth Israel Deaconess Med Ctr - Boston; **Address:** Beth Israel Deaconess Med Ctr, 330 Brookline Ave Stoneman Bldg - rm 932, Boston, MA 02215; **Phone:** 617-667-4159; **Board Cert:** Colon & Rectal Surgery 2006; Surgery 2004; **Med School:** Univ Pennsylvania 1988; **Resid:** Surgery, Graduate Hosp 1993; Colon & Rectal Surgery, Thos Jefferson Univ Hosp 1994

Roberts, Patricia L MD [CRS] - **Spec Exp:** Colon & Rectal Cancer; **Hospital:** Lahey Clin; **Address:** 41 Mall Rd, Burlington, MA 01805; **Phone:** 781-744-8243; **Board Cert:** Surgery 1996; Colon & Rectal Surgery 2003; **Med School:** Boston Univ 1981; **Resid:** Surgery, Boston City Hosp 1986; **Fellow:** Colon & Rectal Surgery, Lahey Clinic 1988; **Fac Appt:** Prof S, Tufts Univ

Schoetz Jr, David J MD [CRS] - **Spec Exp:** Colon & Rectal Cancer; Incontinence-Fecal; **Hospital:** Lahey Clin; **Address:** Lahey Clin Med Ctr, Dept Colon & Rectal Surg, 41 Mall Rd, Burlington, MA 01805-0001; **Phone:** 781-744-8889; **Board Cert:** Surgery 2001; Colon & Rectal Surgery 1983; **Med School:** Med Coll Wisc 1974; **Resid:** Surgery, Boston Univ Med Ctr 1981; Surgery, Boston Univ Med Ctr 1978; **Fellow:** Colon & Rectal Surgery, Lahey Clin 1982; **Fac Appt:** Prof S, Tufts Univ

Shellito, Paul C MD [CRS] - **Spec Exp:** Colon & Rectal Cancer; Anorectal Disorders; **Hospital:** Mass Genl Hosp; **Address:** 15 Parkman St, Ste 460, Boston, MA 02114-3117; **Phone:** 617-724-0365; **Board Cert:** Surgery 2002; Colon & Rectal Surgery 1994; **Med School:** Harvard Med Sch 1977; **Resid:** Surgery, Mass Genl Hosp 1983; Surgery, Auckland Univ Med Sch 1981; **Fellow:** Colon & Rectal Surgery, Univ Minn 1985; **Fac Appt:** Asst Prof S, Harvard Med Sch

Mid Atlantic

Caushaj, Fillor Philip MD [CRS] - **Spec Exp:** Colon & Rectal Cancer; Laparoscopic Surgery; **Hospital:** Geisinger Med Ctr, Geisinger-Wyoming Med Ctr; **Address:** Geisinger Med Ctr, Div Colon & Rectal Surgery, 100 N Academy Ave, Danville, PA 17822; **Phone:** 570-271-6361; **Board Cert:** Colon & Rectal Surgery 1986; Surgery 2004; **Med School:** Johns Hopkins Univ 1979; **Resid:** Surgery, Columbia-Presby Med Ctr 1984; **Fellow:** Colon & Rectal Surgery, Lahey Clinic 1985; **Fac Appt:** Prof S, Temple Univ

Eisenstat, Theodore E MD [CRS] - **Spec Exp:** Colon Cancer; Anorectal Disorders; **Hospital:** Robert Wood Johnson Univ Hosp - New Brunswick, JFK Med Ctr - Edison; **Address:** 3900 Park Ave, Ste 101, Edison, NJ 08820-3032; **Phone:** 732-494-6640; **Board Cert:** Surgery 1974; Colon & Rectal Surgery 1994; **Med School:** NY Med Coll 1968; **Resid:** Surgery, Thomas Jefferson Univ Hosp 1971; Surgery, Pennsylvania Hosp 1973; **Fellow:** Colon & Rectal Surgery, Muhlenberg Med Ctr 1978; **Fac Appt:** Clin Prof S, UMDNJ-RW Johnson Med Sch

Fry, Robert D MD [CRS] - **Spec Exp:** Colon & Rectal Cancer; Anal Cancer; Anorectal Disorders; **Hospital:** Pennsylvania Hosp (page 81), Hosp Univ Penn - UPHS (page 81); **Address:** Pennsylvania Hospital, Div Colon & Rectal Surgery, 700 Spruce St, Ste 305, Philadelphia, PA 19106-4023; **Phone:** 215-829-5333; **Board Cert:** Surgery 2006; Colon & Rectal Surgery 1998; **Med School:** Washington Univ, St Louis 1972; **Resid:** Surgery, Barnes Jewish Hosp 1977; **Fellow:** Colon & Rectal Surgery, Cleveland Clinic 1978; **Fac Appt:** Prof S, Univ Pennsylvania

Goldstein, Scott D MD [CRS] - **Spec Exp:** Colon & Rectal Cancer; Laparoscopic Surgery; **Hospital:** Thomas Jefferson Univ Hosp (page 83); **Address:** 1100 Walnut St, Ste 500, Philadelphia, PA 19107; **Phone:** 215-955-5869; **Board Cert:** Surgery 1984; Colon & Rectal Surgery 1985; **Med School:** SUNY Buffalo 1978; **Resid:** Surgery, Lenox Hill Hosp 1983; Colon & Rectal Surgery, UMDNJ Med Ctr 1984; **Fac Appt:** Assoc Prof S, Thomas Jefferson Univ

Gorfine, Stephen R MD [CRS] - **Spec Exp:** Rectal Cancer; Anal Cancer; **Hospital:** Mount Sinai Med Ctr (page 77), Lenox Hill Hosp; **Address:** 25 E 69th St, New York, NY 10021-4925; **Phone:** 212-517-8600; **Board Cert:** Internal Medicine 1981; Surgery 2007; Colon & Rectal Surgery 1988; **Med School:** Univ Mass Sch Med 1978; **Resid:** Internal Medicine, Mt Sinai Hosp 1981; Surgery, Mt Sinai Hosp 1985; **Fellow:** Colon & Rectal Surgery, Ferguson Hosp 1987; **Fac Appt:** Clin Prof S, Mount Sinai Sch Med

Guillem, Jose MD [CRS] - **Spec Exp:** Colon & Rectal Cancer; Rectal Cancer/Sphincter Preservation; Colon & Rectal Cancer-Hereditary; Peritoneal Mucinous Carcinomatosis; **Hospital:** Meml Sloan-Kettering Cancer Ctr (page 76); **Address:** 1275 York Avenue, New York, NY 10065; **Phone:** 212-639-8278; **Board Cert:** Colon & Rectal Surgery 2005; Surgery 2004; **Med School:** Yale Univ 1983; **Resid:** Surgery, Columbia-Presby Med Ctr 1990; **Fellow:** Colon & Rectal Surgery, Lahey Clinic 1991; **Fac Appt:** Prof CRS, Cornell Univ-Weill Med Coll

Colon & Rectal Surgery

Medich, David MD [CRS] - **Spec Exp:** Colon & Rectal Cancer; **Hospital:** Allegheny General Hosp; **Address:** Allegheny General Hosp, South Tower, 320 E North Ave Fl 5, Pittsburgh, PA 15212; **Phone:** 412-359-3901; **Board Cert:** Surgery 2004; Colon & Rectal Surgery 2006; **Med School:** Ohio State Univ 1987; **Resid:** Surgery, Univ Pittsburgh 1990; **Fellow:** Research, Univ Pittsburgh 1993; Colon & Rectal Surgery, Cleveland Clinic 1994; **Fac Appt:** Assoc Prof CRS, Drexel Univ Coll Med

Milsom, Jeffrey W MD [CRS] - **Spec Exp:** Laparoscopic Surgery; Colon & Rectal Cancer; **Hospital:** NY-Presby Hosp/Weill Cornell (page 79); **Address:** NY Cornell Med Ctr, Div Colorectal Surgery, 1315 York Ave Fl 2, New York, NY 10065-5304; **Phone:** 212-746-6030; **Board Cert:** Colon & Rectal Surgery 1986; **Med School:** Univ Pittsburgh 1979; **Resid:** Surgery, Roosevelt Hosp 1981; Surgery, Univ Virginia Med Ctr 1984; **Fellow:** Colon & Rectal Surgery, Ferguson Hosp 1985; **Fac Appt:** Prof S, Cornell Univ-Weill Med Coll

Rombeau, John L MD [CRS] - **Spec Exp:** Colon & Rectal Cancer; Rectal Cancer/Sphincter Preservation; **Hospital:** Temple Univ Hosp; **Address:** Department of Surgery, 3401 N Broad St, Parkinson Pavilion Fl 4, Philadelphia, PA 19104-5103; **Phone:** 215-707-3133; **Board Cert:** Colon & Rectal Surgery 1977; **Med School:** Loma Linda Univ 1967; **Resid:** Surgery, Good Samaritan Hosp 1971; Surgery, LAC-USC Med Ctr 1975; **Fellow:** Colon & Rectal Surgery, Cleveland Clinic 1976; Nutrition & Metabolism, Brigham & Women's Hosp 1977; **Fac Appt:** Prof S, Temple Univ

Stein, David E MD [CRS] - **Spec Exp:** Colon & Rectal Cancer & Surgery; Laparoscopic Surgery; Anorectal Disorders; **Hospital:** Hahnemann Univ Hosp; **Address:** 245 N 15th St, #4013, Philadelphia, PA 19102; **Phone:** 215-762-1545; **Board Cert:** Surgery 2004; Colon & Rectal Surgery 2004; **Med School:** SUNY Downstate 1997; **Resid:** Surgery, T Jefferson Univ Hosp 2002; **Fellow:** Colon & Rectal Surgery, Cleveland Clinic 2003; **Fac Appt:** Asst Prof S, Drexel Univ Coll Med

Steinhagen, Randolph MD [CRS] - **Spec Exp:** Colostomy Avoidance; Colon & Rectal Cancer; **Hospital:** Mount Sinai Med Ctr (page 77); **Address:** Div Colon & Rectal Surgery, 5 E 98th St Fl 14, Box 1259, New York, NY 10029-6501; **Phone:** 212-241-3547; **Board Cert:** Surgery 2002; Colon & Rectal Surgery 1985; **Med School:** Wayne State Univ 1977; **Resid:** Surgery, Mount Sinai Hosp 1982; **Fellow:** Colon & Rectal Surgery, Cleveland Clinic 1983; **Fac Appt:** Assoc Prof S, Mount Sinai Sch Med

Whelan, Richard L MD [CRS] - **Spec Exp:** Laparoscopic Surgery; Colon & Rectal Cancer; **Hospital:** NY-Presby Hosp/Columbia (page 79); **Address:** 161 Ft Washington Ave, rm 817, New York, NY 10032; **Phone:** 212-342-1155; **Board Cert:** Surgery 1997; Colon & Rectal Surgery 1989; **Med School:** Columbia P&S 1982; **Resid:** Surgery, Columbia Presby Hosp 1987; **Fellow:** Colon & Rectal Surgery, Univ Minn Med Ctr 1988; **Fac Appt:** Assoc Clin Prof S, Columbia P&S

Wong, W Douglas MD [CRS] - **Spec Exp:** Rectal Cancer/Sphincter Preservation; Colon & Rectal Cancer; Anal Disorders & Reconstruction; **Hospital:** Meml Sloan-Kettering Cancer Ctr (page 76); **Address:** 1275 York Ave, Ste C-1067, New York, NY 10065; **Phone:** 212-639-5117; **Board Cert:** Surgery 1997; Colon & Rectal Surgery 2004; **Med School:** Univ Manitoba 1972; **Resid:** Surgery, Univ Manitoba Hosp 1977; **Fellow:** Colon & Rectal Surgery, Univ Minn Med Ctr 1984; **Fac Appt:** Prof S, Cornell Univ-Weill Med Coll

Southeast

Galandiuk, Susan MD [CRS] - **Spec Exp:** Colon & Rectal Cancer; **Hospital:** Univ of Louisville Hosp, Norton Hosp; **Address:** 401 E Chestnut St, Ste 710, Louisville, KY 40202; **Phone:** 502-583-8303; **Board Cert:** Surgery 2008; Colon & Rectal Surgery 2002; **Med School:** Germany 1982; **Resid:** Surgery, Cleveland Clinic Fdtn 1988; **Fellow:** Research, Univ Louisville Hosp 1989; Colon & Rectal Surgery, Mayo Clinic 1990; **Fac Appt:** Prof CRS, Univ Louisville Sch Med

Golub, Richard W MD [CRS] - **Spec Exp:** Colon & Rectal Cancer; Laparoscopic Surgery; **Hospital:** Sarasota Meml Hosp, Doctors Hosp - Sarasota; **Address:** Surgical Specialists, 3333 Cattlemen Rd, Ste 206, Sarasota, FL 34232; **Phone:** 941-341-0042; **Board Cert:** Surgery 2000; Colon & Rectal Surgery 2003; **Med School:** Albert Einstein Coll Med 1984; **Resid:** Surgery, Univ Hosp 1990; **Fellow:** Colon & Rectal Surgery, Grant Medical Center 1991

Mantyh, Christopher MD [CRS] - **Spec Exp:** Colon & Rectal Cancer & Surgery; Rectal Cancer/Sphincter Preservation; Incontinence-Fecal; **Hospital:** Duke Univ Med Ctr; **Address:** 200 Trent Drive, Durham, NC 27710; **Phone:** 919-681-3977; **Board Cert:** Surgery 1999; Colon & Rectal Surgery 2000; **Med School:** Univ Wisc 1991; **Resid:** Surgery, Duke Univ Med Ctr 1998; **Fellow:** Colon & Rectal Surgery, Cleveland Clinic 1999

Marcet, Jorge MD [CRS] - **Spec Exp:** Colon & Rectal Cancer; **Hospital:** Tampa Genl Hosp; **Address:** 1 Tampa General Cir, Ste F145, Tampa, FL 33606; **Phone:** 813-844-4545; **Board Cert:** Surgery 2001; Colon & Rectal Surgery 2003; **Med School:** Cornell Univ-Weill Med Coll 1985; **Resid:** Surgery, St Luke's-Roosevelt Med Ctr 1990; **Fellow:** Colon & Rectal Surgery, Columbia Presby Med Ctr 1990; Colon & Rectal Surgery, St Luke's-Roosevelt Med Ctr 1991; **Fac Appt:** Assoc Prof S, Univ S Fla Coll Med

Nogueras, Juan J MD [CRS] - **Spec Exp:** Colon & Rectal Cancer; Incontinence-Fecal; **Hospital:** Cleveland Clin - Weston (page 70); **Address:** Cleveland Clinic, Dept Colorectal Surgery, 2950 Cleveland Clinic Blvd, Weston, FL 33331; **Phone:** 954-659-5251; **Board Cert:** Surgery 2007; Colon & Rectal Surgery 2003; **Med School:** Jefferson Med Coll 1982; **Resid:** Surgery, Columbia Presby Med Ctr 1987; **Fellow:** Colon & Rectal Surgery, Univ Minn Med Ctr 1991

Vernava III, Anthony M MD [CRS] - **Spec Exp:** Colon & Rectal Cancer; Incontinence-Fecal; **Hospital:** Physicians Regl Med Ctr; **Address:** Medical Surgical Specialists, 6101 Pine Ridge Rd, Naples, FL 34119; **Phone:** 239-348-4400; **Board Cert:** Surgery 2007; Colon & Rectal Surgery 1989; **Med School:** St Louis Univ 1982; **Resid:** Surgery, St Louis Univ Med Ctr 1988; Colon & Rectal Surgery, Univ Minnesota Med Ctr 1989; **Fellow:** Colon & Rectal Surgery, St Marks Hosp 1990

Wexner, Steven MD [CRS] - **Spec Exp:** Colon & Rectal Cancer; Laparoscopic Surgery; **Hospital:** Cleveland Clin - Weston (page 70); **Address:** 2950 Cleveland Clinic Blvd, Weston, FL 33331-3609; **Phone:** 954-659-5278; **Board Cert:** Surgery 2005; Colon & Rectal Surgery 2006; **Med School:** Cornell Univ-Weill Med Coll 1982; **Resid:** Surgery, Roosevelt Hosp 1987; **Fellow:** Colon & Rectal Surgery, Univ Minn 1988; **Fac Appt:** Prof S, Cleveland Cl Coll Med/Case West Res

Midwest

Abcarian, Herand MD [CRS] - **Spec Exp:** Rectal Cancer/Sphincter Preservation; Incontinence-Fecal; **Hospital:** Univ of IL Med Ctr at Chicago, Gottlieb Meml Hosp; **Address:** 675 W North Ave, Ste 406, Melrose Park, IL 60160; **Phone:** 708-450-5075; **Board Cert:** Surgery 1972; Colon & Rectal Surgery 1972; **Med School:** Iran 1965; **Resid:** Surgery, Cook County Hosp 1971; Colon & Rectal Surgery, Cook County Hosp 1972; **Fac Appt:** Prof S, Univ IL Coll Med

Delaney, Conor P MD/PhD [CRS] - **Spec Exp:** Laparoscopic Surgery; Colon & Rectal Cancer; **Hospital:** Univ Hosps Case Med Ctr; **Address:** 11100 Euclid Ave, MS 5047, Cleveland, OH 44106-5047; **Phone:** 216-844-8087; **Board Cert:** Surgery 1998; Colon & Rectal Surgery 1998; **Med School:** Ireland 1989; **Resid:** Surgery, Univ Hosp 1993; Surgery, Univ Hosp 1999; **Fellow:** Research, Univ of Pittsburgh 1995; Colon & Rectal Surgery, Cleveland Clinic 2000; **Fac Appt:** Prof S, Cleveland Cl Coll Med/Case West Res

Colon & Rectal Surgery

Fleshman, James MD [CRS] - **Spec Exp:** Colon & Rectal Cancer; Laparoscopic Surgery; **Hospital:** Barnes-Jewish Hosp, Barnes-Jewish West County Hosp; **Address:** Wash Univ Sch Med, Div Col Rectal Surgery, 660 S Euclid Ave, Box 8109, St Louis, MO 63110; **Phone:** 314-454-7177; **Board Cert:** Colon & Rectal Surgery 1988; Surgery 1996; **Med School:** Washington Univ, St Louis 1980; **Resid:** Surgery, Jewish Hospital 1986; **Fellow:** Colon & Rectal Surgery, Univ Toronto 1987; **Fac Appt:** Prof S, Washington Univ, St Louis

Foley, Eugene F MD [CRS] - **Spec Exp:** Colon & Rectal Cancer; **Hospital:** Univ WI Hosp & Clins; **Address:** Univ WI Hosp & Clins, 600 Highland Ave, Madison, WI 53792-7375; **Phone:** 608-263-7502; **Board Cert:** Surgery 2003; Colon & Rectal Surgery 2005; **Med School:** Harvard Med Sch 1985; **Resid:** Surgery, New England Deaconess Hosp 1991; **Fellow:** Colon & Rectal Surgery, Lahey Clinic 1993; **Fac Appt:** Prof S, Univ Wisc

Kodner, Ira J MD [CRS] - **Spec Exp:** Colon & Rectal Cancer; Laparoscopic Surgery; **Hospital:** Barnes-Jewish Hosp; **Address:** Wash Univ Sch Med, Div Col Rectal Surgery, 660 S Euclid Ave, Box 8109, St Louis, MO 63110; **Phone:** 314-454-7177; **Board Cert:** Surgery 1975; Colon & Rectal Surgery 1975; **Med School:** Washington Univ, St Louis 1967; **Resid:** Surgery, Barnes-Jewish Hosp 1974; **Fellow:** Colon & Rectal Surgery, Cleveland Clinic 1975; **Fac Appt:** Prof S, Washington Univ, St Louis

Lavery, Ian C MD [CRS] - **Spec Exp:** Colon & Rectal Cancer; **Hospital:** Cleveland Clin Fdn (page 70); **Address:** 9500 Euclid Ave, Desk A30, Cleveland, OH 44195; **Phone:** 216-444-6930; **Board Cert:** Colon & Rectal Surgery 1998; **Med School:** Australia 1967; **Resid:** Surgery, Princess Alexandra Hosp 1974; Colon & Rectal Surgery, Cleveland Clinic 1977; **Fac Appt:** Prof S, Case West Res Univ

Ludwig, Kirk A MD [CRS] - **Spec Exp:** Colon & Rectal Cancer & Surgery; Rectal Cancer/Sphincter Preservation; Incontinence-Fecal; Colon & Rectal Cancer-Familial Polyposis; **Hospital:** Froedtert Meml Lutheran Hosp; **Address:** 9200 W Wisconsin Ave, Dept Surgery, Milwaukee, WI 53226; **Phone:** 414-805-5800; **Board Cert:** Surgery 2005; Colon & Rectal Surgery 2007; **Med School:** Univ Cincinnati 1988; **Resid:** Surgery, Med Coll Wisc 1994; **Fellow:** Colon & Rectal Surgery, Cleveland Clinic 1996; **Fac Appt:** Assoc Prof S, Med Coll Wisc

Madoff, Robert D MD [CRS] - **Spec Exp:** Colon & Rectal Cancer; **Hospital:** Univ Minn Med Ctr, Fairview - Univ Campus; **Address:** 516 Delaware St SE, Phillips-Wangensteen Bldg, MMC 88, Minneapolis, MN 55455; **Phone:** 612-624-9708; **Board Cert:** Colon & Rectal Surgery 2002; **Med School:** Columbia P&S 1979; **Resid:** Surgery, Univ Minn Hosps 1987; **Fellow:** Colon & Rectal Surgery, Univ Minn Hosps 1988; **Fac Appt:** Prof S, Univ Minn

Nelson, Heidi MD [CRS] - **Spec Exp:** Colon & Rectal Cancer; Gastrointestinal Cancer; **Hospital:** Mayo Med Ctr & Clin - Rochester, Rochester Methodist Hosp; **Address:** Mayo Clinic, Gonda 9 South, 200 First St SW, Rochester, MN 55905; **Phone:** 507-284-3329; **Board Cert:** Surgery 2007; Colon & Rectal Surgery 1989; **Med School:** Univ Wash 1981; **Resid:** Surgery, Oregon Hlth Sci Univ Hosp 1987; Colon & Rectal Surgery, Oregon Hlth Sci Univ Hosp 1985; **Fellow:** Colon & Rectal Surgery, Mayo Clinic 1988; **Fac Appt:** Prof S, Mayo Med Sch

Pemberton, John H MD [CRS] - **Spec Exp:** Colon & Rectal Cancer; **Hospital:** St Mary's Hosp - Rochester, Rochester Methodist Hosp; **Address:** Mayo Clinic, Div Colon & Rectal Surg, 200 First St SW, Gonda 9-S, Rochester, MN 55905; **Phone:** 507-284-2359; **Board Cert:** Surgery 2001; Colon & Rectal Surgery 1985; **Med School:** Tulane Univ 1976; **Resid:** Surgery, Mayo Clinic 1983; **Fellow:** Colon & Rectal Surgery, Mayo Clinic 1984; **Fac Appt:** Prof S, Mayo Med Sch

Rafferty, Janice F MD [CRS] - **Spec Exp:** Colon & Rectal Cancer; Anal Disorders & Reconstruction; **Hospital:** Univ Hosp - Cincinnati, Christ Hospital; **Address:** U of Cincinnati, Colon & Rectal Surgery, 2123 Auburn Ave, Ste 524, Cincinnati, OH 45219; **Phone:** 513-929-0104; **Board Cert:** Colon & Rectal Surgery 2008; Surgery 2004; **Med School:** Ohio State Univ 1988; **Resid:** Surgery, Univ CincinnatiHosp 1995; Colon & Rectal Surgery, Barnes Jewish Hosp 1996; **Fac Appt:** Assoc Prof S, Univ Cincinnati

Rothenberger, David A MD [CRS] - **Spec Exp:** Colon & Rectal Cancer; **Hospital:** Univ Minn Med Ctr, Fairview - Univ Campus; **Address:** Univ Minnesota Med Ctr, Dept Surg, 516 Delaware St SE MMC 88, Minneapolis, MN 55455; **Phone:** 612-624-9708; **Board Cert:** Colon & Rectal Surgery 2006; **Med School:** Tufts Univ 1973; **Resid:** Surgery, St Paul-Ramsey Med Ctr 1978; **Fellow:** Colon & Rectal Surgery, Univ Minnesota Hosps 1979; **Fac Appt:** Prof S, Univ Minn

Saclarides, Theodore J MD [CRS] - **Spec Exp:** Rectal Cancer/Sphincter Preservation; Laparoscopic Surgery; **Hospital:** Rush Univ Med Ctr, Rush N Shore Med Ctr; **Address:** University Surgeons, 1725 W Harrison St, Ste 810, Chicago, IL 60612-3832; **Phone:** 312-942-6543; **Board Cert:** Surgery 2007; Colon & Rectal Surgery 1989; **Med School:** Univ Miami Sch Med 1982; **Resid:** Surgery, Rush Univ Med Ctr 1987; **Fellow:** Colon & Rectal Surgery, Mayo Clinic 1988; **Fac Appt:** Prof S, Rush Med Coll

Senagore, Anthony MD [CRS] - **Spec Exp:** Laparoscopic Surgery; Colon & Rectal Cancer; Anorectal Disorders; Incontinence-Fecal; **Hospital:** Spectrum Hlth Blodgett Campus; **Address:** Spectrum Health, 100 Michigan St NE, MC 005, Grand Rapids, MI 49503; **Phone:** 616-391-2467; **Board Cert:** Surgery 2006; Colon & Rectal Surgery 2001; Surgical Critical Care 2006; **Med School:** Mich State Univ 1981; **Resid:** Surgery, Butterworth Hosp 1987; Colon & Rectal Surgery, Ferguson Hosp 1989; **Fac Appt:** Prof S, Med Univ Ohio at Toledo

Stryker, Steven J MD [CRS] - **Spec Exp:** Colon & Rectal Cancer; Laparoscopic Surgery; **Hospital:** Northwestern Meml Hosp; **Address:** 676 N Saint Clair St, Ste 1525A, Chicago, IL 60611-2862; **Phone:** 312-943-5427; **Board Cert:** Surgery 2004; Colon & Rectal Surgery 1986; **Med School:** Northwestern Univ 1978; **Resid:** Surgery, Northwestern Meml Hosp 1983; **Fellow:** Colon & Rectal Surgery, Mayo Clinic 1985; **Fac Appt:** Clin Prof S, Northwestern Univ

Wolff, Bruce G MD [CRS] - **Spec Exp:** Colon & Rectal Cancer; **Hospital:** Mayo Med Ctr & Clin - Rochester; **Address:** Mayo Clinic, Gonda 9 South, 200 First St SW, Rochester, MN 55905; **Phone:** 507-284-3329; **Board Cert:** Surgery 2000; Colon & Rectal Surgery 2001; **Med School:** Duke Univ 1973; **Resid:** Surgery, NY Hosp-Cornell Med Ctr 1981; **Fellow:** Colon & Rectal Surgery, Mayo Clinic 1982; **Fac Appt:** Prof S, Mayo Med Sch

Great Plains and Mountains

Thorson, Alan G MD [CRS] - **Spec Exp:** Colon & Rectal Cancer; Laparoscopic Surgery; Incontinence-Fecal; Ileal Pouch Anal Anastomosis; **Hospital:** Nebraska Meth Hosp, Archbishop Bergan Mercy Med Ctr; **Address:** 9850 Nicholas St, Ste 100, Omaha, NE 68114-2191; **Phone:** 402-343-1122; **Board Cert:** Colon & Rectal Surgery 1999; **Med School:** Univ Nebr Coll Med 1979; **Resid:** Surgery, Univ Nebraska Affil Hosp 1984; Colon & Rectal Surgery, Univ Minn Affil Hosp 1985; **Fac Appt:** Assoc Clin Prof S, Creighton Univ

Colon & Rectal Surgery

Southwest

Adkins, Terrance P MD [CRS] - **Spec Exp:** Colon & Rectal Cancer; **Hospital:** Tucson Med Ctr; **Address:** Southwestern Surgery Assoc, 1951 N Wilmot Rd Bldg 2, Tucson, AZ 85712; **Phone:** 520-795-5845; **Board Cert:** Surgery 2001; Colon & Rectal Surgery 2004; **Med School:** Univ Tex SW, Dallas 1985; **Resid:** Surgery, Univ Utah Med Ctr 1991; **Fellow:** Colon & Rectal Surgery, Univ Texas Med Ctr 1992; **Fac Appt:** Asst Clin Prof S, Univ Ariz Coll Med

Bailey, H Randolph MD [CRS] - **Spec Exp:** Rectal Cancer/Sphincter Preservation; Incontinence-Fecal; **Hospital:** Methodist Hosp - Houston, St Luke's Episcopal Hosp-Houston; **Address:** Colon & Rectal Clinic, Smith Twr, 6550 Fannin St, Ste 2307, Houston, TX 77030-2717; **Phone:** 713-790-9250; **Board Cert:** Surgery 1974; Colon & Rectal Surgery 2004; **Med School:** Univ Tex SW, Dallas 1968; **Resid:** Surgery, Hermann Hosp-Univ Tex Med Sch 1973; **Fellow:** Colon & Rectal Surgery, Ferguson-Droste Hosp 1974; **Fac Appt:** Clin Prof S, Univ Tex, Houston

Beck, David E MD [CRS] - **Spec Exp:** Colon & Rectal Cancer; Minimally Invasive Surgery; **Hospital:** Ochsner Fdn Hosp, Summit Hosp-Baton Rouge; **Address:** Ochsner Clinic Fdn, Colorectal Surgery, 1514 Jefferson Hwy, 4th Fl, rm 04 East, New Orleans, LA 70121-2429; **Phone:** 504-842-4060; **Board Cert:** Colon & Rectal Surgery 1987; **Med School:** Univ Miami Sch Med 1979; **Resid:** Surgery, Wilford Hall USAF Med Ctr 1984; **Fellow:** Colon & Rectal Surgery, Cleveland Clinic Fdn 1986; **Fac Appt:** Assoc Clin Prof S, Louisiana State U, New Orleans

Efron, Jonathan E MD [CRS] - **Spec Exp:** Colon & Rectal Cancer; Incontinence-Fecal; Anorectal Disorders; **Hospital:** Mayo Clinic - Scottsdale; **Address:** Mayo Clinic, Concourse B, 13400 E Shea Blvd, Scottsdale, AZ 85259; **Phone:** 480-342-2697; **Board Cert:** Surgery 1999; Colon & Rectal Surgery 2000; **Med School:** Univ MD Sch Med 1993; **Resid:** Surgery, LIJ Medical Ctr 1999; **Fellow:** Colon & Rectal Surgery, Cleveland Clinic 2000; Research, Cleveland Clinic 2001; **Fac Appt:** Assoc Prof S, Mayo Med Sch

Heppell, Jacques P MD [CRS] - **Spec Exp:** Colon & Rectal Cancer; Anorectal Disorders; **Hospital:** Mayo Clinic - Phoenix; **Address:** Mayo Clinic, GENS/CB/Distribution 13, 5777 E Mayo Blvd, Phoenix, AZ 85054; **Phone:** 480-342-2697; **Board Cert:** Surgery 2004; Colon & Rectal Surgery 1995; **Med School:** Univ Montreal 1974; **Resid:** Surgery, Univ Montreal Med Ctr 1979; **Fellow:** Colon & Rectal Surgery, Mayo Clinic 1983; **Fac Appt:** Prof S, Mayo Med Sch

Huber Jr, Philip J MD [CRS] - **Spec Exp:** Colon & Rectal Cancer; **Hospital:** Med City Dallas Hosp, Presby Hosp of Dallas; **Address:** 7777 Forest Lane, Ste C-204, Dallas, TX 75230; **Phone:** 972-566-6115; **Board Cert:** Surgery 1997; Colon & Rectal Surgery 1993; **Med School:** Columbia P&S 1972; **Resid:** Surgery, Parkland Hosp 1977; Colon & Rectal Surgery, Presby Hosp 1978

West Coast and Pacific

Beart Jr, Robert W MD [CRS] - **Spec Exp:** Colon & Rectal Cancer; **Hospital:** USC Norris Cancer Hosp, USC Univ Hosp; **Address:** USC Comprehensive Cancer Center, Topping Tower Suite 7418, 1441 Eastlake Ave, Los Angeles, CA 90033; **Phone:** 323-865-3690; **Board Cert:** Colon & Rectal Surgery 1995; **Med School:** Harvard Med Sch 1971; **Resid:** Surgery, Univ Colo Med Ctr 1976; Colon & Rectal Surgery, Mayo Clinic 1978; **Fellow:** Transplant Surgery, Univ Colo Med Ctr 1975; **Fac Appt:** Prof S, USC Sch Med

Chiu, Yanek S MD [CRS] - **Hospital:** CA Pacific Med Ctr - Pacific Campus; **Address:** 3838 California St, Ste 616, San Francisco, CA 94118; **Phone:** 415-668-0411; **Board Cert:** Colon & Rectal Surgery 1997; **Med School:** Boston Univ 1971; **Resid:** Surgery, Boston Med Ctr 1976; **Fellow:** Colon & Rectal Surgery, Mayo Clinic 1978; **Fac Appt:** Assoc Clin Prof CRS, UCSF

Sokol, Thomas P MD [CRS] - **Spec Exp:** Colon & Rectal Cancer & Surgery; Incontinence-Fecal; **Hospital:** Cedars-Sinai Med Ctr, Century City Hosp; **Address:** 8737 Beverly Blvd, Ste 402, Los Angeles, CA 90048-1828; **Phone:** 310-854-3580; **Board Cert:** Colon & Rectal Surgery 2008; **Med School:** Ros Franklin Univ/Chicago Med Sch 1980; **Resid:** Surgery, Habor UCLA Med Ctr 1985; **Fellow:** Colon & Rectal Surgery, Carle Fdn Hosp/Univ Ill 1986; **Fac Appt:** Assoc Clin Prof S, UCLA

Stamos, Michael J MD [CRS] - **Spec Exp:** Rectal Cancer/Sphincter Preservation; Laparoscopic Surgery; Colon & Rectal Cancer; Anorectal Disorders; **Hospital:** UC Irvine Med Ctr; **Address:** UC Irvine Med Ctr, Div Colon & Rectal Surg, 333 City Blvd W, Ste 850, Orange, CA 92868-2993; **Phone:** 888-717-4463; **Board Cert:** Surgery 2000; Colon & Rectal Surgery 2003; **Med School:** Case West Res Univ 1985; **Resid:** Surgery, Jackson Meml Hosp 1990; Colon & Rectal Surgery, Ochsner Clinic 1991; **Fac Appt:** Prof S, UC Irvine

Welton, Mark L MD [CRS] - **Spec Exp:** Colon & Rectal Cancer; Anal Cancer; **Hospital:** Stanford Univ Med Ctr; **Address:** Advanced Medical Center, 875 Blake Wilbur Drive, Stanford, CA 94305-5655; **Phone:** 650-723-5461; **Board Cert:** Surgery 2000; Colon & Rectal Surgery 2005; **Med School:** UCLA 1984; **Resid:** Surgery, UCLA Med Ctr 1992; **Fellow:** Colon & Rectal Surgery, Barnes Jewish Hosp 1993; **Fac Appt:** Assoc Prof S, Stanford Univ

Cleveland Clinic

National Leader in Colorectal Cancer

At the Cleveland Clinic Taussig Cancer Institute, more than 250 cancer specialists, researchers, nurses and technicians are dedicated to developing and applying the latest and most effective medical techniques to achieve the long-term survival and improve the quality of life for 7,500 new cancer patients every year. Because of our patient-centered care, leading-edge treatments, innovative research, 350 clinical trials and state-of-the-art medical technologies, *U.S.News & World Report* has ranked Cleveland Clinic's cancer program one of the top cancer centers in the nation.

Special Assistance for Our Out-of-State Patients

Cleveland Clinic Global Patient Services offers a complimentary Medical Concierge service for patients who travel to Cleveland Clinic from outside of Ohio. We can help coordinate medical appointments, assist with travel needs and more. **For more information, call 800.223.2273, ext. 55580, or email medicalconcierge@ccf.org.**

Taussig Cancer Institute's leading oncologists work closely with a multi-disciplinary team of specialists from the Digestive Disease Institute to provide patients with innovative diagnostic techniques, the best clinical or surgical options, clinical trials, novel therapies and genetic counseling to treat colorectal cancer. **To schedule an appointment or get a second opinion, call 866.223.8100 today or visit clevelandclinic.org/colorectalTCD.**

As one of the largest centers in the nation, the Digestive Disease Institute performs up to 10 laparoscopic intestinal resections a week. Even though colon surgery is one of the more difficult procedures to perform laparoscopically, the latest research suggests that this minimally invasive procedure offers an equally good outcome compared to open surgery when the laparoscopic surgery is performed by an experienced surgeon.

In cooperation with the Taussig Cancer Institute, the Digestive Disease Institute became the first in the nation to integrate its departments of Colorectal Surgery, Gastroenterology & Hepatology, Hepatopancreatobiliary and Transplant Surgery and Nutrition Services. This integration provides unprecedented patient care, multidisciplinary education and collaborative research. In addition, the David G. Jagelman Inherited Colorectal Cancer Registries, the largest registries in the U.S. for inherited forms of colorectal cancer, is part of the Digestive Disease Institute.

The Cleveland Clinic's digestive disease program has been ranked #2 in the nation since 2003, by *U.S.News and World Report's* "America's Best Hospitals" Survey.

To schedule an appointment or for more information about Cleveland Clinic Taussig Cancer Institute, call 866.223.8100 or visit clevelandclinic.org/colorectalTCD.

Cleveland Clinic Taussig Cancer Institute | Cleveland, OH

Cancer Institute

NYU LANGONE MEDICAL CENTER

Dermatology

A dermatologist is trained to diagnose and treat pediatric and adult patients with benign and malignant disorders of the skin, mouth, external genitalia, hair and nails, as well as a number of sexually transmitted diseases. The dermatologist has had additional training and experience in the diagnosis and treatment of skin cancers, melanomas, moles and other tumors of the skin, the management of contact dermatitis and other allergic and non-allergic skin disorders, and in the recognition of the skin manifestations of systemic (including internal malignancy) and infectious diseases.

Dermatologists may have special training in dermatopathology and in the surgical techniques used in dermatology. They also have expertise in the management of cosmetic disorders of the skin such as hair loss and scars, and the skin changes associated with aging.

Training Required: Four years

DERMATOLOGY

New England

Del Giudice, Stephen M MD [D] - **Spec Exp:** Skin Cancer; **Hospital:** Concord Hospital; **Address:** Dartmouth Hitchcock Concord-Dermatology, 253 Pleasant St, Concord, NH 03301; **Phone:** 603-226-6119; **Board Cert:** Dermatology 1987; **Med School:** Tufts Univ 1981; **Resid:** Dermatology, Yale-New Haven Hosp 1987

Edelson, Richard L MD [D] - **Spec Exp:** Cutaneous Lymphoma; **Hospital:** Yale-New Haven Hosp; **Address:** 2 Church St S, Ste 305, New Haven, CT 06519; **Phone:** 203-789-1249; **Board Cert:** Dermatology 1977; **Med School:** Yale Univ 1970; **Resid:** Dermatology, Mass Genl Hosp 1972; Dermatology, Natl Inst Hlth 1975; **Fac Appt:** Prof D, Yale Univ

Fewkes, Jessica L MD [D] - **Spec Exp:** Mohs' Surgery; Skin Cancer-Head & Neck; Melanoma-Head & Neck; **Hospital:** Mass Eye & Ear Infirmary, Mass Genl Hosp; **Address:** Mass Eye & Ear Infirmary, 243 Charles St Fl 9, Boston, MA 02114; **Phone:** 617-573-3789; **Board Cert:** Dermatology 1982; **Med School:** UCSF 1978; **Resid:** Dermatology, Mass Genl Hosp 1982; **Fellow:** Chemosurgery, Duke Univ Med Ctr 1983; **Fac Appt:** Asst Prof D, Harvard Med Sch

Gilchrest, Barbara MD [D] - **Spec Exp:** Melanoma; Skin Cancer; **Hospital:** Boston Med Ctr; **Address:** Boston Med Ctr- Dermatolgy Dept, 720 Harrison Ave, Boston, MA 02118-2394; **Phone:** 617-638-7420; **Board Cert:** Internal Medicine 1975; Dermatology 1978; **Med School:** Harvard Med Sch 1971; **Resid:** Internal Medicine, Boston City Hosp 1973; Dermatology, Harvard Med Sch 1976; **Fellow:** Photo Biology, Harvard Med Sch 1975; **Fac Appt:** Prof D, Boston Univ

Kupper, Thomas S MD [D] - **Spec Exp:** Melanoma; Cutaneous Lymphoma; Skin Cancer; **Hospital:** Brigham & Women's Hosp, Dana-Farber Cancer Inst; **Address:** Brigham & Women's Hosp, Dept Dermatology, 77 Avenue Louis Pasteur, Ste 671, Boston, MA 02115; **Phone:** 617-525-5550; **Board Cert:** Dermatology 1989; **Med School:** Yale Univ 1981; **Resid:** Surgery, Yale-New Haven Hosp 1983; Dermatology, Yale-New Haven Hosp 1989; **Fac Appt:** Prof D, Harvard Med Sch

Leffell, David J MD [D] - **Spec Exp:** Mohs' Surgery; Melanoma; Skin Cancer; Skin Laser Surgery; **Hospital:** Yale-New Haven Hosp; **Address:** Yale New Haven Hosp-Dept Dermatology, 40 Temple St, Ste 5A, PO Box 208059, New Haven, CT 06520; **Phone:** 203-785-3466; **Board Cert:** Internal Medicine 1984; Dermatology 1987; **Med School:** McGill Univ 1981; **Resid:** Internal Medicine, New York Hosp 1984; Dermatology, Yale-New Haven Hosp 1986; **Fellow:** Dermatology, Yale-New Haven Hosp 1987; Dermatologic Surgery, Univ Michigan Med Ctr 1988; **Fac Appt:** Prof D, Yale Univ

Maloney, Mary MD [D] - **Spec Exp:** Mohs' Surgery; Skin Laser Surgery; **Hospital:** UMass Memorial Med Ctr; **Address:** Univ Mass Med Ctr, Dept Derm, 281 Lincoln St Fl 4, Worcester, MA 01605-2138; **Phone:** 508-334-5962; **Board Cert:** Dermatology 1982; **Med School:** Univ VT Coll Med 1977; **Resid:** Internal Medicine, Hartford Hospital 1979; Dermatology, Dartmouth-Hitchcock Med Ctr 1982; **Fellow:** Dermatologic Surgery, UCSF Med Ctr 1983; **Fac Appt:** Prof D, Univ Mass Sch Med

McDonald, Charles J MD [D] - **Spec Exp:** Cutaneous Lymphoma; Melanoma; **Hospital:** Rhode Island Hosp, Miriam Hosp; **Address:** Rhode Island Hosp, Dept Dermatology, 593 Eddy St, APC-10, Providence, RI 02903-4923; **Phone:** 401-444-7959; **Board Cert:** Dermatology 1966; **Med School:** Howard Univ 1960; **Resid:** Internal Medicine, Hosp St Raphael 1963; Dermatology, Yale New Haven Hosp 1965; **Fellow:** Clinical Oncology, Yale New Haven Hosp 1966; **Fac Appt:** Prof D, Brown Univ

Mihm Jr, Martin C MD [D] - **Spec Exp:** Melanoma; Dermatopathology; **Hospital:** Mass Genl Hosp; **Address:** Mass General Hosp, 55 Fruit St, Warren Bldg 825, Boston, MA 02114-2926; **Phone:** 617-724-1350; **Board Cert:** Dermatology 1969; Dermatopathology 1974; Anatomic Pathology 1974; **Med School:** Univ Pittsburgh 1961; **Resid:** Internal Medicine, Mt Sinai Hosp 1964; Dermatology, Mass Genl Hosp 1967; **Fellow:** Anatomic Pathology, Mass Genl Hosp 1972; **Fac Appt:** Clin Prof Path, Harvard Med Sch

Neel, Victor A MD/PhD [D] - **Spec Exp:** Mohs' Surgery; Skin Cancer; **Hospital:** Mass Genl Hosp; **Address:** 50 Staniford St, Ste 270, Boston, MA 02114; **Phone:** 617-726-1869; **Board Cert:** Dermatology 2000; **Med School:** Cornell Univ-Weill Med Coll 1995; **Resid:** Pediatrics, Rhode Island Hosp 1997; Dermatology, Rhode Island Hosp 2000; **Fellow:** Mohs Surgery, UCLA Med Ctr 2001

Olbricht, Suzanne M MD [D] - **Spec Exp:** Skin Cancer; Mohs' Surgery; **Hospital:** Lahey Clin; **Address:** Lahey Clinic, 41 Mall Rd, Burlington, MA 01805; **Phone:** 781-744-8348; **Board Cert:** Dermatology 1983; Internal Medicine 1979; **Med School:** Baylor Coll Med 1976; **Resid:** Internal Medicine, Mass General Hosp 1979; Dermatology, Mass General Hosp 1983; **Fellow:** Mohs Surgery, Mass General Hosp 1991; **Fac Appt:** Assoc Prof D, Harvard Med Sch

Sober, Arthur MD [D] - **Spec Exp:** Melanoma; Skin Cancer; **Hospital:** Mass Genl Hosp; **Address:** Mass General Hospital, 50 Staniford St, Ste 200, Boston, MA 02114; **Phone:** 617-726-2914; **Board Cert:** Dermatology 1975; Internal Medicine 1974; **Med School:** Geo Wash Univ 1968; **Resid:** Internal Medicine, Beth Israel Hosp 1970; Dermatology, Mass General Hosp 1974; **Fellow:** Immunology, Peter Bent Brigham Hosp 1976; **Fac Appt:** Prof D, Harvard Med Sch

Mid Atlantic

Bickers, David MD [D] - **Spec Exp:** Skin Cancer; Photodynamic Therapy; **Hospital:** NY-Presby Hosp/Columbia (page 79); **Address:** 16 E 60th St, Ste 300, New York, NY 10022-1002; **Phone:** 212-326-8465; **Board Cert:** Dermatology 1974; **Med School:** Univ VA Sch Med 1967; **Resid:** Dermatology, NYU Med Ctr 1973; **Fellow:** Pharmacology, Rockefeller Univ Hosp 1974; **Fac Appt:** Prof D, Columbia P&S

Braun III, Martin MD [D] - **Spec Exp:** Mohs' Surgery; Skin Cancer; **Hospital:** G Washington Univ Hosp; **Address:** 2112 F St NW, Ste 701, Washington, DC 20037; **Phone:** 202-293-7618; **Board Cert:** Dermatology 1977; Dermatopathology 1982; **Med School:** Univ MD Sch Med 1970; **Resid:** Dermatology, Univ Mich Med Ctr 1976; **Fellow:** Mohs Surgery, Precept w/ Dr Frederic Mohs 1975; **Fac Appt:** Clin Prof D, Geo Wash Univ

Brodland, David MD [D] - **Spec Exp:** Mohs' Surgery; Skin Cancer; Reconstructive Surgery-Skin; **Hospital:** UPMC Shadyside, Jefferson Hosp - Pittsburgh; **Address:** South Hills Med Bldg, 575 Coal Valley Rd, Ste 360, Clairton, PA 15025; **Phone:** 412-466-9400; **Board Cert:** Dermatology 1989; **Med School:** Southern IL Univ 1985; **Resid:** Dermatology, Mayo Grad Sch Med 1989; **Fellow:** Mohs Surgery, John A Zitelli MD 1990; **Fac Appt:** Asst Clin Prof D, Univ Pittsburgh

Bystryn, Jean-Claude MD [D] - **Spec Exp:** Melanoma; Skin Cancer; **Hospital:** NYU Langone Med Ctr (page 80); **Address:** 530 1st Ave, Ste 7F, New York, NY 10016; **Phone:** 212-889-3846; **Board Cert:** Dermatology 1970; Clinical & Laboratory Dematologic Immunology 1985; **Med School:** NYU Sch Med 1962; **Resid:** Internal Medicine, Montefiore Hosp 1964; Dermatology, NYU Med Ctr 1969; **Fellow:** Immunology, New York Univ 1972; **Fac Appt:** Prof D, NYU Sch Med

Dermatology

Dzubow, Leonard M MD [D] - **Spec Exp:** Mohs' Surgery; Skin Cancer; **Address:** 101 Chesley Drive, Media, PA 19063; **Phone:** 484-621-0082; **Board Cert:** Internal Medicine 1978; Dermatology 2006; **Med School:** Univ Pennsylvania 1975; **Resid:** Internal Medicine, Hosp Univ Penn 1978; Dermatology, NYU-Skin Cancer Unit 1980; **Fellow:** Mohs Surgery, NYU-Skin Cancer Unit 1981; **Fac Appt:** Prof D, Univ Pennsylvania

Geronemus, Roy MD [D] - **Spec Exp:** Skin Laser Surgery; Mohs' Surgery; Skin Cancer; **Hospital:** NYU Langone Med Ctr (page 80), New York Eye & Ear Infirm (page 78); **Address:** 317 E 34 St, Ste 11N, New York, NY 10016-4974; **Phone:** 212-686-7306; **Board Cert:** Dermatology 1983; **Med School:** Univ Miami Sch Med 1979; **Resid:** Dermatology, NYU-Skin Cancer Unit 1983; **Fellow:** Mohs Surgery, NYU-Skin Cancer Unit 1984; **Fac Appt:** Clin Prof D, NYU Sch Med

Granstein, Richard D MD [D] - **Spec Exp:** Autoimmune Disease; Skin Cancer; **Hospital:** NY-Presby Hosp/Weill Cornell (page 79); **Address:** 1305 York Ave Fl 9, New York, NY 10021; **Phone:** 646-962-7546; **Board Cert:** Dermatology 1983; Clinical & Laboratory Dermatologic Immunology 1985; **Med School:** UCLA 1978; **Resid:** Dermatology, Mass Genl Hosp 1981; **Fellow:** Research, Natl Cancer Inst 1982; Dermatology, Mass Genl Hosp 1983; **Fac Appt:** Prof D, Cornell Univ-Weill Med Coll

Halpern, Allan C MD [D] - **Spec Exp:** Skin Cancer; Melanoma; Melanoma Early Detection/Prevention; **Hospital:** Meml Sloan-Kettering Cancer Ctr (page 76); **Address:** 1275 York Avenue, New York, NY 10065; **Phone:** 212-610-0766; **Board Cert:** Internal Medicine 1984; Dermatology 1988; **Med School:** Albert Einstein Coll Med 1981; **Resid:** Internal Medicine, Montefiore Hosp 1985; Dermatology, Hosp Univ Penn 1989; **Fellow:** Epidemiology, Hosp Univ Penn 1989; **Fac Appt:** Assoc Prof Med, Cornell Univ-Weill Med Coll

Kriegel, David MD [D] - **Spec Exp:** Mohs' Surgery; Skin Laser Surgery; **Hospital:** Mount Sinai Med Ctr (page 77); **Address:** 250 W 57th St, Ste 825, New York, NY 10107-0809; **Phone:** 212-489-6669; **Board Cert:** Dermatology 2003; **Med School:** Boston Univ 1987; **Resid:** Dermatology, New England Med Ctr 1991; **Fellow:** Mohs Surgery, Stony Brook Univ Hosp 1993; **Fac Appt:** Assoc Prof D, Mount Sinai Sch Med

Lebwohl, Mark MD [D] - **Spec Exp:** Skin Cancer; Cutaneous Lymphoma; Melanoma; **Hospital:** Mount Sinai Med Ctr (page 77); **Address:** 5 E 98th St Fl 5, New York, NY 10029-6501; **Phone:** 212-241-9728; **Board Cert:** Internal Medicine 1981; Dermatology 1983; **Med School:** Harvard Med Sch 1978; **Resid:** Internal Medicine, Mt Sinai Hosp 1981; **Fellow:** Dermatology, Mt Sinai Hosp 1983; **Fac Appt:** Prof D, Mount Sinai Sch Med

Lessin, Stuart R MD [D] - **Spec Exp:** Melanoma; Skin Cancer; Cutaneous Lymphoma; Melanoma Risk Assessment; **Hospital:** Fox Chase Cancer Ctr (page 72); **Address:** Fox Chase Cancer Ctr, Dept Dermatology, 333 Cottman Ave, Philadelphia, PA 19111; **Phone:** 215-728-2570; **Board Cert:** Dermatology 1986; **Med School:** Temple Univ 1982; **Resid:** Dermatology, Hosp Univ Penn 1986; **Fellow:** Molecular Biology, Wistar Inst 1987; **Fac Appt:** Prof D, Temple Univ

Miller, Stanley J MD [D] - **Spec Exp:** Skin Cancer; Mohs' Surgery; Melanoma; **Hospital:** Johns Hopkins Hosp; **Address:** Charles Towson Bldg, 1104 Kenilworth Drive, Ste 201, Towson, MD 21204; **Phone:** 443-279-0340; **Board Cert:** Dermatology 1989; **Med School:** Univ VT Coll Med 1984; **Resid:** Dermatology, UCSD Med Ctr 1989; **Fellow:** Dermatologic Surgery, Univ Penn 1991; **Fac Appt:** Prof D, Johns Hopkins Univ

Nigra, Thomas P MD [D] - **Spec Exp:** Skin Cancer; Lymphoma; **Hospital:** Washington Hosp Ctr, Natl Rehab Hosp; **Address:** Dermatology Assocs, 110 Irving St NW, 2B44, Washington, DC 20010; **Phone:** 202-877-6227; **Board Cert:** Dermatology 1973; **Med School:** Univ Pennsylvania 1967; **Resid:** Dermatology, Mass Genl Hosp 1973; Dermatology, Natl Insts of Health 1971; **Fac Appt:** Clin Prof D, Geo Wash Univ

Ramsay, David L MD [D] - **Spec Exp:** Cutaneous Lymphoma; Skin Cancer; **Hospital:** NYU Langone Med Ctr (page 80); **Address:** 530 1st Ave, Ste 7G, New York, NY 10016-6402; **Phone:** 212-683-6283; **Board Cert:** Dermatology 1974; **Med School:** Indiana Univ 1969; **Resid:** Dermatology, NYU Med Ctr 1973; **Fellow:** Dermatology, Univ Ill Hosp 1973; **Fac Appt:** Clin Prof D, NYU Sch Med

Rigel, Darrell S MD [D] - **Spec Exp:** Melanoma; Skin Cancer; **Hospital:** NYU Langone Med Ctr (page 80), Mount Sinai Med Ctr (page 77); **Address:** 35 E 35th Street, Ste 208, New York, NY 10016-3823; **Phone:** 212-684-5964; **Board Cert:** Dermatology 1983; **Med School:** Geo Wash Univ 1978; **Resid:** Dermatology, NYU Med Ctr 1982; **Fellow:** Dermatologic Surgery, NYU Med Ctr 1983; **Fac Appt:** Clin Prof D, NYU Sch Med

Robins, Perry MD [D] - **Spec Exp:** Mohs' Surgery; Skin Cancer; Melanoma; **Hospital:** NYU Langone Med Ctr (page 80), Bellevue Hosp Ctr; **Address:** 345 E 37 St, Ste 209, New York, NY 10016; **Phone:** 212-263-7222; **Med School:** Germany 1961; **Resid:** Dermatology, VA Med Ctr 1964; **Fellow:** Dermatology, NYU Med Ctr 1967; **Fac Appt:** Prof Emeritus D, NYU Sch Med

Rook, Alain H MD [D] - **Spec Exp:** Cutaneous Lymphoma; **Hospital:** Hosp Univ Penn - UPHS (page 81); **Address:** Dept Dermatology, 3400 Spruce St Maloney Bldg Fl 2, Philadelphia, PA 19104; **Phone:** 215-662-7610; **Board Cert:** Internal Medicine 1979; Nephrology 1980; Dermatology 2001; **Med School:** Univ Mich Med Sch 1975; **Resid:** Internal Medicine, McGill Univ Med Ctr 1977; Dermatology, Hosp Univ Penn 1989; **Fellow:** Nephrology, McGill Univ Med Ctr 1979; Immunology, NIH 1986; **Fac Appt:** Prof D, Univ Pennsylvania

Zitelli, John MD [D] - **Spec Exp:** Mohs' Surgery; Skin Cancer; Melanoma; **Hospital:** UPMC Shadyside, Jefferson Hosp - Pittsburgh; **Address:** Shadyside Med Ctr, 5200 Centre Ave, Ste 303, Pittsburgh, PA 15232-1312; **Phone:** 412-681-9400; **Board Cert:** Dermatology 1980; **Med School:** Univ Pittsburgh 1976; **Resid:** Dermatology, Univ Hlth Ctr Hosp 1979; **Fellow:** Mohs Surgery, Univ Wisconsin 1980; **Fac Appt:** Assoc Clin Prof D, Univ Pittsburgh

Southeast

Amonette, Rex A MD [D] - **Spec Exp:** Skin Cancer; Mohs' Surgery; **Address:** Memphis Dermatology Clinic, 1455 Union Ave, Memphis, TN 38104-6727; **Phone:** 901-726-6655; **Board Cert:** Dermatology 1974; **Med School:** Univ Ark 1966; **Resid:** Dermatology, Univ Tenn Med Ctr 1971; **Fellow:** Mohs Surgery, NYU Med Ctr 1972; **Fac Appt:** Clin Prof D, Univ Tenn Coll Med, Memphis

Cook, Jonathan L MD [D] - **Spec Exp:** Skin Cancer; Mohs' Surgery; Reconstructive Surgery-Skin; **Hospital:** Duke Univ Med Ctr; **Address:** Duke Univ Med Ctr, Box 3915, Durham, NC 27710; **Phone:** 919-684-6805; **Board Cert:** Dermatology 2005; **Med School:** Med Univ SC 1992; **Resid:** Dermatology, Emory Univ Hosp 1996; **Fellow:** Dermatologic Surgery, Hosp Univ Penn 1997; **Fac Appt:** Prof D, Duke Univ

Eichler, Craig J MD [D] - **Spec Exp:** Skin Cancer; **Hospital:** Physicians Regl Med Ctr; **Address:** 6101 Pine Ridge Rd, Naples, FL 34119-3900; **Phone:** 239-348-4335; **Board Cert:** Dermatology 2003; **Med School:** Univ Fla Coll Med 1989; **Resid:** Dermatology, Univ Texas Med Branch 1993

Dermatology

Elmets, Craig A MD [D] - **Spec Exp:** Skin Cancer; Photodynamic Therapy; Melanoma; **Hospital:** Univ of Ala Hosp at Birmingham, VA Med Ctr; **Address:** Univ of Alabama-Birmingham-Derm Dept, 1530 3 Ave S EFH Bldg - rm 414, Birmingham, AL 35294; **Phone:** 205-996-7546; **Board Cert:** Internal Medicine 1978; Dermatology 1980; Clinical & Laboratory Dematologic Immunology 1989; **Med School:** Univ Iowa Coll Med 1975; **Resid:** Internal Medicine, Kansas Med Ctr 1978; Dermatology, Univ Iowa Hosps 1980; **Fellow:** Immunological Dermatology, Univ Texas Hlth Sci Ctr 1982; **Fac Appt:** Prof D, Univ Alabama

Fenske, Neil A MD [D] - **Spec Exp:** Skin Cancer; Melanoma; **Hospital:** H Lee Moffitt Cancer Ctr & Research Inst, Tampa Genl Hosp; **Address:** 12901 Bruce B Downs Blvd, MDC-33, Tampa, FL 33612-4742; **Phone:** 813-974-2920; **Board Cert:** Dermatology 1977; Dermatopathology 1984; **Med School:** St Louis Univ 1973; **Resid:** Dermatology, Wisc Hlth Sci Ctr 1977; **Fac Appt:** Prof Med, Univ S Fla Coll Med

Flowers, Franklin P MD [D] - **Spec Exp:** Mohs' Surgery; Dermatopathology; **Hospital:** Shands at Univ of FL; **Address:** Shands Healthcare, PO Box 100383, Gainesville, FL 32610-0383; **Phone:** 352-265-8001; **Board Cert:** Dermatology 1976; Dermatopathology 1981; **Med School:** Univ Fla Coll Med 1971; **Resid:** Dermatology, Ohio State Univ 1975; **Fellow:** Mohs Surgery, Univ Alabama 1993; **Fac Appt:** Prof Med, Univ Fla Coll Med

Garrett, Algin MD [D] - **Spec Exp:** Skin Cancer; Mohs' Surgery; **Hospital:** Med Coll of VA Hosp; **Address:** Stonypoint Medical Park, 9000 Stonypoint Pkwy Fl 2, Richmond, VA 23235; **Phone:** 804-560-8991; **Board Cert:** Dermatology 1983; **Med School:** Penn State Univ-Hershey Med Ctr 1978; **Resid:** Internal Medicine, VA Med Ctr 1980; Dermatology, Med Col VA 1983; **Fellow:** Mohs Surgery, Cleveland Clinic Found 1988; **Fac Appt:** Prof D, Va Commonwealth Univ Sch Med

Green, Howard A MD [D] - **Spec Exp:** Mohs' Surgery; Skin Cancer; **Hospital:** St Mary's Med Ctr - W Palm Bch; **Address:** 120 Butler St, Ste A, West Palm Beach, FL 33407-6106; **Phone:** 561-659-1510; **Board Cert:** Internal Medicine 1988; Dermatology 2004; **Med School:** Boston Univ 1985; **Resid:** Internal Medicine, Jefferson Univ Hosp 1988; Dermatology, Harvard Affil Hosps 1992; **Fellow:** Mohs Surgery, Boston Univ Med Ctr 1993

Grichnik, James M MD/PhD [D] - **Spec Exp:** Melanoma; Skin Cancer; **Hospital:** Univ of Miami Hosp & Clins/Sylvester Comp Canc Ctr (page 82); **Address:** Univ Miami, UMHC-Sylvester CCC, 1475 NW 12th Ave, D1, Miami, FL 33136; **Phone:** 305-243-6045; **Board Cert:** Dermatology 2003; **Med School:** Harvard Med Sch 1990; **Resid:** Dermatology, Duke Univ Med Ctr 1994; **Fac Appt:** Assoc Prof D, Duke Univ

Johr, Robert MD [D] - **Spec Exp:** Pigmented Lesions; Melanoma; **Hospital:** Univ of Miami Hosp & Clins/Sylvester Comp Canc Ctr (page 82), Boca Raton Comm Hosp; **Address:** 1050 NW 15th St, Ste 201A, Boca Raton, FL 33486-1341; **Phone:** 561-368-4545; **Board Cert:** Dermatology 1981; **Med School:** Mexico 1975; **Resid:** Dermatology, Roswell Park Cancer Ctr 1977; Dermatology, Metro Med Ctr/Case Western Reserve 1979; **Fac Appt:** Clin Prof D, Univ Miami Sch Med

Leshin, Barry MD [D] - **Spec Exp:** Skin Cancer; Mohs' Surgery; **Address:** 125 Sunnynoll Ct, Ste 100, Winston-Salem, NC 27106; **Phone:** 336-724-2434; **Board Cert:** Dermatology 1985; **Med School:** Univ Tex, Houston 1981; **Resid:** Dermatology, Univ Iowa Hosp 1985; **Fellow:** Dermatologic Surgery, Univ Iowa Hosp 1986; **Fac Appt:** Clin Prof PlS, Wake Forest Univ

Olsen, Elise A MD [D] - **Spec Exp:** Cutaneous Lymphoma; **Hospital:** Duke Univ Med Ctr; **Address:** Duke Univ Med Ctr, Box 3294, Durham, NC 27710; **Phone:** 919-684-3432; **Board Cert:** Dermatology 1983; **Med School:** Baylor Coll Med 1978; **Resid:** Internal Medicine, Univ NC Meml Hosp 1980; Dermatology, Duke Univ Med Ctr 1983; **Fac Appt:** Prof D, Duke Univ

Sobel, Stuart MD [D] - **Spec Exp:** Skin Cancer; **Hospital:** Meml Regl Hosp, Joe Di Maggio Chldns Hosp; **Address:** 4340 Sheridan St, Ste 101, Hollywood, FL 33021-3511; **Phone:** 954-983-5533; **Board Cert:** Dermatology 1977; **Med School:** Tufts Univ 1972; **Resid:** Dermatology, Mt Sinai Hosp 1976

Sokoloff, Daniel O MD [D] - **Spec Exp:** Skin Cancer; **Hospital:** St Mary's Med Ctr - W Palm Bch, Good Sam Med Ctr - W Palm Beach; **Address:** 4475 Med Ctr Way, Ste 2, 1000 45th St, Ste 1, West Palm Beach, FL 33407-2416; **Phone:** 561-863-1000; **Board Cert:** Dermatology 1982; **Med School:** Geo Wash Univ 1977; **Resid:** Dermatology, Baylor Coll Med 1982

Thiers, Bruce H MD [D] - **Spec Exp:** Cutaneous Lymphoma; Skin Cancer; **Hospital:** MUSC Med Ctr; **Address:** MUSC Dept Dermatology, 135 Rutledge Ave Fl 11, MS 578, Charleston, SC 29425; **Phone:** 843-792-9784; **Board Cert:** Dermatology 1978; **Med School:** SUNY Buffalo 1974; **Resid:** Dermatology, SUNY Buffalo Med Ctr 1978; **Fac Appt:** Prof D, Med Univ SC

Midwest

Arpey, Christopher J MD [D] - **Spec Exp:** Mohs' Surgery; **Hospital:** Univ Iowa Hosp & Clinics; **Address:** UIHC Dept Dermatology, 200 Hawkins Drive, 300 EMRB, Iowa City, IA 52242-1009; **Phone:** 319-356-2856; **Board Cert:** Dermatology 2001; Internal Medicine 1989; **Med School:** Univ Rochester 1986; **Resid:** Internal Medicine, Univ Iowa Hosps & Clinics 1989; Dermatology, Univ Hosps 1992; **Fellow:** Mohs Surgery, Univ Iowa Hosps & Clinics 1994; **Fac Appt:** Prof D, Univ Iowa Coll Med

Bailin, Philip L MD [D] - **Spec Exp:** Mohs' Surgery; Skin Laser Surgery; Skin Cancer; **Hospital:** Cleveland Clin Fdn (page 70); **Address:** Cleveland Clinic, Dept Dermatology, 9500 Euclid Ave, Desk A61, Cleveland, OH 44195-5032; **Phone:** 216-444-2115; **Board Cert:** Dermatology 1975; **Med School:** Northwestern Univ 1968; **Resid:** Dermatology, Cleveland Clin Fdn 1974; **Fellow:** Dermatopathology, Armed Forces Inst Pathology 1975; Mohs Surgery, Univ Wisc Hosp & Clin

Cornelius, Lynne A MD [D] - **Spec Exp:** Melanoma; **Hospital:** Barnes-Jewish Hosp; **Address:** Washington Univ Dept Dermatology, 660 S Euclid, Box 8123, St Louis, MO 63110; **Phone:** 314-362-2643; **Board Cert:** Dermatology 1989; **Med School:** Univ MO-Columbia Sch Med 1984; **Resid:** Dermatology, Barnes Jewish Hosp-Wash Univ 1989; **Fellow:** Immunological Dermatology, Emory Univ Med Ctr 1992; **Fac Appt:** Assoc Prof D, Washington Univ, St Louis

Hanke, C William MD [D] - **Spec Exp:** Mohs' Surgery; Skin Laser Surgery; Photodynamic Therapy; **Hospital:** St Vincent Carmel Hosp, Clarian Hlth Ptrs (page 74); **Address:** Laser & Skin Surgery Ctr of Indiana, 13400 N Meridian St, Ste 290, Carmel, IN 46032-1486; **Phone:** 317-660-4900; **Board Cert:** Dermatology 1978; Dermatopathology 1982; **Med School:** Univ Iowa Coll Med 1971; **Resid:** Dermatology, Cleveland Clinic 1978; Dermatopathology, Indiana Univ 1982; **Fellow:** Cutaneous Oncology, Cleveland Clinic 1979; **Fac Appt:** Clin Prof D, Indiana Univ

Hruza, George J MD [D] - **Spec Exp:** Skin Laser Surgery; Mohs' Surgery; **Hospital:** St Luke's Hosp - Chesterfield, MO, St Louis Univ Hosp; **Address:** Laser & Derm Surg Ctr, 1001 Chesterfield Pkwy E, Ste 101, St Louis, MO 63017; **Phone:** 314-878-3839; **Board Cert:** Dermatology 1986; **Med School:** NYU Sch Med 1982; **Resid:** Dermatology, NYU Med Ctr-Skin Cancer Unit 1986; **Fellow:** Laser Surgery, Mass Genl Hosp-Harvard 1987; Mohs Surgery, Univ Wisc Affil Hosp 1988; **Fac Appt:** Assoc Clin Prof D, St Louis Univ

Dermatology

Johnson, Timothy M MD [D] - **Spec Exp:** Melanoma; Mohs' Surgery; **Hospital:** Univ Michigan Hlth Sys; **Address:** Univ Michigan Dermatology, 1910 Taubman Ctr, 1500 E Medical Center Drive, Ann Arbor, MI 48109-5314; **Phone:** 734-936-4190; **Board Cert:** Dermatology 1988; **Med School:** Univ Tex, Houston 1984; **Resid:** Dermatology, Univ Texas Med Ctr 1988; **Fellow:** Cutaneous Oncology, Univ Mich Med Ctr 1989; Mohs Surgery, Univ Oregon Hlth Sci Ctr 1990; **Fac Appt:** Prof D, Univ Mich Med Sch

Lim, Henry W MD [D] - **Spec Exp:** Cutaneous Lymphoma; Skin Cancer; **Hospital:** Henry Ford Hosp; **Address:** Henry Ford Hosp, Dept Derm, 3031 W Grand Blvd, Ste 800, Detroit, MI 48202-3141; **Phone:** 313-916-4060; **Board Cert:** Dermatology 2005; Clinical & Laboratory Dematologic Immunology 1985; **Med School:** SUNY Downstate 1975; **Resid:** Dermatology, NYU Med Ctr 1979; **Fellow:** Immunological Dermatology, NYU Med Ctr 1980; **Fac Appt:** Prof Path, Wayne State Univ

Lowe, Lori MD [D] - **Spec Exp:** Dermatopathology; Skin Cancer; **Hospital:** Univ Michigan Hlth Sys; **Address:** Univ Michigan Dept Pathology, 1301 Catherine Rd, M3261-Med Sci I, Ann Arbor, MI 48109-5602; **Phone:** 734-764-4460; **Board Cert:** Dermatology 1990; Dermatopathology 1991; **Med School:** Univ Tex, Houston 1985; **Resid:** Dermatology, Univ Tex Hlth Sci Ctr 1990; **Fellow:** Dermatopathology, Univ Colo Hlth Sci Ctr 1991; **Fac Appt:** Prof D, Univ Mich Med Sch

Neuburg, Marcelle MD [D] - **Spec Exp:** Mohs' Surgery; Skin Cancer; Pigmented Lesions; **Hospital:** Froedtert Meml Lutheran Hosp; **Address:** Dept Dermatology, 9200 W Wisconsin Ave, Milwaukee, WI 53226; **Phone:** 414-805-5300; **Board Cert:** Internal Medicine 1985; Dermatology 1988; **Med School:** Oregon Hlth Sci Univ 1982; **Resid:** Internal Medicine, Georgetown Univ Hosp 1985; Dermatology, Boston Univ Sch Med Ctr 1988; **Fellow:** Mohs Surgery, Tufts New England Med Ctr 1990; **Fac Appt:** Prof D, Med Coll Wisc

Otley, Clark C MD [D] - **Spec Exp:** Mohs' Surgery; Skin Cancer; Skin Cancer in Transplant Patients; **Hospital:** Mayo Med Ctr & Clin - Rochester; **Address:** Mayo Clinic, 200 First St SW, Rochester, MN 55905; **Phone:** 507-284-3579; **Board Cert:** Dermatology 2004; **Med School:** Duke Univ 1991; **Resid:** Dermatology, Mass Genl Hosp 1995; **Fellow:** Dermatologic Surgery, Mayo Clinic 1996; **Fac Appt:** Assoc Prof D, Mayo Med Sch

Wheeland, Ronald MD [D] - **Spec Exp:** Skin Laser Surgery; Mohs' Surgery; **Hospital:** Univ of Missouri Hosp & Clins; **Address:** Univ Missouri, Dept Dermatology, One Hospital Drive, Columbia, MO 65212; **Phone:** 573-882-4800 x2; **Board Cert:** Dermatology 1977; Dermatopathology 1978; **Med School:** Univ Ariz Coll Med 1973; **Resid:** Dermatology, Univ Ok Hlth Sci Ctr 1977; **Fellow:** Dermatopathology, Univ Ok Hlth Sci Ctr 1978; Dermatologic Surgery, Cleveland Clin Fnd 1984; **Fac Appt:** Prof D, Univ MO-Columbia Sch Med

Wood, Gary S MD [D] - **Spec Exp:** Cutaneous Lymphoma; Melanoma; Skin Cancer; **Hospital:** Univ WI Hosp & Clins, VA Hospital, Madison; **Address:** Univ Wisconsin Health, Dept Dermatology, 1 S Park St Fl 7, Madison, WI 53715-1375; **Phone:** 608-287-2620; **Board Cert:** Anatomic Pathology 1983; Dermatology 1986; Dermatopathology 1987; **Med School:** Univ IL Coll Med 1979; **Resid:** Anatomic Pathology, Stanford Univ Med Ctr 1983; Dermatology, Stanford Univ Med Ctr 1985; **Fellow:** Immunopathology, Stanford Univ Med Ctr 1981; **Fac Appt:** Prof D, Univ Wisc

Great Plains and Mountains

Bowen, Glen M MD [D] - **Spec Exp:** Melanoma; Cutaneous Lymphoma; Clinical Trials; Mohs' Surgery; **Hospital:** Univ Utah Hosps and Clins, Cottonwood Hosp & Med Ctr; **Address:** Huntsman Cancer Inst, 500 N Medical Drive, rm 4A330, Salt Lake City, UT 84132; **Phone:** 801-585-0197; **Board Cert:** Dermatology 2005; **Med School:** Univ Utah 1990; **Resid:** Dermatology, Univ Michigan Med Ctr 1993; **Fellow:** Immunological Dermatology, Univ Michigan Med Ctr 1995; Mohs Surgery, Univ Utah 2001; **Fac Appt:** Assoc Prof D, Univ Utah

Southwest

Butler, David F MD [D] - **Spec Exp:** Skin Cancer; **Hospital:** Scott & White Mem Hosp; **Address:** Scott White Meml Hosp, Dept Dermatology, 409 W Adams St, Temple, TX 76501; **Phone:** 254-742-3724; **Board Cert:** Dermatology 1985; **Med School:** Univ Tex Med Br, Galveston 1980; **Resid:** Dermatology, Walter Reed Army Med Ctr 1985; **Fac Appt:** Assoc Prof D, Texas Tech Univ

Carney, John M MD [D] - **Spec Exp:** Mohs' Surgery; Skin Cancer; **Hospital:** UAMS Med Ctr; **Address:** Southwest Med Arts Bldg, 11321 Interstate 30, Ste 201, Little Rock, AR 72209; **Phone:** 501-455-4700; **Board Cert:** Dermatology 1984; **Med School:** Northwestern Univ 1979; **Resid:** Dermatology, Univ Hosps 1984; **Fellow:** Physiology, Harvard Med Sch 1985; Dermatologic Surgery, Univ Tenn Med Ctr 1986

Duvic, Madeleine MD [D] - **Spec Exp:** Cutaneous Lymphoma; Skin Cancer; **Hospital:** UT MD Anderson Cancer Ctr, St Luke's Episcopal Hosp-Houston; **Address:** MD Anderson Cancer Ctr, Dept Dermatology, 1515 Holcombe Blvd, Unit 434, Houston, TX 77030; **Phone:** 713-745-1113; **Board Cert:** Dermatology 1981; Internal Medicine 1982; **Med School:** Duke Univ 1977; **Resid:** Dermatology, Duke Univ Med Ctr 1980; Internal Medicine, Duke Univ Med Ctr 1982; **Fellow:** Geriatric Medicine, Duke Univ Med Ctr 1984; **Fac Appt:** Prof D, Univ Tex, Houston

Lim, Katherine MD [D] - **Spec Exp:** Mohs' Surgery; Skin Cancer; **Address:** Mayo Clinic, Dept Dermatology, 13400 E Shea Blvd, Scottsdale, AZ 85259-5499; **Phone:** 480-301-6479; **Board Cert:** Dermatology 1996; **Med School:** Northwestern Univ 1992; **Resid:** Dermatology, Mayo Clinic 1996; **Fellow:** Mohs Surgery, Mayo Clinic 1997

Orengo, Ida F MD [D] - **Spec Exp:** Melanoma; Mohs' Surgery; **Hospital:** St Luke's Episcopal Hosp-Houston, DeBakey VA Med Ctr-Houston; **Address:** Baylor College of Medicine, 6620 Main St, Ste 1425, Houston, TX 77030; **Phone:** 713-798-6925; **Board Cert:** Dermatology 2001; **Med School:** Harvard Med Sch 1988; **Resid:** Dermatology, Baylor Coll Med 1991; **Fac Appt:** Assoc Prof D, Baylor Coll Med

Taylor, R Stan MD [D] - **Spec Exp:** Mohs' Surgery; Melanoma; Skin Cancer; **Hospital:** UT Southwestern Med Ctr at Dallas, Parkland Meml Hosp - Dallas; **Address:** Univ Tex SW Med Sch, Dept Derm, 5323 Harry Hines Blvd, MC 9192, Dallas, TX 75390-7208; **Phone:** 214 645 8950; **Board Cert:** Dermatology 1989; **Med School:** Univ Tex Med Br, Galveston 1985; **Resid:** Dermatology, Univ Mich Med Ctr 1989; **Fellow:** Immunological Dermatology, Univ Mich 1990; Mohs Surgery, Oregon Hlth Sci Univ 1991; **Fac Appt:** Prof D, Univ Tex SW, Dallas

West Coast and Pacific

Bennett, Richard G MD [D] - **Spec Exp:** Mohs' Surgery; Skin Cancer; **Hospital:** UCLA Ronald Reagan Med Ctr, USC Univ Hosp; **Address:** 1301 20th St, Ste 570, Santa Monica, CA 90404-2080; **Phone:** 310-315-0171; **Board Cert:** Dermatology 1975; **Med School:** Case West Res Univ 1970; **Resid:** Dermatology, Hosp Univ Penn 1974; **Fellow:** Chemosurgery, NYU Med Ctr 1977; **Fac Appt:** Clin Prof D, UCLA

Berg, Daniel MD [D] - **Spec Exp:** Skin Cancer; Mohs' Surgery; Skin Laser Surgery; **Hospital:** Univ Wash Med Ctr; **Address:** 4225 Roosevelt Way NE, Seattle, WA 98105; **Phone:** 206-598-6647; **Board Cert:** Dermatology 1999; **Med School:** Univ Toronto 1985; **Resid:** Internal Medicine, Sunnybrook Med Ctr 1988; Dermatology, Duke Univ Med Ctr 1991; **Fellow:** Dermatologic Surgery, Univ Toronto 1992; Dermatologic Surgery, Univ British Columbia 1994; **Fac Appt:** Prof D, Univ Wash

Dermatology

Glogau, Richard G MD [D] - **Spec Exp:** Skin Laser Surgery; Mohs' Surgery; **Hospital:** UCSF Med Ctr; **Address:** 350 Parnassus Ave, Ste 400, San Francisco, CA 94117; **Phone:** 415-564-1261; **Board Cert:** Dermatology 1978; Dermatopathology 1982; **Med School:** Harvard Med Sch 1973; **Resid:** Dermatology, UCSF Med Ctr 1977; **Fellow:** Chemosurgery, UCSF Med Ctr 1978; **Fac Appt:** Clin Prof D, UCSF

Greenway, Hubert T MD [D] - **Spec Exp:** Skin Cancer; Mohs' Surgery; Melanoma; **Hospital:** Scripps Green Hosp; **Address:** Scripps Clinic, Div Mohs' Surgery, 10666 N Torrey Pines Rd, MS 112A, La Jolla, CA 92037; **Phone:** 858-554-8646; **Board Cert:** Dermatology 1982; **Med School:** Med Coll GA 1974; **Resid:** Dermatology, Naval Hosp 1982; **Fellow:** Mohs Surgery, Univ Wisconsin Med Ctr 1981

Kim, Youn-Hee MD [D] - **Spec Exp:** Cutaneous Lymphoma; Skin Cancer; **Hospital:** Stanford Univ Med Ctr; **Address:** Stanford Outpatient Med Ctr, 450 Broadway, Redwood City, CA 94063; **Phone:** 650-723-6316; **Board Cert:** Dermatology 1989; **Med School:** Stanford Univ 1984; **Resid:** Dermatology, Metropolitan Hospital 1989

Swanson, Neil A MD [D] - **Spec Exp:** Skin Cancer; **Hospital:** OR Hlth & Sci Univ, VA Medical Center - Portland; **Address:** Oregon HSU, Center for Health & Healing, 3303 SW Bond Ave, CH16D, Portland, OR 97239; **Phone:** 503-418-3376; **Board Cert:** Dermatology 1980; **Med School:** Univ Rochester 1976; **Resid:** Dermatology, Univ Michigan Med Ctr 1979; **Fellow:** Dermatology, UCSF Med Ctr 1980; **Fac Appt:** Prof D, Oregon Hlth Sci Univ

Swetter, Susan M MD [D] - **Spec Exp:** Melanoma; Melanoma Early Detection/Prevention; Skin Cancer; **Hospital:** Stanford Univ Med Ctr, VA Hlth Care Sys - Palo Alto; **Address:** Stanford Univ Med Ctr, Dept Dermatology, 900 Blake Wilbur Dr, W0069, MC 5334, Stanford, CA 94305; **Phone:** 650-723-0119; **Board Cert:** Dermatology 2001; **Med School:** Univ Pennsylvania 1990; **Resid:** Dermatology, Stanford Univ Med Ctr 1994; **Fac Appt:** Assoc Prof D, Stanford Univ

NYU Cancer Institute

NYU LANGONE MEDICAL CENTER

Endocrinology, Diabetes & Metabolism

a subspecialty of Internal Medicine

An internist who concentrates on disorders of the internal (en-docrine) glands such as the thyroid and adrenal glands. This special-ist also deals with disorders such as diabetes, metabolic and nutritional disorders, pituitary diseases, menstrual and sexual problems.

Training Required: Three years in internal medicine plus additional training and examination for certification in endocrinology, dia-betes, and metabolism.

ENDOCRINOLOGY, DIABETES & METABOLISM

New England

Levine, Robert A MD [EDM] - **Spec Exp:** Thyroid Cancer; Thyroid Disorders; Thyroid Ultrasound; **Hospital:** St Joseph Hosp; **Address:** Thyroid Center of New Hampshire, 5 Coliseum Ave, Nashua, NH 03060; **Phone:** 603-881-7141; **Board Cert:** Internal Medicine 1984; Endocrinology, Diabetes & Metabolism 1987; **Med School:** Univ Conn 1981; **Resid:** Internal Medicine, Mt Auburn Hosp 1984; **Fellow:** Endocrinology, Yale Univ 1987

Mid Atlantic

Ball, Douglas W MD [EDM] - **Spec Exp:** Thyroid Cancer; **Hospital:** Johns Hopkins Hosp; **Address:** Sidney Kimmel Cancer Ctr, 1830 E Monument St, Ste 333, Baltimore, MD 21287; **Phone:** 410-955-8964; **Board Cert:** Internal Medicine 1987; **Med School:** Geo Wash Univ 1984; **Resid:** Internal Medicine, Univ Pittsburgh 1987; **Fellow:** Endocrinology, Diabetes & Metabolism, Johns Hopkins Hosp 1991; **Fac Appt:** Assoc Prof Med, Johns Hopkins Univ

Ladenson, Paul W MD [EDM] - **Spec Exp:** Thyroid Disorders; Thyroid Cancer; **Hospital:** Johns Hopkins Hosp; **Address:** Johns Hopkins Hosp, Div Endocrinology & Metabolism, 1830 E Monument St, rm 333, Baltimore, MD 21287; **Phone:** 410-955-3663; **Board Cert:** Internal Medicine 1978; Endocrinology, Diabetes & Metabolism 1981; **Med School:** Harvard Med Sch 1975; **Resid:** Internal Medicine, Mass Genl Hosp 1978; **Fellow:** Endocrinology, Diabetes & Metabolism, Mass Genl Hosp 1980; **Fac Appt:** Prof Med, Johns Hopkins Univ

Snyder, Peter J MD [EDM] - **Spec Exp:** Pituitary Tumors; **Hospital:** Hosp Univ Penn - UPHS (page 81); **Address:** Univ Pennsylvania Med Group, 3400 Civic Center Blvd, Philadelphia, PA 19104; **Phone:** 215-662-2300; **Board Cert:** Internal Medicine 1972; Endocrinology, Diabetes & Metabolism 1972; **Med School:** Harvard Med Sch 1965; **Resid:** Internal Medicine, Beth Israel Hosp 1967; Internal Medicine, Beth Israel Hosp 1970; **Fellow:** Endocrinology, Diabetes & Metabolism, Hosp Univ Penn 1971; **Fac Appt:** Prof Med, Univ Pennsylvania

Tuttle, R Michael MD [EDM] - **Spec Exp:** Thyroid Cancer; **Hospital:** Meml Sloan-Kettering Cancer Ctr (page 76); **Address:** 1275 York Avenue, New York, NY 10065; **Phone:** 800-525-2225; **Board Cert:** Endocrinology, Diabetes & Metabolism 2004; **Med School:** Univ Louisville Sch Med 1987; **Resid:** Internal Medicine, DD Eisenhower Army Med Ctr 1990; **Fellow:** Endocrinology, Diabetes & Metabolism, Madigan Army Med Ctr 1993; **Fac Appt:** Assoc Prof Med, Cornell Univ-Weill Med Coll

Wartofsky, Leonard MD [EDM] - **Spec Exp:** Thyroid Cancer; Thyroid Disorders; **Hospital:** Washington Hosp Ctr; **Address:** 110 Irving St NW, Ste 2A62, Washington, DC 20010-2975; **Phone:** 202-877-3109; **Board Cert:** Internal Medicine 1971; Endocrinology, Diabetes & Metabolism 1972; **Med School:** Geo Wash Univ 1964; **Resid:** Internal Medicine, Barnes Jewish Hosp 1966; Internal Medicine, Montefiore Med Ctr 1967; **Fellow:** Endocrinology, Diabetes & Metabolism, Boston City Hosp 1969; **Fac Appt:** Prof Med, Georgetown Univ

Southeast

Ain, Kenneth B MD [EDM] - **Spec Exp:** Thyroid Cancer; Thyroid Disorders; **Hospital:** Univ of Kentucky Chandler Hosp, VA Med Ctr - Lexington; **Address:** Thyroid Oncology Program, rm MN524, 800 Rose St, Lexington, KY 40536-0298; **Phone:** 859-323-3778; **Board Cert:** Internal Medicine 1984; Endocrinology, Diabetes & Metabolism 1987; **Med School:** Brown Univ 1981; **Resid:** Internal Medicine, Hahnemann Univ Hosp 1984; **Fellow:** Endocrinology, Univ Chicago 1986; Thyroid Oncology, NIDDK, Natl Inst Hlth 1990; **Fac Appt:** Prof Med, Univ KY Coll Med

Earp III, H Shelton MD [EDM] - **Spec Exp:** Cancer-Hormonal Influences; **Hospital:** Univ NC Hosps; **Address:** UNC Lineberger Comprehensive Cancer Center, 450 West Drive, Fl 1 - rm 10-012, Chapel Hill, NC 27599; **Phone:** 919-966-3036; **Board Cert:** Internal Medicine 1976; Endocrinology, Diabetes & Metabolism 1977; **Med School:** Univ NC Sch Med 1970; **Resid:** Internal Medicine, NC Memorial Hosp 1975; **Fellow:** Endocrinology, Diabetes & Metabolism, Univ North Carolina Hosp 1977; **Fac Appt:** Prof Med, Univ NC Sch Med

Koch, Christian A MD [EDM] - **Spec Exp:** Endocrine Cancers; Thyroid Cancer; **Hospital:** Univ Mississippi Med Ctr; **Address:** 2500 N State St, Jackson, MS 39216; **Phone:** 601-984-5525; **Board Cert:** Internal Medicine 1999; Endocrinology, Diabetes & Metabolism 2000; **Med School:** Germany 1991; **Resid:** Internal Medicine, Ohio State Univ Hosp 1997; **Fellow:** Endocrinology, Natl Inst Hlth 2001; **Fac Appt:** Prof Med, Univ Miss

Midwest

Clutter, William E MD [EDM] - **Spec Exp:** Endocrine Cancers; **Hospital:** Barnes-Jewish Hosp, Washington Univ Med Ctr; **Address:** Washington Univ, Dept Internal Medicine, 4921 Parkview Pl Fl 5 - Ste C, St Louis, MO 63110; **Phone:** 314-362-3500; **Board Cert:** Internal Medicine 1978; Endocrinology, Diabetes & Metabolism 1981; **Med School:** Ohio State Univ 1975; **Resid:** Internal Medicine, Barnes Jewish Hosp 1978; **Fellow:** Endocrinology, Diabetes & Metabolism, Barnes Jewish Hosp 1980; **Fac Appt:** Prof Med, Washington Univ, St Louis

Kloos, Richard MD [EDM] - **Spec Exp:** Thyroid Cancer; **Hospital:** Ohio St Univ Med Ctr; **Address:** 446 McCampbell Hall, 1581 Dodd Drive, Columbus, OH 43210; **Phone:** 614-292-3800; **Board Cert:** Nuclear Medicine 2005; Internal Medicine 2002; Endocrinology, Diabetes & Metabolism 2005; **Med School:** Case West Res Univ 1989; **Resid:** Internal Medicine, Metrohealth MC 1992; **Fellow:** Endocrinology, Diabetes & Metabolism, Univ Michigan 1995; Nuclear Medicine, Univ Michigan 1996; **Fac Appt:** Assoc Prof Med, Ohio State Univ

Kopp, Peter A MD [EDM] - **Spec Exp:** Thyroid Cancer; **Hospital:** Northwestern Meml Hosp; **Address:** Northwestern Meml Hospital, 675 N St Clair St, Ste 14-100, Chicago, IL 60611; **Phone:** 312-695-7970; **Board Cert:** Internal Medicine 2003; Endocrinology, Diabetes & Metabolism 2004; **Med School:** Switzerland 1985; **Resid:** Internal Medicine, Regl Hosp 1992; Endocrinology, Diabetes & Metabolism, Univ Berne 1990; **Fellow:** Endocrinology, Diabetes & Metabolism, Northwestern Univ Hosp 1997; **Fac Appt:** Assoc Prof Med, Northwestern Univ-Feinberg Sch Med

Great Plains and Mountains

Ridgway, E Chester MD [EDM] - **Spec Exp:** Thyroid Cancer; **Hospital:** Univ Colorado Hosp, VA Med Ctr; **Address:** UCHSC at Fitzsimons, Div Endocrinology, 1635 Aurora Court, Box 6510, MS F732, Aurora, CO 80045; **Phone:** 720-848-2650; **Board Cert:** Internal Medicine 1972; Endocrinology 1973; **Med School:** Univ Colorado 1968; **Resid:** Internal Medicine, Mass Genl Hosp 1970; **Fellow:** Endocrinology, Mass Genl Hosp 1972; **Fac Appt:** Prof Med, Univ Colorado

Endocrinology, Diabetes & Metabolism

Southwest

Robbins, Richard J MD [EDM] - **Spec Exp:** Thyroid Cancer; Pituitary Tumors; **Hospital:** Methodist Hosp - Houston; **Address:** The Methodist Hosp, 6550 Fannin St, Ste 1001, Houston, TX 77030; **Phone:** 713-441-6640; **Board Cert:** Internal Medicine 1978; Endocrinology, Diabetes & Metabolism 1983; **Med School:** Creighton Univ 1975; **Resid:** Internal Medicine, NY Hosp-Cornell Med Ctr 1978; **Fellow:** Endocrinology, New England Med Ctr 1981; **Fac Appt:** Prof Med, Cornell Univ-Weill Med Coll

Rubenfeld, Sheldon MD [EDM] - **Spec Exp:** Thyroid Cancer; **Hospital:** St Luke's Episcopal Hosp-Houston, Methodist Hosp - Houston; **Address:** 7515 S Main St, Ste 690, Houston, TX 77030; **Phone:** 713-795-5750; **Board Cert:** Internal Medicine 1976; Endocrinology, Diabetes & Metabolism 1979; **Med School:** Georgetown Univ 1971; **Resid:** Internal Medicine, Baylor Affil Hosps 1976; **Fellow:** Endocrinology, Baylor Affil Hosps 1978; **Fac Appt:** Clin Prof Med, Baylor Coll Med

Sherman, Steven I MD [EDM] - **Spec Exp:** Thyroid Cancer; Endocrine Cancers; **Hospital:** UT MD Anderson Cancer Ctr; **Address:** MD Anderson Cancer Ctr, 1515 Holcombe Blvd, Unit 435, Houston, TX 77030; **Phone:** 713-792-2840; **Board Cert:** Internal Medicine 1988; Endocrinology, Diabetes & Metabolism 2007; **Med School:** Johns Hopkins Univ 1985; **Resid:** Internal Medicine, Johns Hopkins Hosp 1988; **Fellow:** Endocrinology, Diabetes & Metabolism, Johns Hopkins Hosp 1991; **Fac Appt:** Prof Med, Baylor Coll Med

Waguespack, Steven G MD [EDM] - **Spec Exp:** Thyroid Cancer; Pituitary Tumors; Adrenal Tumors & Disorders; **Hospital:** UT MD Anderson Cancer Ctr; **Address:** MD Anderson Cancer Ctr, Dept Endocrine Neoplasia & Hormonal Disorders, 1400 Pressler St. Unit 1461, Houston, TX 77030; **Phone:** 713-563-4400; **Board Cert:** Internal Medicine 1998; Endocrinology, Diabetes & Metabolism 2002; Pediatric Endocrinology 2003; **Med School:** Univ Tex, Houston 1994; **Resid:** Internal Medicine & Pediatrics, Indiana Univ Hosp 1998; **Fellow:** Endocrinology, Indiana Univ Hosp 2002

West Coast and Pacific

Darwin, Christine H MD [EDM] - **Spec Exp:** Pituitary Tumors; **Hospital:** UCLA Ronald Reagan Med Ctr; **Address:** 200 UCLA Medical Plaza, Ste 365A, Box 951693, Los Angeles, CA 90095-7065; **Phone:** 310-794-5584; **Med School:** India 1980; **Resid:** Internal Medicine, UC Irvine Med Ctr 1987; **Fellow:** Endocrinology, VA Hosp 1988; Endocrinology, USC Med Ctr 1993; **Fac Appt:** Assoc Prof Med, UCLA

Fitzgerald, Paul A MD [EDM] - **Spec Exp:** Thyroid Cancer; Paraganglioma; Pheochromocytoma; Pituitary Tumors; **Hospital:** UCSF Med Ctr; **Address:** 350 Parnassus Ave, Ste 710, San Francisco, CA 94117; **Phone:** 415-665-1136; **Board Cert:** Internal Medicine 1975; Endocrinology, Diabetes & Metabolism 1981; **Med School:** Jefferson Med Coll 1972; **Resid:** Internal Medicine, Presby Med Ctr-Univ Colo 1975; **Fellow:** Endocrinology, Diabetes & Metabolism, UCSF Med Ctr 1978; **Fac Appt:** Clin Prof Med, UCSF

Heber, David MD [EDM] - **Spec Exp:** Nutrition & Cancer Prevention; Nutrition & Disease Prevention/Control; **Hospital:** UCLA Ronald Reagan Med Ctr; **Address:** 900 Veteran Ave, Rm 12-217, UCLA Center for Human Nutrition, Los Angeles, CA 90095-1742; **Phone:** 310-206-1987; **Board Cert:** Internal Medicine 1976; Endocrinology, Diabetes & Metabolism 1977; **Med School:** Harvard Med Sch 1973; **Resid:** Internal Medicine, LAC Harbor Genl Hosp 1975; **Fellow:** Endocrinology, Diabetes & Metabolism, LAC Harbor Genl Hosp 1978; **Fac Appt:** Prof Med, UCLA

Hoffman, Andrew R MD [EDM] - **Spec Exp:** Pituitary Tumors; **Hospital:** Stanford Univ Med Ctr, VA Hlth Care Sys - Palo Alto; **Address:** 300 Pastur Drive, rm MC5303, Stanford, CA 94305; **Phone:** 650-723-6961; **Board Cert:** Internal Medicine 1979; Endocrinology 1981; **Med School:** Stanford Univ 1976; **Resid:** Internal Medicine, Mass Genl Hosp 1978; **Fellow:** Pharmacology, Mass Genl Hosp 1980; Endocrinology, Diabetes & Metabolism, Mass Genl Hosp 1982; **Fac Appt:** Prof Med, Stanford Univ

Kandeel, Fouad MD/PhD [EDM] - **Spec Exp:** Thyroid Cancer; Endocrine Cancers; **Hospital:** City of Hope Natl Med Ctr & Beckman Rsch (page 69); **Address:** City of Hope, Diabetes Department, 1500 E Duarte Rd, Duarte, CA 91010; **Phone:** 626-256-4673 x62251; **Med School:** Egypt 1969; **Resid:** Internal Medicine, Birmingham & Midland Hosp for Women; Endocrinology, Diabetes & Metabolism, Queen Elizabeth Hosp; **Fac Appt:** Assoc Clin Prof Med, UCLA

Melmed, Shlomo MD [EDM] - **Spec Exp:** Pituitary Tumors; **Hospital:** Cedars-Sinai Med Ctr; **Address:** Cedars Sinai Med Ctr, 8700 Beverly Blvd, Ste 2015, Los Angeles, CA 90048; **Phone:** 310-423-4691; **Board Cert:** Internal Medicine 1979; Endocrinology, Diabetes & Metabolism 1983; **Med School:** South Africa 1970; **Resid:** Internal Medicine, Sheba Med Ctr 1976; **Fellow:** Endocrinology, Diabetes & Metabolism, Wadsworth VA Hosp 1980; **Fac Appt:** Prof Med, UCLA

Gastroenterology

a subspecialty of Internal Medicine

An internist who specializes in diagnosis and treatment of diseases of the digestive organs including the stomach, bowels, liver, and gallbladder. This specialist treats conditions such as abdominal pain, ulcers, diarrhea, cancer and jaundice and performs complex diagnostic and therapeutic procedures using endoscopes to see internal organs.

Training Required: Three years in internal medicine plus additional training and examination for certification in gastroenterology.

GASTROENTEROLOGY

New England

Levine, Joel B MD [Ge] - **Spec Exp:** Colon & Rectal Cancer Detection; Colonoscopy; **Hospital:** Univ of Conn Hlth Ctr, John Dempsey Hosp; **Address:** Univ Connecticut Health Center, Colon Cancer Prevention Program, 263 Farmington Ave, Farmington, CT 06030-2813; **Phone:** 860-679-4567; **Board Cert:** Internal Medicine 1973; Gastroenterology 1977; **Med School:** SUNY Downstate 1969; **Resid:** Internal Medicine, Univ Chicago Hosps 1971; Internal Medicine, Mass Genl Hosp 1974; **Fellow:** Gastroenterology, Mass Genl Hosp 1977; **Fac Appt:** Prof Med, Univ Conn

Mason, Joel B MD [Ge] - **Spec Exp:** Nutrition & Cancer Prevention; **Hospital:** Tufts Med Ctr; **Address:** Tufts Med Ctr #239, 800 Washington St, Boston, MA 02111-1513; **Phone:** 617-636-5623; **Board Cert:** Internal Medicine 1984; Gastroenterology 1987; **Med School:** Univ Chicago-Pritzker Sch Med 1981; **Resid:** Internal Medicine, Univ Iowa Hosps 1984; **Fellow:** Gastroenterology, Univ Chicago Hosps 1986; Nutrition, Univ Chicago Hosps 1986; **Fac Appt:** Assoc Prof Med, Tufts Univ

Mid Atlantic

Canto, Marcia MD [Ge] - **Spec Exp:** Endoscopy; Endoscopic Ultrasound; Pancreatic Cancer-Early Detection; **Hospital:** Johns Hopkins Hosp; **Address:** Dept of Med, Gastroenterology, 1830 E Monument St, rm 426, Baltimore, MD 21205; **Phone:** 410-614-5388; **Board Cert:** Internal Medicine 1989; **Med School:** Philippines 1985; **Resid:** Internal Medicine, SUNY Hlth Sci Ctr 1991; **Fellow:** Gastroenterology, SUNY Hlth Sci Ctr 1993; **Fac Appt:** Assoc Prof Med, Johns Hopkins Univ

Gerdes, Hans MD [Ge] - **Spec Exp:** Endoscopy; Endoscopic Ultrasound; Barrett's Esophagus; Gastrointestinal Cancer; **Hospital:** Meml Sloan-Kettering Cancer Ctr (page 76); **Address:** 1275 York Avenue, New York, NY 10065; **Phone:** 800-525-2225; **Board Cert:** Internal Medicine 1987; Gastroenterology 1989; **Med School:** Cornell Univ-Weill Med Coll 1983; **Resid:** Internal Medicine, New York Hosp 1986; **Fellow:** Gastroenterology, Meml Sloan Kettering Cancer Ctr 1989

Goggins, Michael MD [Ge] - **Spec Exp:** Pancreatic Cancer-Early Detection; **Hospital:** Johns Hopkins Hosp; **Address:** Johns Hopkins Univ Sch Med, 1550 Orleans St, CRB-2 St, rm 342, Baltimore, MD 21231; **Phone:** 410-955-3511; **Med School:** Ireland 1988; **Resid:** Internal Medicine, St James's Hosp 1990; **Fellow:** Gastroenterology, St James's Hosp 1992; **Fac Appt:** Assoc Prof Med, Johns Hopkins Univ

Greenwald, Bruce D MD [Ge] - **Spec Exp:** Endoscopic Ultrasound; Barrett's Esophagus; Esophageal Cancer; Clinical Trials; **Hospital:** Univ of MD Med Ctr; **Address:** Univ of Maryland Hosp, Gastroenterology, 22 S Greene St Fl 3 - rm N3W62, Baltimore, MD 21201-1544; **Phone:** 410-328-8731; **Board Cert:** Internal Medicine 2000; Gastroenterology 2000; **Med School:** Univ MD Sch Med 1987; **Resid:** Internal Medicine, Univ of Virginia Hosp 1990; **Fellow:** Gastroenterology, Univ of Maryland Hosp 1992; **Fac Appt:** Assoc Prof Med, Univ MD Sch Med

Haluszka, Oleh MD [Ge] - **Spec Exp:** Pancreatic/Biliary Endoscopy (ERCP); Gastrointestinal Cancer; Endoscopic Ultrasound; Endoscopy; **Hospital:** Fox Chase Cancer Ctr (page 72); **Address:** Fox Chase Cancer Ctr, 333 Cottman Ave, Ste C307, Philadelphia, PA 19111; **Phone:** 215-214-1424; **Board Cert:** Internal Medicine 1987; Gastroenterology 2001; **Med School:** Uniformed Srvs Univ, Bethesda 1982; **Resid:** Internal Medicine, US Naval Hosp 1987; **Fellow:** Gastroenterology, US Naval Hosp 1990; Endoscopy, Med Coll Wisconsin 1993; **Fac Appt:** Assoc Clin Prof Med, Temple Univ

Itzkowitz, Steven H MD [Ge] - **Spec Exp:** Colon & Rectal Cancer; Colon & Rectal Cancer Detection; **Hospital:** Mount Sinai Med Ctr (page 77); **Address:** 5 E 98th St, Box 1625, New York, NY 10029-6501; **Phone:** 212-241-4299; **Board Cert:** Internal Medicine 1982; Gastroenterology 1985; **Med School:** Mount Sinai Sch Med 1979; **Resid:** Internal Medicine, Bellevue Hosp/NYU Med Ctr 1982; **Fellow:** Gastroenterology, UCSF Med Ctr 1984; **Fac Appt:** Prof Med, Mount Sinai Sch Med

Kastenberg, David M MD [Ge] - **Spec Exp:** Gastrointestinal Cancer; Colon & Rectal Cancer Detection; Nutrition & Cancer Prevention; **Hospital:** Thomas Jefferson Univ Hosp (page 83); **Address:** Jefferson Univ Hosps, 132 S 10th St Main Bldg - Ste 480, Dept Gastroenterology, Phildelphia, PA 19107; **Phone:** 215-955-8900; **Board Cert:** Internal Medicine 2000; Gastroenterology 2000; **Med School:** NYU Sch Med 1987; **Resid:** Internal Medicine, Temple Univ Hosp 1990; **Fellow:** Gastroenterology, Thomas Jefferson Univ Hosp 1992; **Fac Appt:** Asst Clin Prof Med, Jefferson Med Coll

Kochman, Michael L MD [Ge] - **Spec Exp:** Endoscopy; Pancreatic/Biliary Endoscopy (ERCP); Gastrointestinal Cancer; **Hospital:** Hosp Univ Penn - UPHS (page 81); **Address:** Hosp Univ Penn, Div Gastroenterology, 3400 Spruce St, 3 Dulles, Philadelphia, PA 19104-4206; **Phone:** 215-349-8222; **Board Cert:** Internal Medicine 1989; Gastroenterology 2003; **Med School:** Univ IL Coll Med 1986; **Resid:** Internal Medicine, Univ Illinois Med Ctr 1990; **Fellow:** Gastroenterology, Univ Michigan Med Ctr 1993; **Fac Appt:** Prof Med, Univ Pennsylvania

Kurtz, Robert C MD [Ge] - **Spec Exp:** Pancreatic Cancer(Familial); Gastrointestinal Cancer; Endoscopy; Nutrition & Cancer Prevention/Control; **Hospital:** Meml Sloan-Kettering Cancer Ctr (page 76); **Address:** 1275 York Avenue, New York, NY 10065; **Phone:** 800-525-2225; **Board Cert:** Internal Medicine 1971; Gastroenterology 1977; **Med School:** Jefferson Med Coll 1968; **Resid:** Internal Medicine, NY Hosp/Meml Sloan Kettering Cancer Ctr 1971; **Fellow:** Gastroenterology, Meml Sloan Kettering Cancer Ctr 1973; **Fac Appt:** Prof Med, Cornell Univ-Weill Med Coll

Lightdale, Charles J MD [Ge] - **Spec Exp:** Barrett's Esophagus; Gastrointestinal Cancer; Endoscopic Ultrasound; **Hospital:** NY-Presby Hosp/Columbia (page 79); **Address:** Columbia-Presby Med Ctr, Irving Pavilion, 161 Fort Washington Ave, rm 812, New York, NY 10032-3713; **Phone:** 212-305-3423; **Board Cert:** Internal Medicine 1972; Gastroenterology 1973; **Med School:** Columbia P&S 1966; **Resid:** Internal Medicine, Yale-New Haven Hosp 1968; Internal Medicine, NY Hosp-Cornell 1969; **Fellow:** Gastroenterology, NY Hosp-Cornell 1973; **Fac Appt:** Prof Med, Columbia P&S

Okolo III, Patrick I MD [Ge] - **Spec Exp:** Liver Cancer; Pancreatic Cancer; Gastrointestinal Cancer; Clinical Trials; **Hospital:** Johns Hopkins Hosp; **Address:** 3001 S Hanover St, Ste Gruehn 300, Baltimore, MD 21225; **Phone:** 410-350-8209; **Board Cert:** Internal Medicine 2004; Gastroenterology 2008; **Med School:** Nigeria 1988; **Resid:** Internal Medicine, Indiana Univ Med Ctr 1994; **Fellow:** Gastroenterology, John Hopkins Hosp 1997; **Fac Appt:** Assoc Prof Med, Johns Hopkins Univ

Pochapin, Mark B MD [Ge] - **Spec Exp:** Pancreatic Cancer; Endoscopic Ultrasound; Colon & Rectal Cancer Detection; Colon Cancer; **Hospital:** NY-Presby Hosp/Weill Cornell (page 79); **Address:** The Jay Monahan Ctr for GI Hlth, 1315 York Ave, New York, NY 10021; **Phone:** 212-746-4014; **Board Cert:** Gastroenterology 2004; **Med School:** Cornell Univ-Weill Med Coll 1988; **Resid:** Internal Medicine, NY Hosp-Cornell Med Ctr 1991; **Fellow:** Gastroenterology, Montefiore Med Ctr 1993; **Fac Appt:** Assoc Clin Prof Med, Cornell Univ-Weill Med Coll

Shike, Moshe MD [Ge] - **Spec Exp:** Gastrointestinal Cancer; Nutrition & Cancer Prevention; Endoscopy; **Hospital:** Meml Sloan-Kettering Cancer Ctr (page 76); **Address:** 1275 York Avenue, New York, NY 10065; **Phone:** 800-525-2225; **Board Cert:** Internal Medicine 1977; Gastroenterology 1981; **Med School:** Israel 1975; **Resid:** Internal Medicine, Mt Auburn Hosp 1977; **Fellow:** Gastroenterology, Toronto Genl Hosp 1981; **Fac Appt:** Prof Med, Cornell Univ-Weill Med Coll

Gastroenterology

Slivka, Adam MD/PhD [Ge] - **Spec Exp:** Pancreatic Cancer; **Hospital:** UPMC Presby, Pittsburgh; **Address:** Digestive Disorders Center, 200 Lothrop St, 3rd Fl-PUH, Pittsburgh, PA 15213; **Phone:** 412-647-8666; **Board Cert:** Internal Medicine 2002; Gastroenterology 1995; **Med School:** Mount Sinai Sch Med 1988; **Resid:** Internal Medicine, Brigham & Womens Hosp 1991; **Fellow:** Gastroenterology, Brigham & Womens Hosp 1994; **Fac Appt:** Assoc Prof Med, Univ Pittsburgh

Smoot, Duane Thomas MD [Ge] - **Spec Exp:** Colon & Rectal Cancer Detection; Gastrointestinal Cancer; **Hospital:** Howard Univ Hosp; **Address:** Howard Univ Hosp, Med, Div Gastroenterology, Ste 5100, 2041 Georgia Ave NW Tower Bldg, Washington, DC 20060; **Phone:** 202-865-6620; **Board Cert:** Internal Medicine 1987; Gastroenterology 2003; **Med School:** Howard Univ 1983; **Resid:** Internal Medicine, Univ MD Hosp 1986; **Fellow:** Gastroenterology, Univ MD Hosp 1989; **Fac Appt:** Prof Med, Howard Univ

Waye, Jerome MD [Ge] - **Spec Exp:** Endoscopy; Colon Cancer; Colonoscopy; **Hospital:** Mount Sinai Med Ctr (page 77), Lenox Hill Hosp; **Address:** 650 Park Ave, New York, NY 10021-6115; **Phone:** 212-439-7779; **Board Cert:** Internal Medicine 1965; Gastroenterology 1970; **Med School:** Boston Univ 1958; **Resid:** Internal Medicine, Mt Sinai Hosp 1961; **Fellow:** Gastroenterology, Mt Sinai Hosp 1962; **Fac Appt:** Clin Prof Med, Mount Sinai Sch Med

Weinberg, David Seth MD [Ge] - **Spec Exp:** Colonoscopy; Cancer Risk Assessment; Cancer Prevention; Endoscopy; **Hospital:** Fox Chase Cancer Ctr (page 72); **Address:** Fox Chase Cancer Ctr-Dept GI, 333 Cottman Ave, Ste P3047, Philadelphia, PA 19111; **Phone:** 215-214-1424; **Board Cert:** Gastroenterology 2006; **Med School:** Cornell Univ-Weill Med Coll 1989; **Resid:** Internal Medicine, Beth Israel Hosp 1992; **Fellow:** Gastroenterology, Hosp U Penn 1995; Epidemiology, Hosp U Penn 1995

Winawer, Sidney J MD [Ge] - **Spec Exp:** Colon Cancer; Cancer Prevention; **Hospital:** Meml Sloan-Kettering Cancer Ctr (page 76); **Address:** 1275 York Avenue, New York, NY 10065; **Phone:** 800-525-2225; **Board Cert:** Internal Medicine 1965; Gastroenterology 1973; **Med School:** SUNY Downstate 1956; **Resid:** Internal Medicine, VA Hosp 1961; Internal Medicine, Maimonides Hosp 1962; **Fellow:** Gastroenterology, Boston City Hosp 1964; **Fac Appt:** Prof Med, Cornell Univ-Weill Med Coll

Southeast

Barkin, Jamie S MD [Ge] - **Spec Exp:** Gastrointestinal Cancer; Endoscopy; **Hospital:** Mount Sinai Med Ctr - Miami, Univ of Miami Hosp & Clins/Sylvester Comp Canc Ctr (page 82); **Address:** Mount Sinai Medical Center, Gumenick Bldg, 4300 Alton Rd, Ste 2522, Miami Beach, FL 33140-2800; **Phone:** 305-674-2240; **Board Cert:** Internal Medicine 1973; Gastroenterology 1975; **Med School:** Univ Miami Sch Med 1970; **Resid:** Internal Medicine, Univ Miami Hosp 1973; **Fellow:** Gastroenterology, Univ Miami Hosp 1975; **Fac Appt:** Prof Med, Univ Miami Sch Med

Eloubeidi, Mohamad A MD [Ge] - **Spec Exp:** Gastrointestinal Cancer; Colon & Rectal Cancer; Pancreatic Cancer; Endoscopic Ultrasound; **Hospital:** Univ of Ala Hosp at Birmingham; **Address:** 1530 3rd Ave S, Ste LHRB-406, Birmingham, AL 35294-0007; **Phone:** 205-934-7955; **Board Cert:** Internal Medicine 2006; Gastroenterology 2000; **Med School:** Lebanon 1993; **Resid:** Internal Medicine, Duke Univ Med Ctr 1996; **Fellow:** Gastroenterology, Duke Univ Med Ctr 1999; Advanced Endoscopy, Med Univ South Carolina 2000; **Fac Appt:** Assoc Prof Med, Univ Alabama

Estores, David MD [Ge] - **Spec Exp:** Barrett's Esophagus; **Hospital:** H Lee Moffitt Cancer Ctr & Research Inst; **Address:** Ctr for Swallowing Disorders, 12901 Bruce B Downs Blvd, MDC 72, Tampa, FL 33612-4742; **Phone:** 813-974-3374; **Board Cert:** Internal Medicine 1989; Gastroenterology 2001; **Med School:** Philippines 1985; **Resid:** Internal Medicine, St Lukes Hosp 1989; **Fellow:** Gastroenterology, Univ Pittsburgh-Presby Hosp 1992

Hoffman, Brenda J MD [Ge] - **Spec Exp:** Endoscopic Ultrasound; Gastrointestinal Cancer; Colon & Rectal Cancer-Familial Polyposis; **Hospital:** MUSC Med Ctr; **Address:** MUSC Digestive Disease Center, 25 Courteney Drive, rm MS7100A, MSC290, Charleston, SC 29425; **Phone:** 843-792-6999; **Board Cert:** Internal Medicine 1986; Gastroenterology 1989; **Med School:** Univ KY Coll Med 1983; **Resid:** Internal Medicine, MUSC Med Ctr 1987; **Fellow:** Gastroenterology, MUSC Med Ctr 1989; **Fac Appt:** Prof Med, Univ SC Sch Med

Porayko, Michael K MD [Ge] - **Spec Exp:** Transplant Medicine-Liver; **Hospital:** Vanderbilt Univ Med Ctr; **Address:** GI Clinic, 1301 Medical Center Drive, Ste 1660, Nashville, TN 37232; **Phone:** 615-322-0128; **Board Cert:** Internal Medicine 1984; Gastroenterology 1987; Transplant Hepatology 2006; **Med School:** Univ IL Coll Med 1981; **Resid:** Internal Medicine, Michigan State Univ affil Hosps 1984; **Fellow:** Gastroenterology, Lahey Clin & New England Deaconess Hosp 1987; Hepatology, Mayo Clinic 1988; **Fac Appt:** Assoc Prof Med, Vanderbilt Univ

Midwest

Brown, Kimberly A MD [Ge] - **Spec Exp:** Transplant Medicine-Liver; Liver Cancer; **Hospital:** Henry Ford Hosp; **Address:** Henry Ford Hosp, Dept Gastroenterology, 2799 W Grand Blvd K-747 Bldg Fl 7, Detroit, MI 48202-2608; **Phone:** 313-916-8632; **Board Cert:** Internal Medicine 1988; Gastroenterology 2002; Transplant Hepatology 2006; **Med School:** Wayne State Univ 1985; **Resid:** Internal Medicine, Univ Michigan Med Ctr 1989; **Fellow:** Gastroenterology, Univ Michigan Med Ctr 1992

Crippin, Jeffrey S MD [Ge] - **Spec Exp:** Transplant Medicine-Liver; Gastrointestinal Cancer; **Hospital:** Barnes-Jewish Hosp; **Address:** Barnes Jewish Hosp, Div Gastroenterology, 660 S Euclid Ave Campus Box 8124, St Louis, MO 63110; **Phone:** 314-454-8160; **Board Cert:** Internal Medicine 1987; Gastroenterology 2001; Transplant Hepatology 2006; **Med School:** Univ Kans 1984; **Resid:** Internal Medicine, Kansas Univ Med Ctr 1988; **Fellow:** Gastroenterology, Mayo Clinic 1991; **Fac Appt:** Assoc Prof Med, Washington Univ, St Louis

Di Bisceglie, Adrian M MD [Ge] - **Spec Exp:** Liver Cancer; **Hospital:** St Louis Univ Hosp; **Address:** St Louis Univ Hosp, Dept. Gastroenterology, 3635 Vista Ave, PO Box 15250, St Louis, MO 63110-0250; **Phone:** 314-577-8764; **Board Cert:** Internal Medicine 2002; Gastroenterology 2002; **Med School:** South Africa 1977; **Resid:** Internal Medicine, Baragwanath Hosp 1984; **Fellow:** Hepatology, Natl Inst Hlth 1988; **Fac Appt:** Prof Med, St Louis Univ

Goldberg, Michael J MD [Ge] - **Spec Exp:** Colon Cancer; Pancreatic/Biliary Endoscopy (ERCP); Pancreatic Cancer; **Hospital:** Evanston/Northshore Univ Hlth Syst, Glenbrook/NorthShore Univ Hlth Syst; **Address:** 2650 Ridge Ave, Ste G-208, Evanston, IL 60201; **Phone:** 847-657-1900; **Board Cert:** Internal Medicine 1978; Gastroenterology 1981; **Med School:** Univ IL Coll Med 1975; **Resid:** Internal Medicine, Univ Illinois Hosp 1978; **Fellow:** Gastroenterology, Tufts-New England Med Ctr 1980; **Fac Appt:** Assoc Clin Prof Med, Northwestern Univ

Rex, Douglas K MD [Ge] - **Spec Exp:** Endoscopy; Endoscopic Ultrasound; Colon & Rectal Cancer Detection; **Hospital:** Indiana Univ Hosp (page 74); **Address:** 550 N University Blvd, Ste 4100, Indianapolis, IN 46202; **Phone:** 317-278-9763; **Board Cert:** Internal Medicine 1985; Gastroenterology 1987; **Med School:** Indiana Univ 1980; **Resid:** Internal Medicine, Indiana Univ Med Ctr 1982; Internal Medicine, Indiana Univ Hosp 1985; **Fellow:** Gastroenterology, Indiana Univ Med Ctr 1984; **Fac Appt:** Prof Med, Indiana Univ

Gastroenterology

Waxman, Irving MD [Ge] - **Spec Exp:** Gastrointestinal Cancer; Pancreatic Cancer; Endoscopy; **Hospital:** Univ of Chicago Med Ctr; **Address:** University of Chicago Hospitals, 5758 S Maryland Ave, MC 9028, Chicago, IL 60637; **Phone:** 773-702-1459; **Board Cert:** Internal Medicine 1988; Gastroenterology 2003; **Med School:** Mexico 1985; **Resid:** Internal Medicine, New Eng Deaconess Hosp 1988; **Fellow:** Gastroenterology, Georgetown Univ Med Ctr 1991; Endoscopy, Univ Academic Med Ctr 1991; **Fac Appt:** Prof Med, Univ Chicago-Pritzker Sch Med

Great Plains and Mountains

Burt, Randall W MD [Ge] - **Spec Exp:** Colon Cancer; Colon & Rectal Cancer-Familial Polyposis; **Hospital:** Univ Utah Hosps and Clins; **Address:** Huntsman Cancer Institute, 2000 Circle of Hope, Salt Lake City, UT 84112; **Phone:** 801-585-3281; **Board Cert:** Internal Medicine 1977; Gastroenterology 1979; **Med School:** Univ Utah 1974; **Resid:** Internal Medicine, Barnes Hosp 1977; **Fellow:** Gastroenterology, Univ Utah Med Ctr 1979; **Fac Appt:** Prof Med, Univ Utah

Southwest

Boland, C Richard MD [Ge] - **Spec Exp:** Colon & Rectal Cancer Detection; Cancer Genetics; **Hospital:** Baylor Univ Medical Ctr; **Address:** GI Cancer Research Lab H-250, 3500 Gaston Ave, Dallas, TX 75246; **Phone:** 214-820-2692; **Board Cert:** Internal Medicine 1978; Gastroenterology 1981; **Med School:** Yale Univ 1973; **Resid:** Internal Medicine, USPHS Hosp 1978; **Fellow:** Gastroenterology, UCSF Med Ctr 1981; **Fac Appt:** Clin Prof Med, Univ Tex SW, Dallas

Bresalier, Robert MD [Ge] - **Spec Exp:** Gastrointestinal Cancer; **Hospital:** UT MD Anderson Cancer Ctr; **Address:** MD Anderson Canc Ctr, GI Med & Nutrition, 1515 Holcombe Blvd - Unit 436, Houston, TX 77030-4009; **Phone:** 713-745-4340; **Board Cert:** Internal Medicine 1981; Gastroenterology 1983; **Med School:** Univ Chicago-Pritzker Sch Med 1978; **Resid:** Internal Medicine, Barnes Hosp-Washington Univ 1981; **Fellow:** Gastroenterology, UCSF Med Ctr 1983; **Fac Appt:** Prof Med, Univ Tex, Houston

Fleischer, David MD [Ge] - **Spec Exp:** Barrett's Esophagus; Esophageal Cancer; **Hospital:** Mayo Clinic - Scottsdale; **Address:** Mayo Clinic - Scottsdale, 13400 E Shea Blvd, Div Gastroenterology 2A, Scottsdale, AZ 85259; **Phone:** 480-301-8484; **Board Cert:** Internal Medicine 1975; Gastroenterology 1977; **Med School:** Vanderbilt Univ 1970; **Resid:** Internal Medicine, Metro General Hosp 1975; **Fellow:** Gastroenterology, LA Co Harbor-UCLA Med Ctr 1977; **Fac Appt:** Prof Med, Mayo Med Sch

West Coast and Pacific

Gish, Robert MD [Ge] - **Spec Exp:** Liver Cancer; Transplant Medicine-Liver; Clinical Trials; **Hospital:** CA Pacific Med Ctr - Pacific Campus; **Address:** 2340 Clay St Fl 3, San Francisco, CA 94115; **Phone:** 415-600-1020; **Board Cert:** Internal Medicine 1984; Gastroenterology 1987; Transplant Hepatology 2006; **Med School:** Univ Kans 1980; **Resid:** Internal Medicine, UCSD Med Ctr 1983; **Fellow:** Gastroenterology, UCLA Med Ctr 1988; **Fac Appt:** Assoc Clin Prof Med, UCSF

Lenz, Heinz J MD [Ge] - **Spec Exp:** Gastrointestinal Cancer; Colon & Rectal Cancer; **Hospital:** USC Univ Hosp; **Address:** 1441 East Lake Ave, NOR 3456, Los Angeles, CA 90033; **Phone:** 323-865-3955; **Board Cert:** Internal Medicine 2000; Gastroenterology 2000; **Med School:** Germany 1981; **Resid:** Internal Medicine, Univ Hamburg Affil Hosp 1987; Internal Medicine, UC San Diego Med Ctr 1989; **Fellow:** Gastroenterology, UC San Diego Med Ctr 1990; **Fac Appt:** Prof Med, USC-Keck School of Medicine

NYU Cancer Institute

NYU LANGONE MEDICAL CENTER

Looking for information on our expert physicians?
1-212-731-5000

NYU Clinical Cancer Center
160 East 34th Street
New York, New York 10016
www.nyuci.org/atcd

NYU Langone Medical Center
550 First Avenue
(at 31st Street)
New York, New York 10016
www.nyumc.org/atcd

Stephen D. Hassenfeld Children's Center for Cancer and Blood Disorders
160 East 32nd Street
New York, New York 10016
www.nyumc.org/hassenfeld

A Collaborative Approach
The NYU Cancer Institute, an NCI designated center, is a "matrix cancer center" without walls operating within the larger NYU Langone Medical Center. With over 175 members and a research funding base of over $81 million, this structure strengthens our capabilities to forge collaborations across medical and scientific disciplines, which translates to comprehensive care for our patients and discoveries that will influence the future of this disease.

Renowned Expertise
Team members' compassion and expertise help patients better manage the symptoms of their disease as well as their special needs. Our highly skilled Magnet™ nursing team not only plays a pivotal role in coordinating direct patient care, but is also a source of invaluable patient education.

A Patient-Focused Setting
The NYU Clinical Cancer Center, with over 70 faculty members from various disciplines at the New York University School of Medicine, is the principal outpatient facility of the Cancer Institute and serves as home for our patients and their caregivers. The center and its multidisciplinary team of experts provide access to the latest treatment options and clinical trials along with a variety of programs in cancer prevention, screening, diagnostics, genetic counseling, and supportive services. When it comes to kids and cancer, the Stephen D. Hassenfeld Children's Center for Cancer and Blood Disorders offers not just innovation but insight. As a leading member of the NCI-sponsored Children's Oncology Group, our physicians are known for developing new ways to treat childhood cancer. Our affiliation with Bellevue Hospital, the oldest public hospital in the country, affords clinically distinctive opportunities to learn and care for patients with cancer by observing its presentation and behavior in a variety of patient groups.

Hematology/Medical Oncology

a subspecialty of Internal Medicine

Hematology: An internist with additional training who specializes in diseases of the blood, spleen and lymph glands. This specialist treats conditions such as anemia, clotting disorders, sickle cell disease, hemophilia, leukemia and lymphoma.

Medical Oncology: An internist who specializes in the diagnosis and treatment of all types of cancer and other benign and malignant tumors. This specialist decides on and administers chemotherapy for malignancy, as well as consulting with surgeons and radiotherapists on other treatments for cancer.

Training Required: Three years in internal medicine plus additional training and examination for certification in hematology or medical oncology.

HEMATOLOGY

New England

Anderson, Kenneth C MD [Hem] - **Spec Exp:** Multiple Myeloma; Hematologic Malignancies; **Hospital:** Dana-Farber Cancer Inst, Brigham & Women's Hosp; **Address:** 44 Binney St Mayer Bldg - rm 557, Dana-Farber Cancer Inst, Div Hematology, Boston, MA 02115; **Phone:** 617-632-2144; **Board Cert:** Internal Medicine 1980; **Med School:** Johns Hopkins Univ 1977; **Resid:** Internal Medicine, Johns Hopkins Hosp 1980; **Fellow:** Hematology & Oncology, Dana Farber Cancer Inst 1983; **Fac Appt:** Prof Med, Harvard Med Sch

Comenzo, Raymond MD [Hem] - **Spec Exp:** Plasma Cell Disorders; **Hospital:** Tufts Med Ctr; **Address:** 800 Washington St, Box 826, Boston, MA 02111; **Phone:** 617-636-6454; **Board Cert:** Internal Medicine 1989; Hematology 2004; Blood Banking Transfusion Medicine 1992; **Med School:** Boston Univ 1986; **Resid:** Internal Medicine, Boston City Hosp 1989; **Fellow:** Hematology & Oncology, New Engl Med Ctr 1991

Dezube, Bruce J MD [Hem] - **Spec Exp:** AIDS Related Cancers; Clinical Trials; **Hospital:** Beth Israel Deaconess Med Ctr - Boston; **Address:** BIDMC-Division of Hematology/Oncology, 330 Brookline Ave, MASCO 414, Boston, MA 02215; **Phone:** 617-632-9258; **Board Cert:** Internal Medicine 1986; Medical Oncology 1989; Hematology 1988; **Med School:** Tufts Univ 1983; **Resid:** Internal Medicine, New England Med Ctr 1986; **Fellow:** Hematology & Oncology, Beth Israel Deaconess Hosp 1989; **Fac Appt:** Assoc Prof Med, Harvard Med Sch

Ellman, Leonard MD [Hem] - **Spec Exp:** Multiple Myeloma; Leukemia; **Hospital:** Mass Genl Hosp; **Address:** Mass Genl Hosp, 15 Parkman St, rm 516, Boston, MA 02114; **Phone:** 617-726-3448; **Board Cert:** Internal Medicine 1972; Hematology 1974; **Med School:** Harvard Med Sch 1967; **Resid:** Internal Medicine, Mass Genl Hosp 1969; **Fellow:** Hematology, Natl Inst Hlth 1971; **Fac Appt:** Assoc Prof Med, Harvard Med Sch

Meehan, Kenneth MD [Hem] - **Spec Exp:** Bone Marrow Transplant; **Hospital:** Dartmouth - Hitchcock Med Ctr; **Address:** Norris Cotton Cancer Ctr, Dartmouth-Hitchcock Med Ctr, 1 Medical Center Drive, Lebanon, NH 03756; **Phone:** 603-650-4628; **Board Cert:** Internal Medicine 1989; Hematology 2004; **Med School:** Georgetown Univ 1986; **Resid:** Internal Medicine, Georgetown Univ 1989; **Fellow:** Hematology & Oncology, Dartmouth-Hitchcock Med Ctr 1992; **Fac Appt:** Assoc Prof Med, Dartmouth Med Sch

Miller, Kenneth B MD [Hem] - **Spec Exp:** Bone Marrow Transplant; Leukemia; Myelodysplastic Syndromes; **Hospital:** Tufts Med Ctr; **Address:** Dept Medicine, 750 Washington St, Box 245, Boston, MA 02211; **Phone:** 617-636-2600; **Board Cert:** Internal Medicine 1976; Hematology 1980; **Med School:** NY Med Coll 1972; **Resid:** Internal Medicine, NYU Med Ctr/VA Hosp 1976; Internal Medicine, NYU Med Ctr 1976; **Fellow:** Hematology, New England Med Ctr 1979; **Fac Appt:** Prof Med, Tufts Univ

Spitzer, Thomas R MD [Hem] - **Spec Exp:** Bone Marrow Transplant; Leukemia; **Hospital:** Mass Genl Hosp; **Address:** Mass Genl Hosp-Bone Marrow Tranplant Program, 55 Fruit St, Emerson Pl, Ste 118, Boston, MA 02114; **Phone:** 617-724-1124; **Board Cert:** Internal Medicine 1977; Medical Oncology 1983; Hematology 1984; **Med School:** Univ Rochester 1974; **Resid:** Internal Medicine, NYew York Hosp-Cornell Med Ctr 1977; Internal Medicine, Mem Sloan Kettering Cancer Ctr 1977; **Fellow:** Hematology & Oncology, Case West Res Univ 1983; **Fac Appt:** Prof Med, Harvard Med Sch

Stone, Richard M MD [Hem] - **Spec Exp:** Leukemia; **Hospital:** Dana-Farber Cancer Inst, Brigham & Women's Hosp; **Address:** Dana Farber Cancer Inst, Adult Leukemia Program, 44 Binney St, Ste M1B17, Boston, MA 02115-6084; **Phone:** 617-632-2214; **Board Cert:** Internal Medicine 1984; Medical Oncology 1987; Hematology 1988; **Med School:** Harvard Med Sch 1981; **Resid:** Internal Medicine, Brigham & Womens Hosp 1984; **Fellow:** Medical Oncology, Dana Farber Cancer Inst 1987; **Fac Appt:** Prof Med, Harvard Med Sch

Mid Atlantic

Baer, Maria R MD [Hem] - **Spec Exp:** Leukemia; Myelodysplastic Syndromes; Myeloprolifera-tive Disorders; **Hospital:** Univ of MD Med Ctr; **Address:** Univ Maryland, Greenebaum Cancer Ctr, 22 S Greene St, rm S9D04, Baltimore, MD 21201; **Phone:** 410-328-7904; **Board Cert:** Internal Medicine 1983; Hematology 1984; **Med School:** Johns Hopkins Univ 1979; **Resid:** Internal Medi-cine, Vanderbilt Univ Hosp 1982; **Fellow:** Hematology, Vanderbilt Univ Hosp 1984; **Fac Appt:** Prof Med, Univ MD Sch Med

Cheson, Bruce D MD [Hem] - **Spec Exp:** Leukemia; Hematologic Malignancies; **Hospital:** Georgetown Univ Hosp; **Address:** GUMC - Lombardi Cancer Ctr, 3800 Reservoir Rd NW, Podium B, Washington, DC 20007; **Phone:** 202-444-7932; **Board Cert:** Internal Medicine 1974; Hematology 1976; **Med School:** Tufts Univ 1971; **Resid:** Internal Medicine, Univ Virginia Hosp 1974; **Fellow:** Hematology, New England Med Ctr Hosp 1976

Gewirtz, Alan M MD [Hem] - **Spec Exp:** Leukemia; Gene Therapy; **Hospital:** Hosp Univ Penn - UPHS (page 81); **Address:** Perelman Ctr for Advanced Medicine Fl 2, 3400 Civic Center Blvd, Philadelphia, PA 19104; **Phone:** 215-615-5858; **Board Cert:** Internal Medicine 1979; Medical On-cology 1981; Hematology 1982; **Med School:** SUNY Buffalo 1976; **Resid:** Internal Medicine, Mt Sinai Hosp 1979; **Fellow:** Medical Oncology, Yale-New Haven Hosp 1981; Hematology, Yale-New Haven Hosp 1982; **Fac Appt:** Prof Med, Univ Pennsylvania

Goldberg, Jack MD [Hem] - **Spec Exp:** Leukemia; Lymphoma; Breast Cancer; Bone Marrow Transplant; **Hospital:** Penn Presby Med Ctr - UPHS (page 81), Virtua West Jersey Hosp - Voorhees; **Address:** 409 Route 70 E, Cherry Hill, NJ 08034; **Phone:** 856-429-1519; **Board Cert:** Internal Medicine 1976; Hematology 1980; Medical Oncology 1989; **Med School:** SUNY Upstate Med Univ 1973; **Resid:** Internal Medicine, Boston Univ Hosp 1975; **Fellow:** Hematology & Oncology, SUNY Syracuse Med Ctr 1977; **Fac Appt:** Clin Prof Med, Univ Pennsylvania

Kempin, Sanford J MD [Hem] - **Spec Exp:** Bleeding/Coagulation Disorders; Leukemia; Lym-phoma; **Hospital:** St Vincent Cath Med Ctrs - Manhattan; **Address:** St Vincents Cancer Ctr, 325 W 15th St, New York, NY 10011; **Phone:** 212-604-6068; **Board Cert:** Internal Medicine 1976; Med-ical Oncology 1977; Hematology 1978; **Med School:** Belgium 1971; **Resid:** Internal Medicine, Lemuel Shattuck Hosp 1972; **Fellow:** Hematology, St Jude Chldns Hosp 1975; Medical Oncology, Meml Sloan Kettering Cancer Ctr 1976; **Fac Appt:** Asst Prof Med, NY Med Coll

Kessler, Craig M MD [Hem] - **Spec Exp:** Bleeding/Coagulation Disorders; Hematologic Ma-lignancies; **Hospital:** Georgetown Univ Hosp; **Address:** GUMC, Lombardi Cancer Ctr, 3800 Reser-voir Rd NW, Washington, DC 20007; **Phone:** 202-444-8676; **Board Cert:** Internal Medicine 1976; Hematology 1980; **Med School:** Tulane Univ 1973; **Resid:** Internal Medicine, Ochsner Fdn Hosp 1976; **Fellow:** Hematology, Johns Hopkins Hosp 1978; **Fac Appt:** Prof Med, Georgetown Univ

Hematology

Kopel, Samuel MD [Hem] - **Spec Exp:** Hematologic Malignancies; Solid Tumors; **Hospital:** Maimonides Med Ctr (page 75); **Address:** MMC Hematology/Oncology, 6300 8th Ave, Brooklyn, NY 11220; **Phone:** 718-765-2600; **Board Cert:** Internal Medicine 1975; Hematology 1978; Medical Oncology 1979; **Med School:** Italy 1972; **Resid:** Internal Medicine, Jewish Hosp 1975; **Fellow:** Hematology & Oncology, Mt Sinai Med Ctr 1978; **Fac Appt:** Asst Prof Med, SUNY Downstate

Mangan, Kenneth F MD [Hem] - **Spec Exp:** Bone Marrow Transplant; **Hospital:** Temple Univ Hosp; **Address:** Temple BMT Program, Friends Hall Physicians Bldg, 7604 Central Ave, Lower Level, Philadelphia, PA 19111-2499; **Phone:** 215-214-3129; **Board Cert:** Internal Medicine 1976; Hematology 1978; **Med School:** Geo Wash Univ 1973; **Resid:** Internal Medicine, G Washington Univ Hosps 1976; **Fellow:** Hematology, Tufts-New England Med Ctr 1977

Marks, Stanley M MD [Hem] - **Spec Exp:** Leukemia; Lymphoma; **Hospital:** UPMC Shadyside; **Address:** 5115 Center Ave Fl 3, Pittsburgh, PA 15232; **Phone:** 412-235-1020; **Board Cert:** Internal Medicine 1976; Hematology 1978; **Med School:** Univ Pittsburgh 1973; **Resid:** Internal Medicine, Presby Univ Hosp 1976; **Fellow:** Hematology & Oncology, Peter Bent Brigham Hosp 1978; **Fac Appt:** Assoc Clin Prof Med, Drexel Univ Coll Med

Mears, John Gregory MD [Hem] - **Spec Exp:** Lymphoma; Leukemia; Multiple Myeloma; Breast Cancer; **Hospital:** NY-Presby Hosp/Columbia (page 79); **Address:** 161 Ft Washington Ave, Ste 923, New York, NY 10032; **Phone:** 212-305-3506; **Board Cert:** Internal Medicine 1976; Hematology 1978; **Med School:** Columbia P&S 1973; **Resid:** Internal Medicine, Boston Univ Med Ctr 1975; **Fellow:** Hematology & Oncology, Columbia-Presby Med Ctr 1978; **Fac Appt:** Clin Prof Med, Columbia P&S

Millenson, Michael M MD [Hem] - **Spec Exp:** Leukemia & Lymphoma; Hematologic Malignancies; **Hospital:** Fox Chase Cancer Ctr (page 72); **Address:** Fox Chase Cancer Center, 7701 Burholme Ave, Ste C307, Philadelphia, PA 19111; **Phone:** 215-728-2600; **Board Cert:** Internal Medicine 1987; Medical Oncology 2000; Hematology 2000; **Med School:** Temple Univ 1984; **Resid:** Internal Medicine, Temple Univ Hosp 1987; **Fellow:** Hematology & Oncology, Beth Israel Hosp 1991

Nimer, Stephen D MD [Hem] - **Spec Exp:** Bone Marrow Transplant; Myelodysplastic Syndromes; Leukemia; Stem Cell Transplant; **Hospital:** Meml Sloan-Kettering Cancer Ctr (page 76); **Address:** 1275 York Avenue, New York, NY 10065; **Phone:** 800-525-2225; **Board Cert:** Internal Medicine 1982; Hematology 1986; Medical Oncology 1985; **Med School:** Univ Chicago-Pritzker Sch Med 1979; **Resid:** Internal Medicine, UCLA Med Ctr 1982; **Fellow:** Hematology & Oncology, UCLA Med Ctr 1986; **Fac Appt:** Prof Med, Cornell Univ-Weill Med Coll

Porter, David L MD [Hem] - **Spec Exp:** Leukemia; Bone Marrow Transplant; Lymphoma; **Hospital:** Hosp Univ Penn - UPHS (page 81); **Address:** Perelman Ctr for Advanced Medicine Fl 2, 3400 Civic Center Blvd, Philadelphia, PA 19104; **Phone:** 215-615-5858; **Board Cert:** Hematology 2006; **Med School:** Brown Univ 1987; **Resid:** Internal Medicine, Univ Hosp 1990; **Fellow:** Hematology & Oncology, Brigham & Womens Hosp 1992; **Fac Appt:** Assoc Prof Med, Univ Pennsylvania

Rai, Kanti MD [Hem] - **Spec Exp:** Leukemia; Lymphoma; Multiple Myeloma; **Hospital:** Long Island Jewish Med Ctr; **Address:** 410 Lakeville Rd, Ste 212, New Hyde Park, NY 10042; **Phone:** 718-470-4050; **Board Cert:** Pediatrics 1959; **Med School:** India 1955; **Resid:** Pediatrics, Lincoln Hosp 1958; Pediatrics, North Shore Univ Hosp 1959; **Fellow:** Hematology, LI Jewish Med Ctr 1960; **Fac Appt:** Prof Med, Albert Einstein Coll Med

Raphael, Bruce MD [Hem] - **Spec Exp:** Lymphoma; Leukemia; Multiple Myeloma; **Hospital:** NYU Langone Med Ctr (page 80), NY Downtown Hosp; **Address:** 160 E 34th Street Ave Fl 7, NYU Clinical Cancer Ctr, New York, NY 10016-6402; **Phone:** 212-731-5185; **Board Cert:** Internal Medicine 1978; Hematology 1980; Medical Oncology 1981; **Med School:** McGill Univ 1975; **Resid:** Internal Medicine, Jewish Genl Hosp 1977; **Fellow:** Medical Oncology, Meml Sloan Kettering Cancer Ctr 1978; Hematology, NYU Med Ctr 1980; **Fac Appt:** Assoc Prof Med, NYU Sch Med

Roodman, G David MD [Hem] - **Spec Exp:** Multiple Myeloma; **Hospital:** UPMC Shadyside, VA Pittsburgh Hlth Care Sys; **Address:** VA Pittsburgh Healthcare System, R&D 151-U, rm 2E113, University Drive C, Pittsburgh, PA 15240; **Phone:** 412-692-4724; **Board Cert:** Internal Medicine 1978; Hematology 1980; **Med School:** Univ KY Coll Med 1973; **Resid:** Internal Medicine, Univ Minnesota Hosp 1978; **Fellow:** Hematology, Univ Minnesota Hosp 1980; **Fac Appt:** Prof Med, Univ Pittsburgh

Rowley, Scott D MD [Hem] - **Spec Exp:** Stem Cell Transplant; Bone Marrow Transplant; **Hospital:** Hackensack Univ Med Ctr (page 73); **Address:** 360 Essex St, Ste 303, Hackensack, NJ 07601; **Phone:** 201-336-8297; **Board Cert:** Internal Medicine 1981; Medical Oncology 1983; Hematology 1984; **Med School:** Univ Mass Sch Med 1978; **Resid:** Internal Medicine, Rhode Island Hosp 1981; **Fellow:** Hematology & Oncology, Rhode Island Hosp 1984; **Fac Appt:** Assoc Prof Med, UMDNJ-NJ Med Sch, Newark

Savage, David G MD [Hem] - **Spec Exp:** Stem Cell Transplant; Multiple Myeloma; Lymphoma; **Hospital:** NY-Presby Hosp/Columbia (page 79); **Address:** 177 Fort Washington Ave, Millstein Bldg Fl 6 - rm 435, New York, NY 10032; **Phone:** 212-305-9783; **Board Cert:** Internal Medicine 1977; Hematology 1982; Medical Oncology 1985; **Med School:** Columbia P&S 1974; **Resid:** Internal Medicine, Harlem Hosp/Columbia Presby Med Ctr 1977; **Fellow:** Hematology & Oncology, Harlem Hosp/Columbia Presby Med Ctr 1979; **Fac Appt:** Assoc Prof Med, Columbia P&S

Schuster, Michael W MD [Hem] - **Spec Exp:** Bone Marrow Transplant; **Hospital:** NY-Presby Hosp/Weill Cornell (page 79); **Address:** NY Weill Cornell Medical Ctr, 525 E 68th St, Starr 341, New York, NY 10021; **Phone:** 212-746-2119; **Board Cert:** Internal Medicine 1984; Hematology 1986; **Med School:** Dartmouth Med Sch 1980; **Resid:** Internal Medicine, New Eng Deaconess Hosp 1983; **Fellow:** Hematology & Oncology, Beth Israel Med Ctr 1987; **Fac Appt:** Assoc Prof Med, Cornell Univ-Weill Med Coll

Slease, Robert B MD [Hem] - **Spec Exp:** Hematologic Malignancies; Hodgkin's Disease; Stem Cell Transplantation; Clinical Trials; **Hospital:** Christiana Care Hlth Svs; **Address:** Christiana Care Hlth Svs, Div Hematology, 4735 Ogletown-Stanton Rd, Ste S-2225, Newark, DE 19713; **Phone:** 302-737-7700; **Board Cert:** Internal Medicine 1975; Hematology 1978; **Med School:** Univ Kans 1972; **Resid:** Internal Medicine, Natl Naval Med Ctr 1975; **Fellow:** Hematology, Natl Naval Med Ctr 1977; **Fac Appt:** Clin Prof Med, Jefferson Med Coll

Spivak, Jerry L MD [Hem] - **Spec Exp:** Myeloproliferative Disorders; Leukemia; **Hospital:** Johns Hopkins Hosp; **Address:** 720 Rutland Ave Bldg Ross - Ste 1025, Baltimore, MD 21205; **Phone:** 410-614-0167; **Board Cert:** Internal Medicine 1971; Hematology 1974; **Med School:** Cornell Univ-Weill Med Coll 1964; **Resid:** Internal Medicine, Johns Hopkins Hosp 1966; Internal Medicine, Johns Hopkins Hosp 1972; **Fellow:** Hematology, Natl Cancer Inst 1968; Hematology, Johns Hopkins Hosp 1971; **Fac Appt:** Prof Med, Johns Hopkins Univ

Wisch, Nathaniel MD [Hem] - **Spec Exp:** Lymphoma; Breast Cancer; Leukemia; Anemia-Cancer Related; **Hospital:** Lenox Hill Hosp, Mount Sinai Med Ctr (page 77); **Address:** 12 E 86th St, New York, NY 10028-0506; **Phone:** 212-861-6660; **Board Cert:** Internal Medicine 1965; Hematology 1972; Medical Oncology 1977; **Med School:** Northwestern Univ 1958; **Resid:** Internal Medicine, VA Hosp 1960; Internal Medicine, Montefiore Hosp 1961; **Fellow:** Hematology, Mount Sinai Hosp 1962; **Fac Appt:** Clin Prof Med, Mount Sinai Sch Med

Hematology

Zalusky, Ralph MD [Hem] - **Spec Exp:** Leukemia; Lymphoma; **Hospital:** Beth Israel Med Ctr - Petrie Division (page 71); **Address:** Beth Israel Med Ctr, First Ave at 16th St, New York, NY 10003; **Phone:** 212-420-4185; **Board Cert:** Internal Medicine 1964; Hematology 1972; **Med School:** Boston Univ 1957; **Resid:** Internal Medicine, Duke Univ Med Ctr 1962; **Fellow:** Hematology, Boston Med Ctr 1961; **Fac Appt:** Prof Med, Albert Einstein Coll Med

Southeast

Bigelow, Carolyn L MD [Hem] - **Spec Exp:** Bone Marrow Transplant; **Hospital:** Univ Mississippi Med Ctr; **Address:** Univ Mississippi Med Ctr-Div Hematology, 2500 N State St, Jackson, MS 39216; **Phone:** 601-984-5615; **Board Cert:** Internal Medicine 1982; Hematology 1988; **Med School:** Univ Miss 1979; **Resid:** Internal Medicine, Univ Mississippi Med Ctr 1982; **Fellow:** Hematology & Oncology, Univ Washington Med Ctr 1987; **Fac Appt:** Prof Med, Univ Miss

Djulbegovic, Benjamin MD [Hem] - **Spec Exp:** Multiple Myeloma; Lymphoma; Myeloproliferative Disorders; **Hospital:** Univ of S FL - Tampa, H Lee Moffitt Cancer Ctr & Research Inst; **Address:** 12901 Bruce B Downs Blvd, MDC 02, Tampa, FL 33612; **Phone:** 813-396-9178; **Board Cert:** Internal Medicine 2002; Hematology 2004; **Med School:** Bosnia 1976; **Resid:** Internal Medicine, Univ Med Ctr 1983; Internal Medicine, Univ Louisville Med Ctr 1988; **Fellow:** Univ Manchester 1985; Hematology & Oncology, Univ Louisville 1990; **Fac Appt:** Prof Med, Univ S Fla Coll Med

Files, Joe C MD [Hem] - **Spec Exp:** Bone Marrow Transplant; Stem Cell Transplant; Leukemia; **Hospital:** Univ Mississippi Med Ctr; **Address:** Univ Miss Med Ctr-Div Hematology, 2500 N State St, Jackson, MS 39216; **Phone:** 601-984-5615; **Board Cert:** Internal Medicine 1976; Hematology 1980; **Med School:** Univ Miss 1972; **Resid:** Internal Medicine, Univ Miss Med Ctr 1976; **Fellow:** Hematology, Univ Wash Sch Med 1979; **Fac Appt:** Prof Med, Univ Miss

Greer, John P MD [Hem] - **Spec Exp:** Leukemia & Lymphoma; Myelodysplastic Syndromes; Stem Cell Transplant; **Hospital:** Vanderbilt Univ Med Ctr; **Address:** 2665 The Vanderbilt Clinic, 1301 22nd Ave S, Nashville, TN 37232-5505; **Phone:** 615-936-1803; **Board Cert:** Pediatrics 1985; Internal Medicine 1979; Hematology 1984; Medical Oncology 1985; **Med School:** Vanderbilt Univ 1976; **Resid:** Internal Medicine, Tulane Univ Med Ctr 1979; Pediatrics, Med Coll Virginia 1981; **Fellow:** Hematology & Oncology, Vanderbilt Univ Med Ctr 1984; **Fac Appt:** Prof Med, Vanderbilt Univ

Lin, Weei-Chin MD/PhD [Hem] - **Spec Exp:** Hematologic Malignancies; **Hospital:** Univ of Ala Hosp at Birmingham; **Address:** Univ of Alabama, 1530 3rd Ave S, Ste 520A, Birmingham, AL 35294; **Phone:** 205-934-3980; **Board Cert:** Hematology 1999; Medical Oncology 1999; **Med School:** Taiwan 1986; **Resid:** Internal Medicine, Duke Univ Med Ctr 1996; **Fellow:** Hematology & Oncology, Duke Univ Med Ctr 1999; **Fac Appt:** Assoc Prof Med, Univ Alabama

List, Alan F MD [Hem] - **Spec Exp:** Myelodysplastic Syndromes; Leukemia; **Hospital:** H Lee Moffitt Cancer Ctr & Research Inst; **Address:** 12902 Magnolia Drive, MCC-VP, Tampa, FL 33612-9497; **Phone:** 813-745-6086; **Board Cert:** Internal Medicine 1983; Medical Oncology 1985; Hematology 1986; **Med School:** Univ Pennsylvania 1980; **Resid:** Internal Medicine, Good Samaritan Hosp 1983; Oncology, Vanderbilt Univ Med Ctr 1985; **Fellow:** Hematology, Vanderbilt Univ Med Ctr 1986

Powell, Bayard L MD [Hem] - **Spec Exp:** Leukemia; Myelodysplastic Syndromes; **Hospital:** Wake Forest Univ Baptist Med Ctr (page 84); **Address:** Wake Forest Univ Baptist Med Ctr, Med Ctr Blvd-Cancer Center, Winston-Salem, NC 27157-1082; **Phone:** 336-716-7970; **Board Cert:** Internal Medicine 1983; Medical Oncology 1985; **Med School:** Univ NC Sch Med 1980; **Resid:** Internal Medicine, NC Baptist Hosp 1983; **Fellow:** Hematology & Oncology, Wake Forest Univ Sch Med 1986; **Fac Appt:** Prof Med, Wake Forest Univ

Rosenblatt, Joseph D MD [Hem] - **Spec Exp:** Lymphoma; Leukemia; Multiple Myeloma; **Hospital:** Univ of Miami Hosp & Clins/Sylvester Comp Canc Ctr (page 82), Jackson Meml Hosp (page 82); **Address:** Sylvester Comprehensive Cancer Ctr, 1475 NW 12th Ave, D8-4, Ste 3300, Miami, FL 33136; **Phone:** 305-243-4909; **Board Cert:** Internal Medicine 1983; Medical Oncology 1985; **Med School:** UCLA 1980; **Resid:** Internal Medicine, UCLA Med Ctr 1983; **Fellow:** Hematology & Oncology, UCLA Med Ctr 1986; **Fac Appt:** Prof Med, Univ Miami Sch Med

Schwartzberg, Lee S MD [Hem] - **Spec Exp:** Breast Cancer; Lung Cancer; Stem Cell Transplant; **Hospital:** Baptist Memorial Hospital - Memphis; **Address:** The West Clinic, 100 N Humphreys Blvd, Memphis, TN 38120; **Phone:** 901-683-0055; **Board Cert:** Internal Medicine 1983; Hematology 1986; Medical Oncology 1985; **Med School:** NY Med Coll 1980; **Resid:** Internal Medicine, North Shore Univ Hosp 1983; Internal Medicine, Meml Sloan Kettering Cancer Ctr 1985; **Fellow:** Hematology & Oncology, Meml Sloan Kettering Cancer Ctr 1984; Hematology & Oncology, Meml Sloan Kettering Cancer Ctr 1987; **Fac Appt:** Assoc Prof Med, Univ Tenn Coll Med, Memphis

Solberg, Lawrence MD/PhD [Hem] - **Spec Exp:** Bone Marrow Transplant; Myeloproliferative Disorders; **Hospital:** Mayo - Jacksonville, Rochelle Comm Hosp; **Address:** Mayo Clinic-Dept Hem-Onc, 4500 San Pablo Rd Fl 8, Jacksonville, FL 32224; **Phone:** 904-953-7292; **Board Cert:** Internal Medicine 1978; Hematology 1980; **Med School:** St Louis Univ 1975; **Resid:** Internal Medicine, Mayo Clinic 1978; **Fellow:** Hematology, Mayo Clinic 1980; **Fac Appt:** Prof Med, Mayo Med Sch

Zuckerman, Kenneth S MD [Hem] - **Spec Exp:** Myeloproliferative Disorders; Leukemia; Lymphoma; **Hospital:** H Lee Moffitt Cancer Ctr & Research Inst, Tampa Genl Hosp; **Address:** H Lee Moffitt Cancer Ctr, 12902 Magnolia Drive, FOB3, Tampa, FL 33612-9416; **Phone:** 813-745-8090; **Board Cert:** Internal Medicine 1975; Hematology 1978; **Med School:** Ohio State Univ 1972; **Resid:** Internal Medicine, Ohio State Univ Hosps 1975; **Fellow:** Hematology, Brigham Hosp/Harvard Univ 1978; **Fac Appt:** Prof Med, Univ S Fla Coll Med

Midwest

Baron, Joseph M MD [Hem] - **Spec Exp:** Lymphoma; Myeloproliferative Disorders; **Hospital:** Univ of Chicago Med Ctr; **Address:** 5758 S Maryland Ave, MC 9015, Chicago, IL 60637-1463; **Phone:** 773-702-6149; **Board Cert:** Internal Medicine 1969; Hematology 1972; Medical Oncology 1975; **Med School:** Univ Chicago-Pritzker Sch Med 1962; **Resid:** Internal Medicine, Univ Chicago Hosps 1964; Internal Medicine, Univ Chicago Hosps 1968; **Fellow:** Hematology, Univ Chicago Hosps 1968; **Fac Appt:** Assoc Prof Med, Univ Chicago-Pritzker Sch Med

Bockenstedt, Paula MD [Hem] - **Spec Exp:** Bleeding/Coagulation Disorders; Leukemia; **Hospital:** Univ Michigan Hlth Sys; **Address:** Div Hematology, 1500 E Med Ctr Dr, MIB, rm C-344, Ann Arbor, MI 48109-8048; **Phone:** 734-647-8921; **Board Cert:** Internal Medicine 1981; Hematology 1984; **Med School:** Harvard Med Sch 1978; **Resid:** Internal Medicine, Brigham-Womens Hosp 1981; **Fellow:** Hematology, Brigham-Womens Hosp 1984; **Fac Appt:** Assoc Clin Prof Med, Univ Mich Med Sch

Byrd, John C MD [Hem] - **Spec Exp:** Leukemia-Chronic Lymphocytic; **Hospital:** Arthur G James Cancer Hosp & Research Inst; **Address:** Bl02 Starling-Loving Hall, 320 W 10th Ave, Columbus, OH 43210; **Phone:** 614-293-3196; **Board Cert:** Hematology 2007; **Med School:** Univ Ark 1991; **Resid:** Internal Medicine, Walter Reed AMC 1994; **Fellow:** Hematology & Oncology, Walter Reed AMC 1997; **Fac Appt:** Assoc Prof Med, Ohio State Univ

Hematology

Copelan, Edward A MD [Hem] - **Spec Exp:** Leukemia; Myelodysplastic Syndromes; Bone Marrow Transplant; Multiple Myeloma; **Hospital:** Cleveland Clin Fdn (page 70); **Address:** Cleveland Clinic Fdn, 9500 Euclid Ave, MC R35, Cleveland, OH 44195; **Phone:** 216-445-5647; **Board Cert:** Internal Medicine 1980; Hematology 1982; Medical Oncology 1983; **Med School:** Tufts Univ 1977; **Resid:** Internal Medicine, Ohio State Univ Hosp 1980; **Fellow:** Hematology & Oncology, Ohio State Univ Hosp 1983; Bone Marrow Transplant, UCLA Med Ctr

Di Persio, John MD/PhD [Hem] - **Spec Exp:** Bone Marrow Transplant; Hematologic Malignancies; Leukemia; **Hospital:** Barnes-Jewish Hosp; **Address:** Wash Univ Sch Med, Sect Bone Marrow Transplant & Leukemia, 660 S Euclid Ave, Box 8007, St Louis, MO 63110; **Phone:** 314-454-8306; **Board Cert:** Internal Medicine 1984; Medical Oncology 1987; Hematology 1988; **Med School:** Univ Rochester 1980; **Resid:** Internal Medicine, Parkland Meml Hosp 1984; **Fellow:** Hematology & Oncology, UCLA Med Ctr 1987; **Fac Appt:** Prof Med, Washington Univ, St Louis

Erba, Harry P MD/PhD [Hem] - **Spec Exp:** Leukemia; Myelodysplastic Syndromes; Lymphoma; **Hospital:** Univ Michigan Hlth Sys; **Address:** Univ Michigan Medical Ctr, 1500 E Medical Center Dr, B1-358 Cancer Ctr, Ann Arbor, MI 48109-5848; **Phone:** 734-647-8901; **Board Cert:** Internal Medicine 2004; Hematology 2004; Medical Oncology 2005; **Med School:** Stanford Univ 1988; **Resid:** Internal Medicine, Brigham & Womens Hosp 1990; **Fellow:** Hematology & Oncology, Brigham & Womens Hosp 1993; **Fac Appt:** Assoc Prof Med, Univ Mich Med Sch

Farag, Sherif S MD/PhD [Hem] - **Spec Exp:** Multiple Myeloma; Leukemia & Lymphoma; Bone Marrow Transplant; Stem Cell Transplant; **Hospital:** Indiana Univ Hosp (page 74); **Address:** 980 W Walnut St, Walther Hall, R3-C400, Indianapolis, IN 46202; **Phone:** 317-274-0843; **Med School:** Australia 1995; **Resid:** Internal Medicine, Univ Melbourne Med Ctr; **Fellow:** Hematology & Oncology, Roswell Park Cancer Inst; **Fac Appt:** Assoc Prof Med, Indiana Univ

Flynn, Patrick MD [Hem] - **Spec Exp:** Hematologic Malignancies; Colon & Rectal Cancer; Clinical Trials; Breast Cancer; **Hospital:** Abbott - Northwestern Hosp, Fairview Southdale Hosp; **Address:** 800 E 28th St, Piper Bldg, Ste 405, Minneapolis, MN 55407; **Phone:** 612-863-8585; **Board Cert:** Internal Medicine 1978; Medical Oncology 1981; Hematology 1982; **Med School:** Univ Minn 1975; **Resid:** Internal Medicine, Hennepin Co Med Ctr 1978; **Fellow:** Hematology & Oncology, Univ Minnesota Hosp 1981

Gaynor, Ellen MD [Hem] - **Spec Exp:** Lymphoma; Genitourinary Cancer; Breast Cancer; **Hospital:** Loyola Univ Med Ctr; **Address:** Loyola Univ Med Ctr, Dept Hematology, 2160 S First Ave Bldg 112 - rm 108, Maywood, IL 60153-3328; **Phone:** 708-327-3214; **Board Cert:** Internal Medicine 1982; Hematology 1986; Medical Oncology 1985; **Med School:** Univ Wisc 1978; **Resid:** Internal Medicine, Loyola Univ Med Ctr 1982; **Fellow:** Medical Oncology, Loyola Univ Med Ctr 1981; Hematology & Oncology, Univ Chicago Hosp 1984; **Fac Appt:** Prof Med, Loyola Univ-Stritch Sch Med

Gertz, Morie MD [Hem] - **Spec Exp:** Multiple Myeloma; Waldenstrom's Macroglobulinemia; Plasma Cell Disorders; **Hospital:** Mayo Med Ctr & Clin - Rochester, Rochester Methodist Hosp; **Address:** 200 SW 1st St Fl W10, Rochester, MN 55905; **Phone:** 507-284-2511; **Board Cert:** Internal Medicine 1979; Hematology 1982; Medical Oncology 1983; **Med School:** Loyola Univ-Stritch Sch Med 1975; **Resid:** Internal Medicine, St Lukes Hosp 1979; **Fellow:** Hematology & Oncology, Mayo Clin 1982; **Fac Appt:** Prof Med, Mayo Med Sch

Godwin, John MD [Hem] - **Spec Exp:** Leukemia in Elderly; Head & Neck Cancer; Lymphoma; Lung Cancer; **Hospital:** St John's Hosp - Springfield, Memorial Med Ctr-Springfield; **Address:** SIU School Medicine, Simmons Cooper Cancer Inst, PO Box 19678, Springfield, IL 62794; **Phone:** 217-545-5817; **Board Cert:** Internal Medicine 1981; Hematology 1986; **Med School:** Univ Alabama 1978; **Resid:** Internal Medicine, Baylor Coll Med 1981; Internal Medicine, Baylor Coll Med 1982; **Fellow:** Hematology, Baylor Coll Med 1983; Hematology, North Carolina Meml Hosp 1985; **Fac Appt:** Prof Med, Southern IL Univ

Gordon, Leo I MD [Hem] - **Spec Exp:** Lymphoma, Non-Hodgkin's; Hodgkin's Disease; Bone Marrow Transplant; **Hospital:** Northwestern Meml Hosp; **Address:** 676 N St Clair St, Ste 850, Chicago, IL 60611-3124; **Phone:** 312-695-4546; **Board Cert:** Internal Medicine 1976; Hematology 1978; Medical Oncology 1979; **Med School:** Univ Cincinnati 1973; **Resid:** Internal Medicine, Univ Chicago Hosps 1976; **Fellow:** Hematology, Univ Minnesota Hosps 1978; Hematology & Oncology, Univ Chicago Hosps 1979; **Fac Appt:** Prof Med, Northwestern Univ

Gregory, Stephanie A MD [Hem] - **Spec Exp:** Lymphoma; Leukemia; Plasma Cell Disorders; Multiple Myeloma; **Hospital:** Rush Univ Med Ctr; **Address:** 1725 W Harrison St, Ste 834, Rush Professional Office Bldg, Chicago, IL 60612-3861; **Phone:** 312-942-5982; **Board Cert:** Internal Medicine 1972; Hematology 1972; **Med School:** Med Coll PA Hahnemann 1965; **Resid:** Internal Medicine, Rush/Presby-St Luke's Med Ctr 1969; **Fellow:** Hematology, Rush/Presby-St Luke's Med Ctr 1972; **Fac Appt:** Prof Med, Rush Med Coll

Greipp, Philip R MD [Hem] - **Spec Exp:** Multiple Myeloma; **Hospital:** Mayo Med Ctr & Clin - Rochester; **Address:** Mayo Clinic, Div Hematology, 200 First St SW Mayo Bldg Fl W-10, Rochester, MN 55905-0001; **Phone:** 507-284-3159; **Board Cert:** Internal Medicine 1974; Hematology 1994; **Med School:** Georgetown Univ 1968; **Resid:** Internal Medicine, Mayo Clinic 1973; **Fellow:** Hematology, Mayo Clinic 1975; **Fac Appt:** Prof Med, Mayo Med Sch

Grever, Michael R MD [Hem] - **Spec Exp:** Hematologic Malignancies; Leukemia; Drug Development; Clinical Trials; **Hospital:** Ohio St Univ Med Ctr; **Address:** 215 Means Hall, 1654 Upham Drive, Columbus, OH 43210; **Phone:** 614-293-8724; **Board Cert:** Internal Medicine 1975; Hematology 1988; Medical Oncology 1979; **Med School:** Univ Pittsburgh 1971; **Resid:** Internal Medicine, Univ of Pittsburgh 1974; **Fellow:** Hematology & Oncology, Ohio State Univ 1978; **Fac Appt:** Prof Med, Ohio State Univ

Habermann, Thomas M MD [Hem] - **Spec Exp:** Lymphoma; Hodgkin's Disease; Leukemia; **Hospital:** Mayo Med Ctr & Clin - Rochester; **Address:** Mayo Clinic, 200 1st St SW, Rochester, MN 55905; **Phone:** 507-284-3159; **Board Cert:** Internal Medicine 1982; Hematology 1984; **Med School:** Creighton Univ 1979; **Resid:** Internal Medicine, Mayo Clinic 1982; **Fellow:** Hematology, Mayo Clinic 1985; **Fac Appt:** Prof Med, Mayo Med Sch

Juckett, Mark B MD [Hem] - **Spec Exp:** Bone Marrow Transplant; **Hospital:** Univ WI Hosp & Clins; **Address:** 600 Highland Ave, Ste H4/534, 2817 New Pinery Rd, Portage, WI 53901; **Phone:** 608-745-5660; **Board Cert:** Internal Medicine 2001; Hematology 2004; Medical Oncology 2005; **Med School:** Univ Louisville Sch Med 1987; **Resid:** Internal Medicine, Univ Minnesota 1990; **Fellow:** Hematology & Oncology, Univ Minnesota 1992; **Fac Appt:** Assoc Prof Med, Univ Wisc

Kraut, Eric H MD [Hem] - **Spec Exp:** Hematologic Malignancies; Leukemia; Drug Development; Clinical Trials; **Hospital:** Ohio St Univ Med Ctr; **Address:** B405 Starling Loving Hall, 320 W 10th Ave, Columbus, OH 43210; **Phone:** 614-293-2887; **Board Cert:** Internal Medicine 1975; Hematology 1978; Medical Oncology 1977; **Med School:** Temple Univ 1972; **Resid:** Internal Medicine, Univ Pittsburgh 1975; **Fellow:** Hematology & Oncology, Ohio State Univ Hosp 1977; **Fac Appt:** Prof Med, Ohio State Univ

Kuriakose, Philip MD [Hem] - **Spec Exp:** Leukemia; **Hospital:** Henry Ford Hosp; **Address:** Henry Ford Hosp, Hematology/Oncology, 2799 W Grand Blvd, Detroit, MI 48202; **Phone:** 313-916-1841; **Board Cert:** Internal Medicine 1999; Medical Oncology 2002; Hematology 2002; **Med School:** India 1990; **Resid:** Internal Medicine, Christian Med Coll 1992; Internal Medicine, Henry Ford Hosp 1994; **Fellow:** Hematology & Oncology, Mayo Clinic 1995

Hematology

Kuzel, Timothy M MD [Hem] - **Spec Exp:** Kidney Cancer; Melanoma; Cutaneous Lymphoma; **Hospital:** Northwestern Meml Hosp; **Address:** Northwestern Meml Hosp, 675 N St Clair, Ste 21-100, Chicago, IL 60611; **Phone:** 312-695-0990; **Board Cert:** Internal Medicine 1987; Hematology 2000; Medical Oncology 1989; **Med School:** Univ Mich Med Sch 1984; **Resid:** Internal Medicine, McGraw MC-Northwestern Univ 1987; **Fellow:** Hematology & Oncology, McGraw MC-Northwestern Univ 1990; **Fac Appt:** Prof Med, Northwestern Univ

Larson, Richard A MD [Hem] - **Spec Exp:** Leukemia & Lymphoma; Bone Marrow Transplant; Myelodysplastic Syndromes; **Hospital:** Univ of Chicago Med Ctr; **Address:** Univ Chicago Hosps, 5841 S Maryland Ave, MC 2115, Chicago, IL 60637; **Phone:** 773-702-6149; **Board Cert:** Internal Medicine 1980; Hematology 1982; Medical Oncology 1983; **Med School:** Stanford Univ 1977; **Resid:** Internal Medicine, Univ Chicago Hosps 1980; **Fellow:** Hematology & Oncology, Univ Chicago Hosps 1983; **Fac Appt:** Prof Med, Univ Chicago-Pritzker Sch Med

Laughlin, Mary J MD [Hem] - **Spec Exp:** Bone Marrow Transplant; **Hospital:** Univ Hosps Case Med Ctr; **Address:** 2103 Cornell Rd, WRB 2-129, Cleveland, OH 44106; **Phone:** 216-844-5182; **Board Cert:** Internal Medicine 2003; Hematology 2004; **Med School:** SUNY Buffalo 1988; **Resid:** Internal Medicine, Duke Univ Med Ctr 1991; **Fellow:** Hematology & Oncology, Duke Univ Med Ctr 1992; Bone Marrow Transplant, Rosewell Park Cancer Inst 1994; **Fac Appt:** Assoc Prof Med, Case West Res Univ

Lazarus, Hillard M MD [Hem] - **Spec Exp:** Bone Marrow Transplant; Stem Cell Transplant; Leukemia; **Hospital:** Univ Hosps Case Med Ctr; **Address:** 11100 Euclid Ave, Cleveland, OH 44106-5065; **Phone:** 216-844-3629; **Board Cert:** Internal Medicine 1977; Medical Oncology 1979; Hematology 1980; **Med School:** Univ Rochester 1974; **Resid:** Internal Medicine, Univ Hosps 1977; **Fellow:** Hematology & Oncology, Univ Hosps 1979; **Fac Appt:** Prof Med, Case West Res Univ

Litzow, Mark R MD [Hem] - **Spec Exp:** Bone Marrow Transplant; Leukemia; **Hospital:** Mayo Med Ctr & Clin - Rochester; **Address:** Mayo Clinic, Div Hematology, 200 First St SW, Rochester, MN 55905; **Phone:** 507-284-0923; **Board Cert:** Internal Medicine 1983; Hematology 1988; Medical Oncology 1989; **Med School:** Univ Chicago-Pritzker Sch Med 1980; **Resid:** Internal Medicine, Mayo Clinic 1984; **Fellow:** Medical Oncology, Mayo Clinic 1990; **Fac Appt:** Asst Prof Med, Mayo Med Sch

Maciejewski, Jaroslaw P MD/PhD [Hem] - **Spec Exp:** Anemia-Aplastic; Hematologic Malignancies; Stem Cell Transplant; **Hospital:** Cleveland Clin Fdn (page 70); **Address:** Cleveland Clinic, 9500 Euclid Ave, Desk R40, Cleveland, OH 44195; **Phone:** 216-445-5962; **Board Cert:** Internal Medicine 1999; Hematology 2001; **Med School:** Germany 1990; **Resid:** Internal Medicine, Univ Nevada Med Ctr 1997; **Fellow:** Hematology, Natl Inst Hlth 2000; **Fac Appt:** Prof Med, Case West Res Univ

McGlave, Philip B MD [Hem] - **Spec Exp:** Leukemia; Bone Marrow Transplant; **Hospital:** Univ Minn Med Ctr, Fairview - Univ Campus; **Address:** Univ Minn, Dept Med - Div Hem/Onc, Mayo Mail Code 480, 420 Delaware St SE, Minneapolis, MN 55455; **Phone:** 612-626-2446; **Board Cert:** Internal Medicine 1977; Hematology 1980; **Med School:** Univ IL Coll Med 1974; **Resid:** Internal Medicine, Univ Minnesota Med Ctr 1977; **Fellow:** Hematology & Oncology, Univ Minnesota Med Ctr 1980; **Fac Appt:** Prof Med, Univ Minn

Nand, Sucha MD [Hem] - **Spec Exp:** Myelodysplastic Syndromes; Myeloproliferative Disorders; Leukemia; Lymphoma, Non-Hodgkin's; **Hospital:** Loyola Univ Med Ctr; **Address:** Cardinal Bernardin Cancer Ctr, 2160 S First Ave Bldg 112 - rm 342, Maywood, IL 60153-3304; **Phone:** 708-327-3217; **Board Cert:** Internal Medicine 1979; Medical Oncology 1981; Hematology 1982; **Med School:** India 1971; **Resid:** Physical Medicine & Rehabilitation, Northwestern Meml Hosp 1976; Internal Medicine, North Chicago VA Hosp 1978; **Fellow:** Medical Oncology, Northwestern Meml Hosp 1981; **Fac Appt:** Prof Med, Loyola Univ-Stritch Sch Med

Porcu, Pierluigi MD [Hem] - **Spec Exp:** Lymphoma; Lymphoma, Non-Hodgkin's; Immunotherapy; **Hospital:** Ohio St Univ Med Ctr; **Address:** 320 W 10th Ave, B320 Starling Loving Hall, Columbus, OH 43210; **Phone:** 614-293-9273; **Board Cert:** Hematology 1999; Medical Oncology 1999; **Med School:** Italy 1987; **Resid:** Internal Medicine, Indiana Univ Hosp 1996; **Fellow:** Hematology & Oncology, Indiana Univ Hosp 1999; **Fac Appt:** Asst Prof Med, Ohio State Univ

Singhal, Seema MD [Hem] - **Spec Exp:** Multiple Myeloma; **Hospital:** Northwestern Meml Hosp; **Address:** 675 N St Claire St, Ste 21-100, Chicago, IL 60611; **Phone:** 312-695-0990; **Board Cert:** Internal Medicine 2005; **Med School:** India 1989; **Resid:** Internal Medicine, King Edward Meml Hosp 1991; Hematology, King Edward Meml Hosp 1991; **Fellow:** Bone Marrow Transplant, Hadassah Univ Hosp 1992; **Fac Appt:** Prof Med, Northwestern Univ

Stiff, Patrick J MD [Hem] - **Spec Exp:** Bone Marrow Transplant; Lymphoma, Non-Hodgkin's; Leukemia; **Hospital:** Loyola Univ Med Ctr; **Address:** Cardinal Bernadin Cancer Ctr, 2160 S First Ave Bldg 112 - rm 255, Maywood, IL 60153; **Phone:** 708-327-3304; **Board Cert:** Internal Medicine 1978; Medical Oncology 1981; Hematology 1982; **Med School:** Loyola Univ-Stritch Sch Med 1975; **Resid:** Internal Medicine, Cleveland Clinic Fdn 1978; **Fellow:** Hematology & Oncology, Meml Sloan Kettering Cancer Ctr 1981; **Fac Appt:** Prof Med, Loyola Univ-Stritch Sch Med

Sweetenham, John MD [Hem] - **Spec Exp:** Leukemia; Lymphoma; **Hospital:** Cleveland Clin Fdn (page 70); **Address:** Cleveland Clinic, Taussig Cancer Inst, 9500 Euclid Ave, MC R35, Cleveland, OH 44195; **Phone:** 216-445-6707; **Med School:** England, UK 1980; **Resid:** Internal Medicine, Royal United Hosp 1984; **Fellow:** Hematology & Oncology, Univ Southampton 1989; **Fac Appt:** Prof Med, Univ Colorado

Tallman, Martin S MD [Hem] - **Spec Exp:** Bone Marrow Transplant; Leukemia; Lymphoma; **Hospital:** Northwestern Meml Hosp; **Address:** 675 N St Clair St, Ste 21-100, Chicago, IL 60611; **Phone:** 312-695-0990; **Board Cert:** Internal Medicine 1983; Medical Oncology 1987; Hematology 1988; **Med School:** Ros Franklin Univ/Chicago Med Sch 1980; **Resid:** Internal Medicine, Evanston Hosp 1983; **Fellow:** Medical Oncology, Fred Hutchinson Cancer Ctr 1987; **Fac Appt:** Prof Med, Northwestern Univ

van Besien, Koen W MD [Hem] - **Spec Exp:** Lymphoma; Stem Cell Transplant; **Hospital:** Univ of Chicago Med Ctr; **Address:** Stem Cell Transplant Program, 5841 S Maryland Ave, MC 2115, Chicago, IL 60637; **Phone:** 773-702-4400; **Board Cert:** Internal Medicine 2005; Medical Oncology 2005; Hematology 2006; **Med School:** Belgium 1984; **Resid:** Internal Medicine, Univ Leuven Med Ctr 1987; **Fellow:** Hematology & Oncology, Indiana Univ Med Ctr 1990; **Fac Appt:** Prof Med, Univ Chicago-Pritzker Sch Med

Winter, Jane N MD [Hem] - **Spec Exp:** Lymphoma, Non-Hodgkin's; Hodgkin's Disease; Bone Marrow Transplant; **Hospital:** Northwestern Meml Hosp; **Address:** Northwestern Univ - Div Hem/Oncology, 675 N St Clair St, Ste 21-100, Chicago, IL 60611; **Phone:** 312-695-0990; **Board Cert:** Internal Medicine 1980; Hematology 1982; Medical Oncology 1983; **Med School:** Univ Pennsylvania 1977; **Resid:** Internal Medicine, Univ Chicago Hosps 1980; **Fellow:** Hematology & Oncology, Columbia Presby Hosp 1981; Hematology & Oncology, Northwestern Univ 1983; **Fac Appt:** Prof Med, Northwestern Univ

Hematology

Great Plains and Mountains

Vose, Julie M MD [Hem] - **Spec Exp:** Lymphoma; **Hospital:** Nebraska Med Ctr; **Address:** 987680 Nebraska Med Ctr, Emile @ 42nd St, Omaha, NE 68198-7680; **Phone:** 402-559-5600; **Board Cert:** Internal Medicine 1987; Medical Oncology 2000; Hematology 2000; **Med School:** Univ Nebr Coll Med 1984; **Resid:** Internal Medicine, Univ Nebraska Med Ctr 1987; **Fellow:** Hematology & Oncology, Univ Nebraska Med Ctr 1990; **Fac Appt:** Prof Med, Univ Nebr Coll Med

Southwest

Barlogie, Bart MD/PhD [Hem] - **Spec Exp:** Bone Marrow Transplant; Plasma Cell Disorders; Multiple Myeloma; **Hospital:** UAMS Med Ctr; **Address:** UAMS-Myeloma Inst Rsch & Therapy, 4301 West Markham St, Slot 816, Little Rock, AR 72205; **Phone:** 501-526-2873; **Med School:** Germany 1969; **Resid:** Internal Medicine, Univ Muenster Med Sch; **Fellow:** Medical Oncology, MD Anderson Cancer Ctr-Tumor Inst 1976; **Fac Appt:** Prof Med, Univ Ark

Brenner, Malcolm K MD/PhD [Hem] - **Spec Exp:** Gene Therapy; Bone Marrow Transplant; **Hospital:** Methodist Hosp - Houston, Texas Chldns Hosp; **Address:** 6621 Fannin St, rm 3-3320, Houston, TX 77030; **Phone:** 832-824-4671; **Med School:** England, UK 1975; **Resid:** Internal Medicine, Cambridge Univ 1979; **Fellow:** Immunology, Clinical Rsch Ctr 1984; Hematology & Oncology, Royal Free Hosp 1986; **Fac Appt:** Prof Med, Baylor Coll Med

Champlin, Richard E MD [Hem] - **Spec Exp:** Bone Marrow Transplant; Stem Cell Transplant; Leukemia & Lymphoma; **Hospital:** UT MD Anderson Cancer Ctr; **Address:** MD Anderson Cancer Ctr, Stem Cell Transplantation Ctr, 1515 Holcombe Blvd, Box 0423, Houston, TX 77030; **Phone:** 713-792-6100; **Board Cert:** Internal Medicine 1978; Hematology 1980; Medical Oncology 1981; **Med School:** Univ Chicago-Pritzker Sch Med 1975; **Resid:** Internal Medicine, LA Co Harbor/UCLA Med Ctr 1978; **Fellow:** Hematology & Oncology, LA Co Harbor/UCLA Med Ctr 1980; **Fac Appt:** Prof Med, Univ Tex, Houston

Cobos, Everardo MD [Hem] - **Spec Exp:** Bone Marrow Transplant; **Hospital:** Univ Med Ctr-Lubbock; **Address:** Texas Tech Univ Med Sch, Dept Med, 3601 4th St, MS 9410, Lubbock, TX 79430; **Phone:** 806-775-8600; **Board Cert:** Internal Medicine 1985; Medical Oncology 1987; Hematology 1988; **Med School:** Univ Tex, San Antonio 1981; **Resid:** Internal Medicine, Letterman Army Med Ctr 1985; **Fellow:** Hematology & Oncology, Letterman Army Med Ctr 1988; **Fac Appt:** Prof Med, Texas Tech Univ

Cooper, Barry MD [Hem] - **Spec Exp:** Leukemia; Lymphoma; **Hospital:** Baylor Univ Medical Ctr; **Address:** 3535 Worth St, Ste 200, Dallas, TX 75246-2096; **Phone:** 214-370-1002; **Board Cert:** Internal Medicine 1974; Medical Oncology 1977; Hematology 1978; **Med School:** Johns Hopkins Univ 1971; **Resid:** Internal Medicine, Johns Hopkins Hosp 1973; **Fellow:** Metabolism, Natl Inst of Health 1975; Hematology, Peter Bent Brigham Hosp 1977; **Fac Appt:** Clin Prof Med, Univ Tex SW, Dallas

Emanuel, Peter D MD [Hem] - **Spec Exp:** Lymphoma; Leukemia; Hodgkin's Disease; Multiple Myeloma; **Hospital:** UAMS Med Ctr; **Address:** 4301 W Markham, Slot 623, Little Rock, AR 72205; **Phone:** 501-526-2272; **Board Cert:** Internal Medicine 1988; **Med School:** Univ Wisc 1985; **Resid:** Internal Medicine, Univ Alabama Hosp 1988; **Fellow:** Hematology & Oncology, Univ Alabama 1991; **Fac Appt:** Prof Med, Univ Ark

Fonseca, Rafael MD [Hem] - **Spec Exp:** Multiple Myeloma; **Hospital:** Mayo Clinic - Scottsdale; **Address:** 13400 E Shea Blvd, MCCRB 3-001, Scottsdale, AZ 85259; **Phone:** 480-301-4280; **Board Cert:** Hematology 1998; **Med School:** Mexico 1991; **Resid:** Internal Medicine, Jackson Meml Hosp 1994; **Fellow:** Hematology & Oncology, Mayo Clinic 1998; **Fac Appt:** Assoc Prof Med, Mayo Med Sch

Kantarjian, Hagop M MD [Hem] - **Spec Exp:** Leukemia; **Hospital:** UT MD Anderson Cancer Ctr; **Address:** 1400 Holcombe Blvd, Unit 428, Houston, TX 77030; **Phone:** 713-792-7026; **Board Cert:** Internal Medicine 1983; Medical Oncology 1985; **Med School:** Amer Univ Beirut 1979; **Resid:** Internal Medicine, Univ Tex MD Anderson Cancer Ctr 1983; **Fellow:** Hematology & Oncology, Univ Tex MD Anderson Cancer Ctr 1983; **Fac Appt:** Prof Med, Univ Tex, Houston

Keating, Michael MD [Hem] - **Spec Exp:** Leukemia; **Hospital:** UT MD Anderson Cancer Ctr; **Address:** MD Anderson Cancer Ctr, 1400 Holcombe Blvd, Unit 428, Houston, TX 77030-4000; **Phone:** 713-745-2376; **Med School:** Australia 1966; **Resid:** Internal Medicine, St Vincents Hosp 1973; **Fellow:** Hematology, MD Anderson Cancer Ctr 1975; **Fac Appt:** Prof Med, Univ Tex, Houston

Lyons, Roger M MD [Hem] - **Spec Exp:** Leukemia & Lymphoma; Multiple Myeloma; Myelodysplastic Syndromes; **Hospital:** SW TX Meth Hosp, Methodist Spec & Transpl Hosp; **Address:** 4411 Medical Drive, Ste 100, San Antonio, TX 78229-3325; **Phone:** 210-595-5300; **Board Cert:** Internal Medicine 1981; Hematology 1982; **Med School:** Canada 1967; **Resid:** Internal Medicine, Winnipeg Genl Hosp 1969; Internal Medicine, Barnes-Wohl Hosps 1972; **Fellow:** Hematology, Washington Univ Hosps 1975; **Fac Appt:** Clin Prof Med, Univ Tex, San Antonio

Maddox, Anne Marie MD [Hem] - **Spec Exp:** Hematologic Malignancies; Lung Cancer; Head & Neck Cancer; Clinical Trials; **Hospital:** UAMS Med Ctr; **Address:** Univ Arkansas Med Ctr, 4301 W Markham St, Slot 74-5, Little Rock, AR 72205; **Phone:** 501-686-8530; **Board Cert:** Internal Medicine 1979; Medical Oncology 1985; Hematology 2004; **Med School:** Dalhousie Univ 1975; **Resid:** Internal Medicine, Univ Toronto 1978; **Fellow:** Medical Oncology, TX MD Anderson Cancer Ctr 1982; **Fac Appt:** Prof, Univ Ark

Munker, Reinhold MD [Hem] - **Spec Exp:** Leukemia & Lymphoma; Bone Marrow Transplant; Hematologic Malignancies; **Hospital:** Louisiana State Univ Hosp; **Address:** LSUHSC Shreveport, Feist-Weiller Cancer Ctr, 1501 Kings Hwy, Shreveport, LA 71130; **Phone:** 318-813-1016; **Board Cert:** Internal Medicine 2004; Hematology 2006; **Med School:** Germany 1979; **Resid:** Internal Medicine, Universit%otsklinikum Gro?hadern 1989; **Fellow:** Hematology & Oncology, Universit%otsklinikum Gro?hadern 1993; Blood Banking, Universit%otsklinikum Gro?hadern 1997; **Fac Appt:** Assoc Prof Med, Louisiana State U, Shrevport

Strauss, James F MD [Hem] - **Spec Exp:** Bleeding/Coagulation Disorders; Leukemia; Lymphoma; **Hospital:** Presby Hosp of Dallas; **Address:** Texas Oncology at Presbyterian, 8220 Walnut Hill Ln Bldg 2 - Ste 700, Dallas, TX 75231; **Phone:** 214-739-4175; **Board Cert:** Internal Medicine 1976; Hematology 1978; Medical Oncology 1981; **Med School:** NYU Sch Med 1972; **Resid:** Internal Medicine, Baylor Univ Medical Ctr 1976; **Fellow:** Hematology, Univ Texas SW Medical Ctr 1977

Yeager, Andrew M MD [Hem] - **Spec Exp:** Bone Marrow & Stem Cell Transplant; Graft vs Host Disease; Leukemia; **Hospital:** Univ Med Ctr - Tucson; **Address:** Arizona Cancer Ctr, 1515 N Campbell Ave, Ste 2956, Tucson, AZ 85724-0001; **Phone:** 520-626-0662; **Board Cert:** Pediatrics 1979; Pediatric Hematology-Oncology 1980; **Med School:** Johns Hopkins Univ 1975; **Resid:** Pediatrics, Johns Hopkins Hosp 1978; Pediatrics, Johns Hopkins Hosp 1982; **Fellow:** Pediatric Hematology-Oncology, Johns Hopkins Hosp 1980; **Fac Appt:** Prof Med, Univ Ariz Coll Med

Hematology

West Coast and Pacific

Damon, Lloyd E MD [Hem] - **Spec Exp:** Leukemia; Lymphoma; Stem Cell Transplant; **Hospital:** UCSF Med Ctr; **Address:** UCSF Comprehensive Cancer Ctr, 400 Parnassus Ave, Ste A502, San Francisco, CA 94143; **Phone:** 415-353-2421; **Board Cert:** Internal Medicine 1985; Medical Oncology 1987; Hematology 1988; **Med School:** Univ Mich Med Sch 1982; **Resid:** Internal Medicine, UCSF Med Ctr 1985; **Fellow:** Hematology & Oncology, UCSF Med Ctr 1988; **Fac Appt:** Prof Med, UCSF

Forman, Stephen J MD [Hem] - **Spec Exp:** Lymphoma; Leukemia; Bone Marrow Transplant; **Hospital:** City of Hope Natl Med Ctr & Beckman Rsch (page 69); **Address:** City Hope National Medical Ctr, 1500 E Duarte Rd, rm 3002, Duarte, CA 91010-3012; **Phone:** 626-256-4673 x62403; **Board Cert:** Internal Medicine 1977; **Med School:** USC Sch Med 1974; **Resid:** Internal Medicine, LAC-Harbor-UCLA Med Ctr 1976; **Fellow:** Hematology, LAC-USC Med Ctr 1978; Hematology, City of Hope Med Ctr 1979; **Fac Appt:** Clin Prof Med, USC Sch Med

Heinrich, Michael C MD [Hem] - **Spec Exp:** Hematologic Malignancies; Sarcoma; Gastrointestinal Stromal Tumors; **Hospital:** VA Medical Center - Portland, OR Hlth & Sci Univ; **Address:** 3710 SW US Veteran's Hospital Rd, Portland, OR 97239; **Phone:** 503-220-8262 x51169; **Board Cert:** Internal Medicine 1987; Hematology 2000; Medical Oncology 2001; **Med School:** Johns Hopkins Univ 1984; **Resid:** Internal Medicine, Oreg Hlth Scis Univ 1988; **Fellow:** Hematology & Oncology, Oreg Hlth Scis Univ 1991; **Fac Appt:** Prof Med, Oregon Hlth Sci Univ

Kipps, Thomas J MD/PhD [Hem] - **Spec Exp:** Leukemia; Lymphoma, Non-Hodgkin's; **Hospital:** UCSD Med Ctr; **Address:** Moores UCSD Cancer Ctr, 3855 Health Sciences Drive, La Jolla, CA 92093; **Phone:** 858-822-5635; **Board Cert:** Internal Medicine 1982; Hematology 1984; **Med School:** Harvard Med Sch 1979; **Resid:** Internal Medicine, Stanford Univ Med Ctr 1981; **Fellow:** Hematology & Oncology, Stanford Univ Med Ctr 1984; **Fac Appt:** Prof Med, UCSD

Levine, Alexandra M MD [Hem] - **Spec Exp:** Lymphoma; AIDS Related Cancers; **Hospital:** City of Hope Natl Med Ctr & Beckman Rsch (page 69); **Address:** 1500 E Duarte Rd, Needleman 213, Duarte, CA 91010; **Phone:** 626-471-7213; **Med School:** USC Sch Med 1971; **Resid:** Internal Medicine, LAC-USC Med Ctr 1974; **Fellow:** Hematology & Oncology, Grady Meml Hosp-Emory Univ 1975; Hematology, LAC-USC Med Ctr 1978; **Fac Appt:** Prof Med, USC Sch Med

Lill, Michael MD [Hem] - **Spec Exp:** Lymphoma; Stem Cell Transplant; Hematologic Malignancies; **Hospital:** Cedars-Sinai Med Ctr; **Address:** Cedars-Sinai Med Ctr-Outpt Cancer Ctr, 8700 Beverly Blvd, Ste AC 1070, Los Angeles, CA 90048; **Phone:** 310-423-1160; **Med School:** Australia 1982; **Resid:** Internal Medicine, Sir Charles Gairdner Hospital 1985; **Fellow:** Hematology, Royal Perth Hospital 1988; **Fac Appt:** Prof Med, UCLA

Linenberger, Michael MD [Hem] - **Spec Exp:** Bone Marrow Transplant; Leukemia & Lymphoma; Multiple Myeloma; **Hospital:** Univ Wash Med Ctr; **Address:** 825 Eastlake Ave E, MS G6-800, Seattle, WA 98109; **Phone:** 206-288-1260; **Board Cert:** Internal Medicine 1985; Hematology 1988; **Med School:** Univ Kans 1982; **Resid:** Internal Medicine, Rhode Island Hosp 1985; **Fellow:** Hematology, Univ Wash Med Ctr 1989; **Fac Appt:** Assoc Prof Med, Univ Wash

Linker, Charles A MD [Hem] - **Spec Exp:** Leukemia; Bone Marrow Transplant; Multiple Myeloma; **Hospital:** UCSF Med Ctr, St Francis Memorial Hosp; **Address:** 400 Parnassus Ave, Ste A502, San Francisco, CA 94143; **Phone:** 415-353-2421; **Board Cert:** Internal Medicine 1978; Hematology 1980; Medical Oncology 1981; **Med School:** Stanford Univ 1974; **Resid:** Internal Medicine, Stanford Univ Hosp 1978; **Fellow:** Hematology & Oncology, UCSF Med Ctr 1981; **Fac Appt:** Clin Prof Med, UCSF

Maziarz, Richard MD [Hem] - **Spec Exp:** Leukemia; Immunotherapy; Bone Marrow Transplant; Lymphoma; **Hospital:** OR Hlth & Sci Univ; **Address:** OHSU Ctr Hematologic Malignancies, 3181 SW Sam Jackson Park Rd, UHN 73C, Portland, OR 97239; **Phone:** 503-494-4601; **Board Cert:** Internal Medicine 1982; Hematology 1988; Medical Oncology 1989; **Med School:** Harvard Med Sch 1979; **Resid:** Internal Medicine, Univ Hosp 1982; **Fellow:** Hematology & Oncology, Brigham & Womens Hosp 1988; **Fac Appt:** Prof Med, Oregon Hlth Sci Univ

Mitchell, Beverly S MD [Hem] - **Spec Exp:** Hematologic Malignancies; Leukemia; Lymphoma; **Hospital:** Stanford Univ Med Ctr; **Address:** Stanford Cancer Center, 800 Welch Rd, Ste 280, MC 5-5796, Stanford, CA 94305-5402; **Phone:** 650-736-7716; **Board Cert:** Internal Medicine 1973; Hematology 1978; **Med School:** Harvard Med Sch 1969; **Resid:** Internal Medicine, Univ Washington Med Ctr 1972; **Fellow:** Metabolism, Univ Zurich 1975; Hematology & Oncology, Univ Michigan 1977; **Fac Appt:** Prof Med, Stanford Univ

Nademanee, Auayporn P MD [Hem] - **Spec Exp:** Lymphoma; Hematologic Malignancies; Clinical Trials; **Hospital:** City of Hope Natl Med Ctr & Beckman Rsch (page 69); **Address:** City of Hope Med Ctr-Dept Hematology, 1500 Duarte Rd, Duarte, CA 91010; **Phone:** 626-256-4673 x62691; **Board Cert:** Hematology 1982; Medical Oncology 1983; Internal Medicine 1978; **Med School:** Thailand 1973; **Resid:** Internal Medicine, Touro Infirm-Tulane Univ 1978; **Fellow:** Hematology & Oncology, Sepulveda VA Hosp 1980; Hematology & Oncology, USC Med Ctr 1981; **Fac Appt:** Prof Med, UCLA

Negrin, Robert S MD [Hem] - **Spec Exp:** Bone Marrow Transplant; **Hospital:** Stanford Univ Med Ctr; **Address:** BMT Program, 300 Pasteur Drive, rm H3249, MC 5623, Stanford, CA 94305; **Phone:** 650-723-0822; **Board Cert:** Internal Medicine 1987; Hematology 2007; **Med School:** Harvard Med Sch 1984; **Resid:** Internal Medicine, Stanford Univ Hosp 1987; **Fellow:** Hematology, Stanford Univ Hosp 1990; **Fac Appt:** Prof Med, Stanford Univ

O'Donnell, Margaret R MD [Hem] - **Spec Exp:** Leukemia; Clinical Trials; **Hospital:** City of Hope Natl Med Ctr & Beckman Rsch (page 69); **Address:** City of Hope National Med Ctr, 1500 E Duarte Rd, MOB-rm 3001, Duarte, CA 91010; **Phone:** 626-359-8111 x62405; **Board Cert:** Internal Medicine 1978; Hematology 1980; Medical Oncology 1979; **Med School:** Med Coll PA 1974; **Resid:** Internal Medicine, Montreal Genl Hosp 1976; Hematology, Royal Victoria Hosp-Montreal 1977; **Fellow:** Hematology & Oncology, Fred Hutchinson Cancer Ctr 1979

Saven, Alan MD [Hem] - **Spec Exp:** Leukemia; Lymphoma; **Hospital:** Scripps Green Hosp; **Address:** Scripps Green Hosp, 10666 N Torrey Pines Rd, MS 312, La Jolla, CA 92037; **Phone:** 858-554-9489; **Board Cert:** Internal Medicine 1987; Medical Oncology 1989; **Med School:** South Africa 1982; **Resid:** Internal Medicine, Albert Einstein Med Ctr 1986; **Fellow:** Hematology & Oncology, Scripps Clinic 1987

Schiller, Gary J MD [Hem] - **Spec Exp:** Leukemia; **Hospital:** UCLA Ronald Reagan Med Ctr; **Address:** 10833 Le Conte Ave, rm 42-121 CHS, Los Angeles, CA 90095; **Phone:** 310-825-5513; **Board Cert:** Internal Medicine 1987; Medical Oncology 1989; Hematology 2000; **Med School:** USC Sch Med 1984; **Resid:** Internal Medicine, UCLA Med Ctr 1987; **Fellow:** Hematology & Oncology, UCLA Med Ctr 1990; **Fac Appt:** Prof Med, UCLA

Snyder, David S MD [Hem] - **Spec Exp:** Leukemia; Bone Marrow Transplant; **Hospital:** City of Hope Natl Med Ctr & Beckman Rsch (page 69); **Address:** 1500 E Duarte Rd, rm 003, Duarte, CA 91010-3012; **Phone:** 626-256-4673; **Board Cert:** Internal Medicine 1980; Hematology 1984; **Med School:** Harvard Med Sch 1977; **Resid:** Internal Medicine, Beth Israel Hosp 1980; **Fellow:** Immunology, Harvard Med Sch 1982; Hematology & Oncology, New England Med Ctr 1984

MEDICAL ONCOLOGY

New England

Antin, Joseph H MD [Onc] - **Spec Exp:** Bone Marrow Transplant; Stem Cell Transplant; Leukemia; **Hospital:** Brigham & Women's Hosp, Dana-Farber Cancer Inst; **Address:** 44 Binney St, rm D1B20, Boston, MA 02115-6013; **Phone:** 617-632-3667; **Board Cert:** Internal Medicine 1981; Medical Oncology 1983; Hematology 1984; **Med School:** Cornell Univ-Weill Med Coll 1978; **Resid:** Internal Medicine, Peter Bent Brigham Hosp 1981; **Fellow:** Hematology & Oncology, Brigham & Womens Hosp/Dana Farber 1984; **Fac Appt:** Prof Med, Harvard Med Sch

Atkins, Michael B MD [Onc] - **Spec Exp:** Melanoma; Kidney Cancer; Immunotherapy; **Hospital:** Beth Israel Deaconess Med Ctr - Boston; **Address:** Beth Israel Deaconess Med Ctr, Cancer Clinical Trials 375 Longwood Ave, Masco Bldg Fl 4 - Ste 412, Boston, MA 02215; **Phone:** 617-632-9250; **Board Cert:** Internal Medicine 1983; Medical Oncology 1987; **Med School:** Tufts Univ 1980; **Resid:** Internal Medicine, New England Med Ctr 1983; **Fellow:** Hematology & Oncology, New England Med Ctr 1987; **Fac Appt:** Prof Med, Harvard Med Sch

Bubley, Glenn J MD [Onc] - **Spec Exp:** Prostate Cancer; **Hospital:** Beth Israel Deaconess Med Ctr - Boston; **Address:** Beth Israel Deaconess Med Ctr, 330 Brookline Ave, Shapiro Bldg Fl 9, Boston, MA 02215; **Phone:** 617-735-2062; **Board Cert:** Internal Medicine 1980; Medical Oncology 1983; **Med School:** Mich State Univ 1977; **Resid:** Internal Medicine, St Francis Hosp 1980; **Fellow:** Hematology & Oncology, Beth Israel Deaconess Med Ctr 1983; **Fac Appt:** Assoc Prof Med, Harvard Med Sch

Burstein, Harold J MD [Onc] - **Spec Exp:** Breast Cancer; **Hospital:** Dana-Farber Cancer Inst, Brigham & Women's Hosp; **Address:** Dana Farber Cancer Inst, 44 Binney St, Ste Mayer 2, Boston, MA 02115; **Phone:** 617-632-4587; **Board Cert:** Medical Oncology 2000; **Med School:** Harvard Med Sch 1994; **Resid:** Internal Medicine, Mass Genl Hosp 1996; **Fellow:** Medical Oncology, Dana Farber Cancer Inst 1999; **Fac Appt:** Asst Prof Med, Harvard Med Sch

Canellos, George P MD [Onc] - **Spec Exp:** Lymphoma; Leukemia; Breast Cancer; **Hospital:** Dana-Farber Cancer Inst, Brigham & Women's Hosp; **Address:** 44 Binney St, Boston, MA 02115; **Phone:** 617-632-3470; **Board Cert:** Internal Medicine 1967; Hematology 1972; Medical Oncology 1973; **Med School:** Columbia P&S 1960; **Resid:** Internal Medicine, Mass Genl Hosp 1963; Internal Medicine, Mass Genl Hosp 1966; **Fellow:** Medical Oncology, Natl Cancer Inst 1965; Hematology, Hammersmith Hosp 1967; **Fac Appt:** Prof Med, Harvard Med Sch

Cannistra, Stephen A MD [Onc] - **Spec Exp:** Gynecologic Cancer; **Hospital:** Beth Israel Deaconess Med Ctr - Boston, Dana-Farber Cancer Inst; **Address:** Beth Israel Deaconess Med Ctr, 330 Brookline Ave, KS 158, Boston, MA 02215; **Phone:** 617-667-1909; **Board Cert:** Internal Medicine 1982; Medical Oncology 1985; **Med School:** Brown Univ 1979; **Resid:** Internal Medicine, Johns Hopkins Hosp 1982; **Fellow:** Medical Oncology, Dana-Farber Cancer Inst 1985; **Fac Appt:** Prof Med, Harvard Med Sch

Chabner, Bruce A MD [Onc] - **Spec Exp:** Colon & Rectal Cancer; Breast Cancer; **Hospital:** Mass Genl Hosp; **Address:** Mass General Hospital, 55 Fruit St, Lawrence House 214, Boston, MA 02114; **Phone:** 617-724-3200; **Board Cert:** Internal Medicine 1971; Medical Oncology 1973; **Med School:** Harvard Med Sch 1965; **Resid:** Internal Medicine, Peter Bent Brigham Hosp 1967; Internal Medicine, Yale-New Haven Hosp 1970; **Fellow:** Medical Oncology, Natl Inst Hlth 1969; **Fac Appt:** Prof Med, Harvard Med Sch

Chu, Edward MD [Onc] - **Spec Exp:** Colon & Rectal Cancer; Gastrointestinal Cancer; Clinical Trials; **Hospital:** Yale-New Haven Hosp, VA Conn Hlthcre Sys; **Address:** Yale Cancer Ctr, 333 Cedar St, Room WWW221, New Haven, CT 06520-8032; **Phone:** 203-785-6879; **Board Cert:** Internal Medicine 1986; Medical Oncology 1989; **Med School:** Brown Univ 1983; **Resid:** Internal Medicine, Roger Williams Hosp 1987; **Fellow:** Hematology & Oncology, Natl Cancer Inst 1990; Internal Medicine, Natl Cancer Inst 1992; **Fac Appt:** Prof Med, Yale Univ

Come, Steven E MD [Onc] - **Spec Exp:** Breast Cancer; Hodgkin's Disease; **Hospital:** Beth Israel Deaconess Med Ctr - Boston, Dana-Farber Cancer Inst; **Address:** Beth Israel Deaconess Hosp, 330 Brookline Ave, Ste CC913, Boston, MA 02215-5400; **Phone:** 617-667-4599; **Board Cert:** Internal Medicine 1975; Medical Oncology 1979; **Med School:** Harvard Med Sch 1972; **Resid:** Internal Medicine, Beth Israel Hosp 1977; **Fellow:** Medical Oncology, Natl Cancer Inst 1976; **Fac Appt:** Assoc Prof Med, Harvard Med Sch

Demetri, George D MD [Onc] - **Spec Exp:** Sarcoma; Bone Tumors; **Hospital:** Dana-Farber Cancer Inst; **Address:** Dana Farber Cancer Inst, 44 Binney St, D1212, Boston, MA 02115; **Phone:** 617-632-3985; **Board Cert:** Internal Medicine 1986; Medical Oncology 1989; **Med School:** Stanford Univ 1983; **Resid:** Internal Medicine, Univ Wash Med Ctr 1986; **Fellow:** Medical Oncology, Dana Farber Cancer Inst 1989; **Fac Appt:** Assoc Prof Med, Harvard Med Sch

DeVita Jr, Vincent T MD [Onc] - **Spec Exp:** Lymphoma Consultation; Hodgkin's Disease Consultation; **Hospital:** Yale-New Haven Hosp; **Address:** Yale Cancer Ctr, 333 Cedar St, rm WWW-211B, New Haven, CT 06520-8028; **Phone:** 203-737-1010; **Board Cert:** Internal Medicine 1974; Hematology 1972; Medical Oncology 1973; **Med School:** Geo Wash Univ 1961; **Resid:** Internal Medicine, Geo Wash Hosp 1963; Internal Medicine, Yale-New Haven Hosp 1966; **Fellow:** Medical Oncology, Natl Cancer Inst 1965; **Fac Appt:** Prof Med, Yale Univ

Erban III, John K MD [Onc] - **Spec Exp:** Breast Cancer; Hematologic Malignancies; Stem Cell Transplant; **Hospital:** Mass Genl Hosp; **Address:** Mass Genl Hosp, Yawkey Center, Ste 9A, 55 Fruit St, Boston, MA 02114; **Phone:** 617-726-6500; **Board Cert:** Internal Medicine 1984; Medical Oncology 1989; Hematology 1999; **Med School:** Tufts Univ 1981; **Resid:** Internal Medicine, Hosp Univ Penn 1984; **Fellow:** Hematology & Oncology, New England Med Ctr 1990; **Fac Appt:** Assoc Prof Med, Harvard Med Sch

Fuchs, Charles S MD [Onc] - **Spec Exp:** Gastrointestinal Cancer; **Hospital:** Dana-Farber Cancer Inst, Brigham & Women's Hosp; **Address:** 44 Binney St, Dana 1220, Boston, MA 02115; **Phone:** 617-632-5840; **Board Cert:** Internal Medicine 1989; Medical Oncology 2002; **Med School:** Harvard Med Sch 1986; **Resid:** Internal Medicine, Brigham & Womens Hosp 1989; **Fellow:** Hematology & Oncology, Dana Farber Cancer Inst 1992; **Fac Appt:** Assoc Prof Med, Harvard Med Sch

Garber, Judy E MD [Onc] - **Spec Exp:** Breast Cancer; **Hospital:** Dana-Farber Cancer Inst, Brigham & Women's Hosp; **Address:** Dana Farber Cancer Inst, 44 Binney St, Smith 210, Boston, MA 02115; **Phone:** 617-632-5770; **Board Cert:** Internal Medicine 1984; Medical Oncology 1987; Hematology 1988; **Med School:** Yale Univ 1981; **Resid:** Internal Medicine, Brigham & Womens Hosp 1984; **Fellow:** Medical Oncology, Dana Farber Cancer Inst 1988; Epidemiology, Dana Farber Cancer Inst 1990; **Fac Appt:** Assoc Prof Med, Harvard Med Sch

Garnick, Marc B MD [Onc] - **Spec Exp:** Prostate Cancer; Urologic Cancer; **Hospital:** Beth Israel Deaconess Med Ctr - Boston; **Address:** Beth Israel Deaconess Medical Ctr, SCC9, 330 Brookline Ave, Boston, MA 02215; **Phone:** 617-735-2062; **Board Cert:** Internal Medicine 1976; Medical Oncology 1979; **Med School:** Univ Pennsylvania 1972; **Resid:** Internal Medicine, Hosp Univ Penn 1974; **Fellow:** Research, Natl Inst Hlth 1976; Medical Oncology, Dana-Farber Cancer Inst 1978; **Fac Appt:** Clin Prof Med, Harvard Med Sch

Medical Oncology

Grunberg, Steven M MD [Onc] - **Spec Exp:** Lung Cancer; Head & Neck Cancer; **Hospital:** Fletcher Allen Health Care- Med Ctr Campus; **Address:** FAHC Division of Hematology/Oncology, 89 Beaumont Ave, Given Bldg, E214, Burlington, VT 05405; **Phone:** 802-847-8400; **Board Cert:** Internal Medicine 1978; Medical Oncology 1983; **Med School:** Cornell Univ-Weill Med Coll 1975; **Resid:** Internal Medicine, Mofitt Hosp-U Calif 1978; **Fellow:** Medical Oncology, Sidney Farber Cancer Ctr 1981; **Fac Appt:** Prof Med, Univ VT Coll Med

Hammond, Denis B MD [Onc] - **Spec Exp:** Breast Cancer; Prostate Cancer; **Hospital:** Elliot Hosp, Catholic Med Ctr; **Address:** NH Oncology, 200 Technology Drive, Hooksett, NH 03106; **Phone:** 603-622-6484; **Board Cert:** Internal Medicine 1977; Hematology 1978; **Med School:** Tufts Univ 1973; **Resid:** Internal Medicine, SUNY Buffalo Affil Hosps 1976; **Fellow:** Hematology, Mass Genl Hosp 1977; Medical Oncology, Dartmouth Med Sch 1978

Johnson, Bruce E MD [Onc] - **Spec Exp:** Lung Cancer; Thoracic Cancers; Merkel Cell Carcinoma; **Hospital:** Dana-Farber Cancer Inst, Brigham & Women's Hosp; **Address:** Lowe Ctr Thoracic Oncology, 44 Binney St, Ste D-1234, Boston, MA 02115; **Phone:** 617-632-6875; **Board Cert:** Internal Medicine 1982; Medical Oncology 1985; **Med School:** Univ Minn 1979; **Resid:** Internal Medicine, Univ Chicago Hosps 1982; **Fellow:** Medical Oncology, Natl Cancer Inst 1985; **Fac Appt:** Assoc Prof Med, Harvard Med Sch

Kantoff, Philip W MD [Onc] - **Spec Exp:** Genitourinary Cancer; Prostate Cancer; **Hospital:** Dana-Farber Cancer Inst, Brigham & Women's Hosp; **Address:** 44 Binney St Fl 11, Boston, MA 02115; **Phone:** 617-632-1914; **Board Cert:** Internal Medicine 1982; Medical Oncology 1989; **Med School:** Brown Univ 1979; **Resid:** Internal Medicine, NYU/Bellevue Hosp 1983; **Fellow:** Gene Therapy Research, NIH 1986; **Fac Appt:** Prof Med, Harvard Med Sch

Kaufman, Peter A MD [Onc] - **Spec Exp:** Breast Cancer; Clinical Trials; **Hospital:** Dartmouth - Hitchcock Med Ctr; **Address:** Dept Hematology-Oncology, One Medical Center Drive, Lebanon, NH 03756; **Phone:** 603-653-6181; **Board Cert:** Internal Medicine 1986; Medical Oncology 1989; **Med School:** NYU Sch Med 1983; **Resid:** Internal Medicine, Duke Univ Med Ctr 1986; **Fellow:** Hematology & Oncology, Duke Univ Med Ctr 1989; **Fac Appt:** Assoc Prof Med, Dartmouth Med Sch

Kelly, William K DO [Onc] - **Spec Exp:** Prostate Cancer; Genitourinary Cancer; Solid Tumors; **Hospital:** Yale-New Haven Hosp; **Address:** Yale Physicians Bldg - 2nd FL, 800 Howard Ave, New Haven, CT 06510; **Phone:** 203-785-4191; **Board Cert:** Medical Oncology 2003; **Med School:** Philadelphia Coll Osteo Med 1986; **Resid:** Internal Medicine, Montefiore Med Ctr 1990; **Fellow:** Hematology & Oncology, Meml Sloan Kettering Cancer Ctr 1993; **Fac Appt:** Assoc Prof Med, Yale Univ

Lacy, Jill MD [Onc] - **Spec Exp:** Colon & Rectal Cancer; Brain Tumors; Gastrointestinal Cancer; Pancreatic Cancer; **Hospital:** Yale-New Haven Hosp; **Address:** Yale Univ Sch Med-Div Medical Oncology, 333 Cedar St, PO Box 208032, New Haven, CT 06520-8032; **Phone:** 203-785-4191; **Board Cert:** Internal Medicine 1982; Medical Oncology 2005; **Med School:** Yale Univ 1978; **Resid:** Internal Medicine, Yale-New Haven Hosp 1981; **Fellow:** Medical Oncology, Yale-New Haven Hosp 1985; **Fac Appt:** Assoc Prof Med, Yale Univ

Legare, Robert D MD [Onc] - **Spec Exp:** Breast Cancer; Breast Cancer Risk Assessment; **Hospital:** Women & Infants Hosp of RI; **Address:** Women & Infants Hospital, 101 Dudeley St, Providence, RI 02905; **Phone:** 401-453-7520; **Board Cert:** Internal Medicine 2005; Hematology 2006; Medical Oncology 2008; **Med School:** Tufts Univ 1990; **Resid:** Internal Medicine, Yale-New Haven Hosp 1992; **Fellow:** Hematology & Oncology, Brigham & Women's Hosp 1996; **Fac Appt:** Asst Prof Med, Brown Univ

Mathew, Paul MD [Onc] - **Spec Exp:** Prostate Cancer; **Hospital:** Tufts Med Ctr; **Address:** 800 Washington St, Box 245, Boston, MA 02111; **Phone:** 617-636-8483; **Board Cert:** Internal Medicine 2000; Medical Oncology 2003; Hematology 2004; **Med School:** Chile 1985; **Resid:** Internal Medicine, Cook Co Hos 1990; **Fellow:** Hematology & Oncology, Mayo Clinic 1994; **Fac Appt:** Assoc Prof Med, Boston Univ

Matulonis, Ursula A MD [Onc] - **Spec Exp:** Gynecologic Cancer; Ovarian Cancer; Breast Cancer; Drug Development; **Hospital:** Dana-Farber Cancer Inst; **Address:** Gynecologic Oncology Program, Dana Farber Cancer Institute, 44 Binney St, Ste Dana 1210, Boston, MA 02115; **Phone:** 617-632-2334; **Board Cert:** Internal Medicine 2000; Medical Oncology 2000; **Med School:** Albany Med Coll 1987; **Resid:** Internal Medicine, Univ Pittsburgh Hosp 1990; **Fellow:** Medical Oncology, Dana Farber Cancer Inst 1993; **Fac Appt:** Asst Prof Med, Harvard Med Sch

Nadler, Lee M MD [Onc] - **Spec Exp:** Lymphoma; **Hospital:** Dana-Farber Cancer Inst, Brigham & Women's Hosp; **Address:** Dana Farber Cancer Inst, 44 Binney St, SM 339A, Boston, MA 02115; **Phone:** 617-632-3331; **Board Cert:** Internal Medicine 1976; **Med School:** Harvard Med Sch 1973; **Resid:** Internal Medicine, Columbia-Presby Hosp 1975; **Fellow:** Medical Oncology, Natl Cancer Inst 1977; Medical Oncology, Dana-Farber Cancer Inst 1978; **Fac Appt:** Prof Med, Harvard Med Sch

Oh, William K MD [Onc] - **Spec Exp:** Genitourinary Cancer; Prostate Cancer; Testicular Cancer; **Hospital:** Dana-Farber Cancer Inst, Brigham & Women's Hosp; **Address:** Dana-Farber Cancer Institute, 44 Binney St # D1230, Boston, MA 02115-6013; **Phone:** 617-632-4524; **Board Cert:** Medical Oncology 1998; **Med School:** NYU Sch Med 1992; **Resid:** Internal Medicine, Brigham & Womens Hosp 1995; **Fellow:** Medical Oncology, Dana-Farber Cancer Inst 1997; **Fac Appt:** Assoc Prof Med, Harvard Med Sch

Posner, Marshall R MD [Onc] - **Spec Exp:** Head & Neck Cancer; Skin Cancer-Head & Neck; **Hospital:** Dana-Farber Cancer Inst, Beth Israel Deaconess Med Ctr - Boston; **Address:** Dana-Farber Cancer Inst, Head & Neck Cancer Ctr, 44 Binney St, rm G430, Boston, MA 02115; **Phone:** 617-632-3090; **Board Cert:** Internal Medicine 1978; Medical Oncology 1981; **Med School:** Tufts Univ 1975; **Resid:** Internal Medicine, Boston City Hosp 1978; **Fellow:** Oncology, Dana-Farber Cancer Inst 1981; **Fac Appt:** Assoc Prof Med, Harvard Med Sch

Schnipper, Lowell E MD [Onc] - **Spec Exp:** Breast Cancer; Lymphoma; **Hospital:** Beth Israel Deaconess Med Ctr - Boston; **Address:** Beth Israel Deaconess Med Ctr, 330 Brookline Ave, RABB 430, Boston, MA 02215; **Phone:** 617-667-1198; **Board Cert:** Internal Medicine 1973; Medical Oncology 1983; **Med School:** SUNY Downstate 1968; **Resid:** Internal Medicine, Yale-New Haven Hosp 1970; Medical Oncology, Natl Cancer Inst 1973; **Fellow:** Hematology & Oncology, Barnes Jewish Hosp 1974; **Fac Appt:** Prof Med, Harvard Med Sch

Shulman, Lawrence N MD [Onc] - **Spec Exp:** Breast Cancer; **Hospital:** Dana-Farber Cancer Inst; **Address:** Dana-Farber Cancer Inst, 44 Binney St, rm Dana-1608, Boston, MA 02115; **Phone:** 617-632-2277; **Board Cert:** Internal Medicine 1978; Medical Oncology 1981; Hematology 1982; **Med School:** Harvard Med Sch 1975; **Resid:** Internal Medicine, Beth Israel Hosp 1977; **Fellow:** Hematology & Oncology, Beth Israel Hosp 1980; **Fac Appt:** Assoc Prof Med, Harvard Med Sch

Smith, Matthew R MD/PhD [Onc] - **Spec Exp:** Prostate Cancer; **Hospital:** Mass Genl Hosp; **Address:** Mass Genl Hosp, Hematology/Oncology, 55 Fruit St, Yawkey 7E, Boston, MA 02114; **Phone:** 617-724-5257; **Board Cert:** Medical Oncology 1997; **Med School:** Duke Univ 1992; **Resid:** Internal Medicine, Brigham & Women's Hosp 1994; **Fellow:** Medical Oncology, Dana Farber Cancer Inst 1997; **Fac Appt:** Assoc Prof Med, Harvard Med Sch

Medical Oncology

Soiffer, Robert J MD [Onc] - **Spec Exp:** Stem Cell Transplant; Bone Marrow Transplant; Leukemia; Lymphoma; **Hospital:** Dana-Farber Cancer Inst, Brigham & Women's Hosp; **Address:** Dana-Farber Cancer Inst, 44 Binney St, Dana 1B11, Boston, MA 02115; **Phone:** 617-632-4731; **Board Cert:** Internal Medicine 1986; Medical Oncology 1989; **Med School:** NYU Sch Med 1983; **Resid:** Internal Medicine, Brigham & Women's Hosp 1986; **Fellow:** Medical Oncology, Brigham & Women's Hosp 1989; **Fac Appt:** Clin Prof Med, Harvard Med Sch

Strauss, Gary M MD [Onc] - **Spec Exp:** Melanoma; **Hospital:** Tufts Med Ctr; **Address:** Tufts Medical Ctr, 800 Washington St, Box 245, Boston, MA 02111; **Phone:** 617-636-5627; **Board Cert:** Internal Medicine 1975; Medical Oncology 1979; Hematology 1980; **Med School:** Yale Univ 1972; **Resid:** Internal Medicine, Boston City Hosp 1976; **Fellow:** Medical Oncology, Natl Cancer Inst 1976; Hematology & Oncology, Mass General Hosp 1979

Taplin, Mary-Ellen MD [Onc] - **Spec Exp:** Prostate Cancer; Genitourinary Cancer; **Hospital:** Dana-Farber Cancer Inst, Brigham & Women's Hosp; **Address:** Dana Farber Cancer Inst, 44 Binney St, rm D1230, Boston, MA 02115; **Phone:** 617-632-3237; **Board Cert:** Internal Medicine 1989; Hematology 2006; Medical Oncology 2003; **Med School:** Univ Mass Sch Med 1986; **Resid:** Internal Medicine, Univ Mass Med Ctr 1990; **Fellow:** Hematology & Oncology, Beth Israel Deaconess Hosp 1993; **Fac Appt:** Assoc Prof Med

Treon, Steven P MD/PhD [Onc] - **Spec Exp:** Waldenstrom's Macroglobulinemia; Multiple Myeloma; **Hospital:** Dana-Farber Cancer Inst; **Address:** Dana-Farber Cancer Inst, 44 Binney St, Ste Dana 1B, Boston, MA 02115; **Phone:** 617-632-2681; **Med School:** Boston Univ 1993; **Resid:** Internal Medicine, Boston Univ Med Ctr 1995; **Fellow:** Hematology & Oncology, Mass Genl Hosp 1996; Research, Dana Farber Cancer Inst 1997; **Fac Appt:** Assoc Prof Med, Harvard Med Sch

Weisberg, Tracey MD [Onc] - **Spec Exp:** Breast Cancer; **Hospital:** Maine Med Ctr; **Address:** 100 Campus Drive, Unit 108, Scarborough, ME 04074; **Phone:** 207-885-7600; **Board Cert:** Internal Medicine 1987; Medical Oncology 1989; **Med School:** SUNY Stony Brook 1983; **Resid:** Internal Medicine, Mount Sinai Hosp 1985; Internal Medicine, Hartford Hosp 1986; **Fellow:** Medical Oncology, Yale Univ Hosp 1988

Winer, Eric P MD [Onc] - **Spec Exp:** Breast Cancer; **Hospital:** Dana-Farber Cancer Inst, Brigham & Women's Hosp; **Address:** Dana Farber Cancer Inst, 44 Binney St Fl 9th, Boston, MA 02115; **Phone:** 617-582-7933; **Board Cert:** Internal Medicine 1987; Medical Oncology 1989; **Med School:** Yale Univ 1983; **Resid:** Internal Medicine, Yale-New Haven Hosp 1987; **Fellow:** Hematology & Oncology, Duke Univ 1989; **Fac Appt:** Assoc Prof Med, Harvard Med Sch

Mid Atlantic

Adler, Kenneth R MD [Onc] - **Spec Exp:** Breast Cancer; Myeloproliferative Disorders; Lymphoma; **Hospital:** Morristown Mem Hosp; **Address:** 100 Madison Ave Fl 2, Box 1089, Morristown, NJ 07962; **Phone:** 973-538-5210; **Board Cert:** Internal Medicine 1976; Hematology 1978; **Med School:** Albany Med Coll 1973; **Resid:** Internal Medicine, Albany Med Ctr 1976; **Fellow:** Hematology & Oncology, Albany Med Ctr 1978; **Fac Appt:** Asst Clin Prof Med, UMDNJ-NJ Med Sch, Newark

Ahlgren, James D MD [Onc] - **Spec Exp:** Gastrointestinal Cancer; **Hospital:** G Washington Univ Hosp; **Address:** Geo Wash Univ Med Ctr, Div Hem/Oncology, 2150 Pennsylvania Ave NW, Ste 3-428, Washington, DC 20037-3201; **Phone:** 202-741-2478; **Board Cert:** Internal Medicine 1980; Medical Oncology 1989; **Med School:** Georgetown Univ 1977; **Resid:** Internal Medicine, Georgetown Univ Hosp 1979; **Fellow:** Medical Oncology, Georgetown Univ Hosp 1981; **Fac Appt:** Prof Med, Geo Wash Univ

Aisner, Joseph MD [Onc] - **Spec Exp:** Lung Cancer; Solid Tumors; **Hospital:** Robert Wood Johnson Univ Hosp - New Brunswick; **Address:** Cancer Inst of New Jersey, 195 Little Albany St, rm 2006, New Brunswick, NJ 08903-2681; **Phone:** 732-235-6777; **Board Cert:** Internal Medicine 1973; Medical Oncology 1975; **Med School:** Wayne State Univ 1970; **Resid:** Internal Medicine, Georgetown Univ Hosp 1972; **Fellow:** Medical Oncology, Natl Cancer Inst 1975

Algazy, Kenneth M MD [Onc] - **Spec Exp:** Lung Cancer; Mesothelioma; Hematologic Malignancies; **Hospital:** Hosp Univ Penn - UPHS (page 81), VA Med Ctr; **Address:** Hosp Univ Pennsylvania, 3400 Spruce St, 12 Penn Tower, Philadelphia, PA 19104; **Phone:** 215-614-1858; **Board Cert:** Internal Medicine 1972; Hematology 1974; Medical Oncology 1979; **Med School:** Temple Univ 1969; **Resid:** Internal Medicine, Univ Rochester-Strong Meml Hosp 1972; **Fellow:** Hematology & Oncology, Johns Hopkins Med Ctr 1974; **Fac Appt:** Clin Prof Med, Univ Pennsylvania

Ambinder, Richard F MD/PhD [Onc] - **Spec Exp:** Lymphoma; Hodgkin's Disease; AIDS Related Cancers; **Hospital:** Johns Hopkins Hosp; **Address:** Cancer Research Bldg, 1650 Orleans St, rm CRB 389, Baltimore, MD 21231; **Phone:** 410-955-8964; **Board Cert:** Internal Medicine 1982; Medical Oncology 1985; **Med School:** Johns Hopkins Univ 1979; **Resid:** Internal Medicine, Johns Hopkins Hosp 1981; **Fellow:** Internal Medicine, Johns Hopkins Hosp 1982; Medical Oncology, Johns Hopkins Hosp 1985; **Fac Appt:** Prof Med, Johns Hopkins Univ

Argiris, Athanassios MD [Onc] - **Spec Exp:** Lung Cancer; Head & Neck Cancer; Clinical Trials; **Hospital:** UPMC Presby, Pittsburgh, UPMC Shadyside; **Address:** UPMC Presbyterian Cancer Ctr, 5115 Centre Ave Fl 2, Pittsburgh, PA 15232; **Phone:** 412-692-4724; **Board Cert:** Internal Medicine 1997; Medical Oncology 2000; **Med School:** Greece 1990; **Resid:** Internal Medicine, Beth Israel Med Ctr 1997; **Fellow:** Medical Oncology, Yale-New Haven Hosp 2000; **Fac Appt:** Assoc Prof Med, Univ Pittsburgh

Arlen, Philip M MD [Onc] - **Spec Exp:** Prostate Cancer-Vaccine Therapy; Vaccine Therapy-Clinical Trials Only; Clinical Trials Only; **Hospital:** Natl Inst of Hlth - Clin Ctr, Natl Naval Med Ctr; **Address:** National Cancer Inst, MSC 1750, 10 Center Drive Bldg 10 - rm 5B52, Bethesda, MD 20892-1750; **Phone:** 301-496-0629; **Board Cert:** Medical Oncology 1998; **Med School:** Med Coll GA 1991; **Resid:** Internal Medicine, Georgia Baptist Hlth Care Syst 1994; **Fellow:** Hematology & Oncology, Emory Univ Med Ctr 1994; NCI/NIH 1999

Attas, Lewis MD [Onc] - **Spec Exp:** Breast Cancer; Lymphoma; Bleeding/Coagulation Disorders; **Hospital:** Englewood Hosp & Med Ctr, Holy Name Hosp; **Address:** 25 Rockwood Pl Fl 1, Englewood, NJ 07631-4957; **Phone:** 201-568-5250; **Board Cert:** Internal Medicine 1985; Medical Oncology 1987; Hematology 1988; **Med School:** Mount Sinai Sch Med 1982; **Resid:** Internal Medicine, Montefiore Hosp Med Ctr 1985; **Fellow:** Hematology & Oncology, North Shore Univ Hosp 1988; **Fac Appt:** Assoc Clin Prof Med, Mount Sinai Sch Med

Axelrod, Rita S MD [Onc] - **Spec Exp:** Head & Neck Cancer; Lung Cancer; Complementary Medicine; **Hospital:** Thomas Jefferson Univ Hosp (page 83); **Address:** Thomas Jefferson Univ Hosp, 111 S 11th St, Ste 4240, Gibbon Bldg, Philadelphia, PA 19107; **Phone:** 215-955-8874; **Board Cert:** Internal Medicine 1976; Medical Oncology 1977; Hematology 1978; **Med School:** NYU Sch Med 1970; **Resid:** Internal Medicine, Med Coll Georgia Hosps 1973; **Fellow:** Hematology & Oncology, Hosp Univ Penn 1975; **Fac Appt:** Assoc Prof Med, Thomas Jefferson Univ

Bashevkin, Michael MD [Onc] - **Spec Exp:** Solid Tumors; Hematologic Malignancies; **Hospital:** Maimonides Med Ctr (page 75); **Address:** 1660 E 14st St, Ste 501, Brooklyn, NY 11229; **Phone:** 718-382-8500 x501; **Board Cert:** Internal Medicine 1976; Hematology 1978; Medical Oncology 1979; **Med School:** SUNY Downstate 1973; **Resid:** Internal Medicine, VA Med Ctr 1976; Hematology & Oncology, Maimonides Med Ctr 1979

Medical Oncology

Belani, Chandra P MD [Onc] - **Spec Exp:** Lung Cancer; Drug Discovery; **Hospital:** Penn State Milton S Hershey Med Ctr; **Address:** Penn State Hershey Cancer Ctr, 500 University Drive, MC H072, Hershey, PA 17033; **Phone:** 717-531-1078; **Board Cert:** Internal Medicine 1986; Medical Oncology 1987; **Med School:** India 1978; **Resid:** Internal Medicine, SMS Med Hosp 1981; Internal Medicine, Good Samaritan/Univ MD Hosps 1984; **Fellow:** Hematology & Oncology, Univ Maryland Hosp 1987; **Fac Appt:** Prof Med, Univ Pittsburgh

Biggs, David D MD [Onc] - **Spec Exp:** Breast Cancer; Kidney Cancer; Melanoma; Skin Cancer; **Hospital:** Christiana Care Hlth Svs; **Address:** Med. Onc. Hem. Consultants, 4701 Ogletown-Stanton Rd, Ste 3400, Newark, DE 19713; **Phone:** 302-366-1200; **Board Cert:** Internal Medicine 1988; Hematology 2002; Medical Oncology 2001; **Med School:** Univ Kans 1984; **Resid:** Internal Medicine, Med Coll Wisconsin 1989; **Fellow:** Hematology & Oncology, Hosp Univ Penn 1991; **Fac Appt:** Asst Clin Prof Med

Bosl, George MD [Onc] - **Spec Exp:** Testicular Cancer; **Hospital:** Meml Sloan-Kettering Cancer Ctr (page 76); **Address:** 1275 York Avenue, New York, NY 10065; **Phone:** 800-525-2225; **Board Cert:** Internal Medicine 1976; Medical Oncology 1979; **Med School:** Creighton Univ 1973; **Resid:** Internal Medicine, NY Hosp 1975; Internal Medicine, Meml Sloan-Kettering Cancer Ctr 1977; **Fellow:** Medical Oncology, Univ Minn Hosps 1979; **Fac Appt:** Prof Med, Cornell Univ-Weill Med Coll

Brufsky, Adam M MD/PhD [Onc] - **Spec Exp:** Breast Cancer; **Hospital:** Magee-Womens Hosp - UPMC, UPMC Presby, Pittsburgh; **Address:** Univ Pitt Cancer Inst/Magee-Women's Hosp, 300 Halket St, Ste 4628, Pittsburgh, PA 15213; **Phone:** 412-641-4530; **Board Cert:** Internal Medicine 2004; Medical Oncology 2005; **Med School:** Univ Conn 1990; **Resid:** Internal Medicine, Brigham & Womens Hosp 1992; **Fellow:** Medical Oncology, Dana Farber Cancer Inst 1995; Medical Microbiology, Brigham & Womens Hosp 1995; **Fac Appt:** Asst Prof Med, Univ Pittsburgh

Carabasi, Matthew H MD [Onc] - **Spec Exp:** Bone Marrow Transplant; Stem Cell Transplant; **Hospital:** Thomas Jefferson Univ Hosp (page 83); **Address:** Jefferson Univ Hosp, 111 S 11th St, Gibbon Bldg - Ste 4240, Philadelphia, PA 19107; **Phone:** 215-955-8874; **Board Cert:** Internal Medicine 1983; Medical Oncology 1987; **Med School:** Jefferson Med Coll 1980; **Resid:** Internal Medicine, Hahnemann MC Hosp 1984; **Fellow:** Hematology & Oncology, Meml Sloan-Kettering Cancer Ctr 1988; Research, Meml Sloan-Kettering Cancer Ctr 1989; **Fac Appt:** Assoc Prof Med, Jefferson Med Coll

Carducci, Michael A MD [Onc] - **Spec Exp:** Urologic Cancer; Drug Discovery & Development; Vaccine Therapy; Clinical Trials; **Hospital:** Johns Hopkins Hosp; **Address:** Sidney Kimmel Cancer Ctr, 1650 Orleans St 1M59 BB Bldg, Baltimore, MD 21231; **Phone:** 410-614-3977; **Board Cert:** Internal Medicine 2001; Medical Oncology 2005; **Med School:** Wayne State Univ 1988; **Resid:** Internal Medicine, Univ Colorado Hlth Sci Ctr 1992; **Fellow:** Medical Oncology, Johns Hopkins Hosp 1995; **Fac Appt:** Prof Med, Johns Hopkins Univ

Chachoua, Abraham MD [Onc] - **Spec Exp:** Lung Cancer; **Hospital:** NYU Langone Med Ctr (page 80); **Address:** NYU Clinical Cancer Ctr, 160 E 34th St Fl 8, New York, NY 10016; **Phone:** 212-731-5388; **Med School:** Australia 1978; **Resid:** Internal Medicine, Alfred Hosp 1982; **Fellow:** Hematology & Oncology, Alfred Hosp 1985; Hematology & Oncology, NYU Med Ctr 1988; **Fac Appt:** Asst Prof Med, NYU Sch Med

Chanan-Khan, Asher A MD [Onc] - **Spec Exp:** Multiple Myeloma; Leukemia; **Hospital:** Roswell Park Cancer Inst; **Address:** Roswell Park Cancer Inst, Elm & Carlton Sts, Buffalo, NY 14263; **Phone:** 716-845-3221; **Board Cert:** Medical Oncology 2001; Hematology 2004; **Med School:** Pakistan 1993; **Resid:** Internal Medicine, Harlem Hosp Ctr 1997; **Fellow:** Hematology & Oncology, NYU Med Ctr 1999; **Fac Appt:** Asst Prof Med, SUNY Buffalo

Chapman, Paul B MD [Onc] - **Spec Exp:** Melanoma; Immunotherapy; Vaccine Therapy; **Hospital:** Meml Sloan-Kettering Cancer Ctr (page 76); **Address:** 1275 York Avenue, New York, NY 10065; **Phone:** 646-888-2378; **Board Cert:** Internal Medicine 1984; Medical Oncology 1987; **Med School:** Cornell Univ-Weill Med Coll 1981; **Resid:** Internal Medicine, Univ Chicago Hosps 1984; **Fellow:** Medical Oncology, Meml Sloan-Kettering Cancer Ctr 1987; **Fac Appt:** Prof Med, Cornell Univ-Weill Med Coll

Claxton, David F MD [Onc] - **Spec Exp:** Leukemia; Bone Marrow Transplant; Hematologic Malignancies; **Hospital:** Penn State Milton S Hershey Med Ctr; **Address:** MS Hershey Med Ctr, Medical Oncology, 500 University Drive, MC HO46, Hershey, PA 17033; **Phone:** 717-531-8677; **Board Cert:** Internal Medicine 1984; Medical Oncology 2004; **Med School:** McGill Univ 1978; **Resid:** Internal Medicine, Royal Victoria Hosp 1984; **Fellow:** Hematology, Royal Victoria Hosp 1986; Medical Oncology, UTMD Anderson Cancer Ctr 1989; **Fac Appt:** Assoc Prof Med, Penn State Univ-Hershey Med Ctr

Cohen, Philip MD [Onc] - **Spec Exp:** Breast Cancer; **Hospital:** Georgetown Univ Hosp; **Address:** Georgetown Univ Hosp, Lombardi Cancer Ctr, 3800 Reservoir Rd NW, Washington, DC 20007; **Phone:** 202-444-2198; **Board Cert:** Internal Medicine 1973; Medical Oncology 1975; Hematology 1976; **Med School:** Harvard Med Sch 1970, **Resid:** Internal Medicine, Mass Genl Hosp 1972; **Fellow:** Medical Oncology, Natl Cancer Inst 1974; **Fac Appt:** Assoc Prof Med, Geo Wash Univ

Cohen, Roger MD [Onc] - **Spec Exp:** Drug Discovery & Development; Clinical Trials; Thyroid Cancer; Lung Cancer; **Hospital:** Fox Chase Cancer Ctr (page 72); **Address:** Fox Chase Cancer Ctr, 333 Cottman Ave, Ste C307, Philadelphia, PA 19111; **Phone:** 215-728-2570; **Board Cert:** Internal Medicine 1984; Medical Oncology 1993; Hematology 1986; **Med School:** Harvard Med Sch 1980; **Resid:** Internal Medicine, Mt Sinai Hosp 1982; **Fellow:** Research, Sloan Kettering Cancer Inst 1985; Hematology, Mt Sinai Hosp 1986

Cohen, Seymour M MD [Onc] - **Spec Exp:** Breast Cancer; Melanoma; Lung Cancer; Merkel Cell Carcinoma; **Hospital:** Mount Sinai Med Ctr (page 77); **Address:** 1150 5th Ave, New York, NY 10128; **Phone:** 212-249-9141; **Board Cert:** Internal Medicine 1971; Medical Oncology 1973; **Med School:** Univ Pittsburgh 1962; **Resid:** Internal Medicine, Montefiore Med Ctr 1964; Internal Medicine, Mount Sinai Med Ctr 1965; **Fellow:** Hematology, Mount Sinai Med Ctr 1966; Hematology & Oncology, LI Jewish Hosp 1969; **Fac Appt:** Assoc Clin Prof Med, Mount Sinai Sch Med

Coleman, Morton MD [Onc] - **Spec Exp:** Leukemia & Lymphoma; Hodgkin's Disease; Multiple Myeloma; Waldenstrom's Macroglobulinemia; **Hospital:** NY-Presby Hosp/Weill Cornell (page 79); **Address:** 407 E 70th St, FL 3, New York, NY 10021-5302; **Phone:** 212-517-5900; **Board Cert:** Internal Medicine 1971; Hematology 1972; Medical Oncology 1973; **Med School:** Med Coll VA 1963; **Resid:** Internal Medicine, Grady Meml Hosp-Emory 1965; Internal Medicine, NY Hosp-Cornell 1968; **Fellow:** Hematology & Oncology, NY Hosp-Cornell 1970; **Fac Appt:** Clin Prof Med, Cornell Univ-Weill Med Coll

Cullen, Kevin MD [Onc] - **Spec Exp:** Head & Neck Cancer; **Hospital:** Univ of MD Med Ctr; **Address:** Univ Md Greenbaum Cancer Ctr, 22 S Greene St, rm N9E22, Baltimore, MD 21201; **Phone:** 410-328-5506; **Board Cert:** Internal Medicine 1986; Medical Oncology 1989; **Med School:** Harvard Med Sch 1983; **Resid:** Internal Medicine, Beth Israel Hosp 1986; Internal Medicine, Hammersmith Hosp 1985; **Fellow:** Medical Oncology, Natl Cancer Inst 1988

Medical Oncology

Czuczman, Myron S MD [Onc] - **Spec Exp:** Lymphoma; Multiple Myeloma; Leukemia; **Hospital:** Roswell Park Cancer Inst; **Address:** Roswell Park Cancer Inst, Elm & Carlton Sts, Buffalo, NY 14263; **Phone:** 716-845-7695; **Board Cert:** Internal Medicine 1988; **Med School:** Penn State Univ-Hershey Med Ctr 1985; **Resid:** Internal Medicine, North Shore Univ Hosp 1988; **Fellow:** Hematology & Oncology, Meml Sloan-Kettering Cancer Ctr 1992; **Fac Appt:** Assoc Prof Med, SUNY Buffalo

Daly, Mary B MD/PhD [Onc] - **Spec Exp:** Breast Cancer; Breast Cancer Risk Assessment; Cancer Prevention; Ovarian Cancer Risk Assessment; **Hospital:** Fox Chase Cancer Ctr (page 72); **Address:** Fox Chase Cancer Ctr, 333 Cottman Ave, P1054, Philadelphia, PA 19111; **Phone:** 215-728-2791; **Board Cert:** Internal Medicine 1981; Medical Oncology 1983; **Med School:** Univ NC Sch Med 1978; **Resid:** Internal Medicine, Univ Texas Hlth Sci Ctr 1981; **Fellow:** Medical Oncology, Univ Texas Hlth Sci Ctr 1983; **Fac Appt:** Clin Prof Med, Temple Univ

Davidson, Nancy E MD [Onc] - **Spec Exp:** Breast Cancer; **Hospital:** UPMC Shadyside, Magee-Womens Hosp - UPMC; **Address:** Univ Pittsburgh Cancer Inst, 5150 Centre Ave, Ste 500, Pittsburgh, PA 15232; **Phone:** 412-623-3205; **Board Cert:** Internal Medicine 1982; Medical Oncology 1985; **Med School:** Harvard Med Sch 1979; **Resid:** Internal Medicine, Johns Hopkins Hosp 1982; **Fellow:** Medical Oncology, Natl Cancer Inst 1986; **Fac Appt:** Prof Med, Univ Pittsburgh

Dawson, Nancy MD [Onc] - **Spec Exp:** Prostate Cancer; Kidney Cancer; Bladder Cancer; **Hospital:** Georgetown Univ Hosp; **Address:** Lombardi Cancer Ctr, Georgetown Univ Hosp, 3800 Reservoir Rd NW, Washington, DC 20007; **Phone:** 202-444-9094; **Board Cert:** Internal Medicine 1982; Hematology 1984; Medical Oncology 1985; **Med School:** Georgetown Univ 1979; **Resid:** Internal Medicine, Walter Reed AMC 1982; **Fellow:** Hematology & Oncology, Walter Reed AMC 1985; **Fac Appt:** Prof Med, Georgetown Univ

Dickler, Maura MD [Onc] - **Spec Exp:** Breast Cancer; **Hospital:** Meml Sloan-Kettering Cancer Ctr (page 76); **Address:** 1275 York Avenue, New York, NY 10065; **Phone:** 800-525-2225; **Board Cert:** Medical Oncology 1998; **Med School:** Univ Chicago-Pritzker Sch Med 1991; **Resid:** Internal Medicine, Univ Chicago Hosps 1994; **Fellow:** Medical Oncology, Meml Sloan Kettering Cancer Ctr 1998; **Fac Appt:** Asst Prof Med, Cornell Univ-Weill Med Coll

Donehower, Ross Carl MD [Onc] - **Spec Exp:** Pancreatic Cancer; Colon Cancer; Prostate Cancer; **Hospital:** Johns Hopkins Hosp; **Address:** Hopkins Kimmel Cancer Ctr, 1650 Orleans St, CRB-I, rm 187, Baltimore, MD 21231-1000; **Phone:** 410-955-8964; **Board Cert:** Internal Medicine 1977; Medical Oncology 1979; **Med School:** Univ Minn 1974; **Resid:** Internal Medicine, Johns Hopkins Hosp 1976; **Fellow:** Medical Oncology, Natl Inst Hlth 1980; **Fac Appt:** Prof Med, Johns Hopkins Univ

Doroshow, James H MD [Onc] - **Spec Exp:** Drug Discovery & Development; Colon Cancer; Breast Cancer; **Hospital:** Natl Inst of Hlth - Clin Ctr; **Address:** National Cancer Institute, Div Cancer Treatment & Diagnosis, 31 Center, Bldg 31-rm 3A44, Bethesda, MD 20892-2440; **Phone:** 301-496-4291; **Board Cert:** Internal Medicine 1976; Medical Oncology 1977; **Med School:** Harvard Med Sch 1973; **Resid:** Internal Medicine, Mass Genl Hosp 1975; **Fellow:** Medical Oncology, Natl Cancer Inst 1978

Dutcher, Janice P MD [Onc] - **Spec Exp:** Kidney Cancer; Melanoma; Breast Cancer; **Hospital:** Montefiore Med Ctr - Div. North, Montefiore Med Ctr - Div. Moses; **Address:** 600 E 233rd St, 600 E 233rd St, Bronx, NY 10466-2697; **Phone:** 718-304-7219; **Board Cert:** Internal Medicine 1978; Medical Oncology 1983; **Med School:** UC Davis 1975; **Resid:** Internal Medicine, Rush Presbyterian Med Ctr 1978; **Fellow:** Medical Oncology, National Cancer Inst 1981; **Fac Appt:** Prof Med, NY Med Coll

Edelman, Martin J MD [Onc] - **Spec Exp:** Thoracic Cancers; Lung Cancer; Drug Discovery & Development; **Hospital:** Univ of MD Med Ctr; **Address:** Greenebaum Cancer Ctr-Univ MD, 22 S Greene St, rm N9808, Baltimore, MD 21201; **Phone:** 410-328-2703; **Board Cert:** Internal Medicine 1986; Medical Oncology 1989; **Med School:** Albany Med Coll 1982; **Resid:** Internal Medicine, Naval Hosp 1986; **Fellow:** Hematology & Oncology, Naval Hosp 1990; **Fac Appt:** Prof Med, Univ MD Sch Med

Eisenberger, Mario MD [Onc] - **Spec Exp:** Prostate Cancer; **Hospital:** Johns Hopkins Hosp; **Address:** 1650 Orleans St, rm 1M51, Baltimore, MD 21231; **Phone:** 410-614-3511; **Board Cert:** Internal Medicine 1976; Medical Oncology 1979; **Med School:** Brazil 1972; **Resid:** Internal Medicine, Michael Reese Hosp 1975; **Fellow:** Hematology, Michael Reese Hosp 1976; Medical Oncology, Jackson Meml Hosp/Univ Miami 1979; **Fac Appt:** Prof Med, Johns Hopkins Univ

Ettinger, David S MD [Onc] - **Spec Exp:** Lung Cancer; Sarcoma; Clinical Trials; **Hospital:** Johns Hopkins Hosp; **Address:** Bunting Blaustein Cancer Rsrch Bldg, 1650 Orleans St, rm G88, Baltimore, MD 21231-1000; **Phone:** 410-955-8847; **Board Cert:** Internal Medicine 1976; Medical Oncology 1977; **Med School:** Univ Louisville Sch Med 1967; **Resid:** Internal Medicine, Mayo Grad Schl 1971; **Fellow:** Medical Oncology, Johns Hopkins Hosp 1975; **Fac Appt:** Prof Med, Johns Hopkins Univ

Fanucchi, Michael P MD [Onc] - **Spec Exp:** Sarcoma; Aerodigestive Tract Cancer; Lung Cancer; **Hospital:** St Vincent Cath Med Ctrs - Manhattan; **Address:** 325 W 15th St, New York, NY 10011; **Phone:** 212-604-6011; **Board Cert:** Internal Medicine 1980; Medical Oncology 1985; **Med School:** Columbia P&S 1977; **Resid:** Internal Medicine, Bronx Muni Hosp Ctr 1981; **Fellow:** Medical Oncology, Meml Sloan-Kettering Cancer Ctr 1984; **Fac Appt:** Assoc Prof Med, Emory Univ

Fine, Howard Alan MD [Onc] - **Spec Exp:** Brain Tumors; **Hospital:** Natl Inst of Hlth - Clin Ctr; **Address:** NIH/NCI/NOB, Bloch Building 82, Rm 225 MSC 8202, 9030 Old Georgetown Rd, Bethesda, MD 20892-0001; **Phone:** 301-402-6298; **Board Cert:** Internal Medicine 1987; Medical Oncology 1989; **Med School:** Mount Sinai Sch Med 1984; **Resid:** Internal Medicine, Hosp Univ Penn 1987; **Fellow:** Medical Oncology, Dana Farber Cancer Ctr 1990

Fine, Robert MD [Onc] - **Spec Exp:** Pancreatic Cancer; Drug Development; Brain Tumors; Clinical Trials; **Hospital:** NY-Presby Hosp/Columbia (page 79); **Address:** Columbia Univ Comprehensive Cancer Ctr, 650 W 168th St, rm BB 20-05, New York, NY 10032; **Phone:** 212-305-1168; **Board Cert:** Internal Medicine 1983; Medical Oncology 1985; **Med School:** Univ Chicago-Pritzker Sch Med 1979; **Resid:** Internal Medicine, Stanford Univ Med Ctr 1982; **Fellow:** Medical Oncology, National Cancer Inst 1988; **Fac Appt:** Assoc Prof Med, Columbia P&S

Fisher, Richard I MD [Onc] - **Spec Exp:** Lymphoma; Hodgkin's Disease; **Hospital:** Univ of Rochester Strong Meml Hosp; **Address:** James P Wilmot Cancer Ctr, 601 Elmwood Ave, Box 704, Rochester, NY 14642; **Phone:** 585-275-5823; **Board Cert:** Internal Medicine 1973; Medical Oncology 1977; **Med School:** Harvard Med Sch 1970; **Resid:** Internal Medicine, Mass Genl Hosp 1972; **Fac Appt:** Prof Med, Univ Rochester

Flomenberg, Neal MD [Onc] - **Spec Exp:** Bone Marrow Transplant; Stem Cell Transplant; Leukemia & Lymphoma; **Hospital:** Thomas Jefferson Univ Hosp (page 83); **Address:** Thomas Jefferson Univ Hosp, 125 S 9th St, Ste 801, Philadelphia, PA 19107; **Phone:** 215-955-0356; **Board Cert:** Internal Medicine 1979; Medical Oncology 1981; Hematology 1982; **Med School:** Jefferson Med Coll 1976; **Resid:** Internal Medicine, Montefiore Med Ctr 1979; **Fellow:** Hematology & Oncology, Meml Sloan Kettering Cancer Ctr 1982; **Fac Appt:** Clin Prof Med, Thomas Jefferson Univ

Medical Oncology

Forastiere, Arlene A MD [Onc] - **Spec Exp:** Esophageal Cancer; Head & Neck Cancer; **Hospital:** Johns Hopkins Hosp; **Address:** Bunting Blaustein Cancer Research Bldg, 1650 Orleans St, rm G90, Baltimore, MD 21231; **Phone:** 410-955-8964; **Board Cert:** Internal Medicine 1978; Medical Oncology 1981; **Med School:** NY Med Coll 1975; **Resid:** Internal Medicine, Albert Einstein Med Ctr 1977; Internal Medicine, Univ Conn Health Ctr 1978; **Fellow:** Medical Oncology, Meml Sloan Kettering Cancer Ctr 1980; **Fac Appt:** Prof Med, NY Med Coll

Fox, Kevin R MD [Onc] - **Spec Exp:** Breast Cancer; **Hospital:** Hosp Univ Penn - UPHS (page 81); **Address:** 3400 Spruce St, 14 Penn Tower, Philadelphia, PA 19104; **Phone:** 215-662-7469; **Board Cert:** Internal Medicine 1985; Medical Oncology 1987; **Med School:** Johns Hopkins Univ 1981; **Resid:** Internal Medicine, Johns Hopkins Hosp 1984; **Fellow:** Hematology & Oncology, Hosp Univ Penn 1987; **Fac Appt:** Prof Med, Univ Pennsylvania

Friedberg, Jonathan MD [Onc] - **Spec Exp:** Lymphoma; Hodgkin's Disease; **Hospital:** Univ of Rochester Strong Meml Hosp; **Address:** James P Wilmot Cancer Ctr, 601 Elmwood Ave, Box 704, Rochester, NY 14642-8704; **Phone:** 585-275-4911; **Board Cert:** Internal Medicine 1997; Hematology 2000; Medical Oncology 2000; **Med School:** Harvard Med Sch 1994; **Resid:** Internal Medicine, Mass Genl Hosp 1997; Hematology & Oncology, Dana-Farber/Partners Cancer Ctr 1999; **Fac Appt:** Asst Prof Med, Univ Rochester

Gabrilove, Janice MD [Onc] - **Spec Exp:** Myelodysplastic Syndromes; Leukemia; Hematologic Malignancies; Myeloproliferative Disorders; **Hospital:** Mount Sinai Med Ctr (page 77); **Address:** Mount Sinai Med Ctr, One Gustave L Levy Pl, Box 1079, Dept Hem Onc, New York, NY 10029-6574; **Phone:** 212-241-9650; **Board Cert:** Internal Medicine 1980; Medical Oncology 1983; **Med School:** Mount Sinai Sch Med 1977; **Resid:** Internal Medicine, Columbia-Presby Med Ctr 1980; **Fellow:** Hematology & Oncology, Meml Sloan-Kettering Cancer Ctr 1983; **Fac Appt:** Prof Med, Mount Sinai Sch Med

Gelmann, Edward P MD [Onc] - **Spec Exp:** Prostate Cancer; Testicular Cancer; **Hospital:** NY-Presby Hosp/Columbia (page 79); **Address:** Columbia Univ Med Ctr, Milstein Hosp Bldg 6-435, 177 Fort Washington Ave, New York, NY 10032; **Phone:** 212-305-8602; **Board Cert:** Internal Medicine 1979; Medical Oncology 1981; **Med School:** Stanford Univ 1976; **Resid:** Internal Medicine, Univ Chicago Hosps 1978; **Fellow:** Medical Oncology, National Cancer Inst 1981; **Fac Appt:** Prof Med, Columbia P&S

Geyer Jr, Charles E MD [Onc] - **Spec Exp:** Breast Cancer; **Hospital:** Allegheny General Hosp; **Address:** Allegheny Cancer Ctr, 320 E North Ave Fl 3, Pittsburgh, PA 15212; **Phone:** 412-359-6147; **Board Cert:** Internal Medicine 1983; Medical Oncology 1987; **Med School:** Texas Tech Univ 1980; **Resid:** Internal Medicine, Baylor Affil Hosps 1983; **Fellow:** Medical Oncology, Baylor Affil Hosps 1985

Glick, John H MD [Onc] - **Spec Exp:** Breast Cancer; Hodgkin's Disease; Lymphoma, Non-Hodgkin's; **Hospital:** Hosp Univ Penn - UPHS (page 81); **Address:** Abramson Cancer Ctr of Univ Penn, 3400 Spruce St, 1218 Penn Tower, Philadelphia, PA 19104; **Phone:** 215-662-6065; **Board Cert:** Internal Medicine 1973; Medical Oncology 1975; **Med School:** Columbia P&S 1969; **Resid:** Internal Medicine, Presbyterian Hosp 1971; **Fellow:** Medical Oncology, Natl Cancer Inst 1973; Medical Oncology, Stanford Univ 1974; **Fac Appt:** Prof Med, Univ Pennsylvania

Goldstein, Lori J MD [Onc] - **Spec Exp:** Breast Cancer; **Hospital:** Fox Chase Cancer Ctr (page 72); **Address:** Fox Chase Cancer Ctr, Dept Med Oncology, 333 Cottman Ave, Philadelphia, PA 19111; **Phone:** 215-728-2689; **Board Cert:** Internal Medicine 1985; Medical Oncology 2002; **Med School:** SUNY Upstate Med Univ 1982; **Resid:** Internal Medicine, Presby Univ Hosp 1985; **Fellow:** Medical Oncology, Natl Cancer Inst/NIH 1990

Goy, Andre MD [Onc] - **Spec Exp:** Lymphoma; Hodgkin's Disease; **Hospital:** Hackensack Univ Med Ctr (page 73); **Address:** 20 Prospect Ave, Ste 400, Hackensack, NJ 07601; **Phone:** 201-996-5900; **Med School:** France 1988; **Resid:** Internal Medicine, Grenoble Univ Med Ctr 1992; **Fellow:** Hematology & Oncology, Grenoble Univ Med Ctr 1993

Grana, Generosa MD [Onc] - **Spec Exp:** Breast Cancer; Cancer Genetics; Cancer Prevention; **Hospital:** Cooper Univ Hosp, Virtua West Jersey Hosp - Voorhees; **Address:** 900 Centennial Blvd, Ste M, Voorhees, NJ 08043; **Phone:** 856-325-6740; **Board Cert:** Internal Medicine 1988; Medical Oncology 2001; **Med School:** Northwestern Univ 1985; **Resid:** Internal Medicine, Temple Univ Hosp 1988; **Fellow:** Hematology & Oncology, Fox Chase Cancer Ctr 1992; **Fac Appt:** Assoc Prof Med, UMDNJ-RW Johnson Med Sch

Grossbard, Michael L MD [Onc] - **Spec Exp:** Lymphoma; Breast Cancer; Gastrointestinal Cancer; **Hospital:** St Luke's - Roosevelt Hosp Ctr - Roosevelt Div (page 71), Beth Israel Med Ctr - Petrie Division (page 71); **Address:** 1000 10th Ave Fl 11 - Ste C02, New York, NY 10019; **Phone:** 212-523-5419; **Board Cert:** Internal Medicine 1989; Medical Oncology 2001; **Med School:** Yale Univ 1986; **Resid:** Internal Medicine, Mass Genl Hosp 1989; **Fellow:** Medical Oncology, Dana Farber Cancer Inst 1991; **Fac Appt:** Clin Prof Med, Columbia P&S

Grossman, Stuart MD [Onc] - **Spec Exp:** Brain Tumors; Neuro-Oncology; Pain-Cancer; **Hospital:** Johns Hopkins Hosp; **Address:** Cancer Research Bldg 2, rm 1M16, 1551 Orleans St, Baltimore, MD 21231; **Phone:** 410-955-8837; **Board Cert:** Internal Medicine 1976; Medical Oncology 1983; **Med School:** Univ Rochester 1973; **Resid:** Internal Medicine, Strong Meml Hosp 1976; **Fellow:** Medical Oncology, Johns Hopkins Hosp 1981; **Fac Appt:** Prof Med, Johns Hopkins Univ

Gulley, James L MD/PhD [Onc] - **Spec Exp:** Prostate Cancer-Vaccine Therapy; Vaccine Therapy-Clinical Trials Only; Clinical Trials Only; **Hospital:** Natl Inst of Hlth - Clin Ctr; **Address:** NIH Cancer Research Ctr, MSC 1750, 10 Center Drive Bldg 10 - rm 5B52, Bethesda, MD 20892; **Phone:** 301-435-2956; **Board Cert:** Internal Medicine 1999; Medical Oncology 2000; **Med School:** Loma Linda Univ 1995; **Resid:** Internal Medicine, Emory Univ Med Ctr 1998; **Fellow:** Medical Oncology, Natl Cancer Inst 2000

Haas, Naomi S Balzer MD [Onc] - **Spec Exp:** Genitourinary Cancer; Kidney Cancer; Clinical Trials; **Hospital:** Hosp Univ Penn - UPHS (page 81); **Address:** Abramson Cancer Ctr, 12 Penn Tower, 3400 Spruce St, Philadelphia, PA 19104; **Phone:** 215-615-5121; **Board Cert:** Internal Medicine 1988; Medical Oncology 2005; **Med School:** NE Ohio Univ 1985; **Resid:** Internal Medicine, Abington Meml Hosp 1988; **Fellow:** Hematology & Oncology, Fox Chase Cancer Ctr 1989

Haller, Daniel G MD [Onc] - **Spec Exp:** Gastrointestinal Cancer; Colon & Rectal Cancer; Cancer Prevention; **Hospital:** Hosp Univ Penn - UPHS (page 81); **Address:** Hosp Univ Penn, Div Hematology/Oncology, 3400 Spruce St, 12 Penn Tower, Philadelphia, PA 19104; **Phone:** 215-662-6318; **Board Cert:** Internal Medicine 1976; Medical Oncology 1979; **Med School:** Univ Pittsburgh 1973; **Resid:** Internal Medicine, Georgetown Univ Hosp 1976; **Fellow:** Medical Oncology, Georgetown Univ Hosp 1978; **Fac Appt:** Prof Med, Univ Pennsylvania

Himelstein, Andrew L MD [Onc] - **Spec Exp:** Leukemia & Lymphoma; Palliative Care; **Hospital:** Christiana Hospital; **Address:** Med. Onc. Hem. Consultants, PA, 4701 Ogletown-Stanton Rd, Ste 3400, Newark, DE 19713; **Phone:** 302-366-1200; **Board Cert:** Internal Medicine 1988; Medical Oncology 2000; Hematology 2000; **Med School:** Washington Univ, St Louis 1985; **Resid:** Internal Medicine, Mt Sinai Hosp 1988; **Fellow:** Hematology & Oncology, Colum-Presby Univ Hosp 1991

Medical Oncology

Hochster, Howard S MD [Onc] - **Spec Exp:** Gastrointestinal Cancer; Gynecologic Cancer; Colon & Rectal Cancer; **Hospital:** NYU Langone Med Ctr (page 80); **Address:** NYU Cancer Institute, 160 E 34 St Fl 9, New York, NY 10016; **Phone:** 212-731-5100; **Board Cert:** Internal Medicine 1983; Medical Oncology 1985; Hematology 1986; **Med School:** Yale Univ 1980; **Resid:** Internal Medicine, NYU Med Ctr 1983; **Fellow:** Hematology & Oncology, NYU Med Ctr 1985; Medical Oncology, Jules Bordet Inst 1986; **Fac Appt:** Prof Med, NYU Sch Med

Hogan, Thomas F MD [Onc] - **Spec Exp:** Genitourinary Cancer; Kidney Cancer; Urologic Cancer; **Hospital:** WV Univ Hosp - Ruby Memorial; **Address:** WVU HSC-Dept Med-Hem/Onc, 1 Med Ctr Drive, P.O. Box 9162, Morgantown, WV 26506; **Phone:** 304-293-4500; **Board Cert:** Anatomic Pathology 1997; Internal Medicine 1975; Medical Oncology 1977; **Med School:** Med Coll VA 1972; **Resid:** Internal Medicine, Jefferson Hosp 1975; **Fellow:** Medical Oncology, Univ Wisconsin 1977; **Fac Appt:** Prof Med, W VA Univ

Holland, James F MD [Onc] - **Spec Exp:** Breast Cancer; Colon Cancer; Lung Cancer; Pancreatic Cancer; **Hospital:** Mount Sinai Med Ctr (page 77); **Address:** Ruttenberg Cancer Ctr, Div Med Oncology, 1 Gustave L Levy Pl, Box 1129, New York, NY 10029-6500; **Phone:** 212-241-4495; **Board Cert:** Internal Medicine 1955; **Med School:** Columbia P&S 1947; **Resid:** Internal Medicine, Columbia-Presby Hosp 1949; **Fellow:** Medical Oncology, Francis Delafield Hosp 1953; **Fac Appt:** Prof Med, Mount Sinai Sch Med

Horwitz, Steven MD [Onc] - **Spec Exp:** Lymphoma, Cutaneous T Cell (CTCL); **Hospital:** Meml Sloan-Kettering Cancer Ctr (page 76); **Address:** Meml Sloan-Kettering Cancer Ctr, 1275 York Ave, New York, NY 10021; **Phone:** 212-639-3045; **Board Cert:** Medical Oncology 2001; **Med School:** Case West Res Univ 1993; **Resid:** Internal Medicine, Strong Memorial Hosp 1996; **Fellow:** Medical Oncology, Stanford Univ Med Ctr 1999

Hudes, Gary R MD [Onc] - **Spec Exp:** Prostate Cancer; Genitourinary Cancer; Kidney Cancer; **Hospital:** Fox Chase Cancer Ctr (page 72); **Address:** 333 Cottman Ave, rm C307, Philadelphia, PA 19111; **Phone:** 215-728-3889; **Board Cert:** Internal Medicine 1982; Hematology 1984; Medical Oncology 1985; **Med School:** SUNY Downstate 1979; **Resid:** Internal Medicine, Graduate Hosp 1982; **Fellow:** Hematology & Oncology, Presby-Univ Penn Med Ctr 1985

Hudis, Clifford A MD [Onc] - **Spec Exp:** Breast Cancer; **Hospital:** Meml Sloan-Kettering Cancer Ctr (page 76); **Address:** 1275 York Avenue, New York, NY 10065; **Phone:** 800-525-2225; **Board Cert:** Internal Medicine 1986; Medical Oncology 2001; **Med School:** Med Coll PA Hahnemann 1983; **Resid:** Internal Medicine, Hosp Med Coll Penn 1986; **Fellow:** Medical Oncology, Meml Sloan Kettering Cancer Ctr 1991; **Fac Appt:** Prof Med, Cornell Univ-Weill Med Coll

Ilson, David H MD [Onc] - **Spec Exp:** Esophageal Cancer; Colon & Rectal Cancer; Mesothelioma; Unknown Primary Cancer; **Hospital:** Meml Sloan-Kettering Cancer Ctr (page 76); **Address:** 1275 York Avenue, New York, NY 10065; **Phone:** 800-525-2225; **Board Cert:** Internal Medicine 1989; Medical Oncology 2002; **Med School:** NYU Sch Med 1986; **Resid:** Internal Medicine, Bellevue-NYU Sch Med 1989; **Fellow:** Medical Oncology, Meml Sloan Kettering Hosp 1992; **Fac Appt:** Assoc Prof Med, Cornell Univ-Weill Med Coll

Isaacs, Claudine J MD [Onc] - **Spec Exp:** Breast Cancer; Breast Cancer Risk Assessment; **Hospital:** Georgetown Univ Hosp; **Address:** Lombardi Cancer Ctr, Podium B, 3800 Reservoir Rd NW, Washington, DC 20007; **Phone:** 202-444-3677; **Board Cert:** Internal Medicine 2002; Medical Oncology 2003; **Med School:** McGill Univ 1987; **Resid:** Internal Medicine, Montreal Genl Hosp 1990; Hematology & Oncology, McGill Univ Hosp 1992; **Fellow:** Medical Oncology, Georgetown Univ Med Ctr 1993; **Fac Appt:** Assoc Prof Med, Georgetown Univ

Jurcic, Joseph G MD [Onc] - **Spec Exp:** Leukemia; Myelodysplastic Syndromes; Clinical Trials; **Hospital:** Meml Sloan-Kettering Cancer Ctr (page 76); **Address:** 1275 York Avenue, New York, NY 10065; **Phone:** 800-525-2225; **Board Cert:** Internal Medicine 2001; Medical Oncology 2005; Hematology 1998; **Med School:** Univ Pennvania 1988; **Resid:** Internal Medicine, Barnes Hosp 1991; **Fellow:** Hematology & Oncology, Meml Sloan Kettering Cancer Ctr 1994; **Fac Appt:** Assoc Prof Med, Cornell Univ-Weill Med Coll

Karp, Judith MD [Onc] - **Spec Exp:** Leukemia; Clinical Trials; Myelodysplastic Syndromes; **Hospital:** Johns Hopkins Hosp; **Address:** 1650 Orleans St, CRB1 Bldg - rm 289, Baltimore, MD 21287; **Phone:** 410-502-7726; **Board Cert:** Internal Medicine 1976; **Med School:** Stanford Univ 1971; **Resid:** Internal Medicine, John Hopkins Hosp 1974; **Fellow:** Medical Oncology, John Hopkins Hosp 1977; **Fac Appt:** Prof Med, Johns Hopkins Univ

Kelsen, David MD [Onc] - **Spec Exp:** Gastrointestinal Cancer; Neuroendocrine Tumors; Unknown Primary Cancer; Merkel Cell Carcinoma; **Hospital:** Meml Sloan-Kettering Cancer Ctr (page 76); **Address:** 1275 York Avenue, New York, NY 10065; **Phone:** 212-639-8470; **Board Cert:** Internal Medicine 1976; Medical Oncology 1979; **Med School:** Hahnemann Univ 1972; **Resid:** Internal Medicine, Temple Univ Hosp 1976; **Fellow:** Medical Oncology, Meml Sloan Kettering Cancer Ctr 1978; **Fac Appt:** Prof Med, Cornell Univ Weill Med Coll

Kemeny, Nancy MD [Onc] - **Spec Exp:** Colon Cancer; Rectal Cancer; Liver Cancer; **Hospital:** Meml Sloan-Kettering Cancer Ctr (page 76); **Address:** 1275 York Avenue, New York, NY 10065; **Phone:** 800-525-2225; **Board Cert:** Internal Medicine 1974; Medical Oncology 1981; **Med School:** UMDNJ-NJ Med Sch, Newark 1971; **Resid:** Internal Medicine, St Luke's Hosp 1974; **Fellow:** Medical Oncology, Mem Sloan Kettering Cancer Ctr 1976; **Fac Appt:** Prof Med, Cornell Univ-Weill Med Coll

Kirkwood, John M MD [Onc] - **Spec Exp:** Melanoma; Immunotherapy; **Hospital:** UPMC Presby, Pittsburgh, UPMC Shadyside; **Address:** Hillman Cancer Research Pavilion, 5117 Centre Ave, Ste 1.32, Pittsburgh, PA 15213-1862; **Phone:** 412-623-7707; **Board Cert:** Internal Medicine 1976; Medical Oncology 1981; **Med School:** Yale Univ 1973; **Resid:** Internal Medicine, Yale-New Haven Hosp 1976; **Fellow:** Medical Oncology, Dana Farber Cancer Inst 1979; **Fac Appt:** Prof Med, Univ Pittsburgh

Kris, Mark G MD [Onc] - **Spec Exp:** Lung Cancer; Mediastinal Tumors; Thymoma; Thoracic Cancers; **Hospital:** Meml Sloan-Kettering Cancer Ctr (page 76); **Address:** 1275 York Avenue, New York, NY 10065; **Phone:** 212-639-7590; **Board Cert:** Internal Medicine 1980; Medical Oncology 1983; **Med School:** Cornell Univ-Weill Med Coll 1977; **Resid:** Internal Medicine, NY Hosp 1980; **Fellow:** Medical Oncology, Meml Sloan Kettering Cancer Ctr 1983; **Fac Appt:** Prof Med, Cornell Univ-Weill Med Coll

Langer, Corey J MD [Onc] - **Spec Exp:** Lung Cancer; Head & Neck Cancer; Mesothelioma; Thoracic Cancers; **Hospital:** Hosp Univ Penn - UPHS (page 81); **Address:** Hospital U Penn, Abramson Cancer Ctr, Div Hem/Oncology, 16 Penn Tower, 3400 Spruce St, Philadelphia, PA 19104; **Phone:** 215-615-5121; **Board Cert:** Internal Medicine 1984; Hematology 1986; Medical Oncology 1987; **Med School:** Boston Univ 1981; **Resid:** Internal Medicine, Graduate Hosp 1984; Hematology & Oncology, Presby Hosp 1986; **Fellow:** Medical Oncology, Fox Chase Cancer Ctr 1987; **Fac Appt:** Prof Med, Univ Pennsylvania

Levine, Ellis G MD [Onc] - **Spec Exp:** Breast Cancer; Testicular Cancer; Bladder Cancer; Prostate Cancer; **Hospital:** Roswell Park Cancer Inst; **Address:** Roswell Park Cancer Inst, Elm & Carlton St, Buffalo, NY 14263-0001; **Phone:** 716-845-8547; **Board Cert:** Internal Medicine 1982; Medical Oncology 1985; **Med School:** Univ Pittsburgh 1979; **Resid:** Internal Medicine, Univ Minn Hosps 1982; **Fellow:** Medical Oncology, Univ Minn Hosps 1984; **Fac Appt:** Assoc Prof Med, SUNY Buffalo

Medical Oncology

Levy, Michael H MD/PhD [Onc] - **Spec Exp:** Pain Management; Palliative Care; Pain-Cancer; Ethics; **Hospital:** Fox Chase Cancer Ctr (page 72); **Address:** Fox Chase Cancer Ctr, Div Med Oncology, 333 Cottman Ave, Ste C307, Philadelphia, PA 19111; **Phone:** 215-728-3637; **Board Cert:** Internal Medicine 1979; Medical Oncology 1981; **Med School:** Jefferson Med Coll 1976; **Resid:** Internal Medicine, Mt Sinai Med Ctr 1978; Internal Medicine, Hosp Univ Penn 1979; **Fellow:** Hematology & Oncology, Hosp Univ Penn 1981

Livingston, Philip O MD [Onc] - **Spec Exp:** Melanoma; Vaccine Therapy; Immunotherapy; **Hospital:** Meml Sloan-Kettering Cancer Ctr (page 76); **Address:** 1275 York Avenue, New York, NY 10065; **Phone:** 800-525-2225; **Board Cert:** Internal Medicine 1980; Allergy & Immunology 1974; Rheumatology 1974; Medical Oncology 1981; **Med School:** Harvard Med Sch 1969; **Resid:** Internal Medicine, North Shore Hosp-Cornell 1971; **Fellow:** Immunology, NYU Med Ctr 1973; Medical Oncology, Meml Sloan Kettering Cancer Inst 1977; **Fac Appt:** Prof Med, Cornell Univ-Weill Med Coll

Marshall, John L MD [Onc] - **Spec Exp:** Gastrointestinal Cancer; Drug Development; **Hospital:** Georgetown Univ Hosp; **Address:** Lombardi Cancer Ctr, Podium A, 3800 Reservoir Rd NW, Washington, DC 20007; **Phone:** 202-444-7064; **Board Cert:** Internal Medicine 2001; Medical Oncology 2003; **Med School:** Univ Louisville Sch Med 1988; **Resid:** Internal Medicine, Georgetown Univ Hosp 1991; **Fellow:** Medical Oncology, Georgetown Univ Hosp 1993; **Fac Appt:** Assoc Prof Med, Georgetown Univ

Maslak, Peter G MD [Onc] - **Spec Exp:** Leukemia; Stem Cell Transplant; Myelodysplastic Syndromes; Clinical Trials; **Hospital:** Meml Sloan-Kettering Cancer Ctr (page 76); **Address:** 1275 York Avenue, New York, NY 10065; **Phone:** 800-525-2225; **Board Cert:** Internal Medicine 1987; Hematology 2000; Medical Oncology 1989; **Med School:** Mount Sinai Sch Med 1984; **Resid:** Internal Medicine, Univ Michigan Med Ctr 1987; **Fellow:** Hematology & Oncology, Meml Sloan Kettering Cancer Ctr 1990

Masters, Gregory A MD [Onc] - **Spec Exp:** Lung Cancer; Esophageal Cancer; Thoracic Cancers; **Hospital:** Christiana Hospital; **Address:** Medical Oncology-Hematology Consultants, Graham Cancer Ctr, 4701 Ogletown-Stanton Rd, Ste 2200, Newark, DE 19713; **Phone:** 302-366-1200; **Board Cert:** Internal Medicine 2003; Medical Oncology 2005; **Med School:** Northwestern Univ 1990; **Resid:** Internal Medicine, Hosp Univ Penn 1993; **Fellow:** Medical Oncology, Univ Chicago Hosps 1995; **Fac Appt:** Assoc Prof Med, Thomas Jefferson Univ

McGuire III, William P MD [Onc] - **Spec Exp:** Gynecologic Cancer; Ovarian Cancer; Breast Cancer; **Hospital:** Franklin Square Hosp; **Address:** Harry & Jeanette Weinberg Cancer Inst, 9103 Franklin Square Drive, Ste 2200, Baltimore, MD 21287; **Phone:** 443-777-7826; **Board Cert:** Internal Medicine 1974; Medical Oncology 1981; **Med School:** Baylor Coll Med 1971; **Resid:** Internal Medicine, Yale-New Haven Hosp 1973; **Fac Appt:** Clin Prof Med, Univ MD Sch Med

Miller, Vincent A MD [Onc] - **Spec Exp:** Lung Cancer; Drug Development; **Hospital:** Meml Sloan-Kettering Cancer Ctr (page 76); **Address:** Memorial Sloan-Kettering Cancer Ctr, 1275 York Ave, New York, NY 10065; **Phone:** 800-525-2225; **Board Cert:** Internal Medicine 2002; Medical Oncology 2005; **Med School:** UMDNJ-NJ Med Sch, Newark 1987; **Resid:** Internal Medicine, Thos Jefferson Univ Hosp 1991; **Fellow:** Medical Oncology, Meml Sloan Kettering Cancer Ctr 1994; **Fac Appt:** Assoc Prof Med, Cornell Univ-Weill Med Coll

Mintzer, David M MD [Onc] - **Spec Exp:** Breast Cancer; Gastrointestinal Cancer; Head & Neck Cancer; **Hospital:** Pennsylvania Hosp (page 81); **Address:** 230 W Washington Square Fl 2, Philadelphia, PA 19106; **Phone:** 215-829-6088; **Board Cert:** Internal Medicine 1980; Hematology 1982; Medical Oncology 1983; **Med School:** Jefferson Med Coll 1977; **Resid:** Internal Medicine, Pennsylvania Hosp 1980; **Fellow:** Hematology, Jefferson Med Coll 1982; Medical Oncology, Meml Sloan Kettering Cancer Ctr 1984; **Fac Appt:** Assoc Clin Prof Med, Univ Pennsylvania

Moore, Anne MD [Onc] - **Spec Exp:** Breast Cancer; **Hospital:** NY-Presby Hosp/Weill Cornell (page 79); **Address:** Weill Cornell Breast Ctr, 425 E 61st St Fl 8, New York, NY 10065; **Phone:** 212-821-0654; **Board Cert:** Internal Medicine 1973; Hematology 1976; Medical Oncology 2008; **Med School:** Columbia P&S 1969; **Resid:** Internal Medicine, Cornell Univ Med Ctr 1973; **Fellow:** Medical Oncology, Rockefeller Univ 1973; **Fac Appt:** Prof Med, Cornell Univ-Weill Med Coll

Motzer, Robert J MD [Onc] - **Spec Exp:** Kidney Cancer; Testicular Cancer; Prostate Cancer; **Hospital:** Meml Sloan-Kettering Cancer Ctr (page 76); **Address:** 1275 York Avenue, New York, NY 10065; **Phone:** 800-525-2225; **Board Cert:** Internal Medicine 1984; Medical Oncology 1987; **Med School:** Univ Mich Med Sch 1981; **Resid:** Internal Medicine, Meml Sloan Kettering Cancer Ctr 1984; **Fellow:** Medical Oncology, Meml Sloan Kettering Cancer Ctr 1987; **Fac Appt:** Assoc Prof Med, Cornell Univ-Weill Med Coll

Muggia, Franco MD [Onc] - **Spec Exp:** Gynecologic Cancer; **Hospital:** NYU Langone Med Ctr (page 80); **Address:** NYU Clinical Cancer Ctr, 160 E 34th St Fl 8, New York, NY 10016; **Phone:** 212-731-5433; **Board Cert:** Internal Medicine 1968; Medical Oncology 1973; Hematology 1974; **Med School:** Cornell Univ-Weill Med Coll 1961; **Resid:** Internal Medicine, Hartford Hosp 1964; Internal Medicine, Francis A Delafield Hosp 1966; **Fac Appt:** Prof Med, NYU Sch Med

Nissenblatt, Michael MD [Onc] - **Spec Exp:** Breast Cancer; Colon Cancer; Hereditary Cancer; Lymphoma; **Hospital:** Robert Wood Johnson Univ Hosp - New Brunswick, St Peter's Univ Hosp; **Address:** 205 Easton Ave, New Brunswick, NJ 08901-1722; **Phone:** 732-828-9570; **Board Cert:** Internal Medicine 1976; Medical Oncology 1979; **Med School:** Columbia P&S 1973; **Resid:** Internal Medicine, Johns Hopkins Hosp 1976; **Fellow:** Medical Oncology, Johns Hopkins Hosp 1978; **Fac Appt:** Clin Prof Med, Robert W Johnson Med Sch

Norton, Larry MD [Onc] - **Spec Exp:** Breast Cancer; **Hospital:** Meml Sloan-Kettering Cancer Ctr (page 76); **Address:** 1275 York Avenue, New York, NY 10065; **Phone:** 800-525-2225; **Board Cert:** Internal Medicine 1975; Medical Oncology 1977; **Med School:** Columbia P&S 1972; **Resid:** Internal Medicine, Bronx Muni Hosp 1974; **Fellow:** Medical Oncology, Natl Cancer Inst 1977; **Fac Appt:** Prof Med, Cornell Univ-Weill Med Coll

O'Reilly, Eileen M MD [Onc] - **Spec Exp:** Pancreatic Cancer; Liver Cancer; Biliary Cancer; Neuroendocrine Tumors; **Hospital:** Meml Sloan-Kettering Cancer Ctr (page 76), NY-Presby Hosp/Weill Cornell (page 79); **Address:** 1275 York Avenue, Meml Sloan-Kettering Cancer Ctr, New York, NY 10065; **Phone:** 212-639-6672; **Med School:** Ireland 1990; **Resid:** Internal Medicine, St Vincent's Hosp 1994; **Fellow:** Hematology, St Vincent's Hosp 1995; Medical Oncology, Memorial-Sloan Kettering Cancer Ctr 1997; **Fac Appt:** Assoc Prof Med, Cornell Univ-Weill Med Coll

Offit, Kenneth MD [Onc] - **Spec Exp:** Cancer Genetics; Breast Cancer; Lymphoma; **Hospital:** Meml Sloan-Kettering Cancer Ctr (page 76); **Address:** 1275 York Avenue, New York, NY 10065; **Phone:** 800-525-2225; **Board Cert:** Internal Medicine 1985; Medical Oncology 1987; **Med School:** Harvard Med Sch 1982; **Resid:** Internal Medicine, Lenox Hill Hosp 1985; **Fellow:** Hematology & Oncology, Meml Sloan Kettering Cancer Ctr 1988; **Fac Appt:** Prof Med, Cornell Univ-Weill Med Coll

Oratz, Ruth MD [Onc] - **Spec Exp:** Breast Cancer; Ovarian Cancer; **Hospital:** NYU Langone Med Ctr (page 80); **Address:** 345 E 37th St, Ste 202, New York, NY 10016; **Phone:** 212-400-4904; **Board Cert:** Internal Medicine 1985; Medical Oncology 1989; **Med School:** Albert Einstein Coll Med 1982; **Resid:** Internal Medicine, NYU Med Ctr 1982; **Fellow:** Medical Oncology, NYU Med Ctr 1985; **Fac Appt:** Assoc Clin Prof Med, NYU Sch Med

Medical Oncology

Oster, Martin W MD [Onc] - **Spec Exp:** Breast Cancer; Gastrointestinal Cancer; Head & Neck Cancer; **Hospital:** NY-Presby Hosp/Columbia (page 79); **Address:** NY Presby Hosp-Columbia Presby Med Ctr, 161 Fort Washington Ave, New York, NY 10032-3713; **Phone:** 212-305-8231; **Board Cert:** Internal Medicine 1974; Medical Oncology 1975; **Med School:** Columbia P&S 1971; **Resid:** Internal Medicine, Mass Genl Hosp 1973; **Fellow:** Medical Oncology, Natl Cancer Inst/NIH 1976; **Fac Appt:** Assoc Clin Prof Med, Columbia P&S

Pasmantier, Mark W MD [Onc] - **Spec Exp:** Lung Cancer; Ovarian Cancer; Breast Cancer; Lymphoma; **Hospital:** NY-Presby Hosp/Weill Cornell (page 79); **Address:** 407 E 70th St Fl 3, New York, NY 10021-5302; **Phone:** 212-517-5900; **Board Cert:** Internal Medicine 1972; Hematology 1974; Medical Oncology 1975; **Med School:** NYU Sch Med 1966; **Resid:** Internal Medicine, Harlem Hosp 1970; **Fellow:** Hematology, Montefiore Med Ctr 1971; Medical Oncology, NY Hosp 1972; **Fac Appt:** Clin Prof Med, Cornell Univ-Weill Med Coll

Pecora, Andrew L MD [Onc] - **Spec Exp:** Stem Cell Transplant; Myelodysplastic Syndromes; Melanoma; Immunotherapy; **Hospital:** Hackensack Univ Med Ctr (page 73); **Address:** The Cancer Ctr-Hackensack Univ Med Ctr, 20 Prospect Ave, Ste 400, Hackensack, NJ 07601; **Phone:** 201-996-5900; **Board Cert:** Internal Medicine 1986; Hematology 1988; Medical Oncology 1989; **Med School:** UMDNJ-NJ Med Sch, Newark 1983; **Resid:** Internal Medicine, New York Hosp 1986; **Fellow:** Hematology & Oncology, Meml Sloan Kettering Cancer Ctr 1988; **Fac Appt:** Prof Med, UMDNJ-NJ Med Sch, Newark

Perry, David J MD [Onc] - **Spec Exp:** Gastrointestinal Cancer; Lung Cancer; Genitourinary Cancer; Clinical Trials; **Hospital:** Washington Hosp Ctr; **Address:** Washington Hosp Ctr-Dept Med Oncology, 110 Irving St NW Fl 2nd - rm CI-2151, Washington, DC 20010; **Phone:** 202-877-2843; **Board Cert:** Internal Medicine 1979; Hematology 1982; Medical Oncology 1981; **Med School:** Univ Pennsylvania 1974; **Resid:** Internal Medicine, Walter Reed AMC 1979; **Fellow:** Hematology & Oncology, Walter Reed AMC 1979; **Fac Appt:** Assoc Prof Med, Eastern VA Med Sch

Petrylak, Daniel P MD [Onc] - **Spec Exp:** Genitourinary Cancer; Prostate Cancer; Bladder Cancer; Kidney Cancer; **Hospital:** NY-Presby Hosp/Columbia (page 79); **Address:** 161 Fort Washington Ave, New York, NY 10032-3729; **Phone:** 212-305-1731; **Board Cert:** Internal Medicine 2001; Medical Oncology 2003; **Med School:** Case West Res Univ 1985; **Resid:** Internal Medicine, Jacobi Med Ctr 1988; **Fellow:** Oncology, Meml-Sloan Kettering Cancer Ctr 1991; **Fac Appt:** Assoc Prof Med, Columbia P&S

Pfister, David G MD [Onc] - **Spec Exp:** Head & Neck Cancer; Laryngeal Cancer; Thyroid Cancer; Skin Cancer; **Hospital:** Meml Sloan-Kettering Cancer Ctr (page 76); **Address:** 1275 York Avenue, New York, NY 10065; **Phone:** 800-525-2225; **Board Cert:** Internal Medicine 1985; Medical Oncology 1989; **Med School:** Univ Pennsylvania 1982; **Resid:** Internal Medicine, Hosp Univ Penn 1985; **Fellow:** Epidemiology, Yale-New Haven Hosp 1987; Hematology & Oncology, Meml Sloan Kettering Cancer Ctr 1989; **Fac Appt:** Prof Med, Cornell Univ-Weill Med Coll

Raptis, George MD [Onc] - **Spec Exp:** Breast Cancer; **Hospital:** Mount Sinai Med Ctr (page 77); **Address:** 1190 5th Ave, Box 1132, New York, NY 10029; **Phone:** 212-241-6756; **Board Cert:** Medical Oncology 2003; **Med School:** Mount Sinai Sch Med 1987; **Resid:** Internal Medicine, Mt Sinai Med Ctr 1990; **Fellow:** Hematology & Oncology, Meml Sloan-Kettering Canc Ctr 1993; **Fac Appt:** Assoc Prof Med, Mount Sinai Sch Med

Remick, Scot C MD [Onc] - **Spec Exp:** AIDS Related Cancers; Clinical Trials; Drug Development; Thyroid Cancer; **Hospital:** WV Univ Hosp - Ruby Memorial; **Address:** WVU Mary Babb Randolph Cancer Ctr, Box 9300, Morgantown, WV 26506-9300; **Phone:** 304-598-4552; **Board Cert:** Internal Medicine 1985; Medical Oncology 1988; **Med School:** NY Med Coll 1982; **Resid:** Internal Medicine, Johns Hopkins Hosp 1985; **Fellow:** Medical Oncology, Univ Wisconsin Clin Cancer Ctr 1988; **Fac Appt:** Prof Med, W VA Univ

Ruggiero, Joseph T MD [Onc] - **Spec Exp:** Colon Cancer; Breast Cancer; **Hospital:** NY-Presby Hosp/Weill Cornell (page 79); **Address:** 428 E 72nd St, Ste 300, New York, NY 10021-4635; **Phone:** 212-746-2083; **Board Cert:** Internal Medicine 1980; Hematology 1982; Medical Oncology 1983; **Med School:** NYU Sch Med 1977; **Resid:** Internal Medicine, New York Hosp 1980; **Fellow:** Hematology & Oncology, New York Hosp/Cornell 1983; **Fac Appt:** Assoc Clin Prof Med, Cornell Univ-Weill Med Coll

Saltz, Leonard B MD [Onc] - **Spec Exp:** Colon & Rectal Cancer; Gastrointestinal Cancer & Rare Tumors; Liver Cancer; Neuroendocrine Tumors; **Hospital:** Meml Sloan-Kettering Cancer Ctr (page 76); **Address:** 1275 York Avenue, New York, NY 10065; **Phone:** 646-497-9053; **Board Cert:** Internal Medicine 1986; Hematology 1988; Medical Oncology 1989; **Med School:** Yale Univ 1983; **Resid:** Internal Medicine, New Yor Hosp 1986; **Fellow:** Hematology & Oncology, New York Hosp-Cornell/Rockefeller Univ 1987; **Fac Appt:** Prof Med, Cornell Univ-Weill Med Coll

Scheinberg, David MD/PhD [Onc] - **Spec Exp:** Leukemia; Immunotherapy; Vaccine Therapy; **Hospital:** Meml Sloan-Kettering Cancer Ctr (page 76); **Address:** 1275 York Avenue, New York, NY 10065; **Phone:** 800-525-2225; **Board Cert:** Internal Medicine 1986; Medical Oncology 2005; **Med School:** Johns Hopkins Univ 1983; **Resid:** Internal Medicine, NY Hosp-Cornell Med Ctr 1985; **Fellow:** Medical Oncology, Meml Sloan Kettering Cancer Ctr 1987; **Fac Appt:** Prof Med, Cornell Univ-Weill Med Coll

Scher, Howard MD [Onc] - **Spec Exp:** Genitourinary Cancer; Prostate Cancer; Bladder Cancer; **Hospital:** Meml Sloan-Kettering Cancer Ctr (page 76); **Address:** 1275 York Avenue, New York, NY 10065; **Phone:** 800-525-2225; **Board Cert:** Internal Medicine 1979; Medical Oncology 1985; **Med School:** NYU Sch Med 1976; **Resid:** Internal Medicine, Bellevue Hosp 1980; **Fellow:** Medical Oncology, Meml Sloan Kettering Cancer Ctr 1983; **Fac Appt:** Prof Med, Cornell Univ-Weill Med Coll

Schilder, Russell J MD [Onc] - **Spec Exp:** Gynecologic Cancer; Hematologic Malignancies; Drug Development; Clinical Trials; **Hospital:** Fox Chase Cancer Ctr (page 72); **Address:** Fox Chase Cancer Center, 333 Cottman Ave, Philadelphia, PA 19111; **Phone:** 215-728-4300; **Board Cert:** Internal Medicine 1986; Hematology 1988; Medical Oncology 1989; **Med School:** Univ Miami Sch Med 1983; **Resid:** Internal Medicine, Temple Univ Hosp 1986; **Fellow:** Hematology & Oncology, Fox Chase Cancer Ctr 1989; **Fac Appt:** Prof Med, Temple Univ

Schuchter, Lynn M MD [Onc] - **Spec Exp:** Melanoma; Breast Cancer; Clinical Trials; **Hospital:** Hosp Univ Penn - UPHS (page 81); **Address:** Univ Penn/Abramson Cancer Ctr, 3400 Spruce St, 16 Penn Tower, Philadelphia, PA 19104-4206; **Phone:** 215-662-7907; **Board Cert:** Internal Medicine 1985; Medical Oncology 1989; **Med School:** Ros Franklin Univ/Chicago Med Sch 1982; **Resid:** Internal Medicine, Michael Reese Hosp 1985; **Fellow:** Medical Oncology, Johns Hopkins Hosp 1989; **Fac Appt:** Prof Med, Univ Pennsylvania

Selvaggi, Kathy J MD [Onc] - **Spec Exp:** Palliative Care; Pain-Cancer; **Hospital:** Allegheny General Hosp; **Address:** West Penn Allegheny Health System, 4815 Liberty Ave, Ste 435, Pittsburgh, PA 15224; **Phone:** 412-578-1112; **Board Cert:** Internal Medicine 1989; Medical Oncology 2005; **Med School:** Penn State Univ-Hershey Med Ctr 1985; **Resid:** Internal Medicine, UPMC Shadyside Hosp 1989; **Fellow:** Medical Oncology, UPMC Shadyside Hosp 1992

Shields, Peter G MD [Onc] - **Spec Exp:** Hematologic Malignancies; **Hospital:** Georgetown Univ Hosp; **Address:** Lombardi Cancer Ctr, 3800 Reservoir Rd NW, First Floor, Washington, DC 20007; **Phone:** 202-444-9495; **Board Cert:** Internal Medicine 1986; Medical Oncology 1989; **Med School:** Mount Sinai Sch Med 1983; **Resid:** Internal Medicine, George Washington Univ Hosp 1986; **Fellow:** Hematology & Oncology, George Washington Univ Hosp 1990; **Fac Appt:** Prof Med, Georgetown Univ

Medical Oncology

Sidransky, David MD [Onc] - **Spec Exp:** Head & Neck Cancer; **Hospital:** Johns Hopkins Hosp; **Address:** 1550 Orleans St, rm 5-N03, Baltimore, MD 21231; **Phone:** 410-502-5153; **Board Cert:** Internal Medicine 1988; **Med School:** Baylor Coll Med 1984; **Resid:** Internal Medicine, Baylor Coll Med 1988; **Fellow:** Medical Oncology, Johns Hopkins Hosp 1992; **Fac Appt:** Prof Oto, Johns Hopkins Univ

Silverman, Lewis R MD [Onc] - **Spec Exp:** Myelodysplastic Syndromes; Leukemia & Lymphoma; Multiple Myeloma; **Hospital:** Mount Sinai Med Ctr (page 77); **Address:** 1190 5th Ave, Ruttenberg Treatment Ctr, New York, NY 10029; **Phone:** 212-241-6756; **Board Cert:** Internal Medicine 1981; Medical Oncology 1987; **Med School:** Belgium 1978; **Resid:** Internal Medicine, Metro Hospital 1980; Internal Medicine, Montefiore Med Ctr 1981; **Fellow:** Hematology, Montefiore Med Ctr 1982; Neoplastic Diseases, Mt Sinai Med Ctr 1984; **Fac Appt:** Assoc Prof Med, Mount Sinai Sch Med

Simon, George R MD [Onc] - **Spec Exp:** Mesothelioma; Lung Cancer; **Hospital:** Fox Chase Cancer Ctr (page 72); **Address:** Fox Chase Cancer Ctr, 333 Cottman Ave, Philadelphia, PA 19111; **Phone:** 215-728-2570; **Board Cert:** Internal Medicine 2007; Medical Oncology 2007; Hematology 1999; **Med School:** India 1986; **Resid:** Internal Medicine, St Joseph's Hosp 1995; **Fellow:** Hematology & Oncology, Univ Colorado Hlth Sciences Ctr 1997

Smith, Mitchell R MD/PhD [Onc] - **Spec Exp:** Lymphoma; Leukemia; Hodgkin's Disease; Multiple Myeloma; **Hospital:** Fox Chase Cancer Ctr (page 72); **Address:** Fox Chase Cancer Center, 333 Cottman Ave, Ste C307, Philadelphia, PA 19111; **Phone:** 215-728-2570; **Board Cert:** Internal Medicine 1985; Medical Oncology 1987; Hematology 1988; **Med School:** Case West Res Univ 1979; **Resid:** Pathology, Barnes Jewish Hosp 1983; Internal Medicine, Barnes Jewish Hosp 1984; **Fellow:** Medical Oncology, Meml Sloan-Ketter Cancer Ctr 1988

Speyer, James MD [Onc] - **Spec Exp:** Ovarian Cancer; Breast Cancer; Cardiac Toxicity in Cancer Therapy; **Hospital:** NYU Langone Med Ctr (page 80); **Address:** NYU Clinical Cancer Center, 160 E 34th St Fl 8, New York, NY 10016-4750; **Phone:** 212-731-5432; **Board Cert:** Internal Medicine 1977; Hematology 1978; Medical Oncology 1979; **Med School:** Johns Hopkins Univ 1974; **Resid:** Internal Medicine, Columbia-Presby Med Ctr 1976; Hematology, Columbia-Presby Med Ctr 1977; **Fellow:** Medical Oncology, Natl Cancer Inst 1979; **Fac Appt:** Prof Med, NYU Sch Med

Spriggs, David R MD [Onc] - **Spec Exp:** Ovarian Cancer; Drug Development; Uterine Cancer; **Hospital:** Meml Sloan-Kettering Cancer Ctr (page 76); **Address:** 1275 York Avenue, New York, NY 10065; **Phone:** 800-525-2225; **Board Cert:** Internal Medicine 1981; Medical Oncology 2006; **Med School:** Univ Wisc 1977; **Resid:** Internal Medicine, Columbia-Presby Hosp 1981; **Fellow:** Medical Oncology, Dana-Farber Cancer Inst 1985; **Fac Appt:** Prof Med, Cornell Univ-Weill Med Coll

Stadtmauer, Edward A MD [Onc] - **Spec Exp:** Bone Marrow & Stem Cell Transplant; Leukemia; Multiple Myeloma; **Hospital:** Hosp Univ Penn - UPHS (page 81); **Address:** Abramson Cancer Ctr, Univ of Penn, 2 PCAM, 34th & Cancer Ctr Blvd, Philadelphia, PA 19104; **Phone:** 215-662-7910; **Board Cert:** Internal Medicine 1986; Hematology 1988; Medical Oncology 1989; **Med School:** Univ Pennsylvania 1983; **Resid:** Internal Medicine, Bronx Muni Hosp 1986; **Fellow:** Hematology & Oncology, Hosp Univ Penn 1989; **Fac Appt:** Assoc Prof Med, Univ Pennsylvania

Stoopler, Mark MD [Onc] - **Spec Exp:** Lung Cancer; Esophageal Cancer; Unknown Primary Cancer; **Hospital:** NY-Presby Hosp/Columbia (page 79); **Address:** 161 Fort Washington Ave, Ste 936, New York, NY 10032-3713; **Phone:** 212-305-8230; **Board Cert:** Internal Medicine 1978; Medical Oncology 1981; **Med School:** Cornell Univ-Weill Med Coll 1975; **Resid:** Internal Medicine, North Shore Univ Hosp 1978; Internal Medicine, Meml Hosp 1978; **Fellow:** Medical Oncology, Meml-Sloan Kettering Cancer Ctr 1980; **Fac Appt:** Assoc Clin Prof Med, Columbia P&S

Straus, David J MD [Onc] - **Spec Exp:** Lymphoma; Multiple Myeloma; **Hospital:** Meml Sloan-Kettering Cancer Ctr (page 76); **Address:** 1275 York Avenue, New York, NY 10065; **Phone:** 212-639-8365; **Board Cert:** Internal Medicine 1972; Hematology 1976; Medical Oncology 1977; **Med School:** Marquette Sch Med 1969; **Resid:** Internal Medicine, Montefiore Med Ctr 1972; Medical Oncology, Meml Sloan Kettering Cancer Ctr 1977; **Fellow:** Hematology, Beth Israel Hosp 1973; **Fac Appt:** Prof Med, Cornell Univ-Weill Med Coll

Sun, Weijing MD [Onc] - **Spec Exp:** Gastrointestinal Cancer; Pancreatic Cancer; **Hospital:** Hosp Univ Penn - UPHS (page 81); **Address:** Hosp of the Univ of Pennsylvania, Division of Hematology-Oncology, 3400 Spruce St, 15 Penn Tower, Philadelphia, PA 19104; **Phone:** 215-662-6319; **Board Cert:** Internal Medicine 1998; Medical Oncology 2001; **Med School:** China 1982; **Resid:** Internal Medicine, Loyola U Med Ctr 1998; **Fellow:** Hematology & Oncology, Hosp Univ Penn 2001; **Fac Appt:** Assoc Prof Med, Univ Pennsylvania

Swain, Sandra MD [Onc] - **Spec Exp:** Breast Cancer; **Hospital:** Washington Hosp Ctr; **Address:** Washington Cancer Inst, 110 Irving St NW, Washington, DC 20010; **Phone:** 202-877-8112; **Board Cert:** Internal Medicine 1983; Medical Oncology 1985; **Med School:** Univ Fla Coll Med 1980; **Resid:** Internal Medicine, Vanderbilt Univ Affil Hosp 1980; **Fellow:** Medical Oncology, NIH-Natl Cancer Inst 1986; **Fac Appt:** Assoc Prof Med, Georgetown Univ

Tagawa, Scott T MD [Onc] - **Spec Exp:** Prostate Cancer; Bladder Cancer; Kidney Cancer; Urologic Cancer; **Hospital:** NY-Presby Hosp/Weill Cornell (page 79); **Address:** NY Presby-Cornell Medical Ctr, 525 E 68th St, Starr Bldg - Ste 341, New York, NY 10065; **Phone:** 212-746-5360; **Board Cert:** Internal Medicine 2001; Medical Oncology 2005; Hematology 2006; **Med School:** USC-Keck School of Medicine 1998; **Resid:** Internal Medicine, USC Med Ctr 2001; **Fellow:** Medical Oncology, USC Med Ctr 2003; Hematology, USC Med Ctr 2004

Tepler, Jeffrey MD [Onc] - **Spec Exp:** Breast Cancer; Leukemia & Lymphoma; Multiple Myeloma; **Hospital:** NY-Presby Hosp/Weill Cornell (page 79); **Address:** 310 E 72nd St, New York, NY 10021; **Phone:** 212-650-1780; **Board Cert:** Internal Medicine 1985; Medical Oncology 1987; Hematology 1988; **Med School:** Yale Univ 1982; **Resid:** Internal Medicine, NY Hosp 1985; **Fellow:** Hematology & Oncology, NY Hosp 1988; **Fac Appt:** Asst Clin Prof Med, Cornell Univ-Weill Med Coll

Tkaczuk, Katherine H MD [Onc] - **Spec Exp:** Breast Cancer; **Hospital:** Univ of MD Med Ctr; **Address:** Univ MD Cancer Ctr, 22 3 Greene St, rm S9D12, Baltimore, MD 21201; **Phone:** 410-328-7904; **Board Cert:** Internal Medicine 1989; Medical Oncology 2001; **Med School:** Poland 1984; **Resid:** Internal Medicine, St Agnes Hosp 1989; **Fellow:** Hematology & Oncology, Univ Maryland Cancer Ctr 1992; **Fac Appt:** Assoc Prof Med, Univ MD Sch Med

Toppmeyer, Deborah L MD [Onc] - **Spec Exp:** Breast Cancer; Hereditary Cancer; **Hospital:** Robert Wood Johnson Univ Hosp - New Brunswick; **Address:** Cancer Inst of New Jersey, 195 Little Albany St, New Brunswick, NJ 08903-2681; **Phone:** 732-235-6777; **Board Cert:** Internal Medicine 1988; Medical Oncology 2006; **Med School:** Albany Med Coll 1985; **Resid:** Internal Medicine, Univ Pittsburgh Hlth Ctr Hosp 1988; **Fellow:** Medical Oncology, Dana Farber Cancer Inst 1993; **Fac Appt:** Assoc Prof Med, Robert W Johnson Med Sch

Trump, Donald L MD [Onc] - **Spec Exp:** Prostate Cancer; Genitourinary Cancer; Drug Discovery & Development; **Hospital:** Roswell Park Cancer Inst; **Address:** Elm & Carlton St, Buffalo, NY 14263; **Phone:** 716-845-3499; **Board Cert:** Internal Medicine 1973; Medical Oncology 1977; **Med School:** Johns Hopkins Univ 1970; **Resid:** Internal Medicine, Johns Hopkins Hosp 1975; **Fellow:** Medical Oncology, Johns Hopkins Hosp 1974; **Fac Appt:** Prof Med, SUNY Buffalo

Medical Oncology

Vaughn, David J MD [Onc] - **Spec Exp:** Testicular Cancer; Bladder Cancer; Prostate Cancer; Genitourinary Cancer; **Hospital:** Hosp Univ Penn - UPHS (page 81), Penn Presby Med Ctr - UPHS (page 81); **Address:** Hosp Univ of Pennsylvania-16 Penn Tower, 3400 Spruce St, Philadelphia, PA 19104; **Phone:** 215-349-8140; **Board Cert:** Medical Oncology 2003; **Med School:** Harvard Med Sch 1987; **Resid:** Internal Medicine, NY Hosp-Cornell Med Ctr 1990; **Fellow:** Hematology & Oncology, Hosp U Penn 1993; **Fac Appt:** Assoc Prof Med, Univ Pennsylvania

von Mehren, Margaret MD [Onc] - **Spec Exp:** Sarcoma; Melanoma; Immunotherapy; Gastrointestinal Stromal Tumors; **Hospital:** Fox Chase Cancer Ctr (page 72); **Address:** Fox Chase Cancer Ctr, Dept Med Oncology, 333 Cottman Ave, Philadelphia, PA 19111-2434; **Phone:** 215-728-2570; **Board Cert:** Medical Oncology 1997; **Med School:** Albany Med Coll 1989; **Resid:** Internal Medicine, NYU Med Ctr 1993; **Fellow:** Hematology & Oncology, Fox Chase Cancer Ctr 1996; **Fac Appt:** Assoc Prof Med, Temple Univ

Waintraub, Stanley MD [Onc] - **Spec Exp:** Breast Cancer; Gynecologic Cancer; Bleeding/Coagulation Disorders; **Hospital:** Hackensack Univ Med Ctr (page 73), Holy Name Hosp; **Address:** Northern NJ Cancer Associates, 20 Prospect Ave, Fl 4, Hackensack, NJ 07601-1997; **Phone:** 201-996-5900; **Board Cert:** Internal Medicine 1980; Hematology 1982; Medical Oncology 1983; **Med School:** NY Med Coll 1977; **Resid:** Internal Medicine, Metropolitan Hosp Ctr 1980; **Fellow:** Hematology, Montefiore Hosp Med Ctr 1982; Medical Oncology, Meml Sloan Kettering Cancer Ctr 1983; **Fac Appt:** Asst Clin Prof Med, UMDNJ-NJ Med Sch, Newark

Weiner, Louis M MD [Onc] - **Spec Exp:** Gastrointestinal Cancer; Immunotherapy; Liver Cancer; **Hospital:** Georgetown Univ Hosp; **Address:** Lombardi Cancer Ctr, Georgetown Univ, Research Bldg - rm E501, 3970 Reservoir Rd NW, Washington, DC 20057; **Phone:** 202-687-2110; **Board Cert:** Internal Medicine 1980; Medical Oncology 1985; **Med School:** Mount Sinai Sch Med 1977; **Resid:** Internal Medicine, Med Ctr Hosp Vermont 1981; **Fellow:** Hematology & Oncology, New England Med Ctr 1984; **Fac Appt:** Prof Med, Georgetown Univ

Wolff, Antonio C MD [Onc] - **Spec Exp:** Breast Cancer; Drug Development; **Hospital:** Johns Hopkins Hosp; **Address:** 1650 Orleans St, rm 189, crb-1 Bldg, Baltimore, MD 21231; **Phone:** 410-614-4192; **Board Cert:** Internal Medicine 2000; Medical Oncology 2000; **Med School:** Brazil 1986; **Resid:** Internal Medicine, Mt Sinai Med Ctr 1991; **Fellow:** Hematology & Oncology, Washington Univ Med Ctr 1992; Medical Oncology, Johns Hopkins Hosp 1995; **Fac Appt:** Assoc Prof Med, Johns Hopkins Univ

Zelenetz, Andrew D MD/PhD [Onc] - **Spec Exp:** Lymphoma; **Hospital:** Meml Sloan-Kettering Cancer Ctr (page 76); **Address:** 1275 York Avenue, New York, NY 10065; **Phone:** 800-525-2225; **Med School:** Harvard Med Sch 1984; **Resid:** Internal Medicine, Stanford Univ Med Ctr 1986; **Fellow:** Medical Oncology, Stanford Univ Med Ctr 1991; **Fac Appt:** Asst Prof Med, Cornell Univ-Weill Med Coll

Southeast

Antonia, Scott J MD/PhD [Onc] - **Spec Exp:** Kidney Cancer; Lung Cancer; **Hospital:** H Lee Moffitt Cancer Ctr & Research Inst; **Address:** H Lee Moffitt Cancer Ctr, 12902 Magnolia Drive, Tampa, FL 33612; **Phone:** 813-979-3883; **Board Cert:** Internal Medicine 2002; Medical Oncology 2006; **Med School:** Univ Conn 1989; **Resid:** Internal Medicine, Yale-New Haven Hosp 1991; **Fellow:** Medical Oncology, Yale-New Haven Hosp 1994; **Fac Appt:** Assoc Prof Med, Univ S Fla Coll Med

Arteaga, Carlos L MD [Onc] - **Spec Exp:** Breast Cancer; **Hospital:** Vanderbilt Univ Med Ctr, VA Med Ctr - Nashville; **Address:** Vanderbilt-Ingram Cancer Ctr, 2220 Pierce Ave, 777-PRB, Nashville, TN 37232-6838; **Phone:** 615-936-3524; **Board Cert:** Internal Medicine 1984; Medical Oncology 1989; **Med School:** Ecuador 1980; **Resid:** Internal Medicine, Grady Meml Hosp 1984; **Fellow:** Hematology & Oncology, Univ Texas Hlth Sci Ctr 1987; **Fac Appt:** Prof Med, Vanderbilt Univ

Balducci, Lodovico MD [Onc] - **Spec Exp:** Genitourinary Cancer; Breast Cancer; **Hospital:** H Lee Moffitt Cancer Ctr & Research Inst, Tampa Genl Hosp; **Address:** H Lee Moffitt Cancer Ctr, 12902 Magnolia Drive, Tampa, FL 33612; **Phone:** 813-745-8658; **Board Cert:** Internal Medicine 1987; Hematology 1978; Medical Oncology 1979; **Med School:** Italy 1968; **Resid:** Internal Medicine, Univ Miss Med Ctr 1976; Hematology & Oncology, Univ Miss Med Ctr 1979; **Fellow:** Internal Medicine, A Gemelli Genl Hosp 1970; **Fac Appt:** Prof Med, Univ S Fla Coll Med

Benedetto, Pasquale W MD [Onc] - **Spec Exp:** Genitourinary Cancer; Bladder Cancer; Kidney Cancer; Pancreatic Cancer; **Hospital:** Univ of Miami Hosp & Clins/Sylvester Comp Canc Ctr (page 82), Jackson Meml Hosp (page 82); **Address:** Sylvester Comp Cancer Ctr, Med Oncology, 1475 NW 12th Ave, Ste 3310, Locator D8-4, Miami, FL 33136; **Phone:** 305-243-4909; **Board Cert:** Internal Medicine 1979; Medical Oncology 1981; Hematology 1982; **Med School:** Cornell Univ-Weill Med Coll 1976; **Resid:** Internal Medicine, Johns Hopkins Hosp 1979; **Fellow:** Medical Oncology, Meml Sloan Kettering Cancer Ctr 1981; **Fac Appt:** Prof Med, Univ Miami Sch Med

Berlin, Jordan D MD [Onc] - **Spec Exp:** Gastrointestinal Cancer; Pancreatic Cancer; Liver Cancer; **Hospital:** Vanderbilt Univ Med Ctr; **Address:** 777 Preston Research Building, Nashville, TN 37232-0001; **Phone:** 615-322-6053; **Board Cert:** Internal Medicine 2002; Medical Oncology 2005; **Med School:** Univ IL Coll Med 1989; **Resid:** Internal Medicine, Univ Cincinnati 1992; **Fellow:** Medical Oncology, Univ Wisconsin 1995; **Fac Appt:** Assoc Prof Med, Vanderbilt Univ

Bernard, Stephen MD [Onc] - **Spec Exp:** Gastrointestinal Cancer; Palliative Care; Clinical Trials; **Hospital:** Univ NC Hosps; **Address:** Univ North Carolina Sch Med, 170 Manning Drive, CB 7305, Chapel Hill, NC 27599; **Phone:** 919-966-0000; **Board Cert:** Internal Medicine 1987; Medical Oncology 1979; Hospice & Palliative Medicine 2004; **Med School:** Univ NC Sch Med 1973; **Resid:** Internal Medicine, Columbia-Presby Med Ctr 1976; **Fellow:** Hematology & Oncology, Wash Univ Hosps 1978; **Fac Appt:** Prof Med, Univ NC Sch Med

Bolger, Graeme B MD [Onc] - **Spec Exp:** Prostate Cancer; Testicular Cancer; **Hospital:** Univ of Ala Hosp at Birmingham; **Address:** 1530 3rd Ave S, Ste FOT-1105, Birmingham, AL 35294; **Phone:** 205-934-2992; **Board Cert:** Internal Medicine 1984; Medical Oncology 2000; **Med School:** McGill Univ 1981; **Resid:** Internal Medicine, Johns Hopkins Hosp 1984; **Fellow:** Medical Oncology, Fred Hutchinson Cancer Rsch 1985; Oncology, Meml Sloan-Kettering Cancer Ctr 1992; **Fac Appt:** Assoc Prof Med, Univ Alabama

Boston, Barry MD [Onc] - **Spec Exp:** Gastrointestinal Cancer; Genitourinary Cancer; Prostate Cancer; **Hospital:** St Francis Hosp - Memphis, Methodist Univ Hosp - Memphis; **Address:** Univ of Tennessee Cancer Inst, 7945 Wolf River Blvd, Ste 300, Germantown, TN 38138; **Phone:** 901-752-6131; **Board Cert:** Internal Medicine 1974; Medical Oncology 1977; **Med School:** Louisiana State U, New Orleans 1971; **Resid:** Internal Medicine, Univ Tenn Hosp-VA Hosp 1973; Hematology, Univ Tenn Hosp-VA Hosp 1973; **Fellow:** Medical Oncology, Yale-New Haven Hosp 1975; **Fac Appt:** Assoc Prof Med, Univ Tenn Coll Med, Memphis

Medical Oncology

Brescia, Frank J MD [Onc] - **Spec Exp:** Palliative Care; Breast Cancer; Gastrointestinal Cancer; Ethics; **Hospital:** Roper Hosp, MUSC Med Ctr; **Address:** Low Country Hematology & Oncology, 900 Bowman Drive, Mount Pleasant, SC 29464; **Phone:** 843-881-5844; **Board Cert:** Internal Medicine 1974; Medical Oncology 1975; **Med School:** UMDNJ-NJ Med Sch, Newark 1968; **Resid:** Internal Medicine, North Shore Univ Hosp 1970; **Fellow:** Medical Oncology, Meml Sloan Kettering Cancer Ctr 1974; **Fac Appt:** Prof Med, Med Univ SC

Burris III, Howard A MD [Onc] - **Spec Exp:** Drug Development; Drug Discovery; Breast Cancer; **Hospital:** Centennial Med Ctr, Baptist Hosp - Nashville; **Address:** 250 25th Ave N Atrium Bldg - Ste 100, Nashville, TN 37203; **Phone:** 615-329-7276; **Board Cert:** Internal Medicine 1988; Medical Oncology 2001; **Med School:** Univ S Ala Coll Med 1985; **Resid:** Internal Medicine, Brooke Army Med Ctr 1988; **Fellow:** Medical Oncology, Brooke Army Med Ctr 1991

Butler, William M MD [Onc] - **Spec Exp:** Breast Cancer; Prostate Cancer; Lung Cancer; Clinical Trials; **Hospital:** Palmetto Richland Mem Hosp; **Address:** SC Oncology Associates, 166 Stoneridge St, Columbia, SC 29210; **Phone:** 803-461-3000; **Board Cert:** Internal Medicine 1975; Hematology 1980; Medical Oncology 1979; **Med School:** Tulane Univ 1972; **Resid:** Internal Medicine, Charity Hosp 1975; **Fellow:** Hematology & Oncology, Walter Reed AMC 1980; **Fac Appt:** Clin Prof Med, Univ SC Sch Med

Carbone, David MD/PhD [Onc] - **Spec Exp:** Lung Cancer; **Hospital:** Vanderbilt Univ Med Ctr; **Address:** Vanderbilt-Ingram Cancer Ctr, 685 Preston Rsch Bldg, 2200 Pierce Ave, Nashville, TN 37232-6838; **Phone:** 615-936-1279; **Board Cert:** Internal Medicine 1988; Medical Oncology 2001; **Med School:** Johns Hopkins Univ 1985; **Resid:** Internal Medicine, Johns Hopkins Hosp 1988; **Fellow:** Oncology, Natl Cancer Inst 1991; **Fac Appt:** Prof Med, Vanderbilt Univ

Carey, Lisa A MD [Onc] - **Spec Exp:** Breast Cancer; **Hospital:** Univ NC Hosps; **Address:** Univ North Carolina-Div Hem/Onc, Campus Box 7305, 3009 Old Clinic Bldg, Chapel Hill, NC 27599; **Phone:** 919-966-4431; **Board Cert:** Internal Medicine 2003; Medical Oncology 2007; **Med School:** Johns Hopkins Univ 1990; **Resid:** Internal Medicine, Johns Hopkins Hosp 1993; **Fellow:** Oncology, Johns Hopkins Hosp 1996; **Fac Appt:** Asst Prof Med, Univ NC Sch Med

Carpenter Jr, John T MD [Onc] - **Spec Exp:** Breast Cancer; **Hospital:** Univ of Ala Hosp at Birmingham; **Address:** Univ Alabama Birmingham, 1530 3rd Ave S, Birmingham, AL 35294-3300; **Phone:** 205-934-2084; **Board Cert:** Internal Medicine 1972; Hematology 1981; Medical Oncology 1975; **Med School:** Tulane Univ 1968; **Resid:** Internal Medicine, Grady Meml Hosp 1971; **Fellow:** Hematology & Oncology, Emory Univ 1973; **Fac Appt:** Prof Med, Univ Alabama

Chao, Nelson Jen An MD [Onc] - **Spec Exp:** Bone Marrow Transplant; Lymphoma; Leukemia; **Hospital:** Duke Univ Med Ctr; **Address:** Duke Univ Med Ctr, Box 3961, Durham, NC 27710; **Phone:** 919-668-1002; **Board Cert:** Internal Medicine 1984; Medical Oncology 1987; **Med School:** Yale Univ 1981; **Resid:** Internal Medicine, Stanford Univ Med Ctr 1984; **Fellow:** Oncology, Stanford Univ Med Ctr 1987; **Fac Appt:** Prof Med, Duke Univ

Colon-Otero, Gerardo MD [Onc] - **Spec Exp:** Ovarian Cancer; Breast Cancer; Hematologic Malignancies; **Hospital:** Mayo - Jacksonville, St Luke's Hosp - Jacksonville; **Address:** Mayo Clinic Jacksonville, 4500 San Pablo Rd S, Jacksonville, FL 32224-1865; **Phone:** 904-953-2000; **Board Cert:** Internal Medicine 1982; Hematology 1984; Medical Oncology 1985; **Med School:** Puerto Rico 1979; **Resid:** Internal Medicine, Mayo Clinic 1982; **Fellow:** Hematology, Mayo Clinic 1984; Medical Oncology, Univ Va Med Ctr 1986; **Fac Appt:** Assoc Prof Med, Mayo Med Sch

Conry, Robert M MD [Onc] - **Spec Exp:** Melanoma; Lung Cancer; Colon & Rectal Cancer; Sarcoma; **Hospital:** Univ of Ala Hosp at Birmingham; **Address:** The Kirklin Clinic At Acton Rd, 2145 Bonner Way, Birmingham, AL 35243; **Phone:** 205-978-0250; **Board Cert:** Hematology 2001; **Med School:** Univ Alabama 1987; **Resid:** Internal Medicine, Univ Alabama Hosp 1990; **Fellow:** Medical Oncology, Univ Alabama Hosp 1993; **Fac Appt:** Assoc Prof Med, Univ Alabama

Crawford, Jeffrey MD [Onc] - **Spec Exp:** Lung Cancer; **Hospital:** Duke Univ Med Ctr; **Address:** Duke Univ Med Ctr, Box 3476, Durham, NC 27710-0001; **Phone:** 919-668-6688; **Board Cert:** Internal Medicine 1977; Hematology 1980; Medical Oncology 1981; **Med School:** Ohio State Univ 1974; **Resid:** Internal Medicine, Duke Univ Med Ctr 1977; **Fellow:** Hematology & Oncology, Duke Univ Med Ctr 1981; **Fac Appt:** Prof Med, Duke Univ

De Simone, Philip MD [Onc] - **Spec Exp:** Colon Cancer; Pancreatic Cancer; **Hospital:** Univ of Kentucky Chandler Hosp; **Address:** UKMC Markey Cancer Ctr, 800 Rose St, rm 134, Whitney-Hendrickson bldg, Lexington, KY 40536; **Phone:** 859-323-8043; **Board Cert:** Internal Medicine 1972; Hematology 1974; **Med School:** Univ VT Coll Med 1967; **Resid:** Internal Medicine, Univ Kentucky Hosp 1972; **Fellow:** Hematology & Oncology, Univ Kentucky Hosp 1974; **Fac Appt:** Prof Med, Univ KY Coll Med

Dunphy, Frank R MD [Onc] - **Spec Exp:** Lung Cancer; Head & Neck Cancer; **Hospital:** Duke Univ Med Ctr; **Address:** Duke Univ Med Ctr, Box 3685, Durham, NC 27710; **Phone:** 919-668-6688; **Board Cert:** Internal Medicine 1984; Hematology 1986; Medical Oncology 1989; **Med School:** Louisiana State U, New Orleans 1979; **Resid:** Internal Medicine, Lousiana St Univ Hosp 1983; **Fellow:** Hematology & Oncology, Louisiana St Univ Hosp 1985; **Fac Appt:** Assoc Prof Med, Duke Univ

Flinn, Ian W MD/PhD [Onc] - **Spec Exp:** Hematologic Malignancies; Lymphoma; Bone Marrow Transplant; Clinical Trials; **Hospital:** Centennial Med Ctr; **Address:** Tennessee Oncology, 250 25th Ave N, Ste 412, Nashville, TN 37203; **Phone:** 615-986-7600; **Board Cert:** Hematology 2007; Medical Oncology 2008; **Med School:** Johns Hopkins Univ 1990; **Resid:** Internal Medicine, Univ Michigan Med Ctr 1993; **Fellow:** Hematology & Oncology, Johns Hopkins Univ Hosps 1993

Forero, Andres MD [Onc] - **Spec Exp:** Lymphoma; **Hospital:** Univ of Ala Hosp at Birmingham; **Address:** 615 18th St S, Birmingham, AL 35233; **Phone:** 205-934-9999; **Med School:** Colombia 1982; **Resid:** Internal Medicine, Javeriana Univ 1987; **Fellow:** Medical Oncology, Javeriana Univ 1991; **Fac Appt:** Assoc Prof Med, Univ Alabama

Fracasso, Paula M MD/PhD [Onc] - **Spec Exp:** Gynecologic Cancer; Breast Cancer; **Hospital:** Univ Virginia Med Ctr; **Address:** Dept Medicine, Div Hem/Onc, PO Box 800716, Charlottesville, VA 22908; **Phone:** 434-243-6143; **Board Cert:** Internal Medicine 1987; Medical Oncology 2003; **Med School:** Yale Univ 1984; **Resid:** Internal Medicine, Beth Israel Hosp 1987; **Fellow:** Cancer Research, Mass Inst Tech 1989; Hematology & Oncology, Tufts-New England Med Ctr 1991; **Fac Appt:** Prof Med, Univ VA Sch Med

Garst, Jennifer L MD [Onc] - **Spec Exp:** Lung Cancer; Thoracic Cancers; Cancer Survivors-Late Effects of Therapy; **Hospital:** Duke Univ Med Ctr; **Address:** Reg Cancer Care Ctr, 4411 Ben Franklin Blvd, Durham, NC 27704; **Phone:** 919-477-0047; **Board Cert:** Internal Medicine 2008; **Med School:** Med Coll GA 1990; **Resid:** Internal Medicine, Univ SW Texas Hosp 1993; **Fellow:** Hematology & Oncology, Duke Univ Med Ctr 1996; **Fac Appt:** Assoc Prof Med, Duke Univ

Gockerman, Jon Paul MD [Onc] - **Spec Exp:** Leukemia; Lymphoma; **Hospital:** Duke Univ Med Ctr; **Address:** Duke Univ Med Ctr, 1 Trent Drive, rm 25153, Box 3872, Morris Bldg, Durham, NC 27710; **Phone:** 919-684-8964; **Board Cert:** Internal Medicine 1972; Hematology 1974; Medical Oncology 1973; **Med School:** Univ Chicago-Pritzker Sch Med 1967; **Resid:** Internal Medicine, Duke Univ Med Ctr 1969; **Fellow:** Hematology & Oncology, Duke Univ Med Ctr 1971

Medical Oncology

Goldberg, Richard M MD [Onc] - **Spec Exp:** Stomach Cancer; Esophageal Cancer; Pancreatic Cancer; Neuroendocrine Tumors; **Hospital:** Univ NC Hosps; **Address:** Division of Hematology/Oncology, CB 7305, 3009 Old Clinic Bldg SW, Chapel Hill, NC 27599-0001; **Phone:** 919-843-7711; **Board Cert:** Internal Medicine 1982; Medical Oncology 1985; **Med School:** SUNY Upstate Med Univ 1979; **Resid:** Internal Medicine, Emory Univ Med Ctr 1982; **Fellow:** Medical Oncology, Georgetown Univ Med Ctr 1984; **Fac Appt:** Prof Med, Univ NC Sch Med

Graham II, Mark L MD [Onc] - **Spec Exp:** Breast Cancer; Breast Cancer Genetics; **Hospital:** WakeMed Cary; **Address:** Waverly Hematology/Oncology, 300 Ashville Ave, Ste 310, Cary, NC 27518; **Phone:** 919-233-8585; **Board Cert:** Internal Medicine 1989; **Med School:** Mayo Med Sch 1982; **Resid:** Internal Medicine, Duke Univ Med Ctr 1985; **Fellow:** Medical Oncology, Univ CO Hlth Sci Ctr 1990; Medical Oncology, Mayo Clinic 1991; **Fac Appt:** Assoc Clin Prof Med, Univ NC Sch Med

Greco, F Anthony MD [Onc] - **Spec Exp:** Lung Cancer; Unknown Primary Cancer; **Hospital:** Centennial Med Ctr; **Address:** Sarah Cannon Research Inst, 250 25th Ave N Atrium Bldg - Ste 100, Nashville, TN 37203; **Phone:** 615-320-5090; **Board Cert:** Internal Medicine 1975; Medical Oncology 1977; **Med School:** W VA Univ 1972; **Resid:** Internal Medicine, Univ West Virginia Hosp 1974; **Fellow:** Medical Oncology, Natl Cancer Inst 1976

Grosh, William W MD [Onc] - **Spec Exp:** Melanoma; Sarcoma; Neuroendocrine Tumors; **Hospital:** Univ Virginia Med Ctr; **Address:** UVA Health System, Div Hem/Oncology, PO Box 800716, Charlottesville, VA 22908; **Phone:** 434-924-1904; **Board Cert:** Internal Medicine 1978; Medical Oncology 1985; **Med School:** Columbia P&S 1974; **Resid:** Internal Medicine, Vanderbilt Univ Med Ctr 1977; **Fellow:** Medical Oncology, Vanderbilt Univ Med Ctr 1983; **Fac Appt:** Assoc Prof Med, Univ VA Sch Med

Hande, Kenneth R MD [Onc] - **Spec Exp:** Drug Discovery; Sarcoma; Carcinoid Tumors; **Hospital:** Vanderbilt Univ Med Ctr, VA Med Ctr - Nashville; **Address:** Vanderbilt Univ Med Ctr, 777 Preston Research Building, Nashville, TN 37232-6307; **Phone:** 615-322-4967; **Board Cert:** Internal Medicine 1975; Medical Oncology 1977; **Med School:** Johns Hopkins Univ 1972; **Resid:** Internal Medicine, Barnes Hosp 1974; **Fellow:** Medical Oncology, Natl Cancer Inst 1977; **Fac Appt:** Prof Med, Vanderbilt Univ

Hurd, David MD [Onc] - **Spec Exp:** Lymphoma; Leukemia; Bone Marrow Transplant; **Hospital:** Wake Forest Univ Baptist Med Ctr (page 84); **Address:** Wake Forest Sch Med, Comp Cancer Ctr, Medical Center Boulevard, Winston-Salem, NC 27157-1082; **Phone:** 336-713-5440; **Board Cert:** Internal Medicine 1977; Medical Oncology 1981; **Med School:** Univ IL Coll Med 1974; **Resid:** Internal Medicine, Univ Minn Hosp 1977; **Fellow:** Medical Oncology, Univ Minn Hosp 1979; **Fac Appt:** Prof Med, Wake Forest Univ

Jahanzeb, Mohammad MD [Onc] - **Spec Exp:** Breast Cancer; Lung Cancer; **Hospital:** Boca Raton Comm Hosp; **Address:** 21020 State Rd 7, Boca Raton, FL 33428; **Phone:** 561-883-7600; **Board Cert:** Medical Oncology 2003; Hematology 2005; **Med School:** Pakistan 1986; **Resid:** Internal Medicine, New Britain Genl Hosp 1990; **Fellow:** Hematology & Oncology, Washington Univ 1993

Jillella, Anand MD [Onc] - **Spec Exp:** Bone Marrow Transplant; Leukemia; Lymphoma; Multiple Myeloma; **Hospital:** Med Coll of GA Hosp and Clin (MCG Health Inc); **Address:** Med Coll Ga - BMT Program, 1120 15th St, BAA 5407, Augusta, GA 30912-3125; **Phone:** 706-721-2505; **Board Cert:** Medical Oncology 1997; **Med School:** India 1985; **Resid:** Internal Medicine, Med Coll Georgia 1992; **Fellow:** Medical Oncology, Yale-New Haven Hosp 1996; **Fac Appt:** Prof Med, Med Coll GA

Johnson, David H MD [Onc] - **Spec Exp:** Lung Cancer; Breast Cancer; Drug Development; **Hospital:** Vanderbilt Univ Med Ctr; **Address:** Vanderbilt Univ Med Ctr, Div Med Onc, 2220 Pierce Ave, 777 PRB, Nashville, TN 37232-0021; **Phone:** 615-322-6053; **Board Cert:** Internal Medicine 1979; Medical Oncology 2008; **Med School:** Med Coll GA 1976; **Resid:** Internal Medicine, Univ South Alabama Med Ctr 1979; Internal Medicine, Med Coll Georgia Hosps 1980; **Fellow:** Medical Oncology, Vanderbilt Univ Med Ctr 1983; **Fac Appt:** Prof Med, Vanderbilt Univ

Khuri, Fadlo MD [Onc] - **Spec Exp:** Lung Cancer; Head & Neck Cancer; **Hospital:** Emory Univ Hosp, Grady Hlth Sys; **Address:** Winship Cancer Institute, 1365 Clifton Rd NE, C Bldg Fl 2, Atlanta, GA 30322; **Phone:** 404-778-1900; **Board Cert:** Medical Oncology 2008; **Med School:** Columbia P&S 1989; **Resid:** Internal Medicine, Boston City Hosp 1992; **Fellow:** Medical Oncology, New England Med Ctr-Tufts 1995; **Fac Appt:** Prof Hem & Onc, Emory Univ

Kraft, Andrew S MD [Onc] - **Spec Exp:** Prostate Cancer; Sarcoma; Drug Development; Clinical Trials; **Hospital:** MUSC Med Ctr; **Address:** 86 Jonathan Lucas St, PO BOX 250955, Charleston, SC 29425; **Phone:** 843-792-8284; **Board Cert:** Internal Medicine 1980; Medical Oncology 1985; **Med School:** Univ Pennsylvania 1975; **Resid:** Internal Medicine, Mt Sinai Hosp 1979; **Fellow:** Medical Oncology, Natl Cancer Inst 1983; **Fac Appt:** Prof Med, Med Univ SC

Kucuk, Omer MD [Onc] - **Spec Exp:** Genitourinary Cancer; Nutrition in Cancer Therapy; Prostate Cancer; Nutrition & Cancer Prevention/Control; **Hospital:** Emory Univ Hosp; **Address:** Winship Cancer Inst, 1365C Clifton Rd, Ste 2110, Atlanta, GA 30322; **Phone:** 404-778-1900; **Board Cert:** Internal Medicine 1978; Hematology 1984; Medical Oncology 1989; **Med School:** Turkey 1975; **Resid:** Internal Medicine, St Francis Hosp 1978; **Fellow:** Hematology & Oncology, Northwestern Univ 1981; **Fac Appt:** Prof Hem & Onc, Emory Univ

Kvols, Larry K MD [Onc] - **Spec Exp:** Gastrointestinal Cancer; Carcinoid Tumors; Neuroendocrine Tumors; **Hospital:** H Lee Moffitt Cancer Ctr & Research Inst; **Address:** H Lee Moffitt Cancer Ctr & Research Inst, 12902 Magnolia Drive, WCB-GI Program, Tampa, FL 33612-9497; **Phone:** 813-745-7257; **Board Cert:** Internal Medicine 1976; Medical Oncology 1977; **Med School:** Baylor Coll Med 1970; **Resid:** Internal Medicine, Johns Hopkins Hosp 1972; **Fellow:** Hematology & Oncology, Johns Hopkins Hosp 1973; **Fac Appt:** Prof Med, Mayo Med Sch

Lawson, David H MD [Onc] - **Spec Exp:** Melanoma; **Hospital:** Emory Univ Hosp; **Address:** Winship Cancer Institute, 1365 Clifton Rd NE C Bldg, Atlanta, GA 30322; **Phone:** 404-778-1900; **Board Cert:** Internal Medicine 1977; Medical Oncology 1979; **Med School:** Emory Univ 1974; **Resid:** Internal Medicine, Emory Univ Hosps 1977; **Fellow:** Medical Oncology, Emory Univ Hosps 1979; **Fac Appt:** Assoc Prof Med, Emory Univ

Lesser, Glenn J MD [Onc] - **Spec Exp:** Neuro-Oncology; Brain Tumors; **Hospital:** Wake Forest Univ Baptist Med Ctr (page 84); **Address:** Wake Forest Univ-Div Hematolgy/Oncology, Medical Center Blvd, Winston-Salem, NC 27157-1082; **Phone:** 336-716-9527; **Board Cert:** Medical Oncology 2007; **Med School:** Penn State Univ-Hershey Med Ctr 1987; **Resid:** Internal Medicine, NC Baptist Hosp/Bowman Gray Sch Med 1991; **Fellow:** Medical Oncology, Johns Hopkins Hosp 1994; **Fac Appt:** Assoc Prof Med, Wake Forest Univ

Lilenbaum, Rogerio MD [Onc] - **Spec Exp:** Lung Cancer; **Hospital:** Mount Sinai Med Ctr - Miami; **Address:** Mount Sinai Cancer Ctr, 4306 Alton Rd, Ste 3, Miami, FL 33140-2840; **Phone:** 305-535-3310; **Board Cert:** Internal Medicine 2005; Hematology 1998; Medical Oncology 2007; **Med School:** Brazil 1986; **Resid:** Internal Medicine, Univ Hosp-Rio de Janeiro 1989; **Fellow:** Hematology & Oncology, Washington Univ Sch Med 1992; Oncology, UCSD 1994; **Fac Appt:** Assoc Clin Prof Med, Univ Miami Sch Med

Medical Oncology

Limentani, Steven A MD [Onc] - **Spec Exp:** Breast Cancer; Multiple Myeloma; Clinical Trials; **Hospital:** Carolinas Med Ctr; **Address:** 1100 S Tryon St, Ste 400, Charlotte, NC 28203; **Phone:** 704-446-9046; **Board Cert:** Internal Medicine 1989; Medical Oncology 2001; Hematology 2002; **Med School:** Tufts Univ 1986; **Resid:** Internal Medicine, New England Deaconess Hosp 1989; **Fellow:** Hematology & Oncology, New England Med Ctr 1992; **Fac Appt:** Clin Prof Med, Univ NC Sch Med

Lippman, Marc E MD [Onc] - **Spec Exp:** Breast Cancer; **Hospital:** Univ of Miami Hosp & Clins/Sylvester Comp Canc Ctr (page 82); **Address:** Leonard M Miller Sch Med, Dept Med, 1430 NW 11th Ave, MTSL, Ste 1001, Miami, FL 33136; **Phone:** 305-243-9120; **Board Cert:** Internal Medicine 1987; Endocrinology 1975; Medical Oncology 1977; **Med School:** Yale Univ 1968; **Resid:** Internal Medicine, Johns Hopkins Hosp 1970; **Fellow:** Medical Oncology, Natl Cancer Inst 1973; Endocrinology, Yale-New Haven Hosp 1974; **Fac Appt:** Prof Med, Univ Mich Med Sch

Lossos, Izidore MD [Onc] - **Spec Exp:** Lymphoma; Hodgkin's Disease; Leukemia; **Hospital:** Univ of Miami Hosp & Clins/Sylvester Comp Canc Ctr (page 82), Jackson Meml Hosp (page 82); **Address:** Univ Miami - Sylvester Comp Cancer Ctr, 1475 NW 12th Ave, D8-4, Miami, FL 33136; **Phone:** 305-243-4785; **Med School:** Israel 1987; **Resid:** Internal Medicine, Hadassah Univ Hosp 1995; **Fellow:** Hematology & Oncology, Hadassah Univ Hosp 1997; Medical Oncology, Stanford Univ 2001; **Fac Appt:** Prof Med, Univ Miami Sch Med

Lyckholm, Laurel J MD [Onc] - **Spec Exp:** Neuro-Oncology; **Hospital:** Med Coll of VA Hosp; **Address:** Med Coll of VA, Div Hem/Onc, PO Box 980230, Richmond, VA 23298; **Phone:** 804-828-9723; **Board Cert:** Internal Medicine 1989; Medical Oncology 2003; Hematology 2004; **Med School:** Creighton Univ 1985; **Resid:** Internal Medicine, Creighton Univ 1989; **Fellow:** Hematology & Oncology, Univ IA Coll Med 1992; **Fac Appt:** Assoc Prof Med, Med Coll VA

Lyman, Gary H MD [Onc] - **Spec Exp:** Breast Cancer; **Hospital:** Duke Univ Med Ctr; **Address:** Duke Comprehensive Cancer Center, Hock Plaza, 2424 Erwin Rd, Ste 602 - rm 6038, Box 3645, Durham, NC 27710; **Phone:** 919-681-1736; **Board Cert:** Internal Medicine 1987; Medical Oncology 1977; Hematology 1978; **Med School:** SUNY Buffalo 1972; **Resid:** Internal Medicine, Univ North Carolina Hosp 1974; **Fellow:** Medical Oncology, Roswell Park Meml Inst 1976; Biostatistics, Harvard Med Sch 1982; **Fac Appt:** Prof Med, Duke Univ

Lynch Jr, James W MD [Onc] - **Spec Exp:** Lymphoma; Immunotherapy; Lung Cancer; **Hospital:** Shands at Univ of FL; **Address:** Shands Hlthcare, Div Hematology/Oncology, PO Box 100383, Gainesville, FL 32610-0383; **Phone:** 352-265-0725; **Board Cert:** Internal Medicine 1987; Medical Oncology 2001; **Med School:** Eastern VA Med Sch 1984; **Resid:** Internal Medicine, Univ Florida 1987; **Fellow:** Medical Oncology, Natl Cancer Inst 1991; **Fac Appt:** Prof Med, Univ Fla Coll Med

Marcom, Paul K MD [Onc] - **Spec Exp:** Breast Cancer; Clinical Trials; Cancer Genetics; **Hospital:** Duke Univ Med Ctr; **Address:** Duke Univ Med Ctr, Box 3147, Seeley G Mudd Bldg, Ste 461, Durham, NC 27710; **Phone:** 919-684-3877; **Board Cert:** Internal Medicine 2003; Medical Oncology 2005; **Med School:** Baylor Coll Med 1989; **Resid:** Internal Medicine, Duke Univ Med Ctr 1992; Hematology & Oncology, Duke Univ Med Ctr 1995; **Fac Appt:** Assoc Prof Med, Duke Univ

Miller, Antonius A MD [Onc] - **Spec Exp:** Lung Cancer; **Hospital:** Wake Forest Univ Baptist Med Ctr (page 84); **Address:** Wake Forest Baptist Med Ctr, Comp Cancer Ctr, 3rd Fl (Hem/Onc), Medical Center Boulevard, Winston-Salem, NC 27157; **Phone:** 336-713-4392; **Med School:** Germany 1977; **Resid:** Internal Medicine, Univ Essen Med Sch 1979; **Fellow:** Hematology & Oncology, UT MD Anderson Cancer Ctr 1981; **Fac Appt:** Prof Med, Wake Forest Univ

Miller, Donald M MD/PhD [Onc] - **Spec Exp:** Melanoma; Lung Cancer; **Hospital:** Univ of Louisville Hosp; **Address:** 529 S Jackson St, Louisville, KY 40202; **Phone:** 502-562-4790; **Board Cert:** Internal Medicine 1979; **Med School:** Duke Univ 1973; **Resid:** Internal Medicine, Peter Bent Brigham Hosp 1975; **Fellow:** Internal Medicine, Peter Bent Brigham Hosp 1978; Medical Oncology, Natl Cancer Inst 1979; **Fac Appt:** Prof Med, Univ Louisville Sch Med

Moore, Joseph O MD [Onc] - **Spec Exp:** Leukemia; Hodgkin's Disease; Lymphoma, Non-Hodgkin's; Neuroendocrine Tumors; **Hospital:** Duke Univ Med Ctr; **Address:** Duke Univ Med Ctr, Box 3872, Durham, NC 27710; **Phone:** 919-684-8964; **Board Cert:** Internal Medicine 1975; Medical Oncology 1977; **Med School:** Johns Hopkins Univ 1970; **Resid:** Internal Medicine, Johns Hopkins Hosp 1975; **Fellow:** Hematology & Oncology, Duke Univ 1977; **Fac Appt:** Prof Med, Duke Univ

Muss, Hyman B MD [Onc] - **Spec Exp:** Breast Cancer; **Hospital:** Univ NC Hosps; **Address:** Div of Hem/Onc, Physicians Office Bldg, 170 Manning Drive Fl 3 - rm 3120, Box 7305, Chapel Hill, NC 27599-7305; **Phone:** 919-966-0840; **Board Cert:** Internal Medicine 1973; Hematology 1974; Medical Oncology 1975; **Med School:** SUNY Downstate 1968; **Resid:** Internal Medicine, Peter Bent Brigham Hosp 1971; **Fellow:** Hematology & Oncology, Peter Bent Brigham Hosp 1974

Nabell, Lisle M MD [Onc] - **Spec Exp:** Breast Cancer; Head & Neck Cancer; **Hospital:** Univ of Ala Hosp at Birmingham; **Address:** Univ of Alabama, 1530 3rd Ave S, Ste WTI237, Birmingham, AL 35294; **Phone:** 205-934-3061; **Board Cert:** Internal Medicine 2000; Medical Oncology 2000; **Med School:** Univ NC Sch Med 1987; **Resid:** Internal Medicine, Univ Alabama Hosp 1990; **Fellow:** Hematology & Oncology, Univ Alabama Hosp 1992; **Fac Appt:** Assoc Prof Med, Univ Alabama

O'Regan, Ruth M MD [Onc] - **Spec Exp:** Breast Cancer; Breast Cancer Risk Assessment; Cancer Prevention; Clinical Trials; **Hospital:** Emory Univ Hosp; **Address:** Emory Univ Winship Cancer Inst, 1365C Clifton Rd, Ste 4005, Atlanta, GA 30322; **Phone:** 404-778-1900; **Board Cert:** Internal Medicine 1999; Medical Oncology 2000; **Med School:** Ireland 1988; **Resid:** Internal Medicine, Med Coll Wisconsin 1995; Medical Oncology, Northwestern Univ Hosp 1999; **Fellow:** Medical Oncology, Northwestern Univ Hosp 1998; **Fac Appt:** Assoc Prof Med, Emory Univ

Pasche, Boris C MD/PhD [Onc] - **Spec Exp:** Cancer Genetics; Gastrointestinal Cancer; **Hospital:** Univ of Ala Hosp at Birmingham; **Address:** 2000 Morris Ave, Ste 1610, Birmingham, AL 35203; **Phone:** 205-934-9591; **Board Cert:** Medical Oncology 2008; Hematology 1999; **Med School:** Sweden 1986; **Resid:** Internal Medicine, NY Hosp/Cornell Med Ctr 1994; **Fellow:** Hematology & Oncology, Meml Sloan Kettering Cancer Ctr 1996; **Fac Appt:** Assoc Prof Med, Northwestern Univ

Perez, Edith A MD [Onc] - **Spec Exp:** Breast Cancer; Breast Cancer Risk Assessment; Clinical Trials; **Hospital:** Mayo - Jacksonville; **Address:** Mayo Clinic-Jacksonville, 4500 San Pablo Rd Davis Bldg Fl 8, Jacksonville, FL 32224; **Phone:** 904-953-7283; **Board Cert:** Internal Medicine 1983; Hematology 1986; Medical Oncology 1987; **Med School:** Univ Puerto Rico 1979; **Resid:** Internal Medicine, Loma Linda Univ Med Ctr 1982; **Fellow:** Hematology & Oncology, Martinez VA Hosp/UC Davis 1987; **Fac Appt:** Prof Med, Mayo Med Sch

Posey III, James A MD [Onc] - **Spec Exp:** Gastrointestinal Cancer; Colon Cancer; Liver Cancer; Biliary Cancer; **Hospital:** Univ of Ala Hosp at Birmingham; **Address:** 1806 6th Ave S, NP-2540U, Birmingham, AL 35294-3300; **Phone:** 205-934-0916; **Board Cert:** Medical Oncology 1997; **Med School:** Howard Univ 1991; **Resid:** Internal Medicine, Georgetown Univ Med Ctr 1994; **Fellow:** Hematology & Oncology, Georgetown Univ Med Ctr 1997; **Fac Appt:** Assoc Prof Med, Univ Alabama

Medical Oncology

Robert, Nicholas J MD [Onc] - **Spec Exp:** Breast Cancer; **Hospital:** Inova Fairfax Hosp; **Address:** 8503 Arlington Blvd, Ste 400, Fairfax, VA 22031; **Phone:** 703-280-5390; **Board Cert:** Internal Medicine 1978; Anatomic Pathology 1979; Medical Oncology 1981; Hematology 1984; **Med School:** McGill Univ 1974; **Resid:** Internal Medicine, Royal Victoria Hosp 1976; Pathology, Mass Genl Hosp 1979; **Fellow:** Hematology, Peter Bent Brigham Hosp 1980; Medical Oncology, Dana Farber Cancer Inst 1981

Robert-Vizcarrondo, Francisco MD [Onc] - **Spec Exp:** Lung Cancer; Mesothelioma; Drug Development; Clinical Trials; **Hospital:** Univ of Ala Hosp at Birmingham; **Address:** 1802 6th Ave S, rm NP-2555D, Birmingham, AL 35294-0001; **Phone:** 205-934-5077; **Board Cert:** Internal Medicine 1973; Medical Oncology 1975; Hematology 1976; **Med School:** Puerto Rico 1969; **Resid:** Internal Medicine, Univ PR Hosp 1972; Hematology, Univ PR Hosp 1974; **Fellow:** Medical Oncology, Univ AL Hosp at Birmingham 1976; **Fac Appt:** Prof Med, Univ Alabama

Romond, Edward H MD [Onc] - **Spec Exp:** Breast Cancer; **Hospital:** Univ of Kentucky Chandler Hosp; **Address:** Univ Kentucky Med Ctr, Div Hematology/Oncology, CC413 Markey Cancer Center, Lexington, KY 40536-0093; **Phone:** 859-323-8043; **Board Cert:** Internal Medicine 1980; Hematology 1984; Medical Oncology 1983; **Med School:** Univ KY Coll Med 1977; **Resid:** Internal Medicine, Michigan State Univ Hosps 1980; **Fellow:** Hematology & Oncology, Michigan State Univ 1983; **Fac Appt:** Prof Med, Univ KY Coll Med

Roth, Bruce J MD [Onc] - **Spec Exp:** Prostate Cancer; Bladder Cancer; Testicular Cancer; **Hospital:** Vanderbilt Univ Med Ctr; **Address:** Vanderbilt Ingram Cancer Center, 777 Preston Research Bldg, Nashville, TN 37232-6307; **Phone:** 615-343-4070; **Board Cert:** Internal Medicine 1983; Medical Oncology 1985; **Med School:** St Louis Univ 1980; **Resid:** Internal Medicine, Indiana Univ Med Ctr 1983; **Fellow:** Hematology & Oncology, Indiana Univ Med Ctr 1986; **Fac Appt:** Prof Med, Vanderbilt Univ

Schwartz, Michael A MD [Onc] - **Spec Exp:** Breast Cancer; Lymphoma; Colon Cancer; **Hospital:** Mount Sinai Med Ctr - Miami, Miami Heart Inst; **Address:** 4306 Alton Rd Fl 3, Miami Beach, FL 33140; **Phone:** 305-535-3310; **Board Cert:** Internal Medicine 1989; Medical Oncology 2004; Hematology 2004; **Med School:** UMDNJ-RW Johnson Med Sch 1986; **Resid:** Internal Medicine, Mt Sinai Medical Ctr 1989; **Fellow:** Hematology & Oncology, Meml Sloan Kettering Cancer Ctr 1992; **Fac Appt:** Asst Clin Prof Med, Univ Miami Sch Med

Serody, Jonathan S MD [Onc] - **Spec Exp:** Breast Cancer Vaccine Therapy; Clinical Trials; Lymphoma; **Hospital:** Univ NC Hosps; **Address:** Lineberger Comprehensive Cancer Ctr, 450 West Drive, CB 7295, Chapel Hill, NC 27599-7295; **Phone:** 919-966-8644; **Board Cert:** Internal Medicine 1989; Hematology 2007; **Med School:** Univ VA Sch Med 1986; **Resid:** Internal Medicine, Univ NC Med Ctr 1989; **Fellow:** Hematology, Univ NC Med Ctr 1992; Bone Marrow Transplant, Fred Hutchinson Transplant Program 1993; **Fac Appt:** Assoc Prof Med, Univ NC Sch Med

Shea, Thomas MD [Onc] - **Spec Exp:** Bone Marrow Transplant; Lymphoma; Leukemia; **Hospital:** Univ NC Hosps; **Address:** Univ N Carolina, Dept Medicine, 170 Manning Drive, CB 7305, Chapel Hill, NC 27599; **Phone:** 919-966-7746; **Board Cert:** Internal Medicine 1982; Hematology 1984; Medical Oncology 1985; **Med School:** Univ NC Sch Med 1978; **Resid:** Internal Medicine, Beth Israel Deaconess Med Ctr 1982; **Fellow:** Hematology & Oncology, Beth Israel Deaconess Med Ctr 1985; Bone Marrow Transplant, Dana Farber Cancer Inst 1988; **Fac Appt:** Prof Med, Univ NC Sch Med

Sherman, Carol A MD [Onc] - **Spec Exp:** Lung Cancer; Thoracic Cancers; **Hospital:** MUSC Med Ctr; **Address:** 96 Jonathan Lucas St, Ste CSB-903, Charleston, SC 29425; **Phone:** 843-792-9621; **Board Cert:** Internal Medicine 1987; Medical Oncology 1989; **Med School:** Univ Mass Sch Med 1984; **Resid:** Internal Medicine, Univ Mass Med Ctr 1987; **Fellow:** Hematology & Oncology, Univ Mass Med Ctr 1989; **Fac Appt:** Assoc Prof Med, Med Univ SC

Shin, Dong Moon MD [Onc] - **Spec Exp:** Head & Neck Cancer; Cancer Prevention; Mesothelioma; Thymoma; **Hospital:** Emory Univ Hosp; **Address:** Emory Winship Cancer Inst, 1365 C Clifton Rd NE, Ste 3090, Atlanta, GA 30322; **Phone:** 404-778-5990; **Board Cert:** Internal Medicine 1985; Medical Oncology 1989; **Med School:** South Korea 1975; **Resid:** Internal Medicine, Cook Co Hosp 1985; **Fellow:** Medical Oncology, Univ Texas MD Anderson Cancer Ctr 1986; **Fac Appt:** Prof Med, Emory Univ

Smith, Thomas Joseph MD [Onc] - **Spec Exp:** Breast Cancer; Palliative Care; **Hospital:** Med Coll of VA Hosp; **Address:** Med Coll Va, Div Hem/Onc, PO Box 980230, Richmond, VA 23298-0230; **Phone:** 804-828-9992; **Board Cert:** Internal Medicine 1982; Medical Oncology 1987; Hospice & Palliative Medicine 2003; **Med School:** Yale Univ 1979; **Resid:** Internal Medicine, Hosp Univ Penn 1982; **Fellow:** Medical Oncology, Med Coll Virginia 1987; **Fac Appt:** Prof Med, Med Coll VA

Socinski, Mark A MD [Onc] - **Spec Exp:** Lung Cancer; **Hospital:** Univ NC Hosps; **Address:** UNC Chapel Hill, Div Hem/Onc, 170 Manning Drive, CB 7305, Chapel Hill, NC 27599-7305; **Phone:** 919-966-0000; **Board Cert:** Internal Medicine 1988; Medical Oncology 2002; **Med School:** Univ VT Coll Med 1984; **Resid:** Internal Medicine, Beth Israel Hosp 1986; **Fellow:** Medical Oncology, Dana-Farber Cancer Inst 1989; **Fac Appt:** Assoc Prof Med, Univ NC Sch Med

Sosman, Jeffrey MD [Onc] - **Spec Exp:** Kidney Cancer; Melanoma; Drug Discovery; **Hospital:** Vanderbilt Univ Med Ctr; **Address:** Vanderbilt Ingram Cancer Ctr, 777 Preston Research Bldg, Nashville, TN 37232-6307; **Phone:** 615-322-4967; **Board Cert:** Anatomic Pathology 1985; Internal Medicine 1987; Medical Oncology 1989; **Med School:** Albert Einstein Coll Med 1981; **Resid:** Anatomic Pathology, Univ Chicago Hosps 1985; Internal Medicine, Univ Wisconsin Hosp 1986; **Fellow:** Medical Oncology, Univ Wisconsin 1989; **Fac Appt:** Clin Prof Med, Vanderbilt Univ

Sotomayor, Eduardo M MD [Onc] - **Spec Exp:** Lymphoma; Gene Therapy; Vaccine Therapy; Clinical Trials; **Hospital:** H Lee Moffitt Cancer Ctr & Research Inst; **Address:** H Lee Moffitt Cancer Inst, 12902 Magnolia Drive, MRC 3 East, Ste 3056D, Tampa, FL 33612; **Phone:** 813-745-1387; **Med School:** Peru 1988; **Resid:** Internal Medicine, Univ Miami Sch Med 1995; **Fellow:** Immunology, Univ Miami Sch Med 1989; Oncology, Johns Hopkins Hosp 1998; **Fac Appt:** Assoc Prof Med, Univ S Fla Coll Med

Stone, Joel MD [Onc] - **Spec Exp.** Lung Cancer; Breast Cancer; **Hospital:** St Vincent's Med Ctr - Jacksonville; **Address:** St Vincent's Med Ctr, 2 Shircliff Way, Ste 800, Jacksonville, FL 32204; **Phone:** 904-388-2619; **Board Cert:** Internal Medicine 1977; Medical Oncology 1979; **Med School:** Univ VA Sch Med 1974; **Resid:** Internal Medicine, Univ KY Med Ctr 1977; **Fellow:** Hematology & Oncology, Emory Univ 1979

Sutton, Linda Marie MD [Onc] - **Spec Exp:** Breast Cancer; Palliative Care; **Hospital:** Duke Univ Med Ctr; **Address:** University Tower, 3100 Tower Blvd, Ste 600, Durham, NC 27707; **Phone:** 919-419-5005; **Board Cert:** Internal Medicine 2002; Medical Oncology 2003; **Med School:** Univ Mass Sch Med 1987; **Resid:** Internal Medicine, Montefiore Med Ctr 1990; **Fellow:** Hematology & Oncology, Duke Univ Med Ctr 1993

Thigpen, James T MD [Onc] - **Spec Exp:** Gynecologic Cancer; Breast Cancer; Lung Cancer; **Hospital:** Univ Mississippi Med Ctr; **Address:** Univ Mississippi Med Ctr, Div Med Onc, 2500 N State St, Jackson, MS 39216; **Phone:** 601-984-5590; **Board Cert:** Internal Medicine 1972; Hematology 1974; Medical Oncology 1975; **Med School:** Univ Miss 1969; **Resid:** Internal Medicine, Univ Miss Med Ctr 1971; **Fellow:** Hematology & Oncology, Univ Miss Med Ctr 1973; **Fac Appt:** Prof Med, Univ Miss

Medical Oncology

Torti, Frank M MD [Onc] - **Spec Exp:** Prostate Cancer; Urologic Cancer; **Hospital:** Wake Forest Univ Baptist Med Ctr (page 84); **Address:** Wake Forest Med Ctr-Comp Cancer Ctr, Medical Center Blvd, Winston-Salem, NC 27157-1082; **Phone:** 336-716-7971; **Board Cert:** Internal Medicine 1978; Medical Oncology 1979; **Med School:** Harvard Med Sch 1974; **Resid:** Internal Medicine, Beth Israel Hosp 1976; **Fellow:** Medical Oncology, Stanford Univ Med Ctr 1979; **Fac Appt:** Prof Med, Wake Forest Univ

Troner, Michael MD [Onc] - **Spec Exp:** Head & Neck Cancer; Urologic Cancer; **Hospital:** Baptist Hosp of Miami; **Address:** 8940 N Kendall Drive, Ste 300, East Tower, Miami, FL 33176-2132; **Phone:** 305-595-2141; **Board Cert:** Internal Medicine 1972; Medical Oncology 1973; **Med School:** SUNY Downstate 1968; **Resid:** Internal Medicine, Univ Maryland Hosp 1971; **Fellow:** Medical Oncology, Univ Miami Med Ctr 1973; **Fac Appt:** Assoc Clin Prof Med, Univ Miami Sch Med

Vance, Ralph MD [Onc] - **Spec Exp:** Lung Cancer; **Hospital:** Univ Mississippi Med Ctr; **Address:** Univ Mississippi Med Ctr, Div Med Onc, 2500 N State St, Jackson, MS 39216; **Phone:** 601-984-5590; **Med School:** Univ Miss 1972; **Resid:** Internal Medicine, Univ Hosp; **Fellow:** Hematology & Oncology, Univ Hosp; **Fac Appt:** Prof Med, Univ Miss

Vaughan, William P MD [Onc] - **Spec Exp:** Bone Marrow Transplant; Breast Cancer; **Hospital:** Univ of Ala Hosp at Birmingham; **Address:** 1900 University Blvd, rm 541, Tinsley Harrison Twr, Birmingham, AL 35294; **Phone:** 205-934-1908; **Board Cert:** Internal Medicine 1975; Medical Oncology 1979; **Med School:** Univ Conn 1972; **Resid:** Internal Medicine, Univ Chicago Hosps 1975; **Fellow:** Oncology, Johns Hopkins Hosp 1977; **Fac Appt:** Prof Med, Univ Alabama

Weber, Jeffrey S MD/PhD [Onc] - **Spec Exp:** Melanoma; **Hospital:** H Lee Moffitt Cancer Ctr & Research Inst; **Address:** H Lee Moffitt Cancer Ctr, 12902 Magnolia Ave, MS SRB-2, Tampa, FL 33612; **Phone:** 813-745-2691; **Board Cert:** Internal Medicine 1983; Medical Oncology 1987; **Med School:** NYU Sch Med 1980; **Resid:** Internal Medicine, UCSD Med Ctr 1983; **Fellow:** Medical Oncology, Natl Cancer Inst 1990; **Fac Appt:** Assoc Prof Med, USC Sch Med

Weiss, Geoffrey R MD [Onc] - **Spec Exp:** Gastrointestinal Cancer; Genitourinary Cancer; Melanoma; **Hospital:** Univ Virginia Med Ctr; **Address:** Univ Virginia Hlth System, Div Hem/Onc, PO Box 800716, Charlottesville, VA 22908-0716; **Phone:** 434-243-0066; **Board Cert:** Internal Medicine 1977; Medical Oncology 1981; **Med School:** St Louis Univ 1974; **Resid:** Internal Medicine, Temple Univ Hosp 1978; **Fellow:** Medical Oncology, Dana Farber Cancer Inst 1982; **Fac Appt:** Prof Med, Univ VA Sch Med

Williams, Michael E MD [Onc] - **Spec Exp:** Lymphoma; Multiple Myeloma; Leukemia; **Hospital:** Univ Virginia Med Ctr; **Address:** UVA Hlth System, Div Hem/Oncology, PO Box 800716, Charlottesville, VA 22908-0716; **Phone:** 434-924-9637; **Board Cert:** Internal Medicine 1982; Medical Oncology 1987; Hematology 1988; **Med School:** Univ Cincinnati 1979; **Resid:** Internal Medicine, Univ Virginia Med Ctr 1983; **Fellow:** Hematology & Oncology, Univ Virginia Med Ctr 1986; **Fac Appt:** Prof Med, Univ VA Sch Med

Wingard, John R MD [Onc] - **Spec Exp:** Bone Marrow Transplant; Leukemia; Multiple Myeloma; Lymphoma; **Hospital:** Shands at Univ of FL; **Address:** 1376 Mowry Rd, rm 458, Box 103633, Gainesville, FL 32610; **Phone:** 352-265-0062; **Board Cert:** Internal Medicine 1977; Medical Oncology 1983; **Med School:** Johns Hopkins Univ 1973; **Resid:** Internal Medicine, Memphis City Hosps 1976; Internal Medicine, VA Hosp 1977; **Fellow:** Medical Oncology, Johns Hopkins Hosp 1979; **Fac Appt:** Prof Med, Univ Fla Coll Med

Yunus, Furhan MD [Onc] - **Spec Exp:** Multiple Myeloma; Lymphoma; **Hospital:** Methodist Univ Hosp - Memphis, Regional Med Ctr - Memphis; **Address:** Univ TN Cancer Inst, 1331 Union Ave, Ste 800, Memphis, TN 38104; **Phone:** 901-725-1785; **Board Cert:** Medical Oncology 2008; **Med School:** Pakistan 1986; **Resid:** Internal Medicine, Methodist Hosp 1993; **Fellow:** Hematology & Oncology, Univ Ariz Coll Med Affil Hosp 1995; **Fac Appt:** Asst Prof Med, Univ Tenn Coll Med, Memphis

Midwest

Adelstein, David J MD [Onc] - **Spec Exp:** Head & Neck Cancer; Esophageal Cancer; Lung Cancer; **Hospital:** Cleveland Clin Fdn (page 70); **Address:** Cleveland Clinic Fdn, Taussig Cancer Ctr, 9500 Euclid Ave, R35, Cleveland, OH 44195; **Phone:** 216-444-9310; **Board Cert:** Internal Medicine 1978; Medical Oncology 1981; Hematology 1982; **Med School:** NYU Sch Med 1975; **Resid:** Internal Medicine, Univ Hosps Cleveland 1978; **Fellow:** Hematology & Oncology, Univ Hosps Cleveland 1981; **Fac Appt:** Prof Med, Cleveland Cl Coll Med/Case West Res

Albain, Kathy S MD [Onc] - **Spec Exp:** Breast Cancer; Lung Cancer; Cancer Survivors-Late Effects of Therapy; **Hospital:** Loyola Univ Med Ctr; **Address:** Loyola Univ Med Ctr, 2160 S First Ave, Bldg 112 - Ste 109, Maywood, IL 60153-5590; **Phone:** 708-327-3102; **Board Cert:** Internal Medicine 1981; Medical Oncology 1983; **Med School:** Univ Mich Med Sch 1978; **Resid:** Internal Medicine, Univ Illinois Med Ctr 1981; **Fellow:** Hematology & Oncology, Univ Chicago Hosps 1984; **Fac Appt:** Prof Med, Loyola Univ-Stritch Sch Med

Albertini, Mark R MD [Onc] - **Spec Exp:** Melanoma; Melanoma-Metastatic; **Hospital:** Univ WI Hosp & Clins; **Address:** Univ Wisconsin Medical Oncology, 600 Highland Ave, K6-930 CSC, Madison, WI 53792; **Phone:** 608-265-1700; **Board Cert:** Internal Medicine 1987; Medical Oncology 2002; **Med School:** Univ VT Coll Med 1984; **Resid:** Internal Medicine, Univ Wisc Hosps Clins 1987; **Fellow:** Medical Oncology, Univ Wisconsin 1991; **Fac Appt:** Assoc Prof Med, Univ Wisc

Anderson, Joseph M MD [Onc] - **Spec Exp:** Breast Cancer; Palliative Care; Neuro-Oncology; **Hospital:** Henry Ford Hosp; **Address:** 2799 W Grand Blvd, Ste K13, Detroit, MI 48202; **Phone:** 313-916-1854; **Board Cert:** Internal Medicine 1985; Medical Oncology 1989; **Med School:** Univ Mich Med Sch 1982; **Resid:** Internal Medicine, Henry Ford Hosp 1986; **Fellow:** Medical Oncology, Henry Ford Hosp 1988

Benson III, Al B MD [Onc] - **Spec Exp:** Colon Cancer; Carcinoid Tumors; Pancreatic Cancer; **Hospital:** Northwestern Meml Hosp, Jesse A Brown VA Med Ctr; **Address:** 675 N St Clair St, Ste 21-100, Chicago, IL 60611; **Phone:** 312-695-0990; **Board Cert:** Internal Medicine 1979; Medical Oncology 1983; **Med School:** SUNY Buffalo 1976; **Resid:** Internal Medicine, Univ Wisc Hosps 1979; **Fellow:** Medical Oncology, Univ Wisc Hosps 1984; **Fac Appt:** Prof Med, Northwestern Univ

Bitran, Jacob D MD [Onc] - **Spec Exp:** Breast Cancer; Bone Marrow Transplant; Lung Cancer; **Hospital:** Adv Luth Genl Hosp, Rush N Shore Med Ctr; **Address:** Lutheran Genl Cancer Care Specialists, 1700 Luther Lane, Park Ridge, IL 60068-1270; **Phone:** 866-611-1991; **Board Cert:** Internal Medicine 1974; Hematology 1986; Medical Oncology 1977; **Med School:** Univ IL Coll Med 1971; **Resid:** Pathology, Rush Presby St Lukes Hosp 1973; Internal Medicine, Michael Reese Hosp 1975; **Fellow:** Hematology & Oncology, Univ Chicago Hosps 1977; **Fac Appt:** Prof Med, Ros Franklin Univ/Chicago Med Sch

Medical Oncology

Bolwell, Brian J MD [Onc] - **Spec Exp:** Bone Marrow Transplant; Hematologic Malignancies; **Hospital:** Cleveland Clin Fdn (page 70); **Address:** 9500 Euclid Ave, Desk R32, Cleveland, OH 44195; **Phone:** 216-444-6922; **Board Cert:** Internal Medicine 1985; Medical Oncology 1987; **Med School:** Case West Res Univ 1981; **Resid:** Internal Medicine, Univ Hosp 1984; **Fellow:** Hematology & Oncology, Hosp Univ Penn 1987; **Fac Appt:** Prof Med, Cleveland Cl Coll Med/Case West Res

Bonomi, Philip D MD [Onc] - **Spec Exp:** Lung Cancer; Thymoma; Mesothelioma; **Hospital:** Rush Univ Med Ctr; **Address:** 1725 W Harrison St, Ste 821, Chicago, IL 60612; **Phone:** 312-942-3312; **Board Cert:** Internal Medicine 1975; Medical Oncology 1977; **Med School:** Univ IL Coll Med 1970; **Resid:** Internal Medicine, Geisinger Med Ctr 1972; Internal Medicine, Geisinger Med Ctr 1975; **Fellow:** Medical Oncology, Rush Presby-St Luke's Med Ctr 1977; **Fac Appt:** Prof Med, Rush Med Coll

Borden, Ernest C MD [Onc] - **Spec Exp:** Melanoma; Immunotherapy; Sarcoma; Vaccine Therapy; **Hospital:** Cleveland Clin Fdn (page 70); **Address:** 9500 Euclid Ave, Desk R40, Cleveland, OH 44195; **Phone:** 216-444-8183; **Board Cert:** Internal Medicine 1973; Medical Oncology 1975; **Med School:** Duke Univ 1966; **Resid:** Internal Medicine, Hosp Univ Penn 1968; **Fellow:** Medical Oncology, Johns Hopkins Hosp 1973; **Fac Appt:** Prof Med, Cleveland Cl Coll Med/Case West Res

Bricker, Leslie J MD [Onc] - **Spec Exp:** Palliative Care; **Hospital:** Henry Ford Hosp; **Address:** Henry Ford Hospital, 2799 W Grand Blvd, CFP 5, Detroit, MI 48202; **Phone:** 313-916-1859; **Board Cert:** Internal Medicine 1980; Hematology 1982; Medical Oncology 1983; Hospice & Palliative Medicine 2008; **Med School:** Wayne State Univ 1977; **Resid:** Internal Medicine, Sinai Hosp 1980; **Fellow:** Hematology & Oncology, Univ Mich Hosp 1983; **Fac Appt:** Assoc Prof Med, Wayne State Univ

Brockstein, Bruce E MD [Onc] - **Spec Exp:** Head & Neck Cancer; Sarcoma; Melanoma; **Hospital:** Evanston/Northshore Univ Hlth Syst, Highland Park/North Shore Univ Hlth Syst; **Address:** Evanston Northwestern Healthcare, Div Hematology/Oncology, 2650 Ridge Ave, rm 5134, Evanston, IL 60201; **Phone:** 847-570-2515; **Board Cert:** Internal Medicine 2003; Medical Oncology 2005; **Med School:** Univ Chicago-Pritzker Sch Med 1990; **Resid:** Internal Medicine, Hosp Univ Penn 1993; **Fellow:** Hematology & Oncology, Univ Chicago Hosps 1996; **Fac Appt:** Assoc Prof Med, Northwestern Univ

Buckner, Jan Craig MD [Onc] - **Spec Exp:** Brain Tumors; Neuro-Oncology; **Hospital:** Mayo Med Ctr & Clin - Rochester; **Address:** Mayo Clinic, 200 First St SW, Rochester, MN 55905; **Phone:** 507-284-4320; **Board Cert:** Internal Medicine 1983; Medical Oncology 1985; **Med School:** Univ NC Sch Med 1980; **Resid:** Internal Medicine, Butterworth Hosp 1983; **Fellow:** Medical Oncology, Mayo Clinic 1985; **Fac Appt:** Prof Med, Mayo Med Sch

Budd, George T MD [Onc] - **Spec Exp:** Breast Cancer; **Hospital:** Cleveland Clin Fdn (page 70); **Address:** Cleveland Clinic, Taussig Cancer Ctr, 9500 Euclid Ave, Desk R35, Cleveland, OH 44195; **Phone:** 216-444-6480; **Board Cert:** Internal Medicine 1980; Medical Oncology 1983; **Med School:** Univ Kans 1976; **Resid:** Internal Medicine, Cleveland Clinic 1980; **Fellow:** Hematology & Oncology, Cleveland Clinic 1982

Burt, Richard K MD [Onc] - **Spec Exp:** Autoimmune Disease; **Hospital:** Northwestern Meml Hosp; **Address:** Div Immunotherapy, 750 N Lakeshore Drive, rm 649, Chicago, IL 60611; **Phone:** 312-908-0059; **Board Cert:** Internal Medicine 1989; **Med School:** St Louis Univ 1984; **Resid:** Internal Medicine, Baylor Coll Med 1988; **Fellow:** Medical Oncology, Natl Inst Hlth Clin Ctr 1991; Hematology, Nat Inst Hlth Clin Ctr 1993; **Fac Appt:** Assoc Prof Med, Northwestern Univ

Chapman, Robert A MD [Onc] - **Spec Exp:** Lung Cancer; **Hospital:** Henry Ford Hosp; **Address:** 2799 W Grand Blvd, Fl K13, Detroit, MI 48202; **Phone:** 313-916-1841; **Board Cert:** Internal Medicine 1985; Medical Oncology 1989; **Med School:** Cornell Univ-Weill Med Coll 1976; **Resid:** Internal Medicine, Henry Ford Hosp 1979; **Fellow:** Medical Oncology, Meml Sloan Kettering Cancer Ctr 1981

Chitambar, Christopher R MD [Onc] - **Spec Exp:** Lymphoma; Leukemia; Breast Cancer; **Hospital:** Froedtert Meml Lutheran Hosp; **Address:** Div Neoplastic Disease, 9200 W Wisconsin Ave, Milwaukee, WI 53226-3522; **Phone:** 414-805-4600; **Board Cert:** Internal Medicine 1980; Hematology 1982; Medical Oncology 1983; **Med School:** India 1977; **Resid:** Internal Medicine, Brackenridge Hosp 1980; **Fellow:** Hematology & Oncology, Univ CO Hlth Sci Ctr 1983; **Fac Appt:** Prof Med, Med Coll Wisc

Clamon, Gerald H MD [Onc] - **Spec Exp:** Lung Cancer; Drug Development; **Hospital:** Univ Iowa Hosp & Clinics; **Address:** Univ Iowa Hosps & Clins, Dept Internal Med, 200 Hawkins Drive, rm 5970 JPP, Iowa City, IA 52242; **Phone:** 319-356-1932; **Board Cert:** Internal Medicine 1976; Medical Oncology 1979; **Med School:** Washington Univ, St Louis 1971; **Resid:** Internal Medicine, Barnes Hosp 1976; **Fellow:** Natl Cancer Inst 1974; Medical Oncology, Univ Iowa Hosp & Clinics 1977; **Fac Appt:** Prof Med, Univ Iowa Coll Med

Clark, Joseph I MD [Onc] - **Spec Exp:** Kidney Cancer; Melanoma; Head & Neck Cancer; **Hospital:** Loyola Univ Med Ctr, Hines VA Hosp; **Address:** Cardinal Bernardin Cancer Ctr, Loyola Univ Med Ctr, 2160 S 1st Ave, rm 346, Maywood, IL 60153-5500; **Phone:** 708-327-3236; **Board Cert:** Internal Medicine 2002; Medical Oncology 2006; **Med School:** Loyola Univ-Stritch Sch Med 1989; **Resid:** Internal Medicine, Loyola Univ Med Ctr/Hines VA Hosp 1992; **Fellow:** Hematology & Oncology, Fox Chase Cancer Ctr/Temple Univ Hosp 1995; **Fac Appt:** Prof Med, Loyola Univ-Stritch Sch Med

Cleary, James F MD [Onc] - **Spec Exp:** Palliative Care; Head & Neck Cancer; **Hospital:** Univ WI Hosp & Clins; **Address:** K6546 CSC, 600 Highland Ave, Madison, WI 53792; **Phone:** 608-263-8090; **Med School:** Australia 1984; **Resid:** Internal Medicine, Royal Adelaide Hosp 1987; **Fellow:** Medical Oncology, Royal Adelaide Hosp 1990; **Fac Appt:** Assoc Prof Med, Univ Wisc

Clinton, Steven K MD/PhD [Onc] - **Spec Exp:** Genitourinary Cancer; Prostate Cancer; Nutrition & Cancer Prevention/Control; **Hospital:** Ohio St Univ Med Ctr; **Address:** 4434 Starling Loving Hall, 320 W 10th Ave, Columbus, OH 43210; **Phone:** 614-293-7560; **Board Cert:** Internal Medicine 1987; **Med School:** Univ IL Coll Med 1984; **Resid:** Internal Medicine, Univ Chicago Hosps 1987; **Fellow:** Medical Oncology, Dana Farber Cancer Inst/Harvard 1991; **Fac Appt:** Assoc Prof Med, Ohio State Univ

Cobleigh, Melody A MD [Onc] - **Spec Exp:** Breast Cancer; **Hospital:** Rush Univ Med Ctr; **Address:** Rush Univ Med Ctr, 1725 W Harrison St, Ste 821, Chicago, IL 60612-3828; **Phone:** 312-942-5904; **Board Cert:** Internal Medicine 1979; Medical Oncology 1981; **Med School:** Rush Med Coll 1976; **Resid:** Internal Medicine, Rush Presby-St Lukes Med Ctr 1979; **Fellow:** Medical Oncology, Indiana Univ 1981; **Fac Appt:** Prof Med, Rush Med Coll

Daugherty, Christopher K MD [Onc] - **Spec Exp:** Leukemia & Lymphoma; Stem Cell Transplant; **Hospital:** Univ of Chicago Med Ctr; **Address:** University of Chicago Hospitals, 5758 S Maryland Ave, MC 2115, Chicago, IL 60637; **Phone:** 773-702-6149; **Med School:** Indiana Univ 1989; **Resid:** Internal Medicine, Indiana Univ 1993; **Fellow:** Hematology & Oncology, Univ Chicago Hosps 1997; Medical Ethics, Univ Chicago Hosps

Medical Oncology

Davis, Mellar P MD [Onc] - **Spec Exp:** Palliative Care; Lung Cancer (advanced); **Hospital:** Cleveland Clin Fdn (page 70); **Address:** Cleveland Clin Fdn, 9500 Euclid Ave, Desk R35, Cleveland, OH 44195-0002; **Phone:** 216-445-4622; **Board Cert:** Internal Medicine 1980; Hematology 1982; Medical Oncology 1983; Hospice & Palliative Medicine 2004; **Med School:** Ohio State Univ 1977; **Resid:** Internal Medicine, Riverside Methodist Hosp 1979; **Fellow:** Hematology, Mayo Clinic 1981; Medical Oncology, Mayo Clinic 1982

Dreicer, Robert MD [Onc] - **Spec Exp:** Prostate Cancer; Kidney Cancer; Bladder Cancer; Testicular Cancer; **Hospital:** Cleveland Clin Fdn (page 70); **Address:** Cleveland Clinic, Taussig Cancer Ctr, 9500 Euclid Ave, Desk R35, Cleveland, OH 44195; **Phone:** 216-445-4623; **Board Cert:** Internal Medicine 1986; Medical Oncology 1989; **Med School:** Univ Tex, Houston 1983; **Resid:** Internal Medicine, Ind Univ Med Ctr 1986; **Fellow:** Medical Oncology, Univ Wisconsin Hosp 1989; **Fac Appt:** Prof Med, Cleveland Cl Coll Med/Case West Res

Einhorn, Lawrence H MD [Onc] - **Spec Exp:** Testicular Cancer; Lung Cancer; Urologic Cancer; **Hospital:** Indiana Univ Hosp (page 74); **Address:** 535 Barnhill Drive, rm 473, Indianapolis, IN 46202; **Phone:** 317-278-0054; **Board Cert:** Internal Medicine 1972; Medical Oncology 1975; **Med School:** UCLA 1967; **Resid:** Internal Medicine, Indiana Univ Hosp 1969; **Fellow:** Medical Oncology, Indiana Univ Hosp 1972; **Fac Appt:** Prof Med, Indiana Univ

Ellis, Matthew J MD/PhD [Onc] - **Spec Exp:** Breast Cancer; **Hospital:** Barnes-Jewish Hosp; **Address:** Washington University, 660 S Euclid Ave, Box 8056, St Louis, MO 63110; **Phone:** 314-747-1171; **Board Cert:** Internal Medicine 2004; Medical Oncology 2005; **Med School:** England, UK 1984; **Fellow:** Research, Georgetown Univ Med Ctr 1992; Medical Oncology, Georgetwon Univ Med Ctr 1994; **Fac Appt:** Prof Med, Washington Univ, St Louis

Eng, Charis MD [Onc] - **Spec Exp:** Breast Cancer; Ovarian Cancer; Cancer Genetics; **Hospital:** Cleveland Clin Fdn (page 70); **Address:** Cleveland Clinic Foundation, 9500 Euclid Ave, MC NE50, Cleveland, OH 44195; **Phone:** 216-444-3440; **Board Cert:** Internal Medicine 1991; Medical Oncology 1997; **Med School:** Univ Chicago-Pritzker Sch Med 1988; **Resid:** Internal Medicine, Beth Israel Hosp 1991; **Fellow:** Medical Oncology, Dana-Farber Cancer Inst 1995

Ensminger, William D MD/PhD [Onc] - **Spec Exp:** Gastrointestinal Cancer; Liver Cancer; Clinical Trials; **Hospital:** Univ Michigan Hlth Sys; **Address:** 1150 W Med Ctr Drive, Med Sci II Rm #4742, Ann Arbor, MI 48109-5633; **Phone:** 734-764-5468; **Board Cert:** Internal Medicine 1976; Medical Oncology 1979; **Med School:** Harvard Med Sch 1973; **Resid:** Internal Medicine, Beth Israel Hosp 1975; **Fellow:** Medical Oncology, Dana Farber Cancer Inst 1977; **Fac Appt:** Prof Med, Univ Mich Med Sch

Fleming, Gini F MD [Onc] - **Spec Exp:** Breast Cancer; Gynecologic Cancer; **Hospital:** Univ of Chicago Med Ctr; **Address:** Univ Chicago Hospitals, 5841 S Maryland MC2115, Chicago, IL 60637-1470; **Phone:** 773-839-7924; **Board Cert:** Internal Medicine 1988; Medical Oncology 2001; Hematology 2002; **Med School:** Univ IL Coll Med 1985; **Resid:** Internal Medicine, Univ Chicago Hosps 1988; **Fellow:** Hematology & Oncology, Univ Chicago 1992; **Fac Appt:** Prof Med, Univ Chicago-Pritzker Sch Med

Gerson, Stanton MD [Onc] - **Spec Exp:** Leukemia; Lymphoma, Non-Hodgkin's; Stem Cell Transplant; **Hospital:** Univ Hosps Case Med Ctr; **Address:** Ireland Cancer Ctr, 11000 Euclid Ave, 1 WEARN 151, Cleveland, OH 44106-5065; **Phone:** 216-844-1232; **Board Cert:** Internal Medicine 1980; Medical Oncology 1983; Hematology 1982; **Med School:** Harvard Med Sch 1977; **Resid:** Internal Medicine, Hosp Univ Penn 1980; **Fellow:** Hematology & Oncology, Hosp Univ Penn 1983; **Fac Appt:** Prof Med, Case West Res Univ

Golomb, Harvey MD [Onc] - **Spec Exp:** Lung Cancer; Leukemia; Lymphoma; **Hospital:** Univ of Chicago Med Ctr; **Address:** Univ of Chicago Hospital, 5758 S Maryland Ave, MC 9015, Chicago, IL 60637-1463; **Phone:** 773-702-6115; **Board Cert:** Internal Medicine 1975; Medical Oncology 1979; **Med School:** Univ Pittsburgh 1968; **Resid:** Internal Medicine, Johns Hopkins Hosp 1972; Clinical Genetics, Johns Hopkins Hosp 1973; **Fellow:** Hematology & Oncology, Univ Chicago Hosps 1975; **Fac Appt:** Prof Med, Univ Chicago-Pritzker Sch Med

Gradishar, William J MD [Onc] - **Spec Exp:** Breast Cancer; **Hospital:** Northwestern Meml Hosp; **Address:** 676 N St Claire St, Ste 21-100, Chicago, IL 60611; **Phone:** 312-695-0990; **Board Cert:** Internal Medicine 1985; Medical Oncology 1989; **Med School:** Univ IL Coll Med 1982; **Resid:** Internal Medicine, Michael Reese Hosp 1985; **Fellow:** Hematology & Oncology, Univ Chicago Hosps 1990; **Fac Appt:** Prof Med, Northwestern Univ

Gruber, Stephen B MD/PhD [Onc] - **Spec Exp:** Cancer Genetics; Colon & Rectal Cancer; Melanoma; **Hospital:** Univ Michigan Hlth Sys; **Address:** 109 Zina Pitcher Pl, Ann Arbor, MI 48109-2200; **Phone:** 734-615-9712; **Board Cert:** Internal Medicine 1995; Medical Oncology 1998; **Med School:** Univ Pennsylvania 1992; **Resid:** Internal Medicine, Hosp Univ Penn 1994; **Fellow:** Medical Oncology, Johns Hopkins Hosp 1997; Clinical Genetics, Univ Michigan Hlth Sys 1999; **Fac Appt:** Assoc Prof Med, Univ Mich Med Sch

Hartmann, Lynn Carol MD [Onc] - **Spec Exp:** Ovarian Cancer; **Hospital:** Mayo Med Ctr & Clin - Rochester; **Address:** Mayo Clinic Gonda 10 South, 200 First St SW, Rochester, MN 55905; **Phone:** 507-284-3903; **Board Cert:** Internal Medicine 1986; Medical Oncology 1989; **Med School:** Northwestern Univ 1983; **Resid:** Internal Medicine, Univ Ia Hosps/Clinics 1986; **Fellow:** Medical Oncology, Mayo Clinic 1989; **Fac Appt:** Prof Med, Mayo Med Sch

Hayes, Daniel F MD [Onc] - **Spec Exp:** Breast Cancer; **Hospital:** Univ Michigan Hlth Sys; **Address:** Univ Michigan Comprehensive Cancer Ctr, 6312 CCC SPC, 5942, Ann Arbor, MI 48109-5942; **Phone:** 734-615-6725; **Board Cert:** Internal Medicine 1982; Medical Oncology 1985; **Med School:** Indiana Univ 1979; **Resid:** Internal Medicine, Parkland Meml Hosp 1982; **Fellow:** Medical Oncology, Dana Farber Cancer Inst 1985; **Fac Appt:** Prof Med, Univ Mich Med Sch

Hoffman, Philip C MD [Onc] - **Spec Exp:** Lung Cancer; Breast Cancer; Esophageal Cancer; **Hospital:** Univ of Chicago Med Ctr, Little Company of Mary Hosp & Hlth Care Ctrs; **Address:** 5841 3 Maryland Ave, MC 2115, Chicago, IL 60637 1417; **Phone:** 773-834-7424; **Board Cert:** Internal Medicine 1975; Hematology 1980; Medical Oncology 1981; **Med School:** Jefferson Med Coll 1972; **Resid:** Internal Medicine, Hosp Univ Penn 1975; **Fellow:** Hematology & Oncology, Univ Chicago Hosps 1980; **Fac Appt:** Prof Med, Univ Chicago-Pritzker Sch Med

Hussain, Maha H MD [Onc] - **Spec Exp:** Prostate Cancer; Bladder Cancer; Testicular Cancer; Genitourinary Cancer; **Hospital:** Univ Michigan Hlth Sys; **Address:** Univ Michigan Cancer Ctr, 1500 E Medical Ctr Drive, rm 7310, Ann Arbor, MI 48109; **Phone:** 734-936-8906; **Board Cert:** Internal Medicine 1986; Medical Oncology 1989; **Med School:** Iraq 1980; **Resid:** Internal Medicine, Wayne State Univ Affil Hosps 1986; **Fellow:** Medical Oncology, Wayne State Univ Affil Hosps 1989; **Fac Appt:** Prof Med, Univ Mich Med Sch

Ingle, James N MD [Onc] - **Spec Exp:** Breast Cancer; **Hospital:** Rochester Methodist Hosp, Mayo Med Ctr & Clin - Rochester; **Address:** Mayo Clinic, 200 First St SW, Gonda Bldg Fl 10, Rochester, MN 55905-0001; **Phone:** 507-284-8432; **Board Cert:** Internal Medicine 1974; Medical Oncology 1975; **Med School:** Johns Hopkins Univ 1971; **Resid:** Internal Medicine, Johns Hopkins Hosp 1976; Medical Oncology, Natl Cancer Inst 1975; **Fac Appt:** Prof Med, Mayo Med Sch

Medical Oncology

Kalaycio, Matt E MD [Onc] - **Spec Exp:** Leukemia; Bone Marrow Transplant; **Hospital:** Cleveland Clin Fdn (page 70); **Address:** Taussig Cancer Ctr, 9500 Euclid Ave, Desk R35, Cleveland, OH 44195; **Phone:** 216-444-3705; **Board Cert:** Internal Medicine 2002; Hematology 2004; Medical Oncology 2005; **Med School:** W VA Univ 1988; **Resid:** Internal Medicine, Mercy Hosp 1991; **Fellow:** Hematology & Oncology, Cleveland Clinic 1994; **Fac Appt:** Prof Med, Cleveland Cl Coll Med/Case West Res

Kalemkerian, Gregory MD [Onc] - **Spec Exp:** Lung Cancer; Mesothelioma; Thymoma; **Hospital:** Univ Michigan Hlth Sys; **Address:** 1500 E Medical Center Dr, C350MIB, Ann Arbor, MI 48109-0848; **Phone:** 734-232-6046; **Board Cert:** Internal Medicine 1988; Medical Oncology 2001; **Med School:** Northwestern Univ 1985; **Resid:** Internal Medicine, Northwestern Meml Hosp 1988; **Fac Appt:** Prof Med, Univ Mich Med Sch

Kaminski, Mark S MD [Onc] - **Spec Exp:** Lymphoma; Bone Marrow Transplant; Drug Development; Clinical Trials; **Hospital:** Univ Michigan Hlth Sys; **Address:** Univ Michigan Cancer Ctr, 1500 E Medical Ctr Drive, rm 4316, Ann Arbor, MI 48109-0936; **Phone:** 734-936-5310; **Board Cert:** Internal Medicine 1981; Medical Oncology 1983; **Med School:** Stanford Univ 1978; **Resid:** Internal Medicine, Barnes Hosp 1981; **Fellow:** Medical Oncology, Stanford Univ Med Ctr 1985; **Fac Appt:** Prof Med, Univ Mich Med Sch

Kindler, Hedy Lee MD [Onc] - **Spec Exp:** Mesothelioma; Pancreatic Cancer; Colon & Rectal Cancer; **Hospital:** Univ of Chicago Med Ctr; **Address:** Univ of Chicago Hospital, 5841 S Maryland Ave, MC 2115, Chicago, IL 60637-1470; **Phone:** 773-834-7424; **Board Cert:** Internal Medicine 2002; Medical Oncology 2005; **Med School:** SUNY Buffalo 1985; **Resid:** Internal Medicine, UCLA Med Ctr 1992; **Fellow:** Medical Oncology, Meml Sloan Kettering Cancer Ctr 1995; **Fac Appt:** Assoc Prof Med, Univ Chicago-Pritzker Sch Med

Loehrer, Patrick J MD [Onc] - **Spec Exp:** Gastrointestinal Cancer; Thymoma; Genitourinary Cancer; **Hospital:** Indiana Univ Hosp (page 74); **Address:** Indiana Cancer Pavilion, 535 Barnhill Drive, rm 473, Indianapolis, IN 46202-5112; **Phone:** 317-278-7418; **Board Cert:** Internal Medicine 1981; Medical Oncology 2006; **Med School:** Rush Med Coll 1978; **Resid:** Internal Medicine, Rush-Presby-St Lukes Hosp 1981; **Fellow:** Medical Oncology, Indiana Univ 1983; **Fac Appt:** Prof Med, Indiana Univ

Loprinzi, Charles L MD [Onc] - **Spec Exp:** Breast Cancer; **Hospital:** Mayo Med Ctr & Clin - Rochester; **Address:** Mayo Clinic, Dept Med Oncology, 200 First St SW, Rochester, MN 55905-0001; **Phone:** 507-284-4137; **Board Cert:** Internal Medicine 1982; Medical Oncology 1985; **Med School:** Oregon Hlth Sci Univ 1979; **Resid:** Internal Medicine, Maricopa Co Hosp 1982; **Fellow:** Medical Oncology, Univ Wisconsin Med Ctr 1984; **Fac Appt:** Prof Med, Mayo Med Sch

Markowitz, Sanford D MD [Onc] - **Spec Exp:** Colon & Rectal Cancer; Hereditary Cancer; **Hospital:** Univ Hosps Case Med Ctr; **Address:** Ireland Cancer Ctr, 11100 Euclid Ave Fl 6, Cleveland, OH 44106; **Phone:** 216-844-6966; **Board Cert:** Internal Medicine 1984; Medical Oncology 1987; **Med School:** Yale Univ 1980; **Resid:** Internal Medicine, Univ Chicago Hosp 1984; **Fellow:** Medical Oncology, Natl Cancer Inst 1986; **Fac Appt:** Prof Med, Case West Res Univ

Olopade, Olufunmilayo I F MD [Onc] - **Spec Exp:** Breast Cancer; Hereditary Cancer; Breast Cancer Genetics; **Hospital:** Univ of Chicago Med Ctr; **Address:** Univ Chicago Hospital, 5841 S Maryland Ave, MC 2115, Section, Hematology-Oncology, Chicago, IL 60637-1470; **Phone:** 773-702-6149; **Board Cert:** Internal Medicine 1986; Hematology 2001; Medical Oncology 1989; **Med School:** Nigeria 1980; **Resid:** Internal Medicine, Cook Co Hosp 1986; **Fellow:** Hematology & Oncology, Univ Chicago Hosps 1991; **Fac Appt:** Prof Med, Univ Chicago-Pritzker Sch Med

Peereboom, David M MD [Onc] - **Spec Exp:** Neuro-Oncology; Brain Tumors; Drug Development; **Hospital:** Cleveland Clin Fdn (page 70); **Address:** Cleveland Clinic Taussig Cancer Ctr, 9500 Euclid Ave, MC R35, Cleveland, OH 44195; **Phone:** 216-445-6068; **Board Cert:** Internal Medicine 1989; Medical Oncology 2004; **Med School:** Med Coll VA 1986; **Resid:** Internal Medicine, Univ Hosp of Cleveland 1990; **Fellow:** Medical Oncology, Johns Hopkins Hosp 1993

Perry, Michael C MD [Onc] - **Spec Exp:** Lung Cancer; Breast Cancer; **Hospital:** Univ of Missouri Hosp & Clins; **Address:** Ellis Fischel Cancer Ctr, 115 Business Loop 70 W, DC 116.71, rm 524, Columbia, MO 65203-3299; **Phone:** 573-882-4979; **Board Cert:** Internal Medicine 1987; Hematology 1974; Medical Oncology 1975; **Med School:** Wayne State Univ 1970; **Resid:** Internal Medicine, Mayo Grad Sch 1972; **Fellow:** Hematology, Mayo Grad Sch 1974; Medical Oncology, Mayo Grad Sch 1975; **Fac Appt:** Prof Med, Univ MO-Columbia Sch Med

Peterson, Bruce MD [Onc] - **Spec Exp:** Lymphoma; Leukemia; **Hospital:** Univ Minn Med Ctr, Fairview - Univ Campus; **Address:** Univ of Minnesota, MMC 480, 420 Delaware St SE, Minneapolis, MN 55455; **Phone:** 612-625-5411; **Board Cert:** Internal Medicine 1974; Medical Oncology 1977; **Med School:** Univ Minn 1971; **Resid:** Internal Medicine, Fletcher Allen Hlthcare 1973; Internal Medicine, Fairview-Univ Med Ctr 1974; **Fellow:** Medical Oncology, Fairview-Univ Med Ctr 1977; **Fac Appt:** Prof Med, Univ Minn

Picus, Joel MD [Onc] - **Spec Exp:** Pancreatic Cancer; Prostate Cancer; Colon Cancer; Bladder Cancer; **Hospital:** Barnes-Jewish Hosp; **Address:** Washington University School of Medicine, Dept Medicine, 660 S Euclid Ave Campus Box 8056, St Louis, MO 63110; **Phone:** 314-362-5737; **Board Cert:** Internal Medicine 1987; Medical Oncology 1989; **Med School:** Harvard Med Sch 1984; **Resid:** Internal Medicine, Duke Univ Med Ctr 1987; **Fellow:** Hematology & Oncology, UCSF Med Ctr 1991; **Fac Appt:** Assoc Prof Med, Washington Univ, St Louis

Pienta, Kenneth J MD [Onc] - **Spec Exp:** Prostate Cancer; **Hospital:** Univ Michigan Hlth Sys; **Address:** Cancer Center/Geriatrics Center, 1500 E Medical Center Drive, rm 7303 CCC, Ann Arbor, MI 48109-5946; **Phone:** 734-647-3421; **Board Cert:** Internal Medicine 2001; Medical Oncology 2001; **Med School:** Johns Hopkins Univ 1986; **Resid:** Internal Medicine, Univ Chicago Hosps 1988; **Fellow:** Medical Oncology, Johns Hopkins Hosp 1991; **Fac Appt:** Prof Med, Univ Mich Med Sch

Pohlman, Brad L MD [Onc] - **Spec Exp:** Lymphoma; Lymphoma, Non Hodgkin's; Bone Marrow Transplant; **Hospital:** Cleveland Clin Fdn (page 70); **Address:** Cleveland Clinic Fdn, 9500 Euclid Ave R35, Cleveland, OH 44195; **Phone:** 216-445-6070; **Board Cert:** Internal Medicine 1988; **Med School:** Indiana Univ 1985; **Resid:** Internal Medicine, Univ Wisconsin Hosp 1988; **Fellow:** Hematology, Univ Minnesota Hosp 1992

Raghavan, Derek MD/PhD [Onc] - **Spec Exp:** Prostate Cancer; Testicular Cancer; Bladder Cancer; Genitourinary Cancer; **Hospital:** Cleveland Clin Fdn (page 70); **Address:** Cleveland Clinic Taussig Cancer Inst, 9500 Euclid Ave, MC R35, Cleveland, OH 44195; **Phone:** 216-445-6888; **Med School:** Australia 1974; **Resid:** Internal Medicine, Royal Prince Alfred Hosp 1977; **Fellow:** Medical Oncology, Royal Prince Alfred Hosp 1979; Medical Oncology, Royal Marsden Hosp 1980; **Fac Appt:** Prof Med, Cleveland Cl Coll Med/Case West Res

Ratain, Mark J MD [Onc] - **Spec Exp:** Solid Tumors; Drug Discovery & Development; **Hospital:** Univ of Chicago Med Ctr; **Address:** Univ Chicago Med Ctr, 5841 S Maryland Ave, MC 211, Chicago, IL 60637; **Phone:** 773-702-6149; **Board Cert:** Internal Medicine 1983; Hematology 1986; Medical Oncology 1985; **Med School:** Yale Univ 1980; **Resid:** Internal Medicine, Johns Hopkins Hosp 1983; **Fellow:** Hematology & Oncology, Univ Chicago 1986; **Fac Appt:** Prof Med, Univ Chicago-Pritzker Sch Med

Medical Oncology

Richards, Jon M MD/PhD [Onc] - **Spec Exp:** Testicular Cancer; Prostate Cancer; Melanoma; **Hospital:** Adv Luth Genl Hosp, Rush N Shore Med Ctr; **Address:** Center for Advanced Care, 1700 Luther Ln Fl 2, Park Ridge, IL 60068; **Phone:** 847-268-8200; **Board Cert:** Internal Medicine 1998; Medical Oncology 2007; **Med School:** Cornell Univ-Weill Med Coll 1983; **Resid:** Internal Medicine, Univ Chicago Hosp 1985; **Fellow:** Hematology & Oncology, Univ Chicago Hosp 1988; **Fac Appt:** Asst Prof Med, Univ IL Coll Med

Rosen, Steven T MD [Onc] - **Spec Exp:** Hematologic Malignancies; Breast Cancer; Lymphoma; **Hospital:** Northwestern Meml Hosp; **Address:** Northwestern Univ, 303 E Chicago Ave, Lurie 3-125, Chicago, IL 60611-3013; **Phone:** 312-695-0990; **Board Cert:** Internal Medicine 1979; Medical Oncology 1981; Hematology 1984; **Med School:** Northwestern Univ 1976; **Resid:** Internal Medicine, Northwestern Univ Hosp 1979; **Fellow:** Medical Oncology, Natl Cancer Inst 1981; **Fac Appt:** Prof Med, Northwestern Univ

Ruckdeschel, John C MD [Onc] - **Spec Exp:** Lung Cancer; Mesothelioma; **Hospital:** Karmanos Cancer Inst; **Address:** Barbara Ann Karmanos Cancer Inst, 4100 John R, Detroit, MI 48201; **Phone:** 313-576-8670; **Board Cert:** Internal Medicine 1976; Medical Oncology 1977; **Med School:** Albany Med Coll 1971; **Resid:** Internal Medicine, Johns Hopkins Hosp 1972; Internal Medicine, Beth Israel Hosp 1976; **Fellow:** Medical Oncology, Natl Cancer Inst 1975

Salgia, Ravi MD/PhD [Onc] - **Spec Exp:** Lung Cancer; Mesothelioma; Thoracic Cancers; **Hospital:** Univ of Chicago Med Ctr; **Address:** University Chicago Hosps, 5841 S Maryland Ave, MC 2115, Chicago, IL 60637; **Phone:** 773-702-4400; **Board Cert:** Medical Oncology 2006; **Med School:** Loyola Univ-Stritch Sch Med 1987; **Resid:** Internal Medicine, Johns Hopkins Hosp 1990; **Fellow:** Medical Oncology, Dana-Farber Cancer Inst 1993; **Fac Appt:** Assoc Prof Med, Univ IL Coll Med

Schiffer, Charles A MD [Onc] - **Spec Exp:** Leukemia; Lymphoma; Multiple Myeloma; **Hospital:** Karmanos Cancer Inst, Harper Univ Hosp; **Address:** Karmanos Cancer Inst, Cancer Research Ctr, 4100 John R, 4 CRC-Hudson Webber, Detroit, MI 48201; **Phone:** 313-576-8737; **Board Cert:** Internal Medicine 1972; Medical Oncology 1973; **Med School:** NYU Sch Med 1968; **Resid:** Internal Medicine, Bellevue-NY VA Hosp-NYU 1972; **Fellow:** Medical Oncology, Natl Cancer Inst 1974; **Fac Appt:** Prof Med, Wayne State Univ

Schilsky, Richard MD [Onc] - **Spec Exp:** Gastrointestinal Cancer; Pancreatic Cancer; Drug Development; **Hospital:** Univ of Chicago Med Ctr; **Address:** Univ Chicago- Bio Sciences Div, 5841 S Maryland Ave, MC 2115, Chicago, IL 60637; **Phone:** 773-834-3914; **Board Cert:** Internal Medicine 1978; Medical Oncology 1979; **Med School:** Univ Chicago-Pritzker Sch Med 1975; **Resid:** Internal Medicine, Univ Texas 1977; **Fellow:** Medical Oncology, Natl Cancer Inst 1980; **Fac Appt:** Prof Med, Univ Chicago-Pritzker Sch Med

Schwartz, Burton S MD [Onc] - **Spec Exp:** Lymphoma; Breast Cancer; **Hospital:** Abbott - Northwestern Hosp; **Address:** 800 E 28th St, Piper Bldg, Ste 405, Minneapolis, MN 55407; **Phone:** 612-863-8585; **Board Cert:** Internal Medicine 1980; Hematology 1976; Medical Oncology 1977; **Med School:** Meharry Med Coll 1968; **Resid:** Internal Medicine, Michael Reese Hosp 1971; **Fellow:** Hematology, Univ Minn Hosp 1976; **Fac Appt:** Clin Prof Med, Univ Minn

Shapiro, Charles L MD [Onc] - **Spec Exp:** Breast Cancer; **Hospital:** Arthur G James Cancer Hosp & Research Inst; **Address:** Starling Loving Hall, rm B420, 320 W 10th Ave, Columbus, OH 43210; **Phone:** 614-293-6401; **Board Cert:** Internal Medicine 1987; Medical Oncology 2005; **Med School:** SUNY Buffalo 1984; **Resid:** Internal Medicine, Temple Univ Hosp 1987; **Fellow:** Medical Oncology, Dana Farber Cancer Inst 1991; **Fac Appt:** Assoc Prof Med, Ohio State Univ

Silverman, Paula MD [Onc] - **Spec Exp:** Breast Cancer; **Hospital:** Univ Hosps Case Med Ctr; **Address:** Univ Hosp Cleveland, Ireland Cancer Ctr, 11100 Euclid Ave Bolwell Bldg Fl 6, Cleveland, OH 44106; **Phone:** 216-844-8510; **Board Cert:** Internal Medicine 1984; Medical Oncology 1989; **Med School:** Case West Res Univ 1981; **Resid:** Internal Medicine, Univ Hosps 1984; **Fellow:** Hematology & Oncology, Case Western Reserve Univ 1987; **Fac Appt:** Assoc Prof Med, Case West Res Univ

Sledge Jr, George W MD [Onc] - **Spec Exp:** Breast Cancer; **Hospital:** Indiana Univ Hosp (page 74); **Address:** 535 Barnhill Drive, rm 473, Indianapolis, IN 46202; **Phone:** 317-274-0920; **Board Cert:** Internal Medicine 1980; Medical Oncology 1983; **Med School:** Tulane Univ 1977; **Resid:** Internal Medicine, St Louis Univ 1980; **Fellow:** Medical Oncology, Univ Texas 1983; **Fac Appt:** Prof Med, Indiana Univ

Stadler, Walter M MD [Onc] - **Spec Exp:** Kidney Cancer; Bladder Cancer; Prostate Cancer; Testicular Cancer; **Hospital:** Univ of Chicago Med Ctr; **Address:** Div Hem/Onc, 5841 S Maryland Ave, MC 2115, Chicago, IL 60637; **Phone:** 773-834-7424; **Board Cert:** Internal Medicine 2002; Medical Oncology 2003; **Med School:** Yale Univ 1988; **Resid:** Internal Medicine, Michael Reese Hosp 1991; **Fellow:** Medical Oncology, Univ Chicago Hosps 1994; **Fac Appt:** Prof Med, Univ Chicago-Pritzker Sch Med

Triozzi, Pierre L MD [Onc] - **Spec Exp:** Melanoma; Vaccine Therapy; Clinical Trials; **Hospital:** Cleveland Clin Fdn (page 70); **Address:** Cleveland Clinic Fdn, 9500 Euclid Ave, MC R40, Cleveland, OH 44195; **Phone:** 216-445-5141; **Board Cert:** Internal Medicine 1983; Medical Oncology 1987; Hematology 1988; **Med School:** Ohio State Univ 1980; **Resid:** Internal Medicine, Duke Univ Med Ctr 1983; **Fellow:** Hematology & Oncology, Duke Univ Med Ctr 1987; **Fac Appt:** Prof Med, Case West Res Univ

Urba, Susan G MD [Onc] - **Spec Exp:** Head & Neck Cancer; **Hospital:** Univ Michigan Hlth Sys; **Address:** Comp Cancer Ctr & Geriatrics Ctr, 1500 E Med Ctr Drive, rm 4214, Ann Arbor, MI 48109-0922; **Phone:** 734-647-8902; **Board Cert:** Internal Medicine 1986; Medical Oncology 2002; **Med School:** Univ Mich Med Sch 1983; **Resid:** Internal Medicine, Univ Mich Med Ctr 1986; **Fellow:** Hematology & Oncology, Univ Mich Med Ctr 1988; **Fac Appt:** Assoc Prof Med, Univ Mich Med Sch

Von Roenn, Jamie H MD [Onc] - **Spec Exp:** Palliative Care; AIDS Related Cancers; Breast Cancer; **Hospital:** Northwestern Meml Hosp; **Address:** 675 N St Clair, Ste 21-100, Chicago, IL 60611; **Phone:** 312-695-6180; **Board Cert:** Internal Medicine 1983; Medical Oncology 1985; Hospice & Palliative Medicine 2003; **Med School:** Rush Med Coll 1980; **Resid:** Internal Medicine, Rush-Presby-St Lukes Hosp 1983; **Fellow:** Medical Oncology, Rush-Presby-St Lukes Hosp 1985; **Fac Appt:** Prof Med, Northwestern Univ

Wade, James C MD [Onc] - **Spec Exp:** Infections in Cancer Patients; Bone Marrow Transplant; Leukemia; **Hospital:** Froedtert Meml Lutheran Hosp; **Address:** 9200 W Wisconsin Ave, CLCC4193, Milwaukee, WI 53226-3522; **Phone:** 414-805-4693; **Board Cert:** Internal Medicine 1977; Infectious Disease 1982; Medical Oncology 1981; **Med School:** Univ Utah 1974; **Resid:** Internal Medicine, Johns Hopkins Hosp 1977; **Fellow:** Medical Oncology, Natl Cancer Inst/NIH 1979; Infectious Disease, Univ Wash/Fred Hutchinson Cancer Rsch Ctr 1982; **Fac Appt:** Prof Med, Med Coll Wisc

Weiner, George J MD [Onc] - **Spec Exp:** Lymphoma; Leukemia; Immunotherapy; **Hospital:** Univ Iowa Hosp & Clinics; **Address:** Holden Comprehensive Cancer Center, 200 Hawkins Drive Bldg 5970JPP, Iowa City, IA 52242; **Phone:** 319-356-1932; **Board Cert:** Internal Medicine 1985; Hematology 1988; Medical Oncology 1987; **Med School:** Ohio State Univ 1981; **Resid:** Medical Oncology, Med Coll Ohio 1984; **Fellow:** Hematology & Oncology, Univ Mich Med Ctr 1987; **Fac Appt:** Prof Med, Univ Iowa Coll Med

Medical Oncology

Weissman, David E MD [Onc] - **Spec Exp:** Palliative Care; Pain-Cancer; **Hospital:** Froedtert Meml Lutheran Hosp; **Address:** Med Coll Wisc, Dept Hem/Onc, 9200 W Wisconsin Ave, Milwaukee, WI 53226-3596; **Phone:** 414-805-6800; **Board Cert:** Internal Medicine 1983; Medical Oncology 1985; **Med School:** UCSD 1980; **Resid:** Internal Medicine, UCSD Univ Hosp 1983; **Fellow:** Medical Oncology, Johns Hopkins Hosp 1985; **Fac Appt:** Prof Med, Univ Wisc

Wicha, Max S MD [Onc] - **Spec Exp:** Breast Cancer; Stem Cell Transplant; **Hospital:** Univ Michigan Hlth Sys; **Address:** Comp Cancer Ctr & Geriatrics Ctr, 1500 E Med Ctr Dr, rm 6302 CC, Ann Arbor, MI 48109-5942; **Phone:** 734-936-1831; **Board Cert:** Internal Medicine 1977; Medical Oncology 1983; **Med School:** Stanford Univ 1974; **Resid:** Internal Medicine, Univ Chicago Hosp 1977; **Fellow:** Medical Oncology, Natl Inst Hlth 1980; **Fac Appt:** Prof Med, Univ Mich Med Sch

Wilding, George MD [Onc] - **Spec Exp:** Prostate Cancer; Kidney Cancer; Genitourinary Cancer; Drug Discovery & Development; **Hospital:** Univ WI Hosp & Clins; **Address:** 1111 Highland Ave, Ste 7057WIMR, Madison, WI 53705; **Phone:** 608-263-8610; **Board Cert:** Internal Medicine 1983; Medical Oncology 1985; **Med School:** Univ Mass Sch Med 1980; **Resid:** Internal Medicine, Univ Mass Med Ctr 1983; **Fellow:** Medical Oncology, Natl Cancer Inst 1985; **Fac Appt:** Prof Med, Univ Wisc

Worden, Francis P MD [Onc] - **Spec Exp:** Head & Neck Cancer; Palliative Care; Clinical Trials; **Hospital:** Univ Michigan Hlth Sys; **Address:** Cancer Center & Geriatric Center, 1500 E Medical Center Drive, rm 4214, Ann Arbor, MI 48109; **Phone:** 734-647-8902; **Board Cert:** Medical Oncology 2000; **Med School:** Indiana Univ 1993; **Resid:** Internal Medicine & Pediatrics, Detroit Med Ctr 1997; **Fellow:** Medical Oncology, Detroit Med Ctr 1920; **Fac Appt:** Asst Clin Prof Med, Univ Mich Med Sch

Yee, Douglas MD [Onc] - **Spec Exp:** Breast Cancer; **Hospital:** Univ Minn Med Ctr, Fairview - Univ Campus; **Address:** Univ Minnesota Cancer Ctr, 420 Delaware St SE, MMC 806, Minneapolis, MN 55455; **Phone:** 612-625-5411; **Board Cert:** Internal Medicine 1984; Medical Oncology 1987; **Med School:** Univ Chicago-Pritzker Sch Med 1981; **Resid:** Internal Medicine, Univ NC Med Ctr 1984; **Fellow:** Medical Oncology, NIH-Clin Ctr 1987; **Fac Appt:** Prof Med, Univ Minn

Great Plains and Mountains

Akerley, Wallace MD [Onc] - **Spec Exp:** Lung Cancer; Clinical Trials; **Hospital:** Univ Utah Hosps and Clins; **Address:** Huntsman Cancer Inst, 2000 Circle of Hope, rm 2165, Salt Lake City, UT 84112; **Phone:** 801-585-0100; **Board Cert:** Internal Medicine 1984; Medical Oncology 1987; Hematology 1988; **Med School:** Brown Univ 1981; **Resid:** Internal Medicine, USC Medical Ctr 1985; **Fellow:** Medical Oncology, USC Medical Ctr 1986; Hematology, Norris Cotton Cancer Ctr/Dartmouth 1988; **Fac Appt:** Prof Med, Univ Utah

Armitage, James MD [Onc] - **Spec Exp:** Lymphoma; Bone Marrow Transplant; **Hospital:** Nebraska Med Ctr; **Address:** 987680 Nebraska Medical Center, Omaha, NE 68198-7680; **Phone:** 402-559-7290; **Board Cert:** Internal Medicine 1976; Medical Oncology 1977; Hematology 1984; **Med School:** Univ Nebr Coll Med 1973; **Resid:** Internal Medicine, Univ Nebraska Med Ctr 1975; **Fellow:** Hematology & Oncology, Univ Iowa Hosp 1977; **Fac Appt:** Prof Med, Univ Nebr Coll Med

Beatty, Patrick G MD [Onc] - **Spec Exp:** Hematologic Malignancies; Lymphoma; **Hospital:** St Patrick Hospital - Missoula; **Address:** PO Box 7877, Missoula, MT 59807; **Phone:** 406-728-2539; **Board Cert:** Internal Medicine 1980; Medical Oncology 1985; **Resid:** Internal Medicine, Vanderbilt Univ Med Ctr 1979; **Fellow:** Oncology, Univ Washington Hosps 1982

Bierman, Philip J MD [Onc] - **Spec Exp:** Lymphoma; Bone Marrow Transplant; **Hospital:** Nebraska Med Ctr; **Address:** Nebraska Medical Ctr, Dept Hem/Oncology, 987680 Nebraska Medical Ctr, Omaha, NE 68198-7680; **Phone:** 402-559-5520; **Board Cert:** Internal Medicine 1982; Medical Oncology 1985; Hematology 1986; **Med School:** Univ MO-Kansas City 1979; **Resid:** Internal Medicine, Univ Nebraska Med Ctr 1983; **Fellow:** Medical Oncology, Univ Nebraska Med Ctr 1985; Hematology, City of Hope Natl Med Ctr 1986; **Fac Appt:** Assoc Prof Med, Univ Nebr Coll Med

Bunn Jr, Paul A MD [Onc] - **Spec Exp:** Lung Cancer; Clinical Trials; **Hospital:** Univ Colorado Hosp, Vail Valley Med Ctr; **Address:** Univ Colorado Hosp Cancer Ctr, 1665 Aurora Ct, Ste MS F-704, 1665 Aurora Court, Aurora, CO 80045-0510; **Phone:** 303-724-4499; **Board Cert:** Internal Medicine 1974; Medical Oncology 1975; **Med School:** Cornell Univ-Weill Med Coll 1971; **Resid:** Internal Medicine, Moffitt Hosp/ UCSF Med Ctr 1973; **Fellow:** Medical Oncology, Natl Cancer Inst 1976; **Fac Appt:** Prof Med, Univ Colorado

Buys, Saundra S MD [Onc] - **Spec Exp:** Breast Cancer; Breast Cancer Risk Assessment; Breast Cancer Genetics; **Hospital:** Univ Utah Hosps and Clins; **Address:** Huntsman Cancer Institute, 2000 Circle of Hope, Ste 210, Salt Lake City, UT 84112; **Phone:** 801-585-3525; **Board Cert:** Internal Medicine 1982; Medical Oncology 1985; Hematology 1984; **Med School:** Tufts Univ 1979; **Resid:** Internal Medicine, Univ Utah Hosps 1982; **Fellow:** Hematology & Oncology, Univ Utah Hosps 1985; **Fac Appt:** Prof Med, Univ Utah

Cowan, Kenneth H MD/PhD [Onc] - **Spec Exp:** Breast Cancer; **Hospital:** Nebraska Med Ctr; **Address:** Eppley Cancer Center, 986805 Nebraska Medical Ctr, Omaha, NE 68198-6805; **Phone:** 402-559-4238; **Board Cert:** Internal Medicine 1978; Medical Oncology 1981; **Med School:** Case West Res Univ 1974; **Resid:** Internal Medicine, Parkland Meml Hosp 1977

Dakhil, Shaker MD [Onc] - **Spec Exp:** Leukemia; Mesothelioma; Lymphoma; **Hospital:** Univ of Kansas Hosp; **Address:** Cancer Center Kansas, 818 N Emporia, Ste 403, Wichita, KS 67214; **Phone:** 316-262-4467; **Board Cert:** Internal Medicine 1978; Medical Oncology 1981; **Med School:** Lebanon 1976; **Resid:** Internal Medicine, Wayne State Univ Hosp 1978; **Fellow:** Hematology & Oncology, Univ Michigan Sch Med 1981; **Fac Appt:** Assoc Clin Prof Med, Univ Kans

Eckhardt, S Gail MD [Onc] - **Spec Exp:** Gastrointestinal Cancer; Drug Development; **Hospital:** Univ Colorado Hosp; **Address:** Univ Colorado Hosp Cancer Ctr, PO Box 6510, MS F-704, 1665 Aurora Court, Aurora, CO 00045 0510; **Phone:** 720-848-0300; **Board Cert:** Internal Medicine 1988; Medical Oncology 2006; **Med School:** Univ Tex Med Br, Galveston 1985; **Resid:** Internal Medicine, Univ Virginia Med Ctr 1988; **Fellow:** Research, Scripps Clinic 1989; Medical Oncology, UCSD Med Ctr 1992; **Fac Appt:** Prof Med, Univ Colorado

Elias, Anthony D MD [Onc] - **Spec Exp:** Breast Cancer; **Hospital:** Univ Colorado Hosp; **Address:** UCH Breast Ctr, Anschutz OPD Pavillion, 1635 Aurora Ct, MS F724, Aurora, CO 80045; **Phone:** 720-848-1030; **Board Cert:** Internal Medicine 1983; Medical Oncology 1985; **Med School:** NYU Sch Med 1980; **Resid:** Internal Medicine, Johns Hopkins Hsop 1983; **Fellow:** Medical Oncology, Dana-Farber Cancer Inst 1983; **Fac Appt:** Assoc Prof Med, Univ Colorado

Fabian, Carol J MD [Onc] - **Spec Exp:** Breast Cancer; Breast Cancer Risk Assessment; **Hospital:** Univ of Kansas Hosp; **Address:** Univ Kansas Med Ctr, Div Clinical Onc, 2330 Shawnee Mission Pkwy, Ste 1102, MS 5015, Kansas City, KS 66160-7418; **Phone:** 913-588-7791; **Board Cert:** Internal Medicine 1976; Medical Oncology 1977; **Med School:** Univ Kans 1972; **Resid:** Internal Medicine, Wesley Med Ctr 1975; **Fellow:** Medical Oncology, Univ Kansas Med Ctr 1977; **Fac Appt:** Prof Med, Univ Kans

Medical Oncology

Glode, L Michael MD [Onc] - **Spec Exp:** Prostate Cancer; Genitourinary Cancer; **Hospital:** Univ Colorado Hosp; **Address:** U Colo Hlth Scis Ctr, Div Med Oncology, PO Box 6510, MS F710, Aurora, CO 80045-0510; **Phone:** 720-848-0170; **Board Cert:** Internal Medicine 1975; Medical Oncology 1981; **Med School:** Washington Univ, St Louis 1972; **Resid:** Internal Medicine, Univ Texas SW Med Sch 1973; Immunology, Natl Inst Hlth 1976; **Fellow:** Medical Oncology, Dana Farber Cancer Inst 1978; **Fac Appt:** Prof Med, Univ Colorado

Grem, Jean L MD [Onc] - **Spec Exp:** Colon & Rectal Cancer; Pancreatic Cancer; Stomach Cancer; Esophageal Cancer; **Hospital:** Nebraska Med Ctr; **Address:** 987680 Nebraska Medical Ctr, Omaha, NE 68198-7680; **Phone:** 402-559-6210; **Board Cert:** Internal Medicine 1983; Medical Oncology 1985; **Med School:** Jefferson Med Coll 1980; **Resid:** Internal Medicine, Univ Iowa Hosps & Clinics 1983; **Fellow:** Medical Oncology, Univ Wisc Clin Cancer Ctr 1986; **Fac Appt:** Prof Med, Univ Nebr Coll Med

Hauke, Ralph J MD [Onc] - **Spec Exp:** Urologic Cancer; Clinical Trials; Testicular Cancer; Prostate Cancer; **Hospital:** Methodist Hosp - Omaha, Alegent Hlth - Bergan Mercy Med Ctr; **Address:** 8303 Dodge St, Ste 250, Omaha, NE 68114; **Phone:** 402-354-8124; **Board Cert:** Medical Oncology 2001; **Med School:** Panama 1990; **Resid:** Internal Medicine, Univ Nebraska Med Ctr 1996; **Fellow:** Medical Oncology, Univ Nebraska Med Ctr 2001; **Fac Appt:** Assoc Prof Med, Univ Nebr Coll Med

Kane, Madeleine A MD/PhD [Onc] - **Spec Exp:** Head & Neck Cancer; Gastrointestinal Cancer; Neuroendocrine Tumors; **Hospital:** Univ Colorado Hosp, VA Med Ctr; **Address:** Univ Colorado Hosp Cancer Ctr, PO Box 6510, MS F-704, 1665 Aurora Court, Aurora, CO 80045; **Phone:** 720-848-0300; **Board Cert:** Internal Medicine 1981; Medical Oncology 1983; Hematology 1986; **Med School:** Univ Miami Sch Med 1978; **Resid:** Internal Medicine, Stanford Univ Med Ctr 1981; **Fellow:** Hematology & Oncology, Univ Colo Hlth Sci Ctr 1984; **Fac Appt:** Prof Med, Univ Colorado

Kelly, Karen Lee MD [Onc] - **Spec Exp:** Lung Cancer; **Hospital:** Univ of Kansas Hosp; **Address:** Univ Kansas Cancer Ctr, 4030 Robinson, MS #1027, 3901 Rainbow Blvd, Kansas City, KS 66160; **Phone:** 913-588-4761; **Board Cert:** Internal Medicine 1987; Medical Oncology 2003; **Med School:** Univ Kans 1984; **Resid:** Internal Medicine, Univ Colo Hlth Sci Ctr 1987; **Fellow:** Medical Oncology, Univ Colo Hlth Sci Ctr 1990; **Fac Appt:** Assoc Prof Med, Univ Colorado

Samuels, Brian L MD [Onc] - **Spec Exp:** Sarcoma; **Hospital:** Kootenai Med Ctr; **Address:** North Idaho Cancer Center, 700 W Ironwood Drive, Ste 103, Coeur D'Alene, ID 83814; **Phone:** 208-666-3800; **Board Cert:** Internal Medicine 1984; Medical Oncology 1987; **Med School:** Zimbabwe 1976; **Resid:** Internal Medicine, Albert Einstein Med Ctr 1981; Internal Medicine, Albert Einstein Med Ctr 1984; **Fellow:** Hematology & Oncology, Univ Chicago Hosps 1988

Ward, John H MD [Onc] - **Spec Exp:** Breast Cancer; Gastrointestinal Cancer; **Hospital:** Univ Utah Hosps and Clins; **Address:** Huntsman Cancer Inst, 2000 Circle of Hope, Ste 2100, Salt Lake City, UT 84112-5550; **Phone:** 801-585-0255; **Board Cert:** Internal Medicine 1979; Medical Oncology 1981; Hematology 1982; **Med School:** Univ Utah 1976; **Resid:** Internal Medicine, Duke Univ Med Ctr 1979; **Fellow:** Hematology & Oncology, Univ Utah 1982; **Fac Appt:** Prof Med, Univ Utah

Southwest

Abbruzzese, James L MD [Onc] - **Spec Exp:** Gastrointestinal Cancer; Pancreatic Cancer; Clinical Trials; **Hospital:** UT MD Anderson Cancer Ctr; **Address:** Univ Tex MD Anderson Cancer Ctr, 1515 Holcombe Blvd, Unit 426, Houston, TX 77030; **Phone:** 713-792-2828; **Board Cert:** Internal Medicine 1981; Medical Oncology 1983; **Med School:** Univ Chicago-Pritzker Sch Med 1978; **Resid:** Internal Medicine, Johns Hopkins Hosp 1981; **Fellow:** Medical Oncology, Dana-Farber Cancer Inst 1983; **Fac Appt:** Prof Med, Univ Tex, Houston

Ahmann, Frederick R MD [Onc] - **Spec Exp:** Prostate Cancer; Testicular Cancer; Bladder Cancer; **Hospital:** Univ Med Ctr - Tucson; **Address:** Arizona Cancer Ctr, 1515 N Campbell Ave, Box 245024, Tucson, AZ 85724; **Phone:** 520-694-2873; **Board Cert:** Internal Medicine 1977; Medical Oncology 1981; **Med School:** Univ MO-Columbia Sch Med 1974; **Resid:** Internal Medicine, Georgetown Univ Med Ctr 1977; **Fellow:** Medical Oncology, Univ Med Ctr 1980; **Fac Appt:** Prof Med, Univ Ariz Coll Med

Ajani, Jaffer A MD [Onc] - **Spec Exp:** Gastrointestinal Cancer; Esophageal Cancer; Stomach Cancer; Neuroendocrine Tumors; **Hospital:** UT MD Anderson Cancer Ctr; **Address:** Univ Tex MD Anderson Cancer Ctr, Faculty Ctr Unit 426, Houston, TX 77230; **Phone:** 713-792-2828; **Board Cert:** Internal Medicine 1979; Medical Oncology 1983; **Med School:** India 1971; **Resid:** Family Medicine, Penn Stae Univ-Altoona 1977; Internal Medicine, Tulane Univ Sch Med 1980; **Fellow:** Medical Oncology, MD Anderson Cancer Ctr 1983; **Fac Appt:** Prof Med, Univ Tex, Houston

Alberts, David S MD [Onc] - **Spec Exp:** Cancer Prevention; Ovarian Cancer; **Hospital:** Univ Med Ctr - Tucson; **Address:** Arizona Cancer Center, 1515N Campbell Ave, PO Box 245024, Tucson, AZ 85724; **Phone:** 520-626-7685; **Board Cert:** Internal Medicine 1973; Medical Oncology 1973; **Med School:** Univ VA Sch Med 1966; **Resid:** Medical Oncology, Natl Cancer Inst-NIH 1969; Internal Medicine, Univ Minn Hosps 1971; **Fellow:** Clinical Pharmacology, UC San Francisco 1974; **Fac Appt:** Prof Med, Univ Ariz Coll Med

Anthony, Lowell B MD [Onc] - **Spec Exp:** Gastrointestinal Cancer; Carcinoid Tumors; Neuroendocrine Tumors; **Hospital:** LSU Interim Public Hosp; **Address:** 200 W Esplanade, Ste 200, Kenner, LA 70065; **Phone:** 504-464-8500; **Board Cert:** Internal Medicine 1983; Medical Oncology 1989; **Med School:** Vanderbilt Univ 1979; **Resid:** Internal Medicine, Vanderbilt Univ Med Ctr 1982; **Fellow:** Medical Oncology, Vanderbilt Univ Med Ctr 1985; **Fac Appt:** Assoc Prof Med, Louisiana State U, New Orleans

Arun, Banu K MD [Onc] - **Spec Exp:** Breast Cancer; Cancer Prevention; Clinical Trials; **Hospital:** UT MD Anderson Cancer Ctr; **Address:** 1515 Holcombe Blvd, Unit 1354, Houston, TX 77030; **Phone:** 713-792-2817; **Med School:** Turkey 1990; **Resid:** Internal Medicine, Univ Istanbul 1994; **Fellow:** Hematology & Oncology, Lombardi Cancer Ctr-Georgetown Univ 1997; **Fac Appt:** Assoc Prof Med, Univ Tex, Houston

Benjamin, Robert S MD [Onc] - **Spec Exp:** Sarcoma; **Hospital:** UT MD Anderson Cancer Ctr; **Address:** UT MD Anderson Cancer Ctr, 1515 Holcombe Blvd, Unit 450, Houston, TX 77030; **Phone:** 713-792-3626; **Board Cert:** Internal Medicine 1973; Medical Oncology 1973; **Med School:** NYU Sch Med 1968; **Resid:** Internal Medicine, Bellevue Hosp Ctr-NYU 1970; **Fellow:** Medical Oncology, Baltimore Cancer Rsch Ctr 1972; **Fac Appt:** Prof Med, Univ Tex, Houston

Bergsagel, Peter Leif MD [Onc] - **Spec Exp:** Multiple Myeloma; Hematologic Malignancies; **Hospital:** Mayo Clinic - Scottsdale; **Address:** 13400 E Shea Blvd, Scottsdale, AZ 85259; **Phone:** 480-301-8335; **Board Cert:** Internal Medicine 1987; Medical Oncology 1989; **Med School:** Univ Toronto 1984; **Resid:** Internal Medicine, Stanford Univ Med Ctr 1986; Internal Medicine, Sunnybrook Med Ctr 1987; **Fellow:** Medical Oncology, NIH Natl Cancer Inst 1990; **Fac Appt:** Prof Med, Mayo Med Sch

Medical Oncology

Bruera, Eduardo MD [Onc] - **Spec Exp:** Palliative Care; **Hospital:** UT MD Anderson Cancer Ctr; **Address:** 1515 Holcombe Blvd, Unit 8, Houston, TX 77030; **Phone:** 713-792-6085; **Med School:** Argentina 1979; **Resid:** Internal Medicine, Hospital Privado; **Fellow:** Medical Oncology, Cross Cancer Inst; **Fac Appt:** Prof Med, Univ Tex, Houston

Buzdar, Aman U MD [Onc] - **Spec Exp:** Breast Cancer; **Hospital:** UT MD Anderson Cancer Ctr; **Address:** UT MD Anderson Canc Ctr, Dept Breast Oncology, PO Box 301429, Unit 1354, Houston, TX 77030; **Phone:** 713-792-2817; **Board Cert:** Internal Medicine 1975; Medical Oncology 1979; **Med School:** Pakistan 1967; **Resid:** Internal Medicine, Norwalk Hosp 1973; Internal Medicine, Lakewood Hosp 1971; **Fellow:** Hematology, Norwalk Hosp 1974; Oncology, MD Anderson Cancer Ctr 1975; **Fac Appt:** Prof Med, Univ Tex, Houston

Camoriano, John MD [Onc] - **Spec Exp:** Lymphoma; Breast Cancer; Bone Marrow Transplant; Myeloproliferative Disorders; **Hospital:** Mayo Clinic - Scottsdale; **Address:** Mayo Clinic - Scottsdale, 13400 E Shea Blvd Fl 3, Scottsdale, AZ 85259; **Phone:** 480-301-8335; **Board Cert:** Internal Medicine 1985; Hematology 1988; Medical Oncology 1989; **Med School:** Univ Nebr Coll Med 1982; **Resid:** Internal Medicine, Univ OK 1985; **Fellow:** Hematology & Oncology, Mayo Grad Sch Med 1989; **Fac Appt:** Asst Prof Med, Mayo Med Sch

Chang, Jenny C N MD [Onc] - **Spec Exp:** Breast Cancer; Clinical Trials; **Hospital:** Methodist Hosp - Houston; **Address:** One Baylor Plaza, MS BCM600, Houston, TX 77030; **Phone:** 713-798-1034; **Board Cert:** Internal Medicine 2004; **Med School:** England, UK 1989; **Resid:** Internal Medicine 1993; **Fellow:** Medical Oncology, Royal Marsden Hosp 1997; **Fac Appt:** Assoc Prof Med, Baylor Coll Med

Fay, Joseph W MD [Onc] - **Spec Exp:** Bone Marrow Transplant; Melanoma; Leukemia & Lymphoma; **Hospital:** Baylor Univ Medical Ctr; **Address:** 3535 Worth St, Sammons Tower, Suite 500, Dallas, TX 75246; **Phone:** 214-370-1500; **Board Cert:** Internal Medicine 1975; Medical Oncology 1977; Hematology 1978; **Med School:** Ohio State Univ 1972; **Resid:** Internal Medicine, Duke Med Ctr 1974; Oncology, Natl Cancer Institute 1976; **Fellow:** Hematology, Duke Med Ctr 1977; **Fac Appt:** Clin Prof Med, Univ Tex SW, Dallas

Fitch, Tom R MD [Onc] - **Spec Exp:** Breast Cancer; Sarcoma; Cancer Prevention; Palliative Care; **Hospital:** Mayo Clinic - Scottsdale; **Address:** Mayo Clinic - Scottsdale, 13400 E Shea Blvd Fl 3, Scottsdale, AZ 85259; **Phone:** 480-301-8335; **Board Cert:** Internal Medicine 1985; Medical Oncology 1987; Hematology 1988; **Med School:** Univ Kans 1982; **Resid:** Internal Medicine, Univ Michigan Med Ctr 1985; **Fellow:** Hematology & Oncology, Mayo Clinic 1988; **Fac Appt:** Asst Prof Med, Mayo Med Sch

Fossella, Frank V MD [Onc] - **Spec Exp:** Lung Cancer; **Hospital:** UT MD Anderson Cancer Ctr; **Address:** Dept Thoracic Head/Neck Med Oncol, Unit 432, 1400 Holcombe Blvd, Houston, TX 77030; **Phone:** 713-792-6363; **Board Cert:** Internal Medicine 1985; Medical Oncology 1987; **Med School:** Baylor Coll Med 1982; **Resid:** Internal Medicine, Baylor Coll Med 1985; **Fellow:** Medical Oncology, Baylor Coll Med 1987; **Fac Appt:** Prof Med, Univ Tex, Houston

Glisson, Bonnie S MD [Onc] - **Spec Exp:** Head & Neck Cancer; Lung Cancer; **Hospital:** UT MD Anderson Cancer Ctr; **Address:** 1515 Holcombe Blvd, Unit 432, Houston, TX 77030; **Phone:** 713-792-6363; **Board Cert:** Internal Medicine 1982; Medical Oncology 1985; **Med School:** Ohio State Univ 1979; **Resid:** Internal Medicine, Univ Va Med Ctr 1982; **Fellow:** Medical Oncology, Univ Fla Health Sci Ctr 1985; **Fac Appt:** Prof Med, Univ Tex, Houston

Haley, Barbara MD [Onc] - **Spec Exp:** Breast Cancer; **Hospital:** UT Southwestern Med Ctr at Dallas; **Address:** 5323 Harry Hines Blvd, Dallas, TX 75390-8852; **Phone:** 214-648-4180; **Board Cert:** Internal Medicine 1979; Hematology 1984; **Med School:** Univ Tex SW, Dallas 1976; **Resid:** Internal Medicine, Parkland Meml Hosp 1979; **Fellow:** Hematology & Oncology, Parkland Meml Hosp 1981; **Fac Appt:** Prof Med, Univ Tex SW, Dallas

Herbst, Roy S MD/PhD [Onc] - **Spec Exp:** Lung Cancer; Head & Neck Cancer; Breast Cancer; Drug Development; **Hospital:** UT MD Anderson Cancer Ctr; **Address:** Thoracic/Head & Neck Med Onc - Unit 432, UT MD Anderson Cancer Ctr, PO Box 301402, Houston, TX 77230-1402; **Phone:** 713-792-6363; **Board Cert:** Medical Oncology 2007; **Med School:** Cornell Univ-Weill Med Coll 1991; **Resid:** Internal Medicine, Brigham & Women's Hosp 1994; **Fellow:** Medical Oncology, Dana Farber Cancer Inst 1996; **Fac Appt:** Assoc Prof Med, Univ Tex, Houston

Hong, Waun Ki MD [Onc] - **Spec Exp:** Lung Cancer; Head & Neck Cancer; Thoracic Cancers; **Hospital:** UT MD Anderson Cancer Ctr; **Address:** Dept Thoracic Head/Neck, Unit 432, 1400 Holcombe Blvd, Houston, TX 77030; **Phone:** 713-792-6363; **Board Cert:** Internal Medicine 1976; Medical Oncology 1979; **Med School:** South Korea 1967; **Resid:** Internal Medicine, Boston VA Hosp 1973; **Fellow:** Medical Oncology, Meml Sloan-Kettering Cancer Ctr 1975; **Fac Appt:** Prof Med, Univ Tex, Houston

Hortobagyi, Gabriel N MD [Onc] - **Spec Exp:** Breast Cancer; Clinical Trials; Gene Therapy; **Hospital:** UT MD Anderson Cancer Ctr; **Address:** UT MD Anderson Cancer Ctr, Dept Breast Oncology, PO Box 301429, Unit 1354, Houston, TX 77030-1439; **Phone:** 713-792-2817; **Board Cert:** Internal Medicine 1975; Medical Oncology 1977; **Med School:** Colombia 1970; **Resid:** Internal Medicine, St Lukes Hosp 1974; **Fellow:** Medical Oncology, MD Anderson Cancer Ctr 1976; **Fac Appt:** Prof Med

Hutchins, Laura F MD [Onc] - **Spec Exp:** Breast Cancer; Melanoma; **Hospital:** UAMS Med Ctr; **Address:** Univ Arkansas Med Scis, Dept Hem/Onc, 4301 W Markham St, MS 721-5, Little Rock, AR 72205-7101; **Phone:** 501-686-8511; **Board Cert:** Internal Medicine 1980; Hematology 1984; Medical Oncology 1987; **Med School:** Univ Ark 1977; **Resid:** Internal Medicine, Univ Ark Affil Hosp 1980; **Fellow:** Hematology & Oncology, Univ Arkansas 1983; **Fac Appt:** Prof Med, Univ Ark

Karp, Daniel D MD [Onc] - **Spec Exp:** Lung Cancer; **Hospital:** UT MD Anderson Cancer Ctr; **Address:** 1515 Holcombe Blvd, Unit 432, Houston, TX 77030-4009; **Phone:** 713-792-6363; **Board Cert:** Internal Medicine 1976; Hematology 1980; Medical Oncology 1981; **Med School:** Duke Univ 1973; **Resid:** Internal Medicine, Dartmouth-Hitchcock Med Ctr 1976; **Fellow:** Hematology, Dartmouth-Hitchcock Med Ctr 1978; Medical Oncology, Dana Farber Cancer Inst 1979; **Fac Appt:** Prof Med, Univ Tex, Houston

Kies, Merrill S MD [Onc] - **Spec Exp:** Head & Neck Cancer; Lung Cancer; **Hospital:** UT MD Anderson Cancer Ctr; **Address:** Dept Thoracic, Head & Neck Oncology, 1515 Holcombe Blvd, Unit 432, Houston, TX 77030; **Phone:** 713-792-6363; **Board Cert:** Internal Medicine 1976; Medical Oncology 1979; **Med School:** Loyola Univ-Stritch Sch Med 1973; **Resid:** Internal Medicine, Walter Reed AMC 1976; **Fellow:** Medical Oncology, Brooke AMC 1978; **Fac Appt:** Prof Med, Univ Tex, Houston

Kwak, Larry W MD/PhD [Onc] - **Spec Exp:** Lymphoma; Multiple Myeloma; Vaccine Therapy; Immunotherapy; **Hospital:** UT MD Anderson Cancer Ctr; **Address:** MD Anderson Cancer Ctr, Dept Lymphoma/Myeloma, 1515 Holcombe Blvd, Unit 429, Houston, TX 77030; **Phone:** 713-745-4244; **Board Cert:** Internal Medicine 1987; Medical Oncology 1989; **Med School:** Northwestern Univ 1982; **Resid:** Internal Medicine, Stanford Univ Hosp 1987; **Fellow:** Oncology, Stanford Univ Hosp 1989

Medical Oncology

Lippman, Scott M MD [Onc] - **Spec Exp:** Cancer Prevention; Lung Cancer; Head & Neck Cancer; **Hospital:** UT MD Anderson Cancer Ctr; **Address:** UT MD Anderson Cancer Ctr, 1515 Holcombe Blvd, Box 432, Houston, TX 77030-1439; **Phone:** 713-745-5439; **Board Cert:** Internal Medicine 1987; Hematology 1988; Medical Oncology 1989; **Med School:** Johns Hopkins Univ 1981; **Resid:** Internal Medicine, Harbor-UCLA Med Ctr 1983; **Fellow:** Hematology, Stanford Univ Med Ctr 1985; Hematology & Oncology, Univ Ariz Hlth Scis Ctr 1987; **Fac Appt:** Prof Med, Univ Tex, Houston

Livingston, Robert B MD [Onc] - **Spec Exp:** Bone Marrow Transplant; Breast Cancer; Lung Cancer; **Hospital:** Univ Med Ctr - Tucson; **Address:** University Medical Center, 3838 N Campbell Ave, Tucson, AZ 85719; **Phone:** 520-694-2873; **Board Cert:** Internal Medicine 1972; Medical Oncology 1973; **Med School:** Univ Okla Coll Med 1965; **Resid:** Internal Medicine, Univ Oklahoma Med Ctr 1971; **Fellow:** Medical Oncology, Univ Texas Cancer Ctr 1973; **Fac Appt:** Prof Med, Univ Wash

Logothetis, Christopher J MD [Onc] - **Spec Exp:** Prostate Cancer; Bladder Cancer; **Hospital:** UT MD Anderson Cancer Ctr; **Address:** UT MD Anderson Cancer Ctr, Dept GU Onc, Unit 1374, Box 301439, Houston, TX 77230-1439; **Phone:** 713-745-7020; **Board Cert:** Internal Medicine 1978; Medical Oncology 1981; **Med School:** Greece 1974; **Resid:** Internal Medicine, Univ Texas 1979; **Fellow:** Hematology & Oncology, Univ Tex-MD Anderson Cancer Ctr 1981; **Fac Appt:** Prof Med, Univ Tex, Houston

Markman, Maurie MD [Onc] - **Spec Exp:** Ovarian Cancer; Gynecologic Cancer; Drug Development; Palliative Care; **Hospital:** UT MD Anderson Cancer Ctr; **Address:** Univ Texas MD Anderson Cancer Ctr, 1515 Holcombe Blvd, Box 1435, Houston, TX 77030-4009; **Phone:** 713-745-7140; **Board Cert:** Internal Medicine 1977; Hematology 1982; Medical Oncology 1981; **Med School:** NYU Sch Med 1974; **Resid:** Internal Medicine, Bellevue Hosp Ctr 1978; **Fellow:** Medical Oncology, Johns Hopkins Hosp 1980; **Fac Appt:** Prof Med, Univ Tex, Houston

Miller, Thomas P MD [Onc] - **Spec Exp:** Lymphoma; **Hospital:** Univ Med Ctr - Tucson; **Address:** Arizona Cancer Ctr, 1515 N Campbell Ave, PO Box 245024, Tucson, AZ 85724; **Phone:** 520-626-2667; **Board Cert:** Internal Medicine 1977; Medical Oncology 1981; **Med School:** Univ IL Coll Med 1972; **Resid:** Internal Medicine, Univ Illinois Hosps 1977; **Fellow:** Hematology & Oncology, Univ Med Ctr 1980; **Fac Appt:** Prof Med, Univ Ariz Coll Med

Nemunaitis, John G MD [Onc] - **Spec Exp:** Cancer Genetics; Vaccine Therapy; Lung Cancer; **Hospital:** Baylor Univ Medical Ctr; **Address:** Mary Crowley Med Rsch Ctr, 3535 Worth St, Ste 302, Dallas, TX 75246; **Phone:** 214-370-1870; **Board Cert:** Internal Medicine 1987; **Med School:** Case West Res Univ 1982; **Resid:** Internal Medicine, Boston City Hosp 1985; **Fellow:** Hematology & Oncology, Fred Hutchinson Cancer Rsch Ctr 1989

Northfelt, Donald W MD [Onc] - **Spec Exp:** Breast Cancer; Colon & Rectal Cancer; Lung Cancer; **Hospital:** Mayo Clinic - Scottsdale; **Address:** Mayo Clinic Scottsdale, 13400 E Shea Blvd Fl 3, Scottsdale, AZ 85259; **Phone:** 480-301-8335; **Board Cert:** Internal Medicine 1988; Medical Oncology 2001; **Med School:** Univ Minn 1985; **Resid:** Internal Medicine, UCLA Med Ctr 1988; **Fellow:** Hematology & Oncology, UCSF Med Ctr 1991; **Fac Appt:** Assoc Prof Med, Mayo Med Sch

O'Brien, Susan M MD [Onc] - **Spec Exp:** Leukemia; Lymphoma; **Hospital:** UT MD Anderson Cancer Ctr; **Address:** Univ Texas MD Anderson Cancer Ctr, Dept Leukemia, Unit 428, Box 301439, Houston, TX 77230; **Phone:** 713-792-7305; **Board Cert:** Internal Medicine 1983; Medical Oncology 1987; **Med School:** UMDNJ-NJ Med Sch, Newark 1980; **Resid:** Internal Medicine, UMDNJ Med Ctr 1983; **Fellow:** Medical Oncology, Univ TX MD Anderson Med Ctr 1987; **Fac Appt:** Prof Med, Univ Tex, Houston

O'Shaughnessy, Joyce A MD [Onc] - **Spec Exp:** Breast Cancer; **Hospital:** Baylor Univ Medical Ctr; **Address:** US Oncology, 3535 Worth St, Ste 600, Dallas, TX 75246; **Phone:** 214-370-1000; **Board Cert:** Internal Medicine 1985; Medical Oncology 1987; **Med School:** Yale Univ 1982; **Resid:** Internal Medicine, Mass Genl Hosp 1985; **Fellow:** Medical Oncology, National Cancer Inst 1988

Orlowski, Robert Z MD/PhD [Onc] - **Spec Exp:** Multiple Myeloma; Lymphoma, Non-Hodgkin's; Leukemia; Clinical Trials; **Hospital:** UT MD Anderson Cancer Ctr; **Address:** MD Anderson Cancer Ctr, Lymphoma & Myeloma Clinic, 1515 Holcombe Blvd, Box 429, Houston, TX 77030; **Phone:** 713-792-3510; **Med School:** Yale Univ 1991; **Resid:** Internal Medicine, Barnes Hosp/Wash Univ 1994; **Fellow:** Hematology & Oncology, Johns Hopkins Hosp 1998

Osborne, Charles K MD [Onc] - **Spec Exp:** Breast Cancer; **Hospital:** Methodist Hosp - Houston; **Address:** 1 Baylor Plaza, MS BCM600, Houston, TX 77030; **Phone:** 713-798-1641; **Board Cert:** Internal Medicine 1975; Medical Oncology 1977; **Med School:** Univ MO-Columbia Sch Med 1972; **Resid:** Internal Medicine, Johns Hopkins Hosp 1974; **Fellow:** Medical Oncology, Natl Cancer Inst 1977; **Fac Appt:** Prof Med, Baylor Coll Med

Papadopoulos, Nicholas E MD [Onc] - **Spec Exp:** Melanoma; **Hospital:** UT MD Anderson Cancer Ctr; **Address:** 1515 Holcombe Blvd, Unit 430, Houston, TX 77030; **Phone:** 713-792-2828; **Med School:** Greece 1966; **Resid:** Internal Medicine, Baylor Coll Med 1976; **Fellow:** Medical Oncology, MD Anderson Cancer Ctr 1978; **Fac Appt:** Assoc Prof Med, Univ Tex, Houston

Patel, Shreyaskumar MD [Onc] - **Spec Exp:** Sarcoma; **Hospital:** UT MD Anderson Cancer Ctr; **Address:** 1515 Holcombe Blvd, Box 0450, Houston, TX 77030; **Phone:** 713-792-3626; **Board Cert:** Internal Medicine 1987; Medical Oncology 2000; **Med School:** India 1983; **Resid:** Internal Medicine, Wayne State Univ 1987; **Fellow:** Medical Oncology, Mayo Clinic 1990

Patt, Yehuda Z MD [Onc] - **Spec Exp:** Liver Cancer; Biliary Cancer; Colon & Rectal Cancer; Gastrointestinal Cancer; **Hospital:** Univ NM Hlth & Sci Ctr; **Address:** Univ New Mexico CRTC, Div Hem/Onc, 900 Camino de Salud NE, MSC 084630, Albuquerque, NM 87131-0001; **Phone:** 505-272-5837; **Board Cert:** Internal Medicine 1982; Medical Oncology 1987; **Med School:** Israel 1967; **Resid:** Internal Medicine, Tel Aviv Sheba Med Ctr 1974; **Fellow:** Medical Oncology, UT MD Anderson Cancer Ctr 1977; **Fac Appt:** Prof Med, Univ New Mexico

Pisters, Katherine M W MD [Onc] - **Spec Exp:** Lung Cancer; **Hospital:** UT MD Anderson Cancer Ctr; **Address:** UT MD Anderson Cancer Ctr, 1414 Holcombe Blvd, Houston, TX 77030; **Phone:** 713-792-6110; **Board Cert:** Internal Medicine 1988; Medical Oncology 2002; **Med School:** Univ Western Ontario 1985; **Resid:** Internal Medicine, N Shore Univ Hosp 1988; **Fellow:** Medical Oncology, Meml Sloan Kettering Cancer Ctr 1991; **Fac Appt:** Prof Med, Univ Tex, Houston

Romaguera, Jorge MD [Onc] - **Spec Exp:** Lymphoma; **Hospital:** UT MD Anderson Cancer Ctr; **Address:** 1515 Holcombe Blvd, Box 0429, Houston, TX 77030; **Phone:** 713-745-4246; **Board Cert:** Internal Medicine 1988; Medical Oncology 1989; **Med School:** Univ Puerto Rico 1982; **Resid:** Internal Medicine, Univ Hosp 1985; **Fellow:** Hematology & Oncology, Univ Hosp 1987

Ross, Helen J MD [Onc] - **Spec Exp:** Lung Cancer; Mesothelioma; Esophageal Cancer; **Hospital:** Mayo Clinic - Scottsdale; **Address:** Mayo Clinic, 13400 E Shea Blvd, Scottsdale, AZ 85259; **Phone:** 480-301-8335; **Board Cert:** Internal Medicine 1987; Medical Oncology 1989; **Med School:** UCLA 1984; **Resid:** Internal Medicine, Cedars Sinai Med Ctr 1987; **Fellow:** Medical Oncology, UCLA Med Ctr 1989; **Fac Appt:** Assoc Prof Med, Mayo Med Sch

Medical Oncology

Saiki, John H MD [Onc] - **Hospital:** Univ NM Hlth & Sci Ctr; **Address:** Univ of New Mexico Cancer Ctr, 900 Camino de Salud NE, MSC 084630, Albuquerque, NM 87131-0001; **Phone:** 505-272-8740; **Board Cert:** Internal Medicine 1970; Medical Oncology 1973; **Med School:** McGill Univ 1961; **Resid:** Internal Medicine, Univ New Mexico 1968; Hematology, Univ New Mexico 1969; **Fellow:** Medical Oncology, MD Anderson Hosp 1970; **Fac Appt:** Prof Emeritus Med, Univ New Mexico

Schiller, Joan H MD [Onc] - **Spec Exp:** Lung Cancer; **Hospital:** UT Southwestern Med Ctr at Dallas; **Address:** Univ Texas SW, 5323 Harry Hines Blvd, Dallas, TX 75390-8852; **Phone:** 214-648-4180; **Board Cert:** Internal Medicine 1983; Medical Oncology 1987; **Med School:** Univ IL Coll Med 1980; **Resid:** Internal Medicine, Northwestern Meml Hosp 1983; **Fellow:** Medical Oncology, Univ Wisconsin Hosp 1986; **Fac Appt:** Prof Med, Univ Wisc

Stopeck, Alison T MD [Onc] - **Spec Exp:** Breast Cancer; Breast Cancer Risk Assessment; **Hospital:** Univ Med Ctr - Tucson; **Address:** 1515 N Campbell Ave, PO Box 245024, Tucson, AZ 85724; **Phone:** 520-626-2816; **Board Cert:** Internal Medicine 1988; Medical Oncology 2002; Hematology 2002; **Med School:** Columbia P&S 1985; **Resid:** Internal Medicine, Columbia-Presby Med Ctr 1988; **Fellow:** Hematology & Oncology, New York Hosp 1991; **Fac Appt:** Assoc Prof Med, Univ Ariz Coll Med

Valero, Vicente MD [Onc] - **Spec Exp:** Breast Cancer; **Hospital:** UT MD Anderson Cancer Ctr, LBJ General Hosp; **Address:** Univ Texas MD Anderson Cancer Ctr, 1515 Holcombe Blvd, Unit 1354, Houston, TX 77030; **Phone:** 713-792-2817; **Board Cert:** Internal Medicine 1985; Medical Oncology 1987; Hematology 1988; **Med School:** Mexico 1980; **Resid:** Internal Medicine, Univ Cincinnati Med Ctr 1985; Hematology & Oncology, Univ Cincinnati Med Ctr 1987; **Fellow:** Hematology & Oncology, Univ Texas Med Br 1988; **Fac Appt:** Prof Med, Univ Tex, Houston

Varadhachary, Gauri MD [Onc] - **Spec Exp:** Unknown Primary Cancer; Pancreatic Cancer; **Hospital:** UT MD Anderson Cancer Ctr; **Address:** 1515 Holcombe Blvd, Box 426, Houston, TX 77030; **Phone:** 713-792-2828; **Board Cert:** Internal Medicine 2004; Hematology 1998; Medical Oncology 2008; **Med School:** India 1991; **Resid:** Internal Medicine, Greater Baltimore Med Ctr 1995; **Fellow:** Hematology & Oncology, Baylor Univ 1998

Verschraegen, Claire F MD [Onc] - **Spec Exp:** Ovarian Cancer; Drug Discovery; Mesothelioma; **Hospital:** Univ NM Hlth & Sci Ctr; **Address:** UNM Cancer Research & Treatment Ctr, 900 Camino de Salud NE, rm MS C084630, Albuquerque, NM 87131-0001; **Phone:** 505-272-6760; **Board Cert:** Internal Medicine 2000; Medical Oncology 2000; **Med School:** Belgium 1982; **Resid:** Internal Medicine, Bordet 1985; Internal Medicine, Univ Texas 1991; **Fellow:** Cancer Research, Stehlin Fdn for Cancer Research 1988; Oncology, MD Anderson Cancer Ctr 1994; **Fac Appt:** Prof Med, Univ New Mexico

Von Burton, Gary MD [Onc] - **Spec Exp:** Breast Cancer; Sarcoma; Brain Tumors; **Hospital:** Louisiana State Univ Hosp; **Address:** LSUHSC-Shreveport, Feist-Weiller Cancer Ctr, 1501 Kings Hwy, PO Box 33932, Shreveport, LA 71130; **Phone:** 318-675-5972; **Board Cert:** Internal Medicine 1981; Medical Oncology 1983; **Med School:** Univ Utah 1978; **Resid:** Internal Medicine, Duke Univ Med Ctr 1981; **Fellow:** Hematology & Oncology, Duke Univ Med Ctr 1983; **Fac Appt:** Prof Med, Louisiana State U, Shrevport

Von Hoff, Daniel D MD [Onc] - **Spec Exp:** Pancreatic Cancer; Breast Cancer; Drug Discovery; **Hospital:** Scottsdale Hlthcare - Shea; **Address:** Translational Genomics Research Inst, 445 N 5th St, Ste 600, Phoenix, AZ 85004; **Phone:** 602-343-8492; **Board Cert:** Internal Medicine 1976; Medical Oncology 1979; **Med School:** Columbia P&S 1973; **Resid:** Internal Medicine, UCSF Med Ctr 1975; **Fac Appt:** Prof Med, Univ Ariz Coll Med

Willson, James KV MD [Onc] - **Spec Exp:** Gastrointestinal Cancer; Colon Cancer; Pancreatic Cancer; **Hospital:** UT Southwestern Med Ctr at Dallas; **Address:** 5323 Harry Hines Blvd, Dallas, TX 75390-8590; **Phone:** 214-645-4673; **Board Cert:** Internal Medicine 1980; Medical Oncology 1981; **Med School:** Univ Alabama 1976; **Resid:** Internal Medicine, Johns Hopkins Hosp 1978; **Fellow:** Medical Oncology, Natl Cancer Inst-NIH 1980; **Fac Appt:** Prof Med, Univ Tex SW, Dallas

West Coast and Pacific

Abrams, Donald I MD [Onc] - **Spec Exp:** AIDS Related Cancers; **Hospital:** San Francisco Genl Hosp; **Address:** Positive Hlth Program-SF Genl Hosp, 995 Potrero Ave, Bldg 80, Ward 84, San Francisco, CA 94110; **Phone:** 415-476-4082 x444; **Board Cert:** Internal Medicine 1980; Medical Oncology 1983; **Med School:** Stanford Univ 1977; **Resid:** Internal Medicine, Kaiser Fdn Hosp 1980; **Fellow:** Medical Oncology, UCSF Cancer Rsch 1982; **Fac Appt:** Clin Prof Med, UCSF

Appelbaum, Frederick R MD [Onc] - **Spec Exp:** Bone Marrow Transplant; Leukemia; **Hospital:** Univ Wash Med Ctr; **Address:** 1100 Fairview Ave N, rm D5-310, PO Box 19024, Seattle, WA 98109; **Phone:** 206-288-1024; **Board Cert:** Internal Medicine 1975; Medical Oncology 1977; **Med School:** Tufts Univ 1972; **Resid:** Internal Medicine, Univ Michigan Med Ctr 1974; **Fellow:** Medical Oncology, Natl Cancer Inst 1976; **Fac Appt:** Prof Med, Univ Wash

Back, Anthony MD [Onc] - **Spec Exp:** Palliative Care; Gastrointestinal Cancer; **Hospital:** Univ Wash Med Ctr; **Address:** Seattle Cancer Care Alliance, 825 Eastlake Ave E, Seattle, WA 98109; **Phone:** 206-288-6478; **Board Cert:** Internal Medicine 1987; Medical Oncology 2001; **Med School:** Harvard Med Sch 1984; **Resid:** Internal Medicine, Univ Washington Med Ctr 1988; **Fellow:** Oncology, Univ Washington Med Ctr 1991; **Fac Appt:** Prof Med, Univ Wash

Ball, Edward D MD [Onc] - **Spec Exp:** Bone Marrow & Stem Cell Transplant; Leukemia & Lymphoma; Multiple Myeloma; Immunotherapy; **Hospital:** UCSD Med Ctr; **Address:** 3855 Health Sciences Dr, #0960, La Jolla, CA 92093; **Phone:** 858-822-6600; **Board Cert:** Internal Medicine 1979; Medical Oncology 1983; Hematology 2000; **Med School:** Case West Res Univ 1976; **Resid:** Internal Medicine, Hartford Hosp 1979; **Fellow:** Hematology & Oncology, Univ Hosps Cleveland 1981; Hematology & Oncology, Dartmouth-Hitchcock Hosp 1982; **Fac Appt:** Prof Med, UCSD

Beer, Tomasz M MD [Onc] - **Spec Exp:** Prostate Cancer; **Hospital:** OR Hlth & Sci Univ; **Address:** 3303 SW Bond Ave, CH14R, Portland, OR 97239; **Phone:** 503-494-6594; **Board Cert:** Medical Oncology 2000; **Med School:** Johns Hopkins Univ 1991; **Resid:** Internal Medicine, Oreg Hlth Scis Univ 1994; Internal Medicine, Oreg Hlth Scis Univ 1996; **Fellow:** Hematology & Oncology, Oreg Hlth Scis Univ 1999; **Fac Appt:** Assoc Prof Med, Oregon Hlth Sci Univ

Bensinger, William I MD [Onc] - **Spec Exp:** Multiple Myeloma; Stem Cell Transplant; **Hospital:** Univ Wash Med Ctr; **Address:** Fred Hutchinson Cancer Research Ctr, 1100 Fairview Ave N, MS DS-390, Seattle, WA 98109-1024; **Phone:** 206-288-1024; **Board Cert:** Internal Medicine 1978; Medical Oncology 1979; **Med School:** Northwestern Univ 1973; **Resid:** Internal Medicine, Univ Wash Hosps 1978; **Fellow:** Medical Oncology, Univ Wash Hosps 1979; **Fac Appt:** Assoc Prof Med, Univ Wash

Carlson, Robert W MD [Onc] - **Spec Exp:** Breast Cancer; **Hospital:** Stanford Univ Med Ctr; **Address:** Stanford Comprehensive Cancer Ctr, 875 Blake Wilbur Drive, MC 5826, Stanford, CA 94305; **Phone:** 650-498-6000; **Board Cert:** Internal Medicine 1981; Medical Oncology 1983; **Med School:** Stanford Univ 1978; **Resid:** Internal Medicine, Barnes Hosp 1980; Internal Medicine, Stanford Univ Hosp 1981; **Fellow:** Medical Oncology, Stanford Univ Hosp 1983; **Fac Appt:** Prof Med, Stanford Univ

Medical Oncology

Chap, Linnea MD [Onc] - **Spec Exp:** Breast Cancer; **Hospital:** St John's Hlth Ctr, Santa Monica; **Address:** Premier Oncology, 2020 Santa Monica Blvd, Ste 600, Santa Monica, CA 90404-2023; **Phone:** 310-633-8400; **Board Cert:** Medical Oncology 2005; **Med School:** Univ Chicago-Pritzker Sch Med 1988; **Resid:** Internal Medicine, Northwestern Meml Hosp 1991; **Fellow:** Hematology & Oncology, UCLA Med Ctr 1992

Chlebowski, Rowan T MD/PhD [Onc] - **Spec Exp:** Breast Cancer; **Hospital:** LAC - Harbor - UCLA Med Ctr; **Address:** 1124 W Carson St J3 Bldg, Torrance, CA 90502; **Phone:** 310-222-2218; **Board Cert:** Internal Medicine 1980; Medical Oncology 1981; **Med School:** Case West Res Univ 1974; **Resid:** Internal Medicine, MetroHealth Med Ctr 1976; Medical Oncology, LAC-USC Med Ctr 1979; **Fac Appt:** Prof Med, UCLA

Chow, Warren A MD [Onc] - **Spec Exp:** Sarcoma-Soft Tissue; Sarcoma; **Hospital:** City of Hope Natl Med Ctr & Beckman Rsch (page 69); **Address:** 1500 E Duarte Rd, Duarte, CA 91010; **Phone:** 626-359-8111; **Board Cert:** Internal Medicine 1989; Medical Oncology 2003; Hematology 2004; **Med School:** Ros Franklin Univ/Chicago Med Sch 1986; **Resid:** Internal Medicine, Cedars-Sinai Med Ctr 1990; **Fellow:** Hematology & Oncology, City of Hope Med Ctr 1992; Molecular Genetics, City of Hope Med Ctr 1994; **Fac Appt:** Assoc Prof Med

Crocenzi, Todd MD [Onc] - **Spec Exp:** Gastrointestinal Cancer; **Hospital:** Providence Portland Med Ctr; **Address:** 4805 NE Glisan, Ste 6N40, Portland, OR 97213; **Phone:** 503-215-5696; **Board Cert:** Medical Oncology 2004; **Med School:** Jefferson Med Coll 1994; **Resid:** Internal Medicine, Univ MD Med Ctr 1997; **Fellow:** Hematology & Oncology, Dartmouth Hitchcock Med Ctr 2004; Immunology, Dartmouth Hitchcock Med Ctr 2005

Daud, Adil I MD [Onc] - **Spec Exp:** Melanoma; Skin Cancer; Drug Development; **Hospital:** UCSF Med Ctr; **Address:** 1600 Divisadero St, Box 1706, San Francisco, CA 94115; **Phone:** 415-353-9900; **Board Cert:** Hematology 2000; Medical Oncology 2000; **Med School:** India 1987; **Resid:** Internal Medicine, Indiana Univ; **Fellow:** Hematology & Oncology, Meml Sloan Kettering Cancer Ctr

Deeg, H. Joachim MD [Onc] - **Spec Exp:** Bone Marrow Failure Disorders; Hematologic Malignancies; **Hospital:** Univ Wash Med Ctr; **Address:** Fred Hutchinson Cancer Research Center, 1100 Fairview Avenue N, D1-100, Box 19024, Seattle, WA 98109-1024; **Phone:** 206-667-5985; **Board Cert:** Internal Medicine 1976; Medical Oncology 1979; **Med School:** Germany 1972; **Fac Appt:** Prof Med, Univ Wash

Disis, Mary Lenora MD [Onc] - **Spec Exp:** Breast Cancer; Ovarian Cancer; Clinical Trials; **Hospital:** Univ Wash Med Ctr; **Address:** Univ Washington, Tumor Vaccine Group, 815 Mercer St, Seattle, WA 98109; **Phone:** 206-543-8557; **Board Cert:** Internal Medicine 1989; Medical Oncology 2008; **Med School:** Univ Nebr Coll Med 1986; **Resid:** Internal Medicine, Univ Illinois Med Ctr 1990; **Fellow:** Medical Oncology, Fred Hutchinson Cancer Ctr 1993; **Fac Appt:** Assoc Prof Med, Univ Wash

Druker, Brian J MD [Onc] - **Spec Exp:** Leukemia; **Hospital:** OR Hlth & Sci Univ; **Address:** 3181 SW Sam Jackson Park Rd, MC L592, Portland, OR 97239-3098; **Phone:** 503-494-5058; **Board Cert:** Internal Medicine 1984; Medical Oncology 1987; **Med School:** UCSD 1981; **Resid:** Internal Medicine, Barnes Jewish Hosp 1984; **Fellow:** Medical Oncology, Dana-Farber Cancer Inst 1987; **Fac Appt:** Prof Med, Oregon Hlth Sci Univ

Ellis, Georgiana K MD [Onc] - **Spec Exp:** Breast Cancer; Clinical Trials; **Hospital:** Univ Wash Med Ctr; **Address:** Univ Washington Sch Med, Div Oncology, SCCA 825 Eastlake Ave E, Box 358081, MS G3-630, Seattle, WA 98109-1023; **Phone:** 206-288-6989; **Board Cert:** Internal Medicine 1985; Medical Oncology 1987; **Med School:** Univ Wash 1982; **Resid:** Internal Medicine, Univ Washington Med Ctr 1985; **Fellow:** Medical Oncology, Univ Washington Med Ctr 1988; **Fac Appt:** Assoc Prof Med, Univ Wash

Estey, Elihu H MD [Onc] - **Spec Exp:** Leukemia; Myelodysplastic Syndromes; Clinical Trials; **Hospital:** Univ Wash Med Ctr; **Address:** Seattle Cancer Care Alliance, 825 Eastlake Ave E, UW Box 3587710, Seattle, WA 98109; **Phone:** 206-288-7176; **Board Cert:** Internal Medicine 1975; Medical Oncology 1981; **Med School:** Johns Hopkins Univ 1972; **Resid:** Internal Medicine, Bellevue Hosp Ctr 1975; **Fellow:** Medical Oncology, MD Anderson Cancer Ctr 1978

Figlin, Robert A MD [Onc] - **Spec Exp:** Urologic Cancer; Kidney Cancer; Immunotherapy; **Hospital:** City of Hope Natl Med Ctr & Beckman Rsch (page 69); **Address:** Med Oncology & Therapeutics Research, 1500 E Duarte Rd, Duarte, CA 91010; **Phone:** 626-256-4673; **Board Cert:** Internal Medicine 1979; Medical Oncology 1983; **Med School:** Med Coll PA Hahnemann 1976; **Resid:** Internal Medicine, Cedars Sinai Med Ctr 1980; **Fellow:** Hematology & Oncology, UCLA Ctr Hlth Sci 1982; **Fac Appt:** Prof Med, UCLA

Fisher Jr, George A MD/PhD [Onc] - **Spec Exp:** Gastrointestinal Cancer; Pancreatic Cancer; **Hospital:** Stanford Univ Med Ctr; **Address:** Stanford Comp Cancer Ctr, GI Onc, 875 Blake Wilbur Drive, MC 5826, Stanford, CA 94305; **Phone:** 650-723-7621; **Board Cert:** Medical Oncology 1997; **Med School:** Stanford Univ 1987; **Resid:** Internal Medicine, Stanford Univ Med Ctr 1991; **Fellow:** Medical Oncology, Stanford Univ Med Ctr 1993; **Fac Appt:** Assoc Prof Med, Stanford Univ

Ford, James M MD [Onc] - **Spec Exp:** Gastrointestinal Cancer; Colon & Rectal Cancer; Cancer Genetics; **Hospital:** Stanford Univ Med Ctr; **Address:** Stanford Comp Cancer Ctr, 875 Blake Wilbur Drive, Ste Clinic B, Stanford, CA 94305-5820; **Phone:** 650-723-7621; **Board Cert:** Medical Oncology 2005; **Med School:** Yale Univ 1989; **Resid:** Internal Medicine, Stanford Univ Med Ctr 1991; **Fellow:** Medical Oncology, Stanford Univ Med Ctr 1994; **Fac Appt:** Assoc Prof Med, Stanford Univ

Forscher, Charles A MD [Onc] - **Spec Exp:** Bone Tumors; Sarcoma-Soft Tissue; **Hospital:** Cedars Sinai Med Ctr, UCLA Ronald Reagan Med Ctr; **Address:** Outpatient Cancer Ctr, Lower Level, 8700 Beverly Blvd, rm AC1042D, Los Angeles, CA 90040, **Phone:** 310 423 8045; **Board Cert:** Internal Medicine 1981; Hematology 1986; Medical Oncology 1987; **Med School:** Albert Einstein Coll Med 1978; **Resid:** Internal Medicine, Montefiore Med Ctr 1981; **Fellow:** Hematology, Montefiore Med Ctr 1983; Neoplastic Diseases, Mt Sinai Med Ctr 1985; **Fac Appt:** Clin Prof Med, UCLA

Gandara, David R MD [Onc] - **Spec Exp:** Lung Cancer; **Hospital:** UC Davis Med Ctr; **Address:** UC Davis Cancer Ctr, 4501 X St, Sacramento, CA 95817; **Phone:** 916-734-5959; **Board Cert:** Internal Medicine 1976; Medical Oncology 1979; **Med School:** Univ Tex Med Br, Galveston 1973; **Resid:** Internal Medicine, Madigan Med Ctr 1976; **Fellow:** Hematology & Oncology, Letterman AMC 1978; **Fac Appt:** Asst Prof Med, UC Davis

Ganz, Patricia A MD [Onc] - **Spec Exp:** Breast Cancer; Cancer Survivors-Late Effects of Therapy; **Hospital:** UCLA Ronald Reagan Med Ctr; **Address:** UCLA, Cancer Prev/Control Rsch, A2-125 CHS, 650 Charles Young Drive S, Box 956900, Los Angeles, CA 90095-6900; **Phone:** 310-206-1404; **Board Cert:** Internal Medicine 1976; Medical Oncology 1979; **Med School:** UCLA 1973; **Resid:** Internal Medicine, UCLA Med Ctr 1976; **Fellow:** Hematology, UCLA Med Ctr 1978; **Fac Appt:** Prof Med, UCLA

Medical Oncology

Glaspy, John A MD [Onc] - **Spec Exp:** Breast Cancer; Melanoma; Lymphoma; **Hospital:** UCLA Ronald Reagan Med Ctr; **Address:** 100 UCLA Medical Plaza, Ste 550, Los Angeles, CA 90095; **Phone:** 310-794-4955; **Board Cert:** Internal Medicine 1982; Medical Oncology 1985; Hematology 1986; **Med School:** UCLA 1979; **Resid:** Internal Medicine, UCLA Med Ctr 1982; **Fellow:** Hematology & Oncology, UCLA Med Ctr 1984; **Fac Appt:** Prof Med, UCLA

Gold, Philip J MD [Onc] - **Spec Exp:** Gastrointestinal Cancer; **Hospital:** Swedish Med Ctr - Seattle; **Address:** Swedish Cancer Inst, 1221 Madison St Fl 2, Seattle, WA 98104; **Phone:** 206-386-2121; **Board Cert:** Internal Medicine 2005; Medical Oncology 2007; **Med School:** Univ Miami Sch Med 1991; **Resid:** Internal Medicine, Univ of Washington Med Ctr 1994; **Fellow:** Medical Oncology, Fred Hutchinson Cancer Rsch Ctr 1997

Gralow, Julie MD [Onc] - **Spec Exp:** Breast Cancer; **Hospital:** Univ Wash Med Ctr; **Address:** Seattle Cancer Care Alliance, 825 Eastlake Ave E, MS G3-630, Seattle, WA 98109; **Phone:** 206-288-7222; **Board Cert:** Medical Oncology 2005; **Med School:** USC Sch Med 1988; **Resid:** Internal Medicine, Brigham & Women's Hosp 1991; **Fellow:** Oncology, Univ Wash Med Ctr 1994; **Fac Appt:** Assoc Prof Med, Univ Wash

Higano, Celestia MD [Onc] - **Spec Exp:** Genitourinary Cancer; Prostate Cancer; Bladder Cancer; Testicular Cancer; **Hospital:** Univ Wash Med Ctr; **Address:** Seattle Cancer Care Alliance, 825 Eastlake Ave E, PO Box 19024, Seattle, WA 98109; **Phone:** 206-288-7222; **Board Cert:** Internal Medicine 1982; Medical Oncology 1985; **Med School:** Univ Mass Sch Med 1979; **Resid:** Internal Medicine, Mayo Clinic 1982; **Fellow:** Oncology, Univ Washington 1985; **Fac Appt:** Assoc Prof Med, Univ Wash

Horning, Sandra J MD [Onc] - **Spec Exp:** Hodgkin's Disease; Bone Marrow & Stem Cell Transplant; Lymphoma; **Hospital:** Stanford Univ Med Ctr; **Address:** Stanford Cancer Center, 875 Blake Wilbur Drive, Clinic C, Palo Alto, CA 94305; **Phone:** 650-723-7621; **Board Cert:** Internal Medicine 1978; Medical Oncology 1981; **Med School:** Univ Iowa Coll Med 1975; **Resid:** Internal Medicine, Strong Meml Hosp 1978; **Fellow:** Medical Oncology, Stanford Univ 1980; **Fac Appt:** Prof Med, Stanford Univ

Jacobs, Charlotte D MD [Onc] - **Spec Exp:** Sarcoma; Unknown Primary Cancer; **Hospital:** Stanford Univ Med Ctr; **Address:** 875 Blake Wilbur Drive, Stanford, CA 94305; **Phone:** 650-498-6000; **Board Cert:** Internal Medicine 1975; Medical Oncology 1977; **Med School:** Washington Univ, St Louis 1972; **Resid:** Internal Medicine, Barnes Hosp 1974; Internal Medicine, UCSF Med Ctr 1975; **Fellow:** Medical Oncology, Stanford Univ 1977; **Fac Appt:** Prof Med, Stanford Univ

Kaplan, Lawrence D MD [Onc] - **Spec Exp:** AIDS Related Cancers; Lymphoma; **Hospital:** UCSF Med Ctr; **Address:** UCSF Medical Center, 400 Parnassus Ave, rm 502, Box 0324, San Francisco, CA 94143-0324; **Phone:** 415-353-2421; **Board Cert:** Internal Medicine 1983; Medical Oncology 1985; **Med School:** UCLA 1980; **Resid:** Internal Medicine, Boston City Hosp 1983; **Fellow:** Hematology & Oncology, UCSF Med Ctr 1985; **Fac Appt:** Clin Prof Med, UCSF

Koczywas, Marianna MD [Onc] - **Spec Exp:** Lung Cancer; **Hospital:** City of Hope Natl Med Ctr & Beckman Rsch (page 69); **Address:** City of Hope National Medical Center, 1500 E Duarte Rd, Duarte, CA 91010; **Phone:** 626-359-8111 x62307; **Board Cert:** Hematology 2000; Medical Oncology 2001; **Med School:** Poland 1984; **Resid:** Internal Medicine, Troczewski City Hosp 1988; Internal Medicine, St Francis Med Ctr 1997; **Fellow:** Hematology & Oncology, City of Hope Natl Med Ctr 2000

Lim, Dean Wee MD [Onc] - **Hospital:** City of Hope Natl Med Ctr & Beckman Rsch (page 69); **Address:** City of Hope-Medical Oncology Dept, 1500 E Duarte Rd, Duarte, CA 91010; **Phone:** 626-256-4673 x69200; **Board Cert:** Internal Medicine 1985; Medical Oncology 1989; **Med School:** Philippines 1980; **Resid:** Internal Medicine, Cabrini Med Ctr 1985; **Fellow:** Hematology & Oncology, St Lukes Roosevelt Hosp 1987; **Fac Appt:** Asst Clin Prof Med, USC-Keck School of Medicine

Maloney, David G MD/PhD [Onc] - **Spec Exp:** Lymphoma; Bone Marrow & Stem Cell Transplant; Vaccine Therapy; **Hospital:** Univ Wash Med Ctr; **Address:** Fred Hutchinson Cancer, Research Ctr Ave, MS D1-100, 1100 Fairview Ave N, Box 19024, Seattle, WA 98109-1024; **Phone:** 206-667-5616; **Board Cert:** Internal Medicine 1988; Medical Oncology 2005; **Med School:** Stanford Univ 1985; **Resid:** Internal Medicine, Brigham & Women's Hosp 1988; **Fellow:** Medical Oncology, Stanford Univ Med Ctr 1994; **Fac Appt:** Prof Med, Univ Wash

Margolin, Kim Allyson MD [Onc] - **Spec Exp:** Melanoma; Kidney Cancer; Germ Cell Tumors; **Hospital:** Univ Wash Med Ctr; **Address:** 825 Eastlake Ave E, PO Box 19024, Seattle, WA 98109; **Phone:** 206-288-7222; **Board Cert:** Internal Medicine 1982; Hematology 1986; Medical Oncology 2006; **Med School:** Stanford Univ 1979; **Resid:** Internal Medicine, Yale-New Haven Hosp 1982; **Fellow:** Hematology & Oncology, UC San Diego Med Ctr 1983; Hematology & Oncology, City of Hope Med Ctr 1985; **Fac Appt:** Prof Med, Univ Wash

Martins, Renato G MD [Onc] - **Spec Exp:** Head & Neck Cancer; Lung Cancer; Mesothelioma; Salivary Gland Tumors; **Hospital:** Univ Wash Med Ctr; **Address:** Seattle Cancer Care Alliance, 825 Eastlake Ave E, MS G4-940, Seattle, WA 98109; **Phone:** 206-288-2048; **Board Cert:** Internal Medicine 2005; Medical Oncology 1998; **Med School:** Brazil 1992; **Resid:** Internal Medicine, Gunderson Clinic 1995; **Fellow:** Medical Oncology, Mass Genl Hosp 1998

Meyskens, Frank MD [Onc] - **Spec Exp:** Cancer Prevention; Melanoma; Sarcoma; **Hospital:** UC Irvine Med Ctr; **Address:** UC Irvine Cancer Ctr, 101 The City Drive Bldg 56 - rm 215, Orange, CA 92868; **Phone:** 714-456-6310; **Board Cert:** Internal Medicine 1975; Medical Oncology 1981; **Med School:** UCSF 1972; **Resid:** Internal Medicine, Moffit-Calif Hosps 1974; **Fellow:** Hematology & Oncology, Natl Cancer Inst 1977; **Fac Appt:** Prof Med, UC Irvine

Mitsuyasu, Ronald T MD [Onc] - **Spec Exp:** AIDS Related Cancers; **Hospital:** UCLA Ronald Reagan Med Ctr; **Address:** 1399 S Roxbury Drive, Ste 100, Los Angeles, CA 90035; **Phone:** 310-557-2273; **Board Cert:** Internal Medicine 1981; **Med School:** UCLA 1978; **Resid:** Internal Medicine, Rush Presby St Lukes Hosp 1981; **Fellow:** Hematology & Oncology, UCLA Med Ctr 1984

Mortimer, Joanne MD [Onc] - **Spec Exp:** Breast Cancer; Clinical Trials; Head & Neck Cancer; **Hospital:** City of Hope Natl Med Ctr & Beckman Rsch (page 69); **Address:** 1500 E Duarte Rd, Duarte, CA 91010; **Phone:** 626-471-9200; **Board Cert:** Internal Medicine 1980; Medical Oncology 1983; **Med School:** Loyola Univ-Stritch Sch Med 1977; **Resid:** Internal Medicine, Cleveland Clinic 1980; **Fellow:** Medical Oncology, Cleveland Clinic 1982

Natale, Ronald B MD [Onc] - **Spec Exp:** Lung Cancer; **Hospital:** Cedars-Sinai Med Ctr; **Address:** Cedars-Sinai Outpatient Comp Cancer Ctr, 8700 Beverly Blvd, Ste AC1042B, Los Angeles, CA 90048; **Phone:** 310-423-1101; **Board Cert:** Internal Medicine 1977; Medical Oncology 1979; **Med School:** Wayne State Univ 1974; **Resid:** Internal Medicine, Wayne State Univ 1977; **Fellow:** Hematology & Oncology, Meml Sloan Kettering 1980; **Fac Appt:** Prof Med, Univ Mich Med Sch

Medical Oncology

Nichols, Craig R MD [Onc] - **Spec Exp:** Testicular Cancer; Hodgkin's Disease; Lymphoma; **Hospital:** Providence Portland Med Ctr; **Address:** Providence Cancer Ctr, Oregon Clinic, 4805 NE Glisan St, Ste 6N40, Portland, OR 97213; **Phone:** 503-215-5696; **Board Cert:** Internal Medicine 1981; Medical Oncology 1985; **Med School:** Oregon Hlth Sci Univ 1978; **Resid:** Internal Medicine, Oschner Fdn Hosp 1981; **Fellow:** Medical Oncology, Indiana Univ 1985; **Fac Appt:** Prof Med, Oregon Hlth Sci Univ

O'Day, Steven J MD [Onc] - **Spec Exp:** Melanoma; Melanoma-Advanced; **Hospital:** St John's Hlth Ctr, Santa Monica; **Address:** 11818 Wilshire Blvd, Ste 200, Los Angeles, CA 90025; **Phone:** 310-231-2121; **Med School:** Johns Hopkins Univ 1988; **Resid:** Internal Medicine, Johns Hopkins Hosp 1991; **Fellow:** Medical Oncology, Dana Farber Cancer Inst 1992; **Fac Appt:** Assoc Clin Prof Med, USC-Keck School of Medicine

Petersdorf, Stephen MD [Onc] - **Spec Exp:** Lymphoma; Myelodysplastic Syndromes; Leukemia; **Hospital:** Univ Wash Med Ctr; **Address:** Seattle Cancer Care Alliance, 825 Eastlake Ave E, MS G3200, Seattle, WA 98109-1023; **Phone:** 206-288-6202; **Board Cert:** Internal Medicine 1986; Hematology 2001; Medical Oncology 2001; **Med School:** Brown Univ 1983; **Resid:** Internal Medicine, Univ Washington Med Ctr 1986; **Fellow:** Hematology & Oncology, Univ Washington Med Ctr 1989; **Fac Appt:** Assoc Prof Med, Univ Wash

Picozzi Jr, Vincent J MD [Onc] - **Spec Exp:** Pancreatic Cancer; **Hospital:** Virginia Mason Med Ctr; **Address:** Virginia Mason Med Ctr, Div Hem/Onc, MS C2-Hem, Seattle, WA 98111; **Phone:** 206-223-6193; **Board Cert:** Internal Medicine 1981; Hematology 1986; Medical Oncology 1987; **Med School:** Stanford Univ 1978; **Resid:** Internal Medicine, Peter Bent Brigham Med Ctr 1981; **Fellow:** Hematology, Stanford Univ Med Ctr 1983; Medical Oncology, Stanford Univ MEd Ctr 1983; **Fac Appt:** Clin Prof Med, Univ Wash

Pinto, Harlan A MD [Onc] - **Spec Exp:** Head & Neck Cancer; Clinical Trials; **Hospital:** Stanford Univ Med Ctr, VA Hlth Care Sys - Palo Alto; **Address:** Stanford Med Ctr Oncology Div, 875 Blake Wilbur Drive, Stanford, CA 94305; **Phone:** 650-723-7621; **Board Cert:** Internal Medicine 1986; Medical Oncology 2002; **Med School:** Yale Univ 1983; **Resid:** Internal Medicine, Mass Genl Hosp 1986; **Fellow:** Medical Oncology, Stanford Univ Med Sch 1991; **Fac Appt:** Assoc Prof Med, Stanford Univ

Prados, Michael MD [Onc] - **Spec Exp:** Neuro-Oncology; Brain Tumors; **Hospital:** UCSF Med Ctr; **Address:** UCSF Med Ctr, Div Neuro-Oncology, 400 Parnassus Ave, rm A-808, San Francisco, CA 94143; **Phone:** 415-353-2966; **Board Cert:** Internal Medicine 1977; **Med School:** Louisiana State U, New Orleans 1974; **Resid:** Internal Medicine, Earl K Long Hosp 1977; **Fac Appt:** Prof NS, UCSF

Press, Oliver W MD/PhD [Onc] - **Spec Exp:** Lymphoma; Bone Marrow Transplant; **Hospital:** Univ Wash Med Ctr; **Address:** 1100 Fairview Ave N, MS D3-19, Seattle, WA 98109; **Phone:** 206-667-1864; **Board Cert:** Internal Medicine 1982; Medical Oncology 1985; **Med School:** Univ Wash 1979; **Resid:** Internal Medicine, Mass Genl Hosp 1982; Internal Medicine, Univ Hosp 1983; **Fellow:** Medical Oncology, Univ Washington 1985; **Fac Appt:** Prof Med, Univ Wash

Quinn, David MD/PhD [Onc] - **Spec Exp:** Testicular Cancer; Prostate Cancer; Kidney Cancer; **Hospital:** USC Norris Cancer Hosp; **Address:** 1441 Eastlake Ave, Ste 3440, Los Angeles, CA 90033; **Phone:** 323-865-3956; **Med School:** Australia 1987; **Resid:** Internal Medicine, St Vincents Hosp 1992; **Fellow:** Medical Oncology, St Vincents Hosp 1995; **Fac Appt:** Asst Prof Med, USC Sch Med

Reid, Tony R MD/PhD [Onc] - **Spec Exp:** Gastrointestinal Cancer; Pancreatic Cancer; Esophageal Cancer; Liver Cancer; **Hospital:** UCSD Med Ctr; **Address:** 3855 Health Sciences Drive, La Jolla, CA 92093; **Phone:** 858-822-6100; **Board Cert:** Medical Oncology 1999; **Med School:** Stanford Univ 1991; **Resid:** Internal Medicine, Stanford Univ Med Ctr 1997; **Fellow:** Oncology, Stanford Univ Med Ctr 1999; Cancer Research, Stanford Univ Med Ctr 2000; **Fac Appt:** Assoc Prof Med, UCSD

Rugo, Hope S MD [Onc] - **Spec Exp:** Breast Cancer; Complementary Medicine; Breast Cancer-Novel Therapies; **Hospital:** UCSF Med Ctr; **Address:** UCSF Comp Cancer Ctr-Breast Care Ctr, 1600 Divisadero St Fl 2, San Francisco, CA 94115; **Phone:** 415-353-7070; **Board Cert:** Internal Medicine 1987; Medical Oncology 1989; **Med School:** Univ Pennsylvania 1984; **Resid:** Internal Medicine, UCSF Med Ctr 1987; **Fellow:** Hematology & Oncology, UCSF Med Ctr 1989; **Fac Appt:** Clin Prof Med, UCSF

Russell, Christy A MD [Onc] - **Spec Exp:** Breast Cancer; **Hospital:** USC Univ Hosp; **Address:** Norris Cancer Ctr, The Breast Ctr, 1441 Eastlake Ave, Los Angeles, CA 90033; **Phone:** 323-865-3371; **Board Cert:** Internal Medicine 1983; Medical Oncology 1985; **Med School:** Med Coll PA Hahnemann 1980; **Resid:** Internal Medicine, Good Sam Med Ctr 1983; **Fellow:** Hematology & Oncology, LAC-USC Med Ctr 1986; **Fac Appt:** Assoc Prof Med, USC Sch Med

Samlowski, Wolfram E MD [Onc] - **Spec Exp:** Kidney Cancer; Melanoma; Immunotherapy; **Address:** Nevada Cancer Institute, One Breakthrough Way, Las Vegas, NV 89135; **Phone:** 702-822-5433; **Board Cert:** Internal Medicine 1981; Medical Oncology 1985; **Med School:** Ohio State Univ 1978; **Resid:** Internal Medicine, Wayne State Univ Affil Hosp 1981; **Fellow:** Hematology & Oncology, Univ Utah Affil Hosp 1984; **Fac Appt:** Prof Hem & Onc, Univ Nevada

Sandler, Alan MD [Onc] - **Spec Exp:** Lung Cancer; Sarcoma; **Hospital:** OR Hlth & Sci Univ; **Address:** 3181 SW Sam Jackson Park Rd, MC L586, Portland, OR 97239; **Phone:** 503-494-5586; **Board Cert:** Medical Oncology 2006; **Med School:** Rush Med Coll 1987; **Resid:** Internal Medicine, Yale-New Haven Hosp 1990; **Fellow:** Medical Oncology, Yale Univ 1993; **Fac Appt:** Prof Med, Oregon Hlth Sci Univ

Shibata, Stephen I MD [Onc] - **Spec Exp:** Gastrointestinal Cancer; Clinical Trials; **Hospital:** City of Hope Natl Med Ctr & Beckman Rsch (page 69); **Address:** City of Hope Cancer Ctr, 1500 E Duarte Rd, Duarte, CA 91010; **Phone:** 626-359-8111 x62307; **Board Cert:** Internal Medicine 1988; Medical Oncology 1991; **Med School:** UC Irvine 1985; **Resid:** Internal Medicine, St Mary Med Ctr 1988; **Fellow:** Medical Oncology, City of Hope Cancer Ctr 1990; Bone Marrow Transplant, City of Hope Cancer Ctr 1991; **Fac Appt:** Assoc Prof Med

Sikic, Branimir I MD [Onc] - **Spec Exp:** Unknown Primary Cancer; Clinical Trials; **Hospital:** Stanford Univ Med Ctr; **Address:** Stanford Comp Cancer Ctr, 875 Blake Wilbur Drive, Clinic C, Palo Alto, CA 94305; **Phone:** 650-723-7621; **Board Cert:** Internal Medicine 1975; Medical Oncology 1979; **Med School:** Ros Franklin Univ/Chicago Med Sch 1972; **Resid:** Internal Medicine, Georgetown Univ Hosp 1975; **Fellow:** Medical Oncology, Natl Cancer Inst 1978; Medical Oncology, Georgetown Univ Hosp 1979; **Fac Appt:** Prof Med, Stanford Univ

Small, Eric J MD [Onc] - **Spec Exp:** Prostate Cancer; Vaccine Therapy; Genitourinary Cancer; **Hospital:** UCSF Med Ctr; **Address:** UCSF Urologic Oncology Practice, 1600 Divisadero St Fl 3, San Francisco, CA 94115-1711; **Phone:** 415-353-7171; **Board Cert:** Internal Medicine 1988; Medical Oncology 2001; **Med School:** Case West Res Univ 1985; **Resid:** Internal Medicine, Beth Israel Hosp 1988; **Fellow:** Hematology & Oncology, Cancer Research Inst/UCSF 1991; **Fac Appt:** Prof Med, UCSF

Medical Oncology

Stewart, Forrest M MD [Onc] - **Spec Exp:** Unknown Primary Cancer; Sarcoma; **Hospital:** Univ Wash Med Ctr; **Address:** Seattle Cancer Care Alliance, 825 Eastlake Ave E, Box 19023, Seattle, WA 98109; **Phone:** 206-288-7222; **Board Cert:** Internal Medicine 1980; Hematology 1982; Medical Oncology 1985; **Med School:** Indiana Univ 1977; **Resid:** Internal Medicine, Indiana Univ Med Ctr 1980; Medical Oncology, Indiana Univ Med Ctr 1981; **Fellow:** Hematology, Univ Virginia Med Ctr 1983; **Fac Appt:** Prof Med, Univ Wash

Stockdale, Frank E MD/PhD [Onc] - **Spec Exp:** Breast Cancer; **Hospital:** Stanford Univ Med Ctr; **Address:** Stanford Univ Medical Ctr, 875 Blake Wilbur Drive, Stanford, CA 94305-5826; **Phone:** 650-723-6449; **Med School:** Univ Pennsylvania 1963; **Resid:** Internal Medicine, Stanford Univ Med Ctr 1967; Hematology & Oncology, Stanford Univ Med Ctr; **Fac Appt:** Prof Emeritus Med, Stanford Univ

Tempero, Margaret MD [Onc] - **Spec Exp:** Pancreatic Cancer; Gastrointestinal Cancer; **Hospital:** UCSF Med Ctr; **Address:** UCSF, Multi-Disciplinary Practice, 1600 Divisadero St Fl 4 - rm 4202, San Francisco, CA 94115; **Phone:** 415-353-9888; **Board Cert:** Internal Medicine 1980; Medical Oncology 1983; Hematology 1984; **Med School:** Univ Nebr Coll Med 1977; **Resid:** Internal Medicine, Univ Nebraska Hosp 1980; **Fellow:** Medical Oncology, Univ Nebraska 1982

Thompson, John A MD [Onc] - **Spec Exp:** Melanoma; **Hospital:** Univ Wash Med Ctr; **Address:** Seattle Cancer Care Alliance, 825 Eastlake Ave E, MS G4-200, Seattle, WA 98109-1023; **Phone:** 206-288-2015; **Board Cert:** Internal Medicine 1982; Medical Oncology 1985; **Med School:** Univ Alabama 1979; **Resid:** Internal Medicine, Univ Wash Med Ctr 1982; **Fellow:** Medical Oncology, Univ Washington 1985

Tripathy, Debasish MD [Onc] - **Spec Exp:** Breast Cancer; Clinical Trials; **Hospital:** USC Norris Cancer Hosp; **Address:** USC Norris Cancer Ctr, 1441 Eastlake Ave, Ste 3447, Los Angeles, CA 90033; **Phone:** 323-865-3105; **Board Cert:** Internal Medicine 1988; Medical Oncology 2001; **Med School:** Duke Univ 1985; **Resid:** Internal Medicine, Duke Univ Med Ctr 1988; **Fellow:** Hematology & Oncology, USCF Med Ctr 1991; **Fac Appt:** Prof Med, Univ SC Sch Med

Twardowski, Przemyslaw MD [Onc] - **Spec Exp:** Genitourinary Cancer; **Hospital:** City of Hope Natl Med Ctr & Beckman Rsch (page 69); **Address:** 1500 E Duarte Rd, Duarte, CA 91010; **Phone:** 626-256-4673; **Board Cert:** Medical Oncology 1998; Hematology 1998; **Med School:** Univ MO-Columbia Sch Med 1990; **Resid:** Internal Medicine, Northwestern Meml Hosp 1994; **Fellow:** Hematology & Oncology, Northwestern Meml Hosp 1996; **Fac Appt:** Asst Prof Med, UCLA

Urba, Walter J MD/PhD [Onc] - **Spec Exp:** Breast Cancer; **Hospital:** Providence Portland Med Ctr; **Address:** Providence Oncology, 4805 NE Glisan Rd, Ste 6N40, Portland, OR 97213; **Phone:** 503-215-5696; **Board Cert:** Internal Medicine 1985; Medical Oncology 1987; **Med School:** Univ Miami Sch Med 1981; **Resid:** Internal Medicine, Morristown Meml Hosp 1983; **Fellow:** Medical Oncology, Natl Cancer Inst 1986; **Fac Appt:** Assoc Clin Prof Med, Oregon Hlth Sci Univ

Venook, Alan P MD [Onc] - **Spec Exp:** Gastrointestinal Cancer; Colon & Rectal Cancer; Liver Cancer; **Hospital:** UCSF Med Ctr; **Address:** UCSF Comprehensive Cancer Ctr, Multi Disciplinary Practice, 1600 Divisadero St Fl 4 - rm 4202, San Francisco, CA 94115; **Phone:** 415-353-9888; **Board Cert:** Internal Medicine 1985; Medical Oncology 1987; Hematology 1988; **Med School:** UCSF 1980; **Resid:** Internal Medicine, UC Davis Med Ctr 1985; **Fellow:** Hematology & Oncology, UCSF Med Ctr 1987; **Fac Appt:** Prof Med

Vescio, Robert A MD [Onc] - **Spec Exp:** Multiple Myeloma; **Hospital:** Cedars-Sinai Med Ctr; **Address:** Cedars Sinai Med Ctr, Dept Hem/Oncology, 8700 Beverly Blvd, Los Angeles, CA 90048; **Phone:** 310-423-1825; **Board Cert:** Internal Medicine 1989; Hematology 2004; Medical Oncology 2003; **Med School:** UCSD 1986; **Resid:** Internal Medicine, UCSD Med Ctr 1989; **Fellow:** Hematology & Oncology, UCLA Med Ctr 1993; **Fac Appt:** Assoc Prof Med, UCLA

Vogelzang, Nicholas J MD [Onc] - **Spec Exp:** Prostate Cancer; Mesothelioma; Kidney Cancer; **Hospital:** Univ Med Ctr - Las Vegas, Summerlin Hosp Med Ctr; **Address:** Nevada Cancer Institute, One Breakthrough Way, Las Vegas, NV 89135; **Phone:** 702-822-5100; **Board Cert:** Internal Medicine 1977; Medical Oncology 1981; **Med School:** Univ IL Coll Med 1974; **Resid:** Internal Medicine, Rush-Presby St Luke's Med Ctr 1977; **Fellow:** Medical Oncology, Univ Minn Med Ctr 1980; **Fac Appt:** Prof Med, Univ Nevada

Volberding, Paul Arthur MD [Onc] - **Spec Exp:** AIDS Related Cancers; **Hospital:** UCSF Med Ctr, VA Med Ctr - San Francisco; **Address:** 4150 Clement St, VAMC 111, San Francisco, CA 94121; **Phone:** 415-750-2203; **Board Cert:** Internal Medicine 1978; Medical Oncology 1981; **Med School:** Univ Minn 1975; **Resid:** Internal Medicine, Univ Utah Med Ctr 1978; **Fellow:** Medical Oncology, UCSF Med Ctr 1981; **Fac Appt:** Prof Med, UCSF

von Gunten, Charles MD/PhD [Onc] - **Spec Exp:** Palliative Care; **Hospital:** San Diego Hospice; **Address:** San Diego Hospice, 4311 Third Ave, San Diego, CA 92103; **Phone:** 619-688-1600; **Board Cert:** Internal Medicine 2002; Medical Oncology 2003; Hospice & Palliative Medicine 2001; **Med School:** Univ Colorado 1988; **Resid:** Internal Medicine, Northwestern Univ 1991; **Fellow:** Medical Oncology, Northwestern Univ 1993; **Fac Appt:** Assoc Clin Prof Med, UCSD

Wierman, Ann MD [Onc] - **Spec Exp:** Breast Cancer; Lymphoma; Lung Cancer; **Hospital:** Univ Med Ctr - Las Vegas; **Address:** 2851 N Tenaya Way, Ste 101, Las Vegas, NV 89128; **Phone:** 702-735-7154; **Board Cert:** Internal Medicine 2002; Medical Oncology 2007; Hematology 1998; **Med School:** Baylor Coll Med 1989; **Resid:** Internal Medicine, Baylor Hosps 1992; Internal Medicine, Ben Taub Genl Hosp 1993; **Fellow:** Hematology & Oncology, Univ CO Hlth Sci Ctr 1996; **Fac Appt:** Assoc Clin Prof Med, Univ Nevada

Yen, Yun MD/PhD [Onc] - **Spec Exp:** Liver Cancer; Biliary Cancer; **Hospital:** City of Hope Natl Med Ctr & Beckman Rsch (page 69); **Address:** City of Hope Comprehensive Cancer Ctr, 1500 E Duarte Rd, Duarte, CA 91010; **Phone:** 626-359-8111 x62307; **Board Cert:** Medical Oncology 2003; **Med School:** Taiwan 1982; **Resid:** Internal Medicine, St Luke's Hosp 1990; **Fellow:** Hematology & Oncology, Yale-New Haven Hosp 1993; **Fac Appt:** Prof Med, USC Sch Med

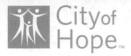

1500 East Duarte Road
Duarte, CA 91010
800-826-HOPE cityofhope.org

City of Hope is a recognized worldwide leader for its compassionate patient care, innovative science and translational research, which rapidly turn laboratory breakthroughs into promising new therapies. One of only 40 National Cancer Institute-designated Comprehensive Cancer Centers nationwide and a founding member of the National Comprehensive Cancer Network, City of Hope is ranked as one of "America's Best Hospitals" in cancer and urology by *U.S.News & World Report*.

ACADEMIC AND CLINICAL AFFILIATIONS

As an independent academic institution, City of Hope enables its researchers to pursue all avenues of scientific inquiry while encouraging collaboration with other researchers and institutions around the world. This helps to speed the development of novel cancer therapies. City of Hope's Graduate School of Biological Sciences also provides a fertile academic environment to prepare future scientists for careers in academia, medical and industrial fields.

MEDICAL STAFF

Guided by a humanistic approach to medicine, nationally recognized physicians and nurses lead collaborative treatment teams that address the whole patient, not just the disease, including emotional, psychological, spiritual and nutritional needs.

PIONEERING, COMPREHENSIVE MEDICAL CARE

City of Hope's Helford Clinical Research Hospital integrates the best of science and human caring in one state-of-the-art facility. There, lifesaving research and superior clinical care join forces as multidisciplinary teams of medical professionals pool their knowledge to bring promising new therapies to patients quickly, safely and effectively.

PHYSICIAN REFERRAL

City of Hope welcomes patient referrals from physicians throughout the world. Referring physicians are encouraged to contact our specialists directly or call 800-826-HOPE.

CENTER OF EXCELLENCE: HEMATOLOGY

In 1976, City of Hope was one of the first medical centers in the nation to successfully perform bone marrow transplantation for leukemia. Today, with more than 9,000 bone marrow and stem cell transplants performed, the Division of Hematology and Hematopoietic Cell Transplantation conducts one of the largest and most successful transplant programs in the world, with innovative protocols for patients with a variety of hematologic cancers and other diseases.

To learn more, visit cityofhope.org/HCT

Cleveland Clinic

Unsurpassed Treatments for Leukemia and Lymphoma

At Cleveland Clinic Taussig Cancer Institute, more than 250 cancer specialists, researchers, nurses and technicians are dedicated to developing and applying the latest and most effective medical techniques to achieve the long-term survival and improve the quality of life for 7,500 new cancer patients every year. Because of our patient-centered care, leading-edge treatments, innovative research, 350 clinical trials and state-of-the-art medical technologies, *U.S.News & World Report* has ranked Cleveland Clinic's cancer program one of the top cancer centers in the nation.

Unsurpassed treatment

The Taussig Cancer Institute is a national leader in caring for and treating patients with leukemia, lymphoma and myeloma. For example, our Bone Marrow Transplant outcomes are unsurpassed by any program in the world. We have one of the most experienced teams in the nation, having performed more than 3,000 bone marrow transplant procedures since 1977. **To schedule an appointment or get a second opinion, call 866.223.8100 today or visit clevelandclinic.org/bloodcancersTCD.**

Discovering new drugs

In addition to providing patients with a wide range of the latest treatments, Taussig Cancer Institute oncologists and researchers are on the cutting edge of developing new therapies and discovering new drugs. The Cleveland Clinic Center for Hematological Oncology Molecular Therapeutics operates six research laboratories focusing on drug discovery and development. The Taussig Cancer Institute's experimental hematopoiesis unit is working to improve diagnosis and therapy of hematologic disorders, including bone marrow failure syndromes and leukemia.

Streamlining drug development

To increase access and participation in clinical trials among adult blood cancer patients, the Leukemia and Lymphoma Society and Cleveland Clinic Taussig Cancer Institute launched a groundbreaking partnership called The Clinical Trial Center for Hematologic Malignancies. The partnership will accelerate the process of developing and delivering new, more advanced drugs for leukemia, lymphoma and myeloma. Trials will all be conducted by a single clinical center with access to a large volume of patients at Cleveland Clinic's main campus and regional hospitals.

To schedule an appointment or for more information about the Cleveland Clinic Taussig Cancer Institute, call 866.223.8100 or visit clevelandclinic.org/bloodcancersTCD.

Cleveland Clinic Taussig Cancer Institute | Cleveland, OH

Cleveland Clinic

Get More Cancer Information and Support

Taussig Cancer Institute – Cancer Answer Line

The Cleveland Clinic Taussig Cancer Institute's Cancer Answer Line is here to help you understand your cancer diagnosis and available treatment options. The Cancer Answer Line is staffed by two clinical nurse specialists and their staff can provide information and answer questions about cancer. If desired, appointments can be scheduled with one of the expert physicians at the Cleveland Clinic. The Cancer Answer Line is operational from 8:00am – 4:30pm, Monday – Friday.

To schedule an appointment or for more information about cancer, call 1.866.223.8100 or visit clevelandclinic.org/cancer TCD

Special Assistance for Our Out-of-State Patients

Cleveland Clinic Global Patient Services offers a complimentary Medical Concierge service for patients who travel to Cleveland Clinic from outside Ohio. We can help coordinate medical appointments, assist with travel needs and more. **For more information, call 800.223.2273, ext. 55580, or email medicalconcierge@ccf.org.**

If your care brings you to the Cleveland Clinic Taussig Cancer Institute, please visit the Patient Resource Center in the northeast corner of the building. It is a place for patients as well as their friends and families to come for cancer information and resources including

- Free cancer information pamphlets
- Computer terminals that can be used for conducting internet searches
- Conference area where you can sit with a nurse and ask questions
- Listings and registrations for support groups and other patient programs
- Listings of resources such as wigs, transportation, and lodging

The Patient Resource Center is open from 8:00 a.m. – 4:30 p.m., Monday – Friday.

CARES

The Scott Hamilton CARES Initiative (CARES) was founded in 1999 as a partnership between Scott Hamilton, Olympic ice-skating champion and cancer survivor, and the Cleveland Clinic Taussig Cancer Center where he was treated. CARES was created to promote cancer awareness while raising significant funds for cancer research.

Key components of CARES include:

4th Angel Mentoring Program – a free phone based program designed to match newly diagnosed patients with trained volunteers who are also cancer survivors. Emphasizing one-on-one contact, individuals are paired according to various demographics including age, cancer type and treatments in an effort to empower both patients and volunteers with knowledge, awareness and hope. In addition, the 4th Angel Caregiver Mentoring program is designed to match a caregiver of a cancer survivor to a current cancer patient caregiver. A 4th Angel Caregiver Mentor uses her/his experience to help others cope with the difficult caregiver role.

Chemocare.com – a unique website designed to help patients better understand the chemotherapy experience. As the first website of its kind in the United States, Chemocare.com is written in easy-to-understand language, both English and Spanish, and outlines everything patients and their families need to know about chemotherapy, side effects and their management.

To learn more about CARES, visit clevelandclinic.org/cancer/scottcaresTCD

Cleveland Clinic Taussig Cancer Institute | 9500 Euclid Avenue / AC311 | Cleveland, OH

202   Sponsored Page

THE JOHN THEURER CANCER CENTER
HACKENSACK UNIVERSITY MEDICAL CENTER

20 Prospect Avenue
Hackensack, New Jersey 07601
phone 201-996-5900 • fax 201-996-3452

www.humc.com

JOHN THEURER
CANCERCENTER
AT HACKENSACK UNIVERSITY MEDICAL CENTER

New Jersey's Largest Cancer Center – The John Theurer Cancer Center at Hackensack University Medical Center is New Jersey's largest and most comprehensive cancer program and one of the top 10 in the nation in patient volume. Each week, more than 150 new patients come to the cancer center seeking services that are widely recognized for their innovation and attention to patients' needs and concerns. With one of the largest Blood and Marrow Transplantation Programs in the nation, the cancer center offers patients the most advanced treatments available.

Vision and Focus – The Cancer Center's mission is to provide the highest quality cancer care, diagnosis, treatment, research, management, and preventive services. Fourteen specialized cancer-care teams provide advanced care that combines state-of-the-art technology, skilled medical expertise, research breakthroughs, and compassionate care giving. The Blood and Marrow Transplantation Program has been recognized with a Gold Seal of Approval™ for healthcare quality from the Joint Commission.

Bringing You Tomorrow's Breakthroughs Today™ – Most of today's cancer-care breakthroughs have come about from basic and clinical research into how cancer can be best detected, treated, or managed. Some of the most innovative cancer clinical trials are conducted at the cancer center, spearheaded by internationally renowned award-winning researchers. These trials give patients access to promising investigational medications, treatment protocols, and surgical techniques. This strong research component coupled with its patient care services elevates the John Theurer Cancer Center to a world-class academic medical center.

Finding Answers – The first step in cancer care is to define the illness, determine its location, and find out whether it has spread. At the cancer center, pathologists, radiologists, and other physicians use precise, sophisticated technology to gain answers to these questions. Among the equipment and tests used are a dedicated PET scanner, ultrasonography, nuclear medicine, computerized tomography, magnetic resonance imaging, mammography, and angiography.

Today's Treatment Innovations – Physicians at the cancer center have pioneered some of the most promising treatments for cancer – including peripheral stem cell transplantation. Through its specialized divisions, the cancer center offers patients the most advanced treatment options, including intensity modulated radiation therapy, brachytherapy, stereotactic radiosurgery; the latest chemotherapy medications; innovative adjuvant therapy approaches; and state-of-the-art surgical techniques, including video-assisted thoracic surgery, radioablation therapy, and minimally invasive procedures that reduce pain, lessen side effects, decrease recovery time, and increase patients' mobility.

To receive information about all of the John Theurer Cancer Center's services and 14 specialized divisions, please call 201-996-5900.

LIVING WITH CANCER

The John Theurer Cancer Center provides an outstanding array of aftercare and support services to help patients manage their quality of life. These include:

• Support groups for adults, children, and family members to help them cope with the illness, treatment, and aftercare

• The Integrative Cancer Care Program at The Center for Health and Healing brings together a range of services to address the physical, emotional, and spiritual needs of patients with cancer, their family members, and friends

• The Department of Social Services, provides crisis intervention, financial guidance, stress reduction sessions, psychosocial counseling, referrals to community resources, a floating library, and various educational workshops

• The Hospice Program offers pain- and symptom-relief services, spiritual support, skilled nursing care, social services, and bereavement in both the home and in an inpatient setting

The Indiana University Melvin and Bren Simon Cancer Center reflects the statewide nationally recognized health care delivery system of Clarian Health, supported by the scientific resources of Indiana University School of Medicine (IUSM), the second largest medical school in the United States.

SCIENTIFIC EXCELLENCE
The Indiana University Melvin and Bren Simon Cancer Center, a partnership between Clarian Health and IUSM, is the only National Cancer Institute (NCI)-designated cancer center in Indiana that provides patient care. This designation recognizes IU Simon Cancer Center's scientific excellence and helps fund life-saving research that ultimately benefits patients.

Nearly 40,000 patients turn to IU Simon Cancer Center for cancer care each year, seeking the multidisciplinary team approach pioneered in Indiana by each of our disease-specific clinical care programs. Our team approach combines treatment, research and supportive care expertise for each patient. With both standards of care and clinical trial options, IU Simon Cancer Center offers diagnostic, treatment and prevention regimens that meet the unique needs of each individual patient.

PATIENT/FAMILY FOCUS
Located in the heart of Indianapolis, the IU Simon Cancer Center offers the most advanced care in modern and comfortable facilities. Our CompleteLife program addresses the full spectrum of patient and family needs, including emotional, psychological and spiritual concerns. The benefits to patients are clear — a wide range of innovative treatment options, expert teams of diverse professionals focused on their specific cancer type and attention to all cancer care needs in one setting.

RESEARCH EXPERTISE
The IU Simon Cancer Center's research expertise is known around the world, offering renewed hope for patients and families and new options in cancer care. Researchers and physicians with IU Simon Cancer Center have improved the cure rate of testicular cancer from 10 percent to nearly 95 percent today. Our physicians have gained international recognition for treatment of the following conditions:

- Breast cancer
- Gastrointestinal cancers
- Genitourinary cancer
- Hematologic cancer
- Bone marrow and stem cell transplantation at Riley Hospital for Children and Indiana University Hospital
- Thoracic cancer

To schedule an appointment or for more information, call 888-600-4822 or visit cancer.iu.edu.

Memorial Sloan-Kettering Cancer Center

The Best Cancer Care. Anywhere.

1275 York Avenue
New York, NY 10065
Phone: (212) 639-2000
Physician Referral: (800) 525-2225
www.mskcc.org

Sponsorship: Private, Non-Profit
Beds: 434
Accreditation: Awarded Accreditation from the Joint Commission on Accreditation of Healthcare Organizations (JCAHO)

At Memorial Sloan-Kettering Cancer Center, our sole focus is cancer. Our doctors are among the most skilled and experienced in the world in treating all kinds of cancer. For patients, the knowledge, talent, and expertise of our medical professionals leads to superb patient care, and often, a significant positive impact on the chances that their cancer will be cured or controlled.

SUB-SPECIALIZED MEDICAL EXPERTISE
Patients at MSKCC benefit from individualized treatment plans developed by a team of specialists with an unsurpassed depth and breadth of experience. The teams include surgeons, medical and radiation oncologists, radiologists, pathologists, nurses, and others who are specialists in treating patients with a specific type of cancer. They develop treatment plans that reflect their combined expertise, so that patients who need several different types of therapy will receive the best combination for them.

RESEARCH EXPANDS TREATMENT OPTIONS
One of Memorial Sloan-Kettering's great strengths is the close relationship between scientists and clinicians. Through the constant collaboration between our doctors and research scientists, new drugs and therapies developed in the laboratory can be quickly translated into improved treatment options for patients.

NURSING AND SUPPORTIVE CARE
Our nurses are essential members of the healthcare team. Their expertise, support, encouragement, and deep sense of caring bring tremendous comfort to patients and family members. Our specially trained oncology nurses care for patients throughout their treatment, help manage clinical trials, and educate patients about all aspects of their care.

Specially trained psychiatrists and psychologists help patients deal with the stress, anxiety, and depression that sometimes accompany cancer and its treatment. We also have social workers who ensure that patients who need it receive assistance with needs such as housing and transportation. They offer individual and family counseling, as well as support groups for both inpatients and outpatients. After treatment, the Post-Treatment Resource Program offers patients seminars, lectures, support groups, and practical advice on various issues such as insurance and employment.

INTEGRATIVE MEDICINE
Our Integrative Medicine Service offers a full range of complementary therapies, including massage, reflexology, meditation, music therapy, and acupuncture. These do not replace medical care but are used along with clinical treatments to help patients relieve stress, reduce pain and anxiety, manage symptoms, and promote a feeling of well-being.

INSURANCE
Memorial Sloan-Kettering Cancer Center is in-network with most New York–area insurance plans.

A TRADITION OF EXCELLENCE

From its founding 125 years ago, Memorial Sloan-Kettering Cancer Center has been guided by a clear mission: to offer the best possible care for patients today, and to seek strategies to prevent, control, and ultimately cure cancer in the future. We are proud of our designation as one of the few select National Cancer Institute Comprehensive Cancer Centers and a member of the National Comprehensive Cancer Network.

To see one of our specialized cancer experts, call us at (800) 525-2225.

Physician Referral: (800) 525-2225

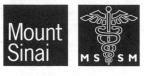

MOUNT SINAI
SCHOOL OF
MEDICINE

THE TISCH CANCER INSTITUTE
AT THE MOUNT SINAI MEDICAL CENTER
One Gustave L. Levy Place
Fifth Avenue and 100th Street
New York, NY 10029-6574
Physician Referral: 1-800-MD-SINAI (637-4624)
www.tischcancerinstitute.org

OVERVIEW
The Tisch Cancer Institute, part of The Mount Sinai Medical Center, is located on the Upper East Side of Manhattan. The Mount Sinai Medical Center was founded in 1852 and encompasses one of the oldest teaching hospitals in the country. In an atmosphere of learning, cutting-edge basic and clinical research, and superb patient care, The Tisch Cancer Institute coordinates a full-service diagnostic and treatment program for cancer patients. Because new treatments are developed at the Institute, patients often have access to these therapies before they are available anywhere else in the world.

A HERITAGE OF BREAKTHROUGHS
Teams of physicians and scientists at The Tisch Cancer Institute at Mount Sinai work together to rapidly translate laboratory research into new patient treatments. Among the advances pioneered at Mount Sinai are the first successful treatment of tumors of the bladder by transurethral electrocoagulation, the first demonstration of how asbestos can cause cancerous changes in the DNA of cells, and the first development of an ultrasound-guided technique to insert radioactive seeds into the prostate to treat prostate cancer.

THE TISCH CANCER INSTITUTE
The Tisch Cancer Institute employs a multidisciplinary treatment approach, providing access to clinical breakthroughs, innovative techniques, leading-edge technologies, and a wide range of diagnostic, therapeutic, and support services for all types of cancer. The Institute treats: head and neck cancer; thoracic cancer (including lung and esophagus); gynecologic cancer; hematological malignancies (including myelodysplastic syndrome and myeloproliferative disorders); brain tumors; and prostate, bladder, kidney, and liver cancer. In addition to surgical treatment, the Institute provides radiation and medical oncology therapies as well as bone marrow transplantation.

The Institute's multidisciplinary treatment approach involves collaboration with colleagues across the Medical Center, drawing upon the knowledge of a vast network of specialists who are outstanding in their fields. These experts consist of award-winning physicians and surgeons specializing in cardiac care, neurology, urology, pediatrics, digestive diseases, obstetrics and gynecology, and other therapeutic areas. Furthermore, Mount Sinai's nursing staff is an important part of the Medical Center's focus on delivering exceptional patient care, and it has received the prestigious Magnet Award for nursing excellence.

THE RUTTENBERG TREATMENT CENTER
The mission of the Ruttenberg Treatment Center at The Mount Sinai Medical Center is to reduce the burden of human cancer through its outstanding interdisciplinary programs in patient care and research, including cancer prevention, treatment, early detection, and education. Oncologists, surgeons, and specialists from across the medical spectrum work together to provide the highest quality care to all cancer patients. The members of the Center—scientists and physicians—are developing cancer therapies and prevention strategies to improve cancer care, and patients at the Center are the first to benefit from these treatments.

Mount Sinai is renowned for its palliative care program, which provides the highest level of care, focusing on the relief of pain, symptoms, and stress in cancer patients in both an inpatient and outpatient setting.

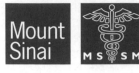

**MOUNT SINAI
SCHOOL OF
MEDICINE**

THE TISCH CANCER INSTITUTE
AT THE MOUNT SINAI MEDICAL CENTER
One Gustave L. Levy Place
Fifth Avenue and 100th Street
New York, NY 10029-6574
Physician Referral: 1-800-MD-SINAI (637-4624)
www.tischcancerinstitute.org

OVERVIEW

The Tisch Cancer Institute, part of The Mount Sinai Medical Center, is located on the Upper East Side of Manhattan. The Mount Sinai Medical Center was founded in 1852 and encompasses one of the oldest teaching hospitals in the country. In an atmosphere of learning, cutting-edge basic and clinical research, and superb patient care, The Tisch Cancer Institute coordinates a full-service diagnostic and treatment program for cancer patients. Because new treatments are developed at the Institute, patients often have access to these therapies before they are available anywhere else in the world.

A HERITAGE OF BREAKTHROUGHS

Teams of physicians and scientists at The Tisch Cancer Institute at Mount Sinai work together to rapidly translate laboratory research into new patient treatments. Among the advances pioneered at Mount Sinai are the first successful treatment of tumors of the bladder by transurethral electrocoagulation, the first demonstration of how asbestos can cause cancerous changes in the DNA of cells, and the first development of an ultrasound-guided technique to insert radioactive seeds into the prostate to treat prostate cancer.

THE TISCH CANCER INSTITUTE

The Tisch Cancer Institute employs a multidisciplinary treatment approach, providing access to clinical breakthroughs, innovative techniques, leading-edge technologies, and a wide range of diagnostic, therapeutic, and support services for all types of cancer. The Institute treats: head and neck cancer; thoracic cancer (including lung and esophagus); gynecologic cancer; hematological malignancies (including myelodysplastic syndrome and myeloproliferative disorders); brain tumors; and prostate, bladder, kidney, and liver cancer. In addition to surgical treatment, the Institute provides radiation and medical oncology therapies as well as bone marrow transplantation.

The Institute's multidisciplinary treatment approach involves collaboration with colleagues across the Medical Center, drawing upon the knowledge of a vast network of specialists who are outstanding in their fields. These experts consist of award-winning physicians and surgeons specializing in cardiac care, neurology, urology, pediatrics, digestive diseases, obstetrics and gynecology, and other therapeutic areas. Furthermore, Mount Sinai's nursing staff is an important part of the Medical Center's focus on delivering exceptional patient care, and it has received the prestigious Magnet Award for nursing excellence.

Mount Sinai is renowned for its palliative care program, which provides the highest level of care, focusing on the relief of pain, symptoms, and stress in cancer patients in both an inpatient and outpatient setting.

THE RUTTENBERG TREATMENT CENTER

The mission of the Ruttenberg Treatment Center at The Mount Sinai Medical Center is to reduce the burden of human cancer through its outstanding interdisciplinary programs in patient care and research, including cancer prevention, treatment, early detection, and education. Oncologists, surgeons, and specialists from across the medical spectrum work together to provide the highest quality care to all cancer patients. The members of the Center—scientists and physicians—are developing cancer therapies and prevention strategies to improve cancer care, and patients at the Center are the first to benefit from these treatments.

⌐ NewYork-Presbyterian
⌐ The University Hospital of Columbia and Cornell
NewYork-Presbyterian Cancer Centers

Affiliated with Columbia University College of Physicians and Surgeons and Weill Cornell Medical College

Herbert Irving Comprehensive Cancer Center	Weill Cornell Cancer Center
At NewYork-Presbyterian Hospital	At NewYork-Presbyterian Hospital
Columbia University Medical Center	Weill Cornell Medical Center
161 Fort Washington Avenue	525 East 68th Street
New York, NY 10032	New York, NY 10065

OVERVIEW:

The NewYork-Presbyterian Cancer Centers are dedicated to understanding cancer and to providing additional and improved therapeutic options to treat cancer. The Cancer Centers:

- Provide state-of-the-art screening, diagnostic, therapeutic and supportive care services.
- Offer cancer-related educational programs and resources to patients, their caregivers, cancer survivors, and the cancer prevention community.
- Conduct peer-reviewed basic, clinical and public health research.

The Cancer Centers, which treat over 6,500 newly diagnosed patients annually, draw on the innovative research excellence and clinical expertise of the NCI-designated Herbert Irving Comprehensive Cancer Center at NewYork-Presbyterian Hospital/Columbia University Medical Center and the Weill Cornell Cancer Center at NewYork-Presbyterian Hospital/Weill Cornell Medical Center. Specialty programs include:

- AIDS-related Malignancies
- Bone Marrow Transplant
- Breast Cancer
- Dermatologic/Skin Cancer
- Esophageal Cancer
- Gastrointestinal Cancers
- Genitourinary Cancers including bladder, kidney and prostate
- Gynecologic Cancers
- Head and Neck Cancers
- Hodgkin's Lymphoma and Non Hodgkin's Lymphoma
- Leukemia
- Myeloma
- Lung Cancer
- Neurological Cancer
- Ophthalmic Cancer
- Pancreatic Cancer
- Pediatric Hematology/Oncology
- Radiation Oncology
- Sarcomas and Mesotheliomas

The Centers research programs are supported by grants from the National Cancer Institute, the National Institutes of Health, other federal agencies, the Leukemia and Lymphoma Society, the Lymphoma Research Foundation, the Avon Breast Cancer Research Foundation, the Komen Breast Cancer Foundation, and other private foundations and philanthropic organizations. Patients have access to over 500 clinical trials.

Physician Referral: For a physician referral call toll free **1-877-NYP-WELL** (1-877-697-9355) or to learn more about our Cancer Centers visit our website at **www.nypcancer.org**

ADVANCED SURGICAL AND THERAPEUTIC SERVICES INCLUDE:

- Double cord transplants and use of mesenchymal stem cells to treat graft vs. host disease
- Sentinel node biopsy to assess spread of breast cancer
- Skin sparing mastectomy and nipple sparing techniques for breast cancer and oncoplastic procedures
- Interventional endoscopy and laparoscopic surgery for colon and other gastrointestinal cancers
- Stereotactic biopsies for breast and brain cancer:
  - Gamma radiation and novel medical therapies for recurrent brain cancer
  - Robotic Prostatectomy for prostate, kidney, bladder, and gynecologic cancers
  - Partial breast radiation using MammoSite balloon brachytherapy
  - State of the art interventional endoscopy
  - Interleukin-2 Vaccine Program
  - Minimally invasive lung sparing surgery and lobectomies for lung cancer
  - Novel therapeutics for lymphomas, leukemias, and myelomas

NYU Cancer Institute
NYU LANGONE MEDICAL CENTER

A Collaborative Approach
The NYU Cancer Institute, an NCI designated center, is a "matrix cancer center" without walls operating within the larger NYU Langone Medical Center. With over 175 members and a research funding base of over $81 million, this structure strengthens our capabilities to forge collaborations across medical and scientific disciplines, which translates to comprehensive care for our patients and discoveries that will influence the future of this disease.

Renowned Expertise
Team members' compassion and expertise help patients better manage the symptoms of their disease as well as their special needs. Our highly skilled Magnet™ nursing team not only plays a pivotal role in coordinating direct patient care, but is also a source of invaluable patient education.

A Patient-Focused Setting
The NYU Clinical Cancer Center, with over 70 faculty members from various disciplines at the New York University School of Medicine, is the principal outpatient facility of the Cancer Institute and serves as home for our patients and their caregivers. The center and its multidisciplinary team of experts provide access to the latest treatment options and clinical trials along with a variety of programs in cancer prevention, screening, diagnostics, genetic counseling, and supportive services. When it comes to kids and cancer, the Stephen D. Hassenfeld Children's Center for Cancer and Blood Disorders offers not just innovation but insight. As a leading member of the NCI-sponsored Children's Oncology Group, our physicians are known for developing new ways to treat childhood cancer. Our affiliation with Bellevue Hospital, the oldest public hospital in the country, affords clinically distinctive opportunities to learn and care for patients with cancer by observing its presentation and behavior in a variety of patient groups.

NYU Cancer Institute
NYU LANGONE MEDICAL CENTER

A Collaborative Approach

The NYU Cancer Institute, an NCI designated center, is a "matrix cancer center" without walls operating within the larger NYU Langone Medical Center. With over 175 members and a research funding base of over $81 million, this structure strengthens our capabilities to forge collaborations across medical and scientific disciplines, which translates to comprehensive care for our patients and discoveries that will influence the future of this disease.

Renowned Expertise

Team members' compassion and expertise help patients better manage the symptoms of their disease as well as their special needs. Our highly skilled Magnet™ nursing team not only plays a pivotal role in coordinating direct patient care, but is also a source of invaluable patient education.

A Patient-Focused Setting

The NYU Clinical Cancer Center, with over 70 faculty members from various disciplines at the New York University School of Medicine, is the principal outpatient facility of the Cancer Institute and serves as home for our patients and their caregivers. The center and its multidisciplinary team of experts provide access to the latest treatment options and clinical trials along with a variety of programs in cancer prevention, screening, diagnostics, genetic counseling, and supportive services. When it comes to kids and cancer, the Stephen D. Hassenfeld Children's Center for Cancer and Blood Disorders offers not just innovation but insight. As a leading member of the NCI-sponsored Children's Oncology Group, our physicians are known for developing new ways to treat childhood cancer. Our affiliation with Bellevue Hospital, the oldest public hospital in the country, affords clinically distinctive opportunities to learn and care for patients with cancer by observing its presentation and behavior in a variety of patient groups.

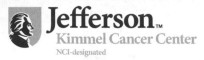

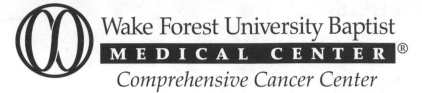

Wake Forest University Baptist
MEDICAL CENTER ®
Comprehensive Cancer Center

Medical Center Boulevard • Winston-Salem, NC 27157 • 336-716-2011
Health On-Call® (Patient access) 1-800-446-2255
PAL® (Physician-to-physician calls) 1-800-277-7654
www.wfubmc.edu/cancer/

TOP RANKINGS

The Comprehensive Cancer Center of Wake Forest University Baptist Medical is among an elite group of only 40 U.S. cancer centers designated by the National Cancer Institute as comprehensive, indicating excellence in research, patient care and education. The comprehensive designation was renewed for an additional five years in late 2006.

RESEARCH ADVANTAGES

Wake Forest Baptist offers more cancer-related clinical trials than any other hospital in western N.C. From gene therapy to vitamin and nutrition studies to new surgical and radiological treatments, patients benefit from the leading edge of cancer knowledge and care. Innovative basic science, public health and clinical research promote new discovery about prevention, detection and treatment of cancers. Wake Forest scientists were first in the world to discover cancer resistant cells in mice.

TECHNOLOGY AND TREATMENT STRENGTHS

Wake Forest University Baptist Medical Center is home to North Carolina's first Gamma Knife, a non-invasive, stereotactic radiosurgical tool used to treat malignant and benign brain tumors once considered inoperable. Operated by one of the nation's most experienced treatment teams, the Gamma Knife painlessly bombards tumors with precisely focused beams of gamma energy—sparing normal tissue—and is performed on an outpatient basis. Extracranial body stereotactic radiosurgery offers new options for cancers in the torso.

Wake Forest Baptist offers an integrated brachytherapy unit (IBU) and highly targeted Intensity Modulated Radiation Therapy (IMRT) for treatment of prostate, brain, lung, head and neck, and gynecological cancers. Other treatment innovations include IPHC (intraperitoneal hyperthermic chemotherapy) for abdominal cavity cancers and radiofrequency ablation for liver malignancies.

MULTIDISCIPLINARY EXPERTISE

Expert, subspecialized oncology teams provide patients a consensus opinion on treatment. Multidisciplinary centers include the Breast Care Center, the Brain Tumor Clinic and the Head and Neck Cancers Multidisciplinary Clinic.

To make an appointment or find a specialist, call Health On-Call® at 1-800-446-2255.

HIGHLIGHTS OF EXCELLENCE

- Western North Carolina's only NCI-designated Comprehensive Cancer Center offers the convenience and comfort of a state-of-the-art Outpatient Cancer Center. The nation's first Cancer Patient Support Group was developed here.

- The Cancer Center's Blood and Marrow Transplant Program operates the nation's second-largest collection site.

- The Hereditary Cancer Program helps patients understand their risk profile for colorectal, breast, ovarian and melanoma cancers.

- Minimally invasive treatments include high dose rate (HDR) brachytherapy for prostate cancer. Lymph node mapping increases chance for lymph-sparing breast surgery.

- Clinical trials testing new methods of drug delivery offer patients with brain tumors potentially more effective treatment while minimizing effects on healthy tissue.

KNOWLEDGE MAKES ALL THE DIFFERENCE.

Neurological Surgery

A neurological surgeon provides the operative and non-operative management (i.e., prevention, diagnosis, evaluation, treatment, critical care and rehabilitation) of disorders of the central, peripheral and autonomic nervous systems, including their supporting structures and vascular supply; the evaluation and treatment of pathological processes which modify function or activity of the nervous system; and the operative and non-operative management of pain. A neurological surgeon treats patients with disorders of the nervous system; disorders of the brain, meninges, skull and their blood supply, including the extracranial carotid and vertebral arteries; disorders of the pituitary gland; disorders of the spinal cord, meninges and vertebral column, including those which may require treatment by spinal fusion or instrumentation; and disorders of the cranial and spinal nerves throughout their distribution.

Training Required: One year minimum of General Surgery followed by five years in Neurological Surgery.

Pediatric Neurological Surgery: The American Board of Pediatric Neurological Surgery (ABPNS) is not a recognized ABMS subspecialty. However, this designation has been included because the certification process is meaningful and rigorous. It is awarded to those doctors who hold a current ABMS certification in Neurological Surgery, have completed a fully accredited one year, post-graduate fellowship in pediatric neurological surgery, and have submitted surgical logs indicating a practice of pediatric neurological surgery for one year, followed by a written examination.

NEUROLOGICAL SURGERY

New England

Black, Peter MD/PhD [NS] - **Spec Exp:** Brain Tumors; Pituitary Tumors; **Hospital:** Brigham & Women's Hosp, Children's Hospital - Boston; **Address:** Brigham & Women's Hosp, Dept Neurosurg, 75 Francis St, Boston, MA 02115-6106; **Phone:** 617-732-6600; **Board Cert:** Neurological Surgery 1984; **Med School:** McGill Univ 1970; **Resid:** Surgery, Mass Genl Hosp 1972; Neurological Surgery, Mass Genl Hosp 1980; **Fellow:** Neurosurgical Oncology, Mass Genl Hosp 1976; **Fac Appt:** Prof NS, Harvard Med Sch

Borges, Lawrence F MD [NS] - **Spec Exp:** Spinal Surgery; Spinal Tumors; **Hospital:** Mass Genl Hosp; **Address:** Mass Genl Hosp, Div Neurosurg Svcs, 55 Fruit St, Ste 1205, Boston, MA 02114-2696; **Phone:** 617-726-6156; **Board Cert:** Neurological Surgery 1986; **Med School:** Johns Hopkins Univ 1977; **Resid:** Neurological Surgery, Mass Genl Hosp 1983; **Fac Appt:** Assoc Prof S, Harvard Med Sch

Cosgrove, G Rees MD [NS] - **Spec Exp:** Brain Tumors; **Hospital:** Lahey Clin, Emerson Hosp; **Address:** Lahey Clinic, 41 Mall Rd, Burlington, MA 01805; **Phone:** 781-744-1990; **Board Cert:** Neurological Surgery 1989; **Med School:** Queens Univ 1980; **Resid:** Neurological Surgery, Montreal Neur Inst 1986; **Fac Appt:** Prof NS, Tufts Univ

David, Carlos MD [NS] - **Spec Exp:** Cerebrovascular Surgery; Skull Base Tumors & Surgery; **Hospital:** Lahey Clin, Emerson Hosp; **Address:** Lahey Clinic, Dept Neurosurgery, 41 Mall Rd, Burlington, MA 01805; **Phone:** 781-744-8643; **Board Cert:** Neurological Surgery 2001; **Med School:** Univ Miami Sch Med 1990; **Resid:** Neurological Surgery, Jackson Memorial Hosp 1995; **Fellow:** Cerebrovascular & Skull Base Surgery, Barrow Neuro Inst 1997; **Fac Appt:** Assoc Clin Prof NS, Tufts Univ

Day, Arthur L MD [NS] - **Spec Exp:** Orbital Tumors/Cancer; Brain Tumors; **Hospital:** Brigham & Women's Hosp, Children's Hospital - Boston; **Address:** Brigham & Womens Hosp, Dept Neurosurgery, 75 Francis St, Boston, MA 02115; **Phone:** 617-732-6600; **Board Cert:** Neurological Surgery 1980; **Med School:** Louisiana State U, New Orleans 1972; **Resid:** Neurological Surgery, Shands-Univ Florida Hosp 1977; **Fellow:** Neurological Pathology, Shands-Univ Florida Hosp 1978; **Fac Appt:** Prof NS, Harvard Med Sch

Duhaime, Ann Christine MD [NS] - **Spec Exp:** Pediatric Neurosurgery; Brain Tumors; **Hospital:** Dartmouth - Hitchcock Med Ctr; **Address:** Chldns Hosp at Dartmouth-Hitchcock Med Ctr, One Medical Center Drive, Lebanon, NH 03756; **Phone:** 603-653-9880; **Board Cert:** Neurological Surgery 1990; Pediatric Neurological Surgery 2005; **Med School:** Univ Pennsylvania 1981; **Resid:** Neurological Surgery, Hosp Univ Penn 1987; **Fellow:** Pediatric Neurological Surgery, Chldns Hosp 1987; **Fac Appt:** Prof S, Dartmouth Med Sch

Goumnerova, Liliana MD [NS] - **Spec Exp:** Pediatric Neurosurgery; Brain Tumors; Endoscopic Surgery/Ventriculoscopy; **Hospital:** Children's Hospital - Boston, Dana-Farber Cancer Inst; **Address:** Chldns Hosp, 300 Longwood Ave, Hunnewell 2, Boston, MA 02115; **Phone:** 617-355-6364; **Board Cert:** Neurological Surgery 1992; Pediatric Neurological Surgery 2006; **Med School:** Canada 1980; **Resid:** Neurological Surgery, Univ Ottawa 1986; **Fellow:** Pediatric Neurological Surgery, Hosp for Sick Chldn 1988; Neurological Science, Univ Penn 1990; **Fac Appt:** Assoc Prof S, Harvard Med Sch

Martuza, Robert L MD [NS] - **Spec Exp:** Brain Tumors; Skull Base Surgery; **Hospital:** Mass Genl Hosp; **Address:** Mass General Hosp, 55 Fruit St, MGH-White 502, Boston, MA 02114; **Phone:** 617-726-8581; **Board Cert:** Neurological Surgery 1983; **Med School:** Harvard Med Sch 1973; **Resid:** Neurological Surgery, Mass Genl Hosp 1980; **Fac Appt:** Prof NS, Harvard Med Sch

Penar, Paul L MD [NS] - **Spec Exp:** Brain & Spinal Tumors; Stereotactic Radiosurgery; Pain-Chronic; **Hospital:** Fletcher Allen Health Care- Med Ctr Campus; **Address:** Fletcher Allen Health Care, 111 Colchester Ave, Burlington, VT 05401; **Phone:** 802-847-4590; **Board Cert:** Neurological Surgery 1989; **Med School:** Univ Mich Med Sch 1981; **Resid:** Neurological Surgery, Yale-New Haven Hosp 1987

Piepmeier, Joseph MD [NS] - **Spec Exp:** Neuro-Oncology; Brain & Spinal Cord Tumors; **Hospital:** Yale-New Haven Hosp; **Address:** Yale Sch Med, Dept Neurosurgery, 333 Cedar St Fl TMP-410, New Haven, CT 06520; **Phone:** 203-785-2791; **Board Cert:** Neurological Surgery 1984; **Med School:** Univ Tenn Coll Med, Memphis 1975; **Resid:** Neurological Surgery, Yale-New Haven Hosp 1982; **Fac Appt:** Prof NS, Yale Univ

Mid Atlantic

Andrews, David MD [NS] - **Spec Exp:** Brain Tumors; Stereotactic Radiosurgery; **Hospital:** Thomas Jefferson Univ Hosp (page 83); **Address:** Thom Jefferson Univ Hosp, Dept Neurosurg, 909 Walnut St Fl 2, Philadelphia, PA 19107 5109; **Phone:** 215-503-7005; **Board Cert:** Neurological Surgery 1992; **Med School:** Univ Colorado 1983; **Resid:** Neurological Surgery, NY Presby Hos-Cornell Med Ctr 1989; **Fellow:** Neuro-Oncology, Meml Sloan Kettering Cancer Ctr 1987; **Fac Appt:** Prof NS, Thomas Jefferson Univ

Bederson, Joshua B MD [NS] - **Spec Exp:** Brain & Spinal Cord Tumors; Pituitary Tumors; Skull Base Tumors; **Hospital:** Mount Sinai Med Ctr (page 77); **Address:** Mount Sinai Med Ctr, 1 Gustave Levy Pl, Box 1136, New York, NY 10029; **Phone:** 212-241-2377; **Board Cert:** Neurological Surgery 1993; **Med School:** UCSF 1984; **Resid:** Neurological Surgery, UCSF Med Ctr 1990; **Fellow:** Neurological Vascular Surgery, Barrow Neur Inst 1990; Neurological Vascular Surgery, Univ Hosp Zurich 1990; **Fac Appt:** Prof NS, Mount Sinai Sch Med

Bilsky, Mark H MD [NS] - **Spec Exp:** Spinal Tumors; Skull Base Tumors; Brain Tumors; Spinal Cord Tumors; **Hospital:** Meml Sloan-Kettering Cancer Ctr (page 76), NY-Presby Hosp/Weill Cornell (page 79); **Address:** 1275 York Avenue, New York, NY 10065; **Phone:** 800-525-2225; **Board Cert:** Neurological Surgery 1999; **Med School:** Emory Univ 1988; **Resid:** Neurological Surgery, NY Hosp-Cornell Med Ctr 1994; **Fellow:** Neuro-Oncology, Louisville Univ Med Ctr 1995; **Fac Appt:** Assoc Prof NS, Cornell Univ-Weill Med Coll

Brem, Henry MD [NS] - **Spec Exp:** Brain & Spinal Cord Tumors; Skull Base Tumors; Pituitary Tumors; **Hospital:** Johns Hopkins Hosp, Johns Hopkins Bayview Med Ctr; **Address:** Johns Hopkins Med Ctr-Dept Neuro Surgery, 600 N Wolfe St Meyer 7 Bldg - rm 113, Baltimore, MD 21287; **Phone:** 410-955-2248; **Board Cert:** Neurological Surgery 1986; **Med School:** Harvard Med Sch 1978; **Resid:** Neurological Surgery, Columbia-Presby Med Ctr 1984; **Fellow:** Neurological Surgery, Johns Hopkins Hosp 1980; **Fac Appt:** Prof NS, Johns Hopkins Univ

Bruce, Jeffrey MD [NS] - **Spec Exp:** Brain Tumors; Pituitary Tumors; Skull Base Surgery; Pineal Tumors; **Hospital:** NY-Presby Hosp/Columbia (page 79); **Address:** NY Presby Hosp, Dept Neurosurgery, 710 W 168th St N1 Bldg Fl 4 - rm 434, New York, NY 10032-3726; **Phone:** 212-305-7346; **Board Cert:** Neurological Surgery 1993; **Med School:** UMDNJ-RW Johnson Med Sch 1983; **Resid:** Neurological Surgery, Columbia-Presby Med Ctr 1990; **Fellow:** Neurological Surgery, Nat Inst Health 1985; **Fac Appt:** Prof NS, Columbia P&S

Neurological Surgery

Carson, Benjamin S MD [NS] - **Spec Exp:** Brain & Spinal Cord Tumors; Pediatric Neurosurgery; **Hospital:** Johns Hopkins Hosp; **Address:** 600 N Wolfe St, Harvey 811, Baltimore, MD 21287-8811; **Phone:** 410-955-7888; **Board Cert:** Neurological Surgery 1988; Pediatric Neurological Surgery 1997; **Med School:** Univ Mich Med Sch 1977; **Resid:** Neurological Surgery, Johns Hopkins Hosp 1983; **Fellow:** Pediatric Neurological Surgery, Queen Elizabeth II Med Ctr 1984; **Fac Appt:** Assoc Prof NS, Johns Hopkins Univ

Chen, Chun Siang MD [NS] - **Spec Exp:** Skull Base Tumors; Skull Base Surgery; Microsurgery; Brain & Spinal Surgery; **Hospital:** Mount Sinai Med Ctr (page 77); **Address:** Mount Sinai Med Ctr, Annenberg Bldg, One Gustave L Levy Pl Fl 8 - rm 10, New York, NY 10029; **Phone:** 212-241-8480; **Med School:** Brazil 1978; **Resid:** Neurological Surgery, Santa Casa de Misericordia of Sao Paulo Med Sch 1983; Neurological Surgery, Mt Sinai Med Ctr 2005; **Fellow:** Skull Base Surgery, St Lukes Roosevelt Hosp 2006; **Fac Appt:** Asst Prof NS, Mount Sinai Sch Med

Di Giacinto, George V MD [NS] - **Spec Exp:** Spinal Surgery; Pain Management; **Hospital:** St Luke's - Roosevelt Hosp Ctr - Roosevelt Div (page 71); **Address:** 425 W 59th St, Ste 4E, New York, NY 10019; **Phone:** 212-523-8500; **Board Cert:** Neurological Surgery 1981; **Med School:** Harvard Med Sch 1970; **Resid:** Neurological Surgery, Columbia-Presby Hosp 1978

Feldstein, Neil A MD [NS] - **Spec Exp:** Pediatric Neurosurgery; Brain Tumors-Pediatric; Craniofacial Surgery-Pediatric; **Hospital:** NY-Presby Hosp/Columbia (page 79); **Address:** Neurological Inst, 710 W 168th St Fl 2 - rm 213, New York, NY 10032; **Phone:** 212-305-1396; **Board Cert:** Neurological Surgery 1995; Pediatric Neurological Surgery 2007; **Med School:** NYU Sch Med 1984; **Resid:** Neurological Surgery, Baylor Coll Med 1989; **Fellow:** Pediatric Neurological Surgery, NYU Med Ctr 1991; **Fac Appt:** Assoc Prof NS, Columbia P&S

Golfinos, John G MD [NS] - **Spec Exp:** Brain Tumors; Stereotactic Radiosurgery; Skull Base Surgery; **Hospital:** NYU Langone Med Ctr (page 80), Lenox Hill Hosp; **Address:** NYU Med Ctr, Dept Neurosurgery, 530 1st Ave, Ste 8R, New York, NY 10016-6402; **Phone:** 212-263-2950; **Board Cert:** Neurological Surgery 1998; **Med School:** Columbia P&S 1988; **Resid:** Neurological Surgery, Barrow Neuro Inst 1995; **Fac Appt:** Assoc Prof NS, NYU Sch Med

Goodrich, James T MD [NS] - **Spec Exp:** Craniofacial Surgery/Reconstruction; Brain Tumors-Pediatric; Pediatric Neurosurgery; **Hospital:** Montefiore Med Ctr - Div. Moses, Jacobi Med Ctr; **Address:** Montefiore Med Ctr, Dept Ped Neurosurgery, 111 E 210th St, Bronx, NY 10467-2401; **Phone:** 718-920-4197; **Board Cert:** Neurological Surgery 1989; Pediatric Neurological Surgery 2007; **Med School:** Columbia P&S 1980; **Resid:** Neurological Surgery, NY Neurological Inst 1986; **Fac Appt:** Prof NS, Albert Einstein Coll Med

Gutin, Philip MD [NS] - **Spec Exp:** Brain Tumors; **Hospital:** Meml Sloan-Kettering Cancer Ctr (page 76), NY-Presby Hosp/Weill Cornell (page 79); **Address:** 1275 York Avenue, New York, NY 10065; **Phone:** 800-525-2225; **Board Cert:** Neurological Surgery 1981; **Med School:** Univ Pennsylvania 1971; **Resid:** Neurological Surgery, UCSF Med Ctr 1979; **Fellow:** Natl Cancer Inst 1976; **Fac Appt:** Prof NS, Cornell Univ-Weill Med Coll

Jallo, George I MD [NS] - **Spec Exp:** Pediatric Neurosurgery; Brain & Spinal Cord Tumors; Minimally Invasive Neurosurgery; **Hospital:** Johns Hopkins Hosp, Johns Hopkins Bayview Med Ctr; **Address:** Johns Hopkins Hosp, Dept of Neurosurgery, 600 N Wolfe St, Ste Harvey 811, Baltimore, MD 21287; **Phone:** 410-955-7851; **Board Cert:** Neurological Surgery 2002; Pediatric Neurological Surgery 2004; **Med School:** Univ VA Sch Med 1991; **Resid:** Neurological Surgery, NYU Med Ctr 1998; **Fellow:** Pediatric Neurological Surgery, Beth Israel Med Ctr 1999; **Fac Appt:** Assoc Prof NS, Johns Hopkins Univ

Judy, Kevin MD [NS] - **Spec Exp:** Brain Tumors; **Hospital:** Hosp Univ Penn - UPHS (page 81), Pennsylvania Hosp (page 81); **Address:** Hosp Univ Penn-Dept Neurosurg, 3400 Spruce St, 3 Silverstein, Philadelphia, PA 19104; **Phone:** 215-662-7854; **Board Cert:** Neurological Surgery 1997; **Med School:** Univ Pittsburgh 1984; **Resid:** Surgery, Mercy Hosp 1986; Neurological Surgery, Johns Hopkins Hosp 1992; **Fellow:** Neurological Surgery, Johns Hopkins Hosp 1991; **Fac Appt:** Assoc Prof NS, Univ Pennsylvania

Kassam, Amin MD [NS] - **Spec Exp:** Skull Base Tumors & Surgery; Cerebrovascular Surgery; Endoscopic Surgery; Minimally Invasive Surgery; **Hospital:** UPMC Presby, Pittsburgh, UPMC Mercy, Pittsburgh; **Address:** Univ Pittsburgh Med Ctr, Dept Neurosurgery, 200 Lothrop St, Ste B400, Pittburgh, PA 15213; **Phone:** 412-647-6778; **Med School:** Univ Toronto 1991; **Resid:** Neurological Surgery, Univ Ottawa Med Ctr 1997; **Fac Appt:** Assoc Prof NS, Univ Pittsburgh

Kobrine, Arthur MD/PhD [NS] - **Spec Exp:** Brain & Spinal Cord Tumors; **Hospital:** Sibley Mem Hosp, Georgetown Univ Hosp; **Address:** 2440 M St NW, Ste 315, Washington, DC 20037-1404; **Phone:** 202-293-7136; **Board Cert:** Neurological Surgery 1976; **Med School:** Northwestern Univ 1968; **Resid:** Neurological Surgery, Northwestern Univ Hosp 1970; Neurological Surgery, Walter Reed Army Hosp 1973; **Fellow:** Physiology, Geo Wash Univ 1979; **Fac Appt:** Clin Prof NS, Georgetown Univ

Kondziolka, Douglas MD [NS] - **Spec Exp:** Brain Tumors-Adult & Pediatric; Brain Tumors-Metastatic; Stereotactic Radiosurgery; **Hospital:** UPMC Presby, Pittsburgh, Chldns Hosp of Pittsburgh - UPMC; **Address:** Univ Pittsburgh Med Ctr, Dept Neurological Surgery, 200 Lothrop St, Ste B400, Pittsburgh, PA 15213; **Phone:** 412-647-9990; **Board Cert:** Neurological Surgery 1994; **Med School:** Univ Toronto 1985; **Resid:** Neurological Surgery, Univ Toronto 1991; **Fellow:** Stereo Neurological Surgery, UPMC Presby Med Ctr 1991; **Fac Appt:** Prof NS, Univ Pittsburgh

Laske, Douglas W MD [NS] - **Spec Exp:** Brain & Spinal Cord Tumors; Stereotactic Radiosurgery; Brain-Tumors Metastatic; **Hospital:** Temple Univ Hosp, Fox Chase Cancer Ctr (page 72); **Address:** Temple Univ Hosp-Dept Neuro-Surgery, 3509 N Broad St, Boyer Pavillio-5th flr, Phildelphia, PA 19140; **Phone:** 215-707-7200; **Board Cert:** Neurological Surgery 1996; **Med School:** Columbia P&S 1985; **Resid:** Neurology, Med Coll Virginia 1991; **Fellow:** Neurosurgical Oncology, Natl Inst Hlth 1995; **Fac Appt:** Assoc Prof NS, Temple Univ

Lavyne, Michael H MD [NS] - **Spec Exp:** Spinal Tumors; **Hospital:** NY-Presby Hosp/Weill Cornell (page 79), Hosp For Special Surgery; **Address:** 110 E 55th St Fl 9, New York, NY 10022; **Phone:** 212-486-9100; **Board Cert:** Neurological Surgery 1982; **Med School:** Cornell Univ-Weill Med Coll 1972; **Resid:** Neurological Surgery, Mass Genl Hosp 1979; **Fellow:** Neurology, Beth Israel Hosp 1974; **Fac Appt:** Clin Prof NS, Cornell Univ-Weill Med Coll

Lunsford, L Dade MD [NS] - **Spec Exp:** Brain Tumors; Stereotactic Radiosurgery; **Hospital:** UPMC Presby, Pittsburgh, Chldns Hosp of Pittsburgh - UPMC; **Address:** UPMC Presbyterian Hosp, 200 Lothrop St, Ste B400, Pittsburgh, PA 15213-2536; **Phone:** 412-647-0953; **Board Cert:** Neurological Surgery 1983; **Med School:** Columbia P&S 1974; **Resid:** Neurological Surgery, Univ Pittsburgh Med Ctr 1980; **Fellow:** Stereo Neurological Surgery, Karolinska Hospital 1981; **Fac Appt:** Prof NS, Univ Pittsburgh

McCormick, Paul C MD [NS] - **Spec Exp:** Spinal Surgery; Spinal Tumors; **Hospital:** NY-Presby Hosp/Columbia (page 79), Valley Hosp; **Address:** 710 W 168th St, Ste 506, New York, NY 10032-2603; **Phone:** 212-305-7976; **Board Cert:** Neurological Surgery 1993; **Med School:** Columbia P&S 1982; **Resid:** Neurological Surgery, Columbia Presby Med Ctr 1989; **Fellow:** Neurological Surgery, Natl Inst Hlth 1984; Spinal Surgery, Med Coll Wisconsin 1990; **Fac Appt:** Prof NS, Columbia P&S

Neurological Surgery

O'Rourke, Donald MD [NS] - **Spec Exp:** Neuro-Oncology; Brain Tumors; **Hospital:** Hosp Univ Penn - UPHS (page 81); **Address:** Hosp Univ Penn - Dept Neurosurg, 3400 Spruce St, 3 Silverstein, Philadelphia, PA 19104; **Phone:** 215-662-3490; **Board Cert:** Neurological Surgery 1998; **Med School:** Univ Pennsylvania 1987; **Resid:** Neurological Surgery, Hosp Univ Penn 1994; **Fac Appt:** Assoc Prof NS, Univ Pennsylvania

Pollack, Ian F MD [NS] - **Spec Exp:** Pediatric Neurosurgery; Brain Tumors; Craniofacial Surgery; Neuro-Oncology; **Hospital:** Chldns Hosp of Pittsburgh - UPMC, UPMC Presby, Pittsburgh; **Address:** Chldns Hosp Pittsburgh, Div Neurosurgery, 3705 Fifth Ave, Ste 3670A, Pittsburgh, PA 15213-2524; **Phone:** 412-692-5881; **Board Cert:** Neurological Surgery 1996; Pediatric Neurological Surgery 2006; **Med School:** Johns Hopkins Univ 1984; **Resid:** Neurological Surgery, Univ Pittsburgh Med Ctr 1991; **Fellow:** Pediatric Neurological Surgery, Hosp Sick Chldn 1992; **Fac Appt:** Prof NS, Univ Pittsburgh

Sen, Chandranath MD [NS] - **Spec Exp:** Brain Tumors; Skull Base Tumors; Skull Base Surgery; **Hospital:** St Luke's - Roosevelt Hosp Ctr - Roosevelt Div (page 71); **Address:** St Lukes Roosevelt Hosp Ctr, Dept Neurosurgery, 1000 10th Ave, Ste 5G-80, New York, NY 10019; **Phone:** 212-523-6720; **Board Cert:** Neurological Surgery 1989; **Med School:** India 1976; **Resid:** Surgery, Univ Wisconsin Hosps 1980; Neurological Surgery, Univ Wisconsin Hosps 1985; **Fellow:** Microsurgery, Univ Pittsburgh Med Ctr 1986

Sisti, Michael B MD [NS] - **Spec Exp:** Brain Tumors; Stereotactic Radiosurgery; **Hospital:** NY-Presby Hosp/Columbia (page 79); **Address:** 710 W 168th St, New York, NY 10032-2603; **Phone:** 212-305-1728; **Board Cert:** Neurological Surgery 1991; **Med School:** Columbia P&S 1981; **Resid:** Neurological Surgery, Neuro Inst-Columbia-Presby Med Ctr 1988; **Fellow:** Neurological Surgery, Natl Inst Hlth 1983; **Fac Appt:** Asst Prof NS, Columbia P&S

Stieg, Philip E MD/PhD [NS] - **Spec Exp:** Skull Base Surgery; Chordomas; **Hospital:** NY-Presby Hosp/Weill Cornell (page 79); **Address:** 525 E 68th St, STARR 651, New York, NY 10021-9800; **Phone:** 212-746-4684; **Board Cert:** Neurological Surgery 1992; **Med School:** Med Coll Wisc 1983; **Resid:** Neurological Surgery, Dallas Chldns Hosp/Parkland Meml Hosp 1988; **Fellow:** Neurological Biology, Karolinska Inst 1988; **Fac Appt:** Prof NS, Cornell Univ-Weill Med Coll

Sutton, Leslie N MD [NS] - **Spec Exp:** Brain Tumors-Pediatric; **Hospital:** Chldns Hosp of Philadelphia, The; **Address:** Childrens Hosp of Phila -Div Neurosurgery, 34th St & Civic Ctr Blvd Wood 6 Bldg, Philadelphia, PA 19104; **Phone:** 215-590-2780; **Board Cert:** Neurological Surgery 1984; Pediatric Neurological Surgery 1996; **Med School:** Univ Pennsylvania 1975; **Resid:** Neurological Surgery, Hosp Univ Penn 1981; **Fac Appt:** Prof NS, Univ Pennsylvania

Turtz, Alan R MD [NS] - **Spec Exp:** Brain Tumors; Pituitary Tumors; Spinal Surgery; Neuro-Endoscopy; **Hospital:** Cooper Univ Hosp; **Address:** 3 Cooper Plaza, Ste 104, Camden, NJ 08103; **Phone:** 856-968-7965; **Board Cert:** Neurological Surgery 1995; **Med School:** Med Coll PA 1986; **Resid:** Neurological Surgery, Med Coll Penn 1992; **Fac Appt:** Assoc Prof NS, UMDNJ-RW Johnson Med Sch

Wisoff, Jeffrey H MD [NS] - **Spec Exp:** Pediatric Neurosurgery; Brain Tumors-Pediatric; **Hospital:** NYU Langone Med Ctr (page 80), Maimonides Med Ctr (page 75); **Address:** 317 E 34th St, Ste 1002, New York, NY 10016-4974; **Phone:** 212-263-6419; **Board Cert:** Neurological Surgery 1990; Pediatric Neurological Surgery 2008; **Med School:** Geo Wash Univ 1978; **Resid:** Neurological Surgery, NYU/Bellevue Hosp 1984; **Fellow:** Pediatric Neurological Surgery, NYU Med Ctr 1985; **Fac Appt:** Assoc Prof NS, NYU Sch Med

Southeast

Asher, Anthony MD [NS] - **Spec Exp:** Brain Tumors; Stereotactic Radiosurgery; **Hospital:** Carolinas Med Ctr, Presby Hosp - Charlotte; **Address:** 225 Baldwin Ave, Charlotte, NC 28204; **Phone:** 704-376-1605; **Board Cert:** Neurological Surgery 1998; **Med School:** Wayne State Univ 1987; **Resid:** Neurological Surgery, Univ Mich Med Ctr 1995; **Fellow:** Surgical Oncology, Natl Cancer Inst 1991

Boop, Frederick A MD [NS] - **Spec Exp:** Pediatric Neurosurgery; Brain Tumors; **Hospital:** Le Bonheur Chldns Med Ctr, Methodist Univ Hosp - Memphis; **Address:** Semmes Murphy Clinic, 1211 Union Ave, Ste 200, Memphis, TN 38104; **Phone:** 901-259-5340; **Board Cert:** Neurological Surgery 1993; Pediatric Neurological Surgery 2005; **Med School:** Univ Ark 1983; **Resid:** Neurological Surgery, Univ Tex Hlth Sci Ctr 1989; Neurological Surgery, Inst Neur/Hosp Sick Chldn 1987; **Fellow:** Epilepsy, Univ Minn 1989; Pediatric Neurological Surgery, Ark Chldns Hosp 1990; **Fac Appt:** Assoc Prof NS, Univ Tenn Coll Med, Memphis

Brem, Steven MD [NS] - **Spec Exp:** Brain Tumors; Pituitary Tumors; Clinical Trials; Neuro-Oncology; **Hospital:** H Lee Moffitt Cancer Ctr & Research Inst; **Address:** H Lee Moffitt Cancer Ctr/Neurosurgery, 12902 Magnolia Drive, Neuro Program, Tampa, FL 33612-9497; **Phone:** 813-745-3056; **Board Cert:** Neurological Surgery 1983; **Med School:** Harvard Med Sch 1972; **Resid:** Neurological Surgery, Massachusetts Genl Hosp 1981; **Fellow:** Oncology, Natl Cancer Inst 1976; **Fac Appt:** Prof NS, Univ S Fla Coll Med

Ewend, Matthew MD [NS] - **Spec Exp:** Brain Tumors; Pituitary Tumors; Pediatric Neurosurgery; **Hospital:** Univ NC Hosps; **Address:** Univ North Carolina Neurosurgery, 3015 Burnett Womack Bldg, CB# 7060, Chapel Hill, NC 27599; **Phone:** 919-966-1374; **Board Cert:** Neurological Surgery 2001; **Med School:** Johns Hopkins Univ 1990; **Resid:** Neurological Surgery, Johns Hopkins Hospital 1994; **Fellow:** Neuro-Oncology, National Institutes of Health 1996; **Fac Appt:** Asst Prof NS, Univ NC Sch Med

Friedman, Allan H MD [NS] - **Spec Exp:** Brain Tumors; Skull Base Tumors; **Hospital:** Duke Univ Med Ctr; **Address:** Duke Univ Med Ctr, DUMC 3807, Durham, NC 27710; **Phone:** 919-681-6421; **Board Cert:** Neurological Surgery 1983; **Med School:** Univ IL Coll Med 1974; **Resid:** Neurological Surgery, Duke Univ Med Ctr 1980; **Fellow:** Vascular Surgery, Univ Western Ontario 1981; **Fac Appt:** Prof S, Duke Univ

Guthrie, Barton L MD [NS] - **Spec Exp:** Brain Tumors; Stereotactic Radiosurgery; **Hospital:** Univ of Ala Hosp at Birmingham; **Address:** Univ Alabama, Div Neurosurg, 510 20th St S, FOT 1038, Birmingham, AL 35294-3410; **Phone:** 205-934-8136; **Board Cert:** Neurological Surgery 1992; **Med School:** Univ Alabama 1980; **Resid:** Neurological Surgery, Mayo Clinic 1988; **Fellow:** Neurological Surgery, Stanford Univ Med Ctr 1988; **Fac Appt:** Assoc Prof NS, Univ Alabama

Heros, Roberto MD [NS] - **Spec Exp:** Cerebrovascular Surgery; Skull Base Surgery; Brain Tumors; **Hospital:** Jackson Meml Hosp (page 82), Univ of Miami Hosp & Clins/Sylvester Comp Canc Ctr (page 82); **Address:** Univ Miami, Dept Neurosurgery, 1095 NW 14th Terrace, Miami, FL 33136; **Phone:** 305-243-4572; **Board Cert:** Neurological Surgery 1979; **Med School:** Univ Tenn Coll Med, Memphis 1968; **Resid:** Surgery, Mass Genl Hosp 1970; Neurological Surgery, Mass Genl Hosp 1976; **Fac Appt:** Prof NS, Univ Miami Sch Med

Markert Jr, James M MD [NS] - **Spec Exp:** Brain Tumors; Stereotactic Radiosurgery; Clinical Trials; **Hospital:** Univ of Ala Hosp at Birmingham; **Address:** Univ Alabama, Div Neurosurgery, 510 20th St S, FOT, rm 1060, Birmingham, AL 35294; **Phone:** 205-975-6985; **Board Cert:** Neurological Surgery 1999; **Med School:** Columbia P&S 1988; **Resid:** Neurological Surgery, Univ Mich Med Ctr 1995; **Fellow:** Neuro-Oncology, Mass Genl Hosp; **Fac Appt:** Prof NS, Univ Alabama

Neurological Surgery

Morrison, Glenn MD [NS] - **Spec Exp:** Pediatric Neurosurgery; Craniofacial Surgery; Spinal Cord Tumors; Brain Tumors-Pediatric; **Hospital:** Miami Children's Hosp, Jackson Meml Hosp (page 82); **Address:** Ambulatory Care Bldg, 3215 SW 62nd Ave, Ste 3109, Miami, FL 33155; **Phone:** 305-662-8386; **Board Cert:** Neurological Surgery 1976; Pediatric Neurological Surgery 1996; **Med School:** Case West Res Univ 1967; **Resid:** Neurological Surgery, Case Western Univ Hosp 1974; **Fac Appt:** Prof NS, Univ Miami Sch Med

Myseros, John S MD [NS] - **Spec Exp:** Pediatric Neurosurgery; Brain Tumors; **Hospital:** Inova Fairfax Hosp for Chldn; **Address:** 8501 Arlington Blvd, Ste 450, Fairfax, VA 22031; **Phone:** 571-226-8330; **Board Cert:** Neurological Surgery 2000; **Med School:** Johns Hopkins Univ 1990; **Resid:** Neurological Surgery, Med Coll Virginia 1996; **Fellow:** Pediatric Neurological Surgery, Hosp for Sick Children 1997; **Fac Appt:** Assoc Prof NS, Geo Wash Univ

Olson, Jeffrey J MD [NS] - **Spec Exp:** Neuro-Oncology; Brain Tumors; Stereotactic Radio-surgery; **Hospital:** Emory Univ Hosp, Emory Univ Hosp Midtown; **Address:** Emory Univ, Dept Neuro-surgery, 1365B Clifton Rd NE, Ste 2200, Atlanta, GA 30322; **Phone:** 404-778-5770; **Board Cert:** Neurological Surgery 1989; **Med School:** Univ Minn 1981; **Resid:** Neurological Surgery, Univ Iowa Hosps & Clinics 1987; **Fellow:** Neurological Surgery, Natl Inst Hlth 1990; **Fac Appt:** Prof NS, Emory Univ

Parent, Andrew D MD [NS] - **Spec Exp:** Pediatric Neurosurgery; Neuroendocrine Tumors; Pituitary Tumors; **Hospital:** Univ Mississippi Med Ctr; **Address:** Univ Miss Med Ctr- Dept Neuro-surgery, 2500 N State St, Jackson, MS 39216-4500; **Phone:** 601-984-5702; **Board Cert:** Neurological Surgery 1981; Pediatric Neurological Surgery 2005; **Med School:** Univ VT Coll Med 1970; **Resid:** Neurological Surgery, Emory Univ 1978; **Fellow:** Neurological Surgery, Univ Tex Med Br 1974; **Fac Appt:** Prof NS, Univ Miss

Reid, William S MD [NS] - **Spec Exp:** Spinal Surgery; Brain & Spinal Cord Tumors; **Hospital:** Univ of Tennesee Mem Hosp; **Address:** 1932 Alcoa Hwy, Bldg C, Ste 280, Knoxville, TN 37920; **Phone:** 865-329-4003; **Board Cert:** Neurological Surgery 1980; **Med School:** Univ Ariz Coll Med 1971; **Resid:** Neurological Surgery, Univ Texas Hlth Sci Ctr 1975; **Fac Appt:** Assoc Clin Prof NS, Univ Tex SW, Dallas

Sampson, John H MD/PhD [NS] - **Spec Exp:** Brain Tumors; Clinical Trials; **Hospital:** Duke Univ Med Ctr; **Address:** Duke Univ Med Ctr, Box 3050, Durham, NC 27710; **Phone:** 919-684-9041; **Board Cert:** Neurological Surgery 2002; **Med School:** Univ Manitoba 1990; **Resid:** Neurological Surgery, Duke Univ Med Ctr 1998; **Fellow:** Neurological Intensive Care, Duke Univ Med Ctr 1999; **Fac Appt:** Assoc Prof S, Duke Univ

Sanford, Robert A MD [NS] - **Spec Exp:** Pediatric Neurosurgery; Brain Tumors-Pediatric; **Hospital:** Le Bonheur Chldns Med Ctr, St Jude Children's Research Hosp; **Address:** 6325 Humphreys Blvd, Memphis, TN 38120; **Phone:** 901-522-7762; **Board Cert:** Neurological Surgery 1976; Pediatric Neurological Surgery 2005; **Med School:** Univ Ark 1967; **Resid:** Neurological Surgery, Univ Minneapolis Med Ctr 1973; **Fac Appt:** Prof NS, Univ Tenn Coll Med, Memphis

Shaffrey, Mark E MD [NS] - **Spec Exp:** Brain Tumors; Clinical Trials; Spinal Cord Tumors; Spinal Tumors; **Hospital:** Univ Virginia Med Ctr; **Address:** UVA Health System, Dept Neurosurgery, PO Box 800212, Charlottesville, VA 22908; **Phone:** 434-924-1843; **Board Cert:** Neurological Surgery 2000; **Med School:** Univ VA Sch Med 1987; **Resid:** Neurological Surgery, Univ Virginia Med Ctr 1991; **Fellow:** Microvascular Physiology, NIH 1992; Neurological Pathology, Univ Virginia Med Ctr 1993; **Fac Appt:** Prof NS, Univ VA Sch Med

Sills Jr, Allen MD [NS] - **Spec Exp:** Brain & Spinal Tumors; Stereotactic Radiosurgery; **Hospital:** Methodist Univ Hosp - Memphis; **Address:** Semmes-Murphey Clinic, 1211 Union Ave, Ste 200, Memphis, TN 38104; **Phone:** 901-259-5340; **Board Cert:** Neurological Surgery 2002; **Med School:** Johns Hopkins Univ 1990; **Resid:** Neurological Surgery, Johns Hopkins Hosp 1994; **Fellow:** Neuro-Oncology, Hunterian Neurosurg Lab/Johns Hopkins 1996; **Fac Appt:** Prof NS, Univ Tenn Coll Med, Memphis

Tatter, Stephen MD/PhD [NS] - **Spec Exp:** Brain Tumors; Pituitary Tumors; Stereotactic Radiosurgery; **Hospital:** Wake Forest Univ Baptist Med Ctr (page 84); **Address:** Wake Forest Univ Sch Med, Dept Neurosurg, Medical Center Blvd, Winston-Salem, NC 27157-1029; **Phone:** 336-716-4047; **Board Cert:** Neurological Surgery 2004; **Med School:** Cornell Univ-Weill Med Coll 1990; **Resid:** Neurological Surgery, Mass Genl Hosp 1996; **Fellow:** Neurological Surgery, Mass Genl Hosp 1997; **Fac Appt:** Assoc Prof NS, Wake Forest Univ

Thompson, Reid C MD [NS] - **Spec Exp:** Neuro-Oncology; Brain & Spinal Cord Tumors; Skull Base Tumors; **Hospital:** Vanderbilt Univ Med Ctr; **Address:** Vanderbilt Univ Med Ctr, Dept Neurosurg, 1500 21st Ave S, Ste 1506, Nashville, TN 37212; **Phone:** 615-322-7417; **Board Cert:** Neurological Surgery 2001; **Med School:** Johns Hopkins Univ 1989; **Resid:** Neurological Surgery, Johns Hopkins Hosp 1995; **Fellow:** Neuro-Oncology, Rsch-Johns Hopkins Hosp 1996; Cerebrovascular Neurosurgery, Stanford Univ Med Ctr 1997; **Fac Appt:** Assoc Prof NS, Vanderbilt Univ

Wharen Jr, Robert E MD [NS] - **Spec Exp:** Brain Tumors; **Hospital:** Mayo - Jacksonville; **Address:** Mayo Clinic, Dept Neurosurgery, 4500 San Pablo Rd, Jacksonville, FL 32224-1865; **Phone:** 904-953-2103; **Board Cert:** Neurological Surgery 1988; **Med School:** Penn State Univ-Hershey Med Ctr 1979; **Resid:** Neurological Surgery, Mayo Clinic 1985; **Fac Appt:** Prof NS, Mayo Med Sch

Young, Byron MD [NS] - **Spec Exp:** Brain Tumors; Stereotactic Radiosurgery; Pituitary Tumors; **Hospital:** Univ of Kentucky Chandler Hosp; **Address:** Div Neurosurgery, MS 101, 800 Rose St, Lexington, KY 40536-0298; **Phone:** 859-323-5861; **Board Cert:** Neurological Surgery 1974; **Med School:** Univ KY Coll Med 1965; **Resid:** Surgery, Vanderbilt Univ Hosp 1967; Neurological Surgery, Vanderbilt Univ Hosp 1971; **Fac Appt:** Prof NS, Univ KY Coll Med

Midwest

Albright, A Leland MD [NS] - **Spec Exp:** Pediatric Neurosurgery; Brain Tumors; **Hospital:** Univ WI Hosp & Clins; **Address:** Dept Neurosurgery, 600 Highland Ave, rm K4/836, Madison, WI 53792; **Phone:** 608-263-9651; **Board Cert:** Neurological Surgery 1981; Pediatric Neurological Surgery 2005; **Med School:** Louisiana State U, New Orleans 1969; **Resid:** Surgery, Wash Hosps 1971; Neurological Surgery, Univ Pittsburgh Med Ctr 1978; **Fellow:** Neurological Surgery, Natl Inst Hlth 1974; Immunopathology, Univ Pittsburgh Med Ctr 1978; **Fac Appt:** Prof NS, Univ Wisc

Bakay, Roy AE MD [NS] - **Spec Exp:** Brain Tumors; **Hospital:** Rush Univ Med Ctr; **Address:** Rush Univ Med Ctr, 1725 W Harrison St, Ste 970, Chicago, IL 60612; **Phone:** 312-942-6644; **Board Cert:** Neurological Surgery 1985; **Med School:** Northwestern Univ 1975; **Resid:** Neurological Surgery, Univ Washington Med Ctr 1981; **Fellow:** Neuronal Plasticity, Natl Inst Hlth 1982; **Fac Appt:** Prof NS, Rush Med Coll

Barnett, Gene H MD [NS] - **Spec Exp:** Brain Tumors; Stereotactic Radiosurgery; **Hospital:** Cleveland Clin Fdn (page 70); **Address:** Cleveland Clinic Brain Tumor Inst, 9500 Euclid Ave, Desk R20, Cleveland, OH 44195; **Phone:** 216-444-5381; **Board Cert:** Neurological Surgery 1990; **Med School:** Case West Res Univ 1980; **Resid:** Neurological Surgery, Cleveland Clinic 1986; **Fellow:** Neurology, Cleveland Clinic 1982; Research, Mass Genl Hosp-Harvard 1987; **Fac Appt:** Prof NS, Cleveland Cl Coll Med/Case West Res

Neurological Surgery

Chandler, William F MD [NS] - **Spec Exp:** Pituitary Surgery; Brain Tumors; **Hospital:** Univ Michigan Hlth Sys; **Address:** 1500 E Med Center Drive, Ste 3470, Tauban Center, Ann Arbor, MI 48109; **Phone:** 734-936-5020; **Board Cert:** Neurological Surgery 1980; **Med School:** Univ Mich Med Sch 1971; **Resid:** Neurological Surgery, Michigan Hosp 1977; **Fac Appt:** Prof NS, Univ Mich Med Sch

Chiocca, E Antonio MD [NS] - **Spec Exp:** Brain Tumors; Spinal Cord Tumors; **Hospital:** Arthur G James Cancer Hosp & Research Inst, Ohio St Univ Med Ctr; **Address:** OSU Med Ctr, Dept Neurosurgery, 410 W 10th Ave, 1021-N Doan Hall, Columbus, OH 43210; **Phone:** 614-293-9312; **Board Cert:** Neurological Surgery 2000; **Med School:** Univ Tex, Houston 1988; **Resid:** Neurological Surgery, Mass Genl Hosp 1995; **Fac Appt:** Prof NS, Ohio State Univ

Cohen, Alan R MD [NS] - **Spec Exp:** Pediatric Neurosurgery; Brain & Spinal Tumors-Pediatric; Minimally Invasive Surgery; **Hospital:** Rainbow Babies & Chldns Hosp, Univ Hosps Case Med Ctr; **Address:** 11100 Euclid Ave, Ste B501, Cleveland, OH 44106; **Phone:** 216-844-5741; **Board Cert:** Neurological Surgery 1991; Pediatric Neurological Surgery 2007; **Med School:** Cornell Univ-Weill Med Coll 1978; **Resid:** Surgery, NYU Medical Ctr 1980; Neurological Surgery, NYU Medical Ctr 1987; **Fellow:** Neurology, Natl Hosp Queen's Square 1982; **Fac Appt:** Prof NS, Case West Res Univ

Dacey Jr, Ralph G MD [NS] - **Spec Exp:** Cerebrovascular Surgery; Brain Tumors; **Hospital:** Barnes-Jewish Hosp, Barnes-Jewish West County Hosp; **Address:** Wash Univ Dept Neurosurgery, 660 S Euclid Ave, Box 8057, St Louis, MO 63110; **Phone:** 314-362-3577; **Board Cert:** Internal Medicine 1978; Neurological Surgery 1985; **Med School:** Univ VA Sch Med 1974; **Resid:** Internal Medicine, Strong Meml Hosp 1977; Neurological Surgery, Univ Virginia Med Ctr 1983; **Fac Appt:** Prof NS, Washington Univ, St Louis

Frim, David M MD/PhD [NS] - **Spec Exp:** Pediatric Neurosurgery; Brain & Spinal Tumors; **Hospital:** Univ of Chicago Med Ctr; **Address:** Univ of Chicago Hosps, Pediatric Neurosurgery, 5841 S Maryland Ave, MC 3026, Chicago, IL 60637-1463; **Phone:** 773-702-2475; **Board Cert:** Neurological Surgery 1998; Pediatric Neurological Surgery 1998; **Med School:** Harvard Med Sch 1988; **Resid:** Neurological Surgery, Mass Genl Hosp 1995; **Fellow:** Pediatric Neurological Surgery, Chldns Hosp 1996; **Fac Appt:** Assoc Prof S, Univ Chicago-Pritzker Sch Med

Greene Jr, Clarence S MD [NS] - **Spec Exp:** Pediatric Neurosurgery; Brain Tumors; **Hospital:** Chldns Mercy Hosps & Clinics; **Address:** 2401 Gillham Rd, Kansas City, MO 64108; **Phone:** 816-234-3000; **Board Cert:** Neurological Surgery 1984; Pediatric Neurological Surgery 2007; **Med School:** Howard Univ 1974; **Resid:** Neurological Surgery, Chldns Hosp 1981; Neurological Surgery, Peter Bent Brigham Hosp 1981; **Fellow:** Pediatric Neurological Surgery, Chldns Hosp 1985; **Fac Appt:** Assoc Clin Prof NS, UC Irvine

Grubb Jr, Robert L MD [NS] - **Spec Exp:** Brain Tumors; Skull Base Tumors; **Hospital:** Barnes-Jewish Hosp, St Louis Chldns Hosp; **Address:** Wash Univ Sch Med, Dept Neurosurgery, 660 S Euclid Ave, Box 8057, St Louis, MO 63110; **Phone:** 314-362-3567; **Board Cert:** Neurological Surgery 1976; **Med School:** Univ NC Sch Med 1965; **Resid:** Surgery, Barnes Jewish Hosp 1967; Neurological Surgery, Barnes Jewish Hosp 1973; **Fellow:** Neurological Surgery, National Inst Health 1969; **Fac Appt:** Prof NS, Washington Univ, St Louis

Guthikonda, Murali MD [NS] - **Spec Exp:** Skull Base Tumors; Pituitary Tumors; Spinal Tumors; **Hospital:** Detroit Med Ctr, Harper Univ Hosp; **Address:** Wayne St U Physicians Grp-Neurosurgery, 4160 John R, Ste 930, Detroit, MI 48201; **Phone:** 313-831-0777; **Board Cert:** Neurological Surgery 1982; **Med School:** India 1971; **Resid:** Surgery, St Elizabeth Hosp 1976; Neurological Surgery, Med Ctr Hosp VT 1980; **Fellow:** Skull Base Surgery, Univ Cincinnati 1993; **Fac Appt:** Assoc Prof NS, Wayne State Univ

Gutierrez, Francisco A MD [NS] - **Spec Exp:** Brain Tumors; Cerebrovascular Surgery; Spinal Surgery; **Hospital:** Northwestern Meml Hosp, Resurrection Med Ctr; **Address:** 7447 W Talcott, Ste 340, Galter Pavilion, Chicago, IL 60631; **Phone:** 773-594-0200; **Board Cert:** Neurological Surgery 1976; **Med School:** Colombia 1965; **Resid:** Neurological Surgery, San Juan de Dios Hosp 1967; Neurological Surgery, Northwestern Meml Hosp 1973; **Fac Appt:** Assoc Prof NS, Northwestern Univ

Kaufman, Bruce A MD [NS] - **Spec Exp:** Pediatric Neurosurgery; Brain & Spinal Cord Tumors; **Hospital:** Chldns Hosp - Wisconsin; **Address:** Chldns Hosp, Dept Neurosurg, 999 N 92nd St, Ste 310, Milwaukee, WI 53226; **Phone:** 414-266-6435; **Board Cert:** Neurological Surgery 1992; Pediatric Neurological Surgery 2006; **Med School:** Case West Res Univ 1982; **Resid:** Neurological Surgery, Univ Hosp Cleveland/Case West Res 1988; **Fellow:** Pediatric Neurological Surgery, Chldns Meml Hosp/Northwestern Univ 1989; **Fac Appt:** Prof NS, Med Coll Wisc

Levy, Robert M MD/PhD [NS] - **Spec Exp:** Stereotactic Radiosurgery; Brain Tumors; Pain-Chronic; **Hospital:** Northwestern Meml Hosp; **Address:** 675 N Saint Clair St, Ste 2210, Galter Bldg Fl 20, Chicago, IL 60611-2922; **Phone:** 312-695-8143; **Board Cert:** Neurological Surgery 1991; **Med School:** Stanford Univ 1981; **Resid:** Neurological Surgery, UCSF Med Ctr 1987; **Fellow:** Neurological Surgery, UCSF Med Ctr 1986; **Fac Appt:** Prof NS, Northwestern Univ

Link, Michael J MD [NS] **Spec Exp:** Skull Base Tumors; Brain Tumors; Cerebrovascular Surgery; **Hospital:** Mayo Med Ctr & Clin - Rochester; **Address:** Mayo Clinic, Dept Neurosurgery, 200 First St SW, Rochester, MN 55905; **Phone:** 507-284-8008; **Board Cert:** Neurological Surgery 2000; **Med School:** Mayo Med Sch 1990; **Resid:** Neurological Surgery, Mayo Clinic 1996; **Fellow:** Cerebrovascular & Skull Base Surgery, Univ Cincinnati/Mayfield Clinic 1998; **Fac Appt:** Assoc Prof NS, Mayo Med Sch

Malik, Ghaus MD [NS] - **Spec Exp:** Cerebrovascular Surgery; Brain & Spinal Cord Tumors; **Hospital:** Henry Ford Hosp, William Beaumont Hosp; **Address:** Henry Ford Hosp, Dept Neurosurg, 2799 W Grand Blvd, Detroit, MI 48202; **Phone:** 313-916-1093; **Board Cert:** Neurological Surgery 1978; **Med School:** Pakistan 1968; **Resid:** Surgery, Henry Ford Hosp 1971; Neurological Surgery, Henry Ford Hosp 1975

Origitano, Thomas MD/PhD [NS] - **Spec Exp:** Skull Base Tumors & Surgery; Cerebrovascular Surgery; Brain Tumors; **Hospital:** Loyola Univ Med Ctr; **Address:** Loyola Univ Med Ctr, Dept Neurosurgery, 2160 S First Ave Bldg 105 - rm 1900, Maywood, IL 60153-3304; **Phone:** 708-216-8920; **Board Cert:** Neurological Surgery 1995; **Med School:** Loyola Univ-Stritch Sch Med 1984; **Resid:** Neurological Surgery, Loyola Univ Med Ctr 1990; **Fac Appt:** Prof NS, Loyola Univ-Stritch Sch Med

Park, Tae Sung MD [NS] - **Spec Exp:** Pediatric Neurosurgery; Neuro-Oncology; **Hospital:** St Louis Chldns Hosp; **Address:** St Louis Children's Hospital, 1 Children's Place, Ste 4-S20, St Louis, MO 63110; **Phone:** 314-454-4629; **Board Cert:** Neurological Surgery 1985; Pediatric Neurological Surgery 2006; **Med School:** Korea 1971; **Resid:** Neurological Surgery, Univ Virginia Hosp 1981; **Fellow:** Pediatric Neurological Surgery, Hosp for Sick Chldn 1983; **Fac Appt:** Prof NS, Washington Univ, St Louis

Raffel, Corey MD/PhD [NS] - **Spec Exp:** Pediatric Neurosurgery; Brain Tumors; Medulloblastoma; **Hospital:** Nationwide Chldn's Hosp; **Address:** Nationwide Chldn's Hosp, Dept Neurosurgery, 700 Children's Drive, Columbus, OH 43205; **Phone:** 614-722-2014; **Board Cert:** Neurological Surgery 1990; Pediatric Neurological Surgery 1996; **Med School:** UCSD 1980; **Resid:** Neurological Surgery, UCSF Med Ctr 1986; **Fellow:** Pediatric Neurological Surgery, Hosp Sick Chldn 1988

Neurological Surgery

Rich, Keith M MD [NS] - **Spec Exp:** Brain Tumors; Stereotactic Radiosurgery; **Hospital:** Barnes-Jewish Hosp; **Address:** Wash Univ Dept Neurosurgery, 660 S Euclid Ave, Box 8057, St Louis, MO 63110; **Phone:** 314-362-3577; **Board Cert:** Neurological Surgery 1987; **Med School:** Indiana Univ 1977; **Resid:** Neurological Surgery, Barnes Jewish Hosp 1982; **Fellow:** Neurological Pharmacology, Barnes Jewish Hosp 1984; **Fac Appt:** Assoc Prof NS, Washington Univ, St Louis

Rock, Jack P MD [NS] - **Spec Exp:** Neuro-Oncology; Pituitary Surgery; Skull Base Surgery; Brain Tumors; **Hospital:** Henry Ford Hosp; **Address:** Henry Ford Hosp, Dept Neurosurg, 2799 W Grand Blvd, Detroit, MI 48202; **Phone:** 313-916-2241; **Board Cert:** Neurological Surgery 1989; **Med School:** Univ Miami Sch Med 1979; **Resid:** Neurological Surgery, New York Hosp-Cornell 1985; **Fellow:** Univ Maryland 1986

Rosenblum, Mark L MD [NS] - **Spec Exp:** Brain Tumors; Spinal Surgery; Neuro-Oncology; **Hospital:** Henry Ford Hosp; **Address:** Henry Ford Hospital, K11, 2799 W Grand Blvd, Detroit, MI 48202; **Phone:** 313-916-1340; **Board Cert:** Neurological Surgery 1982; **Med School:** NY Med Coll 1969; **Resid:** Surgery, UCLA Med Ctr 1973; Neurological Surgery, UCSF Med Ctr 1979; **Fellow:** Neuro-Oncology, NIH/Natl Cancer Inst 1972

Ruge, John MD [NS] - **Spec Exp:** Pediatric Neurosurgery; Brain Tumors; **Hospital:** Adv Luth Genl Hosp; **Address:** Ctr Brain & Spine Surg-Parkside Ctr, 1875 Dempster St, Ste 605, Park Ridge, IL 60068; **Phone:** 847-698-1088; **Board Cert:** Neurological Surgery 1993; **Med School:** Northwestern Univ 1983; **Resid:** Neurological Surgery, Northwestern Meml Hosp 1989; **Fellow:** Pediatric Neurological Surgery, Childrens Hosp 1990; **Fac Appt:** Asst Prof S, Rush Med Coll

Ryken, Timothy C MD [NS] - **Spec Exp:** Brain Tumors; Spinal Surgery; **Hospital:** Covenant Med Ctr; **Address:** Iowa Spine & Brain Institute, 2710 St Francis Drive, Ste 110, Waterloo, IA 50702; **Phone:** 319-272-6700; **Board Cert:** Neurological Surgery 1998; **Med School:** Univ Iowa Coll Med 1988; **Resid:** Neurological Surgery, Univ Iowa 1995; **Fellow:** Cambridge Univ 1996; **Fac Appt:** Assoc Prof NS, Univ Iowa Coll Med

Shapiro, Scott A MD [NS] - **Spec Exp:** Brain Tumors; Pituitary Tumors; **Hospital:** Indiana Univ Hosp (page 74); **Address:** Inidiana Univ, Wishard Memorial Hosp, 1001 W 10th St, Ste EOP323, Indianapolis, IN 46202; **Phone:** 317-630-7625; **Board Cert:** Neurological Surgery 1990; **Med School:** Indiana Univ 1981; **Resid:** Neurological Surgery, Indiana Univ Med Ctr 1987; **Fac Appt:** Prof NS, Indiana Univ

Thompson, B Gregory MD [NS] - **Spec Exp:** Skull Base Tumors & Surgery; **Hospital:** Univ Michigan Hlth Sys; **Address:** Dept Neurosurgery, 3552 Taubman, 1500 E Medical Center Drive, Ann Arbor, MI 48109; **Phone:** 734-936-7493; **Board Cert:** Neurological Surgery 1998; **Med School:** Univ Kans 1986; **Resid:** Neurological Surgery, Univ Pittsburgh 1993; Research, Natl Inst Hlth 1992; **Fellow:** Neurological Surgery, Barrow Neuro Inst 1994; Interventional Radiology, Thomas Jefferson Univ 2005

Tomita, Tadanori MD [NS] - **Spec Exp:** Pediatric Neurosurgery; Brain Tumors-Pediatric; **Hospital:** Children's Mem Hosp, Northwestern Meml Hosp; **Address:** Chldns Meml Hosp, Div Ped Neurosurg, 2300 Children's Plaza, Box 28, Chicago, IL 60614-3363; **Phone:** 773-880-4373; **Board Cert:** Neurological Surgery 1984; Pediatric Neurological Surgery 1996; **Med School:** Japan 1970; **Resid:** Neurological Surgery, Kobe Univ 1974; Neurological Surgery, Northwestern Meml Hosp 1980; **Fellow:** Surgery, Meml Sloan Kettering Canc Ctr 1981; **Fac Appt:** Prof NS, Northwestern Univ

Warnick, Ronald E MD [NS] - **Spec Exp:** Neuro-Oncology; Brain Tumors; **Hospital:** Univ Hosp - Cincinnati, Good Samaritan Hosp - Cincinnati; **Address:** 222 Piedmont Ave, Ste 3100, Cincinnati, OH 45219; **Phone:** 513-475-8629; **Board Cert:** Neurological Surgery 1995; **Med School:** Univ Rochester 1982; **Resid:** Neurological Surgery, NYU Med Ctr 1989; **Fellow:** Neuro-Oncology, UCSF Med Ctr 1991; **Fac Appt:** Prof NS, Univ Cincinnati

Great Plains and Mountains

Cherny, W Bruce MD [NS] - **Spec Exp:** Pediatric Neurosurgery; Brain Tumors; **Hospital:** St. Luke's Reg Med Ctr - Boise; **Address:** 100 E Idaho St, Ste 202, Boise, ID 83712; **Phone:** 208-381-7360; **Board Cert:** Neurological Surgery 2000; **Med School:** Univ Ariz Coll Med 1987; **Resid:** Neurological Surgery, Barrow Neuro Inst/St Joseph's Med Ctr 1994; **Fellow:** Pediatric Neurological Surgery, Primary Chldns Hosp 1995

Couldwell, William MD/PhD [NS] - **Spec Exp:** Brain Tumors; Pituitary Tumors; **Hospital:** Univ Utah Hosps and Clins; **Address:** Univ Utah, Dept Neurological Surgery, 175 N Medical Drive E, Salt Lake City, UT 84132-2303; **Phone:** 801-581-6908; **Board Cert:** Neurological Surgery 1994; **Med School:** McGill Univ 1984; **Resid:** Neurological Surgery, LAC/USC Med Ctr 1989; **Fellow:** Neurological Immunology, Montreal Neur Inst/McGill Univ 1991; Neurological Surgery, CHUV; **Fac Appt:** Prof NS, Univ Utah

Johnson, Stephen D MD [NS] - **Spec Exp:** Skull Base Tumors & Surgery; **Hospital:** Presby - St Luke's Med Ctr; **Address:** Western Neurological Group, 1601 E 19th Ave, Ste 4400, Denver, CO 80218; **Phone:** 303-861-2266; **Board Cert:** Neurological Surgery 1988; **Med School:** Univ Tenn Coll Med, Memphis 1974; **Resid:** Neurological Surgery, Virginia Mason Med Ctr; Neurological Surgery, New York Hosp; **Fellow:** Neurological Surgery, Univ Tennessee; **Fac Appt:** Assoc Prof NS, Univ Colorado

Lillehei, Kevin O MD [NS] - **Spec Exp:** Neuro-Oncology; Pituitary Tumors; **Hospital:** Univ Colorado Hosp, Exempla Lutheran Med Ctr; **Address:** Univ Colorado Hosp, Dept Neurosurgery, 12631 E 17th Ave, Box C307, Aurora, CO 80045; **Phone:** 303-724-2280; **Board Cert:** Neurological Surgery 1989; **Med School:** Univ Minn 1979; **Resid:** Neurological Surgery, Univ Mich Med Ctr 1985; **Fac Appt:** Prof NS, Univ Colorado

Southwest

Al-Mefty, Ossama MD [NS] - **Spec Exp:** Skull Base Surgery; Brain Tumors; Cerebrovascular Surgery; **Hospital:** UAMS Med Ctr, Arkansas Chldns Hosp; **Address:** 4301 W Markham, Slot 507, Little Rock, AR 72205; **Phone:** 501-686-8757; **Board Cert:** Neurological Surgery 1980; **Med School:** Syria 1972; **Resid:** Surgery, Med Coll Ohio 1974; Neurological Surgery, West Va Med Ctr 1978; **Fac Appt:** Prof NS, Univ Ark

De Monte, Franco MD [NS] - **Spec Exp:** Skull Base Tumors & Surgery; Neuro-Oncology; **Hospital:** UT MD Anderson Cancer Ctr; **Address:** UT MD Anderson Cancer Ctr, Dept Neurosurgery, 1515 Holcombe Blvd, Ste 442, Houston, TX 77030; **Phone:** 713-792-2400; **Board Cert:** Neurological Surgery 1995; **Med School:** Canada 1985; **Resid:** Neurological Surgery, Univ Western Ontario 1991; **Fellow:** Skull Base Surgery, Loyola Univ-Stritch Sch Med 1992

Hankinson, Hal L MD [NS] - **Spec Exp:** Brain Tumors; **Hospital:** St Vincent Hosp - Santa Fe; **Address:** 465 St Michael's Drive, Ste 107, Sante Fe, NM 87505; **Phone:** 505-988-3233; **Board Cert:** Neurological Surgery 1977; **Med School:** Tulane Univ 1967; **Resid:** Neurological Surgery, UCSF Med Ctr 1975; **Fac Appt:** Clin Prof NS, Univ New Mexico

Neurological Surgery

Lang Jr, Frederick F MD [NS] - **Spec Exp:** Brain & Spinal Tumors; Neuro-Oncology; **Hospital:** UT MD Anderson Cancer Ctr; **Address:** Univ Texas MD Anderson Cancer Ctr, 1515 Holcombe Blvd, Unit 442, Houston, TX 77030; **Phone:** 713-792-6600; **Board Cert:** Neurological Surgery 2000; **Med School:** Yale Univ 1988; **Resid:** Neurological Surgery, NYU Med Ctr 1995; **Fellow:** Neurosurgical Oncology, MD Anderson Cancer Ctr 1996; **Fac Appt:** Prof NS, Univ Tex, Houston

Mapstone, Timothy B MD [NS] - **Spec Exp:** Brain Tumors-Adult & Pediatric; Pediatric Neurosurgery; **Hospital:** OU Med Ctr, Chldns Hosp OU Med Ctr; **Address:** Univ OK Hlth Sci Ctr, Dept Neurosurgery, 1000 N Lincoln Blvd, Ste 400, Oklahoma City, OK 73104; **Phone:** 405-271-4912; **Board Cert:** Neurological Surgery 1985; Pediatric Neurological Surgery 2005; **Med School:** Case West Res Univ 1977; **Resid:** Neurological Surgery, Univ Hosps 1983; **Fellow:** Research, Case West Reserve Univ; **Fac Appt:** Prof NS, Univ Okla Coll Med

Mickey, Bruce E MD [NS] - **Spec Exp:** Brain Tumors; Skull Base Surgery; **Hospital:** UT Southwestern Med Ctr at Dallas; **Address:** UTSW Med Ctr, Dept Neurosurgery, 5323 Harry Hines Blvd, Dallas, TX 75390-8855; **Phone:** 214-645-2300; **Board Cert:** Neurological Surgery 1987; **Med School:** Univ Tex SW, Dallas 1978; **Resid:** Neurological Surgery, Parkland Meml Hosp 1984; **Fellow:** Research, Righospitalet 1983; **Fac Appt:** Prof NS, Univ Tex SW, Dallas

Sawaya, Raymond MD [NS] - **Spec Exp:** Brain Tumors; **Hospital:** UT MD Anderson Cancer Ctr, Baylor Univ Medical Ctr; **Address:** MD Anderson Cancer Ctr, 1515 Holcombe Blvd, Unit 442, Houston, TX 77030; **Phone:** 713-563-8749; **Board Cert:** Neurological Surgery 1985; **Med School:** Lebanon 1974; **Resid:** Neurological Surgery, Univ Cincinnati Med Ctr 1980; Neurological Surgery, Johns Hopkins Med Ctr 1981; **Fellow:** Neuro-Oncology, Natl Inst Hlth 1982; **Fac Appt:** Prof NS, Univ Tex, Houston

Spetzler, Robert F MD [NS] - **Spec Exp:** Skull Base Tumors & Surgery; Cerebrovascular Surgery; **Hospital:** St Joseph's Hosp & Med Ctr - Phoenix; **Address:** Barrow Neurosurgical Assocs, 2910 N Third Ave, Phoenix, AZ 85013; **Phone:** 602-406-3489; **Board Cert:** Neurological Surgery 1979; **Med School:** Northwestern Univ 1971; **Resid:** Neurological Surgery, UCSF Med Ctr 1976; **Fac Appt:** Prof S, Univ Ariz Coll Med

West Coast and Pacific

Adler Jr, John R MD [NS] - **Spec Exp:** Stereotactic Radiosurgery; Brain Tumors; **Hospital:** Stanford Univ Med Ctr; **Address:** Stanford Univ Med Ctr, Dept Neurosurg, 300 Pasteur Drive R Bldg - rm 205, Stanford, CA 94305-5327; **Phone:** 650-723-5573; **Board Cert:** Neurological Surgery 1990; **Med School:** Harvard Med Sch 1980; **Resid:** Neurological Surgery, Chldns Hosp 1987; Neurological Surgery, Mass Genl Hosp 1985; **Fellow:** Cerebrovascular Disease, Karolinska Inst 1986; **Fac Appt:** Prof NS, Stanford Univ

Apuzzo, Michael L J MD [NS] - **Spec Exp:** Brain Tumors; Stereotactic Radiosurgery; **Hospital:** LAC & USC Med Ctr, USC Norris Cancer Hosp; **Address:** 1420 N San Pablo Street, PMBA106, Los Angeles, CA 90033-1029; **Phone:** 323-226-7421; **Board Cert:** Neurological Surgery 1975; **Med School:** Boston Univ 1965; **Resid:** Neurological Surgery, Hartford Hosp 1970; Neurological Surgery, Hartford Hosp 1973; **Fellow:** Neurological Physiology, Yale Univ Hosp 1972; **Fac Appt:** Prof NS, USC Sch Med

Badie, Behnam MD [NS] - **Spec Exp:** Brain Tumors; **Hospital:** City of Hope Natl Med Ctr & Beckman Rsch (page 69); **Address:** 1500 E Duarte Rd, Duarte, CA 91010; **Phone:** 626-471-7100; **Board Cert:** Neurological Surgery 1998; **Med School:** UCLA 1989; **Resid:** Neurological Surgery, UCLA Med Ctr 1996; **Fac Appt:** Assoc Prof NS, UCLA

Berger, Mitchel S MD [NS] - **Spec Exp:** Brain & Spinal Cord Tumors; Pituitary Tumors; Neuro-Oncology; Pain Management; **Hospital:** UCSF Med Ctr; **Address:** UCSF Med Ctr, Dept Neurosurgery, 505 Parnassus Avenue, M-786, San Francisco, CA 94143-0112; **Phone:** 415-353-3933; **Board Cert:** Neurological Surgery 1991; **Med School:** Univ Miami Sch Med 1979; **Resid:** Neurological Surgery, UCSF Med Ctr 1984; **Fellow:** Neuro-Oncology, UCSF Med Ctr 1985; Pediatric Neurological Surgery, Hosp Sick Chldn 1986; **Fac Appt:** Prof NS, UCSF

Black, Keith L MD [NS] - **Spec Exp:** Brain Tumors; Pituitary Surgery; **Hospital:** Cedars-Sinai Med Ctr; **Address:** Cedars Sinai Med Ctr, Dept Neurosugery, 8631 W 3rd St, Ste 800E, Los Angeles, CA 90048; **Phone:** 310-423-7900; **Board Cert:** Neurological Surgery 1990; **Med School:** Univ Mich Med Sch 1981; **Resid:** Neurological Surgery, Univ Michigan Med Ctr 1987; **Fac Appt:** Prof NS, UCLA-David Geffen Sch Med

Boggan, James E MD [NS] - **Spec Exp:** Skull Base Tumors & Surgery; Pediatric Neurosurgery; **Hospital:** UC Davis Med Ctr; **Address:** Dept Neurological Surgery, 4860 Y St, Ste 3740, Sacramento, CA 95817-2307; **Phone:** 916-734-2371; **Board Cert:** Neurological Surgery 1985; **Med School:** Univ Chicago-Pritzker Sch Med 1976; **Resid:** Neurological Surgery, UCSF Med Ctr 1982; **Fac Appt:** Prof NS, UC Davis

Edwards, Michael S MD [NS] - **Spec Exp:** Brain Tumors-Pediatric; Pediatric Neurosurgery; Stereotactic Radiosurgery; **Hospital:** Lucile Packard Chldn's Hosp; **Address:** Pediatric Neurosurgery, 300 Pasteur Drive, Ste R211, MC 5327, Stanford, CA 94305-5327; **Phone:** 650-497-8775; **Board Cert:** Neurological Surgery 1980; Pediatric Neurological Surgery 2006; **Med School:** Tulane Univ 1970; **Resid:** Neurological Surgery, Oschner Fdn Hosp/Charity Hosp 1977; **Fellow:** Pediatric Neuro-Oncology, UCSF Med Ctr 1978; **Fac Appt:** Prof NS, Stanford Univ

Ellenbogen, Richard MD [NS] - **Spec Exp:** Pediatric Neurosurgery; Brain Tumors; **Hospital:** Chldns Hosp and Regl Med Ctr - Seattle, Univ Wash Med Ctr; **Address:** 4800 Sand Point Way NE, MS W-7729, Seattle, WA 98105; **Phone:** 206-987-2544; **Board Cert:** Neurological Surgery 1992; Pediatric Neurological Surgery 1998; **Med School:** Brown Univ 1983; **Resid:** Neurological Surgery, Brigham Womens Hosp/Childrens Hosp 1989; **Fac Appt:** Prof NS, Univ Wash

Giannotta, Steven L MD [NS] - **Spec Exp:** Skull Base Tumors; **Hospital:** USC Univ Hosp, LAC & USC Med Ctr; **Address:** 1520 San Pablo St, Ste 3800, Los Angeles, CA 90033; **Phone:** 323-442-5720; **Board Cert:** Neurological Surgery 1980; **Med School:** Univ Mich Med Sch 1972; **Resid:** Neurological Surgery, Univ Michigan Med Ctr 1978; **Fac Appt:** Prof NS, USC Sch Med

Harsh IV, Griffith R MD [NS] - **Spec Exp:** Brain & Spinal Cord Tumors; Skull Base Tumors; Pituitary Tumors; Endoscopic Surgery; **Hospital:** Stanford Univ Med Ctr; **Address:** Stanford Center for Advanced Medicine, 875 Blake Wilbur Drive, MC 5826, Stanford, CA 94305; **Phone:** 650-736-9976; **Board Cert:** Neurological Surgery 1989; **Med School:** Harvard Med Sch 1980; **Resid:** Neurological Surgery, UCSF Med Ctr 1986; **Fellow:** Neuro-Oncology, UCSF Med Ctr 1987; **Fac Appt:** Prof NS, Stanford Univ

Liau, Linda M MD/PhD [NS] - **Spec Exp:** Brain Tumors; Neuro-Oncology; **Hospital:** UCLA Ronald Reagan Med Ctr; **Address:** CHS 74-145, Box 956901, 10833 Le Conte Ave, Los Angeles, CA 90095-6901; **Phone:** 310-267-2621; **Board Cert:** Neurological Surgery 2002; **Med School:** Stanford Univ 1991; **Resid:** Neurological Surgery, UCLA Med Ctr 1998; **Fellow:** Neuro-Oncology, UCLA Med Ctr 1998; **Fac Appt:** Prof NS, UCLA

Neurological Surgery

Linskey, Mark E MD [NS] - **Spec Exp:** Brain Tumors; Stereotactic Radiosurgery; Skull Base Surgery; **Hospital:** UC Irvine Med Ctr, Chldns Hosp Orange Co; **Address:** UCI Med Ctr, Dept Neurosurgery-Route 81, 101 The City Drive S Bldg 56 - Ste 400, Orange, CA 92868-3298; **Phone:** 714-456-6392; **Board Cert:** Neurological Surgery 1996; **Med School:** Columbia P&S 1986; **Resid:** Neurological Surgery, Univ Pittsburgh Hlth Ctrs 1993; **Fellow:** Neuro-Oncology, Ludwig Inst Cancer Rsch/Univ Coll London 1994; Neuro-Oncology, Pittsburgh Cancer Inst/Univ Pittsburgh 1992; **Fac Appt:** Assoc Prof NS, UC Irvine

Mamelak, Adam N MD [NS] - **Spec Exp:** Brain Tumors; Spinal Tumors; **Hospital:** Cedars-Sinai Med Ctr, Huntington Memorial Hosp; **Address:** Maxine Dunitz Neurosurgical Institute, 8631 W Third St, Ste 800-East, Los Angeles, CA 90048; **Phone:** 310-423-7900; **Board Cert:** Neurological Surgery 2000; **Med School:** Harvard Med Sch 1990; **Resid:** Neurological Surgery, UCSF Med Ctr 1994; **Fellow:** Epilepsy, UCSF Epilepsy Research Lab 1996

Mayberg, Marc R MD [NS] - **Spec Exp:** Pituitary Surgery; Skull Base Tumors; **Hospital:** Swedish Med Ctr - Seattle; **Address:** Seattle Neuroscience Inst, 550 17th Ave, Ste 500, Seattle, WA 98122; **Phone:** 206-320-2800; **Board Cert:** Neurological Surgery 1988; **Med School:** Mayo Med Sch 1978; **Resid:** Neurological Surgery, Mass Genl Hosp 1984; **Fellow:** Neurological Surgery, Natl Hosp for Nervous Dis 1985

McDermott, Michael W MD [NS] - **Spec Exp:** Brain Tumors; Stereotactic Radiosurgery; Skull Base Tumors; **Hospital:** UCSF Med Ctr; **Address:** UCSF Dept Neurosurgery, 400 Parnassus Ave, rm A808, San Francisco, CA 94143; **Phone:** 415-353-7500; **Board Cert:** Neurological Surgery 2003; **Med School:** Univ Toronto 1982; **Resid:** Neurological Surgery, Univ British Columbia 1988; **Fellow:** Neuro-Oncology, UCSF Med Ctr 1990; **Fac Appt:** Prof NS, UCSF

Neuwelt, Edward A MD [NS] - **Spec Exp:** Neuro-Oncology; Brain Tumors; **Hospital:** OR Hlth & Sci Univ; **Address:** Oregon Hlth Sci Univ, Dept NS, 3181 SW Sam Jackson Pk Rd, MC-L603, Portland, OR 97239; **Phone:** 503-494-5626; **Board Cert:** Neurological Surgery 1980; **Med School:** Univ Colorado 1972; **Resid:** Neurological Surgery, Univ Tex SW Med Sch 1978; **Fellow:** Neuro-Oncology, Natl Canc Inst, NIH 1976; **Fac Appt:** Prof NS, Oregon Hlth Sci Univ

Ott, Kenneth H MD [NS] - **Spec Exp:** Brain Tumors; Stereotactic Radiosurgery; **Hospital:** Scripps Meml Hosp - La Jolla; **Address:** Neurosurgical Medical Clinic, 2100 Fifth Ave, Ste 200, San Diego, CA 92101; **Phone:** 619-297-4481; **Board Cert:** Neurological Surgery 1980; **Med School:** UCSF 1970; **Resid:** Surgery, Mass Genl Hosp 1972; Neurological Surgery, Mass Genl Hosp 1976; **Fac Appt:** Assoc Clin Prof S, UCSD

Sekhar, Laligam N MD [NS] - **Spec Exp:** Brain Tumors; Skull Base Tumors; **Hospital:** Harborview Med Ctr, Univ Wash Med Ctr; **Address:** Harborview Med Ctr, UW Dept Neurosurgery, 325 Ninth Ave, Box 359766, Seattle, WA 98104-2420; **Phone:** 206-744-9300; **Board Cert:** Neurological Surgery 1986; **Med School:** India 1973; **Resid:** Neurology, Univ Cincinnati Med Ctr 1977; Neurology, Univ Pittsburgh Med Ctr 1982; **Fellow:** Skull Base Surgery, Norstadt Krankenhaus 1983; Cerebrovascular Neurosurgery, Univ Zurich Hospital; **Fac Appt:** Prof NS, Univ Wash

Silbergeld, Daniel MD [NS] - **Spec Exp:** Brain Tumors; Brain Tumors-Metastatic; **Hospital:** Univ Wash Med Ctr; **Address:** Univ Wash Med Ctr, Dept Neurosurg, 1959 NE Pacific, Box 356470, Seattle, WA 98195; **Phone:** 206-598-5637; **Board Cert:** Neurological Surgery 1995; **Med School:** Univ Cincinnati 1984; **Resid:** Neurological Surgery, Univ Wash Med Ctr 1990; Research, Univ Wash Med Ctr 1988; **Fellow:** Neuro-Oncology, Univ Wash Med Ctr 1991; Epilepsy, Univ Wash Med Ctr 1991; **Fac Appt:** Assoc Prof NS, Univ Wash

Sun, Peter P MD [NS] - **Spec Exp:** Pediatric Neurosurgery; Congenital Cranial Deformities; Brain Tumors; **Hospital:** Chldns Hosp - Oakland; **Address:** Children's Hospital, Dept Neurosurgery, 744 52nd St, Oakland, CA 94609; **Phone:** 510-428-3319; **Board Cert:** Neurological Surgery 2002; Pediatric Neurological Surgery 2006; **Med School:** Columbia P&S 1991; **Resid:** Neurological Surgery, UC Davis Med Ctr 1994; Neurological Surgery, Yale-New Haven Hosp 1996; **Fellow:** Neurological Surgery, NYU Med Ctr 1997; Pediatric Neurological Surgery, Childrens Hosp 1998; **Fac Appt:** Asst Clin Prof NS, UCSF

Yu, John S MD [NS] - **Spec Exp:** Brain Tumors; Spinal Tumors; Clinical Trials; **Hospital:** Cedars-Sinai Med Ctr; **Address:** Maxine Dunitz Neurosurgical Institute, 8631 W 3rd St, Ste 800-East, Los Angeles, CA 90048; **Phone:** 310-423-7900; **Board Cert:** Neurological Surgery 2002; **Med School:** Harvard Med Sch 1990; **Resid:** Neurological Surgery, Mass General Hosp 1997

Cleveland Clinic

Leading-Edge Treatment for Brain Tumors

At Cleveland Clinic Taussig Cancer Institute, more than 250 cancer specialists, researchers, nurses and technicians are dedicated to developing and applying the latest and most effective medical techniques to achieve the long-term survival and improve the quality of life for 7,500 new cancer patients every year. Because of our patient-centered care, leading-edge treatments, innovative research, 350 clinical trials and state-of-the-art medical technologies, *U.S.News & World Report* has ranked Cleveland Clinic's cancer program one of the top cancer centers in the nation.

The Taussig Cancer Institute and the Brain Tumor and Neuro-Oncology Center collaborate on multidisciplinary teams of leading medical oncologists, radiation oncologists, neuro-oncologists, neurosurgeons, neuroradiologists, neuropathologists and advanced practice nurses to provide all brain cancer patients with comprehensive, individualized treatment strategies to maximize favorable outcomes. **To schedule an appointment or to get a second opinion call 866.223.8100 or visit clevelandclinic.org/braintumorTCD.**

The Center is nationally recognized for its diagnosis and treatment of primary and metastastic tumors of the brain, spine, nerves and their effects on the nervous system. All patients are cared for with the latest advances in surgery, noninvasive radiosurgery, brachytherapy and clinical trials.

Advanced Treatment for Metastatic Disease

The Brain Tumor and Neuro-Oncology Center has the most advanced Gamma Knife® technology. Combined with our medical expertise, the Gamma Knife provides the best nonsurgcial treatment for patients with a wide range of brain tumors including brain metastases. Our Gamma Knife Center has performed more than 2,500 procedures.

Our Stereotactic Spine Radiosurgery Program treats spinal metastases. This technology delivers high doses of conformal radiation and precisely targets spinal tumors, minimizing radiation exposure to nearby healthy tissue. This technique often results in effective pain and/or tumor control.

The Center's patients have the opportunity to participate in anti-cancer agent clinical trials. And our membership in the New Approaches to Brain Tumor Therapy consortium gives our patients access to even more clinical trials, including some that are conducted at just a few centers across the country.

To schedule an appointment or for more information about Cleveland Clinic Taussig Cancer Institute, call 866.223.8100 or visit clevelandclinic.org/braintumorTCD.

Cleveland Clinic Taussig Cancer Institute | Cleveland, OH

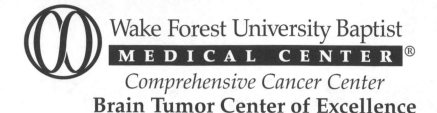

Wake Forest University Baptist
MEDICAL CENTER®
Comprehensive Cancer Center
Brain Tumor Center of Excellence

Medical Center Boulevard • Winston-Salem, NC 27157
PAL® (Physician-to-physician calls) 1-800-277-7654
Health On-Call® (Patient access) 1-800-446-2255
www.wfubmc.edu/cancer/

OVERVIEW

The Brain Tumor Center of Excellence of Wake Forest University was formed in June 2003. With the goal of being a national leader in patient care and research, the Center has built its program with three basic components: an excellent group of clinicians, a world-renowned researcher to direct the Center, and a mission to grow the clinical and basic research programs to a magnitude that would place Wake Forest among the top brain tumor centers in the United States.

RESEARCH

The Brain Tumor Center of Excellence has three areas of research focus:

- Novel therapeutics – identifying innovative treatments that will improve outcome.

- Bioanatomic imaging – identifying the unique signatures of a cancer through non-invasive imaging of tumor biology, chemistry and physiology, thus allowing individual treatment approaches.

- Radiation-induced brain injury – understanding the mechanisms of injury and ways to prevent and treat side effects of brain tumor therapy.

Laboratory researchers are exploring new therapies such as novel chemotherapy drugs, cytotoxins, gene therapy, and radiosensitizers, translating these unique approaches into clinical trials for patients. In addition to studies written and conducted by Comprehensive Cancer Center doctors, clinical trials are also offered from several national Cooperative Groups as well as the pharmaceutical industry. Wake Forest Baptist is one of only 12 centers in the country that is part of the Adult Brain Tumor Consortium. In addition, the clinicians and researchers have one of the most extensive laboratory and clinical research programs in the U.S. for the diagnosis, prevention, and treatment of brain injury resulting from a brain tumor and its treatments, particularly radiation therapy.

MULTIDISCIPLINARY CARE

Offering the region's only multidisciplinary clinic for brain tumor treatment, patients are evaluated by a medical oncologist, neurosurgeon, radiation oncologist and other specialists as needed. The entire clinical neuro-oncology team meets regularly to discuss current patients, as well as cases sent in from around the region, southeast, and nationally/internationally. Recommendations for multidisciplinary care are made and communicated to referring physicians and patients.

For patients who receive their brain tumor care at Wake Forest Baptist, the most sophisticated tools available are used for diagnosis and treatment. Imaging brain tumor and normal brain anatomy using modalities such as magnetic resonance (MR) imaging, MR spectroscopy, functional MR, and combination computed tomography/positron emission tomography (CT/PET) helps the team plan surgical and radiotherapeutic treatments that have the best chance of cure. Image guided surgery, cortical mapping, awake craniotomy, Leksell® Gamma Knife stereotactic radiosurgery, Gliadel® wafer chemotherapy, convection enhanced drug delivery, and GliaSite® brachytherapy are just some of the leading-edge approaches used for brain tumor patients.

To make an appointment or find a specialist at Wake Forest University Baptist Medical Center, call Health On-Call® 1-800-446-2255

KNOWLEDGE MAKES ALL THE DIFFERENCE.

Neurology

A neurologist specializes in the diagnosis and treatment of all types of disease or impaired function of the brain, spinal cord, peripheral nerves, muscles and autonomic nervous system, as well as the blood vessels that relate to these structures.

Training Required: Four years

Certification in the following subspecialty requires additional training and examination.

Child Neurology: A neurologist with special qualifications in child neurology has special skills in the diagnosis and management of neurologic disorders of the neonatal period, infancy, early childhood and adolescence.

Training Required: Five years

Spinal Cord Injury Medicine: A physician who addresses the prevention, diagnosis, treatment and management of traumatic spinal cord injury and non-traumatic etiologies of spinal cord dysfunction by working in an interdisciplinary manner. Care is provided to patients of all ages on a lifelong basis and covers related medical, physical, psychological and vocational disabilities and complications.

Training Required: Five years

Neurology

Mid Atlantic

De Angelis, Lisa M MD [N] - **Spec Exp:** Neuro-Oncology; **Hospital:** Meml Sloan-Kettering Cancer Ctr (page 76); **Address:** 1275 York Avenue, New York, NY 10065; **Phone:** 212-639-7123; **Board Cert:** Neurology 1986; **Med School:** Columbia P&S 1980; **Resid:** Neurology, Neuro Inst-Presby Hosp 1984; **Fellow:** Neuro-Oncology, Neuro Inst-Presby Hosp 1985; Neuro-Oncology, Meml Sloan-Kettering Cancer Ctr 1986; **Fac Appt:** Prof N, Cornell Univ-Weill Med Coll

Glass, Jon MD [N] - **Spec Exp:** Neuro-Oncology; Brain Tumors; Spinal Tumors; **Hospital:** Thomas Jefferson Univ Hosp (page 83); **Address:** 909 Walnut St Fl 2, Philadelphia, PA 19107; **Phone:** 215-503-7005; **Board Cert:** Neurology 1993; **Med School:** SUNY Downstate 1986; **Resid:** Neurology, Boston Univ 1990; **Fellow:** Neuro-Oncology, Mass Genl Hosp 1992; **Fac Appt:** Asst Prof N, NYU Sch Med

Hiesiger, Emile MD [N] - **Spec Exp:** Pain Management; Neuro-Oncology; **Hospital:** NYU Langone Med Ctr (page 80), VA Med Ctr - Manhattan; **Address:** 530 1st Ave, Ste 5A, New York, NY 10016-6402; **Phone:** 212-263-6123; **Board Cert:** Neurology 1983; **Med School:** NY Med Coll 1978; **Resid:** Neurology, NYU Med Ctr 1982; **Fellow:** Neurology, Meml Sloan-Kettering Cancer Ctr 1984; **Fac Appt:** Assoc Clin Prof N, NYU Sch Med

Kunschner, Lara MD [N] - **Spec Exp:** Neuro-Oncology; Brain Tumors; **Hospital:** Allegheny General Hosp; **Address:** 420 E North Ave, Ste 206, Pittsburgh, PA 15212; **Phone:** 412-359-8850; **Board Cert:** Neurology 1999; **Med School:** Univ Pittsburgh 1994; **Resid:** Neurology, Univ Michigan Hosps 1999; **Fellow:** Neuro-Oncology, MD Anderson Cancer Ctr 2000

Laterra, John J MD/PhD [N] - **Spec Exp:** Neuro-Oncology; Brain Tumors; **Hospital:** Johns Hopkins Hosp, Kennedy Krieger Inst; **Address:** Phipps 115, 600 N Wolfe St, Baltimore, MD 21287; **Phone:** 410-614-3853; **Board Cert:** Neurology 1990; **Med School:** Case West Res Univ 1984; **Resid:** Neurology, Univ Mich Hosps 1988; **Fellow:** Research, Johns Hopkins Hosp 1989; **Fac Appt:** Prof N, Johns Hopkins Univ

Posner, Jerome MD [N] - **Spec Exp:** Neuro-Oncology; Brain Tumors; **Hospital:** Meml Sloan-Kettering Cancer Ctr (page 76); **Address:** 1275 York Avenue, New York, NY 10065; **Phone:** 212-639-7047; **Board Cert:** Neurology 1962; **Med School:** Univ Wash 1955; **Resid:** Neurology, Univ WA Affil Hosp 1959; **Fellow:** Biochemistry, Univ WA Affil Hosp 1963; **Fac Appt:** Prof N, Cornell Univ-Weill Med Coll

Rosenfeld, Myrna MD/PhD [N] - **Spec Exp:** Neuro-Oncology; Brain Tumors; **Hospital:** Hosp Univ Penn - UPHS (page 81); **Address:** Hosp Univ Penn, Dept Neurology, 3400 Spruce St, 3W Gates, Philadelphia, PA 19104; **Phone:** 215-746-4707; **Board Cert:** Neurology 1990; **Med School:** Northwestern Univ 1985; **Resid:** Neurology, Northwestern Univ Hosp 1987; Neurology, Univ Hosp Cleveland 1989; **Fellow:** Neuro-Oncology, Meml Sloan Kettering Cancer Ctr; **Fac Appt:** Assoc Prof N, Univ Pennsylvania

Rosenfeld, Steven S MD [N] - **Spec Exp:** Brain Tumors; Gliomas; Neuro-Oncology; **Hospital:** NY-Presby Hosp/Columbia (page 79); **Address:** Neurological Inst of NY-Brain Tumor Ctr, 710 W 168th St, rm 204, New York, NY 10032; **Phone:** 212-305-1718; **Board Cert:** Neurology 1994; **Med School:** Northwestern Univ 1985; **Resid:** Neurology, Duke Univ Med Ctr 1989; **Fellow:** Neuro-Oncology, Duke Univ Med Ctr 1990; **Fac Appt:** Prof N, Columbia P&S

Southeast

Janss, Anna J MD/PhD [N] - **Spec Exp:** Brain Tumors-Pediatric; Clinical Trials; Cancer Survivors-Late Effects of Therapy; **Hospital:** Chldns Hlthcare Atlanta @ Egleston; **Address:** Aflac Cancer & Blood Disorders Ctr, Outpatient Clin, Tower 1 Fl 4, 1405 Clifton Rd NE, Atlanta, GA 30322; **Phone:** 404-785-1200; **Board Cert:** Neurology 1993; **Med School:** Univ Iowa Coll Med 1988; **Resid:** Neurology, Hosp Univ Penn 1992; **Fellow:** Pediatric Neuro-Oncology, Chldns Hosp 1996; **Fac Appt:** Assoc Prof N, Emory Univ

Nabors III, Louis Burt MD [N] - **Spec Exp:** Neuro-Oncology; Brain Tumors; **Hospital:** Univ of Ala Hosp at Birmingham; **Address:** UAB, FOT 1020, 510 20th St S, Birmingham, AL 35294-0001; **Phone:** 205-934-1432; **Board Cert:** Neurology 1999; **Med School:** Univ Tenn Coll Med, Memphis 1991; **Resid:** Neurology, Univ Alabama; **Fellow:** Neuro-Oncology, Univ Alabama; **Fac Appt:** Assoc Prof N, Univ Alabama

Patchell, Roy MD [N] - **Spec Exp:** Neuro-Oncology; Brain Tumors; Spinal Tumors; **Hospital:** Univ of Kentucky Chandler Hosp; **Address:** Univ Kentucky Neurosurgery, Chandler Med Ctr, 800 Rose St, MS 105, Lexington, KY 40536; **Phone:** 859-257-1532; **Board Cert:** Neurology 1984; **Med School:** Univ KY Coll Med 1979; **Resid:** Neurology, Johns Hopkins Hosp 1983; **Fellow:** Neuro-Oncology, Meml Sloan-Kettering Canc Ctr 1985; **Fac Appt:** Prof N, Univ KY Coll Med

Schiff, David MD [N] - **Spec Exp:** Brain Tumors; Spinal Cord Tumors; Neurologic Complications of Cancer; Neuro-Oncology; **Hospital:** Univ Virginia Med Ctr; **Address:** Univ VA, Div of Neuro-Oncology, PO Box 800432, Charlottesville, VA 22908; **Phone:** 434-982-4415; **Board Cert:** Neurology 1994; **Med School:** Harvard Med Sch 1988; **Resid:** Neurology, Harvard Longwood 1992; **Fellow:** Neuro-Oncology, Meml Sloan Kettering Cancer Ctr 1993; Mayo Clinic 1994; **Fac Appt:** Assoc Prof NS, Univ VA Sch Med

Midwest

Barger, Geoffrey R MD [N] - **Spec Exp:** Neuro-Oncology; Brain Tumors; **Hospital:** Harper Univ Hosp; **Address:** Wayne State Univ Hlth Ctr, 4201 St Antoine, Ste 8D-UHC, Detroit, MI 48201; **Phone:** 313-745-4275; **Board Cert:** Neurology 1981; **Med School:** Jefferson Med Coll 1975; **Resid:** Neurology, Penn Hosp 1979; **Fellow:** Neuro-Oncology, Moffitt Hosp & Brain Tumor Ctr/UCSF 1982; **Fac Appt:** Assoc Prof N, Wayne State Univ

Cascino, Terrence L MD [N] - **Spec Exp:** Neuro-Oncology; **Hospital:** Mayo Med Ctr & Clin - Rochester; **Address:** Mayo Clinic, Dept Neurology, 200 1st St SW, Rochester, MN 55905-0001; **Phone:** 507-284-2576; **Board Cert:** Neurology 1984; **Med School:** Loyola Univ-Stritch Sch Med 1972; **Resid:** Neurology, Mayo Clinic 1980; **Fellow:** Neuro-Oncology, Meml Sloan Kettering Cancer Ctr; **Fac Appt:** Assoc Prof N, Mayo Med Sch

Mikkelsen, Tommy MD [N] - **Spec Exp:** Brain Tumors; Gliomas; **Hospital:** Henry Ford Hosp, William Beaumont Hosp; **Address:** Henry Ford Hospital, ER 3096, 2799 W Grand Blvd, Detroit, MI 48202; **Phone:** 313-916-8641; **Board Cert:** Neurology 2008; **Med School:** Univ Calgary 1983; **Resid:** Internal Medicine, Calgary General Hosp 1985; Neurology, Montreal Neurological Inst 1988; **Fellow:** Neuro-Oncology, Royal Victoria Hosp 1990; Neuro-Oncology, Ludwig Inst for Cancer Rsch 1992; **Fac Appt:** Assoc Prof N, Case West Res Univ

Neurology

Newton, Herbert B MD [N] - **Spec Exp:** Neuro-Oncology; Brain & Spinal Tumors; **Hospital:** Ohio St Univ Med Ctr, Arthur G James Cancer Hosp & Research Inst; **Address:** 320 W 10th Ave, Starling Loving Bldg, rm M410, Columbus, OH 43210; **Phone:** 614-293-8930; **Board Cert:** Neurology 1989; **Med School:** SUNY Buffalo 1984; **Resid:** Neurology, Univ Michigan Med Ctr 1988; **Fellow:** Neuro-Oncology, Meml Sloan-Kettering Cancer Ctr 1990; **Fac Appt:** Prof N, Ohio State Univ

Rogers, Lisa R DO [N] - **Spec Exp:** Neuro-Oncology; Brain Tumors; Brain Radiation Toxicity; **Hospital:** Univ Michigan Hlth Sys; **Address:** Univ Michigan, Dept Neurology, 1914 Taubman Center, Ann Arbor, MI 48109-5316; **Phone:** 734-615-2994; **Board Cert:** Neurology 1982; **Med School:** Kirksville Coll Osteo Med 1976; **Resid:** Neurology, Cleveland Clin Fdn 1980; **Fellow:** Neuro-Oncology, Meml-Sloan Kettering Cancer Ctr 1982; **Fac Appt:** Prof N, Univ Mich Med Sch

Vick, Nicholas A MD [N] - **Spec Exp:** Brain Tumors; Neuro-Oncology; **Hospital:** Evanston/Northshore Univ Hlth Syst; **Address:** Evanston Hosp, Dept Neurology, 2650 Ridge Ave, Evanston, IL 60201; **Phone:** 847-570-2570; **Board Cert:** Neurology 1971; **Med School:** Univ Chicago-Pritzker Sch Med 1965; **Resid:** Neurology, Univ Chicago Hosps 1968; **Fellow:** Neurology, Natl Inst Hlth 1970; **Fac Appt:** Prof N, Northwestern Univ

Southwest

Gilbert, Mark R MD [N] - **Spec Exp:** Brain Tumors; Neuro-Oncology; **Hospital:** UT MD Anderson Cancer Ctr; **Address:** Univ Tex MD Anderson Cancer Ctr, 1515 Holcombe Blvd, Unit 431, Houston, TX 77030; **Phone:** 713-792-4008; **Board Cert:** Internal Medicine 1985; Neurology 1990; **Med School:** Johns Hopkins Univ 1982; **Resid:** Internal Medicine, Johns Hopkins Hosp 1985; Neurology, Johns Hopkins Hosp 1988; **Fellow:** Neuro-Oncology, Johns Hopkins Hosp 1988; **Fac Appt:** Assoc Prof N, Univ Tex, Houston

Levin, Victor A MD [N] - **Spec Exp:** Brain Tumors; Neuro-Oncology; Clinical Trials; **Hospital:** UT MD Anderson Cancer Ctr; **Address:** 1515 Holcombe Blvd, Unit #431, Houston, TX 77030-4009; **Phone:** 713-792-8297; **Board Cert:** Neurology 1976; **Med School:** Univ Wisc 1966; **Resid:** Neurology, Mass Genl Hosp 1972; **Fac Appt:** Prof Med, Univ Tex, Houston

Shapiro, William R MD [N] - **Spec Exp:** Neuro-Oncology; **Hospital:** St Joseph's Hosp & Med Ctr - Phoenix; **Address:** Barrow Neurology Clinics, 500 W Thomas Rd, Ste 300, Phoenix, AZ 85013; **Phone:** 602-406-6262; **Board Cert:** Neurology 1969; **Med School:** UCSF 1961; **Resid:** Internal Medicine, Univ Wash Hosp 1963; Neurology, NY Hosp-Cornell Med Ctr 1966; **Fellow:** Neuro-Oncology, Natl Inst Hlth 1969; **Fac Appt:** Prof N, Univ Ariz Coll Med

Yung, Wai-Kwan A MD [N] - **Spec Exp:** Neuro-Oncology; Brain Tumors; **Hospital:** UT MD Anderson Cancer Ctr; **Address:** 1515 Holcombe Blvd, Unit 431, Houston, TX 77030-4017; **Phone:** 713-794-1285; **Board Cert:** Neurology 1980; **Med School:** Univ Chicago-Pritzker Sch Med 1975; **Resid:** Neurology, UCSD Med Ctr 1978; **Fellow:** Neuro-Oncology, Meml Sloan Kettering Cancer Ctr 1981; **Fac Appt:** Prof N, Univ Tex, Houston

West Coast and Pacific

Cloughesy, Timothy F MD [N] - **Spec Exp:** Neuro-Oncology; Brain Tumors; **Hospital:** UCLA Ronald Reagan Med Ctr; **Address:** UCLA Neurological Services, 710 Westwood Plaza, Ste 1-230, Los Angeles, CA 90095; **Phone:** 310-825-5321; **Board Cert:** Neurology 1993; **Med School:** Tulane Univ 1987; **Resid:** Neurology, UCLA Med Ctr 1991; **Fellow:** Neuro-Oncology, Meml Sloan-Kettering Canc Ctr; **Fac Appt:** Clin Prof N, UCLA

Phuphanich, Surasak MD [N] - **Spec Exp:** Neuro-Oncology; Brain Tumors; Spinal Tumors; Lymphoma-Primary CNS; **Hospital:** Cedars-Sinai Med Ctr; **Address:** 8631 W 3rd St, Ste 410E, Los Angeles, CA 90048; **Phone:** 310-423-8100; **Board Cert:** Neurology 1983; **Med School:** Thailand 1975; **Resid:** Neurology, Univ Illinois Med Ctr 1981; **Fellow:** Neuro-Oncology, UCSF Med Ctr 1984

CHILD NEUROLOGY

New England

Mandelbaum, David E MD/PhD [ChiN] - **Spec Exp:** Brain Tumors-Pediatric; **Hospital:** Rhode Island Hosp, Women & Infants Hosp of RI; **Address:** Dept of Neurology, 593 Eddy St George Bldg, Providence, RI 02903; **Phone:** 401-444-5685; **Board Cert:** Child Neurology 1987; Pediatrics 1987; Clinical Neurophysiology 2003; Neurodevelopmental Disabilities 2001; **Med School:** Columbia P&S 1980; **Resid:** Pediatrics, Yale-New Haven Hosp 1982; Neurology, Neuro Inst-Columbia 1983; **Fellow:** Child Neurology, Neuro Inst-Columbia 1985; **Fac Appt:** Prof Ped, Brown Univ

Pomeroy, Scott L MD/PhD [ChiN] - **Spec Exp:** Neuro-Oncology; Brain Tumors; **Hospital:** Children's Hospital - Boston, Dana-Farber Cancer Inst; **Address:** Chldns Hosp, Dept Neurology-Fegan 11, 300 Longwood Ave, Boston, MA 02115; **Phone:** 617-355-6386; **Board Cert:** Pediatrics 2003; Child Neurology 1988; **Med School:** Univ Conn 1982; **Resid:** Pediatrics, Chldns Hosp 1984; Neurology, Barnes Hosp/Washington Univ 1985; **Fellow:** Pediatric Neurology, St Louis Chldns Hosp 1987; Neurological Biology, Washington Univ 1989; **Fac Appt:** Prof N, Harvard Med Sch

Mid Atlantic

Allen, Jeffrey MD [ChiN] - **Spec Exp:** Neuro-Oncology; Brain Tumors; **Hospital:** NYU Langone Med Ctr (page 80); **Address:** Hassenfeld Childrens Ctr, 160 E 32nd St, Ste L3, New York, NY 10016; **Phone:** 212-263-9907; **Board Cert:** Child Neurology 1977; **Med School:** Harvard Med Sch 1969; **Resid:** Pediatrics, Montreal Chldns Hosp 1973; Pediatric Neurology, Montreal Neur Inst/McGill 1976; **Fac Appt:** Prof Ped, NYU Sch Med

Duffner, Patricia K MD [ChiN] - **Spec Exp:** Brain Tumors; Cancer Survivors-Late Effects of Therapy; **Hospital:** Women's & Chldn's Hosp of Buffalo, The; **Address:** Women & Childrens Hosp, Dept Neurology, 219 Bryant St, Buffalo, NY 14222-2006; **Phone:** 716-878-7819; **Board Cert:** Pediatrics 1977; Child Neurology 1979; **Med School:** SUNY Buffalo 1972; **Resid:** Pediatrics, Buffalo Chldns Hosp 1975; **Fellow:** Child Neurology, SUNY Buffalo-Buffalo Chldns Hosp 1978; **Fac Appt:** Prof N, SUNY Buffalo

Packer, Roger J MD [ChiN] - **Spec Exp:** Brain Tumors; **Hospital:** Chldns Natl Med Ctr; **Address:** Chldns Natl Med Ctr, Dept Neurology, 111 Michigan Ave NW, Washington, DC 20010-2978; **Phone:** 202-476-6230; **Board Cert:** Child Neurology 1982; Pediatrics 1982; **Med School:** Northwestern Univ 1976; **Resid:** Pediatrics, Chldns Med Ctr 1978; Neurology, Chldns Hosp-Univ Penn 1981; **Fac Appt:** Prof N, Geo Wash Univ

Phillips, Peter C MD [ChiN] - **Spec Exp:** Brain Tumors; Neuro-Oncology; **Hospital:** Chldns Hosp of Philadelphia, The; **Address:** Childrens Hosp Philadelphia, 34th St & Civic Center Blvd, Philadelphia, PA 19104; **Phone:** 215-590-5188; **Board Cert:** Pediatrics 1985; Child Neurology 1986; **Med School:** Univ Conn 1978; **Resid:** Pediatrics, Chldns Hosp 1980; Pediatric Neurology, Neuro Inst 1983; **Fellow:** Neuro-Oncology, Meml Sloan Kettering Cancer Ctr 1986; **Fac Appt:** Prof N, Univ Pennsylvania

Child Neurology

Midwest

Cohen, Bruce H MD [ChiN] - **Spec Exp:** Brain Tumors; Pain Management; **Hospital:** Cleveland Clin Fdn (page 70); **Address:** Cleveland Clinic, 9500 Euclid Ave, Desk S71, Cleveland, OH 44195; **Phone:** 216-444-9182; **Board Cert:** Pediatrics 2004; Child Neurology 1990; **Med School:** Albert Einstein Coll Med 1982; **Resid:** Pediatrics, Chldns Hosp 1984; Child Neurology, Neurologic Inst-Columbia 1987; **Fellow:** Pediatric Neuro-Oncology, Chldns Hosp 1989

West Coast and Pacific

Chamberlain, Marc C MD [ChiN] - **Spec Exp:** Brain Tumors; Neuro-Oncology; Clinical Trials; **Hospital:** Univ Wash Med Ctr; **Address:** Seattle Cancer Care Alliance, 825 Eastlake Ave E, POB 10923, MS G4940, Seattle, WA 98109-1023; **Phone:** 206-288-8280; **Board Cert:** Pediatrics 1985; Child Neurology 1989; **Med School:** Columbia P&S 1977; **Resid:** Pediatrics, Montefiore Med Ctr 1981; Neurology, UCLA Med Ctr 1983; **Fellow:** Neuro-Oncology, UCSF Med Ctr 1986; **Fac Appt:** Prof N, Univ Wash

Fisher, Paul G MD [ChiN] - **Spec Exp:** Neuro-Oncology; Brain Tumors; **Hospital:** Lucile Packard Chldn's Hosp; **Address:** Stanford Cancer Ctr-Dept Neurology, 875 Blake Wilbur Drive, rm 2220, Stanford, CA 94305; **Phone:** 650-725-8630; **Board Cert:** Pediatrics 2003; Child Neurology 2008; **Med School:** UCSF 1989; **Resid:** Pediatrics, Johns Hopkins Univ Hosp 1991; Neurology, Johns Hopkins Univ Hosp 1994; **Fellow:** Neuro-Oncology, Children's Hosp 1994; **Fac Appt:** Assoc Prof Ped, Stanford Univ

NYU Cancer Institute
NYU LANGONE MEDICAL CENTER

NYU Clinical Cancer Center
160 East 34th Street
New York, New York 10016
www.nyuci.org/atcd

NYU Langone Medical Center
550 First Avenue
(at 31st Street)
New York, New York 10016
www.nyumc.org/atcd

Stephen D. Hassenfeld
Children's Center
for Cancer and Blood
Disorders
160 East 32nd Street
New York, New York 10016
www.nyumc.org/hassenfeld

A Collaborative Approach
The NYU Cancer Institute, an NCI designated center, is a "matrix cancer center" without walls operating within the larger NYU Langone Medical Center. With over 175 members and a research funding base of over $81 million, this structure strengthens our capabilities to forge collaborations across medical and scientific disciplines, which translates to comprehensive care for our patients and discoveries that will influence the future of this disease.

Renowned Expertise
Team members' compassion and expertise help patients better manage the symptoms of their disease as well as their special needs. Our highly skilled Magnet™ nursing team not only plays a pivotal role in coordinating direct patient care, but is also a source of invaluable patient education.

A Patient-Focused Setting
The NYU Clinical Cancer Center, with over 70 faculty members from various disciplines at the New York University School of Medicine, is the principal outpatient facility of the Cancer Institute and serves as home for our patients and their caregivers. The center and its multidisciplinary team of experts provide access to the latest treatment options and clinical trials along with a variety of programs in cancer prevention, screening, diagnostics, genetic counseling, and supportive services. When it comes to kids and cancer, the Stephen D. Hassenfeld Children's Center for Cancer and Blood Disorders offers not just innovation but insight. As a leading member of the NCI-sponsored Children's Oncology Group, our physicians are known for developing new ways to treat childhood cancer. Our affiliation with Bellevue Hospital, the oldest public hospital in the country, affords clinically distinctive opportunities to learn and care for patients with cancer by observing its presentation and behavior in a variety of patient groups.

Obstetrics & Gynecology

An obstetrician/gynecologist possesses special knowledge, skills and professional capability in the medical and surgical care of the female reproductive system and associated disorders. This physician may serve as a consultant to other physicians, and may be a primary physician for some women.

Training Required: Four years plus two years in clinical practice before certification is complete.

Gynecolgic Oncology: An obstetrician/gynecologist who provides consultation and comprehensive management of patients with gynecologic cancer, including those diagnostic and therapeutic procedures necessary for the total care of the patient with gynecologic cancer and resulting complications.

Training Required: Four years plus two years in clinical practice before certification in obstetrics and gynecology is complete plus additional training and examination in gynecologic oncology.

Reproductive Endocrinology/Infertility: An obstetrician/gynecologist who is capable of managing complex problems relating to reproductive endocrinology and infertility.

Training Required: Four years plus two years in clinical practice before certification in obstetrics and gynecology is complete plus additional training and examination in reproductive endocrinology.

GYNECOLOGIC ONCOLOGY

New England

Azodi, Masoud MD [GO] - **Spec Exp:** Laparoscopic Surgery; Ovarian Cancer-Early Detection; Uterine Cancer; **Hospital:** Yale-New Haven Hosp; **Address:** Yale Surgical Oncology, 800 Howard Ave Fl 3, New Haven, CT 06519-1369; **Phone:** 203-785-4013; **Board Cert:** Gynecologic Oncology 2002; Obstetrics & Gynecology 2000; **Med School:** Wright State Univ 1992; **Resid:** Obstetrics & Gynecology, Aultman Hospital 1996; **Fellow:** Obstetrics & Gynecology, Yale-New Haven Hosp 1999; **Fac Appt:** Assoc Prof ObG, Yale Univ

Berkowitz, Ross S MD [GO] - **Spec Exp:** Gynecologic Cancer; **Hospital:** Brigham & Women's Hosp, Dana-Farber Cancer Inst; **Address:** Div OB/GYN Oncology, 75 Francis St, Boston, MA 02115-6110; **Phone:** 617-732-8843; **Board Cert:** Obstetrics & Gynecology 1981; Gynecologic Oncology 1982; **Med School:** Boston Univ 1973; **Resid:** Surgery, Peter Bent Brigham Hosp 1975; Obstetrics & Gynecology, Boston Hosp for Women 1978; **Fellow:** Gynecologic Oncology, Boston Hosp for Women 1980; **Fac Appt:** Prof ObG, Harvard Med Sch

Brewer, Molly A MD [GO] - **Spec Exp:** Ovarian Cancer; **Hospital:** Univ of Conn Hlth Ctr, John Dempsey Hosp; **Address:** Univ Connecticut Hlth Ctr, Div Gyn Oncology, 263 Farmington Ave, MC2875, Farmington, CT 06032-2875; **Phone:** 860-679-2100; **Board Cert:** Obstetrics & Gynecology 2007; Gynecologic Oncology 2007; **Med School:** SUNY Upstate Med Univ 1991; **Resid:** Obstetrics & Gynecology, OR Hlth Scis Univ Hosp 1995; **Fellow:** Gynecologic Oncology, MD Anderson Cancer Ctr 1997

Cain, Joanna M MD [GO] - **Spec Exp:** Ovarian Cancer; Breast Cancer Risk Assessment; Uterine Cancer; Ovarian Cancer-Early Detection; **Hospital:** Women & Infants Hosp of RI; **Address:** Women & Infants Hospital, 101 Dudley St, Providence, RI 02905; **Phone:** 401-274-1122 x1575; **Board Cert:** Obstetrics & Gynecology 2007; Gynecologic Oncology 2007; **Med School:** Creighton Univ 1978; **Resid:** Obstetrics & Gynecology, Univ Washington Med Ctr 1981; **Fellow:** Gynecologic Oncology, Meml Sloan Kettering Cancer Ctr 1983; **Fac Appt:** Prof ObG, Brown Univ

Currie, John L MD [GO] - **Spec Exp:** Gynecologic Cancer; Pelvic Reconstruction; **Hospital:** Hartford Hosp; **Address:** Hartford Hospital, 85 Seymour St Fl 7 - Ste 705, Box 5037, Hartford, CT 06106-5501; **Phone:** 860-545-4341; **Board Cert:** Obstetrics & Gynecology 1991; Gynecologic Oncology 1982; **Med School:** Univ NC Sch Med 1967; **Resid:** Gynecologic Oncology, Hosp Univ Penn 1972; **Fellow:** Gynecologic Oncology, Duke Univ Med Ctr 1980; **Fac Appt:** Prof ObG, Univ Conn

DeMars, Leslie R MD [GO] - **Spec Exp:** Gynecologic Cancer; Laparoscopic Surgery; **Hospital:** Dartmouth - Hitchcock Med Ctr; **Address:** Dartmouth-Hitchcock Med Ctr, Gyn-Oncology, 1 Medical Center Drive, Lebanon, NH 03756; **Phone:** 603-653-3530; **Board Cert:** Obstetrics & Gynecology 2007; Gynecologic Oncology 2007; **Med School:** Univ VT Coll Med 1987; **Resid:** Obstetrics & Gynecology, Univ N Carolina Hosps 1991; **Fellow:** Gynecologic Oncology, Univ N Carolina Hosps 1994; **Fac Appt:** Asst Prof ObG, Dartmouth Med Sch

Granai, Cornelius O MD [GO] - **Spec Exp:** Gynecologic Cancer; Complementary Medicine; International Health; **Hospital:** Women & Infants Hosp of RI, Rhode Island Hosp; **Address:** Womens & Infants Hosp, 101 Dudley St, GYN Oncology Department, Providence, RI 02905; **Phone:** 401-453-7520; **Board Cert:** Obstetrics & Gynecology 2007; Gynecologic Oncology 2007; **Med School:** Univ VT Coll Med 1977; **Resid:** Obstetrics & Gynecology, Hershey Med Ctr 1981; **Fellow:** Gynecologic Oncology, Tufts Univ 1984; **Fac Appt:** Assoc Prof ObG, Brown Univ

Muto, Michael G MD [GO] - **Spec Exp:** Ovarian Cancer; Cervical Cancer; Vulvar & Vaginal Cancer; Robotic Surgery; **Hospital:** Dana-Farber Cancer Inst, Brigham & Women's Hosp; **Address:** Dana Farber Cancer Inst, 44 Binney St Fl 9, Boston, MA 02115; **Phone:** 617-582-7931; **Board Cert:** Gynecologic Oncology 2007; Obstetrics & Gynecology 2007; **Med School:** Univ Mass Sch Med 1983; **Resid:** Obstetrics & Gynecology, Brigham & Women's Hosp 1987; **Fellow:** Gynecologic Oncology, Brigham & Women's Hosp 1990; **Fac Appt:** Assoc Prof ObG, Harvard Med Sch

Rutherford, Thomas J MD [GO] - **Spec Exp:** Ovarian Cancer; Uterine Cancer; Ovarian Cancer-Early Detection; Cervical Cancer; **Hospital:** Yale-New Haven Hosp; **Address:** Yale Univ Sch Med Dept Ob-Gyn, 333 Cedar St, Box 208063, New Haven, CT 06520; **Phone:** 203-785-6301; **Board Cert:** Obstetrics & Gynecology 2007; Gynecologic Oncology 2007; **Med School:** Med Coll OH 1989; **Resid:** Obstetrics & Gynecology, Cooper Hosp 1993; **Fellow:** Gynecologic Oncology, Yale-New Haven Hosp 1995; **Fac Appt:** Assoc Prof ObG, Yale Univ

Santin, Alessandro MD [GO] - **Spec Exp:** Immunotherapy; Ovarian Cancer; **Hospital:** Yale-New Haven Hosp; **Address:** Yale Gynecologic Oncology, 800 Howard Ave, New Haven, CT 06519; **Phone:** 203-737-2280; **Med School:** Italy 1989; **Resid:** Obstetrics & Gynecology, Univ Brescia Sch Med 1993; **Fellow:** Gynecologic Oncology, UC Irvine 1995; Gynecologic Oncology, UAMS Med Ctr 2000; **Fac Appt:** Prof ObG, Yale Univ

Schwartz, Peter E MD [GO] - **Spec Exp:** Ovarian Cancer; Uterine Cancer; Gynecologic Surgery-Complex; Cervical Cancer; **Hospital:** Yale-New Haven Hosp, Hosp of St Raphael; **Address:** Yale Univ Sch Med, Dept Ob/Gyn, 333 Cedar St, rm FMB-316, New Haven, CT 06510-3289; **Phone:** 203-785-4014; **Board Cert:** Obstetrics & Gynecology 1973; Gynecologic Oncology 1979; **Med School:** Albert Einstein Coll Med 1966; **Resid:** Obstetrics & Gynecology, Yale-New Haven Hosp 1970; **Fellow:** Gynecologic Oncology, MD Anderson Cancer Ctr 1975; **Fac Appt:** Prof ObG, Yale Univ

Tarraza, Hector M MD [GO] - **Spec Exp:** Gynecologic Cancer; **Hospital:** Maine Med Ctr; **Address:** 102 Campus Drive, rm 116, Scarborough, ME 04074; **Phone:** 207-883-0069; **Board Cert:** Obstetrics & Gynecology 1998; Gynecologic Oncology 1998; **Med School:** Harvard Med Sch 1981; **Resid:** Obstetrics & Gynecology, Mass Genl Hosp 1985; **Fellow:** Gynecologic Oncology, Mass Genl Hosp 1987; **Fac Appt:** Prof ObG, Univ VT Coll Med

Mid Atlantic

Abbas, Fouad M MD [GO] - **Spec Exp:** Gynecologic Cancer; Ovarian Cancer; Cervical Cancer; **Hospital:** Sinai Hosp - Baltimore; **Address:** Sinai Hosp Baltimore, 2411 W Belvedere Ave, Ste 206, Baltimore, MD 21215; **Phone:** 410-601-9030; **Board Cert:** Obstetrics & Gynecology 2007; Gynecologic Oncology 2007; **Med School:** Univ MD Sch Med 1986; **Resid:** Obstetrics & Gynecology, John Hopkins Hosp 1990; **Fellow:** Gynecologic Oncology, John Hopkins Hosp 1992; **Fac Appt:** Asst Prof ObG, Univ MD Sch Med

Abu-Rustum, Nadeem R MD [GO] - **Spec Exp:** Ovarian Cancer; Uterine Cancer; Cervical Cancer; Vulvar Disease/Cancer; **Hospital:** Meml Sloan-Kettering Cancer Ctr (page 76); **Address:** 1275 York Avenue, New York, NY 10065; **Phone:** 800-525-2225; **Board Cert:** Obstetrics & Gynecology 1998; Gynecologic Oncology 2000; **Med School:** Lebanon 1990; **Resid:** Obstetrics & Gynecology, Greater Baltimore Med Ctr 1994; **Fellow:** Gynecologic Oncology, Meml Sloan-Kettering Cancer Ctr 1997; **Fac Appt:** Assoc Prof ObG, Cornell Univ-Weill Med Coll

Gynecologic Oncology

Barakat, Richard R MD [GO] - **Spec Exp:** Laparoscopic Surgery; Ovarian Cancer; Uterine Cancer; **Hospital:** Meml Sloan-Kettering Cancer Ctr (page 76); **Address:** 1275 York Avenue, New York, NY 10065; **Phone:** 800-525-2225; **Board Cert:** Obstetrics & Gynecology 2006; Gynecologic Oncology 2006; **Med School:** SUNY Hlth Sci Ctr 1985; **Resid:** Obstetrics & Gynecology, Bellevue Hosp 1989; **Fellow:** Gynecologic Oncology, Meml Sloan Kettering Cancer Ctr 1991; **Fac Appt:** Assoc Prof ObG, Cornell Univ-Weill Med Coll

Barnes, Willard MD [GO] - **Spec Exp:** Pelvic Tumors; Gynecologic Cancer; **Hospital:** Georgetown Univ Hosp, Virginia Hosp Ctr - Arlington; **Address:** Georgetown Univ Hosp, Lombardi Cancer Ctr, Dept Gyn Oncology, 3800 Reservoir Rd NW, Washington, DC 20007-2194; **Phone:** 202-444-2114; **Board Cert:** Obstetrics & Gynecology 2007; Gynecologic Oncology 2007; **Med School:** Univ Miss 1979; **Resid:** Obstetrics & Gynecology, Univ Miss Med Ctr 1983; **Fellow:** Gynecologic Oncology, Georgetown Univ Med Ctr 1985; **Fac Appt:** Assoc Prof ObG, Georgetown Univ

Barter, James MD [GO] - **Spec Exp:** Laparoscopic Surgery; Ovarian Cancer; Gynecologic Cancer; **Hospital:** Holy Cross Hospital - Silver Spring, Suburban Hosp; **Address:** 6301 Executive Blvd, Montros Rd, Rockville, MD 20852; **Phone:** 301-770-4967; **Board Cert:** Obstetrics & Gynecology 1997; Gynecologic Oncology 1997; **Med School:** Univ VA Sch Med 1977; **Resid:** Internal Medicine, Univ Kentucky Med Ctr 1979; Obstetrics & Gynecology, Duke Univ Med Ctr 1983; **Fellow:** Gynecologic Oncology, Univ Alabama 1985; **Fac Appt:** Clin Prof ObG, Georgetown Univ

Boice, Charles R MD [GO] - **Spec Exp:** Gynecologic Cancer; Ovarian Cancer; Cervical Cancer; **Hospital:** Univ Wash Med Ctr, Columbia Hosp for Women Med Ctr; **Address:** 10301 Georgia Ave, Ste 205, Silver Springs, MD 20902; **Phone:** 301-592-1600; **Board Cert:** Obstetrics & Gynecology 1981; Gynecologic Oncology 1982; **Med School:** Loma Linda Univ 1973; **Resid:** Obstetrics & Gynecology, Los Angeles Med Ctr 1973; Surgery, City Hope Natl Med Ctr 1978; **Fellow:** Oncology, Univ Texas-MD Anderson Cancer Ctr 1980; **Fac Appt:** Assoc Clin Prof ObG, Univ Wash

Bristow, Robert E MD [GO] - **Spec Exp:** Ovarian Cancer; Cervical Cancer; Uterine Cancer; **Hospital:** Johns Hopkins Hosp; **Address:** Johns Hopkins Hosp, 600 N Wolfe St, Phipps 281, Baltimore, MD 21287; **Phone:** 410-955-8240; **Board Cert:** Obstetrics & Gynecology 1999; Gynecologic Oncology 2003; **Med School:** USC Sch Med 1991; **Resid:** Obstetrics & Gynecology, Johns Hopkins Hosp 1995; **Fellow:** Gynecologic Oncology, UCLA Med Ctr 1998; **Fac Appt:** Assoc Prof ObG, Johns Hopkins Univ

Caputo, Thomas A MD [GO] - **Spec Exp:** Cervical Cancer; Ovarian Cancer; Uterine Cancer; Vulvar Disease/Cancer; **Hospital:** NY-Presby Hosp/Weill Cornell (page 79); **Address:** NY Presby Hosp-Weill Cornell, 525 E 68th St, Ste J130, New York, NY 10021; **Phone:** 212-746-3179; **Board Cert:** Obstetrics & Gynecology 1993; Gynecologic Oncology 1977; **Med School:** UMDNJ-NJ Med Sch, Newark 1965; **Resid:** Obstetrics & Gynecology, Martland Hosp 1969; **Fellow:** Gynecologic Oncology, Emory Univ Hosp 1974; **Fac Appt:** Clin Prof ObG, Cornell Univ-Weill Med Coll

Carlson, John A MD [GO] - **Spec Exp:** Gynecologic Cancer; Ovarian Cancer; Gynecologic Surgery-Complex; **Hospital:** St Peter's Univ Hosp; **Address:** St Peter's Univ Hosp, 254 Easton Ave Cares Bldg, New Brunswick, NJ 08901; **Phone:** 732-937-6003; **Board Cert:** Obstetrics & Gynecology 1981; Gynecologic Oncology 1982; **Med School:** Georgetown Univ 1974; **Resid:** Obstetrics & Gynecology, Hosp Univ Penn 1978; **Fellow:** Gynecologic Oncology, MD Anderson Hosp 1980; **Fac Appt:** Prof ObG, Drexel Univ Coll Med

Coukos, George MD/PhD [GO] - **Spec Exp:** Ovarian Cancer; Gynecologic Cancer; Vaccine Therapy; Clinical Trials; **Hospital:** Hosp Univ Penn - UPHS (page 81); **Address:** Perelman Ctr, Jordan Gynecologic Ctr, 3400 Civic Center Blvd Fl 3 W, Philadelphia, PA 19104; **Phone:** 215-662-3318; **Board Cert:** Obstetrics & Gynecology 2004; Gynecologic Oncology 2004; **Med School:** Italy 1987; **Resid:** Obstetrics & Gynecology, Hosp Univ Penn 1997; **Fellow:** Gynecologic Oncology, Hosp Univ Penn 2000; **Fac Appt:** Assoc Prof ObG, Univ Pennsylvania

Curtin, John P MD [GO] - **Spec Exp:** Uterine Cancer; Ovarian Cancer; Laparoscopic Surgery; **Hospital:** NYU Langone Med Ctr (page 80); **Address:** NYU Clinical Cancer Ctr, 160 E 34th St Fl 4, New York, NY 10016-6402; **Phone:** 212-731-5345; **Board Cert:** Obstetrics & Gynecology 2007; Gynecologic Oncology 2007; **Med School:** Creighton Univ 1979; **Resid:** Obstetrics & Gynecology, Univ Minn Med Ctr 1984; **Fellow:** Gynecologic Oncology, Meml Sloan-Kettering Cancer Ctr 1988; **Fac Appt:** Prof ObG, NYU Sch Med

Dottino, Peter R MD [GO] - **Spec Exp:** Laparoscopic Surgery; Gynecologic Cancer; **Hospital:** Mount Sinai Med Ctr (page 77), Hackensack Univ Med Ctr (page 73); **Address:** 800-A 5th Ave, Ste 405, New York, NY 10021-7215; **Phone:** 212-888-8439; **Board Cert:** Obstetrics & Gynecology 2007; Gynecologic Oncology 2007; **Med School:** Georgetown Univ 1979; **Resid:** Obstetrics & Gynecology, SUNY Downstate Med Ctr 1983; **Fellow:** Gynecologic Oncology, Mt Sinai Hosp 1985

Dunton, Charles J MD [GO] - **Spec Exp:** Ovarian Cancer; Uterine Cancer; Cervical Cancer; Pap Smear Abnormalities; **Hospital:** Lankenau Hosp; **Address:** 100 E Lancaster Ave, Med Office Bldg East, Ste 661, Wynnewood, PA 19096; **Phone:** 610-649-8085; **Board Cert:** Obstetrics & Gynecology 2007; Gynecologic Oncology 2007; **Med School:** Jefferson Med Coll 1980; **Resid:** Obstetrics & Gynecology, Lankenau Hosp 1984; **Fellow:** Gynecologic Oncology, Hosp Univ Penn 1989; **Fac Appt:** Prof ObG, Jefferson Med Coll

Edwards, Robert P MD [GO] - **Spec Exp:** Ovarian Cancer; Gynecologic Cancer; Cervical Cancer; Clinical Trials; **Hospital:** Magee-Womens Hosp - UPMC; **Address:** UPP-Dept Women's Health, 300 Halket St, Ste 0610, Pittsburgh, PA 15213; **Phone:** 412-641-5411; **Board Cert:** Obstetrics & Gynecology 2007; Gynecologic Oncology 2007; **Med School:** Univ Pittsburgh 1984; **Resid:** Obstetrics & Gynecology, Magee WomensHosp-UPMC 1989; **Fellow:** Gynecologic Oncology, Univ Alabama Med Ctr 1993; **Fac Appt:** Prof ObG, Univ Pittsburgh

Fields, Abbie L MD [GO] - **Spec Exp:** Fertility Preservation in Cancer; Robotic Surgery; Cancer Genetics; Pelvic Reconstruction; **Hospital:** Washington Hosp Ctr; **Address:** Washington Hospital Center, 110 Irving St NW, rm 5B-33B, Washington, DC 20010; **Phone:** 202-877-2391; **Board Cert:** Obstetrics & Gynecology 2007; Gynecologic Oncology 2007; **Med School:** Ohio State Univ 1987; **Resid:** Obstetrics & Gynecology, Northwestern Univ 1991; **Fellow:** Gynecologic Oncology, Johns Hopkins Hosp 1993

Fishman, David A MD [GO] - **Spec Exp:** Ovarian Cancer; Ovarian Cancer-Early Detection; Gynecologic Cancer; **Hospital:** Mount Sinai Med Ctr (page 77); **Address:** 1190 Fifth Ave, New York, NY 10029; **Phone:** 212-241-1111; **Board Cert:** Obstetrics & Gynecology 2005; Gynecologic Oncology 2005; **Med School:** Texas Tech Univ 1988; **Resid:** Obstetrics & Gynecology, Yale-New Haven Hosp 1992; **Fellow:** Gynecologic Oncology, Yale-New Haven Hosp 1994; **Fac Appt:** Prof ObG, NYU Sch Med

Giuntoli II, Robert Lawrence MD [GO] - **Spec Exp:** Gynecologic Cancer; Ovarian Cancer; Gestational Trophoblastic Disease; Immunotherapy; **Hospital:** Johns Hopkins Hosp; **Address:** Johns Hopkins Hosp, Div Gyn Onc, 600 N Wolfe St, Phipps #281, Baltimore, MD 21287-1281; **Phone:** 410-502-4245; **Board Cert:** Obstetrics & Gynecology 2005; Gynecologic Oncology 2005; **Med School:** Univ Pennsylvania 1994; **Resid:** Obstetrics & Gynecology, Duke Univ Med Ctr 1998; **Fellow:** Gynecologic Oncology, Mayo Clinic 2002; **Fac Appt:** Asst Prof ObG, Johns Hopkins Univ

Herzog, Thomas J MD [GO] - **Spec Exp:** Cervical Cancer; Gynecologic Cancer; Laparoscopic Surgery; Ovarian Cancer; **Hospital:** NY-Presby Hosp/Columbia (page 79); **Address:** Herbert Irving Pavilion, 161 Fort Washington Ave, 8-837, New York, NY 10032; **Phone:** 212-305-3410; **Board Cert:** Obstetrics & Gynecology 2008; Gynecologic Oncology 2008; **Med School:** Univ Cincinnati 1986; **Resid:** Obstetrics & Gynecology, Good Samaritan Hosp 1990; **Fellow:** Gynecologic Oncology, Barnes Jewish Hosp 1993; **Fac Appt:** Prof ObG, Columbia P&S

Gynecologic Oncology

Kelley III, Joseph L MD [GO] - **Spec Exp:** Breast Cancer; Ovarian Cancer; Cervical Cancer; Gynecologic Cancer; **Hospital:** Magee-Womens Hosp - UPMC; **Address:** UPP-Dept Women's Health, 300 Halket St, Ste 0610, Pittsburgh, PA 15213; **Phone:** 412-641-5411; **Board Cert:** Obstetrics & Gynecology 2007; Gynecologic Oncology 2007; **Med School:** St Louis Univ 1985; **Resid:** Obstetrics & Gynecology, Magee-Womens Hosp 1989; **Fellow:** Gynecologic Oncology, MD Anderson Cancer Ctr 1991; **Fac Appt:** Assoc Prof ObG, Univ Pittsburgh

Koulos, John MD [GO] - **Spec Exp:** Cervical Cancer; Uterine Cancer; Ovarian Cancer; **Hospital:** Beth Israel Med Ctr - Petrie Division (page 71); **Address:** Beth Israel Hosp Cancer Ctr, 10 Union Square E, Ste 4C, New York, NY 10003; **Phone:** 212-844-5729; **Board Cert:** Obstetrics & Gynecology 2006; Gynecologic Oncology 2006; **Med School:** Northwestern Univ 1978; **Resid:** Obstetrics & Gynecology, Northwestern Univ Med Sch 1982; **Fellow:** Gynecologic Oncology, Meml Sloan Kettering Cancer Ctr 1984; **Fac Appt:** Assoc Prof ObG, NY Med Coll

Lele, Shashikant B MD [GO] - **Spec Exp:** Gynecologic Cancer; Ovarian Cancer; **Hospital:** Roswell Park Cancer Inst, Buffalo General Hosp; **Address:** Roswell Park Cancer Inst, Dept Gynecology, Elm & Carlton Sts, Buffalo, NY 14263; **Phone:** 716-845-5776; **Board Cert:** Obstetrics & Gynecology 1976; Gynecologic Oncology 1979; **Med School:** India 1968; **Resid:** Obstetrics & Gynecology, JJ Hosp-Grant Med Ctr 1970; Obstetrics & Gynecology, Mt Sinai Hosp 1973; **Fellow:** Gynecologic Oncology, Roswell Park Cancer Inst 1976; **Fac Appt:** Clin Prof ObG, SUNY Buffalo

Morgan, Mark A MD [GO] - **Spec Exp:** Laparoscopic Surgery; Gynecologic Surgery-Complex; Gynecologic Cancer; Robotic Surgery; **Hospital:** Fox Chase Cancer Ctr (page 72); **Address:** Fox Chase Cancer Ctr-Gyn Oncology, 333 Cottman Ave, Philadelphia, PA 19111; **Phone:** 215-214-1430; **Board Cert:** Obstetrics & Gynecology 2007; Gynecologic Oncology 2007; **Med School:** SUNY Downstate 1982; **Resid:** Obstetrics & Gynecology, Hosp Univ Penn 1986; **Fellow:** Gynecologic Oncology, Hosp Univ Penn 1988

Odunsi, Adekunle O MD/PhD [GO] - **Spec Exp:** Ovarian Cancer; Immunotherapy; Clinical Trials; **Hospital:** Roswell Park Cancer Inst; **Address:** Roswell Park Cancer Inst, Gyn Oncology, Elm and Carlton Streets, Buffalo, NY 14263; **Phone:** 716-845-2300; **Board Cert:** Obstetrics & Gynecology 2004; Gynecologic Oncology 2004; **Med School:** Nigeria 1984; **Resid:** Obstetrics & Gynecology, Rosie Maternity & Addenbrookes Hosps 1990; Obstetrics & Gynecology, Yale-New Haven Hosp 1999; **Fellow:** Gynecologic Oncology, Roswell Park Cancer Inst 2001; **Fac Appt:** Prof ObG, SUNY Buffalo

Randall, Thomas C MD [GO] - **Spec Exp:** Gynecologic Cancer; Pelvic Reconstruction; Robotic Surgery; **Hospital:** Pennsylvania Hosp (page 81); **Address:** Pennsylvania Hospital, Dept OB/GYN, 801 Spruce St Fl 7, Philadelphia, PA 19107; **Phone:** 215-829-2345; **Board Cert:** Obstetrics & Gynecology 2001; Gynecologic Oncology 2002; **Med School:** Johns Hopkins Univ 1987; **Resid:** Obstetrics & Gynecology, Johns Hopkins Hosp 1991; **Fellow:** Gynecologic Oncology, Hosp Univ Penn 1992; **Fac Appt:** Assoc Prof ObG, Univ Pennsylvania

Rosenblum, Norman G MD/PhD [GO] - **Spec Exp:** Ovarian Cancer; Uterine Cancer; Vulvar Disease/Cancer; **Hospital:** Thomas Jefferson Univ Hosp (page 83); **Address:** 834 Chesnut St, Ste 300, Philadelphia, PA 19107-5127; **Phone:** 215-955-6200; **Board Cert:** Obstetrics & Gynecology 2007; Gynecologic Oncology 2007; **Med School:** Jefferson Med Coll 1978; **Resid:** Obstetrics & Gynecology, Hosp Univ Penn 1982; **Fellow:** Gynecologic Oncology, Hosp Univ Penn 1984; **Fac Appt:** Prof ObG, Jefferson Med Coll

Rubin, Stephen C MD [GO] - **Spec Exp:** Gynecologic Cancer; Ovarian Cancer; Cervical Cancer; Uterine Cancer; **Hospital:** Hosp Univ Penn - UPHS (page 81); **Address:** Perelman Center, Jordan Gynecologic Ctr, 3400 Civic Center Blvd Fl 3 W, Philadelphia, PA 19104-4283; **Phone:** 215-662-3318; **Board Cert:** Obstetrics & Gynecology 2005; Gynecologic Oncology 2005; **Med School:** Univ Pennsylvania 1976; **Resid:** Obstetrics & Gynecology, Hosp Univ Penn 1980; **Fellow:** Gynecologic Oncology, Hosp Univ Penn 1982; **Fac Appt:** Prof ObG, Univ Pennsylvania

Southeast

Alvarez, Ronald D MD [GO] - **Spec Exp:** Gynecologic Cancer; Ovarian Cancer; **Hospital:** Univ of Ala Hosp at Birmingham, Brookwood Med Ctr; **Address:** Univ Alabama, Div Gyn Oncology, 619 19th St S, OHB 538, Birmingham, AL 35249-7333; **Phone:** 205-934-4986; **Board Cert:** Obstetrics & Gynecology 2007; Gynecologic Oncology 2007; **Med School:** Louisiana State U, New Orleans 1983; **Resid:** Obstetrics & Gynecology, Univ Alabama Hosp 1987; **Fellow:** Gynecologic Oncology, Univ Alabama Hosp 1990; **Fac Appt:** Assoc Prof ObG, Univ Alabama

Berchuck, Andrew MD [GO] - **Spec Exp:** Ovarian Cancer; Uterine Cancer; **Hospital:** Duke Univ Med Ctr; **Address:** Duke Univ Med Center, DUMC Box 3079, Durham, NC 27710; **Phone:** 919-684-3765; **Board Cert:** Obstetrics & Gynecology 1998; Gynecologic Oncology 1998; **Med School:** Case West Res Univ 1980; **Resid:** Obstetrics & Gynecology, Case Western Resrv 1984; **Fellow:** Gynecology, UT Southwestern 1985, Gynecologic Oncology, Meml Sloan-Kettering 1987; **Fac Appt:** Prof ObG, Duke Univ

Clarke-Pearson, Daniel L MD [GO] - **Spec Exp:** Pelvic Reconstruction; Gynecologic Surgery-Complex; Gynecologic Cancer; **Hospital:** Univ NC Hosps, Wesley Long Comm Hosp; **Address:** Univ of North Carolina, CB #7570, Chapel Hill, NC 27599; **Phone:** 919-966-5280; **Board Cert:** Obstetrics & Gynecology 2006; Gynecologic Oncology 2006; **Med School:** Case West Res Univ 1975; **Resid:** Obstetrics & Gynecology, Duke Univ Med Ctr 1979; **Fellow:** Gynecologic Oncology, Duke Univ Med Ctr 1981; **Fac Appt:** Prof ObG, Univ NC Sch Med

Creasman, William T MD [GO] - **Spec Exp:** Uterine Cancer; Ovarian Cancer; Cervical Cancer; **Hospital:** MUSC Med Ctr; **Address:** Med Univ S Carolina-Dept ObGyn, Charleston, SC 29425; **Phone:** 843-792-4509; **Board Cert:** Obstetrics & Gynecology 1991; Gynecologic Oncology 1974; **Med School:** Baylor Coll Med 1960; **Resid:** Obstetrics & Gynecology, Rochester Med Ctr 1967; **Fellow:** Gynecologic Oncology, Anderson Hosp Tumor Inst 1969; **Fac Appt:** Prof ObG, Med Univ SC

DePriest, Paul D MD [GO] - **Spec Exp:** Ovarian Cancer-Early Detection; Cervical Cancer; Pap Smear Abnormalities; **Hospital:** Univ of Kentucky Chandler Hosp; **Address:** Univ Kentucky Gynecologic Oncology, Whiteney Hendrickson Bldg, 800 Rose St, rm 331E1, Lexington, KY 40536; **Phone:** 859-323-5277; **Board Cert:** Obstetrics & Gynecology 2007; Gynecologic Oncology 2007; **Med School:** Univ KY Coll Med 1985; **Resid:** Obstetrics & Gynecology, Univ Kentucky Med Ctr 1989; **Fellow:** Gynecologic Oncology, Univ Kentucky Med Ctr 1991; **Fac Appt:** Prof ObG, Univ KY Coll Med

Finan, Michael A MD [GO] - **Spec Exp:** Ovarian Cancer; Cervical Cancer; Uterine Cancer; **Hospital:** Univ of S AL Med Ctr, USA Children & Women's Hospital; **Address:** 1660 Springhill Ave, Mobile, AL 36604; **Phone:** 251-665-8000; **Board Cert:** Obstetrics & Gynecology 2007; Gynecologic Oncology 2007; **Med School:** Louisiana State U, New Orleans 1986; **Resid:** Obstetrics & Gynecology, Univ South Fla Affil Hosps 1990; **Fellow:** Gynecologic Oncology, H Lee Moffitt Cancer Ctr 1992; **Fac Appt:** Prof ObG, Univ S Ala Coll Med

Gynecologic Oncology

Fiorica, James V MD [GO] - **Spec Exp:** Gynecologic Cancer; Breast Cancer; Cervical Cancer; **Hospital:** Sarasota Meml Hosp; **Address:** 1888 Hillview St, Sarasota, FL 34239; **Phone:** 941-917-8383; **Board Cert:** Obstetrics & Gynecology 2007; Gynecologic Oncology 2007; **Med School:** Tufts Univ 1982; **Resid:** Obstetrics & Gynecology, Univ South Fla Affil Hosp 1986; **Fellow:** Gynecologic Oncology, Univ South Fla Affil Hosp 1989; Breast Disease, Tufts Univ 1990; **Fac Appt:** Clin Prof ObG, Univ S Fla Coll Med

Fowler Jr, Wesley C MD [GO] - **Spec Exp:** Vulvar Disease/Cancer; DES-Exposed Females; Cancer Prevention; Gynecologic Cancer; **Hospital:** Univ NC Hosps; **Address:** UNC Chapel Hill, Div Ob/Gyn, Campus Box 7572, Chapel Hill, NC 27599-7572; **Phone:** 919-966-7822; **Board Cert:** Obstetrics & Gynecology 1991; Gynecologic Oncology 1979; **Med School:** Univ NC Sch Med 1966; **Resid:** Obstetrics & Gynecology, NC Memorial Hosp 1971; **Fellow:** Gynecologic Oncology, NC Memorial Hosp 1971; **Fac Appt:** Prof ObG, Univ NC Sch Med

Ghamande, Sharad A MD [GO] - **Spec Exp:** Ovarian Cancer; Clinical Trials; **Hospital:** Med Coll of GA Hosp and Clin (MCG Health Inc); **Address:** MCG Health System, 1120 15th St, Augusta, GA 30912; **Phone:** 706-721-6744; **Board Cert:** Obstetrics & Gynecology 2003; Gynecologic Oncology 2003; **Med School:** India 1990; **Resid:** Obstetrics & Gynecology, Boston Univ Hosp 1997; **Fellow:** Gynecologic Oncology, Roswell Park Canc Inst 2000; **Fac Appt:** Assoc Prof ObG, Med Coll GA

Horowitz, Ira R MD [GO] - **Spec Exp:** Laparoscopic Surgery; Ovarian Cancer; Cervical Cancer; **Hospital:** Emory Univ Hosp, Emory Univ Hosp Midtown; **Address:** Emory Clinic, 1365A Clifton Rd NE Fl 4, Atlanta, GA 30322; **Phone:** 404-778-4416; **Board Cert:** Obstetrics & Gynecology 2007; Gynecologic Oncology 2007; **Med School:** Baylor Coll Med 1980; **Resid:** Obstetrics & Gynecology, Baylor Affil Hosp 1984; **Fellow:** Gynecologic Oncology, Johns Hopkins Hosp 1987; **Fac Appt:** Prof ObG, Emory Univ

Kohler, Matthew F MD [GO] - **Spec Exp:** Pelvic Reconstruction; **Hospital:** MUSC Med Ctr; **Address:** MUSC Med Ctr- Women's Hlth Ob/Gyn, 86 Jonathan Lucas St, MS 957, Charleston, SC 29425; **Phone:** 843-792-9300; **Board Cert:** Obstetrics & Gynecology 2007; Gynecologic Oncology 2007; **Med School:** Duke Univ 1987; **Resid:** Obstetrics & Gynecology, Duke Univ Med Ctr 1991; **Fellow:** Gynecologic Oncology, Duke Univ Med Ctr 1994; **Fac Appt:** Assoc Prof ObG, Med Univ SC

Lancaster, Johnathan M MD/PhD [GO] - **Spec Exp:** Ovarian Cancer; Cancer Genetics; Gene Therapy; **Hospital:** H Lee Moffitt Cancer Ctr & Research Inst; **Address:** H Lee Moffitt Cancer Ctr - Gyn Oncology, 12902 Magnolia Drive, MC CGYNPROG, Tampa, FL 33612; **Phone:** 813-745-7272; **Board Cert:** Obstetrics & Gynecology 2008; Gynecologic Oncology 2008; **Med School:** Wales, UK 1997; **Resid:** Obstetrics & Gynecology, Duke Univ Med Ctr 2000; **Fellow:** Gynecologic Oncology, Duke Univ Med Ctr 2003; **Fac Appt:** Asst Prof ObG, Univ S Fla Coll Med

Lentz, Samuel S MD [GO] - **Spec Exp:** Gynecologic Cancer; Pelvic Reconstruction; Incontinence; Incontinence-Fecal; **Hospital:** Wake Forest Univ Baptist Med Ctr (page 84), Forsyth Med Ctr; **Address:** Wake Forest Univ Sch Med, Div Gyn Oncology, Medical Center Blvd, Winston-Salem, NC 27157; **Phone:** 336-716-6673; **Board Cert:** Obstetrics & Gynecology 2007; Gynecologic Oncology 2007; **Med School:** Wake Forest Univ 1978; **Resid:** Obstetrics & Gynecology, NC Baptist Hosp 1982; **Fellow:** Gynecologic Oncology, Mayo Clinic 1989; **Fac Appt:** Prof ObG, Wake Forest Univ

Lucci, Joseph A MD [GO] - **Spec Exp:** Cervical Cancer; **Hospital:** Univ of Miami Hosp (page 82), Jackson Meml Hosp (page 82); **Address:** Univ Miami Dept Ob/Gyn, 1611 NW 12th Ave, Ste 3003, Miami, FL 33136; **Phone:** 305-243-2233; **Board Cert:** Obstetrics & Gynecology 2007; Gynecologic Oncology 2007; **Med School:** Univ Tex, Houston 1984; **Resid:** Obstetrics & Gynecology, St Josephs Hosp 1988; **Fellow:** Gynecologic Oncology, UC Irvine 1992; **Fac Appt:** Clin Prof ObG, Univ Miami Sch Med

Makhija, Sharmila K MD [GO] - **Spec Exp:** Ovarian Cancer; Cervical Cancer; **Hospital:** Emory Univ Hosp; **Address:** The Emory Clinic Bldg A, 1365 Clifton Rd NE Fl 4, Atlanta, GA 30322; **Phone:** 404-778-3401; **Board Cert:** Obstetrics & Gynecology 2007; Gynecologic Oncology 2007; **Med School:** Univ Alabama 1992; **Resid:** Obstetrics & Gynecology, Univ Louisville Hosp 1996; **Fellow:** Gynecologic Oncology, Meml Sloan Kettering Cancer Ctr 1999; **Fac Appt:** Assoc Prof ObG, Emory Univ

Penalver, Manuel A MD [GO] - **Spec Exp:** Gynecologic Cancer; Cervical Cancer; Pelvic Tumors; **Hospital:** Doctors' Hosp, Baptist Hosp of Miami; **Address:** South Florida Gyn Oncology, 5000 University Drive, Ste 3300, Coral Gables, FL 33146; **Phone:** 305-663-7001; **Board Cert:** Obstetrics & Gynecology 2007; Gynecologic Oncology 2007; **Med School:** Univ Miami Sch Med 1977; **Resid:** Obstetrics & Gynecology, Univ Miami/Jackson Meml Hosp 1982; **Fellow:** Gynecologic Oncology, Univ Miami/Jackson Meml Hosp 1984

Poliakoff, Steven R MD [GO] - **Spec Exp:** Ovarian Cancer; Minimally Invasive Surgery; Cancer Genetics; Robotic Surgery; **Hospital:** Mount Sinai Med Ctr - Miami, South Miami Hosp; **Address:** 6280 Sunset Dr, Ste 502, South Miami, FL 33143-4870; **Phone:** 305-596-0870; **Board Cert:** Obstetrics & Gynecology 1983; **Med School:** Univ NC Sch Med 1975; **Resid:** Obstetrics & Gynecology, Johns Hopkins Hosp 1979; **Fellow:** Gynecologic Oncology, Jackson Meml Hosp/Univ Miami 1981

Soper, John T MD [GO] - **Spec Exp:** Gynecologic Cancer; **Hospital:** Univ NC Hosps; **Address:** Univ North Carolina, Dept OB/GYN, Physicians Office Bldg, 101 Manning Drive, Ste B-103, Chapel Hill, NC 27599-7572; **Phone:** 919-966-1195; **Board Cert:** Obstetrics & Gynecology 2007; Gynecologic Oncology 2007; **Med School:** Univ Iowa Coll Med 1978; **Resid:** Obstetrics & Gynecology, Univ Utah Med Ctr 1982; **Fellow:** Gynecologic Oncology, Duke Univ Med Ctr 1985; **Fac Appt:** Prof ObG, Univ NC Sch Med

Spann Jr, Cyril O MD [GO] - **Spec Exp:** Gynecologic Cancer; Ovarian Cancer; **Hospital:** Grady Hlth Sys, Emory Univ Hosp Midtown; **Address:** Dept Gynecology & Obstetrics, 69 Jesse Hill Jr Drive Fl 4, Atlanta, GA 30303; **Phone:** 404-686-8121; **Board Cert:** Obstetrics & Gynecology 2005; Gynecologic Oncology 2005; **Med School:** Meharry Med Coll 1981; **Resid:** Obstetrics & Gynecology, Emory Univ Med Ctr 1985; **Fellow:** Gynecologic Oncology, Univ NC Meml Hosp 1989; **Fac Appt:** Prof ObG, Emory Univ

Taylor Jr, Peyton T MD [GO] - **Spec Exp:** Gynecologic Surgery-Complex; Gynecologic Cancer; **Hospital:** Univ Virginia Med Ctr; **Address:** Univ VA Hlth Sys, Dept Ob/Gyn, PO Box 800712, Charlottesville, VA 22908; **Phone:** 434-924-9933; **Board Cert:** Obstetrics & Gynecology 1994; Gynecologic Oncology 1981; **Med School:** Univ Alabama 1968; **Resid:** Obstetrics & Gynecology, Univ VA Hosp 1970; Obstetrics & Gynecology, Univ VA Hosp 1975; **Fellow:** Surgical Oncology, Natl Cancer Inst 1972; Gynecologic Oncology, Univ Va Hosp 1977; **Fac Appt:** Prof ObG, Univ VA Sch Med

Van Nagell Jr, John R MD [GO] - **Spec Exp:** Ovarian Cancer; Cervical Cancer; **Hospital:** Univ of Kentucky Chandler Hosp; **Address:** UKMC, Dept Ob/Gyn, 800 Rose St, Lexington, KY 40536-0001; **Phone:** 859-323-5553; **Board Cert:** Obstetrics & Gynecology 1973; Gynecologic Oncology 1976; **Med School:** Univ Pennsylvania 1967; **Resid:** Obstetrics & Gynecology, Kentucky Med Ctr 1971; **Fac Appt:** Prof ObG, Univ KY Coll Med

Gynecologic Oncology

Midwest

Belinson, Jerome L MD [GO] - **Spec Exp:** Ovarian Cancer; Cervical Cancer; **Hospital:** Cleveland Clin Fdn (page 70); **Address:** 9500 Euclid Ave, Desk A81, Cleveland, OH 44195; **Phone:** 216-444-7933; **Board Cert:** Obstetrics & Gynecology 1998; Gynecologic Oncology 1980; **Med School:** Univ MO-Columbia Sch Med 1968; **Resid:** Obstetrics & Gynecology, Columbia Presby Med Ctr 1973; **Fellow:** Gynecologic Oncology, Jackson Meml Hosp 1977; **Fac Appt:** Prof ObG, Ohio State Univ

Cliby, William A MD [GO] - **Spec Exp:** Ovarian Cancer; **Hospital:** Mayo Med Ctr & Clin - Rochester; **Address:** Mayo Clinic, 200 First St SW, Rochester, MN 55905; **Phone:** 507-266-9323; **Board Cert:** Obstetrics & Gynecology 2007; Gynecologic Oncology 2007; **Med School:** Univ VT Coll Med 1987; **Resid:** Obstetrics & Gynecology, Duke Univ Med Ctr 1991; **Fellow:** Gynecologic Oncology, Mayo Clinic 1994; Research, Fred Hutchinson Cancer Rsch Ctr; **Fac Appt:** Prof ObG, Mayo Med Sch

Copeland, Larry J MD [GO] - **Spec Exp:** Ovarian Cancer; Uterine Cancer; Gynecologic Cancer; **Hospital:** Arthur G James Cancer Hosp & Research Inst, Ohio St Univ Med Ctr; **Address:** 1654 Upham Drive, Ste 505, Columbus, OH 43210-1250; **Phone:** 614-293-8697; **Board Cert:** Obstetrics & Gynecology 1991; Gynecologic Oncology 1981; **Med School:** Univ Western Ontario 1973; **Resid:** Obstetrics & Gynecology, McMaster Univ Affil Hosps 1977; **Fellow:** Gynecologic Oncology, MD Anderson Cancer Ctr-Univ Tex 1979; **Fac Appt:** Prof ObG, Ohio State Univ

De Geest, Koen MD [GO] - **Spec Exp:** Ovarian Cancer; Uterine Cancer; Clinical Trials; **Hospital:** Univ Iowa Hosp & Clinics; **Address:** Univ Iowa, Div Gynecological Oncology, 200 Hawkins Drive, rm 4630 JCP, Iowa City, IA 52242; **Phone:** 319-356-2015; **Board Cert:** Obstetrics & Gynecology 2007; Gynecologic Oncology 2007; **Med School:** Belgium 1977; **Resid:** Obstetrics & Gynecology, Univ Ghent 1982; **Fellow:** Gynecologic Oncology, Penn State/Hershey Med Ctr 1990; **Fac Appt:** Prof ObG, Univ Iowa Coll Med

Fowler, Jeffrey M MD [GO] - **Spec Exp:** Laparoscopic Surgery; Gynecologic Cancer; Robotic Surgery; Pelvic Reconstruction; **Hospital:** Ohio St Univ Med Ctr; **Address:** Ohio State Univ, Div Gynecologic Oncology, 320 W Tenth Ave, M-210 SLH, Columbus, OH 43210; **Phone:** 614-293-8737; **Board Cert:** Obstetrics & Gynecology 2007; Gynecologic Oncology 2007; **Med School:** Northwestern Univ 1985; **Resid:** Obstetrics & Gynecology, Ohio State Univ Hosp 1989; **Fellow:** Gynecologic Oncology, Cedars-Sinai Med Ctr 1991; **Fac Appt:** Prof ObG, Ohio State Univ

Johnston, Carolyn M MD [GO] - **Spec Exp:** Gynecologic Surgery-Complex; Cervical Cancer; **Hospital:** Univ Michigan Hlth Sys; **Address:** Womens Hosp-Div Gyn Oncology, 1500 E Med Ctr Drive, rm L4510, Ann Arbor, MI 48109-0276; **Phone:** 734-647-8906; **Board Cert:** Obstetrics & Gynecology 2000; Gynecologic Oncology 2000; **Med School:** Yale Univ 1984; **Resid:** Obstetrics & Gynecology, Univ Chicago Hosp 1988; **Fellow:** Gynecologic Oncology, Mt Sinai Hosp 1990; **Fac Appt:** Assoc Clin Prof ObG, Univ Mich Med Sch

Lurain, John R MD [GO] - **Spec Exp:** Gestational Trophoblastic Disease; Uterine Cancer; Ovarian Cancer; Cervical Cancer; **Hospital:** Northwestern Meml Hosp; **Address:** Northwestern Univ Feinberg Sch Med, 250 E Superior St, Ste 05-2168, Chicago, IL 60611-3056; **Phone:** 312-695-0990; **Board Cert:** Obstetrics & Gynecology 1977; Gynecologic Oncology 1981; **Med School:** Univ NC Sch Med 1972; **Resid:** Obstetrics & Gynecology, Univ Pittsburgh Med Ctr 1975; **Fellow:** Gynecologic Oncology, Roswell Park Cancer Inst 1979; **Fac Appt:** Prof ObG, Northwestern Univ

Moore, David H MD [GO] - **Spec Exp:** Cervical Cancer; Ovarian Cancer; Laparoscopic Surgery; Robotic Surgery; **Hospital:** St Francis Hosp; **Address:** Gynecologic Oncology of Indianapolis, 5255 E Stop 11 Rd, Ste 310, Indianapolis, IN 46237; **Phone:** 317-851-2555; **Board Cert:** Obstetrics & Gynecology 2007; Gynecologic Oncology 2007; **Med School:** Indiana Univ 1982; **Resid:** Obstetrics & Gynecology, Indiana Univ Hosp 1986; **Fellow:** Gynecologic Oncology, Univ N Carolina 1988

Mutch, David G MD [GO] - **Spec Exp:** Gynecologic Cancer; Pelvic Reconstruction; **Hospital:** Barnes-Jewish Hosp; **Address:** 4911 Barnes Jewish Hospital Plaza, St Louis, MO 63110; **Phone:** 314-362-3181; **Board Cert:** Obstetrics & Gynecology 2006; Gynecologic Oncology 2006; **Med School:** Washington Univ, St Louis 1980; **Resid:** Obstetrics & Gynecology, Barnes Hosp-Wash Univ 1984; **Fellow:** Gynecologic Oncology, Duke Univ Med Ctr 1987; **Fac Appt:** Prof ObG, Washington Univ, St Louis

Potkul, Ronald MD [GO] - **Spec Exp:** Ovarian Cancer; Cervical Cancer; **Hospital:** Loyola Univ Med Ctr; **Address:** Loyola Univ Med Ctr, 2160 S 1st Ave Bldg 112 - rm 267, Maywood, IL 60153; **Phone:** 708-327-3500; **Board Cert:** Obstetrics & Gynecology 1997; Gynecologic Oncology 1997; **Med School:** Univ Chicago-Pritzker Sch Med 1981; **Resid:** Obstetrics & Gynecology, Univ Chicago Hosps 1985; **Fellow:** Gynecologic Oncology, Georgetown Univ Hosp 1988; **Fac Appt:** Prof ObG, Loyola Univ-Stritch Sch Med

Rader, Janet S MD [GO] - **Spec Exp:** Cervical Cancer; Ovarian Cancer; Uterine Cancer; **Hospital:** Barnes-Jewish Hosp, Missouri Baptist Med Ctr; **Address:** 660 S Euclid Ave, Box 8064, St Louis, MO 63110; **Phone:** 314-362-3181; **Board Cert:** Obstetrics & Gynecology 2007; Gynecologic Oncology 2007; **Med School:** Univ MO-Columbia Sch Med 1983; **Resid:** Obstetrics & Gynecology, Michael Reese Hosp 1987; **Fellow:** Gynecologic Oncology, Johns Hopkins Hosp 1990; **Fac Appt:** Prof ObG, Washington Univ, St Louis

Reynolds, R Kevin MD [GO] - **Hospital:** Univ Michigan Hlth Sys; **Address:** Women's Hosp, Div Gyn Onc, 1500 E Med Ctr Drive, rm L4510, Ann Arbor, MI 48109-0276; **Phone:** 734-764-9106; **Board Cert:** Obstetrics & Gynecology 2007; Gynecologic Oncology 2007; **Med School:** Univ New Mexico 1982; **Resid:** Obstetrics & Gynecology, Univ Vt Hosp 1986; **Fellow:** Gynecologic Oncology, Univ Mich Med Ctr 1991; **Fac Appt:** Asst Prof ObG, Univ Mich Med Sch

Rice, Laurel W MD [GO] - **Spec Exp:** Ovarian Cancer; Uterine Cancer; Cervical Cancer; **Hospital:** Univ WI Hosp & Clins; **Address:** 1 S Park St, Ste 555, Madison, WI 53715; **Phone:** 608-263-3194; **Board Cert:** Obstetrics & Gynecology 2006; Gynecologic Oncology 2006; **Med School:** Univ Colorado 1983; **Resid:** Obstetrics & Gynecology, Brigham-Womens Hosp 1987; **Fellow:** Obstetrics & Gynecology, Brigham-Womens Hosp 1989; **Fac Appt:** Assoc Prof ObG, Univ VA Sch Med

Rose, Peter G MD [GO] - **Spec Exp:** Cervical Cancer; Ovarian Cancer; Uterine Cancer; **Hospital:** Cleveland Clin Fdn (page 70), MetroHealth Med Ctr; **Address:** Cleveland Clinic Fdn, 9500 Euclid Ave A-81, Cleveland, OH 44195; **Phone:** 216-444-1712; **Board Cert:** Obstetrics & Gynecology 2007; Gynecologic Oncology 2007; **Med School:** Boston Univ 1981; **Resid:** Surgery, Vanderbilt Univ Med Ctr 1983; Obstetrics & Gynecology, Ohio State Univ Med Ctr 1986; **Fellow:** Gynecologic Oncology, Roswell Park Med Ctr 1988; **Fac Appt:** Prof ObG, Case West Res Univ

Rotmensch, Jacob MD [GO] - **Spec Exp:** Gynecologic Cancer; Ovarian Cancer; Cervical Cancer; **Hospital:** Rush Univ Med Ctr; **Address:** University Gynecologic Oncology Assocs, 1725 W Harrison St, Ste 829, Chicago, IL 60612; **Phone:** 312-942-6300; **Board Cert:** Obstetrics & Gynecology 2007; Gynecologic Oncology 2007; **Med School:** Meharry Med Coll 1977; **Resid:** Obstetrics & Gynecology, Johns Hopkins Hosp 1981; **Fellow:** Gynecologic Oncology, Johns Hopkins Hosp 1984; **Fac Appt:** Prof ObG, Rush Med Coll

Gynecologic Oncology

Schink, Julian C MD [GO] - **Spec Exp:** Ovarian Cancer; **Hospital:** Northwestern Meml Hosp; **Address:** 675 N St Clair St, Fl 21 - Ste 100, Chicago, IL 60611; **Phone:** 312-695-0990; **Board Cert:** Obstetrics & Gynecology 2000; Gynecologic Oncology 2000; **Med School:** Univ Tex, San Antonio 1982; **Resid:** Obstetrics & Gynecology, Northwestern Univ Med Sch 1986; **Fellow:** Gynecologic Oncology, UCLA Med Ctr 1988; **Fac Appt:** Prof ObG, Northwestern Univ

Smith, Donna M MD [GO] - **Spec Exp:** Cervical Cancer; Ovarian Cancer; **Hospital:** Loyola Univ Med Ctr; **Address:** Cardinal Bernardin Cancer Ctr, Clinic A, 2160 S 1st Ave Bldg 112 - rm 267, Maywood, IL 60153; **Phone:** 708-327-3500; **Board Cert:** Obstetrics & Gynecology 2007; Gynecologic Oncology 2007; **Med School:** Univ MO-Kansas City 1980; **Resid:** Obstetrics & Gynecology, Emory Univ Hosp 1984; **Fellow:** Gynecologic Oncology, Georgetown Univ Med Ctr 1987; **Fac Appt:** Assoc Prof ObG, Loyola Univ-Stritch Sch Med

Stehman, Frederick B MD [GO] - **Spec Exp:** Clinical Trials; Gynecologic Cancer; **Hospital:** Indiana Univ Hosp (page 74), Wishard Hlth Srvs; **Address:** Indiana Univ Hosp, Dept ObGyn, 535 Barnhill, Rt 433, Indianapolis, IN 46202; **Phone:** 317-274-7241; **Board Cert:** Obstetrics & Gynecology 2005; Gynecologic Oncology 2003; **Med School:** Univ Mich Med Sch 1972; **Resid:** Obstetrics & Gynecology, Univ Kansas Med Ctr 1975; Surgery, Univ Kansas Med Ctr 1977; **Fellow:** Gynecologic Oncology, UCLA Med Ctr 1979; **Fac Appt:** Prof ObG, Indiana Univ

Waggoner, Steven MD [GO] - **Spec Exp:** Ovarian Cancer; Cervical Cancer; Uterine Cancer; **Hospital:** Univ Hosps Case Med Ctr; **Address:** Dept Ob/Gyn, Div Gyn Oncology, 11100 Euclid Ave, rm 7136, Cleveland, OH 44106; **Phone:** 216-844-3954; **Board Cert:** Obstetrics & Gynecology 2007; Gynecologic Oncology 2007; **Med School:** Univ Wash 1984; **Resid:** Obstetrics & Gynecology, Univ Chicago Hosps 1988; **Fellow:** Gynecologic Oncology, Georgetown Univ 1991; **Fac Appt:** Prof ObG, Case West Res Univ

Great Plains and Mountains

Davidson, Susan MD [GO] - **Spec Exp:** Gynecologic Cancer; **Hospital:** Univ Colorado Hosp; **Address:** Univ Colorado Hosp, Dept OB/GYN, 12631 E 17th Ave B198-4 Bldg, Box 6511, Denver, CO 80262; **Phone:** 720-848-1060; **Board Cert:** Obstetrics & Gynecology 2007; Gynecologic Oncology 2007; **Med School:** Univ Tex, San Antonio 1984; **Resid:** Obstetrics & Gynecology, Univ Texas Med Ctr 1988; **Fellow:** Gynecologic Oncology, Meml Sloan Kettering Cancer Ctr 1990; **Fac Appt:** Assoc Prof ObG, Univ Colorado

Remmenga, Steven W MD [GO] - **Spec Exp:** Ovarian Cancer; Cervical Cancer; Gynecologic Cancer; **Hospital:** Nebraska Med Ctr; **Address:** Univ Nebraska Med Ctr, Gyne Oncology, 983255 Nebraska Med Ctr, Omaha, NE 68198-3255; **Phone:** 402-559-5068; **Board Cert:** Obstetrics & Gynecology 1998; Gynecologic Oncology 1998; **Med School:** Univ Nebr Coll Med 1981; **Resid:** Obstetrics & Gynecology, Naval Hospital 1986; **Fellow:** Gynecologic Oncology, Walter Reed Army Med Ctr 1990; **Fac Appt:** Assoc Prof ObG, Univ Nebr Coll Med

Soisson, Andrew P MD [GO] - **Spec Exp:** Cervical Cancer; **Hospital:** LDS Hosp, Univ Utah Hosps and Clins; **Address:** Univ Hosp, Div Gyn Oncology, 30 N 1900 E, rm 2B200, Salt Lake City, UT 84132; **Phone:** 801-587-4399; **Board Cert:** Obstetrics & Gynecology 2006; Gynecologic Oncology 2006; **Med School:** Georgetown Univ 1981; **Resid:** Obstetrics & Gynecology, Madigan AMC 1985; **Fellow:** Gynecologic Oncology, Duke Univ Med Ctr 1990; **Fac Appt:** Assoc Prof ObG, Univ Utah

Southwest

Burnett, Alexander F MD [GO] - **Spec Exp:** Laparoscopic Surgery; Fertility Preservation in Cancer; Gynecologic Cancer; **Hospital:** UAMS Med Ctr; **Address:** 4301 W Markham St, Slot 793, Little Rock, AR 72205; **Phone:** 501-296-1099; **Board Cert:** Obstetrics & Gynecology 2007; Gynecologic Oncology 2007; **Med School:** Georgetown Univ 1986; **Resid:** Obstetrics & Gynecology, Georgetown Univ Affil Hosp 1990; **Fellow:** Gynecologic Oncology, Georgetown Univ Affil Hosp 1993; **Fac Appt:** Assoc Prof ObG, Univ Ark

Chambers, Setsuko K MD [GO] - **Spec Exp:** Gynecologic Cancer; Breast Cancer; Ovarian Cancer; **Hospital:** Univ Med Ctr - Tucson; **Address:** 1515 N Campbell Ave, Arizona Cancer Center, Tucson, AZ 85724; **Phone:** 520-626-9285; **Board Cert:** Obstetrics & Gynecology 2007; Gynecologic Oncology 2007; **Med School:** Brown Univ 1980; **Resid:** Obstetrics & Gynecology, Yale-New Haven Hosp 1984; **Fellow:** Gynecologic Oncology, Yale-New Haven Hosp 1986; **Fac Appt:** Prof ObG, Univ Ariz Coll Med

Follen, Michele MD/PhD [GO] - **Spec Exp:** Gynecologic Cancer; Clinical Trials; Cervical Cancer; **Hospital:** UT MD Anderson Cancer Ctr; **Address:** MD Anderson Cancer Ctr, 1515 Holcombe Blvd, Unit 1362, Houston, TX 77030; **Phone:** 713-745-2564; **Board Cert:** Obstetrics & Gynecology 1999; Gynecologic Oncology 1999; **Med School:** Univ Mich Med Sch 1980; **Resid:** Obstetrics & Gynecology, Columbia-Presby Med Ctr 1983; **Fellow:** Gynecologic Oncology, MD Anderson Cancer Ctr 1986; **Fac Appt:** Prof ObG, Univ Tex, Houston

Fromm, Geri-Lynn MD [GO] - **Spec Exp:** Cervical Cancer; Ovarian Cancer; Gestational Trophoblastic Disease; **Hospital:** St Luke's Episcopal Hosp-Houston, Woman's Hosp TX; **Address:** 2223 Dorrington St, Houston, TX 77030; **Phone:** 713-665-0404; **Board Cert:** Obstetrics & Gynecology 2007; Gynecologic Oncology 2007; **Med School:** Northwestern Univ 1981; **Resid:** Obstetrics & Gynecology, Magee Womens Hosp 1985; **Fellow:** Gynecologic Oncology, MD Anderson Cancer Ctr 1987; **Fac Appt:** Assoc Clin Prof ObG, Baylor Coll Med

Gershenson, David M MD [GO] - **Spec Exp:** Ovarian Rare & Borderline Tumors; Uterine Cancer-Serous Carcinoma; Fertility Preservation in Cancer; Sex Cord-Stromal Tumors; **Hospital:** UT MD Anderson Cancer Ctr, St Luke's Episcopal Hosp-Houston; **Address:** Univ Tex MD Anderson Cancer Ctr, PO Box 301439, Houston, TX 77030-1439; **Phone:** 713-745-2565; **Board Cert:** Obstetrics & Gynecology 1991; Gynecologic Oncology 1981; **Med School:** Vanderbilt Univ 1971; **Resid:** Obstetrics & Gynecology, Yale New Haven Hosp 1975; **Fellow:** Gynecologic Oncology, MD Anderson Cancer Ctr 1979; **Fac Appt:** Prof ObG, Univ Tex, Houston

Hatch, Kenneth MD [GO] - **Spec Exp:** Cervical Cancer; **Hospital:** Univ Med Ctr - Tucson, NW Med Ctr; **Address:** Univ Arizona College of Medicine, 1515 N Campbell Ave, rm 1968, Tucson, AZ 85724; **Phone:** 520-626-9285; **Board Cert:** Obstetrics & Gynecology 1993; Gynecologic Oncology 1981; **Med School:** Univ Nebr Coll Med 1971; **Resid:** Obstetrics & Gynecology, Univ AL Med Ctr Birmingham 1976; **Fellow:** Gynecologic Oncology, Univ AL Med Ctr Birmingham 1978; **Fac Appt:** Prof ObG, Univ Ariz Coll Med

Levenback, Charles MD [GO] - **Spec Exp:** Vulvar Disease/Cancer; Cervical Cancer; Gynecologic Cancer; **Hospital:** UT MD Anderson Cancer Ctr; **Address:** PO Box 301439 - Unit 1362, Houston, TX 77230; **Phone:** 713-745-2563; **Board Cert:** Obstetrics & Gynecology 2007; Gynecologic Oncology 2007; **Med School:** Mount Sinai Sch Med 1983; **Resid:** Obstetrics & Gynecology, Albert Einstein Coll Med 1987; **Fellow:** Gynecologic Oncology, Meml Sloan Kettering Cancer Ctr 1989; **Fac Appt:** Prof ObG, Univ Tex, Houston

Gynecologic Oncology

Lu, Karen Hsieh MD [GO] - **Spec Exp:** Ovarian Cancer; Ovarian Cancer-Early Detection; Uterine Cancer; Cancer Genetics; **Hospital:** UT MD Anderson Cancer Ctr; **Address:** Univ of Texas MD Anderson Cancer Ctr, 1515 Holcombe Blvd, Houston, TX 77030; **Phone:** 713-745-8902; **Board Cert:** Obstetrics & Gynecology 2003; Gynecologic Oncology 2003; **Med School:** Yale Univ 1991; **Resid:** Obstetrics & Gynecology, Brigham & Women's Hosp 1994; **Fellow:** Gynecologic Oncology, Brigham & Women's Hosp 1999; **Fac Appt:** Prof ObG, Univ Tex SW, Dallas

Magrina, Javier MD [GO] - **Spec Exp:** Gynecologic Cancer; Robotic Surgery; Minimally Invasive Surgery; **Hospital:** Mayo Clinic - Scottsdale; **Address:** Mayo Clinic, 5779 E Mayo Blvd, Phoenix, AZ 85054; **Phone:** 480-342-2668; **Board Cert:** Obstetrics & Gynecology 1994; Gynecologic Oncology 1982; **Med School:** Spain 1972; **Resid:** Obstetrics & Gynecology, Mayo Clinic 1977; **Fellow:** Gynecologic Oncology, Kansas Med Ctr 1980; **Fac Appt:** Prof ObG, Mayo Med Sch

Sood, Anil K MD [GO] - **Hospital:** UT MD Anderson Cancer Ctr; **Address:** Univ Texas MD Anderson Cancer Ctr, 1515 Holcombe Blvd Ste 440, Houston, TX 77030-4000; **Phone:** 713-745-5266; **Board Cert:** Obstetrics & Gynecology 1999; Gynecologic Oncology 2001; **Med School:** Univ NC Sch Med 1991; **Resid:** Obstetrics & Gynecology, Univ FL 1995; **Fellow:** Gynecologic Oncology, Univ NC Sch Med 1998

Walker, Joan L MD [GO] - **Spec Exp:** Ovarian Cancer; Cervical Cancer; Uterine Cancer; **Hospital:** OU Med Ctr; **Address:** OU Health Science Ctr, Dept Ob/Gyn, PO Box 26901, Oklahoma City, OK 73126; **Phone:** 405-271-8707; **Board Cert:** Obstetrics & Gynecology 2007; Gynecologic Oncology 2007; **Med School:** UCLA 1982; **Resid:** Obstetrics & Gynecology, Hosp Univ Penn 1986; **Fellow:** Gynecologic Oncology, UC-Irvine 1990; **Fac Appt:** Assoc Prof ObG, Univ Okla Coll Med

West Coast and Pacific

Berek, Jonathan S MD [GO] - **Spec Exp:** Ovarian Cancer; Uterine Cancer; Cervical Cancer; Vulvar & Vaginal Cancer; **Hospital:** Stanford Univ Med Ctr; **Address:** Stanford Univ School of Medicine, 300 Pasteur Dr, HH333, Stanford, CA 94305-2296; **Phone:** 650-498-6000; **Board Cert:** Obstetrics & Gynecology 2008; Gynecologic Oncology 2008; **Med School:** Johns Hopkins Univ 1975; **Resid:** Obstetrics & Gynecology, Brigham & Womans Hosp 1979; **Fellow:** Gynecologic Oncology, UCLA Sch Med 1981; **Fac Appt:** Prof ObG, Stanford Univ

Berman, Michael L MD [GO] - **Spec Exp:** Gynecologic Cancer; Cervical Cancer; **Hospital:** UC Irvine Med Ctr, Long Beach Meml Med Ctr; **Address:** Cho Family Comprehensive Cancer Ctr, 101 The City Drive Bldg 56 - Ste 260, Orange, CA 92868-3201; **Phone:** 714-456-8020; **Board Cert:** Obstetrics & Gynecology 2005; Gynecologic Oncology 2005; **Med School:** Geo Wash Univ 1967; **Resid:** Obstetrics & Gynecology, GW Univ Hosp 1969; Obstetrics & Gynecology, LAC-Harbor Hosp 1974; **Fellow:** Gynecologic Oncology, UCLA Med Ctr 1976; **Fac Appt:** Prof ObG, UC Irvine

Carney, Michael E MD [GO] - **Spec Exp:** Gynecologic Cancer; Pelvic Surgery-Complex; Minimally Invasive Surgery; **Hospital:** Kapiolani Med Ctr for Women & Chldn; **Address:** Kapiolani Med Ctr for Women & Children, 1319 Punahou St, Ste 640, Honolulu, HI 96826; **Phone:** 808-983-6090; **Board Cert:** Obstetrics & Gynecology 2002; Gynecologic Oncology 2002; **Med School:** Loyola Univ-Stritch Sch Med 1990; **Resid:** Obstetrics & Gynecology, Duke Univ Med Ctr 1994; **Fellow:** Gynecologic Oncology, Duke Univ Med Ctr 1999; **Fac Appt:** Asst Prof ObG, Univ Hawaii JA Burns Sch Med

Di Saia, Philip J MD [GO] - **Spec Exp:** Ovarian Cancer; Gynecologic Cancer; Cervical Cancer; **Hospital:** UC Irvine Med Ctr; **Address:** 101 The City Drive Bldg 56 - rm 800, Route 80, Orange, CA 92668; **Phone:** 714-456-8000; **Board Cert:** Obstetrics & Gynecology 1983; Gynecologic Oncology 1974; **Med School:** Tufts Univ 1963; **Resid:** Obstetrics & Gynecology, Yale-New Haven Hosp 1967; **Fellow:** Gynecologic Oncology, MD Anderson Hosp 1971; **Fac Appt:** Prof ObG, UC Irvine

Goff, Barbara A MD [GO] - **Spec Exp:** Ovarian Cancer; Uterine Cancer; Cervical Cancer; Gynecologic Surgery-Complex; **Hospital:** Univ Wash Med Ctr; **Address:** Univ Washington, Dept ObGyn, Box 356460, Seattle, WA 98195; **Phone:** 206-288-2273; **Board Cert:** Obstetrics & Gynecology 2007; Gynecologic Oncology 2007; **Med School:** Univ Pennsylvania 1986; **Resid:** Obstetrics & Gynecology, Mass Genl Hosp/Brigham & Womens Hosp 1990; **Fellow:** Gynecologic Oncology, Mass Genl Hosp 1993; **Fac Appt:** Prof ObG, Univ Wash

Greer, Benjamin E MD [GO] - **Spec Exp:** Gynecologic Cancer; **Hospital:** Univ Wash Med Ctr; **Address:** Univ Wash, Dept OB/GYN, Box 356460, Seattle, WA 98195; **Phone:** 206-288-2273; **Board Cert:** Obstetrics & Gynecology 2002; Gynecologic Oncology 2002; **Med School:** Univ Pennsylvania 1966; **Resid:** Obstetrics & Gynecology, Univ Colorado Med Ctr 1970; **Fac Appt:** Prof ObG, Univ Wash

Karlan, Beth Y MD [GO] - **Spec Exp:** Ovarian Cancer; Gynecologic Cancer; **Hospital:** Cedars-Sinai Med Ctr; **Address:** 8700 Beverly Blvd, Ste 290W, Los Angeles, CA 90048; **Phone:** 310-423-3302; **Board Cert:** Obstetrics & Gynecology 1998; Gynecologic Oncology 1998; **Med School:** Harvard Med Sch 1982; **Resid:** Obstetrics & Gynecology, Yale-New Haven Hosp 1986; **Fellow:** Gynecologic Oncology, UCLA 1989; **Fac Appt:** Prof ObG, UCLA

Monk, Bradley J MD [GO] - **Spec Exp:** Gynecologic Surgery-Complex; Cervical Cancer; Ovarian Cancer; Gynecologic Cancer; **Hospital:** UC Irvine Med Ctr; **Address:** UC Irvine Comprehensive Cancer Ctr, 101 The City Drive Bldg 56 - rm 260, Irvine, CA 92868; **Phone:** 714-456-6570; **Board Cert:** Obstetrics & Gynecology 2007; Gynecologic Oncology 2007; **Med School:** Univ Ariz Coll Med 1988; **Resid:** Obstetrics & Gynecology, UCLA Med Ctr 1992; **Fellow:** Gynecologic Oncology, UC Irvine Med Ctr 1995; **Fac Appt:** Assoc Prof ObG, UC Irvine

Muntz, Howard G MD [GO] - **Spec Exp:** Gynecologic Cancer; Ovarian Cancer; Clinical Trials; Gynecologic Surgery-Complex; **Hospital:** Northwest Hosp; **Address:** Women's Cancer Care of Seattle, 1560 N 115th St, Ste 101, Seattle, WA 98133; **Phone:** 206-368-6806; **Board Cert:** Obstetrics & Gynecology 2007; Gynecologic Oncology 2007; **Med School:** Harvard Med Sch 1984; **Resid:** Obstetrics & Gynecology, Brigham & Womens Hosp 1988; **Fellow:** Gynecologic Oncology, Mass General Hosp 1991; **Fac Appt:** Assoc Clin Prof ObG, Univ Wash

Powell, Catherine Bethan MD [GO] - **Spec Exp:** Gynecologic Cancer; Cancer Genetics; **Hospital:** Kaiser Permanente S San Francisco Med Ctr; **Address:** Kaiser Permanente Medical Group Inc, 2238 Geary Blvd Fl 5, San Francisco, CA 94115; **Phone:** 415-833-4199; **Board Cert:** Obstetrics & Gynecology 2007; Gynecologic Oncology 2007; **Med School:** Univ Pennsylvania 1982; **Resid:** Obstetrics & Gynecology, Pennsylvania Hosp 1987; **Fellow:** Gynecologic Oncology, Wash Univ 1990

Smith, Lloyd H MD [GO] - **Spec Exp:** Ovarian Cancer; Uterine Cancer; Vulvar Disease/Cancer; Vaginal Cancer; **Hospital:** UC Davis Med Ctr, Sutter Mem Hospital-Sacramento; **Address:** UC Davis Med Ctr, Dept Ob/Gyn, 4860 Y St, Ste 2500, Sacramento, CA 95817-2307; **Phone:** 916-734-6946; **Board Cert:** Obstetrics & Gynecology 1998; Gynecologic Oncology 1998; **Med School:** UC Davis 1981; **Resid:** Obstetrics & Gynecology, UC Davis Med Ctr 1985; **Fellow:** Gynecologic Oncology, Stanford Univ Hosp 1988; **Fac Appt:** Prof ObG, UC Davis

Gynecologic Oncology

Spirtos, Nicola Michael MD [GO] - **Spec Exp:** Gynecologic Cancer; Ovarian Cancer; **Hospital:** Univ Med Ctr - Las Vegas; **Address:** 3131 La Canada St, Ste 110, Las Vegas, NV 89169; **Phone:** 702-693-6870; **Board Cert:** Obstetrics & Gynecology 1998; Gynecologic Oncology 1998; **Med School:** Northwestern Univ 1980; **Resid:** Obstetrics & Gynecology, Women's Hosp LAC-USC Med Ctr 1984; **Fellow:** Gynecologic Oncology, Stanford Univ Affil Hosp 1987

Stern, Jeffrey L MD [GO] - **Spec Exp:** Laparoscopic Surgery; Vulvar Disease/Cancer; **Hospital:** Alta Bates Summit Med Ctr-Alta Bates Campus; **Address:** Womens Cancer Ctr Northern Calif, 2001 Dwight Way, Berkley, CA 94704; **Phone:** 510-204-5770; **Board Cert:** Obstetrics & Gynecology 1983; Gynecologic Oncology 1984; **Med School:** SUNY Upstate Med Univ 1976; **Resid:** Obstetrics & Gynecology, Johns Hopkins Hosp 1980; **Fellow:** Gynecologic Oncology, USC Med Ctr 1982

Teng, Nelson NH MD/PhD [GO] - **Spec Exp:** Ovarian Cancer; Clinical Trials; **Hospital:** Stanford Univ Med Ctr; **Address:** Dept Gyn Oncology, 875 Blake Wilbur Drive, Stanford, CA 94305-5317; **Phone:** 650-498-8080; **Board Cert:** Obstetrics & Gynecology 2003; Gynecologic Oncology 2003; **Med School:** Univ Miami Sch Med 1977; **Resid:** Obstetrics & Gynecology, UCLA Med Ctr 1981; **Fellow:** Gynecologic Oncology, Stanford Univ Sch Med 1984; **Fac Appt:** Assoc Prof ObG, Stanford Univ

OBSTETRICS & GYNECOLOGY

New England

Cramer, Daniel W MD [ObG] - **Spec Exp:** Ovarian Cancer; Ovarian Cancer-High Risk; **Hospital:** Dana-Farber Cancer Inst, Brigham & Women's Hosp; **Address:** Brigham & Women's Hosp, Ob/Gyn Epidemiology Ctr, 221 Longwood Ave, RFB 366, Boston, MA 02115; **Phone:** 617-732-4895; **Board Cert:** Obstetrics & Gynecology 1979; **Med School:** Univ Colorado 1970; **Resid:** Obstetrics & Gynecology, Boston Womens Hosp 1976; **Fellow:** Public Health, Harvard Med Sch 1982; **Fac Appt:** Prof ObG, Harvard Med Sch

Noller, Kenneth L MD [ObG] - **Spec Exp:** DES-Exposed Females; **Hospital:** Tufts Med Ctr; **Address:** Tufts New England Med Ctr, Box 324, 800 Washington St, Boston, MA 02111; **Phone:** 617-636-2382; **Board Cert:** Obstetrics & Gynecology 1991; **Med School:** Creighton Univ 1970; **Resid:** Obstetrics & Gynecology, Mayo Clinic 1974; **Fac Appt:** Prof ObG, Tufts Univ

Southeast

Morgan, Linda S MD [ObG] - **Spec Exp:** Gynecologic Cancer; **Hospital:** Shands at Univ of FL; **Address:** 25 SW Archer Rd, Gainesville, FL 32610; **Phone:** 352-265-8200; **Board Cert:** Obstetrics & Gynecology 2006; Gynecologic Oncology 2006; **Med School:** Med Coll PA Hahnemann 1975; **Resid:** Obstetrics & Gynecology, Shands Hosp 1979; **Fellow:** Gynecologic Oncology, Mass Genl Hosp 1981; **Fac Appt:** Prof ObG, Univ Fla Coll Med

Midwest

Lipscomb, Gary H MD [ObG] - **Spec Exp:** Cervical Cancer; Pap Smear Abnormalities; **Hospital:** Northwestern Meml Hosp; **Address:** 680 N Lake Shore Drive, Ste 1015, Chicago, IL 60611; **Phone:** 312-695-7382; **Board Cert:** Obstetrics & Gynecology 2007; **Med School:** Univ Tenn Coll Med, Memphis 1981; **Resid:** Obstetrics & Gynecology, Univ Tenn Affil Hosps 1985; **Fac Appt:** Prof ObG, Northwestern Univ

Shulman, Lee P MD [ObG] - **Spec Exp:** Breast Cancer Genetics; Ovarian Cancer Genetics; **Hospital:** Northwestern Meml Hosp, Rush Univ Med Ctr; **Address:** Northwestern Univ, Dept Ob/Gyn, 250 E Superior St, Ste 05-2168, Chicago, IL 60611; **Phone:** 312-472-4683; **Board Cert:** Obstetrics & Gynecology 1999; Clinical Genetics 1990; **Med School:** Cornell Univ-Weill Med Coll 1983; **Resid:** Obstetrics & Gynecology, N Shore Univ Hosp 1987; **Fellow:** Reproductive Genetics, Univ Tenn Med Ctr 1989; **Fac Appt:** Prof ObG, Northwestern Univ

West Coast and Pacific

Parker, William H MD [ObG] - **Spec Exp:** Gynecologic Surgery; Gynecologic Cancer; **Hospital:** St John's Hlth Ctr, Santa Monica; **Address:** 1450 10th St, Ste 404, Santa Monica, CA 90401-2804; **Phone:** 310-451-8144; **Board Cert:** Obstetrics & Gynecology 1981; **Med School:** SUNY Downstate 1974; **Resid:** Obstetrics & Gynecology, UC San Diego 1978; **Fac Appt:** Clin Prof ObG, UCLA

REPRODUCTIVE ENDOCRINOLOGY

New England

Crowley, William F MD [RE] - **Spec Exp:** Fertility Preservation in Cancer; **Hospital:** Mass Genl Hosp; **Address:** Mass Genl Hosp, Reproductive Sci Ctr, 55 Fruit St, Bartlett Hall-Ext 5, Boston, MA 02114; **Phone:** 617-726-5390; **Board Cert:** Internal Medicine 1974; Endocrinology 1977; **Med School:** Tufts Univ 1969; **Resid:** Internal Medicine, Mass Genl Hosp 1971; Internal Medicine, Mass Genl Hosp 1974; **Fellow:** Endocrinology, Mass Genl Hosp 1976; **Fac Appt:** Prof Med, Harvard Med Sch

Ginsburg, Elizabeth MD [RE] - **Spec Exp:** Fertility Preservation in Cancer; **Hospital:** Brigham & Women's Hosp, Dana-Farber Cancer Inst; **Address:** Brigham & Womens Hosp, Reproductive Med, 75 Francis St, Ste 3300, Boston, MA 02115; **Phone:** 617-732-4222; **Board Cert:** Obstetrics & Gynecology 2007; Reproductive Endocrinology 2007; **Med School:** Mount Sinai Sch Med 1985; **Resid:** Obstetrics & Gynecology, Brigham & Womens Hosp 1989; **Fellow:** Reproductive Endocrinology, Brigham & Womens Hosp 1991

Patrizio, Pasquale MD [RE] - **Spec Exp:** Fertility Preservation in Cancer; **Hospital:** Yale-New Haven Hosp; **Address:** Yale Fertility Ctr, Dept OB/GYN, 150 Sargent Drive, New Haven, CT 06511; **Phone:** 203-785-4708; **Board Cert:** Obstetrics & Gynecology 2007; Reproductive Endocrinology 2007; **Med School:** Italy 1983; **Resid:** Obstetrics & Gynecology, Univ Naples 1987; Reproductive Endocrinology, Univ Pisa 1990; **Fellow:** Infertility, UC Irvine 1995; **Fac Appt:** Prof ObG, Yale Univ

Mid Atlantic

Coutifaris, Christos MD/PhD [RE] - **Spec Exp:** Fertility Preservation in Cancer; **Hospital:** Hosp Univ Penn - UPHS (page 81); **Address:** Penn Fertility Care, 3701 Market St Fl 8 - Ste 800, Philadelphia, PA 19104; **Phone:** 215-662-6100; **Board Cert:** Obstetrics & Gynecology 2006; Reproductive Endocrinology 2006; **Med School:** Univ Pennsylvania 1982; **Resid:** Obstetrics & Gynecology, Hosp Univ Penn 1986; **Fellow:** Reproductive Endocrinology, Hosp Univ Penn 1987; **Fac Appt:** Prof ObG, Univ Pennsylvania

Reproductive Endocrinology

Licciardi, Frederick L MD [RE] - **Spec Exp:** Fertility Preservation in Cancer; **Hospital:** NYU Langone Med Ctr (page 80); **Address:** NYU Medical Ctr, 660 First Ave, 5th Fl, New York, NY 10016; **Phone:** 212-263-7754; **Board Cert:** Obstetrics & Gynecology 2007; Reproductive Endocrinology 2007; **Med School:** UMDNJ-Rutgers Med Sch 1986; **Resid:** Obstetrics & Gynecology, St Barnabas Med Ctr 1990; **Fellow:** Reproductive Endocrinology, NY Hosp-Cornell Med Ctr 1992; **Fac Appt:** Assoc Prof ObG, NYU Sch Med

Noyes, Nicole MD [RE] - **Spec Exp:** Fertility Preservation in Cancer; **Hospital:** NYU Langone Med Ctr (page 80); **Address:** NYU Med Ctr, 660 First Ave, 5th FL, New York, NY 10016; **Phone:** 212-263-7981; **Board Cert:** Obstetrics & Gynecology 2007; Reproductive Endocrinology 2007; **Med School:** Univ VT Coll Med 1986; **Resid:** Obstetrics & Gynecology, NY Hosp-Cornell Med Ctr 1990; **Fellow:** Reproductive Endocrinology, NY Hosp-Cornell Med Ctr 1992; **Fac Appt:** Assoc Prof ObG, NYU Sch Med

Rosenwaks, Zev MD [RE] - **Spec Exp:** Fertility Preservation in Cancer; **Hospital:** NY-Presby Hosp/Weill Cornell (page 79); **Address:** Ctr For Reproductive Medicine & Infertility, 1305 York Ave Fl 6, New York, NY 10021-4872; **Phone:** 646-962-3743; **Board Cert:** Obstetrics & Gynecology 1978; Reproductive Endocrinology 1981; **Med School:** SUNY Downstate 1972; **Resid:** Obstetrics & Gynecology, LI Jewish Med Ctr 1976; **Fellow:** Reproductive Endocrinology, Johns Hopkins Hosp 1978; **Fac Appt:** Prof ObG, Cornell Univ-Weill Med Coll

Midwest

Molo, Mary W MD [RE] - **Spec Exp:** Fertility Preservation in Cancer; **Hospital:** Rush Univ Med Ctr; **Address:** 1725 W Harrison St, Ste 408 East, Chicago, IL 60612; **Phone:** 312-997-2229; **Board Cert:** Obstetrics & Gynecology 2007; Reproductive Endocrinology 2007; **Med School:** Southern IL Univ 1982; **Resid:** Obstetrics & Gynecology, Southern Illinois Affil Hosps 1984; Obstetrics & Gynecology, Rush Presby St Lukes Hosp 1987; **Fellow:** Reproductive Endocrinology, Rush Presby St Lukes Hosp 1989; **Fac Appt:** Asst Prof ObG, Rush Med Coll

Cancer Institute

NYU LANGONE MEDICAL CENTER

NYU Cancer Institute
NYU LANGONE MEDICAL CENTER

NYU Clinical Cancer Center
160 East 34th Street
New York, New York 10016
www.nyuci.org/atcd

NYU Langone Medical Center
550 First Avenue
(at 31st Street)
New York, New York 10016
www.nyumc.org/atcd

Stephen D. Hassenfeld
Children's Center
for Cancer and Blood
Disorders
160 East 32nd Street
New York, New York 10016
www.nyumc.org/hassenfeld

A Collaborative Approach
The NYU Cancer Institute, an NCI designated center, is a "matrix cancer center" without walls operating within the larger NYU Langone Medical Center. With over 175 members and a research funding base of over $81 million, this structure strengthens our capabilities to forge collaborations across medical and scientific disciplines, which translates to comprehensive care for our patients and discoveries that will influence the future of this disease.

Renowned Expertise
Team members' compassion and expertise help patients better manage the symptoms of their disease as well as their special needs. Our highly skilled Magnet™ nursing team not only plays a pivotal role in coordinating direct patient care, but is also a source of invaluable patient education.

A Patient-Focused Setting
The NYU Clinical Cancer Center, with over 70 faculty members from various disciplines at the New York University School of Medicine, is the principal outpatient facility of the Cancer Institute and serves as home for our patients and their caregivers. The center and its multidisciplinary team of experts provide access to the latest treatment options and clinical trials along with a variety of programs in cancer prevention, screening, diagnostics, genetic counseling, and supportive services. When it comes to kids and cancer, the Stephen D. Hassenfeld Children's Center for Cancer and Blood Disorders offers not just innovation but insight. As a leading member of the NCI-sponsored Children's Oncology Group, our physicians are known for developing new ways to treat childhood cancer. Our affiliation with Bellevue Hospital, the oldest public hospital in the country, affords clinically distinctive opportunities to learn and care for patients with cancer by observing its presentation and behavior in a variety of patient groups.

Ophthalmology

An ophthalmologist has the knowledge and professional skills needed to provide eye and vision care. Ophthalmologists are medically trained to diagnose, monitor and medically or surgically treat all ocular and visual disorders. This includes problems affecting the eye and its component structures, the eyelids, the orbit and the visual pathways. In so doing, an ophthalmologist prescribes vision services, including glasses and contact lenses.

Training Required: Four years

OPHTHALMOLOGY

New England

Rubin, Peter A D MD [Oph] - **Spec Exp:** Oculoplastic Surgery; Orbital & Eyelid Tumors/Cancer; Eyelid Cancer & Reconstruction; **Hospital:** Beth Israel Deaconess Med Ctr - Boston; **Address:** 44 Washington St, Brookline, MA 02445; **Phone:** 617-232-9600; **Board Cert:** Ophthalmology 1991; **Med School:** Yale Univ 1985; **Resid:** Ophthalmology, Manhattan EET Hosp 1989; **Fellow:** Oculoplastic Surgery, Mass EE Infirm 1990; **Fac Appt:** Assoc Prof Oph, Harvard Med Sch

Mid Atlantic

Abramson, David H MD [Oph] - **Spec Exp:** Eye Tumors/Cancer; Orbital Tumors/Cancer; Retinoblastoma; Melanoma-Choroidal (eye); **Hospital:** Meml Sloan-Kettering Cancer Ctr (page 76); **Address:** 1275 York Avenue, New York, NY 10065; **Phone:** 800-525-2225; **Board Cert:** Ophthalmology 1975; **Med School:** Albert Einstein Coll Med 1969; **Resid:** Ophthalmology, Harkness Eye Inst 1974; **Fellow:** Ocular Oncology, Columbia-Presby Med Ctr 1975; **Fac Appt:** Clin Prof Oph, Cornell Univ-Weill Med Coll

Della Rocca, Robert C MD [Oph] - **Spec Exp:** Orbital Tumors/Cancer; Eyelid Tumors/Cancer; Oculoplastic Surgery; Eyelid Cancer & Reconstruction; **Hospital:** New York Eye & Ear Infirm (page 78), Sound Shore Med Ctr - Westchester; **Address:** 310 E 14th St, South Bldg, rm 319, New York, NY 10003; **Phone:** 212-979-4575; **Board Cert:** Ophthalmology 1975; **Med School:** Creighton Univ 1967; **Resid:** Ophthalmology, NY Eye & Ear Infirm 1973; **Fellow:** Oculoplastic Surgery, Albany Med Ctr

Finger, Paul T MD [Oph] - **Spec Exp:** Eye Tumors/Cancer; Melanoma-Choroidal (eye); Retinoblastoma; Orbital Tumors/Cancer; **Hospital:** New York Eye & Ear Infirm (page 78), NYU Langone Med Ctr (page 80); **Address:** The New York Eye Cancer Ctr, 115 E 61st St, New York, NY 10021-8183; **Phone:** 212-832-8170; **Board Cert:** Ophthalmology 1990; **Med School:** Tulane Univ 1982; **Resid:** Ophthalmology, Manhattan EET Hosp 1986; **Fellow:** Ocular Oncology, N Shore Univ Hosp 1987; **Fac Appt:** Clin Prof Oph, NYU Sch Med

Handa, James T MD [Oph] - **Spec Exp:** Melanoma-Choroidal (eye); Retinoblastoma; **Hospital:** Johns Hopkins Hosp; **Address:** Johns Hopkins-Wilmer Eye Inst, 1550 Orleans St, rm CRB-144, Baltimore, MD 21287; **Phone:** 410-955-3518; **Board Cert:** Ophthalmology 1991; **Med School:** Univ Pennsylvania 1986; **Resid:** Ophthalmology, Wills Eye Hosp 1990; **Fellow:** Retina/Vitreous, Duke Eye Ctr 1992; Ophthalmic Oncololgy, USC Sch Med 1993; **Fac Appt:** Assoc Prof Oph, Johns Hopkins Univ

Iliff, Nicholas T MD [Oph] - **Spec Exp:** Oculoplastic Surgery; Orbital & Eyelid Tumors/Cancer; **Hospital:** Johns Hopkins Hosp; **Address:** Wilmer at Bayview Med Ctr, 4940 Eastern Ave, Baltimore, MD 21224; **Phone:** 410-550-2360; **Board Cert:** Ophthalmology 1978; **Med School:** Johns Hopkins Univ 1972; **Resid:** Ophthalmology, Johns Hopkins-Wilmer Inst 1977; **Fellow:** Retinal Surgery, Johns Hopkins-Wilmer Inst 1978; Oculoplastic & Reconstructive Surgery, Johns Hopkins-Wilmer Inst 1980; **Fac Appt:** Prof Oph, Johns Hopkins Univ

Shields, Carol L MD [Oph] - **Spec Exp:** Orbital Tumors/Cancer; Melanoma-Choroidal (eye); Retinoblastoma; Pediatric Ophthalmology; **Hospital:** Wills Eye Hosp, Jefferson Hosp - Pittsburgh; **Address:** Wills Eye Hosp, Ocular Oncology Service, 840 Walnut St, Ste 1440, Phildelphia, PA 19107; **Phone:** 215-928-3105; **Board Cert:** Ophthalmology 1989; **Med School:** Univ Pittsburgh 1983; **Resid:** Ophthalmology, Willis Eye Hosp 1988; **Fellow:** Ophthalmic Pathology, Willis Eye Hosp 1988; Ophthalmic Oncololgy, Willis Eye Hosp 1989; **Fac Appt:** Prof Oph, Jefferson Med Coll

Shields, Jerry MD [Oph] - **Spec Exp:** Eye Tumors/Cancer; Pediatric Ophthalmology; Retinoblastoma; Melanoma-Choroidal (eye); **Hospital:** Wills Eye Hosp; **Address:** Wills Eye Hosp, Ocular Oncology Service, 840 Walnut St, Ste 1440, Philadelphia, PA 19107; **Phone:** 215-928-3105; **Board Cert:** Ophthalmology 1972; **Med School:** Univ Mich Med Sch 1964; **Resid:** Ophthalmology, Wills Eye Hosp 1970; **Fellow:** Ophthalmology, Wills Eye Hosp 1972; **Fac Appt:** Prof Oph, Thomas Jefferson Univ

Southeast

Dutton, Jonathan J MD/PhD [Oph] - **Spec Exp:** Oculoplastic Surgery; Eye Tumors/Cancer; Melanoma-Choroidal (eye); **Hospital:** Univ NC Hosps; **Address:** Univ North Carolina - Dept Ophthalmology, 130 Mason Farm Rd, 5156 Bioinformatics, CB 7040, Chapel Hill, NC 27599; **Phone:** 919-966-5296; **Board Cert:** Ophthalmology 1983; **Med School:** Washington Univ, St Louis 1977; **Resid:** Ophthalmology, Washington Univ Med Ctr 1982, **Fellow:** Oculoplastic Surgery, Univ Iowa Med Ctr 1983; **Fac Appt:** Prof Oph, Univ NC Sch Med

Grossniklaus, Hans E MD [Oph] - **Spec Exp:** Ophthalmic Pathology; Melanoma-Choroidal (eye); **Hospital:** Emory Univ Hosp; **Address:** Emory Clinic - LF Montgomery Lab, 1365-B Clifton Rd NE, rm BT428, Atlanta, GA 30322; **Phone:** 404-778-4611; **Board Cert:** Ophthalmology 1985; Anatomic Pathology 1987; **Med School:** Ohio State Univ 1980; **Resid:** Ophthalmology, Case West Res Univ Hosp 1984; Pathology, Case West Res Univ Hosp 1987; **Fellow:** Ophthalmological Pathology, Johns Hopkins Hosp 1985; **Fac Appt:** Prof Oph, Emory Univ

Haik, Barrett MD [Oph] - **Spec Exp:** Eye Tumors/Cancer; **Hospital:** St Jude Children's Research Hosp; **Address:** Univ Tenn Med Group, Ophthamology, 930 Madison Ave, Ste 200, Memphis, TN 38103-3452; **Phone:** 901-448-6650; **Board Cert:** Ophthalmology 1981; **Med School:** Louisiana State U, New Orleans 1976; **Resid:** Ophthalmology, Columbia-Presby/Harkness Eye Inst 1980; **Fac Appt:** Prof Oph, Univ Tenn Coll Med, Memphis

Murray, Timothy MD [Oph] - **Spec Exp:** Eye Tumors/Cancer; **Hospital:** Bascom Palmer Eye Inst (page 82); **Address:** Bascom Palmer Eye Inst, 900 NW 17th St, rm 254, Miami, FL 33136-1119; **Phone:** 305-326-6166; **Board Cert:** Ophthalmology 1990; **Med School:** Johns Hopkins Univ 1985; **Resid:** Ophthalmology, UCSF Med Ctr 1989; **Fellow:** Ophthalmology, UCSF 1999; Ophthalmology, Med Coll Wisconsin 1991; **Fac Appt:** Prof Oph, Univ Miami Sch Med

Sternberg Jr, Paul MD [Oph] - **Spec Exp:** Eye Tumors/Cancer; **Hospital:** Vanderbilt Univ Med Ctr, Vanderbilt Children's Hosp; **Address:** Vanderbilt Eye Institute, 2311 Pierce Ave, Nashville, TN 37232-8808; **Phone:** 615-936-1453; **Board Cert:** Ophthalmology 1985; **Med School:** Univ Chicago-Pritzker Sch Med 1979; **Resid:** Ophthalmology, Johns Hopkins Hosp 1983; **Fellow:** Vitreoretinal Surgery, Duke Univ Med Ctr 1984; **Fac Appt:** Prof Oph, Vanderbilt Univ

Tse, David MD [Oph] - **Spec Exp:** Oculoplastic Surgery; Orbital Tumors/Cancer; Eyelid Tumors/Cancer; **Hospital:** Bascom Palmer Eye Inst (page 82), Jackson Meml Hosp (page 82); **Address:** Bascom Palmer Eye Inst, 900 NW 17th St, Miami, FL 33136-1119; **Phone:** 305-326-6086; **Board Cert:** Ophthalmology 2002; **Med School:** Univ Miami Sch Med 1976; **Resid:** Ophthalmology, LAC/USC Med Ctr 1981; **Fellow:** Oculoplastic Surgery, Univ Iowa Hosps 1982; **Fac Appt:** Prof Oph, Univ Miami Sch Med

Ophthalmology

Wilson, Matthew W MD [Oph] - **Spec Exp:** Eye Tumors/Cancer; Retinoblastoma; Melanoma-Choroidal (eye); **Hospital:** St Jude Children's Research Hosp, Methodist Univ Hosp - Memphis; **Address:** Univ Tenn Med Grp, Ophthalmology, 930 Madison Ave, Ste 200, Memphis, TN 38103; **Phone:** 901-448-6650; **Board Cert:** Ophthalmology 2007; **Med School:** Emory Univ 1990; **Resid:** Ophthalmology, Emory Univ Med Ctr 1994; Ophthalmic Pathology, Emory Univ Med Ctr 1995; **Fellow:** Ocular Oncology, Moorfields Eye Hosp 1996; Ophthalmic Plastic & Reconstructive Surgery, Casey Eye Inst 1998; **Fac Appt:** Assoc Prof Oph, Univ Tenn Coll Med, Memphis

Yeatts, R Patrick MD [Oph] - **Spec Exp:** Oculoplastic Surgery; Orbital Tumors/Cancer; Eyelid Tumors/Cancer; Orbital Disease; **Hospital:** Wake Forest Univ Baptist Med Ctr (page 84); **Address:** Wake Forest Univ Eye Ctr, Janeway Clinical Sciences Bldg Fl 6, Medical Ctr Blvd, Winston-Salem, NC 27157; **Phone:** 336-716-4091; **Board Cert:** Ophthalmology 1983; **Med School:** Wake Forest Univ 1978; **Resid:** Ophthalmology, Mayo Clinic 1982; **Fellow:** Oculoplastic & Reconstructive Surgery, Mass Eye & Ear Infirmary 1983; **Fac Appt:** Prof Oph, Wake Forest Univ

Midwest

Albert, Daniel M MD [Oph] - **Spec Exp:** Eye Tumors/Cancer; Ophthalmic Pathology; **Hospital:** Univ WI Hosp & Clins; **Address:** 2880 University Ave, Madison, WI 53705; **Phone:** 608-263-7171; **Board Cert:** Ophthalmology 1969; **Med School:** Univ Pennsylvania 1962; **Resid:** Ophthalmology, Hosp Univ Penn 1966; Neuro-Ophthalmology, Natl Inst Hlth 1968; **Fellow:** Pathology, Armed Forces Inst Path 1969; **Fac Appt:** Prof Oph, Univ Wisc

Augsburger, James MD [Oph] - **Spec Exp:** Eye Tumors/Cancer; Melanoma-Choroidal (eye); Retinoblastoma; **Hospital:** Univ Hosp - Cincinnati, Cincinnati Chldns Hosp Med Ctr; **Address:** Medical Arts Bldg, Ste 1500, 222 Piedmont Ave, rm ML 665-E, Cincinnati, OH 45267-0665; **Phone:** 513-475-7300; **Board Cert:** Ophthalmology 1979; **Med School:** Univ Cincinnati 1974; **Resid:** Ophthalmology, Univ Hosp-Cincinnati 1978; **Fellow:** Ocular Oncology, Wills Eye Hosp 1980; **Fac Appt:** Prof Oph, Univ Cincinnati

Elner, Victor H MD/PhD [Oph] - **Spec Exp:** Browlifts; Eyelid Tumors/Cancer; Orbital Tumors/Cancer; **Hospital:** Univ Michigan Hlth Sys; **Address:** Kellogg Eye Ctr, 1000 Wall St, Ann Arbor, MI 48105; **Phone:** 734-763-9142; **Board Cert:** Ophthalmology 1983; Pathology 1988; **Med School:** Univ Chicago-Pritzker Sch Med 1979; **Resid:** Ophthalmology, Univ Chicago 1982; Pathology, Univ Chicago 1984; **Fellow:** Ophthalmological Pathology, Armed Forces Inst 1985; Ophthalmic Plastic & Reconstructive Surgery, Univ Wisconsin 1987; **Fac Appt:** Prof Oph, Univ Mich Med Sch

Harbour, J William MD [Oph] - **Spec Exp:** Eye Tumors/Cancer; Melanoma-Choroidal (eye); Retinoblastoma; **Hospital:** Barnes-Jewish Hosp, St Louis Chldns Hosp; **Address:** 1600 S Brentwood, Ste 800, St Louis, MO 63144; **Phone:** 314-367-1278 x2156; **Board Cert:** Ophthalmology 2007; **Med School:** Johns Hopkins Univ 1990; **Resid:** Ophthalmology, Wills Eye Hosp 1994; **Fellow:** Retina/Vitreous, Bascom Palmer Eye Inst 1995; Ocular Oncology, UCSF Med Ctr 1996; **Fac Appt:** Prof Oph, Washington Univ, St Louis

Lueder, Gregg T MD [Oph] - **Spec Exp:** Retinoblastoma; Eye Tumors-Pediatric; Pediatric Ophthalmology; **Hospital:** St Louis Chldns Hosp; **Address:** St Louis Children's Hospital, One Children's Pl, Ste 2S89, St Louis, MO 63110; **Phone:** 314-454-6026; **Board Cert:** Ophthalmology 2003; **Med School:** Univ Iowa Coll Med 1985; **Resid:** Pediatrics, St Louis Children's Hosp 1988; Ophthalmology, Univ Iowa Med Ctr 1991; **Fellow:** Pediatric Ophthalmology, Hosp for Sick Children 1993; **Fac Appt:** Assoc Prof Oph, Washington Univ, St Louis

Mieler, William F MD [Oph] - **Spec Exp:** Eye Tumors/Cancer; **Hospital:** Univ of IL Med Ctr at Chicago, Weiss Meml Hosp; **Address:** Univ Chicago, Dept Opth & Vis Sci, 1855 E Taylor St, MS 648, Chicago, IL 60637; **Phone:** 773-702-3838; **Board Cert:** Ophthalmology 1984; **Med School:** Univ Wisc 1979; **Resid:** Ophthalmology, Bascom-Palmer Eye Inst 1983; **Fellow:** Vitreoretinal Surgery & Disease, Med Ctr Wisconsin Eye Inst 1984; Oculoplastic Surgery, Wills Eye Hosp 1986; **Fac Appt:** Prof Oph, Univ IL Coll Med

Nerad, Jeffrey MD [Oph] - **Spec Exp:** Orbital Tumors/Cancer; Eyelid Cancer & Reconstruction; Oculoplastic Surgery; **Address:** Cincinnati Eye Institute, 1945 CEI Drive, Cincinnati, OH 45242; **Phone:** 513-984-5133; **Board Cert:** Ophthalmology 1984; **Med School:** St Louis Univ 1979; **Resid:** Ophthalmology, St Louis Univ Med Ctr 1983; **Fellow:** Oculoplastic & Reconstructive Surgery, Univ Iowa 1984; **Fac Appt:** Prof Oph, Univ Iowa Coll Med

Plager, David A MD [Oph] - **Spec Exp:** Pediatric Ophthalmology; Eye Tumors-Pediatric; Retinoblastoma; **Hospital:** Riley Hosp for Children (page 74); **Address:** Riley Outpatient Ctr-Ophthalmology, 702 Barnhill Drive, Ste 3340, Indianapolis, IN 46202-5133; **Phone:** 317-274-8103; **Board Cert:** Ophthalmology 2006; **Med School:** Indiana Univ 1983; **Resid:** Ophthalmology, Indiana Univ Hosps 1987; **Fellow:** Pediatric Ophthalmology, Chldns Hosp Natl Med Ctr 1988; **Fac Appt:** Prof Oph, Indiana Univ

Pulido, Jose S MD [Oph] - **Spec Exp:** Eye Tumors/Cancer; **Hospital:** Mayo Med Ctr & Clin - Rochester; **Address:** 200 1st St SW, Rochester, MN 55905; **Phone:** 507-284-3721; **Board Cert:** Ophthalmology 1986; **Med School:** Tulane Univ 1981; **Resid:** Ophthalmology, Illinois Eye & Ear Infirm 1986; **Fellow:** Vitreoretinal Surgery & Disease, Bascom-Palmer Eye Inst 1987; Ocular Oncology, Wills Eye Hosp; **Fac Appt:** Prof Oph, Mayo Med Sch

Weingeist, Thomas A MD/PhD [Oph] - **Spec Exp:** Eye Tumors/Cancer; **Hospital:** Univ Iowa Hosp & Clinics; **Address:** Univ Iowa, Dept Ophthalmology, 200 Hawkins Drive, Iowa City, IA 52242; **Phone:** 319-356-2864; **Board Cert:** Ophthalmology 1976; **Med School:** Univ Iowa Coll Med 1972; **Resid:** Ophthalmology, Univ Iowa Hosp 1975; **Fellow:** Vitreoretinal Surgery, Univ Iowa 1976; **Fac Appt:** Prof Oph, Univ Iowa Coll Med

Great Plains and Mountains

Anderson, Richard L MD [Oph] - **Spec Exp:** Orbital & Eyelid Tumors/Cancer; **Hospital:** Salt Lake Regional Med Ctr, Intermountain Shriners Hosp; **Address:** 1002 E South Temple, Ste 308, Salt Lake City, UT 84102-1525; **Phone:** 801-363-3355; **Board Cert:** Ophthalmology 1976; **Med School:** Univ Iowa Coll Med 1971; **Resid:** Ophthalmology, Univ Iowa Hosps-Clins 1975; **Fellow:** Oculoplastic & Reconstructive Surgery, Albany Med Ctr 1975; Oculoplastic & Reconstructive Surgery, UCSF Med Ctr 1976; **Fac Appt:** Prof PlS, Univ Utah

Gigantelli, James W MD [Oph] - **Spec Exp:** Orbital Tumors/Cancer; Eyelid Cancer & Reconstruction; Lymphoma-Ocular (eye); **Hospital:** Nebraska Med Ctr; **Address:** Univ Nebraska Med Ctr, Ophthalmology, 985540 Nebraska Medical Ctr, Omaha, NE 68198-5540; **Phone:** 402-559-4276; **Board Cert:** Ophthalmology 1991; **Med School:** Vanderbilt Univ 1985; **Resid:** Ophthalmology, Baylor Coll Med 1989; **Fellow:** Oculoplastic Surgery, Duke Unv Med Ctr 1990; **Fac Appt:** Assoc Prof Oph, Univ Nebr Coll Med

Ophthalmology

Southwest

Esmaeli-Azad, Bita MD [Oph] - **Spec Exp:** Orbital & Eyelid Tumors/Cancer; Eyelid Cancer & Reconstruction; Oculoplastic Surgery; **Hospital:** UT MD Anderson Cancer Ctr; **Address:** Dept of Head & Neck Surgery, Ophthalmology Section, 1515 Holcombe Blvd, Ste 1445, Houston, TX 77030; **Phone:** 713-792-6523; **Board Cert:** Ophthalmology 2006; **Med School:** Ros Franklin Univ/Chicago Med Sch 1990; **Resid:** Ophthalmology, Univ Michigan Affil Hosp 1994; **Fellow:** Ophthalmic Plastic & Reconstructive Surgery, Univ Toronto Affil Hosp 1996; **Fac Appt:** Assoc Prof Oph, Univ Tex, Houston

Lee, Andrew G MD [Oph] - **Spec Exp:** Neuro-Ophthalmology; Optic Nerve Tumors; **Hospital:** Methodist Hosp - Houston; **Address:** Methodist Hosp, Dept Ophthalmology, 6560 Fannin St, Ste 2100, Houston, TX 77030; **Phone:** 713-441-8821; **Board Cert:** Ophthalmology 2006; **Med School:** Univ VA Sch Med 1989; **Resid:** Ophthalmology, Cullen Eye Inst-Baylor 1993; **Fellow:** Neuro-Ophthalmology, Wilmer Eye Inst-Johns Hopkins 1994; **Fac Appt:** Prof Oph, Univ Iowa Coll Med

Schiffman, Jade S MD [Oph] - **Spec Exp:** Neuro-Ophthalmology; **Hospital:** UT MD Anderson Cancer Ctr; **Address:** MD Anderson Cancer, 1515 Holcombe Blvd Unit 1445, Houston, TX 77035; **Phone:** 713-792-3798; **Board Cert:** Neurology 1983; Ophthalmology 1991; **Med School:** SUNY Upstate Med Univ 1975; **Resid:** Neurology, Univ Miami Affil Hosp 1980; Ophthalmology, Univ California Affil Hosp 1989; **Fellow:** Neuro-Ophthalmology, Univ California Med Ctr 1981; **Fac Appt:** Prof Oph, Univ Tex, Houston

Soparkar, Charles MD [Oph] - **Spec Exp:** Eye Tumors/Cancer; Orbital & Eyelid Tumors/Cancer; Oculoplastic Surgery; **Hospital:** Methodist Hosp - Houston, Texas Chldns Hosp; **Address:** Plastic Eye Surg Assocs, 3730 Kirby Drive, Ste 900, Houston, TX 77098; **Phone:** 713-795-0705; **Board Cert:** Ophthalmology 2007; **Med School:** Univ Mass Sch Med 1990; **Resid:** Ophthalmology, Baylor Affil Hosps 1994; **Fellow:** Ophthalmic Oncololgy, Texas Med Ctr 1995; Ophthalmic Plastic Surgery, Texas Med Ctr 1995; **Fac Appt:** Asst Clin Prof Oph, Baylor Coll Med

West Coast and Pacific

Boxrud, Cynthia Ann MD [Oph] - **Spec Exp:** Oculoplastic Surgery; Eye Tumors/Cancer; **Hospital:** UCLA Ronald Reagan Med Ctr, St John's Hlth Ctr, Santa Monica; **Address:** 2021 Santa Monica Blvd, Ste 700E, Santa Monica, CA 90404-2208; **Phone:** 310-829-9060; **Board Cert:** Ophthalmology 2008; **Med School:** Case West Res Univ 1986; **Resid:** Ophthalmology, NYU-Bellevue Hosp Ctr 1990; **Fellow:** Ophthalmic Oncololgy, New York Hosp-Cornell Med Ctr 1992; Ophthalmic Plastic Surgery, UCLA-Jules Stein Eye Inst 1993; **Fac Appt:** Asst Prof Oph, UCLA

Char, Devron H MD [Oph] - **Spec Exp:** Eye Tumors/Cancer; Oculoplastic Surgery; **Hospital:** CA Pacific Med Ctr - Pacific Campus, UCSF Med Ctr; **Address:** 45 Castro St, Ste 309, San Francisco, CA 94114; **Phone:** 415-522-0700; **Board Cert:** Ophthalmology 1978; **Med School:** Univ Minn 1970; **Resid:** Internal Medicine, Mass Genl Hosp 1972; Ophthalmology, UCSF Med Ctr 1977; **Fellow:** Medical Oncology, Natl Cancer Inst 1974; Ophthalmology, UCSF Med Ctr 1978; **Fac Appt:** Prof Oph, Stanford Univ

Cockerham, Kimberly P MD [Oph] - **Spec Exp:** Orbital Tumors/Cancer; Eyelid Cancer & Reconstruction; Neuro-Ophthalmology; **Hospital:** El Camino Hosp, Stanford Univ Med Ctr; **Address:** 762 Altos Oaks Drive, Ste 2, Los Altos, CA 94024; **Phone:** 650-559-9150; **Board Cert:** Ophthalmology 2004; **Med School:** Geo Wash Univ 1987; **Resid:** Ophthalmology, Walter Reed Army Med Ctr 1992; **Fellow:** Neuro-Ophthalmology, Walter Reed Army Med Ctr 1993; Neuro-Ophthalmology, Allegheny General Hosp 1995

Kim, Jonathan MD [Oph] - **Spec Exp:** Oculoplastic Surgery; Orbital Tumors/Cancer; **Hospital:** Stanford Univ Med Ctr; **Address:** 900 Blake Wilbur Drive, rm W3002, MC 5353, Palo Alto, CA 94304; **Phone:** 650-736-8098; **Board Cert:** Ophthalmology 2000; **Med School:** Univ Iowa Coll Med 1994; **Resid:** Ophthalmology, CA Pacific Med Ctr 1998; **Fellow:** Oculoplastic Surgery, Jules Stein Eye Inst/UCLA Med Ctr 2000; Orbital Surgery, Mass Eye & Ear Infirm 2004

Murphree, A Linn MD [Oph] - **Spec Exp:** Pediatric Ophthalmology; Retinoblastoma; Orbital Tumors/Cancer; **Hospital:** Chldns Hosp - Los Angeles, USC Univ Hosp; **Address:** Chldns Hosp, Div Oph, 4650 Sunset Blvd, MS 88, Los Angeles, CA 90027-6016; **Phone:** 323-361-2347; **Board Cert:** Ophthalmology 1978; **Med School:** Baylor Coll Med 1972; **Resid:** Clinical Genetics, Baylor Heed 1973; Ophthalmology, Baylor Coll Med 1976; **Fellow:** Ophthalmology, Wilmer Inst/Johns Hopkins 1977; **Fac Appt:** Prof Oph, USC Sch Med

O'Brien, Joan M MD [Oph] - **Spec Exp:** Eye Tumors/Cancer; Retinoblastoma; **Hospital:** UCSF Med Ctr; **Address:** UCSF, Dept Ophthalmology, 533 Parnassus Ave Fl 5 - Ste 525, San Francisco, CA 94143; **Phone:** 415-476-3705; **Board Cert:** Ophthalmology 2007; **Med School:** Dartmouth Med Sch 1986; **Resid:** Ophthalmology, Mass Eye & Ear Infirm 1992; **Fellow:** Ophthalmic Pathology, Mass Eye & Ear Infirm 1989; UCSF Med Ctr 1993; **Fac Appt:** Prof Oph, UCSF

Seiff, Stuart R MD [Oph] - **Spec Exp:** Oculoplastic Surgery; Orbital Tumors/Cancer; **Hospital:** UCSF Med Ctr, CA Pacific Med Ctr; **Address:** 2100 Webster St, Ste 214, San Francisco, CA 94115; **Phone:** 415-923-3007; **Board Cert:** Ophthalmology 1986; **Med School:** UCSF 1980; **Resid:** Ophthalmology, UCSF Med Ctr 1984; **Fellow:** Ophthalmic Plastic & Reconstructive Surgery, UCLA Med Ctr 1985; Oculoplastic Surgery, Moorfield's Eye Hosp 1986; **Fac Appt:** Prof Oph, UCSF

Stout, John T MD/PhD [Oph] - **Spec Exp:** Retinoblastoma; **Hospital:** OR Hlth & Sci Univ, Providence St Vincent Med Ctr; **Address:** 3375 SW Terwilliger Blvd, Portland, OR 97239; **Phone:** 503-494-2435; **Board Cert:** Ophthalmology 1999; **Med School:** Baylor Coll Med 1989; **Resid:** Ophthalmology, Doheny Eye Inst 1993; **Fellow:** Ophthalmology, Moorfields Eye Hosp 1994; Retinal Surgery, Doheny Eye Inst 1995; **Fac Appt:** Assoc Prof Oph, Oregon Hlth Sci Univ

Wilson, David Jean MD [Oph] - **Spec Exp:** Eye Tumors/Cancer; Ophthalmic Pathology; **Hospital:** OR Hlth & Sci Univ, Legacy Health System; **Address:** 3375 SW Terwilliger Blvd, Portland, OR 97239; **Phone:** 503-494-7891; **Board Cert:** Ophthalmology 1987; **Med School:** Baylor Coll Med 1981; **Resid:** Ophthalmology, Univ Oregon 1985; **Fellow:** Ophthalmic Pathology, John Hopkins Hosp 1987; Retina/Vitreous, Mass Eye & Ear Infirm 1988; **Fac Appt:** Prof Oph, Oregon Hlth Sci Univ

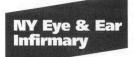

THE NEW YORK EYE AND EAR INFIRMARY

310 East 14th Street
New York, New York 10003
Tel. 212.979.4000   Fax. 212.228.0664
www.nyee.edu

Continuum Health Partners, Inc.

OCULAR TUMOR SERVICE

The Infirmary is a national referral center within the Collaborative Ocular Melanoma Study of the National Eye Institute/National Institutes of Health. New and innovative treatments for patients with eye cancer include radioactive plaques to treat intraocular tumors and chemotherapy for conjunctival neoplasia. Tumors of the eyelids, iris, retina, choroid and optic nerve are also treated by specialists in this service. A multidisciplinary Ocular Tumor Board meets monthly to discuss the most difficult cases and formulate therapeutic options

OTOLARYNGOLOGY/ HEAD & NECK SURGERY

Head & Neck Oncology: A team comprised of board-certified surgeons, medical & radiation oncologists, nutritionists and rehabilitation specialists ensure rapid recovery from complex, life saving surgical procedures and return to daily activities.

Thyroid Center: A unique center concentrates on streamlining the diagnosis and treatment of thyroid diseases and cancers with a highly skilled team of surgeons, endocrinologists and radiologists to manage the patient's care. An area of expertise is cancer resulting from radiation exposure such as that from Chernobyl.

Facial Plastics and Reconstructive Surgery: Treatment of facial tumors, both benign and cancerous, frequently requires expert reconstruction. Designed to restore the function and appearance of the face, these procedures may be required after appropriate treatment of skin cancers or deep tumors.

Otology–Neuro-otology: These rare cancers can be treated by our highly skilled team of surgeons which includes a neuro-otologist and a neuro-surgeon.

Center for the Voice and Swallowing: Program cooperatively staffed by a team of specialists able to diagnose cancer of the vocal cords early and rehabilitate the voice after surgical and radiation treatment.

PATHOLOGY & LABORATORY MEDICINE

The Ocular Pathology Service is the leading laboratory in the Northeast and utilized by ophthalmologists throughout the region. The Infirmary is the site of some of the most promising studies into diseases and cancers of the eye, ear, nose and throat. Among them: cellular markers of oral cancer risk, non-invasive detection of thyroid cancer, basic cell biology of the growth of ocular melanoma cells, and persistence of biomaterials for repair in plastic and reconstructive surgery.

PLASTIC & RECONSTRUCTIVE SURGERY

The Department of Plastic & Reconstructive Surgery treats more than 1,500 patients a year who seek reconstructive surgery of the body as well as facial area as a result of accident, birth defect or cancer, and those who elect cosmetic surgery. It is one of the few hospitals in the region to perform breast reconstruction after mastectomy with newly developed microsurgical techniques for harvesting tissue from patients' lower body to create living, natural and normal-looking breasts, a result which is often preferred to artificial implants.

About
The New York
Eye and Ear Infirmary

Established in 1820, the Infirmary is the oldest continuously operating specialty hospital in the nation and one of the most experienced in terms of the number of patients it treats and complexity of cases.

Each year the Ophthalmology Department performs more than 19,200 surgeries and sees more than 155,000 visits from outpatients. The Otolaryngology Department performs more than 6,000 surgeries and has some 70,000 outpatient visits. A third clinical department, Plastic & Reconstructive Surgery, is a natural complement to the Infirmary's other services with another 1,500 cases a year. Cutting-edge diagnostic tools and state-of-the-art surgical facilities with an experienced, caring staff assure high-tech treatment with a human touch for all.

NYEEI is a teaching affiliate of New York Medical College and a member of Continuum Health Partners, Inc.

**Physician Referral
1.800.449.HOPE (4673)**

Orthopaedic Surgery

An orthopaedic surgeon is trained in the preservation, investigation and restoration of the form and function of the extremities, spine and associated structures by medical, surgical and physical means. An orthopaedic surgeon is involved with the care of patients whose musculoskeletal problems include congenital deformities, trauma, infections, tumors, metabolic disturbances of the musculoskeletal system, deformities, injuries and degenerative diseases of the spine, hands, feet, knee, hip, shoulder and elbow in children and adults. An orthopaedic surgeon is also concerned with primary and secondary muscular problems and the effects of central or peripheral nervous system lesions of the musculoskeletal system.

Training Required: Five years (including general surgery training) plus two years in clinical practice before final certification is achieved.

Note: There are many Orthopaedic Surgeons who are trained in Sports Medicine and prefer to be listed under that heading; some trained in Sports Medicine prefer to be listed under Orthopaedics.

Hand Surgery: A specialist trained in the investigation, preservation and restoration by medical, surgical and rehabilitative means of all structures of the upper extremity directly affecting the form and function of the hand and wrist.

Training Required: Training required for Orthopaedic Surgery certification plus an additional year in hand surgery.

ORTHOPAEDIC SURGERY

New England

Friedlaender, Gary E MD [OrS] - **Spec Exp:** Bone & Soft Tissue Tumors; Tissue Banking; **Hospital:** Yale-New Haven Hosp; **Address:** Dept Orthopedic Surgery, Box 208071, New Haven, CT 06520-8071; **Phone:** 203-737-5656; **Board Cert:** Orthopaedic Surgery 1975; **Med School:** Univ Mich Med Sch 1969; **Resid:** Surgery, Michigan Med Ctr 1971; Orthopaedic Surgery, Yale-New Haven Hosp 1974; **Fellow:** Musculoskeletal Oncology, Mass Genl Hosp 1983; **Fac Appt:** Prof OrS, Yale Univ

Gebhardt, Mark MD [OrS] - **Spec Exp:** Musculoskeletal Tumors; Bone Tumors; **Hospital:** Beth Israel Deaconess Med Ctr - Boston, Children's Hospital - Boston; **Address:** 330 Brookline Ave, Shapiro Bldg Fl 2nd, Boston, MA 02215; **Phone:** 617-667-3940; **Board Cert:** Orthopaedic Surgery 2007; **Med School:** Univ Cincinnati 1975; **Resid:** Surgery, Univ Pittsburg Med Ctr 1977; Orthopaedic Surgery, Harvard Affil Hosps 1982; **Fellow:** Pediatric Orthopaedic Surgery, Boston Chldns Hosp 1983; Orthopaedic Oncology, Mass Genl Hosp 1983; **Fac Appt:** Prof OrS, Harvard Med Sch

Hornicek, Francis J MD/PhD [OrS] - **Spec Exp:** Bone Tumors; Sarcoma; Bone Tumors-Metastatic; Soft Tissue Tumors; **Hospital:** Mass Genl Hosp; **Address:** Orthopaedic Associates, 55 Fruit St, YAW 3700, Boston, MA 02114; **Phone:** 617-724-3700; **Board Cert:** Orthopaedic Surgery 2009; **Med School:** Univ Pittsburgh 1991; **Resid:** Orthopaedic Surgery, Jackson Meml Hosp 1996; **Fellow:** Orthopaedic Oncology, Mass Genl Hosp/Chldns Hosp 1997; **Fac Appt:** Assoc Prof OrS, Harvard Med Sch

Ready, John E MD [OrS] - **Spec Exp:** Bone Cancer; Sarcoma-Soft Tissue; Hip & Knee Replacement in Bone Tumors; **Hospital:** Brigham & Women's Hosp, Dana-Farber Cancer Inst; **Address:** Brigham & Women's Hospital, Dept Orthopaedics, 75 Francis St, Boston, MA 02115; **Phone:** 617-732-5368; **Board Cert:** Orthopaedic Surgery 2002; **Med School:** Dalhousie Univ 1982; **Resid:** Orthopaedic Surgery, Dalhousie Univ Hosp 1987; **Fellow:** Orthopaedic Oncology, St Michael's Hosp 1988; Orthopaedic Oncology, Mass Genl Hosp/Childns Hosp 1989

Springfield, Dempsey MD [OrS] - **Spec Exp:** Bone Tumors; Soft Tissue Tumors; **Hospital:** Mass Genl Hosp; **Address:** 55 Fruit St, Ste YAW 3700, Boston, MA 02114-2621; **Phone:** 617-724-3700; **Board Cert:** Orthopaedic Surgery 2007; **Med School:** Univ Fla Coll Med 1971; **Resid:** Orthopaedic Surgery, Univ Florida/Shands 1978; **Fellow:** Orthopaedic Surgery, Univ Florida/Shands 1979

Weinstein, James DO [OrS] - **Spec Exp:** Pain-Back; Spinal Tumors; **Hospital:** Dartmouth - Hitchcock Med Ctr; **Address:** DHMC, Dept Orthopaedic Surgery, One Medical Ctr Drive, Lebanon, NH 03756; **Phone:** 603-650-2225; **Board Cert:** Orthopaedic Surgery 2002; **Med School:** Chicago Coll Osteo Med 1973; **Resid:** Orthopaedic Surgery, Rush Presby-St Lukes Med Ctr 1983; **Fac Appt:** Prof OrS, Dartmouth Med Sch

Mid Atlantic

Benevenia, Joseph MD [OrS] - **Spec Exp:** Limb Sparing Surgery; Bone Cancer; Sarcoma-Soft Tissue; **Hospital:** UMDNJ-Univ Hosp-Newark; **Address:** 90 Bergen St, Ste 1200, Newark, NJ 07103; **Phone:** 973-972-2153; **Board Cert:** Orthopaedic Surgery 2003; **Med School:** UMDNJ-NJ Med Sch, Newark 1984; **Resid:** Orthopaedic Surgery, UMDNJ-NJ Med Sch Hosp 1988; **Fellow:** Orthopaedic Oncology, Case Western Reserve Univ 1991; **Fac Appt:** Prof OrS, UMDNJ-NJ Med Sch, Newark

Dormans, John P MD [OrS] - **Spec Exp:** Bone Cancer; Pediatric Orthopaedic Surgery; **Hospital:** Chldns Hosp of Philadelphia, The; **Address:** Dept Orthopaedic Surgery, 34th St & Civic Center Blvd, Wood Bldg Fl 2 - rm 2315, Philadelphia, PA 19104-4399; **Phone:** 215-590-1534; **Board Cert:** Orthopaedic Surgery 2002; **Med School:** Indiana Univ 1983; **Resid:** Orthopaedic Surgery, Michigan State Univ Hosps 1988; **Fellow:** Pediatric Orthopaedic Surgery, Hosp for Sick Children 1989; **Fac Appt:** Prof OrS, Univ Pennsylvania

Frassica, Frank J MD [OrS] - **Spec Exp:** Bone Cancer; **Hospital:** Johns Hopkins Hosp, Univ of MD Med Ctr; **Address:** 601 N Caroline St, Ste 5215, Baltimore, MD 21287-0882; **Phone:** 410-955-9300; **Board Cert:** Orthopaedic Surgery 2001; **Med School:** Univ SC Sch Med 1982; **Resid:** Orthopaedic Surgery, Mayo Clinic 1987; **Fellow:** Orthopaedic Oncology, Mayo Clinic 1988; **Fac Appt:** Prof OrS, Johns Hopkins Univ

Healey, John H MD [OrS] - **Spec Exp:** Bone Tumors; Hip & Knee Replacement in Bone Tumors; Sarcoma; Sarcoma-Soft Tissue; **Hospital:** Meml Sloan-Kettering Cancer Ctr (page 76), Hosp For Special Surgery; **Address:** 1275 York Avenue, New York, NY 10065; **Phone:** 800-525-2225; **Board Cert:** Orthopaedic Surgery 2007; **Med School:** Univ VT Coll Med 1978; **Resid:** Orthopaedic Surgery, Hosp Special Surg 1983; **Fellow:** Orthopaedic Oncology, Meml Sloan Kettering Cancer Ctr 1984; Orthopaedic Surgery, Hosp Special Surgery 1984; **Fac Appt:** Prof OrS, Cornell Univ-Weill Med Coll

Kenan, Samuel MD [OrS] - **Spec Exp:** Bone Tumors; **Hospital:** Hosp For Joint Diseases (page 80), NYU Langone Med Ctr (page 80); **Address:** 317 E 34th St Fl 9 - Ste 903, New York, NY 10016; **Phone:** 212-684-5511; **Med School:** Israel 1976; **Resid:** Orthopaedic Surgery, Hadassah Univ Hosp 1984; **Fellow:** Orthopaedic Pathology, Hosp for Joint Diseases 1987; **Fac Appt:** Prof OrS, NYU Sch Med

Lackman, Richard D MD [OrS] - **Spec Exp:** Bone Cancer; Sarcoma; Limb Sparing Surgery; **Hospital:** Hosp Univ Penn - UPHS (page 81), Pennsylvania Hosp (page 81); **Address:** Hosp Univ Penn-Dept Orthopaedic Surg, 301 S 8th St, Garfield Duncan Bldg, Ste 2C, Philadelphia, PA 19104; **Phone:** 215-829-5022; **Board Cert:** Orthopaedic Surgery 1985; **Med School:** Univ Pennsylvania 1977; **Resid:** Orthopaedic Surgery, Hosp Univ Penn 1982; **Fellow:** Orthopaedic Oncology, Mayo Clinic 1983; **Fac Appt:** Assoc Prof OrS, Univ Pennsylvania

Lane, Joseph MD [OrS] - **Spec Exp:** Bone Cancer; **Hospital:** Hosp For Special Surgery, NY-Presby Hosp/Weill Cornell (page 79); **Address:** Hosp for Special Surgery, 535 E 70th St, New York, NY 10021; **Phone:** 212-606-1172; **Board Cert:** Orthopaedic Surgery 1974; **Med School:** Harvard Med Sch 1965; **Resid:** Surgery, Hosp Univ Penn 1967; Orthopaedic Surgery, Hosp Univ Penn 1973; **Fac Appt:** Prof OrS, Cornell Univ-Weill Med Coll

Lee, Francis Y MD/PhD [OrS] - **Spec Exp:** Bone Tumors; Pediatric Orthopaedic Cancers; Pediatric Orthopaedic Surgery; **Hospital:** NY-Presby Hosp/Columbia (page 79); **Address:** 16 E 16th St, New York, NY 10022; **Phone:** 212-305-4565; **Board Cert:** Orthopaedic Surgery 2001; **Med School:** South Korea 1986; **Resid:** Orthopaedic Surgery, NJ Med Ctr 1997; **Fellow:** Orthopaedic Oncology, Harvard Med Sch 1998; Pediatric Orthopaedic Surgery, Hosp for Sick Chldn/Univ Toronto 1999; **Fac Appt:** Asst Prof OrS, Columbia P&S

Malawer, Martin M MD [OrS] - **Spec Exp:** Bone Tumors; Limb Sparing Surgery; Pediatric Orthopaedic Surgery; Sarcoma; **Hospital:** Washington Hosp Ctr; **Address:** Washington Cancer Institute, 110 Irving St NW, Ste C2173, Washington, DC 20010; **Phone:** 202-877-3970; **Board Cert:** Orthopaedic Surgery 1993; **Med School:** NYU Sch Med 1969; **Resid:** Surgery, Bronx Muni Hosp 1972; Orthopaedic Surgery, Bellevue Hosp Ctr 1975; **Fellow:** Orthopaedic Oncology, Shands Hosp-Univ Florida 1978; **Fac Appt:** Prof OrS, Geo Wash Univ

Orthopaedic Surgery

O'Keefe, Regis J MD/PhD [OrS] - **Spec Exp:** Bone & Soft Tissue Tumors; Reconstructive Surgery; **Hospital:** Univ of Rochester Strong Meml Hosp, Highland Hosp of Rochester; **Address:** Univ Rochester, Dept Orthopaedic Surgery, 601 Elmwood Ave, Box 665, Rochester, NY 14642; **Phone:** 585-275-3100; **Board Cert:** Orthopaedic Surgery 2007; **Med School:** Harvard Med Sch 1985; **Resid:** Surgery, New Eng Deaconess Hosp/Harvard 1986; Orthopaedic Surgery, Univ Rochester 1992; **Fellow:** Orthopaedic Oncology, Mass Genl Hosp 1993; **Fac Appt:** Prof S, Univ Rochester

Schmidt, Richard G MD [OrS] - **Spec Exp:** Bone Tumors; Sarcoma-Soft Tissue; Limb Sparing Surgery; Bone Tumors-Metastatic; **Hospital:** Lankenau Hosp, Fox Chase Cancer Ctr (page 72); **Address:** Musculoskeletal Tumor Ctr, 15 N Presidential Blvd, Ste 300, Bala Cynwyd, PA 19004; **Phone:** 610-667-2663; **Board Cert:** Orthopaedic Surgery 1999; **Med School:** Penn State Univ-Hershey Med Ctr 1980; **Resid:** Orthopaedic Surgery, Hosp Univ Penn 1985; **Fellow:** Orthopaedic Oncology, Shands Hosp 1986

Southeast

Berrey, B Hudson MD [OrS] - **Spec Exp:** Musculoskeletal Tumors; Bone Cancer; Soft Tissue Tumors; Sarcoma; **Hospital:** Shands Jacksonville, Wolfson Chldns Hosp; **Address:** Univ Florida Coll Med, Dept Orth Surg, 655 W Eighth St, Jacksonville, FL 32209; **Phone:** 904-244-5942; **Board Cert:** Orthopaedic Surgery 1982; **Med School:** Univ Tex Med Br, Galveston 1977; **Resid:** Orthopaedic Surgery, Tripler Army Med Ctr 1981; **Fellow:** Medical Oncology, Mass Genl Hosp/Harvard 1985; **Fac Appt:** Prof OrS, Univ Fla Coll Med

Kneisl, Jeffrey S MD [OrS] - **Spec Exp:** Bone Cancer; Musculoskeletal Tumors; **Hospital:** Carolinas Med Ctr; **Address:** Carolinas Med Ctr, 1001 Blythe Blvd, Ste 602, Charlotte, NC 28203; **Phone:** 704-355-5982; **Board Cert:** Orthopaedic Surgery 2000; **Med School:** Northwestern Univ 1980; **Resid:** Orthopaedic Surgery, Northwestern Univ 1987; **Fellow:** Orthopaedic Oncology, Univ Chicago 1990

Scarborough, Mark T MD [OrS] - **Spec Exp:** Bone Tumors; Sarcoma; **Hospital:** Shands at Univ of FL; **Address:** Shands Healthcare Univ FL, 3450 Hull Rd, Gainesville, FL 32607; **Phone:** 352-273-7000; **Board Cert:** Orthopaedic Surgery 2003; **Med School:** Univ Fla Coll Med 1985; **Resid:** Orthopaedic Surgery, Univ Texas Med Ctr 1990; **Fellow:** Orthopaedic Surgery, Mass Genl Hosp 1991; **Fac Appt:** Prof OrS, Univ Fla Coll Med

Schwartz, Herbert S MD [OrS] - **Spec Exp:** Bone Tumors-Metastatic; Bone Tumors; Pelvic Surgery-Complex; Musculoskeletal Tumors; **Hospital:** Vanderbilt Univ Med Ctr, Baptist Hosp - Nashville; **Address:** Vanderbilt Orthopaedic Institute, Medical Center East, South Tower, Ste 4200, Nashville, TN 37232-8774; **Phone:** 615-343-8612; **Board Cert:** Orthopaedic Surgery 2007; **Med School:** Univ Chicago-Pritzker Sch Med 1981; **Resid:** Orthopaedic Surgery, Univ Chicago Hosps 1986; **Fellow:** Orthopaedic Oncology, Mayo Clinic 1987; **Fac Appt:** Prof OrS, Vanderbilt Univ

Scully, Sean P MD [OrS] - **Spec Exp:** Bone Cancer; Sarcoma; Musculoskeletal Tumors; **Hospital:** Univ of Miami Hosp & Clins/Sylvester Comp Canc Ctr (page 82), Jackson Meml Hosp (page 82); **Address:** Univ Miami Hospital, 1400 NW 12th Ave, Ste 4035, Miami, FL 33136; **Phone:** 305-325-4683; **Board Cert:** Orthopaedic Surgery 2006; **Med School:** Univ Rochester 1980; **Resid:** Orthopaedic Surgery, Duke Univ Med Ctr 1985; **Fellow:** Orthopaedic Oncology, Mass General Hosp 1987; Research, Natl Inst Health 1988; **Fac Appt:** Prof OrS, Univ Miami Sch Med

Siegel, Herrick J MD [OrS] - **Spec Exp:** Bone Cancer; Sarcoma; Bone Tumors-Metastatic; **Hospital:** Univ of Ala Hosp at Birmingham, UAB Highlands Hosp; **Address:** 1313 13th St S, Birmingham, AL 35205; **Phone:** 205-975-0415; **Board Cert:** Orthopaedic Surgery 2005; **Med School:** NYU Sch Med 1995; **Resid:** Orthopaedic Surgery, USC 2000; **Fellow:** Orthopaedic Oncology, Mayo Clinic 2002; **Fac Appt:** Assoc Prof OrS, Univ Alabama

Walling, Arthur K MD [OrS] - **Spec Exp:** Bone Tumors; Soft Tissue Tumors; **Hospital:** Tampa Genl Hosp; **Address:** Florida Orthopaedic Inst, 13020 Telecom Pkwy N, Tampa, FL 33637; **Phone:** 813-978-9700; **Board Cert:** Orthopaedic Surgery 1982; **Med School:** Creighton Univ 1976; **Resid:** Orthopaedic Surgery, Univ South Florida Affil Hosps 1980; **Fellow:** Surgical Oncology, Univ Florida 1981; **Fac Appt:** Assoc Clin Prof OrS, Univ S Fla Coll Med

Ward, William G MD [OrS] - **Spec Exp:** Bone Tumors; Soft Tissue Tumors; Reconstructive Surgery; **Hospital:** Wake Forest Univ Baptist Med Ctr (page 84); **Address:** Wake Forest Med Ctr, Comprehensive Rehab, 131 Miller St, Winston-Salem, NC 27157; **Phone:** 336-716-8200; **Board Cert:** Orthopaedic Surgery 2004; **Med School:** Duke Univ 1975; **Resid:** Surgery, Duke Univ Med Ctr 1985; Orthopaedic Surgery, Duke Univ Med Ctr 1989; **Fellow:** Sports Medicine, Cleveland Clinic 1990; Orthopaedic Oncology, UCLA Med Ctr 1991; **Fac Appt:** Prof OrS, Wake Forest Univ

Midwest

Biermann, J Sybil MD [OrS] - **Spec Exp:** Sarcoma; Bone Cancer; Multiple Myeloma; Limb Sparing Surgery; **Hospital:** Univ Michigan Hlth Sys; **Address:** Univ Michigan Cancer Ctr, 1500 E Medical Ctr Drive, 7304 CCGC, Ann Arbor, MI 48109-5946; **Phone:** 734-647-8902; **Board Cert:** Orthopaedic Surgery 2006; **Med School:** Stanford Univ 1987; **Resid:** Orthopaedic Surgery, Univ Iowa Hosp 1992; **Fellow:** Orthopaedic Oncology, Univ Chicago Hosps 1993; **Fac Appt:** Assoc Prof OrS, Univ Mich Med Sch

Buckwalter IV, Joseph A MD [OrS] - **Spec Exp:** Bone Cancer; Bone Tumors-Metastatic; **Hospital:** Univ Iowa Hosp & Clinics; **Address:** Univ Iowa Hosps, Dept Orthopaedics, 200 Hawkins Drive, Iowa City, IA 52242; **Phone:** 319-356-2595; **Board Cert:** Orthopaedic Surgery 1980; **Med School:** Univ Iowa Coll Med 1974; **Resid:** Orthopaedic Surgery, Iowa Hosp 1979; **Fac Appt:** Prof OrS, Univ Iowa Coll Med

Cheng, Edward Y MD [OrS] - **Spec Exp:** Bone & Soft Tissue Tumors; Reconstructive Surgery-Adult; **Hospital:** Univ Minn Med Ctr, Fairview - Univ Campus; **Address:** Dept Orthopedic Surgery, Univ Minnesota, 2450 Riverside Ave S, Ste R-200, Minneapolis, MN 55455; **Phone:** 612-273-1177; **Board Cert:** Orthopaedic Surgery 2003; **Med School:** Northwestern Univ 1983; **Resid:** Surgery, Northwestern Univ 1985; Orthopaedic Surgery, Beth Israel Hosp 1989; **Fellow:** Surgical Oncology, Mass Genl Hosp 1990; **Fac Appt:** Prof OrS, Univ Minn

Clohisy, Denis MD [OrS] - **Spec Exp:** Bone Cancer; **Hospital:** Univ Minn Med Ctr, Fairview - Univ Campus; **Address:** Dept Orthopaedic Surgery, 2450 Riverside Ave S, Ste R200, Minneapolis, MN 55454; **Phone:** 612-273-1177; **Board Cert:** Orthopaedic Surgery 2004; **Med School:** Northwestern Univ 1983; **Resid:** Orthopaedic Surgery, Univ Minn 1990; **Fellow:** Pathology, Wash Univ Med Ctr 1987; Musculoskeletal Oncology, Mass Genl Hosp/Harvard 1991; **Fac Appt:** Prof OrS, Univ Minn

Gitelis, Steven MD [OrS] - **Spec Exp:** Bone Cancer; Soft Tissue Tumors; Limb Sparing Surgery; **Hospital:** Rush Univ Med Ctr; **Address:** 1725 W Harrison St, Ste 440, Chicago, IL 60612-3828; **Phone:** 312-563-2600; **Board Cert:** Orthopaedic Surgery 1982; **Med School:** Rush Med Coll 1975; **Resid:** Orthopaedic Surgery, Rush Presby-St Lukes Med Ctr 1980; **Fellow:** Orthopaedic Oncology, Mayo Clinic; **Fac Appt:** Prof OrS, Rush Med Coll

Irwin, Ronald B MD [OrS] - **Spec Exp:** Bone Cancer; Limb Sparing Surgery; Sarcoma-Soft Tissue; **Hospital:** Mount Clemens Regional Med Ctr; **Address:** Mount Clemens Regional Med Ctr, 1080 Harrington Blvd, Ste 201, Mount Clemens, MI 48043; **Phone:** 586-493-7575; **Board Cert:** Orthopaedic Surgery 1979; **Med School:** Univ Mich Med Sch 1971; **Resid:** Orthopaedic Surgery, William Beaumont Hosp 1978; **Fellow:** Orthopaedic Oncology, Mayo Clinic 1978

Orthopaedic Surgery

Joyce, Michael J MD [OrS] - **Spec Exp:** Bone & Soft Tissue Tumors; **Hospital:** Cleveland Clin Fdn (page 70); **Address:** Cleveland Clinic, Dept Orthopaedic Surgery, 9500 Euclid Ave, Desk A41, Cleveland, OH 44195-0001; **Phone:** 216-444-4282; **Board Cert:** Orthopaedic Surgery 1985; **Med School:** Univ Louisville Sch Med 1976; **Resid:** Surgery, Johns Hopkins Hosp 1978; Orthopaedic Surgery, Harvard Combined Program 1981; **Fellow:** Orthopaedic Oncology, Mass General Hosp 1982; Trauma, Univ Toronto-Sunnybrook Hosp 1983; **Fac Appt:** Assoc Clin Prof OrS, Case West Res Univ

McDonald, Douglas J MD [OrS] - **Spec Exp:** Bone & Soft Tissue Tumors; Ewing's Sarcoma; Bone Cancer; **Hospital:** Barnes-Jewish Hosp; **Address:** Ctr Advanced Med, Orthopaedic Surg Ctr, 4921 Parkview Pl Fl 6 - Ste A, Box 8605, St Louis, MO 63110; **Phone:** 314-747-2500; **Board Cert:** Orthopaedic Surgery 2001; **Med School:** Univ Minn 1982; **Resid:** Orthopaedic Surgery, Mayo Clinic 1987; **Fellow:** Orthopaedic Oncology, Mayo Clinic 1988; **Fac Appt:** Prof OrS, Washington Univ, St Louis

Mott, Michael P MD [OrS] - **Spec Exp:** Bone Tumors; Musculoskeletal Tumors; Pediatric Orthopaedic Cancers; **Hospital:** Henry Ford Hosp; **Address:** Henry Ford Hosp, Dept Ortho Surg, 2799 W Grand Blvd Fl 12, Detroit, MI 48202; **Phone:** 313-916-1961; **Board Cert:** Orthopaedic Surgery 2007; **Med School:** Univ Mich Med Sch 1989; **Resid:** Orthopaedic Surgery, Wayne State Univ Affil Hosp 1994; **Fellow:** Musculoskeletal Oncology, Mass Genl Hosp 1995; Orthopaedic Oncology, Wayne State Univ 1996; **Fac Appt:** Assoc Prof OrS, Wayne State Univ

Parsons III, Theodore W MD [OrS] - **Spec Exp:** Bone & Soft Tissue Tumors; Reconstructive Surgery-Adult; **Hospital:** Henry Ford Hosp; **Address:** Henry Ford Hosp, Dept Orthopaedics, 2799 West Grand, Detroit, MI 48202; **Phone:** 313-916-1964; **Board Cert:** Orthopaedic Surgery 2005; **Med School:** Uniformed Srvs Univ, Bethesda 1986; **Resid:** Orthopaedic Surgery, Wilford Hall USAF Med Ctr 1991; **Fellow:** Pediatric Oncology, Boston Chldns Hosp 1992; Orthopaedic Oncology, Mass Genl Hosp 1992; **Fac Appt:** Prof OrS, Wayne State Univ

Peabody, Terrance MD [OrS] - **Spec Exp:** Soft Tissue Tumors; Bone Tumors; Pediatric Orthopaedic Cancers; **Hospital:** Univ of Chicago Med Ctr; **Address:** Univ Chicago Hospital, 5841 S Maryland Ave, MC 3079, Chicago, IL 60637-1463; **Phone:** 773-702-3442; **Board Cert:** Orthopaedic Surgery 2004; **Med School:** UC Irvine 1985; **Resid:** Orthopaedic Surgery, UC Irvine Med Ctr 1990; **Fellow:** Orthopaedic Oncology, Univ Chicago Hosps 1991; **Fac Appt:** Prof S, Univ Chicago-Pritzker Sch Med

Sim, Franklin H MD [OrS] - **Spec Exp:** Sarcoma; Bone Cancer; **Hospital:** Mayo Med Ctr & Clin - Rochester; **Address:** Mayo Clinic, 200 1st St SW, Rochester, MN 55905; **Phone:** 507-284-2511; **Board Cert:** Orthopaedic Surgery 1971; **Med School:** Dalhousie Univ 1965; **Resid:** Orthopaedic Surgery, Mayo Clinic 1970; **Fac Appt:** Prof OrS, Mayo Med Sch

Yasko, Alan MD [OrS] - **Spec Exp:** Pediatric Orthopaedic Surgery; Pediatric Orthopaedic Cancers; Sarcoma; **Hospital:** Northwestern Meml Hosp, Children's Mem Hosp; **Address:** Dept Orthopaedics, 676 N St Clair St, Ste 1350, Chicago, IL 60611; **Phone:** 312-926-4444; **Board Cert:** Orthopaedic Surgery 2004; **Med School:** Northwestern Univ 1984; **Resid:** Orthopaedic Surgery, Case Western 1989; **Fellow:** Orthopaedic Oncology, Meml Sloan Kettering 1991; Metabolic Diseases, Hosp for Special Surgery 1991; **Fac Appt:** Prof S, Northwestern Univ-Feinberg Sch Med

Great Plains and Mountains

Randall, R Lor MD [OrS] - **Spec Exp:** Bone Tumors; Sarcoma-Soft Tissue; Pediatric Orthopaedic Surgery; **Hospital:** Univ Utah Hosps and Clins, Primary Children's Med Ctr; **Address:** Ped Ortho Surg, Primary Chlds Med Ctr, 100 N Medical Drive, Ste 4550, SLC, UT 84113, Salt Lake City, UT 84113; **Phone:** 801-662-5600; **Board Cert:** Orthopaedic Surgery 2001; **Med School:** Yale Univ 1992; **Resid:** Orthopaedic Surgery, UCSF Med Ctr 1997; **Fellow:** Musculoskeletal Oncology, Univ WA Med Ctr 1998; **Fac Appt:** Assoc Prof OrS, Univ Utah

Wilkins, Ross M MD [OrS] - **Spec Exp:** Bone Cancer; **Hospital:** Presby - St Luke's Med Ctr; **Address:** 1601 E 19th Ave, Ste 3300, Denver, CO 80218; **Phone:** 303-837-0072; **Board Cert:** Orthopaedic Surgery 2007; **Med School:** Wayne State Univ 1978; **Resid:** Orthopaedic Surgery, Univ Colorado Med Ctr 1983; **Fellow:** Orthopaedic Oncology, Mayo Clinic 1984

Southwest

Williams, Ronald P MD [OrS] - **Spec Exp:** Bone Tumors; **Hospital:** Univ Hlth Syst-San Antonio; **Address:** Dept of Orthopaedics, 7703 Floyd Curl Drive, MC 7774, San Antonio, TX 78229-3900; **Phone:** 210-567-5125; **Board Cert:** Orthopaedic Surgery 2003; **Med School:** Univ Tex, San Antonio 1984; **Resid:** Orthopaedic Surgery, Univ Kans Sch Med 1989; **Fellow:** Orthopaedic Oncology, Case West Res Univ 1990; **Fac Appt:** Prof OrS, Univ Tex, San Antonio

West Coast and Pacific

Bos, Gary D MD [OrS] - **Spec Exp:** Musculoskeletal Tumors; Sarcoma; Reconstructive Surgery; **Hospital:** Yakima Valley Mem Hosp; **Address:** 16th Avenue Station, 1470 16th Ave, Yakima, WA 98902; **Phone:** 509-574-3300; **Board Cert:** Orthopaedic Surgery 2008; **Med School:** Univ Chicago-Pritzker Sch Med 1978; **Resid:** Orthopaedic Surgery, Case West Reserve 1984; **Fellow:** Orthopaedic Surgery, Case West Reserve 1980; Orthopaedic Oncology, Mayo Clinic 1985

Brien, Earl Warren MD [OrS] - **Spec Exp:** Bone & Soft Tissue Tumors; **Hospital:** Cedars-Sinai Med Ctr; **Address:** 444 S San Vicente Blvd, Ste 603, Los Angeles, CA 90048; **Phone:** 310-423-9887; **Board Cert:** Orthopaedic Surgery 2006; **Med School:** Howard Univ 1986; **Resid:** Orthopaedic Surgery, LAC-King Drew Med Ctr 1992; **Fellow:** Musculoskeletal Disorders, Memorial Sloan Kettering 1993; Metabolic Bone Research, Hosp for Special Surgery 1994

Conrad, Ernest U MD [OrS] - **Spec Exp:** Pediatric Orthopaedic Surgery; Bone Tumors; Sarcoma; **Hospital:** Chldns Hosp and Regl Med Ctr - Seattle, Univ Wash Med Ctr; **Address:** 1959 NE Pacific St, Box 356500, Seattle, WA 98195; **Phone:** 206-543-3690; **Board Cert:** Orthopaedic Surgery 2009; **Med School:** Univ VA Sch Med 1979; **Resid:** Orthopaedic Surgery, Hosp for Special Surgery 1984; **Fellow:** Orthopaedic Oncology, Univ Fla Coll Med 1985; Pediatric Orthopaedic Surgery, Hosp for Sick Chldn 1986; **Fac Appt:** Prof OrS, Univ Wash

Eckardt, Jeffrey J MD [OrS] - **Spec Exp:** Bone Tumors; Soft Tissue Tumors; Limb Sparing Surgery; **Hospital:** Santa Monica - UCLA Med Ctr & Ortho Hosp, UCLA Ronald Reagan Med Ctr; **Address:** UCLA Med Ctr, Dept Ortho Surg/Oncology, 1250 16th St Tower # 745, Santa Monica, CA 90404; **Phone:** 310-319-3816; **Board Cert:** Orthopaedic Surgery 1981; **Med School:** Cornell Univ-Weill Med Coll 1971; **Resid:** Orthopaedic Surgery, UCLA Med Ctr 1979; **Fellow:** Orthopaedic Oncology, Mayo Clinic 1980; **Fac Appt:** Prof OrS, UCLA

Orthopaedic Surgery

Luck Jr, James V MD [OrS] - **Spec Exp:** Musculoskeletal Tumors; **Hospital:** Santa Monica - UCLA Med Ctr & Ortho Hosp; **Address:** 2400 S Flower St, Fl 3, Los Angeles, CA 90007-2660; **Phone:** 213-749-8255; **Board Cert:** Orthopaedic Surgery 2000; **Med School:** USC Sch Med 1967; **Resid:** Orthopaedic Surgery, Orthopaedic Hosp 1973; **Fellow:** Orthopaedic Oncology, Orthopaedic Hosp 1974; Reconstructive Surgery, Rancho Los Amigos 1974; **Fac Appt:** Prof OrS, UCLA

O'Donnell, Richard John MD [OrS] - **Spec Exp:** Bone Cancer; Sarcoma-Soft Tissue; Pediatric Orthopaedic Cancers; **Hospital:** UCSF Med Ctr; **Address:** 1600 Divisadero St Fl 4, San Francisco, CA 94115; **Phone:** 415-885-3800; **Board Cert:** Orthopaedic Surgery 1999; **Med School:** Harvard Med Sch 1989; **Resid:** Orthopaedic Surgery, Mass Genl Hosp 1995; **Fellow:** Musculoskeletal Oncology, Univ WA Med Ctr 1996; **Fac Appt:** Assoc Prof OrS, UCSF

Singer, Daniel I MD [OrS] - **Spec Exp:** Bone Cancer; Hand & Upper Extremity Tumors; **Hospital:** Queen's Med Ctr - Honolulu; **Address:** Queen's Physicians' Office Blg 1, 1380 Lusitana St, Ste 615, Honolulu, HI 96813-2442; **Phone:** 808-521-8109; **Board Cert:** Orthopaedic Surgery 2008; Hand Surgery 2008; **Med School:** Boston Univ 1979; **Resid:** Surgery, Univ Conn Hlth Ctr 1981; Orthopaedic Surgery, Univ Hawaii 1984; **Fellow:** Hand Surgery, Thomas Jefferson Univ Med Ctr 1985; Microvascular Surgery, St Vincent's Hosp 1986; **Fac Appt:** Asst Prof OrS, Univ Hawaii JA Burns Sch Med

HAND SURGERY

Mid Atlantic

Athanasian, Edward MD [HS] - **Spec Exp:** Bone & Soft Tissue Tumors; Hand & Upper Extremity Tumors; **Hospital:** Hosp For Special Surgery, Meml Sloan-Kettering Cancer Ctr (page 76); **Address:** Hospital for Special Surgery, 535 E 70th St, New York, NY 10021; **Phone:** 212-606-1962; **Board Cert:** Orthopaedic Surgery 1997; Hand Surgery 1999; **Med School:** Columbia P&S 1988; **Resid:** Surgery, Beth Israel Hosp 1989; Orthopaedic Surgery, Hosp Special Surgery 1993; **Fellow:** Hand Surgery, Mayo Clinic 1994; Orthopaedic Oncology, Meml Sloan Kettering Cancer Ctr 1995; **Fac Appt:** Asst Prof OrS, Cornell Univ-Weill Med Coll

West Coast and Pacific

Szabo, Robert M MD [HS] - **Spec Exp:** Hand & Upper Extremity Tumors; **Hospital:** UC Davis Med Ctr, Mercy General Hosp - Sacramento; **Address:** UC Davis, Dept Orthopaedics, 4860 Y St, Ste 3800, Sacramento, CA 95817-2307; **Phone:** 916-734-3678; **Board Cert:** Orthopaedic Surgery 2009; Hand Surgery 2009; **Med School:** SUNY Buffalo 1977; **Resid:** Surgery, Mt Sinai Hosp 1979; Orthopaedic Surgery, Mt Sinai Hosp 1982; **Fellow:** Hand Surgery, UCSD Med Ctr 1983; Epidemiology, UC Berkeley 1995; **Fac Appt:** Prof OrS, UC Davis

NYU Cancer Institute
NYU LANGONE MEDICAL CENTER

NYU Clinical Cancer Center
160 East 34th Street
New York, New York 10016
www.nyuci.org/atcd

NYU Langone Medical Center
550 First Avenue
(at 31st Street)
New York, New York 10016
www.nyumc.org/atcd

Stephen D. Hassenfeld
Children's Center
for Cancer and Blood
Disorders
160 East 32nd Street
New York, New York 10016
www.nyumc.org/hassenfeld

A Collaborative Approach
The NYU Cancer Institute, an NCI designated center, is a "matrix cancer center" without walls operating within the larger NYU Langone Medical Center. With over 175 members and a research funding base of over $81 million, this structure strengthens our capabilities to forge collaborations across medical and scientific disciplines, which translates to comprehensive care for our patients and discoveries that will influence the future of this disease.

Renowned Expertise
Team members' compassion and expertise help patients better manage the symptoms of their disease as well as their special needs. Our highly skilled Magnet™ nursing team not only plays a pivotal role in coordinating direct patient care, but is also a source of invaluable patient education.

A Patient-Focused Setting
The NYU Clinical Cancer Center, with over 70 faculty members from various disciplines at the New York University School of Medicine, is the principal outpatient facility of the Cancer Institute and serves as home for our patients and their caregivers. The center and its multidisciplinary team of experts provide access to the latest treatment options and clinical trials along with a variety of programs in cancer prevention, screening, diagnostics, genetic counseling, and supportive services. When it comes to kids and cancer, the Stephen D. Hassenfeld Children's Center for Cancer and Blood Disorders offers not just innovation but insight. As a leading member of the NCI-sponsored Children's Oncology Group, our physicians are known for developing new ways to treat childhood cancer. Our affiliation with Bellevue Hospital, the oldest public hospital in the country, affords clinically distinctive opportunities to learn and care for patients with cancer by observing its presentation and behavior in a variety of patient groups.

Otolaryngology

An otolaryngologist diagnoses and provides medical and/or surgical therapy prevention of diseases, allergies, neoplasms, deformities, disorders and/or injuries of the ears, nose, sinuses, throat, respiratory and upper alimentary systems, face, jaws and the other head and neck systems. Head and neck oncology, facial plastic and reconstructive surgery and the treatment of disorders of hearing and voice are fundamental areas of expertise.

An otolaryngologist-head and neck surgeon provides comprehensive medical and surgical care for patients with diseases and disorders that affect the ears, nose, throat, the respiratory and upper alimentary systems and related structures of the head and neck.

Training Required: Five years. Certification in the following subspecialty requires additional training and examination.

Plastic Surgery within the Head and Neck: An otolaryngologist with additional training in plastic and reconstructive procedures within the head, face, neck and associated structures, including cutaneous head and neck oncology and reconstructioin, management of maxillofacial trauma, soft tissue repair and neural surgery.

This field is diverse and involves a wide range of patients, from the newborn to the aged. While both cosmetic and reconstructive surgeries are practiced, there are many additional procedures which interface with them.

Otolaryngology

New England

Deschler, Daniel G MD [Oto] - **Spec Exp:** Head & Neck Cancer; Head & Neck Reconstruction; Salivary Gland Tumors & Surgery; Voice after Laryngeal Cancer Surgery; **Hospital:** Mass Eye & Ear Infirmary, Mass Genl Hosp; **Address:** Mass Eye & Ear Infirmary, Head & Neck Surgery, 243 Charles St, Boston, MA 02114; **Phone:** 617-573-4100; **Board Cert:** Otolaryngology 1996; **Med School:** Harvard Med Sch 1990; **Resid:** Otolaryngology, UCSF Med Ctr 1995; **Fellow:** Head & Neck Surgical Oncology, Hahneman U Med Ctr 1996; **Fac Appt:** Assoc Prof Oto, Harvard Med Sch

Grillone, Gregory A MD [Oto] - **Spec Exp:** Laryngeal Disorders; Voice Disorders; Laryngeal Cancer; Head & Neck Cancer & Surgery; **Hospital:** Boston Med Ctr; **Address:** Boston Univ Med Ctr, Dept Otolaryngology, 830 Harrison Ave, Boston, MA 02118; **Phone:** 617-638-8124; **Board Cert:** Otolaryngology 1988; **Med School:** Mount Sinai Sch Med 1983; **Resid:** Oncology, Boston Univ Med Ctr 1988; **Fac Appt:** Asst Prof Oto, Boston Univ

Sasaki, Clarence T MD [Oto] - **Spec Exp:** Head & Neck Cancer; Skull Base Surgery; Voice Disorders; Swallowing Disorders; **Hospital:** Yale-New Haven Hosp, Hosp of St Raphael; **Address:** Yale Sch Med, Dept Otolaryngology, 333 Cedar St, Box 208041, New Haven, CT 06520-8041; **Phone:** 203-785-2592; **Board Cert:** Otolaryngology 1973; **Med School:** Yale Univ 1966; **Resid:** Surgery, Mary Hitchcock Hosp 1968; Otolaryngology, Yale-New Haven Hosp 1973; **Fellow:** Head and Neck Surgery, Univ of Milan 1978; Skull Base Surgery, Univ Zurich 1982; **Fac Appt:** Prof Oto, Yale Univ

Zeitels, Steven MD [Oto] - **Spec Exp:** Laryngeal Disorders; Voice Disorders; Laryngeal Cancer; Head & Neck Cancer & Surgery; **Hospital:** Mass Genl Hosp; **Address:** Mass Genl Hosp, 1 Bowdoin Square Fl 11, Boston, MA 02114; **Phone:** 617-726-0218; **Board Cert:** Otolaryngology 1988; **Med School:** Boston Univ 1982; **Resid:** Surgery, Univ Hosp-Boston City Hosp 1983; Otolaryngology, Boston Univ-Tufts Univ 1987; **Fellow:** Head and Neck Surgery, Boston VA Med Ctr 1988; **Fac Appt:** Prof S, Harvard Med Sch

Mid Atlantic

Carrau, Ricardo L MD [Oto] - **Spec Exp:** Skull Base Tumors & Surgery; Nasal & Sinus Cancer & Surgery; Swallowing Disorders; **Hospital:** UPMC Presby, Pittsburgh; **Address:** Eye & Ear Institute, 200 Lothrop St, Ste 500, Pittsburgh, PA 15213; **Phone:** 412-647-2100; **Board Cert:** Otolaryngology 1987; **Med School:** Univ Puerto Rico 1981; **Resid:** Surgery, University Hosp 1984; Head and Neck Surgery, University Hosp 1987; **Fellow:** Head and Neck Oncology, Univ Pittsburgh Med Ctr 1990; **Fac Appt:** Assoc Prof Oto, Univ Pittsburgh

Chalian, Ara A MD [Oto] - **Spec Exp:** Head & Neck Cancer; Head & Neck Reconstruction; Thyroid Cancer; Reconstructive Surgery; **Hospital:** Hosp Univ Penn - UPHS (page 81); **Address:** Hosp Univ Penn, Dept Otolaryngology, 3400 Spruce St, Silverstein Bldg, Philadelphia, PA 19104; **Phone:** 215-349-5559; **Board Cert:** Otolaryngology 1994; **Med School:** Indiana Univ 1988; **Resid:** Surgery, Indiana Univ Hosp 1990; Otolaryngology, Indiana Univ Hosp 1993; **Fellow:** Molecular Biology, Hosp U Penn 1994; Head and Neck Surgery, Hosp U Penn 1995; **Fac Appt:** Assoc Prof Oto, Univ Pennsylvania

Close, Lanny G MD [Oto] - **Spec Exp:** Skull Base Surgery; Head & Neck Cancer; **Hospital:** NY-Presby Hosp/Columbia (page 79); **Address:** 16 E 60th St, Ste 470, New York, NY 10022; **Phone:** 212-326-8475; **Board Cert:** Otolaryngology 1977; **Med School:** Baylor Coll Med 1972; **Resid:** Surgery, Johns Hopkins Hosp 1974; Otolaryngology, Baylor Affil Hosps 1977; **Fellow:** Head and Neck Surgery, MD Anderson Cancer Ctr 1979; **Fac Appt:** Prof Oto, Columbia P&S

Costantino, Peter D MD [Oto] - **Spec Exp:** Skull Base Tumors; Head & Neck Cancer; Cranio-facial Surgery/Reconstruction; **Hospital:** St Luke's - Roosevelt Hosp Ctr - Roosevelt Div (page 71), NY-Presby Hosp/Columbia (page 79); **Address:** 1000 W 10th Ave, Ste 5G-80, New York, NY 10019-1104; **Phone:** 212-523-6756; **Board Cert:** Otolaryngology 1990; Facial Plastic & Reconstr Surgery 2000; **Med School:** Northwestern Univ 1984; **Resid:** Surgery, Northwestern Meml Hosp 1986; Otolaryngology, Northwestern Meml Hosp 1989; **Fellow:** Head and Neck Surgery, Northwestern Meml Hosp 1990; Skull Base Surgery, Univ Pittsburgh 1991; **Fac Appt:** Prof Oto, Columbia P&S

Davidson, Bruce J MD [Oto] - **Spec Exp:** Head & Neck Cancer; Thyroid Disorders; **Hospital:** Georgetown Univ Hosp; **Address:** Georgetown Univ Med Ctr, Dept Otolaryngology-Head & Neck Surgery, 3800 Reservoir Rd NW Gorman Bldg Fl 1, Washington, DC 20007; **Phone:** 202-444-8186; **Board Cert:** Otolaryngology 1993; **Med School:** W VA Univ 1987; **Resid:** Otolaryngology, Georgetown Univ Med Ctr 1992; **Fellow:** Otolaryngology, Memorial Sloan-Kettering Cancer Ctr 1994; **Fac Appt:** Asst Prof Oto, Georgetown Univ

Genden, Eric M MD [Oto] - **Spec Exp:** Head & Neck Cancer & Surgery; Head & Neck Cancer Reconstruction; Airway Reconstruction; Thyroid & Parathyroid Cancer & Surgery; **Hospital:** Mount Sinai Med Ctr (page 77); **Address:** Mt Sinai Dept Otolaryngology, 1 Gustave L Levy Pl, Box 1191, New York, NY 10029; **Phone:** 212-241-9410; **Board Cert:** Otolaryngology 1999; Facial Plastic & Reconstr Surgery 2000; **Med School:** Mount Sinai Sch Med 1992; **Resid:** Otolaryngology, Barnes Jewish Hosp 1998; **Fellow:** Head and Neck Surgery, Mt Sinai Med Ctr 1999; **Fac Appt:** Assoc Prof Oto, Mount Sinai Sch Med

Goldenberg, David MD [Oto] - **Spec Exp:** Head & Neck Cancer & Surgery; Thyroid & Parathyroid Cancer & Surgery; Salivary Gland Tumors & Surgery; **Hospital:** Penn State Milton S Hershey Med Ctr; **Address:** MSHMC-Otolaryngololgy/ENT, 500 University Ave, MC HU25, Hershey, PA 17033-0850; **Phone:** 717-531-5215; **Med School:** Israel 1995; **Resid:** Otolaryngology, Rambam Med Ctr; **Fellow:** Head & Neck Surgical Oncology, Johns Hopkins Med Ctr; **Fac Appt:** Assoc Prof S, Penn State Univ-Hershey Med Ctr

Grandis, Jennifer R MD [Oto] - **Spec Exp:** Head & Neck Cancer; **Hospital:** UPMC Presby, Pittsburgh, Magee-Womens Hosp - UPMC; **Address:** Univ Pittsburgh Med Ctr EELB, 200 Lothrop St, Ste 500, Pittsburgh, PA 15213; **Phone:** 412-647-5280; **Board Cert:** Otolaryngology 1994; **Med School:** Univ Pittsburgh 1987; **Resid:** Otolaryngology, Univ Pittsburgh Med Ctr 1993; **Fac Appt:** Prof Oto, Univ Pittsburgh

Har-El, Gady MD [Oto] - **Spec Exp:** Head & Neck Cancer; Thyroid & Parathyroid Surgery; Skull Base Surgery; **Hospital:** Lenox Hill Hosp, Lenox Hill Hosp (Manh Eye, Ear & Throat Hosp); **Address:** 186 E 76th St Fl 2, New York, NY 10021; **Phone:** 212-434-2323; **Board Cert:** Otolaryngology 1992; **Med School:** Israel 1982; **Resid:** Otolaryngology, SUNY Downstate Med Ctr 1991; **Fac Appt:** Prof Oto, SUNY Hlth Sci Ctr

Hicks Jr, Wesley L MD/DDS [Oto] - **Spec Exp:** Head & Neck Cancer & Surgery; Reconstructive Surgery; **Hospital:** Roswell Park Cancer Inst; **Address:** Roswell Park Cancer Inst, Dept Head & Neck Surgery, Elm & Carlton Sts, Buffalo, NY 14263; **Phone:** 716-845-3158; **Board Cert:** Otolaryngology 1993; **Med School:** SUNY Buffalo 1984; **Resid:** Otolaryngology, Manhattan Eye Ear & Throat Hosp 1988; Otolaryngology, New York Hosp/Meml Sloan Kettering Cancer Ctr 1989; **Fellow:** Head and Neck Surgery, Stanford Univ Med Ctr 1990; **Fac Appt:** Assoc Prof Oto, SUNY Buffalo

Otolaryngology

Hirsch, Barry MD [Oto] - **Spec Exp:** Ear Tumors; Skull Base Tumors; **Hospital:** UPMC Presby, Pittsburgh; **Address:** 200 Lothrop St, Ste 500, Ear Nose Throat Inst, Dept Otolaryngology, Pittsburgh, PA 15213; **Phone:** 412-647-2100; **Board Cert:** Otolaryngology 1982; Neurotology 2005; **Med School:** Univ Pennsylvania 1977; **Resid:** Otolaryngology, Univ Pittsburgh Med Ctr 1982; **Fellow:** Neurotology, Univ Pittsburgh 1985; Neurotology, Univ Zurich 1986; **Fac Appt:** Prof Oto, Univ Pittsburgh

Holliday, Michael J MD [Oto] - **Spec Exp:** Neuro-Otology; Skull Base Surgery; **Hospital:** Johns Hopkins Hosp, Johns Hopkins Bayview Med Ctr; **Address:** Johns Hopkins Hosp-Otology Division, 601 N Caroline St Fl 6, Baltimore, MD 21287; **Phone:** 410-955-3492; **Board Cert:** Otolaryngology 1976; **Med School:** Marquette Sch Med 1969; **Resid:** Otolaryngology, Johns Hopkins Hosp 1976; **Fellow:** Neurotology, Univ Zurich 1979; **Fac Appt:** Assoc Prof Oto, Johns Hopkins Univ

Johnson, Jonas T MD [Oto] - **Spec Exp:** Head & Neck Surgery; Head & Neck Cancer; Parotid Gland Tumors; Thyroid Cancer; **Hospital:** UPMC Montefiore, Magee-Womens Hosp - UPMC; **Address:** Univ Physicians UPMC, Eye & Ear Inst, 200 Lothrop St, Ste 300, Pittsburgh, PA 15213; **Phone:** 412-647-2100; **Board Cert:** Otolaryngology 1977; **Med School:** SUNY Upstate Med Univ 1972; **Resid:** Surgery, Med Coll Virginia Hosps 1974; Otolaryngology, SUNY-Univ Hosp 1977; **Fac Appt:** Prof Oto, Univ Pittsburgh

Keane, William M MD [Oto] - **Spec Exp:** Head & Neck Cancer & Surgery; Thyroid Cancer; **Hospital:** Thomas Jefferson Univ Hosp (page 83); **Address:** Thomas Jefferson Hosp, 925 Chestnut St Fl 6, Philadelphia, PA 19107; **Phone:** 215-955-6760; **Board Cert:** Otolaryngology 1978; **Med School:** Harvard Med Sch 1970; **Resid:** Surgery, Strong Meml Hosp 1972; Otolaryngology, Univ Penn Hosp 1977; **Fac Appt:** Prof Oto, Thomas Jefferson Univ

Kennedy, David W MD [Oto] - **Spec Exp:** Sinus Disorders/Surgery; Skull Base Tumors & Surgery; **Hospital:** Hosp Univ Penn - UPHS (page 81), Pennsylvania Hosp (page 81); **Address:** Hosp Univ Penn, Dept Oto/Head & Neck Surg, 3400 Spruce St Ravdin Bldg Fl 5, Philadelphia, PA 19104-4229; **Phone:** 215-662-6971; **Board Cert:** Otolaryngology 1978; **Med School:** Ireland 1972; **Resid:** Surgery, Johns Hopkins Hosp 1974; Otolaryngology, Johns Hopkins Hosp 1978; **Fac Appt:** Prof Oto, Univ Pennsylvania

Koch, Wayne Martin MD [Oto] - **Spec Exp:** Head & Neck Cancer; Sinus Tumors; **Hospital:** Johns Hopkins Hosp; **Address:** Johns Hopkins Hosp, Dept Otolaryngology, 601 N Caroline St, rm 6221, Baltimore, MD 21287; **Phone:** 410-955-4906; **Board Cert:** Otolaryngology 1987; **Med School:** Univ Pittsburgh 1982; **Resid:** Otolaryngology, Tufts-Boston Univ Hosps 1987; **Fellow:** Surgical Oncology, Johns Hopkins Hosp 1989; **Fac Appt:** Assoc Prof Oto, Johns Hopkins Univ

Kraus, Dennis H MD [Oto] - **Spec Exp:** Head & Neck Cancer; Skull Base Tumors; Thyroid & Parathyroid Surgery; **Hospital:** Meml Sloan-Kettering Cancer Ctr (page 76); **Address:** 1275 York Avenue, New York, NY 10065; **Phone:** 800-525-2225; **Board Cert:** Otolaryngology 1990; **Med School:** Univ Rochester 1985; **Resid:** Surgery, Cleveland Clinic 1987; Otolaryngology, Cleveland Clinic 1990; **Fellow:** Head and Neck Surgery, Meml Sloan Kettering Cancer Ctr 1991; **Fac Appt:** Prof Oto, Cornell Univ-Weill Med Coll

Krespi, Yosef P MD [Oto] - **Spec Exp:** Nasal & Sinus Cancer & Surgery; Head & Neck Cancer & Surgery; **Hospital:** St Luke's - Roosevelt Hosp Ctr - Roosevelt Div (page 71); **Address:** 425 W 59th St Fl 10, New York, NY 10019-1128; **Phone:** 212-262-4444; **Board Cert:** Otolaryngology 1981; **Med School:** Israel 1973; **Resid:** Surgery, Mt Sinai Hosp 1976; Otolaryngology, Mt Sinai Hosp 1980; **Fellow:** Surgery, Northwestern Meml Hosp 1981; **Fac Appt:** Clin Prof Oto, Columbia P&S

Lawson, William MD [Oto] - **Spec Exp:** Sinus Disorders/Surgery; Head & Neck Cancer; Skull Base Surgery; **Hospital:** Mount Sinai Med Ctr (page 77); **Address:** 5 E 98th St Fl 8, Box 1191, New York, NY 10029-6501; **Phone:** 212-241-9410; **Board Cert:** Otolaryngology 1974; **Med School:** NYU Sch Med 1965; **Resid:** Surgery, Bronx VA Hosp 1967; Otolaryngology, Mt Sinai Hosp 1973; **Fellow:** Otolaryngology, Mt Sinai Hosp 1970; **Fac Appt:** Prof Oto, Mount Sinai Sch Med

O'Malley Jr, Bert W MD [Oto] - **Spec Exp:** Head & Neck Cancer; Sinus Tumors; Skull Base Tumors; **Hospital:** Hosp Univ Penn - UPHS (page 81); **Address:** Hosp Univ Penn, Dept Otolaryngology, 3400 Spruce St, 5 Ravdin, Philadelphia, PA 19104; **Phone:** 215-615-4325; **Board Cert:** Otolaryngology 1995; **Med School:** Univ Tex SW, Dallas 1988; **Resid:** Surgery, UTSW Med Ctr/Parkland Meml Hosp 1989; Otolaryngology, Baylor Coll Med 1993; **Fellow:** Head and Neck Oncology, Univ Pittsburgh 1994; Skull Base Surgery, Univ Pittsburgh 1995; **Fac Appt:** Prof Oto, Univ Pennsylvania

Papel, Ira D MD [Oto] - **Spec Exp:** Reconstructive Surgery-Face; Skin Cancer/Facial Reconstruction; **Hospital:** Greater Baltimore Med Ctr, Johns Hopkins Hosp; **Address:** 1838 Greene Tree Rd, Ste 370, Baltimore, MD 21208; **Phone:** 410-486-3400; **Board Cert:** Otolaryngology 1986; Facial Plastic & Reconstr Surgery 1991; **Med School:** Boston Univ 1981; **Resid:** Otolaryngology, Johns Hopkins Hosp 1986; **Fellow:** Facial Plastic Surgery, UCSF Med Ctr 1987; **Fac Appt:** Assoc Prof Oto, Johns Hopkins Univ

Persky, Mark S MD [Oto] - **Spec Exp:** Head & Neck Cancer; Skull Base Tumors; Thyroid Cancer; **Hospital:** Beth Israel Med Ctr - Petrie Division (page 71); **Address:** 10 Union Square East, Ste 4J, New York, NY 10003; **Phone:** 212-844-8648; **Board Cert:** Otolaryngology 1976; **Med School:** SUNY Upstate Med Univ 1972; **Resid:** Otolaryngology, Bellevue Hosp 1976; **Fellow:** Head and Neck Surgery, Beth Israel Med Ctr 1977; **Fac Appt:** Clin Prof Oto, Albert Einstein Coll Med

Rassekh, Christopher MD [Oto] - **Spec Exp:** Laryngeal Cancer-Organ Preservation; Skull Base Tumors; Salivary Gland Tumors & Surgery; **Hospital:** WV Univ Hosp - Ruby Memorial, Monongalia Genl Hosp; **Address:** West Virginia Univ, Dept Otolaryngology, Robin C Byrd Hlth Scis Ctr, Head & Neck Surgery, PO Box 9200, Morgantown, WV 26506-9200; **Phone:** 304-293-3233; **Board Cert:** Otolaryngology 1993; **Med School:** Univ Iowa Coll Med 1986; **Resid:** Otolaryngology, Univ Iowa Med Ctr 1992; **Fellow:** Head and Neck Surgery, Univ Pittsburgh Med Ctr 1993; **Fac Appt:** Assoc Prof Oto, W VA Univ

Schantz, Stimson P MD [Oto] - **Spec Exp:** Head & Neck Surgery; Head & Neck Cancer; Thyroid Cancer; **Hospital:** New York Eye & Ear Infirm (page 78), Beth Israel Med Ctr - Petrie Division (page 71); **Address:** 310 E 14th St Fl 6N, New YorkNew York, NY 10003; **Phone:** 212-979-4535; **Board Cert:** Surgery 2005; **Med School:** Univ Cincinnati 1975; **Resid:** Surgery, Georgetown Univ Med CtrGeorgetown Univ Med Ctr 1982; Otolaryngology, Univ Illinois Eye & Ear Infirm 1980; **Fellow:** Surgical Oncology, MD Anderson Cancer Ctr 1984; **Fac Appt:** Prof Oto, NY Med Coll

Shapshay, Stanley M MD [Oto] - **Spec Exp:** Laryngeal Cancer; **Hospital:** Albany Med Ctr; **Address:** University Ear, Nose & Throat Ctr, 35 Hackett Blvd, Albany, NY 12208-3420; **Phone:** 518-262-5575; **Board Cert:** Otolaryngology 1975; **Med School:** Med Coll VA 1968; **Resid:** Surgery, New England Med Ctr 1971; Otolaryngology, Boston Med Ctr 1975; **Fellow:** Surgery, Serafimer Hosp/Karolinska Med Sch 1972; **Fac Appt:** Prof Oto, Albany Med Coll

Snyderman, Carl H MD [Oto] - **Spec Exp:** Skull Base Tumors & Surgery; Sinus Tumors; Head & Neck Cancer; Endoscopic Surgery; **Hospital:** UPMC Presby, Pittsburgh; **Address:** Eye Ear Inst, Dept of Otolaryngology, 200 Lothrop St, Ste 500, Pittsburgh, PA 15213; **Phone:** 412-647-2100; **Board Cert:** Otolaryngology 1987; **Med School:** Univ Chicago-Pritzker Sch Med 1982; **Resid:** Otolaryngology, Eye-Ear Hosp/Univ Pittsburgh 1987; **Fellow:** Skull Base Surgery, Eye-Ear Hosp/Univ Pittsburgh 1988; **Fac Appt:** Prof Oto, Univ Pittsburgh

Otolaryngology

Strome, Marshall MD [Oto] - **Spec Exp:** Voice Disorders; Head & Neck Cancer; Swallowing Disorders; **Hospital:** St Luke's - Roosevelt Hosp Ctr - St Luke's Hosp (page 71); **Address:** 110 E 59th St, Ste 10A, New York, NY 10022; **Phone:** 212-223-1333; **Board Cert:** Otolaryngology 1970; **Med School:** Univ Mich Med Sch 1964; **Resid:** Surgery, Harper Hosp 1966; Otolaryngology, Univ Michigan Hosp 1970; **Fac Appt:** Prof Oto

Strome, Scott MD [Oto] - **Spec Exp:** Microsurgery; Head & Neck Cancer; Head & Neck Reconstruction; **Hospital:** Univ of MD Med Ctr; **Address:** 16 S Eutaw St, Ste 500, Baltimore, MD 21201; **Phone:** 410-328-6467; **Board Cert:** Otolaryngology 1998; **Med School:** Harvard Med Sch 1991; **Resid:** Otolaryngology, Univ Michigan 1997; **Fellow:** Head and Neck Surgery, Allegheny Genl Hosp 1998; Microvascular Surgery, Allegheny Genl Hosp 1998; **Fac Appt:** Prof Oto, Univ MD Sch Med

Urken, Mark MD [Oto] - **Spec Exp:** Head & Neck Cancer & Surgery; Head & Neck Cancer Reconstruction; Thyroid & Parathyroid Cancer & Surgery; Salivary Gland Tumors; **Hospital:** Beth Israel Med Ctr - Petrie Division (page 71); **Address:** Inst for Head, Neck & Thyroid Cancer, 10 Union Square E, Ste 5B, New York, NY 10003-3314; **Phone:** 212-844-8775; **Board Cert:** Otolaryngology 1986; **Med School:** Univ VA Sch Med 1981; **Resid:** Otolaryngology, Mt Sinai Hosp 1986; **Fellow:** Microvascular Surgery, Mercy Hosp 1987; **Fac Appt:** Prof Oto, Albert Einstein Coll Med

Weinstein, Gregory MD [Oto] - **Spec Exp:** Head & Neck Cancer; Laryngeal Cancer; **Hospital:** Hosp Univ Penn - UPHS (page 81); **Address:** Hosp Univ Penn, Dept Otolaryngology, 3400 Spruce St, 5 Ravdin, Philadelphia, PA 19104; **Phone:** 215-349-5390; **Board Cert:** Otolaryngology 1990; **Med School:** NY Med Coll 1985; **Resid:** Otolaryngology, Univ Iowa Hosp 1990; **Fellow:** Head and Neck Oncology, UC Davis Med Ctr 1991; **Fac Appt:** Assoc Prof Oto, Univ Pennsylvania

Woo, Peak MD [Oto] - **Spec Exp:** Voice Disorders; Laryngeal Cancer; **Hospital:** Mount Sinai Med Ctr (page 77); **Address:** 300 Central Park West, Ste 1-H, New York, NY 10024; **Phone:** 212-580-1004; **Board Cert:** Otolaryngology 1983; **Med School:** Boston Univ 1978; **Resid:** Otolaryngology, Boston Univ Med Ctr 1983; **Fac Appt:** Clin Prof Oto, Mount Sinai Sch Med

Southeast

Browne, J Dale MD [Oto] - **Spec Exp:** Head & Neck Cancer; Thyroid Cancer; Skull Base Surgery; Head & Neck Reconstruction; **Hospital:** Wake Forest Univ Baptist Med Ctr (page 84); **Address:** Wake Forest Baptist Med Ctr, Dept Otolaryngology, Medical Center Blvd, Winston Salem, NC 27103; **Phone:** 336-716-4161; **Board Cert:** Otolaryngology 1987; **Med School:** Med Coll GA 1982; **Resid:** Otolaryngology, NC Baptist Hosp 1987; **Fellow:** Otolaryngology, Univ Hosp 1991; **Fac Appt:** Prof Oto, Wake Forest Univ

Bumpous, Jeffrey MD [Oto] - **Spec Exp:** Head & Neck Cancer; Head & Neck Reconstruction; Thyroid & Parathyroid Cancer & Surgery; **Hospital:** Univ of Louisville Hosp, Norton Hosp; **Address:** 401 E Chestnut St, Ste 710, Louisville, KY 40202-1845; **Phone:** 502-583-8303; **Board Cert:** Otolaryngology 1994; **Med School:** Univ Louisville Sch Med 1988; **Resid:** Otolaryngology, Univ Louisville Hosp 1993; **Fellow:** Head and Neck Surgery, Univ Pittsburgh 1994; **Fac Appt:** Prof Oto, Univ Louisville Sch Med

Cassisi, Nicholas J MD [Oto] - **Spec Exp:** Head & Neck Cancer; **Hospital:** Shands at Univ of FL; **Address:** Shands Healthcare at Univ FL, 1600 SW Archer Rd, Box 100383, Gainesville, FL 32610; **Phone:** 352-265-8989; **Board Cert:** Otolaryngology 1971; **Med School:** Univ Miami Sch Med 1965; **Resid:** Surgery, Jackson Meml Hosp 1967; Otolaryngology, Barnes Hosp-Washington Univ 1971; **Fac Appt:** Prof Oto, Univ Fla Coll Med

Civantos, Francisco J MD [Oto] - **Spec Exp:** Head & Neck Cancer; **Hospital:** Univ of Miami Hosp & Clins/Sylvester Comp Canc Ctr (page 82); **Address:** Sylvester CAncer Ctr, Otolaryngology, 1475 NW 12th Ave, Ste 4027, Miami, FL 33136; **Phone:** 205-243-5276; **Board Cert:** Otolaryngology 1992; **Med School:** Columbia P&S 1986; **Resid:** Otolaryngology, Univ Illinois Coll Med 1991; **Fellow:** Head and Neck Oncology, Vanderbilt Univ 1992; **Fac Appt:** Assoc Prof Oto, Univ Miami Sch Med

Couch, Marion E MD [Oto] - **Spec Exp:** Head & Neck Cancer; Thyroid Cancer; **Hospital:** Univ NC Hosps; **Address:** Univ N Carolina Sch Med, Dept Otolaryngology, CB 7070, Chapel Hill, NC 27599-7070; **Phone:** 919-966-3342; **Board Cert:** Otolaryngology 1997; **Med School:** Rush Med Coll 1990; **Resid:** Surgery, Johns Hopkins Hosp 1991; Otolaryngology, Johns Hopkins Hosp 1995; **Fac Appt:** Assoc Prof Oto, Univ NC Sch Med

Day, Terrence A MD [Oto] - **Spec Exp:** Head & Neck Cancer; Reconstructive Microvascular Surgery; Skull Base Surgery; Facial Plastic & Reconstructive Surgery; **Hospital:** MUSC Med Ctr; **Address:** MUSC, Dept Otolaryngology, 135 Rutledge Ave, Ste 1130, Box MSC550, Charleston, SC 29425; **Phone:** 843-792-0719; **Board Cert:** Otolaryngology 1996; **Med School:** Univ Okla Coll Med 1989; **Resid:** Otolaryngology, LSU Med Ctr 1995; **Fellow:** Head & Neck Surgical Oncology, UC Davis Med Ctr 1996; Maxillofacial Surgery, Univ Hosp 1994; **Fac Appt:** Assoc Prof Oto, Med Univ SC

Goodwin, W Jarrard MD [Oto] - **Spec Exp:** Head & Neck Cancer; **Hospital:** Univ of Miami Hosp & Clins/Sylvester Comp Canc Ctr (page 82), Jackson Meml Hosp (page 82); **Address:** Dept Otolaryngology, 1475 NW 12th Ave, Ste 4037, Miami, FL 33136-1015; **Phone:** 305-243-4387; **Board Cert:** Otolaryngology 1978; **Med School:** Albany Med Coll 1972; **Resid:** Surgery, Univ Miami/Jackson Hosp Meml Hosp 1974; Otolaryngology, Univ Miami/Jackson Hosp 1977; **Fellow:** Head & Neck Surgical Oncology, MD Anderson Hosp 1980; **Fac Appt:** Prof Oto, Univ Miami Sch Med

Lanza, Donald C MD [Oto] - **Spec Exp:** Skull Base Tumors; Sinus Disorders/Surgery; **Hospital:** St Anthony's Hosp - St Petersburg, All Children's Hosp; **Address:** 900 Carillon Pkwy, Ste 200, St. Petersburg, FL 33716-1108; **Phone:** 727-573-0074; **Board Cert:** Otolaryngology 1990; **Med School:** SUNY Hlth Sci Ctr 1985; **Resid:** Surgery, Albany Med Ctr 1987; Otolaryngology, Albany Med Ctr 1990; **Fellow:** Rhinology, Johns Hopkins Univ 1990; Rhinology, Univ Penn 1991

Levine, Paul A MD [Oto] - **Spec Exp:** Head & Neck Cancer; Head & Neck Reconstruction; Skull Base Tumors; **Hospital:** Univ Virginia Med Ctr; **Address:** Dept Otolaryngology, PO Box 800713, Charlottesville, VA 22908; **Phone:** 434-924-5593; **Board Cert:** Otolaryngology 1978; **Med School:** Albany Med Coll 1973; **Resid:** Otolaryngology, Yale-New Haven Hosp 1977; **Fellow:** Head and Neck Surgery, Stanford Med Ctr 1978; **Fac Appt:** Prof Oto, Univ VA Sch Med

McCaffrey, Thomas V MD [Oto] - **Spec Exp:** Head & Neck Cancer; Thyroid Cancer; Tracheal Surgery; **Hospital:** H Lee Moffitt Cancer Ctr & Research Inst, Tampa Genl Hosp; **Address:** H Lee Moffitt Cancer Ctr, Dept Otolaryngology-HNS, 12902 Magnolia Drive, Tampa, FL 33612; **Phone:** 813-745-8463; **Board Cert:** Otolaryngology 1980; **Med School:** Loyola Univ-Stritch Sch Med 1974; **Resid:** Surgery, Mayo Affil Hosps 1976; Otolaryngology, Mayo Affil Hosps 1980; **Fac Appt:** Prof Oto, Univ S Fla Coll Med

Netterville, James L MD [Oto] - **Spec Exp:** Head & Neck Surgery; Head & Neck Cancer; Skull Base Tumors; **Hospital:** Vanderbilt Univ Med Ctr, Vanderbilt Children's Hosp; **Address:** Vanderbilt Univ Med Ctr, Dept Oto, 7209 Med Ctr East, South Twr, 1215 21st Ave S, Nashville, TN 37232-8605; **Phone:** 615-343-8840; **Board Cert:** Otolaryngology 1985; **Med School:** Univ Tenn Coll Med, Memphis 1980; **Resid:** Surgery, Methodist Hosp 1982; Otolaryngology, Univ Tenn Med Ctr 1985; **Fellow:** Surgical Oncology, Univ Iowa 1986; **Fac Appt:** Prof Oto, Vanderbilt Univ

Otolaryngology

Osguthorpe, John D MD [Oto] - **Spec Exp:** Head & Neck Cancer; Thyroid & Parathyroid Cancer & Surgery; Salivary Gland Tumors & Surgery; Laryngeal Cancer; **Hospital:** MUSC Med Ctr, E Cooper Reg Med Ctr; **Address:** MUSC Med Ctr-Dept Otolaryngology, 135 Rutledge Ave, MS S50, Charleston, SC 29425; **Phone:** 843-792-3533; **Board Cert:** Otolaryngology 1978; **Med School:** Univ Utah 1973; **Resid:** Surgery, UCLA Med Ctr 1975; Otolaryngology, UCLA Med Ctr 1978; **Fellow:** Skull Base Surgery, Univ Zurich 1989; **Fac Appt:** Prof Oto, Med Univ SC

Peters, Glenn E MD [Oto] - **Spec Exp:** Thyroid & Parathyroid Cancer & Surgery; **Hospital:** Univ of Ala Hosp at Birmingham; **Address:** UAB Med Ctr, Div of Head & Neck Surgery, 1530 3rd Ave S, Ste BDB 563, Birmingham, AL 35294-0012; **Phone:** 205-934-9767; **Board Cert:** Otolaryngology 1985; **Med School:** Louisiana State U, New Orleans 1980; **Resid:** Surgery, Baptist Med Ctr 1982; Otolaryngology, Univ Alabama Hosp 1984; **Fellow:** Head & Neck Surgical Oncology, Johns Hopkins Hosp 1987; **Fac Appt:** Prof S, Univ Alabama

Pitman, Karen MD [Oto] - **Spec Exp:** Head & Neck Cancer & Surgery; Thyroid & Parathyroid Cancer & Surgery; Sentinel Node Surgery; **Hospital:** Univ Mississippi Med Ctr; **Address:** Univ Mississippi Med Ctr, 2500 N State St, Jackson, MS 39216; **Phone:** 601-984-5160; **Board Cert:** Otolaryngology 1995; **Med School:** Uniformed Srvs Univ, Bethesda 1987; **Resid:** Otolaryngology, Naval Med Ctr 1994; **Fellow:** Head and Neck Oncology, Univ Pittsburgh 1996; **Fac Appt:** Prof Oto, Univ Miss

Stringer, Scott P MD [Oto] - **Spec Exp:** Head & Neck Cancer; Thyroid & Parathyroid Cancer & Surgery; **Hospital:** Univ Mississippi Med Ctr; **Address:** Dept Otolaryngology, 2500 N State St, Jackson, MS 39216-4505; **Phone:** 601-984-5160; **Board Cert:** Otolaryngology 1987; **Med School:** Univ Tex SW, Dallas 1982; **Resid:** Surgery, Univ Tex SW Med Ctr 1984; Otolaryngology, Univ Tex SW Med Ctr 1987; **Fac Appt:** Prof Oto, Univ Miss

Terris, David J MD [Oto] - **Spec Exp:** Thyroid Surgery; Thyroid Cancer; Parathyroid Disease; Minimally Invasive Thyroid Surgery; **Hospital:** Med Coll of GA Hosp and Clin (MCG Health Inc), Doctors Hosp; **Address:** MCG Health System-Dept of Otolaryngology, 1120 15th St, rm BP4109, Augusta, GA 30912; **Phone:** 706-721-4400; **Board Cert:** Otolaryngology 1994; **Med School:** Duke Univ 1988; **Resid:** Surgery, Stanford Univ Med Ctr 1989; Otolaryngology, Stanford Univ Med Ctr 1993; **Fellow:** Head and Neck Surgery, Stanford Univ Med Ctr 1994; **Fac Appt:** Prof Oto, Med Coll GA

Valentino, Joseph MD [Oto] - **Spec Exp:** Head & Neck Cancer; Reconstructive Microvascular Surgery; Thyroid Cancer; **Hospital:** Univ of Kentucky Chandler Hosp; **Address:** 740 S Limestone St, rm B-317, Lexington, KY 40536-0284; **Phone:** 859-257-5405; **Board Cert:** Otolaryngology 1993; **Med School:** UMDNJ-RW Johnson Med Sch 1987; **Resid:** Otolaryngology, Univ Minn 1992; **Fellow:** Otolaryngology, Univ Iowa Coll Med 1993; **Fac Appt:** Assoc Prof Oto, Univ KY Coll Med

Weissler, Mark C MD [Oto] - **Spec Exp:** Head & Neck Cancer; **Hospital:** Univ NC Hosps; **Address:** G106 Physicians Office Bldg, 170 Manning Drive, #CB 7070, Chapel Hill, NC 27599-7070; **Phone:** 919-966-6483; **Board Cert:** Otolaryngology 1985; **Med School:** Boston Univ 1980; **Resid:** Surgery, Mass Genl Hosp 1982; Otolaryngology, Mass Eye & Ear Infirm 1985; **Fellow:** Head and Neck Oncology, Univ Cincinnati 1986; **Fac Appt:** Prof Oto, Univ NC Sch Med

Yarbrough, Wendell G MD [Oto] - **Spec Exp:** Head & Neck Cancer; **Hospital:** Vanderbilt Univ Med Ctr; **Address:** Vanderbilt Otolaryngology, 1215 21st Ave S, Ste 7209, Nashville, TN 37232-8605; **Phone:** 615-343-8840; **Board Cert:** Otolaryngology 1995; **Med School:** Univ NC Sch Med 1989; **Resid:** Otolaryngology, Univ NC Hosps 1994; **Fellow:** Surgical Oncology, Univ NC Hosps 1996; **Fac Appt:** Assoc Prof Oto, Vanderbilt Univ

Midwest

Arts, H Alexander MD [Oto] - **Spec Exp:** Skull Base Tumors & Surgery; Neuro-Otology; **Hospital:** Univ Michigan Hlth Sys; **Address:** Univ Michigan Health Systems, Dept Otolaryngology, 1500 E Medical Ctr Dr, 1904 Taubman Ctr, Ann Arbor, MI 48109; **Phone:** 734-936-8006; **Board Cert:** Otolaryngology 1992; Neurotology 2004; **Med School:** Baylor Coll Med 1983; **Resid:** Surgery, Univ Washington Med Ctr 1985; Otolaryngology, Univ Washington Med Ctr 1990; **Fellow:** Neurotology, Univ Virginia 1991; **Fac Appt:** Prof Oto, Univ Mich Med Sch

Bojrab, Dennis I MD [Oto] - **Spec Exp:** Skull Base Tumors; **Hospital:** Providence Hosp - Southfield, William Beaumont Hosp; **Address:** Michigan Ear Inst, 30055 Northwestern Hwy, Ste 101, Farmington Hills, MI 48334; **Phone:** 248-865-4444; **Board Cert:** Otolaryngology 1985; Neurotology 2005; **Med School:** Indiana Univ 1979; **Resid:** Surgery, Butterworth Hosp 1981; Otolaryngology, Univ Indiana Sch Med 1984; **Fellow:** Skull Base Surgery, Vanderbilt Univ Med Ctr 1985; **Fac Appt:** Prof Oto, Wayne State Univ

Bradford, Carol MD [Oto] - **Spec Exp:** Head & Neck Cancer; Melanoma-Head & Neck; Skin Cancer-Head & Neck; **Hospital:** Univ Michigan Hlth Sys; **Address:** University of Michigan Health System, 1500 E Medical Center Drive, rm 1904-TC, Ann Arbor, MI 48109-0312; **Phone:** 734-936-8029; **Board Cert:** Otolaryngology 1993; **Med School:** Univ Mich Med Sch 1986; **Resid:** Otolaryngology, Univ Michigan Med Ctr 1992; **Fellow:** Head and Neck Surgery, Univ Michigan Med Ctr 1988; **Fac Appt:** Prof Oto, Univ Mich Med Sch

Burkey, Brian MD [Oto] - **Spec Exp:** Parotid Gland Tumors; Head & Neck Cancer; Reconstructive Microvascular Surgery; **Hospital:** Cleveland Clin Fdn (page 70); **Address:** Head & Neck Institute, Desk A71, The Cleveland Clinic, 9500 Euclid Ave, Cleveland, OH 44195; **Phone:** 216-445-8838; **Board Cert:** Otolaryngology 1992; **Med School:** Univ VA Sch Med 1986; **Resid:** Otolaryngology, Univ Mich Med Ctr 1991; **Fellow:** Microsurgery, Ohio State Univ 1991; **Fac Appt:** Assoc Prof Oto, Vanderbilt Univ

Campbell, Bruce H MD [Oto] - **Spec Exp:** Head & Neck Cancer; Thyroid Surgery; **Hospital:** Froedtert Meml Lutheran Hosp, Chldns Hosp - Wisconsin; **Address:** Med Coll Wisc-Dept Oto, 9200 W Wisconsin Ave, Milwaukee, WI 53226; **Phone:** 414-805-5583; **Board Cert:** Otolaryngology 1986; **Med School:** Rush Med Coll 1980; **Resid:** Otolaryngology, Med Coll Wisconsin 1985; **Fellow:** Head and Neck Surgery, MD Anderson Cancer Ctr 1987; **Fac Appt:** Prof Oto, Med Coll Wisc

Funk, Gerry F MD [Oto] - **Spec Exp:** Head & Neck Cancer; Head & Neck Reconstruction; **Hospital:** Univ Iowa Hosp & Clinics; **Address:** UIHC, Dept Otolaryngology, 200 Hawkins Drive, Iowa City, IA 52242-1009; **Phone:** 319-356-2165; **Board Cert:** Otolaryngology 1992; **Med School:** Univ Chicago-Pritzker Sch Med 1986; **Resid:** Surgery, LAC-USC Med Ctr 1987; Otolaryngology, LAC-USC Med Ctr 1991; **Fellow:** Head and Neck Surgery, Univ Iowa Hosp 1992; **Fac Appt:** Prof Oto, Univ Iowa Coll Med

Hartig, Gregory K MD [Oto] - **Spec Exp:** Head & Neck Cancer; Skull Base Tumors; **Hospital:** Univ WI Hosp & Clins; **Address:** 600 Highland Ave, rm K4/720, Madison, WI 53792-7375; **Phone:** 608-263-6190; **Board Cert:** Otolaryngology 1994; **Med School:** Univ Mich Med Sch 1988; **Resid:** Otolaryngology, Univ Mich Med Ctr 1993; **Fellow:** Univ Penn Med Ctr 1994; **Fac Appt:** Prof Oto, Univ Mich Med Sch

Haughey, Bruce H MD [Oto] - **Spec Exp:** Reconstructive Surgery-Face; Head & Neck Cancer; Head & Neck Reconstruction; **Hospital:** Barnes-Jewish Hosp, St Louis Chldns Hosp; **Address:** Barnes Jewish Hosp South, 660 S Euclid Ave, Box 8115, St Louis, MO 63110; **Phone:** 314-362-7509; **Board Cert:** Otolaryngology 1984; **Med School:** New Zealand 1976; **Resid:** Surgery, Univ Auckland 1981; Otolaryngology, Univ Iowa Med Ctr 1984; **Fellow:** Otolaryngology, Univ Iowa Med Ctr 1985; **Fac Appt:** Prof Oto, Washington Univ, St Louis

Otolaryngology

Hoffman, Henry T MD [Oto] - **Spec Exp:** Voice Disorders; Head & Neck Cancer; Salivary Gland Tumors & Surgery; **Hospital:** Univ Iowa Hosp & Clinics; **Address:** Univ Iowa Hosp & Clins-Dept Oto, 200 Hawkins Drive, Iowa City, IA 52242; **Phone:** 319-356-2166; **Board Cert:** Otolaryngology 1985; **Med School:** UCSD 1980; **Resid:** Otolaryngology, Univ Iowa Hosp & Clinics 1985; **Fellow:** Head and Neck Oncology, Univ Michigan Hosp 1989; **Fac Appt:** Clin Prof Oto, Univ Iowa Coll Med

Kern, Robert C MD [Oto] - **Spec Exp:** Head & Neck Cancer; **Hospital:** Northwestern Meml Hosp, Stroger Hosp of Cook Co; **Address:** Northwestern Medical Faculty Fdn, 675 N St Clair St, Ste 15-200, Chicago, IL 60611; **Phone:** 312-695-8182; **Board Cert:** Otolaryngology 1990; **Med School:** Jefferson Med Coll 1985; **Resid:** Otolaryngology, Wayne State Affil Hosp 1990; **Fellow:** Research, Natl Inst Hlth 1991; **Fac Appt:** Prof Oto, Northwestern Univ

Lavertu, Pierre MD [Oto] - **Spec Exp:** Thyroid Cancer; Head & Neck Cancer; Skull Base Tumors; **Hospital:** Univ Hosps Case Med Ctr; **Address:** Univ Hosps, Dept Oto-Head & Neck Surg, 11100 Euclid Ave, Cleveland, OH 44106-5045; **Phone:** 216-844-4773; **Board Cert:** Otolaryngology 1981; **Med School:** Univ Montreal 1976; **Resid:** Otolaryngology, Univ Montreal Med Ctr 1981; **Fellow:** Head and Neck Surgery, Univ Montreal Med Ctr 1982; Head and Neck Surgery, Cleveland Clinic 1983; **Fac Appt:** Prof Oto, Case West Res Univ

Leonetti, John P MD [Oto] - **Spec Exp:** Skull Base Tumors & Surgery; Neuro-Otology; **Hospital:** Loyola Univ Med Ctr; **Address:** Loyola University Medical Ctr, Dept Otolaryngology, 2160 S First Ave Bldg 105 - rm 1870, Maywood, IL 60153; **Phone:** 708-216-4804; **Board Cert:** Otolaryngology 1987; **Med School:** Loyola Univ-Stritch Sch Med 1982; **Resid:** Otolaryngology, Loyola Univ Med Ctr 1987; Research, House Ear Inst 1987; **Fellow:** Neurotology, Barnes Jewish Hosp 1988; **Fac Appt:** Prof Oto, Loyola Univ-Stritch Sch Med

Marentette, Lawrence J MD [Oto] - **Spec Exp:** Skull Base Tumors & Surgery; Facial Plastic & Reconstructive Surgery; **Hospital:** Univ Michigan Hlth Sys; **Address:** Univ Michigan Health Systems, Dept Oto, 1500 E Med Ctr Drive, 1904 Taubman Ctr, Ann Arbor, MI 48109; **Phone:** 734-936-8051; **Board Cert:** Otolaryngology 1981; Facial Plastic & Reconstr Surgery 1995; **Med School:** Wayne State Univ 1976; **Resid:** Otolaryngology, Wayne State Univ 1980; **Fellow:** Maxillofacial Surgery, Univ of Zurich 1985; **Fac Appt:** Prof Oto, Univ Mich Med Sch

Olsen, Kerry D MD [Oto] - **Spec Exp:** Head & Neck Cancer & Surgery; Esthesioneuroblastoma; Salivary Gland Tumors & Surgery; Skull Base Tumors; **Hospital:** Mayo Med Ctr & Clin - Rochester; **Address:** Mayo Clinic, Dept Otolaryngology, 200 1st St SW, Rochester, MN 55905-0001; **Phone:** 507-284-3542; **Board Cert:** Otolaryngology 1981; **Med School:** Mayo Med Sch 1976; **Resid:** Otolaryngology, Mayo Clinic 1981; **Fac Appt:** Prof Oto, Mayo Med Sch

Ozer, Enver MD [Oto] - **Spec Exp:** Head & Neck Cancer; Head & Neck Surgery; **Hospital:** Ohio St Univ Med Ctr; **Address:** 456 W 10th Ave, Ste 4A, Columbus, OH 43210; **Phone:** 614-293-8074; **Med School:** Turkey 1994; **Resid:** Otolaryngology, Marmara Univ Med Sch 1996; Head and Neck Surgery, Marmara Univ Med Sch 2000; **Fellow:** Head and Neck Oncology, Ohio St Univ Med Ctr 2005; **Fac Appt:** Asst Prof Oto, Ohio State Univ

Pelzer, Harold J MD/DDS [Oto] - **Spec Exp:** Head & Neck Cancer; **Hospital:** Northwestern Meml Hosp; **Address:** Northwestern Medical Faculty Fdn, 675 N St Clair St, Ste 15-200, Chicago, IL 60611; **Phone:** 312-695-8182; **Board Cert:** Otolaryngology 1985; **Med School:** Northwestern Univ 1979; **Resid:** Surgery, Northwestern Meml Hosp 1983; **Fellow:** Head and Neck Surgery, Northwestern Meml Hosp 1985; **Fac Appt:** Assoc Prof Oto, Northwestern Univ

Pensak, Myles L MD [Oto] - **Spec Exp:** Skull Base Tumors; **Hospital:** Univ Hosp - Cincinnati, Good Samaritan Hosp - Cincinnati; **Address:** Univ Medical Arts Building, 222 Piedmont Ave, Ste 5200, Cincinnati, OH 45219; **Phone:** 513-475-8400; **Board Cert:** Otolaryngology 1983; Neurotology 2004; **Med School:** NY Med Coll 1978; **Resid:** Surgery, Upstate Med Ctr 1980; Otolaryngology, Yale Univ 1983; **Fellow:** Otology & Neurotology, The Otology Group 1984; **Fac Appt:** Prof Oto, Univ Cincinnati

Petruzzelli, Guy MD/PhD [Oto] - **Spec Exp:** Head & Neck Cancer & Surgery; Skull Base Tumors; Thyroid Cancer; **Hospital:** Rush Univ Med Ctr; **Address:** Rush Univ Med Ctr, 1725 W Harrison St, Ste 218, Chicago, IL 60612; **Phone:** 312-942-6100; **Board Cert:** Otolaryngology 1993; **Med School:** Rush Med Coll 1987; **Resid:** Otolaryngology, Univ Pittsburgh Med Ctr 1992; **Fellow:** Head and Neck Oncology, Univ Pittsburgh Med Ctr 1993; Skull Base Surgery, Univ Pittsburgh Ctr Cranial Base Surg; **Fac Appt:** Prof Oto, Rush Med Coll

Siegel, Gordon J MD [Oto] - **Spec Exp:** Head & Neck Cancer; **Hospital:** Northwestern Meml Hosp; **Address:** 3 E Huron St Fl 1, Chicago, IL 60611-2705; **Phone:** 312-988-7777; **Board Cert:** Otolaryngology 1984; **Med School:** Ros Franklin Univ/Chicago Med Sch 1978; **Resid:** Otolaryngology, Northwestern Univ Affil Hosp 1982; **Fac Appt:** Asst Clin Prof Oto, Northwestern Univ

Teknos, Theodoros N MD [Oto] - **Spec Exp:** Head & Neck Cancer; Thyroid Cancer; Facial Plastic & Reconstructive Surgery; Skull Base Surgery; **Hospital:** Ohio St Univ Med Ctr; **Address:** 456 W 10th Ave, Ste 4A, Columbus, OH 43210; **Phone:** 614-293-8074; **Board Cert:** Otolaryngology 1997; **Med School:** Harvard Med Sch 1991; **Resid:** Otolaryngology, Mass Eye & Ear Hosp 1996; **Fellow:** Head and Neck Surgery, Vanderbilt Univ Med Ctr 1997; **Fac Appt:** Assoc Prof Oto, Univ Mich Med Sch

Wilson, Keith M MD [Oto] - **Spec Exp:** Head & Neck Cancer & Surgery; Voice Disorders; **Hospital:** Univ Hosp - Cincinnati; **Address:** Univ Cincinnati Medical Ctr, 222 Piedmont Ave, Ste 5200, Cincinnati, OH 45219-4222; **Phone:** 513-475-8400; **Board Cert:** Otolaryngology 1992; **Med School:** Cornell Univ-Weill Med Coll 1986; **Resid:** Otolaryngology, St Louis Univ Med Ctr 1991; **Fellow:** Head & Neck Surgical Oncology, Ohio State Med Ctr 1992; **Fac Appt:** Assoc Prof Oto, Univ Cincinnati

Wolf, Gregory T MD [Oto] - **Spec Exp:** Head & Neck Cancer; Laryngeal Cancer; **Hospital:** Univ Michigan Hlth Sys; **Address:** Univ Mich Med Ctr, Dept Oto-HNS, 1500 E Med Ctr, Taubman Ctr, rm 1904, Ann Arbor, MI 48109-0312; **Phone:** 734-936-8029; **Board Cert:** Otolaryngology 1978; **Med School:** Univ Mich Med Sch 1973; **Resid:** Surgery, Georgetown Univ Hosp 1975; Otolaryngology, SUNY Upstate Med Ctr 1978; **Fac Appt:** Prof Oto, Univ Mich Med Sch

Yueh, Bevan MD [Oto] - **Spec Exp:** Head & Neck Cancer; **Hospital:** Univ Minn Med Ctr, Fairview - Univ Campus; **Address:** Dept Otolaryngology/Head & Neck Surgery, MMC 396, 420 Delaware St, Minneapolis, MN 55455-0932; **Phone:** 612-625-2410; **Board Cert:** Otolaryngology 1995; **Med School:** Stanford Univ 1989; **Resid:** Otolaryngology, Johns Hopkins Hosp 1994; **Fellow:** Otolaryngology, Johns Hopkins Hosp 1995; **Fac Appt:** Assoc Prof Oto, Univ Minn

Great Plains and Mountains

Chowdhury, Khalid MD [Oto] - **Spec Exp:** Skull Base Tumors & Surgery; Craniofacial Surgery; **Hospital:** Presby - St Luke's Med Ctr, Chldn's Hosp - Aurora, The; **Address:** Center for Craniofacial Surgery, 1601 E 19th Ave, Ste 3000, Denver, CO 80218; **Phone:** 303-839-5155; **Board Cert:** Otolaryngology 1990; Facial Plastic & Reconstr Surgery 1995; **Med School:** Univ Saskatchewan 1982; **Resid:** Surgery, Univ Saskatchewan Hosp 1985; Otolaryngology, McGill Univ Hosps 1989; **Fellow:** Craniofacial Surgery, Univ Bern Hosp 1990; Facial Plastic & Reconstr Surgery, Univ Bern Hosp 1990; **Fac Appt:** Assoc Prof Oto, Univ Colorado

Otolaryngology

Lydiatt, Daniel D MD/DDS [Oto] - **Spec Exp:** Head & Neck Cancer; **Hospital:** Methodist Hosp - Omaha, Nebraska Med Ctr; **Address:** 981225 Nebraska Medical Ctr, Omaha, NE 68198-1225; **Phone:** 402-559-6500; **Board Cert:** Otolaryngology 1992; **Med School:** Univ Nebr Coll Med 1983; **Resid:** Otolaryngology, Univ Nebraska Med Ctr 1990; **Fellow:** Head and Neck Surgery, MD Anderson Med Ctr 1991; **Fac Appt:** Assoc Prof Oto, Univ Nebr Coll Med

Lydiatt, William M MD [Oto] - **Spec Exp:** Head & Neck Cancer; Thyroid Cancer; Salivary Gland Tumors & Surgery; **Hospital:** Nebraska Med Ctr, Nebraska Meth Hosp; **Address:** 981225 Nebraska Medical Ctr, Omaha, NE 68198-1225; **Phone:** 402-559-6500; **Board Cert:** Otolaryngology 1994; **Med School:** Univ Nebr Coll Med 1988; **Resid:** Otolaryngology, Univ Nebraska Med Ctr 1993; **Fellow:** Head and Neck Surgery, Meml Sloan Kettering Cancer Ctr 1995; **Fac Appt:** Prof Oto, Univ Nebr Coll Med

Song, John I MD [Oto] - **Spec Exp:** Head & Neck Cancer; Skull Base Tumors; Swallowing Disorders; **Hospital:** Univ Colorado Hosp; **Address:** Univ Colorado Hosp, Otolaryngology, 12605 E 16th Ave, MS F737, PO Box 6510, Denver, CO 80219; **Phone:** 720-848-2820; **Board Cert:** Otolaryngology 1998; **Med School:** NYU Sch Med 1991; **Resid:** Otolaryngology, UCLA Med Ctr 1997; **Fellow:** Head and Neck Surgery, Univ PittsburghMed Ctr 1998; **Fac Appt:** Asst Prof Oto, Univ Colorado

Southwest

Clayman, Gary Lee MD/DMD [Oto] - **Spec Exp:** Thyroid Cancer & Surgery; Salivary Gland Tumors & Surgery; Head & Neck Cancer; Thyroid & Parathyroid Surgery; **Hospital:** UT MD Anderson Cancer Ctr; **Address:** Univ TX/MD Anderson Cancer Center, 1515 Holcombe Blvd, Box 1445, Houston, TX 77030-4009; **Phone:** 713-792-8837; **Board Cert:** Otolaryngology 1992; **Med School:** NE Ohio Univ 1986; **Resid:** Surgery, Hennepin Co Med Ctr 1987; Otolaryngology, Univ Minn Med Ctr 1991; **Fellow:** Head and Neck Surgery, MD Anderson Cancer Ctr 1993; **Fac Appt:** Prof Oto, Univ Tex, Houston

Donovan, Donald T MD [Oto] - **Spec Exp:** Head & Neck Cancer; Voice Disorders; Thyroid Disorders; **Hospital:** Methodist Hosp - Houston, St Luke's Episcopal Hosp-Houston; **Address:** 6550 Fannin St, Ste 1701, Houston, TX 77030; **Phone:** 713-798-3380; **Board Cert:** Otolaryngology 1981; **Med School:** Baylor Coll Med 1976; **Resid:** Surgery, Baylor Affil Hosps 1978; Otolaryngology, Baylor Affil Hosps 1981; **Fellow:** Head and Neck Surgery, Columbia-Presby Med Ctr 1982; **Fac Appt:** Prof Oto, Baylor Coll Med

Hanna, Ehab YN MD [Oto] - **Spec Exp:** Skull Base Tumors & Surgery; Head & Neck Cancer & Surgery; **Hospital:** UT MD Anderson Cancer Ctr; **Address:** Univ Tex MD Anderson Cancer Ctr, 1515 Holcombe Blvd, Unit 1445, Houston, TX 77030; **Phone:** 713-745-1815; **Board Cert:** Otolaryngology 1994; **Med School:** Egypt 1982; **Resid:** Otolaryngology, Cleveland Clinic 1989; Otolaryngology, Cleveland Clinic 1993; **Fellow:** Otolaryngology, Univ Pittsburgh Med Ctr 1994; **Fac Appt:** Prof Oto, Univ Tex, Houston

Medina, Jesus E MD [Oto] - **Spec Exp:** Head & Neck Cancer & Surgery; **Hospital:** OU Med Ctr; **Address:** OU Physicians, Dept Otolaryngology, 825 NE 10th St, Ste 4200, Oklahoma City, OK 73104; **Phone:** 405-271-7559; **Board Cert:** Otolaryngology 1980; **Med School:** Peru 1974; **Resid:** Surgery, Wayne St Univ Affil Hosp 1977; Otolaryngology, Wayne St Univ Affil Hosp 1980; **Fellow:** Head and Neck Surgery, Univ Tex Cancer Ctrs 1981; **Fac Appt:** Prof Oto, Univ Okla Coll Med

Myers, Jeffrey N MD/PhD [Oto] - **Spec Exp:** Head & Neck Cancer; Melanoma-Head & Neck; Tongue Cancer; **Hospital:** UT MD Anderson Cancer Ctr; **Address:** Univ Texas MD Anderson Cancer Ctr, 1515 Holcombe Blvd, Box 441, Houston, TX 77030; **Phone:** 713-745-2667; **Board Cert:** Otolaryngology 1997; **Med School:** Univ Pennsylvania 1991; **Resid:** Otolaryngology, Univ Pittsburgh Med Ctr 1996; **Fellow:** Head & Neck Surgical Oncology, MD Anderson Cancer Ctr 1997; **Fac Appt:** Assoc Prof Oto, Univ Tex, Houston

Nuss, Daniel W MD [Oto] - **Spec Exp:** Head & Neck Cancer; Skull Base Tumors & Surgery; **Hospital:** Our Lady of the Lake Regl Med Ctr; **Address:** Our Lady of the Lake Regl Med Ctr, 7777 Hennessy Blvd, Ste 409, Baton Rouge, LA 70808; **Phone:** 225-765-1765; **Board Cert:** Otolaryngology 1987; **Med School:** Louisiana State U, New Orleans 1981; **Resid:** Surgery, Charity Hosp 1983; Otolaryngology, LSU Med Ctr 1987; **Fellow:** Surgical Oncology, MD Anderson Hosp & Tumor Inst 1984; Head and Neck Surgery, Ctr Cranial Base Surg-Univ Pittsburgh 1991; **Fac Appt:** Prof Oto, Louisiana State U, New Orleans

Otto, Randal A MD [Oto] - **Spec Exp:** Head & Neck Cancer; Thyroid & Parathyroid Cancer & Surgery; **Hospital:** Univ Hlth Syst-San Antonio, Audie L Murphy Meml Vets Hosp; **Address:** 7703 Floyd Curl Drive, MS 7777, San Antonio, TX 78229-3900; **Phone:** 210-567-5655; **Board Cert:** Otolaryngology 1987; **Med School:** Univ MO-Columbia Sch Med 1981; **Resid:** Pathology, Queens Med Ctr 1982; Otolaryngology, Univ of Missouri 1987; **Fac Appt:** Prof Oto, Univ Tex, San Antonio

Suen, James Y MD [Oto] - **Spec Exp:** Head & Neck Cancer; Thyroid Cancer; **Hospital:** UAMS Med Ctr, Arkansas Chldns Hosp; **Address:** Univ Hosp Arkansas Med Scis, 4301 W Markham St, Slot 543, Little Rock, AR 72205; **Phone:** 501-686-8224; **Board Cert:** Otolaryngology 1973; **Med School:** Univ Ark 1966; **Resid:** Surgery, Univ Arkansas Med Ctr 1970; Otolaryngology, Univ Arkansas Med Ctr 1973; **Fellow:** Head and Neck Surgery, MD Anderson Cancer Ctr-Tumor Inst 1974; **Fac Appt:** Prof Oto, Univ Ark

Weber, Randal S MD [Oto] - **Spec Exp:** Skin Cancer; Thyroid & Parathyroid Cancer & Surgery; Salivary Gland Tumors & Surgery; Head & Neck Cancer; **Hospital:** UT MD Anderson Cancer Ctr; **Address:** 1515 Holcombe Blvd, Unit 441, Houston, TX 77030-4009; **Phone:** 713-745-0497; **Board Cert:** Otolaryngology 1985; **Med School:** Univ Tenn Coll Med, Memphis 1976; **Resid:** Surgery, Baylor Coll Med 1982; Otolaryngology, Baylor Coll Med 1985; **Fellow:** Head and Neck Surgery, MD Anderson Cancer Ctr 1986; **Fac Appt:** Prof Oto, Univ Tex, Houston

Weber, Samuel C MD [Oto] - **Spec Exp:** Thyroid Cancer; Parathyroid Cancer; Nasal & Sinus Cancer & Surgery; Head & Neck Surgery; **Hospital:** St Luke's Episcopal Hosp-Houston, Methodist Chldns Hosp of South Texas; **Address:** 6624 Fannin St, Ste 1480, Houston, TX 77030-2385; **Phone:** 713-795-5343; **Board Cert:** Otolaryngology 1972; **Med School:** Univ Tenn Coll Med, Memphis 1965; **Resid:** Surgery, Baylor Coll Med 1971; Otolaryngology, Baylor Coll Med 1972; **Fac Appt:** Clin Prof Oto, Univ Tex, San Antonio

West Coast and Pacific

Berke, Gerald S MD [Oto] - **Spec Exp:** Head & Neck Surgery; Head & Neck Cancer; Voice Disorders; Laryngeal Disorders; **Hospital:** UCLA Ronald Reagan Med Ctr; **Address:** 200 UCLA Med Plaza, Ste 550, Los Angeles, CA 90095; **Phone:** 310-825-5179; **Board Cert:** Otolaryngology 1984; **Med School:** USC Sch Med 1978; **Resid:** Otolaryngology, LAC-USC Med Ctr 1979; **Fellow:** Head and Neck Surgery, UCLA Med Ctr 1984; **Fac Appt:** Prof Oto, UCLA

Otolaryngology

Cohen, James I MD [Oto] - **Hospital:** VA Medical Center - Portland; **Address:** Portland VAMC P3-OC, 3710 US Veteran's Hospital Rd, Portland, OR 97239; **Phone:** 503-220-8262; **Board Cert:** Otolaryngology 1984; **Med School:** Univ Manitoba 1978; **Resid:** Surgery, Univ Minn Med Ctr 1980; Otolaryngology, Univ Minn Med Ctr 1984; **Fellow:** Head & Neck Surgical Oncology, MD Anderson Cancer Ctr 1985; **Fac Appt:** Prof Oto, Oregon Hlth Sci Univ

Courey, Mark S MD [Oto] - **Spec Exp:** Swallowing Disorders; Laryngeal Cancer; **Hospital:** UCSF - Mt Zion Med Ctr, UCSF Med Ctr; **Address:** UCSF Voice & Swallowing Ctr, 2330 Post St, Ste 526, San Francisco, CA 94115; **Phone:** 415-885-7700; **Board Cert:** Otolaryngology 1993; **Med School:** SUNY Buffalo 1987; **Resid:** Otolaryngology, SUNY-Buffalo Med Ctr 1992; **Fellow:** Laryngology, Vanderbilt Univ 1993; **Fac Appt:** Prof Oto, UCSF

Donald, Paul MD [Oto] - **Spec Exp:** Skull Base Tumors & Surgery; Head & Neck Cancer; **Hospital:** UC Davis Med Ctr; **Address:** 2521 Stockton Blvd, rm 7200, Sacramento, CA 95817; **Phone:** 916-734-2832; **Board Cert:** Otolaryngology 1973; **Med School:** Univ British Columbia Fac Med 1964; **Resid:** Surgery, St Pauls Hosp 1969; Otolaryngology, Univ Iowa Hosp 1973; **Fac Appt:** Prof Oto, UC Davis

Eisele, David W MD [Oto] - **Spec Exp:** Salivary Gland Tumors & Surgery; Head & Neck Cancer; Thyroid Cancer; **Hospital:** UCSF Med Ctr; **Address:** UCSF, Dept Head & Neck Surgery, 2380 Sutter St Fl 2nd, Box 1703, San Francisco, CA 94115-1703; **Phone:** 415-885-7528; **Board Cert:** Otolaryngology 1988; **Med School:** Cornell Univ-Weill Med Coll 1982; **Resid:** Surgery, Univ Wash Med Ctr 1984; Otolaryngology, Univ Wash Med Ctr 1988; **Fac Appt:** Prof Oto, UCSF

Fee Jr, Willard E MD [Oto] - **Spec Exp:** Head & Neck Cancer; Parotid Gland Tumors; Thyroid Cancer; **Hospital:** Stanford Univ Med Ctr; **Address:** Stanford Cancer Ctr, 875 Lake Wilbur Dr, CC-2227, Stanford, CA 94305-5826; **Phone:** 650-498-6000; **Board Cert:** Otolaryngology 1974; **Med School:** Univ Colorado 1969; **Resid:** Surgery, Wadsworth VA Hosp 1971; Otolaryngology, UCLA Med Ctr 1974; **Fac Appt:** Prof Oto, Stanford Univ

Futran, Neal D MD/DMD [Oto] - **Spec Exp:** Head & Neck Cancer & Surgery; Head & Neck Cancer Reconstruction; Skull Base Tumors & Surgery; **Hospital:** Univ Wash Med Ctr, Harborview Med Ctr; **Address:** U Wash Med Ctr, Oto Office, 1959 NE Pacific St, Box 356515, Seattle, WA 98195-6515; **Phone:** 206-543-3060; **Board Cert:** Otolaryngology 1993; **Med School:** SUNY Downstate 1987; **Resid:** Surgery, Kings Co-SUNY Downstate 1985; Otolaryngology, Univ Rochester Med Ctr 1992; **Fellow:** Microvascular Surgery, Mt Sinai Hosp 1993; **Fac Appt:** Prof Oto, Univ Wash

Jackler, Robert K MD [Oto] - **Spec Exp:** Neuro-Otology; Skull Base Surgery; Ear Tumors; **Hospital:** Stanford Univ Med Ctr; **Address:** Stanford Univ Med Ctr, Dept Head & Neck Surg, 801 Welch Rd, Stanford, CA 94305-5739; **Phone:** 650-725-6500; **Board Cert:** Otolaryngology 1984; Neurotology 2004; **Med School:** Boston Univ 1979; **Resid:** Otolaryngology, UCSF Med Ctr 1984; **Fellow:** Otolaryngology, Oto Med Grp 1985; **Fac Appt:** Prof Oto, Stanford Univ

Kaplan, Michael J MD [Oto] - **Spec Exp:** Head & Neck Surgery; Skull Base Surgery; Head & Neck Cancer; **Hospital:** Stanford Univ Med Ctr; **Address:** Stanford Cancer Ctr, Dept Otolaryngology, 801 Welch Rd Fl 2, Stanford, CA 94305-5739; **Phone:** 650-498-6000; **Board Cert:** Otolaryngology 1982; **Med School:** Harvard Med Sch 1977; **Resid:** Surgery, Beth Israel-Chldns Hosps 1979; Otolaryngology, Mass EE Infirm 1982; **Fellow:** Head and Neck Surgery, Univ Virginia 1984; **Fac Appt:** Prof Oto, Stanford Univ

McMenomey, Sean O MD [Oto] - **Spec Exp:** Skull Base Tumors & Surgery; Head & Neck Surgery; Stereotactic Radiosurgery; **Hospital:** OR Hlth & Sci Univ, Providence St Vincent Med Ctr; **Address:** Oregon Hlth & Sci Univ, Dept Otolaryngology, 3181 SW Sam Jackson Park Rd, MC PV-01, Portland, OR 97239; **Phone:** 503-494-8135; **Board Cert:** Otolaryngology 1993; Neurotology 2004; **Med School:** St Louis Univ 1987; **Resid:** Otolaryngology, Oregon Hlth Sci Ctr 1992; **Fellow:** Otology & Neurotology, Baptist Hosp 1993; **Fac Appt:** Assoc Prof Oto, Oregon Hlth Sci Univ

Rice, Dale MD [Oto] - **Spec Exp:** Head & Neck Cancer; Sinus Disorders/Surgery; **Hospital:** USC Univ Hosp, USC Norris Cancer Hosp; **Address:** USC Keck Sch Med, 1200 N State St, rm 4316, Los Angeles, CA 90033-1029; **Phone:** 323-442-5790; **Board Cert:** Otolaryngology 1976; **Med School:** Univ Mich Med Sch 1968; **Resid:** Surgery, Univ Mich Med Ctr 1970; Otolaryngology, Univ Mich Med Ctr 1976; **Fac Appt:** Prof Oto, USC Sch Med

Shindo, Maisie L MD [Oto] - **Spec Exp:** Head & Neck Cancer & Surgery; Thyroid Cancer; Laryngeal Cancer; Parathyroid Cancer; **Hospital:** OR Hlth & Sci Univ; **Address:** Thyroid & Parathyroid Clinic, 3181 SW Sam Jackson Park Rd, Ste 250, Physicians Pavilion, PV-01, Portland, OR 97239-3098; **Phone:** 503-494-2544; **Board Cert:** Otolaryngology 1989; **Med School:** Univ Saskatchewan 1984; **Resid:** Otolaryngology, LAC-USC Med Ctr 1989; **Fellow:** Head and Neck Surgery, Northwestern Univ 1991; **Fac Appt:** Prof Oto, Oregon Hlth Sci Univ

Singer, Mark I MD [Oto] - **Spec Exp:** Head & Neck Surgery; Head & Neck Cancer; Melanoma; **Hospital:** CA Pacific Med Ctr; **Address:** 2340 Clay St Fl 2, San Francisco, CA 94115; **Phone:** 415-600-2450; **Board Cert:** Otolaryngology 1976; **Med School:** Columbia P&S 1970; **Resid:** Surgery, Northwestern Meml Hosp 1973; Otolaryngology, Northwestern Meml Hosp 1976; **Fellow:** Oncology, Northwestern Meml Hosp 1976

Sinha, Uttam K MD [Oto] - **Spec Exp:** Head & Neck Cancer; Voice Disorders; **Hospital:** USC Univ Hosp, House Ear Inst; **Address:** 1200 N State St, rm 4136, Los Angeles, CA 90033; **Phone:** 323-226-7315; **Board Cert:** Otolaryngology 1998; **Med School:** India 1985; **Resid:** Otolaryngology, LAC-USC Med Ctr 1995; **Fellow:** Microvascular Surgery, Mount Sinai Med Ctr 1996; Laryngology 1997; **Fac Appt:** Assoc Prof Oto, USC Sch Med

Wax, Mark K MD [Oto] - **Spec Exp:** Skull Base Tumors & Surgery; Facial Plastic & Reconstructive Surgery; Head & Neck Cancer; **Hospital:** OR Hlth & Sci Univ; **Address:** Oregon Hlth Scis Univ, Dept Ototlaryngology, 3181 SW Sam Jackson Park Rd, Ste PV-01, Portland, OR 97201; **Phone:** 503-494-5355; **Board Cert:** Otolaryngology 1985; Facial Plastic & Reconstr Surgery 1987; **Med School:** Univ Toronto 1980; **Resid:** Otolaryngology, Univ Toronto 1985; Surgery, Cedars-Sinai Med Ctr 1983; **Fellow:** Head and Neck Surgery, St Michaels Hosp 1991; **Fac Appt:** Prof Oto, Oregon Hlth Sci Univ

Weisman, Robert A MD [Oto] - **Spec Exp:** Head & Neck Cancer; Clinical Trials; Thyroid & Parathyroid Cancer & Surgery; Head & Neck Cancer Reconstruction; **Hospital:** UCSD Med Ctr; **Address:** Moores-UCSD Cancer Center, 3855 Health Sciences Drive, MC 0987, La Jolla, CA 92093-0987; **Phone:** 858-822-6197; **Board Cert:** Otolaryngology 1978; **Med School:** Washington Univ, St Louis 1973; **Resid:** Head and Neck Surgery, UCLA Med Ctr 1978; **Fac Appt:** Prof S, UCSD

Weymuller, Ernest MD [Oto] - **Spec Exp:** Head & Neck Cancer; Sinus Disorders/Surgery; **Hospital:** Univ Wash Med Ctr; **Address:** 1959 NE Pacific St, Box 356161, Seattle, WA 98195-6161; **Phone:** 206-598-4022; **Board Cert:** Otolaryngology 1973; **Med School:** Harvard Med Sch 1966; **Resid:** Surgery, Vanderbilt Univ Hosp 1968; Otolaryngology, Mass Eye and Ear Infirm 1973; **Fac Appt:** Prof Oto, Univ Wash

Pain Medicine

a subspecialty of Anesthesiology, Neurology, Physical Medicine & Rehabilitation or Psychiatry

Some physicians who have their primary board certification in anesthesiology, neurology, physical medicine and rehabilitation, or psychiatry have completed additional training and passed an examination in the subspecialty called pain management. These doctors provide a high level of care, either as a primary physcian or consultant, for patients experiencing problems with acute, chronic and/or cancer pain in both hospital and ambulatory settings.

For more information about the main specialties of these physicians, see Anesthesiology, Neurology, Physical Medicine and Rehabilitation or Psychiatry.

Training Required: Number of years required for primary specialty plus additional one year training and examination.

PAIN MEDICINE

New England

Abrahm, Janet L MD [PM] - **Spec Exp:** Palliative Care; Pain-Cancer; **Hospital:** Dana-Farber Cancer Inst, Brigham & Women's Hosp; **Address:** Dana-Farber Cancer Institute, 44 Binney St, Shields-Warren 420, Boston, MA 02115; **Phone:** 617-632-6464; **Board Cert:** Internal Medicine 1976; Medical Oncology 1981; Hematology 1978; **Med School:** UCSF 1973; **Resid:** Internal Medicine, Mass Genl Hosp 1975; Internal Medicine, Moffitt Hosp-UCSF 1977; **Fellow:** Hematology, Mass Genl Hosp 1976; Hematology & Oncology, Hosp Univ Penn 1980; **Fac Appt:** Assoc Prof Med, Harvard Med Sch

Billings, J Andrew MD [PM] - **Spec Exp:** Palliative Care; Pain Management; Pain-Cancer; **Hospital:** Mass Genl Hosp; **Address:** 55 Fruit St, FND 600, Boston, MA 02114; **Phone:** 617-724-9197; **Board Cert:** Internal Medicine 1975; Hospice & Palliative Medicine 2001; **Med School:** Harvard Med Sch 1972; **Resid:** Internal Medicine, Univ California Hosps 1975; **Fellow:** Internal Medicine, Mass Genl Hosp 1977; **Fac Appt:** Assoc Prof Med, Harvard Med Sch

Mid Atlantic

De Leon-Casasola, Oscar A MD [PM] - **Spec Exp:** Pain-Acute; Pain-Chronic; Pain-Cancer; **Hospital:** Roswell Park Cancer Inst; **Address:** Roswell Park Cancer Inst, Anesthesia/Pain Med, Elm & Carlton Sts, Buffalo, NY 14263; **Phone:** 716-845-4595; **Board Cert:** Anesthesiology 1991; Critical Care Medicine 1993; Pain Medicine 2005; **Med School:** Guatemala 1982; **Resid:** Surgery, SUNY-Downstate Med Ctr 1986; Anesthesiology, Univ Buffalo 1989; **Fac Appt:** Prof Anes, SUNY Buffalo

Diwan, Sudhir MD [PM] - **Spec Exp:** Pain-after Spinal Intervention; Pain-Musculoskeletal; Pain-Neuropathic; Pain-Cancer; **Hospital:** NY-Presby Hosp/Weill Cornell (page 79); **Address:** 1305 York Ave Fl 10, Box 120, New York, NY 10021; **Phone:** 646-962-7246; **Board Cert:** Anesthesiology 2001; Pain Medicine 2002; **Med School:** India 1983; **Resid:** Surgery, St Luke's-Roosevelt Hosp Ctr 1994; Anesthesiology, St Luke's-Roosevelt Hosp Ctr 1997; **Fellow:** Pain Medicine, NY Presby Hosp 1998; **Fac Appt:** Assoc Prof Anes, Cornell Univ-Weill Med Coll

Jain, Subhash MD [PM] - **Spec Exp:** Pain-Cancer; Pain-Neuropathic; Pain-Back; **Hospital:** Beth Israel Med Ctr - Petrie Division (page 71); **Address:** 360 S 72nd St, Ste C, New York, NY 10021; **Phone:** 212-439-6100; **Board Cert:** Anesthesiology 1994; Pain Medicine 1998; **Med School:** India 1968; **Resid:** Surgery, St Vincent Med Ctr 1977; Anesthesiology, New York Hosp 1979; **Fellow:** Pain Medicine, New York Hosp/Meml Sloan Kettering Cancer Ctr 1980; **Fac Appt:** Assoc Prof Anes, Cornell Univ-Weill Med Coll

Kreitzer, Joel MD [PM] - **Spec Exp:** Pain-Back; Pain-Cancer; Pain-Neuropathic; **Hospital:** Mount Sinai Med Ctr (page 77), Mount Sinai Hosp of Queens (page 77); **Address:** Upper East Side Pain Medicine, 1540 York Ave, New York, NY 10028; **Phone:** 212-288-2180; **Board Cert:** Anesthesiology 1990; Pain Medicine 2004; **Med School:** Albert Einstein Coll Med 1985; **Resid:** Anesthesiology, Mt Sinai Hosp 1989; **Fellow:** Pain Medicine, Mt Sinai Hosp 1989; **Fac Appt:** Assoc Clin Prof Anes, Mount Sinai Sch Med

Portenoy, Russell MD [PM] - **Spec Exp:** Pain-Cancer; Palliative Care; **Hospital:** Beth Israel Med Ctr - Petrie Division (page 71); **Address:** Beth Israel Med Ctr, Dept Pain Medicine/Palliative Care, First Ave at 16th St, New York, NY 10003; **Phone:** 212-844-1403; **Board Cert:** Neurology 1985; Hospice & Palliative Medicine 2008; **Med School:** Univ MD Sch Med 1980; **Resid:** Neurology, Montefiore Med Ctr 1984; **Fellow:** Pain Medicine, Meml Sloan-Kettering Cancer Ctr 1985; **Fac Appt:** Prof N, Albert Einstein Coll Med

Staats, Peter MD [PM] - **Spec Exp:** Pain-Cancer; **Hospital:** Riverview Med Ctr, CentraState Med Ctr; **Address:** Metzger Staats Pain Mgmt, 160 Avenue at the Commons, Ste 1, Shrewsbury, NJ 07702; **Phone:** 732-380-0200; **Board Cert:** Anesthesiology 1994; Pain Medicine 2005; **Med School:** Univ Mich Med Sch 1989; **Resid:** Anesthesiology, Johns Hopkins Hosp 1993; **Fellow:** Pain Medicine, Johns Hopkins Hosp 1994

Weinberger, Michael L MD [PM] - **Spec Exp:** Pain-Cancer; Pain-Back; **Hospital:** NY-Presby Hosp/Columbia (page 79); **Address:** 630 W 168th St, PH5, rm 500, New York, NY 10032-3720; **Phone:** 212-305-7114; **Board Cert:** Internal Medicine 1986; Anesthesiology 1990; Pain Medicine 2004; Hospice & Palliative Medicine 2006; **Med School:** Columbia P&S 1983; **Resid:** Internal Medicine, St Vincent's Hosp 1986; Anesthesiology, Columbia-Presby Med Ctr 1989; **Fellow:** Pain Medicine, Meml Sloan Kettering Cancer Ctr 1990; **Fac Appt:** Assoc Prof Anes, Columbia P&S

Southeast

Anghelescu, Doralina L MD [PM] - **Spec Exp:** Pain Management-Pediatric; Pain-Cancer; **Hospital:** St Jude Children's Research Hosp; **Address:** St Jude Chldn's Rsch Hosp, Anesthesiology, 262 Danny Thomas Pl, MS 130, Memphis, TN 38105; **Phone:** 901-495-4034; **Board Cert:** Anesthesiology 1998; Pain Medicine 2001; **Med School:** Romania 1985; **Resid:** Anesthesiology, Univ N Mex Hosp 1997; **Fellow:** Pain Medicine, Chldns Natl Med Ctr 1998; Pain Medicine, Univ NMex Hosp 1999

Rauck, Richard L MD [PM] - **Spec Exp:** Pain-Cancer; **Hospital:** Forsyth Med Ctr, Wake Forest Univ Baptist Med Ctr (page 84); **Address:** Carolinas Pain Institute, 145 Kimel Park Drive, Ste 330, Winston-Salem, NC 27103; **Phone:** 336-765-6181; **Board Cert:** Anesthesiology 1987; Pain Medicine 2005; **Med School:** Bowman Gray 1982; **Resid:** Anesthesiology, Univ Cincinnati Hosp 1985; **Fellow:** Pain Medicine, Univ Cincinnati Hosp 1986; **Fac Appt:** Assoc Prof Anes, Wake Forest Univ

Midwest

Benedetti, Costantino MD [PM] - **Spec Exp:** Pain-Cancer; Palliative Care; Pain-Acute; Pain-Chronic; **Hospital:** Ohio St Univ Med Ctr, Arthur G James Cancer Hosp & Research Inst; **Address:** Ohio State Univ Med Ctr, 300 W 10th Ave, Ste 519, Columbus, OH 43210; **Phone:** 614-293-6599; **Board Cert:** Hospice & Palliative Medicine 1997; **Med School:** Italy 1972; **Resid:** Anesthesiology, Univ Colorado Hosp 1975; Anesthesiology, Univ Wash Med Ctr 1976; **Fellow:** Pain Medicine, Univ Wash Med Ctr 1978; **Fac Appt:** Clin Prof Anes, Ohio State Univ

Huntoon, Marc MD [PM] - **Spec Exp:** Pain-Cancer; Pain-after Spinal Intervention; Palliative Care; **Hospital:** Mayo Med Ctr & Clin - Rochester; **Address:** Mayo Clinic - Pain Medicine, 200 First St SW, Rochester, MN 55905; **Phone:** 507-266-9240; **Board Cert:** Anesthesiology 2003; Pain Medicine 2004; Hospice & Palliative Medicine 2004; **Med School:** Wayne State Univ 1985; **Resid:** Anesthesiology, Naval Hosp Med Ctr 1991; **Fellow:** Pain Medicine, Naval Hosp Med Ctr 1992

Pain Medicine

Swarm, Robert A MD [PM] - **Spec Exp:** Pain-Acute; Pain-Chronic; Pain-Cancer; **Hospital:** Barnes-Jewish Hosp; **Address:** Ctr for Advanced Med-Pain Mngmt Ctr, 4921 Parkview Pl, Ste 10A, MS 90-35-706, St Louis, MO 63110; **Phone:** 314-362-8820; **Board Cert:** Anesthesiology 1990; Pain Medicine 2004; **Med School:** Washington Univ, St Louis 1983; **Resid:** Surgery, Barnes Hosp 1986; Anesthesiology, Barnes Hosp 1989; **Fellow:** Pain Medicine, Univ Sydney; **Fac Appt:** Assoc Prof Anes, Washington Univ, St Louis

Weisman, Steven J MD [PM] - **Spec Exp:** Pain Management-Pediatric; Palliative Care-Pediatric; Pain-Cancer; **Hospital:** Chldns Hosp - Wisconsin; **Address:** Chldns Hosp Wisconsin, 9000 W Wisconsin Ave, MS 792, Milwaukee, WI 53226-3518; **Phone:** 414-266-2775; **Board Cert:** Pediatrics 1982; Pediatric Hematology-Oncology 1984; Anesthesiology 1996; **Med School:** Albert Einstein Coll Med 1978; **Resid:** Pediatrics, Chldns Hosp 1981; Anesthesiology, Univ Conn Hlth Ctr 1994; **Fellow:** Pediatric Hematology-Oncology, Indiana Univ Sch Med 1984; **Fac Appt:** Prof Anes, Med Coll Wisc

Great Plains and Mountains

Fine, Perry G MD [PM] - **Spec Exp:** Pain-Cancer; Palliative Care; Pain-Chronic; **Hospital:** Univ Utah Hosps and Clins; **Address:** 546 S Chipeta Way, Ste 200, Salt Lake City, UT 84108; **Phone:** 801-581-7246; **Board Cert:** Anesthesiology 1985; Pain Medicine 2004; **Med School:** Med Coll VA 1981; **Resid:** Anesthesiology, Univ Utah Hlth Sci Ctr 1984; **Fellow:** Pain Medicine, Univ Toronto 1985; **Fac Appt:** Prof Anes, Univ Utah

Weinstein, Sharon M MD [PM] - **Spec Exp:** Pain-Cancer; Palliative Care; **Hospital:** Univ Utah Hosps and Clins; **Address:** Huntsman Cancer Institute, 2000 Circle of Hope, Salt Lake City, UT 84112; **Phone:** 801-585-0112; **Board Cert:** Neurology 1993; Pain Medicine 2000; **Med School:** Albert Einstein Coll Med 1986; **Resid:** Neurology, Montefiore Med Ctr 1990; **Fellow:** Pain Medicine, Meml Sloan Kettering Cancer Ctr 1991; **Fac Appt:** Assoc Prof Anes, Univ Utah

Southwest

Burton, Allen W MD [PM] - **Spec Exp:** Pain-Cancer; Palliative Care; **Hospital:** UT MD Anderson Cancer Ctr; **Address:** MD Anderson Cancer Ctr, Dept Anesth, 1400 Holcombe Blvd, Unit 409, Houston, TX 77030; **Phone:** 713-745-7246; **Board Cert:** Anesthesiology 1996; Pain Medicine 1998; **Med School:** Baylor Coll Med 1991; **Resid:** Anesthesiology, Brigham & Women's Hosp 1995; **Fellow:** Pain Medicine, U Texas Med Branch Hosp 1998; **Fac Appt:** Assoc Prof Anes, Univ Tex Med Br, Galveston

Driver, Larry C MD [PM] - **Spec Exp:** Pain-Cancer; Palliative Care; **Hospital:** UT MD Anderson Cancer Ctr; **Address:** UT MD Anderson Cancer Ctr, Dept Pain Medicine, 1400 Holcombe Blvd, Unit 409, Houston, TX 77030; **Phone:** 713-745-7246; **Board Cert:** Anesthesiology 1992; Pain Medicine 2002; **Med School:** Univ Tex, San Antonio 1980; **Resid:** Anesthesiology, Univ Colorado Hlth Sci Ctr 1984; **Fellow:** Pain Medicine, MD Anderson Cancer Ctr 1999; **Fac Appt:** Assoc Prof Anes, Univ Tex, Houston

West Coast and Pacific

Audell, Laura G MD [PM] - **Spec Exp:** Pain-Cancer; **Hospital:** Cedars-Sinai Med Ctr; **Address:** 444 S San Vincente, Ste 1101, Los Angeles, CA 90048; **Phone:** 310-423-9600; **Board Cert:** Internal Medicine 1988; Anesthesiology 1988; Pain Medicine 2007; **Med School:** Univ Wash 1982; **Resid:** Internal Medicine, UCLA-Hosps 1985; Anesthesiology, UCLA-Hosps 1987; **Fellow:** Pain Medicine, UCLA-Hosps 1988

Fishman, Scott M MD [PM] - **Spec Exp:** Pain-Cancer; Pain-Chronic; **Hospital:** UC Davis Med Ctr; **Address:** UC Davis Med Ctr, Pain Management Clinic, 4860 Y St, Ste 2700, Sacramento, CA 95817; **Phone:** 916-734-6824; **Board Cert:** Psychiatry 1998; Pain Medicine 1995; **Med School:** Univ Mass Sch Med 1990; **Resid:** Internal Medicine, Greenwich Hosp 1993; Psychiatry, Mass Genl Hosp 1996; **Fellow:** Pain Medicine, Mass Genl Hosp 1995; **Fac Appt:** Prof Anes, UC Davis

Fitzgibbon, Dermot R MD [PM] - **Spec Exp:** Pain-Cancer; **Hospital:** Univ Wash Med Ctr; **Address:** Univ Wash Med Ctr, Dept Anesthesiology, 1959 NE Pacific St, Box 356540, Seattle, WA 98195; **Phone:** 206-598-4260; **Board Cert:** Anesthesiology 1996; Pain Medicine 1998; **Med School:** Ireland 1983; **Resid:** Anesthesiology, St Vincent's Hosp 1992; Anesthesiology, Univ Washington Med Ctr 1995; **Fellow:** Pain Medicine, Univ Wash-Pain Mngmt Clinic 1994; **Fac Appt:** Assoc Prof Anes, Univ Wash

Ready, L Brian MD [PM] - **Spec Exp:** Pain-Cancer; **Hospital:** Allenmore Hosp; **Address:** 1901 S Union Ave, Ste A244, Tacoma, WA 98405; **Phone:** 253-459-6509; **Med School:** Canada 1967; **Resid:** Anesthesiology, Univ Washington Med Ctr 1975

Slatkin, Neal E MD [PM] - **Spec Exp:** Pain-Cancer; Palliative Care; **Hospital:** City of Hope Natl Med Ctr & Beckman Rsch (page 69); **Address:** City of Hope Medical Group, 50 Bellfontane St, Ste 104, Pasadena, CA 91105; **Phone:** 626-396-2900; **Board Cert:** Neurology 1982; Pain Medicine 2000; **Med School:** SUNY Stony Brook 1976; **Resid:** Neurology, Bellevue Hosp Ctr-NYU 1978; Neurology, Med Coll Va 1981; **Fellow:** Neurology, Med Coll Va 1982; Neuro-Oncology, Meml Sloan-Kettering Cancer Ctr 1984; **Fac Appt:** Asst Clin Prof Med, USC-Keck School of Medicine

Wallace, Mark S MD [PM] - **Spec Exp:** Pain-Chronic; Pain-Cancer; Palliative Care; **Hospital:** UCSD Med Ctr; **Address:** 9350 Campus Point Drive, MC 7650, La Jolla, CA 92037; **Phone:** 858-657-6035; **Board Cert:** Anesthesiology 1992; Pain Medicine 2005; **Med School:** Creighton Univ 1987; **Resid:** Anesthesiology, Univ Maryland Hosp 1991; **Fellow:** Pain Medicine, UCSD Med Ctr 1994; **Fac Appt:** Assoc Prof Anes, UCSD

Pathology

A pathologist deals with the causes and nature of disease and contributes to diagnosis, prognosis and treatment through knowledge gained by the laboratory application of the biologic, chemical and physical sciences.

A pathologist uses information gathered from the microscopic examination of tissue specimens, cells and body fluids, and from clinical laboratory tests on body fluids and secretions for the diagnosis, exclusion and monitoring of the disease.

Training Required: Three to four years. Certification in the following subspecialty requires additional training and examination.

Dermatopathology: A dermatopathologist has the expertise to diagnose and monitor diseases of the skin including infectious, immunologic, degenerative and neoplastic diseases. This entails the examination and interpretation of specially prepared tissue sections, cellular scrapings and smears of skin lesions by means of routine and special (electron and fluorescent) microscopes.

PATHOLOGY

New England

Bhan, Atul Kumar MD [Path] - **Spec Exp:** Immunopathology; Liver Pathology; Liver Cancer; **Hospital:** Mass Genl Hosp; **Address:** Mass Genl Hosp, Dept Path, 55 Fruit St, Warren 501, Boston, MA 02114-2620; **Phone:** 617-726-2588; **Board Cert:** Anatomic Pathology 1976; Immunopathology 1985; **Med School:** India 1965; **Resid:** Pathology, Boston Univ Hosp 1971; Pathology, Chldns Univ Hosp 1974; **Fac Appt:** Prof Path, Harvard Med Sch

Connolly, James Leo MD [Path] - **Spec Exp:** Breast Pathology; Breast Cancer; **Hospital:** Beth Israel Deaconess Med Ctr - Boston, Brigham & Women's Hosp; **Address:** Beth Israel Deaconess Med Ctr, Dept Path, 330 Brookline Ave, rm ES 112, Boston, MA 02215-5400; **Phone:** 617-667-4344; **Board Cert:** Anatomic Pathology 1980; **Med School:** Vanderbilt Univ 1974; **Resid:** Anatomic Pathology, Beth Israel Hosp 1978; **Fac Appt:** Prof Path, Harvard Med Sch

DeLellis, Ronald A MD [Path] - **Spec Exp:** Thyroid Cancer; Endocrine Pathology; **Hospital:** Rhode Island Hosp, Miriam Hosp; **Address:** Rhode Island Hospital, Dept Pathology, 593 Eddy St, Providence, RI 02903-4923; **Phone:** 401-444-5154; **Board Cert:** Anatomic Pathology 1972; **Med School:** Tufts Univ 1966; **Resid:** Anatomic Pathology, Natl Inst Hlth 1971; **Fellow:** Pathology, Univ Hosp 1973; **Fac Appt:** Prof Path, Brown Univ

Fletcher, Christopher MD [Path] - **Spec Exp:** Soft Tissue Tumors; Sarcoma; Surgical Pathology; **Hospital:** Brigham & Women's Hosp, Dana-Farber Cancer Inst; **Address:** Brigham & Women's Hospital, Dept Pathology, 75 Francis St, Boston, MA 02115-6110; **Phone:** 617-732-8558; **Med School:** England, UK 1981; **Resid:** Pathology, St Thomas Hosp 1985; **Fellow:** Pathology, St Thomas Hosp 1986; **Fac Appt:** Prof Path, Harvard Med Sch

Harris, Nancy L MD [Path] - **Spec Exp:** Lymphoma; Hematopathology; **Hospital:** Mass Genl Hosp; **Address:** Mass Genl Hosp, Dept Path, 55 Fruit St, Warren 211, Boston, MA 02114; **Phone:** 617-726-5155; **Board Cert:** Anatomic Pathology 1978; Clinical Pathology 1978; **Med School:** Stanford Univ 1970; **Resid:** Pathology, Beth Israel Hosp 1978; **Fellow:** Immunopathology, Mass Genl Hosp 1980; **Fac Appt:** Prof Path, Harvard Med Sch

Mark, Eugene J MD [Path] - **Spec Exp:** Pulmonary Pathology; Cardiac Pathology; **Hospital:** Mass Genl Hosp; **Address:** Mass Genl Hosp, Dept Path, 55 Fruit St, Warren 246, Boston, MA 02114; **Phone:** 617-726-8891; **Board Cert:** Anatomic & Clinical Pathology 1973; Dermatopathology 1975; **Med School:** Harvard Med Sch 1967; **Resid:** Pathology, Mass Genl Hosp 1972; **Fellow:** Pathology, Kantonspital 1966; **Fac Appt:** Prof Path, Harvard Med Sch

Odze, Robert D MD [Path] - **Spec Exp:** Gastrointestinal Pathology; Liver Pathology; Esophageal Cancer; **Hospital:** Brigham & Women's Hosp; **Address:** Brigham & Women's Hosp, Dept Pathology, 75 Francis St, Boston, MA 02115; **Phone:** 617-732-7549; **Board Cert:** Anatomic Pathology 1990; **Med School:** McGill Univ 1984; **Resid:** Surgery, McGill Univ 1987; Pathology, McGill Univ 1990; **Fellow:** Gastrointestinal Pathology, New England Deaconess Med Ctr 1991; **Fac Appt:** Assoc Prof Path, Harvard Med Sch

Schnitt, Stuart J MD [Path] - **Spec Exp:** Breast Pathology; Breast Cancer; **Hospital:** Beth Israel Deaconess Med Ctr - Boston; **Address:** Beth Israel Deaconess Med Ctr, Dept Pathology, 330 Brookline Ave, rm ES 112, Boston, MA 02215-5400; **Phone:** 617-667-4344; **Board Cert:** Anatomic & Clinical Pathology 1983; **Med School:** Albany Med Coll 1979; **Resid:** Anatomic Pathology, Beth Israel Deaconess Med Ctr 1983; **Fellow:** Surgical Pathology, Beth Israel Deaconess Med Ctr 1984; **Fac Appt:** Assoc Prof Path, Harvard Med Sch

Young, Robert H MD [Path] - **Spec Exp:** Ovarian Cancer; Gynecologic Cancer; **Hospital:** Mass Genl Hosp; **Address:** Mass Genl Hosp, Dept Pathology, 55 Fruit St, Warren 215, Boston, MA 02114; **Phone:** 617-726-8892; **Board Cert:** Anatomic Pathology 1980; **Med School:** Ireland 1974; **Resid:** Pathology, Mass Genl Hosp 1979; Pathology, Dublin Univ 1977; **Fac Appt:** Prof Path, Harvard Med Sch

Mid Atlantic

Bagg, Adam MD [Path] - **Spec Exp:** Hematopathology; Leukemia & Lymphoma; Myelodysplastic Syndromes; **Hospital:** Hosp Univ Penn - UPHS (page 81); **Address:** Hosp Univ Penn, Dept Pathology & Lab Med, 3400 Spruce St, Phildelphia, PA 19104; **Phone:** 215-662-4280; **Board Cert:** Clinical Pathology 1992; Hematology 1999; **Med School:** South Africa 1981; **Resid:** Internal Medicine, Univ Witwatersrand 1992; Clinical Pathology, Georgetown Univ 1992; **Fellow:** Hematopathology, Georgetown Univ 1993; **Fac Appt:** Prof Path, Univ Pennsylvania

Brooks, John S MD [Path] - **Spec Exp:** Tumor Pathology; Sarcoma; Bone & Soft Tissue Pathology; **Hospital:** Pennsylvania Hosp (page 81), Hosp Univ Penn - UPHS (page 81); **Address:** Pennsylvania Hospital, Preston 6 FL, 800 Spruce St, Philadelphia, PA 19107; **Phone:** 215-829-3541; **Board Cert:** Anatomic Pathology 1978; Immunopathology 1983; **Med School:** Thomas Jefferson Univ 1974; **Resid:** Pathology, Hosp Univ Penn 1978; **Fellow:** Immunopathology, Hosp Univ Penn 1978; **Fac Appt:** Prof Path, Univ Pennsylvania

Burger, Peter MD [Path] - **Spec Exp:** Brain Tumors; Neuro-Pathology; **Hospital:** Johns Hopkins Hosp; **Address:** Johns Hopkins Hosp-Dept Pathology, 600 N Wolfe St, rm 710, Baltimore, MD 21287; **Phone:** 410-955-8378; **Board Cert:** Anatomic Pathology 1976; Neuropathology 1976; **Med School:** Northwestern Univ 1966; **Resid:** Anatomic Pathology, Duke Univ Med Ctr 1973; **Fellow:** Neuropathology, Duke Univ Med Ctr 1973

Crawford, James M MD/PhD [Path] - **Spec Exp:** Liver Pathology; Gastrointestinal Pathology; Gastrointestinal Cancer; **Hospital:** N Shore Univ Hosp; **Address:** NS-LIJ Laboratories, 10 Nevada Drive, Lake Success, NY 11042-1114; **Phone:** 516-719-1060; **Board Cert:** Anatomic Pathology 1987; **Med School:** Duke Univ 1982; **Resid:** Pathology, Brigham & Women's Hosp 1984; **Fellow:** Gastrointestinal Pathology, Brigham & Women's Hosp 1987; **Fac Appt:** Prof Path, Univ Fla Coll Med

Ehya, Hormoz MD [Path] - **Spec Exp:** Cytopathology; Breast Pathology; Lung Pathology; **Hospital:** Fox Chase Cancer Ctr (page 72); **Address:** Fox Chase Cancer Center, 333 Cottman Ave, rm C427, Philadelphia, PA 19111-2497; **Phone:** 215-728-5389; **Board Cert:** Anatomic Pathology 1979; Cytopathology 1989; **Med School:** Iran 1974; **Resid:** Pathology, Univ Miss Med Ctr 1979; **Fellow:** Cytopathology, Meml Sloan-Kettering Cancer Ctr 1980

Epstein, Jonathan MD [Path] - **Spec Exp:** Bladder Cancer; Prostate Cancer; Urologic Pathology; **Hospital:** Johns Hopkins Hosp; **Address:** 401 N Broadway, Weinberg 2242, Baltimore, MD 21231; **Phone:** 410-955-5043; **Board Cert:** Anatomic Pathology 1986; **Med School:** Boston Univ 1981; **Resid:** Pathology, Johns Hopkins Hosp 1985; **Fellow:** Pathology, Meml Sloan Kettering Cancer Ctr 1984; **Fac Appt:** Prof Path, Johns Hopkins Univ

Fogt, Franz MD/PhD [Path] - **Spec Exp:** Gastrointestinal Pathology; **Hospital:** Penn Presby Med Ctr - UPHS (page 81); **Address:** Presbyterian Medical Ctr, Dept Pathology, 551 Wright Saunders Bldg, Philadelphia, PA 19104; **Phone:** 215-662-8077; **Board Cert:** Anatomic & Clinical Pathology 1995; **Med School:** Germany 1988; **Resid:** Anatomic & Clinical Pathology, New England Deaconess Hosp 1995; **Fellow:** Gastrointestinal Pathology, New England Deaconess Hosp 1996; **Fac Appt:** Assoc Prof Path, Univ Pennsylvania

Pathology

Gottlieb, Geoffrey J MD [Path] - **Spec Exp:** Dermatopathology; Melanoma; **Address:** Ackerman Academy Dermatopathology, 145 E 32nd St Fl 10, New York, NY 10016; **Phone:** 212-889-6225; **Board Cert:** Anatomic Pathology 1979; Dermatopathology 1982; **Med School:** Cornell Univ-Weill Med Coll 1976; **Resid:** Pathology, NY Hosp-Cornell Med Ctr 1979; **Fellow:** Dermatopathology, NYU Med Ctr 1982

Gupta, Prabodh K MD [Path] - **Spec Exp:** Lung Pathology; Cervical Cancer; Fine Needle Aspiration Biopsy; **Hospital:** Hosp Univ Penn - UPHS (page 81); **Address:** Hosp Univ Penn - Cytopathology, 3400 Spruce St, 6 Founders, Philadelphia, PA 19104; **Phone:** 215-662-3238; **Board Cert:** Anatomic Pathology 1975; Cytopathology 1989; **Med School:** India 1965; **Resid:** Pathology, All India Inst Med Scis 1967; **Fellow:** Pathology, Mass Genl Hosp 1968; Cytopathology, Johns Hopkins Hosp 1969; **Fac Appt:** Prof Path, Univ Pennsylvania

Heller, Debra S MD [Path] - **Spec Exp:** Gynecologic Pathology; Pediatric Pathology; Perinatal Pathology; **Hospital:** UMDNJ-Univ Hosp-Newark; **Address:** UMDNJ-NJ Med Sch Dept Pathology, 185 S Orange Ave, Newark, NJ 07101; **Phone:** 973-972-0751; **Board Cert:** Anatomic Pathology 1988; Obstetrics & Gynecology 2008; Pediatric Pathology 1999; **Med School:** NY Med Coll 1977; **Resid:** Obstetrics & Gynecology, Beth Israel Med Ctr 1981; Anatomic Pathology, Mt Sinai Med Ctr 1988; **Fellow:** Pediatric Pathology, Mt Sinai Med Ctr 1987; Gynecologic Pathology, Mt Sinai Med Ctr 1989; **Fac Appt:** Prof Path, UMDNJ-NJ Med Sch, Newark

Hoda, Syed A MD [Path] - **Spec Exp:** Breast Cancer; Surgical Pathology; **Hospital:** NY-Presby Hosp/Weill Cornell (page 79); **Address:** 525 E 68th St, 1028 Starr, New York, NY 10021-4870; **Phone:** 212-746-2700; **Board Cert:** Anatomic & Clinical Pathology 1990; Cytopathology 1991; Pathology 2001; **Med School:** Pakistan 1984; **Resid:** Anatomic & Clinical Pathology, Tulane Univ Affil Hosps 1990; **Fellow:** Cytopathology, Meml Sloan Kettering Cancer Ctr 1991; Pathology, Meml Sloan Kettering Cancer Ctr 1992; **Fac Appt:** Clin Prof Path, Cornell Univ-Weill Med Coll

Hruban, Ralph H MD [Path] - **Spec Exp:** Gastrointestinal Pathology; Pancreatic Cancer; **Hospital:** Johns Hopkins Hosp; **Address:** Johns Hopkins Hosp, Dept Pathology, 401 N Broadway Bldg Weinberg - rm 2242, Baltimore, MD 21231; **Phone:** 410-955-9132; **Board Cert:** Anatomic Pathology 1990; **Med School:** Johns Hopkins Univ 1985; **Resid:** Pathology, Johns Hopkins Hosp 1990; **Fellow:** Meml Sloan Kettering Cancer Ctr 1989; **Fac Appt:** Prof Path, Johns Hopkins Univ

Jaffe, Elaine S MD [Path] - **Spec Exp:** Lymphoma; Hematopathology; **Hospital:** Natl Inst of Hlth - Clin Ctr; **Address:** NIH/NCI - Lab Pathology, 10 Center Drive Bldg 10 - rm 2B42, Bethesda, MD 20892-1500; **Phone:** 301-496-0183; **Board Cert:** Anatomic Pathology 1974; **Med School:** Univ Pennsylvania 1969; **Resid:** Pathology, Clinical Ctr/NIH 1972; **Fellow:** Hematopathology, Natl Cancer Inst 1974; **Fac Appt:** Clin Prof Path, Geo Wash Univ

Jones, Robert V MD [Path] - **Spec Exp:** Neuro-Pathology; Brain Tumors; **Hospital:** Georgetown Univ Hosp; **Address:** GWUMC, Dept Path, 2300 Eye St NW, Ross Hall, Ste 502, Washington, DC 20037; **Phone:** 202-994-3391; **Board Cert:** Anatomic & Clinical Pathology 1981; Neuropathology 1994; **Med School:** Univ VA Sch Med 1977; **Resid:** Anatomic & Clinical Pathology, Walter Reed AMC 1981; **Fellow:** Neurological Pathology, ARmed Forces Inst Path 1990; **Fac Appt:** Assoc Prof Path, Geo Wash Univ

Katzenstein, Anna-Luise A MD [Path] - **Spec Exp:** Lung Cancer; Pulmonary Pathology; **Hospital:** Univ Hosp - SUNY Upstate, Crouse Hosp; **Address:** SUNY Upstate Medical Univ, 766 Irving Ave, Weiskotten, rm 2106, Syracuse, NY 13210; **Phone:** 315-464-7125; **Board Cert:** Anatomic Pathology 1976; **Med School:** Johns Hopkins Univ 1971; **Resid:** Pathology, Univ Hosp 1975; **Fellow:** Surgical Pathology, Barnes Hosp-Wash Univ 1976; **Fac Appt:** Prof Path, SUNY Upstate Med Univ

Knowles, Daniel M MD [Path] - **Spec Exp:** Lymph Node Pathology; Bone Marrow Pathology; Lymphoma; **Hospital:** NY-Presby Hosp/Weill Cornell (page 79); **Address:** Cornell-Weill Med Coll-Dept Pathology, 1300 York Ave, rm C302, New York, NY 10021; **Phone:** 212-746-6464; **Board Cert:** Anatomic Pathology 1978; Immunopathology 1984; **Med School:** Univ Chicago-Pritzker Sch Med 1973; **Resid:** Anatomic Pathology, Columbia-Presby Med Ctr 1975; **Fellow:** Immunopathology, Rockefeller Univ 1977; **Fac Appt:** Prof Path, Cornell Univ-Weill Med Coll

Kurman, Robert J MD [Path] - **Spec Exp:** Gynecologic Pathology; Ovarian Cancer; Uterine Cancer; **Hospital:** Johns Hopkins Hosp; **Address:** Johns Hopkins Hosp, Dept Pathology, 401 N Broadway, Weinberg-2242, Baltimore, MD 21231; **Phone:** 410-955-0471; **Board Cert:** Anatomic Pathology 1972; Obstetrics & Gynecology 1980; **Med School:** SUNY Upstate Med Univ 1968; **Resid:** Pathology, Peter Bent Brigham Hosp/Mass Genl Hosp 1977; Obstetrics & Gynecology, LAC Hosp/USC 1978; **Fellow:** Obstetrics & Gynecology, Harvard Univ 1973; **Fac Appt:** Prof Path, Johns Hopkins Univ

Li Volsi, Virginia A MD [Path] - **Spec Exp:** Endocrine Cancers; Thyroid Cancer; Gynecologic Cancer; **Hospital:** Hosp Univ Penn - UPHS (page 81); **Address:** Hosp Univ Penn - Pathology, 3400 Spruce St 6 Founders Bldg - Ste 6030, Philadelphia, PA 19104; **Phone:** 215-662-6545; **Board Cert:** Anatomic Pathology 1974; **Med School:** Columbia P&S 1969; **Resid:** Anatomic Pathology, Presbyterian Hosp 1974; **Fac Appt:** Prof Path, Univ Pennsylvania

Melamed, Jonathan MD [Path] - **Spec Exp:** Prostate Cancer; Tumor Banking-Prostate; **Hospital:** NYU Langone Med Ctr (page 80); **Address:** NYU Medical Ctr, Dept Pathology, TH-461, 560 First Ave, New York, NY 10016; **Phone:** 212-263-8927; **Board Cert:** Anatomic & Clinical Pathology 1992; **Med School:** South Africa 1985; **Resid:** Pathology, Lenox Hill Hosp 1991; **Fellow:** Pathology, Meml Sloan Kettering Cancer Ctr 1992; Urologic Pathology, Meml Sloan Kettering Cancer Ctr 1993; **Fac Appt:** Assoc Prof Path, NYU Sch Med

Mies, Carolyn MD [Path] - **Spec Exp:** Breast Cancer; **Hospital:** Hosp Univ Penn - UPHS (page 81); **Address:** Hosp Univ Penn-Surgical Pathology, 3400 Spruce St, Founders 6, Philadelphia, PA 19104; **Phone:** 215-662-6503; **Board Cert:** Anatomic Pathology 1984; **Med School:** Rush Med Coll 1980; **Resid:** Pathology, Tufts-New England Med Ctr 1982; Pathology, New England Deaconess Hosp 1984; **Fellow:** Surgical Pathology, Meml Sloan Kettering Cancer Ctr 1986; **Fac Appt:** Assoc Prof Path, Univ Pennsylvania

Montgomery, Elizabeth A MD [Path] - **Spec Exp:** Barrett's Esophagus; Esophageal Cancer; Gastrointestinal Pathology; **Hospital:** Johns Hopkins Hosp; **Address:** Johns Hopkins Univ, Dept Pathology, 401 N Broadway Weinberg Bldg - rm 2242, Baltimore, MD 21231; **Phone:** 410-614-2308; **Board Cert:** Anatomic Pathology 1988; Cytopathology 1994; **Med School:** Geo Wash Univ 1984; **Resid:** Pathology, Walter Reed AMC 1988; **Fac Appt:** Assoc Prof Path, Johns Hopkins Univ

Orazi, Attilio MD [Path] - **Spec Exp:** Hematopathology; Bone Marrow Pathology; Lymph Node Pathology; **Hospital:** NY-Presby Hosp/Weill Cornell (page 79); **Address:** NY Presby-Cornell Medical Ctr, 525 E 68th St, Starr Pavilion, rm 715, New York, NY 10021; **Phone:** 212-746-2050; **Board Cert:** Anatomic Pathology 1997; Hematology 1998; **Med School:** Italy 1979; **Resid:** Internal Medicine, Leicester Royal Infirmary 1982; Histopathology, Northampton Genl Hosp 1983; **Fellow:** Anatomic Pathology, Natl Cancer Inst 1985; **Fac Appt:** Prof Path, Cornell Univ-Weill Med Coll

Patchefsky, Arthur S MD [Path] - **Spec Exp:** Breast Cancer; Pulmonary Pathology; Sarcoma; **Hospital:** Fox Chase Cancer Ctr (page 72); **Address:** Fox Chase Cancer Center, 333 Cottman Ave, rm C4333, Philadelphia, PA 19111; **Phone:** 215-728-5390; **Board Cert:** Anatomic Pathology 1969; **Med School:** Hahnemann Univ 1963; **Resid:** Pathology, John Hopkins Hosp 1966; Pathology, Hosp Univ Penn 1967; **Fellow:** Pathology, Meml Sloan Kettering Cancer Ctr 1968; **Fac Appt:** Prof Path, Thomas Jefferson Univ

Pathology

Reuter, Victor E MD [Path] - **Spec Exp:** Prostate Cancer; Genitourinary Pathology; Bladder Cancer; Urologic Pathology; **Hospital:** Meml Sloan-Kettering Cancer Ctr (page 76); **Address:** Memorial Sloan Kettering Cancer Ctr, Dept Pathology, 1275 York Ave, New York, NY 10021; **Phone:** 212-639-8225; **Board Cert:** Anatomic & Clinical Pathology 1983; **Med School:** Dominican Republic 1978; **Resid:** Anatomic Pathology, Thos Jefferson Univ Hosp 1981; Clinical Pathology, Thos Jefferson Univ Hosp 1983; **Fellow:** Surgical Pathology, Meml Sloan Kettering Cancer Ctr 1985; **Fac Appt:** Prof Path, Cornell Univ-Weill Med Coll

Rosen, Paul P MD [Path] - **Spec Exp:** Breast Pathology; Breast Cancer; **Hospital:** NY-Presby Hosp/Weill Cornell (page 79); **Address:** New York Presbyterian, Dept Pathology, 525 E 68th St, Starr 1031, New York, NY 10065; **Phone:** 212-746-6482; **Board Cert:** Anatomic & Clinical Pathology 1969; Pathology 1998; **Med School:** Columbia P&S 1964; **Resid:** Pathology, Presby Hosp 1966; Pathology, VA Hosp 1968; **Fellow:** Pathology, Meml Hosp Cancer Ctr 1970; **Fac Appt:** Prof Path, Cornell Univ-Weill Med Coll

Rosenblum, Marc K MD [Path] - **Spec Exp:** Neuropathology; Brain Tumors; **Hospital:** Meml Sloan-Kettering Cancer Ctr (page 76); **Address:** 1275 York Avenue, New York, NY 10065; **Phone:** 212-639-5905; **Board Cert:** Anatomic Pathology 1984; Pathology 1998; Neuropathology 1988; **Med School:** Univ Miami Sch Med 1979; **Resid:** Anatomic Pathology, Mt Sinai Med Ctr 1984; **Fellow:** Pathology, Meml Sloan-Kettering Cancer Ctr 1985; Neurological Pathology, Bellevue-NYU Med Ctr 1987; **Fac Appt:** Prof Path, Cornell Univ-Weill Med Coll

Ross, Jeffrey S MD [Path] - **Spec Exp:** Urologic Cancer; Prostate Cancer; Breast Cancer; **Hospital:** Albany Med Ctr; **Address:** Albany Med Coll, Dept Path, 47 New Scotland Ave, MC 81, Albany, NY 12208; **Phone:** 518-262-5471; **Board Cert:** Anatomic & Clinical Pathology 1974; **Med School:** SUNY Buffalo 1970; **Resid:** Pathology, Mass Genl Hosp 1974; **Fellow:** Pathology, Harvard Med Sch 1974; **Fac Appt:** Prof Path, Albany Med Coll

Sanchez, Miguel A MD [Path] - **Spec Exp:** Breast Cancer; Thyroid Cancer; **Hospital:** Englewood Hosp & Med Ctr; **Address:** Englewood Hosp & Med Ctr, Dept Pathology, 350 Engle St, Englewood, NJ 07631-1898; **Phone:** 201-894-3423; **Board Cert:** Anatomic Pathology 1975; Clinical Pathology 1979; Cytopathology 1991; **Med School:** Spain 1969; **Resid:** Pathology, Englewood Hosp 1972; Pathology, Temple Univ 1973; **Fellow:** Pathology, Meml Sloan Kettering Cancer Ctr 1974; Clinical Pathology, St Vincents Hosp 1975; **Fac Appt:** Assoc Prof Path, Mount Sinai Sch Med

Schiller, Alan L MD [Path] - **Spec Exp:** Bone & Joint Pathology; Soft Tissue Pathology; Bone Tumors; **Hospital:** Mount Sinai Med Ctr (page 77); **Address:** Mt Sinai Sch Med, Dept Pathology, 1 Gustave Levy Pl, Box 1194, New York, NY 10029-6500; **Phone:** 212-241-8014; **Board Cert:** Anatomic Pathology 1973; **Med School:** Ros Franklin Univ/Chicago Med Sch 1967; **Resid:** Pathology, Mass Genl Hosp 1972; **Fac Appt:** Prof Path, Mount Sinai Sch Med

Silverberg, Steven G MD [Path] - **Spec Exp:** Gynecologic Pathology; Breast Pathology; Urologic Pathology; Endocrine Pathology; **Hospital:** Univ of MD Med Ctr; **Address:** Univ Maryland Med Ctr, Dept Pathology, 22 S Greene St, Baltimore, MD 21201; **Phone:** 410-328-5072; **Board Cert:** Anatomic Pathology 1969; **Med School:** Johns Hopkins Univ 1962; **Resid:** Pathology, Yale-New Haven Hosp 1965; **Fellow:** Surgical Pathology, Meml Sloan Kettering Cancer Ctr 1966; **Fac Appt:** Prof Path, Univ MD Sch Med

Silverman, Jan F MD [Path] - **Spec Exp:** Breast Cancer; Lung Cancer; Gastrointestinal Pathology; Fine Needle Aspiration Biopsy; **Hospital:** Allegheny General Hosp, West Penn Hosp - Forbes Campus; **Address:** Allegheny Gen Hosp-Dept Lab Medicine, 320 E North Ave, Pittsburgh, PA 15212; **Phone:** 412-359-6886; **Board Cert:** Anatomic & Clinical Pathology 1975; Cytopathology 1989; **Med School:** Med Coll VA 1970; **Resid:** Pathology, Med Coll Virginia 1975; **Fellow:** Surgical Pathology, Med Coll Virginia 1975; **Fac Appt:** Prof Path, Drexel Univ Coll Med

Swerdlow, Steven H MD [Path] - **Spec Exp:** Lymphoma; Hematopathology; Transplant Pathology; **Hospital:** UPMC Presby, Pittsburgh; **Address:** Div Hematopathology, 200 Lothrop St, Ste G-300, Pittsburgh, PA 15213-2536; **Phone:** 412-647-5191; **Board Cert:** Anatomic Pathology 2005; Clinical Pathology 2005; **Med School:** Harvard Med Sch 1975; **Resid:** Pathology, Beth Israel Hosp 1979; **Fellow:** Hematopathology, Vanderbilt Univ 1981; Hematopathology, St Bartholmew's Hosp 1983; **Fac Appt:** Prof Path, Univ Pittsburgh

Tomaszewski, John E MD [Path] - **Spec Exp:** Kidney Pathology; Lung Pathology; Uterine Cancer; Genitourinary Pathology; **Hospital:** Hosp Univ Penn - UPHS (page 81); **Address:** Hosp Univ Penn, Dept Pathology & Lab Med, 3400 Spruce St, 6 Founders Bldg, Ste 6042, Philadelphia, PA 19104; **Phone:** 215-662-6852; **Board Cert:** Anatomic Pathology 1982; Immunopathology 1983; **Med School:** Univ Pennsylvania 1977; **Resid:** Pathology, Hosp Univ Penn 1982; **Fellow:** Surgical Pathology, Hosp Univ Penn 1983; **Fac Appt:** Prof Path, Univ Pennsylvania

Tornos, Carmen MD [Path] - **Spec Exp:** Gynecologic Cancer; Breast Cancer; Ovarian Cancer; **Hospital:** Stony Brook Univ Med Ctr; **Address:** Stony Brook Univ Hosp, Dept Pathology, Level 2, rm 766, Stony Brook, NY 11794; **Phone:** 631-444-2222; **Board Cert:** Anatomic & Clinical Pathology 1989; **Med School:** Spain 1977; **Resid:** Hematology, Ciudad Sanitaria Valle de Hebron 1982; Anatomic & Clinical Pathology, Univ Texas HSC 1989; **Fellow:** Surgical Pathology, MD Anderson Cancer Ctr 1990; **Fac Appt:** Prof Path, SUNY Stony Brook

Travis, William MD [Path] - **Spec Exp:** Pulmonary Pathology; Lung Cancer; **Hospital:** Meml Sloan-Kettering Cancer Ctr (page 76); **Address:** 1275 York Avenue, Pathology Dept, New York, NY 10065; **Phone:** 800-525-2225; **Board Cert:** Anatomic & Clinical Pathology 1985; **Med School:** Univ Fla Coll Med 1981; **Resid:** Anatomic Pathology, New England Deaconess Hosp 1983; Clinical Pathology, Mayo Clinic 1985; **Fellow:** Surgical Pathology, Mayo Clinic 1986

Yousem, Samuel A MD [Path] - **Spec Exp:** Pulmonary Pathology; Transplant-Lung (Pathology); Lung Cancer; **Hospital:** UPMC Presby, Pittsburgh; **Address:** Dept Pathology, A-610, UPMC-Presbyterian Campus, 200 Lothrop St, Pittsburgh, PA 15213; **Phone:** 412-647-6193; **Board Cert:** Anatomic Pathology 1985; Cytopathology 1997; **Med School:** Univ MD Sch Med 1981; **Resid:** Pathology, Stanford Univ Med Ctr 1983; **Fellow:** Surgical Pathology, Stanford Univ Med Ctr 1984; **Fac Appt:** Prof Path, Univ Pittsburgh

Zagzag, David MD/PhD [Path] - **Spec Exp:** Neuropathology; Brain Tumors; Tumor Banking-Brain; **Hospital:** NYU Langone Med Ctr (page 80), Bellevue Hosp Ctr; **Address:** NYU Med Ctr, Dept Pathology, 550 First Ave, Div Neuropathology, NB-4N30, New York, NY 10016; **Phone:** 212-263-6449; **Board Cert:** Anatomic Pathology 1993; Neuropathology 1993; **Med School:** France 1984; **Resid:** Surgical Pathology, NYU Med Ctr 1990; **Fellow:** Neurological Pathology, NYU Med Ctr 1992; **Fac Appt:** Assoc Prof Path, NYU Sch Med

Southeast

Banks, Peter MD [Path] - **Spec Exp:** Hematopathology; Lymphoma; **Hospital:** Carolinas Med Ctr; **Address:** Dept Pathology, 1000 Blythe Blvd, 4th Fl Pathology Lab, Charlotte, NC 28203; **Phone:** 704-355-2251; **Board Cert:** Anatomic Pathology 2008; **Med School:** Harvard Med Sch 1971; **Resid:** Pathology, National Cancer Inst 1974; Pathology, Duke Univ Med Ctr 1975; **Fellow:** Surgical Pathology, Univ Minn Med Ctr 1976; **Fac Appt:** Prof Path, Univ NC Sch Med

Bostwick, David MD [Path] - **Spec Exp:** Urologic Pathology; Prostate Cancer; Bladder Cancer; Gastrointestinal Pathology; **Address:** 4355 Innslake Drive, Glen Allen, VA 23060; **Phone:** 804-967-9225; **Board Cert:** Anatomic Pathology 2003; **Med School:** Univ MD Sch Med 1979; **Resid:** Pathology, Stanford Univ Med Ctr 1981; **Fellow:** Surgical Pathology, Stanford Univ Med Ctr 1984

Pathology

Braylan, Raul MD [Path] - **Spec Exp:** Hematopathology; Leukemia; Lymphoma; **Hospital:** Shands at Univ of FL; **Address:** Univ Florida, Dept Hematopathology, PO Box 100275, Gainesville, FL 32610; **Phone:** 352-265-9900; **Board Cert:** Anatomic Pathology 1972; **Med School:** Argentina 1960; **Resid:** Anatomic Pathology, Mt Sinai Hosp 1965; Anatomic Pathology, Einstein Affil Hosps 1967; **Fellow:** Anatomic Pathology, Meml Sloan Kettering Cancer Hosp 1968; Hematopathology, Univ Chicago Hosps 1973; **Fac Appt:** Prof Path, Univ Fla Coll Med

Cote, Richard J MD [Path] - **Spec Exp:** Lymph Node Pathology; Bladder Cancer; Breast Cancer; **Hospital:** Univ of Miami Hosp (page 82); **Address:** 1611 NW 12th Ave, Holtz Bldg - rm 2046, Miami, FL 33136; **Phone:** 305-585-6103; **Board Cert:** Anatomic Pathology 1987; **Med School:** Univ Chicago-Pritzker Sch Med 1980; **Resid:** Pathology, New York Hosp-Cornell 1987; **Fellow:** Pathology, Meml Sloan-Kettering Cancer Ctr 1990; **Fac Appt:** Prof Path, USC-Keck School of Medicine

Lage, Janice MD [Path] - **Spec Exp:** Gynecologic Pathology; Breast Pathology; **Hospital:** MUSC Med Ctr; **Address:** MUSC Med Ctr, Dept Path, 165 Ashley Ave, Ste 309, Box 250908, Charleston, SC 29425; **Phone:** 843-792-3121; **Board Cert:** Anatomic Pathology 2001; **Med School:** Washington Univ, St Louis 1980; **Resid:** Pathology, Barnes Hosp/Wash Univ 1982; Obstetrics & Gynecology, Barnes Hosp/Wash Univ 1983; **Fellow:** Surgical Pathology, Barnes Hosp/Wash Univ 1984; **Fac Appt:** Prof Path, Med Univ SC

Masood, Shahla MD [Path] - **Spec Exp:** Breast Cancer; Breast Pathology; **Hospital:** Shands Jacksonville; **Address:** Univ of Florida, Dept Pathology, 655 W 8th St, Jacksonville, FL 32209-6511; **Phone:** 904-244-4387; **Board Cert:** Anatomic & Clinical Pathology 1998; Cytopathology 1990; **Med School:** Iran 1973; **Resid:** Anatomic Pathology, Univ Hosp 1977; **Fac Appt:** Prof Path, Univ Fla Coll Med

McCurley, Thomas L MD [Path] - **Spec Exp:** Hematopathology; Immunopathology; **Hospital:** Vanderbilt Univ Med Ctr, VA Med Ctr - Nashville; **Address:** Vanderbilt Univ Hosp, Dept Pathology, 21st & Garland Ave, Nashville, TN 37232-0001; **Phone:** 615-343-9167; **Board Cert:** Anatomic & Clinical Pathology 1981; Immunopathology 1986; Hematology 1999; **Med School:** Vanderbilt Univ 1974; **Resid:** Internal Medicine, UCSF Med Ctr 1976; Pathology, Vanderbilt Univ Med Ctr 1981; **Fellow:** Hematopathology, Vanderbilt Univ 1984; **Fac Appt:** Assoc Prof Path, Vanderbilt Univ

Mills, Stacey E MD [Path] - **Spec Exp:** Breast Pathology; Ear, Nose & Throat Cancer; Surgical Pathology; **Hospital:** Univ Virginia Med Ctr; **Address:** Univ VA Hlth System, Dept Pathology, PO Box 800214, Charlottesville, VA 22908-0214; **Phone:** 434-982-4406; **Board Cert:** Anatomic Pathology 1999; **Med School:** Univ VA Sch Med 1977; **Resid:** Pathology, Univ Virginia Med Ctr 1980; **Fellow:** Pathology, Univ Virginia 1981; **Fac Appt:** Prof Path, Univ VA Sch Med

Nicosia, Santo MD [Path] - **Spec Exp:** Ovarian Cancer; **Hospital:** H Lee Moffitt Cancer Ctr & Research Inst; **Address:** 12901 Bruce B Downs Blvd, MDC Box 11, Tampa, FL 33612-4742; **Phone:** 813-974-3133; **Board Cert:** Anatomic Pathology 1978; Cytopathology 1990; **Med School:** Italy 1967; **Resid:** Anatomic Pathology, Michael Reese Hosp 1972; **Fellow:** Hosp Univ Penn 1973; **Fac Appt:** Prof Path, Univ S Fla Coll Med

Page, David L MD [Path] - **Spec Exp:** Breast Cancer; **Hospital:** Vanderbilt Univ Med Ctr; **Address:** Vanderbilt Univ, 1161 21st Ave S, rm C 3309, Nashville, TN 37232-2561; **Phone:** 615-322-3759; **Board Cert:** Anatomic Pathology 1972; Dermatopathology 1974; **Med School:** Johns Hopkins Univ 1966; **Resid:** Pathology, Mass Genl Hosp 1969; Pathology, Johns Hopkins Hosp 1972; **Fac Appt:** Prof Path, Vanderbilt Univ

Sewell, C Whitaker MD [Path] - **Spec Exp:** Breast Pathology; Surgical Pathology; **Hospital:** Emory Univ Hosp; **Address:** Emory Univ Hosp, Dept Pathology, 1364 Clifton Rd NE, rm H185C, Atlanta, GA 30322; **Phone:** 404-712-5947; **Board Cert:** Anatomic Pathology 1974; Clinical Pathology 1974; **Med School:** Emory Univ 1969; **Resid:** Pathology, Emory Univ Hosp 1974; **Fac Appt:** Prof Path, Emory Univ

Weiss, Sharon A W MD [Path] - **Spec Exp:** Soft Tissue Pathology; Surgical Pathology; Sarcoma; **Hospital:** Emory Univ Hosp; **Address:** Emory Univ Hosp, Dept Pathology, 1364 Clifton Rd NE, rm H176, Atlanta, GA 30322; **Phone:** 404-712-0708; **Board Cert:** Anatomic Pathology 1974; **Med School:** Johns Hopkins Univ 1971; **Resid:** Pathology, Johns Hopkins Hosp 1975; **Fac Appt:** Prof Path, Emory Univ

Midwest

Allred, D Craig MD [Path] - **Spec Exp:** Breast Cancer; Breast Pathology; Breast Cancer Risk Assessment; **Hospital:** Barnes-Jewish Hosp; **Address:** Washington Univ Sch Med, Path & Immunology, 660 S Euclid Ave, Box 8118, St Louis, MO 63110; **Phone:** 314-362-6313; **Board Cert:** Anatomic Pathology 1984; **Med School:** Univ Utah 1979; **Resid:** Anatomic Pathology, Univ Conn Hlth Ctr 1983; **Fellow:** Immunopathology, Univ Conn Hlth Ctr 1982; **Fac Appt:** Prof Path, Baylor Coll Med

Balla, Andre K MD/PhD [Path] - **Spec Exp:** Prostate Cancer; Gynecologic Pathology; Tumor Banking; **Hospital:** Univ of IL Med Ctr at Chicago; **Address:** Univ Illinois Chicago, Dept Path, 840 S Wood St, rm 130, MC 847, Chicago, IL 60612; **Phone:** 312-996-3879; **Board Cert:** Anatomic & Clinical Pathology 1988; **Med School:** Brazil 1972; **Resid:** Pathology, Hahnemann Univ Hosp 1988; **Fellow:** Clinical Immunology, Scripps Clin Rsch Fdn 1981; **Fac Appt:** Prof Path, Univ IL Coll Med

Behm, Frederick G MD [Path] - **Spec Exp:** Hematopathology; **Hospital:** Univ of IL Med Ctr at Chicago; **Address:** Univ Illinois Chicago, Dept Pathology, 130 CSN, MC 847, 840 S Wood St, Chicago, IL 60612-7335; **Phone:** 312-996-3150; **Board Cert:** Anatomic & Clinical Pathology 1980; Hematology 1983; **Med School:** Med Coll Wisc 1974; **Resid:** Pathology, Med Coll Va Hosps 1979; **Fac Appt:** Prof Path, Univ IL Coll Med

Bell, Debra A MD [Path] - **Spec Exp:** Gynecologic Pathology; Ovarian Cancer; **Hospital:** Mayo Med Ctr & Clin - Rochester; **Address:** Mayo Clinic-Pathology Dept, 200 First St SW, Rochester, MN 55905; **Phone:** 507-284-1800; **Board Cert:** Anatomic Pathology 1980; Cytopathology 1989; **Med School:** Albany Med Coll 1976; **Resid:** Pathology, NYU Med Ctr 1981; **Fellow:** Cytopathology, Meml Sloan Kettering Cancer Ctr 1982; **Fac Appt:** Assoc Prof Path, Mayo Med Sch

Cho, Kathleen R MD [Path] - **Spec Exp:** Gynecologic Pathology; Ovarian Cancer; Cervical Cancer; **Hospital:** Univ Michigan Hlth Sys; **Address:** Univ Michigan Med Sch, 109 Zina Pitcher Pl, rm 1506, Ann Arbor, MI 48109-2200; **Phone:** 734-764-1549; **Board Cert:** Anatomic Pathology 1990; **Med School:** Vanderbilt Univ 1984; **Resid:** Pathology, Johns Hopkins Hosp 1988; **Fellow:** Gynecologic Pathology, Johns Hopkins Hosp 1990; **Fac Appt:** Prof Path, Univ Mich Med Sch

Cohen, Michael B MD [Path] - **Spec Exp:** Urologic Cancer; Cytopathology; **Hospital:** Univ Iowa Hosp & Clinics, VA Med Ctr - Iowa City; **Address:** Univ Iowa - Dept Pathology, 200 Hawkins Drive, C670GH, Iowa City, IA 52242; **Phone:** 319-384-9609; **Board Cert:** Anatomic Pathology 2008; Cytopathology 1996; **Med School:** Albany Med Coll 1982; **Resid:** Pathology, UCSF Hosps & Clinics 1986; **Fellow:** Cytopathology, UCSF Hosps & Clinics 1987; **Fac Appt:** Prof Path, Univ Iowa Coll Med

Pathology

Goldblum, John R MD [Path] - **Spec Exp:** Soft Tissue Pathology; Esophageal Cancer; Gastrointestinal Pathology; Sarcoma; **Hospital:** Cleveland Clin Fdn (page 70); **Address:** Cleveland Clinic, Anatomic Pathology L25, 9500 Euclid Ave, Cleveland, OH 44195; **Phone:** 216-444-8238; **Board Cert:** Anatomic Pathology 1993; **Med School:** Univ Mich Med Sch 1989; **Resid:** Anatomic Pathology, Univ Michigan Hosps 1993; **Fac Appt:** Prof Path, Cleveland Cl Coll Med/Case West Res

Greenson, Joel K MD [Path] - **Spec Exp:** Liver Cancer; Gastrointestinal Pathology; Liver Pathology; **Hospital:** Univ Michigan Hlth Sys; **Address:** Univ Michigan Hospitals, Dept Pathology, 1500 E Medical Center Drive, rm 2G332, Ann Arbor, MI 48109-0054; **Phone:** 734-936-6799; **Board Cert:** Anatomic & Clinical Pathology 1988; **Med School:** Univ Mich Med Sch 1984; **Resid:** Pathology, Cedars-Sinai Med Ctr 1988; **Fellow:** Gastrointestinal Pathology, Johns Hopkins Hosp 1990; **Fac Appt:** Prof Path, Univ Mich Med Sch

Kurtin, Paul J MD [Path] - **Spec Exp:** Lymph Node Pathology; Bone Marrow Pathology; Lymphoma; **Hospital:** Mayo Med Ctr & Clin - Rochester; **Address:** Mayo Clinic - Div Hematopathology, 200 First St SW, Hilton 1156A, Rochester, MN 55905; **Phone:** 507-284-4939; **Board Cert:** Anatomic & Clinical Pathology 1983; Hematology 1988; **Med School:** Med Coll Wisc 1979; **Resid:** Anatomic & Clinical Pathology, Vanderbilt Univ Med Ctr 1983; **Fellow:** Hematopathology, Brigham & Women's Hosp 1984; Surgical Pathology, Brigham & Women's Hosp 1986; **Fac Appt:** Prof Path, Mayo Med Sch

Myers, Jeffrey L MD [Path] - **Spec Exp:** Lung Cancer; Lung Pathology; **Hospital:** Univ Michigan Hlth Sys; **Address:** Univ Michigan, 2G332 UH, CCC 1500 E Med Ctr Dr, Fl B1-Rm363, Ann Arbor, MI 48109-5912; **Phone:** 734-647-8902; **Board Cert:** Anatomic Pathology 1986; **Med School:** Washington Univ, St Louis 1981; **Resid:** Anatomic Pathology, Barnes Jewish Hosp 1984; **Fellow:** Surgical Pathology, U Alabama Med Ctr 1985; **Fac Appt:** Prof Path, Univ Mich Med Sch

Nascimento, Antonio G MD [Path] - **Spec Exp:** Bone & Soft Tissue Pathology; Head & Neck Pathology; **Hospital:** Mayo Med Ctr & Clin - Rochester; **Address:** Mayo Clinic - Dept Pathology, 200 First St SW, Rochester, MN 55905; **Phone:** 507-284-1187; **Board Cert:** Anatomic Pathology 1979; **Med School:** Brazil ; **Resid:** Pathology, Univ Mississippi Med Ctr; **Fellow:** Anatomic Pathology, Meml Sloan-Kettering Cancer Ctr; Surgical Pathology, Mayo Clinic

Perry, Arie MD [Path] - **Spec Exp:** Neuro-Pathology; Brain Tumors; **Hospital:** Washington Univ Med Ctr; **Address:** Washington Univ Sch Med, Dept Path-Div Neuropath, Box 8118, 660 S Euclid Ave, St Louis, MO 63110; **Phone:** 314-362-7426; **Board Cert:** Anatomic & Clinical Pathology 1995; Neuropathology 1997; **Med School:** Univ Tex SW, Dallas 1990; **Resid:** Pathology, Univ Tex SW 1994; **Fellow:** Surgical Pathology, Mayo Clinic 1995; Neurological Pathology, Mayo Clinic 1998; **Fac Appt:** Assoc Prof Path, Washington Univ, St Louis

Rubin, Brian P MD [Path] - **Spec Exp:** Bone & Soft Tissue Tumors; Sarcoma; **Hospital:** Cleveland Clin Fdn (page 70); **Address:** Cleveland Clinic, Dept Anatomic Pathology, L25, 9500 Euclid Ave, Cleveland, OH 44195; **Phone:** 216-445-5551; **Board Cert:** Anatomic Pathology 1999; **Med School:** Cornell Univ-Weill Med Coll 1995; **Resid:** Pathology, Brigham & Womens Hosp 2000; **Fac Appt:** Asst Prof Path, Univ Wash

Scheithauer, Bernd W MD [Path] - **Spec Exp:** Brain Tumors; Pituitary Tumors; Neuro-Pathology; **Hospital:** Mayo Med Ctr & Clin - Rochester; **Address:** Dept Pathology, 200 First St SW, Rochester, MN 55905; **Phone:** 507-284-8350; **Board Cert:** Anatomic Pathology 1979; Neuropathology 1979; **Med School:** Loma Linda Univ 1973; **Resid:** Anatomic Pathology, Stanford Univ Med Ctr 1976; Neuropathology, Stanford Univ Med Ctr 1978; **Fellow:** Surgical Pathology, Stanford Univ Med Ctr 1979; **Fac Appt:** Prof Path, Mayo Med Sch

Suster, Saul M MD [Path] - **Spec Exp:** Lung Cancer; Mediastinal Tumors; Surgical Pathology; **Hospital:** Froedtert Meml Lutheran Hosp; **Address:** Med College of Wisconsin, Dept Pathology, Dynacare Lab Bldg, rm 226, 9200 W Wisconsin Ave, Milwaukee, WI 53226; **Phone:** 414-805-6968; **Board Cert:** Anatomic & Clinical Pathology 1988; **Med School:** Ecuador 1976; **Resid:** Anatomic Pathology, Tel Aviv Univ Med Ctr 1984; Anatomic & Clinical Pathology, Mt Sinai Med Ctr 1988; **Fellow:** Surgical Pathology, Yale-New Haven Hosp 1990; **Fac Appt:** Prof Path, Med Coll Wisc

Ulbright, Thomas M MD [Path] - **Spec Exp:** Testicular Cancer; Gynecologic Pathology; **Hospital:** Indiana Univ Hosp (page 74); **Address:** Clarion Pathology Laboratory, 350 W 11th St, rm 4014, Indianapolis, IN 46202; **Phone:** 317-491-6498; **Board Cert:** Anatomic Pathology 1980; **Med School:** Washington Univ, St Louis 1975; **Resid:** Pathology, Barnes Jewish Hosp 1978; Surgical Pathology, Barnes Jewish Hosp 1979; **Fellow:** Gynecologic Pathology, St Johns Mercy Med Ctr 1980; **Fac Appt:** Prof Path, Indiana Univ

Great Plains and Mountains

De Masters, Bette K MD [Path] - **Spec Exp:** Neuro-Pathology; Brain Tumors; **Hospital:** Univ Colorado Hosp, Chldn's Hosp - Aurora, The; **Address:** Univ CO Hlth Sci Ctr, Dept Pathology, Box 6511, MS 8104, Aurora, CO 80045-0508; **Phone:** 303-724-3704; **Board Cert:** Anatomic & Clinical Pathology 1982; Neuropathology 1985; **Med School:** Univ Wisc 1977; **Resid:** Internal Medicine, Presby Hosp 1979; Pathology, Univ Colo Med Sch 1982; **Fellow:** Neurological Pathology, Univ Colo/Univ Kansas 1984; **Fac Appt:** Prof Path, Univ Colorado

Rodgers III, George M MD/PhD [Path] - **Spec Exp:** Hematopathology; Anemia-Cancer Related; **Hospital:** Univ Utah Hosps and Clins; **Address:** Univ Utah Med Ctr - Div Hematology, 30 N 1900 E, rm 5C402, Salt Lake City, UT 84132; **Phone:** 801-585-3229; **Board Cert:** Internal Medicine 1979; Hematology 1982; Pathology 1984; **Med School:** Tulane Univ 1976; **Resid:** Internal Medicine, Baylor Affil Hosps 1979; **Fellow:** Hematology, UCSF Med Ctr 1982; **Fac Appt:** Prof Med, Univ Utah

Thor, Ann D MD [Path] - **Spec Exp:** Breast Cancer; Gynecologic Cancer; **Hospital:** Univ Colorado Hosp; **Address:** Univ CO Hlth Sci Ctr, Dept Pathology, Box 6511, MS B216, Aurora, CO 80045-0508; **Phone:** 303-724-3704; **Board Cert:** Anatomic Pathology 1987; Cytopathology 1989; **Med School:** Vanderbilt Univ 1981; **Resid:** Pathology, Vanderbilt Univ 1983; **Fellow:** Immunopathology, Natl Cancer Inst 1986; Gynecologic Pathology, Mass Genl Hosp 1990; **Fac Appt:** Prof Path, Univ Colorado

Weisenburger, Dennis MD [Path] - **Spec Exp:** Hematopathology; Lymphoma; **Hospital:** Nebraska Med Ctr; **Address:** Univ Nebraska Med Ctr, Dept Pathology, 983135 Nebraska Medical Center, Omaha, NE 68198-3135; **Phone:** 402-559-7688; **Board Cert:** Anatomic & Clinical Pathology 1979; **Med School:** Univ Minn 1974; **Resid:** Anatomic Pathology, Univ Iowa Hosps 1978; **Fellow:** Hematopathology, City of Hope Natl Med Ctr 1980; **Fac Appt:** Prof Path, Univ Nebr Coll Med

Southwest

Bruner, Janet M MD [Path] - **Spec Exp:** Brain Tumors; Neuro-Pathology; **Hospital:** UT MD Anderson Cancer Ctr; **Address:** MD Anderson Cancer Ctr, 1515 Holcombe Blvd, Ste 85, Houston, TX 77030; **Phone:** 713-792-6127; **Board Cert:** Anatomic Pathology 1982; Neuropathology 1984; **Med School:** Med Coll OH 1979; **Resid:** Anatomic & Clinical Pathology, Med Coll Ohio Hosp 1982; **Fellow:** Neurological Pathology, Baylor Coll Med 1984

Pathology

Cagle, Philip MD [Path] - **Spec Exp:** Pulmonary Pathology; Lung Cancer; Mesothelioma; **Hospital:** Methodist Hosp - Houston; **Address:** Methodist Hospital, Dept Pathology, 6565 Fannin St, Ste 227, Houston, TX 77030; **Phone:** 713-441-6478; **Board Cert:** Anatomic & Clinical Pathology 1985; **Med School:** Univ Tenn Coll Med, Memphis 1981; **Fac Appt:** Prof Path, Baylor Coll Med

Foucar, M Kathryn MD [Path] - **Spec Exp:** Leukemia; Lymph Node Pathology; Bone Marrow Pathology; **Hospital:** Univ NM Hlth & Sci Ctr; **Address:** TriCore Reference Lab, Hematopathology, 1001 Woodward Pl NE, Albuquerque, NM 87102; **Phone:** 505-938-8456; **Board Cert:** Anatomic & Clinical Pathology 1978; **Med School:** Ohio State Univ 1974; **Resid:** Anatomic Pathology, Univ NM Health & Sci Ctr 1976; Anatomic Pathology, Univ Minn Med Ctr 1978; **Fellow:** Surgical Pathology, Univ Minn Med Ctr 1979; **Fac Appt:** Prof Path, Univ New Mexico

Grogan, Thomas M MD [Path] - **Spec Exp:** Immunopathology; Lymphoma; **Hospital:** Univ Med Ctr - Tucson; **Address:** AHSC, Dept Pathology, 1501 N Campbell Ave, rm 5211, Tucson, AZ 85724; **Phone:** 520-626-7477; **Board Cert:** Anatomic Pathology 1976; **Med School:** Geo Wash Univ 1971; **Resid:** Pathology, Letterman Army Med Ctr 1976; **Fellow:** Immunopathology, Stanford Univ Sch Med 1979; **Fac Appt:** Prof Path, Univ Ariz Coll Med

Hamilton, Stanley R MD [Path] - **Spec Exp:** Surgical Pathology; Gastrointestinal Pathology; Liver Pathology; **Hospital:** UT MD Anderson Cancer Ctr; **Address:** Univ Texas MD Anderson Cancer Ctr, 1515 Holcombe Blvd, Unit 085, Houston, TX 77030-4009; **Phone:** 713-792-2040; **Board Cert:** Anatomic & Clinical Pathology 1978; **Med School:** Indiana Univ 1973; **Resid:** Pathology, Johns Hopkins Hosp 1978; **Fellow:** St Marks Hosp 1979; **Fac Appt:** Prof Path, Univ Tex, Houston

Kinney, Marsha C MD [Path] - **Spec Exp:** Hematopathology; Lymphoma; Leukemia; **Hospital:** Univ Hlth Syst-San Antonio; **Address:** Univ Tex Hlth & Sci Ctr, Dept Path, 7703 Floyd Curl Drive, MC 775, San Antonio, TX 78229-3900; **Phone:** 210-567-4072; **Board Cert:** Anatomic & Clinical Pathology 1985; Hematology 1998; **Med School:** Univ Tex SW, Dallas 1981; **Resid:** Pathology, Vanderbilt Univ Med Ctr 1985; **Fellow:** Hematopathology, Vanderbilt Univ Med Ctr 1988; **Fac Appt:** Prof Path, Univ Tex, San Antonio

Leslie, Kevin O MD [Path] - **Spec Exp:** Pulmonary Pathology; Lung Cancer; Surgical Pathology; **Hospital:** Mayo Clinic - Scottsdale; **Address:** Mayo Clinic, Scottsdale, 13400 E Shea Blvd, Scottsdale, AZ 85259; **Phone:** 480-301-8021; **Board Cert:** Anatomic & Clinical Pathology 1982; **Med School:** Albert Einstein Coll Med 1976; **Resid:** Anatomic & Clinical Pathology, Univ Colorado Health Sci Ctr 1982; **Fellow:** Surgical Pathology, Stanford Univ Med Ctr 1983; **Fac Appt:** Prof Path, Mayo Med Sch

Moran, Cesar A MD [Path] - **Spec Exp:** Lung Cancer; Mediastinal Tumors; Mesothelioma; **Hospital:** UT MD Anderson Cancer Ctr; **Address:** MD Anderson Cancer Ctr, Dept Pathology, 1515 Holcombe Blvd, rm G1-3738, Houston, TX 77030; **Phone:** 713-792-8134; **Board Cert:** Anatomic Pathology 1992; **Med School:** Guatemala 1981; **Resid:** Anatomic Pathology, Mt Sinai Med Ctr 1988; **Fellow:** Surgical Pathology, Yale-New Haven Med Ctr 1989; **Fac Appt:** Prof Path, Univ Tex, Houston

Prieto, Victor G MD/PhD [Path] - **Spec Exp:** Dermatopathology; Melanoma; Skin Cancer; **Hospital:** UT MD Anderson Cancer Ctr; **Address:** MD Anderson Cancer Ctr, Dept Pathology, 1515 Holcombe Blvd, Box 85, Houston, TX 77030-4000; **Phone:** 713-792-0918; **Board Cert:** Anatomic Pathology 1995; Dermatopathology 1997; **Med School:** Spain 1986; **Resid:** Pathology, New York Hosp-Cornell Med Ctr 1993; **Fellow:** Pathology, Meml Sloan Kettering Cancer Ctr 1995; Dermatopathology, New York Hosp-Cornell Med Ctr 1996; **Fac Appt:** Prof Path, Univ Tex, Houston

Rashid, Asif MD/PhD [Path] - **Spec Exp:** Gastrointestinal Pathology; Liver Pathology; **Hospital:** UT MD Anderson Cancer Ctr; **Address:** MD Anderson Cancer Ctr, Dept Pathology, 1515 Holcombe Blvd, Box 85, Houston, TX 77030; **Phone:** 713-745-1101; **Board Cert:** Anatomic Pathology 1994; **Med School:** Pakistan 1984; **Resid:** Anatomic Pathology, Mass Genl Hosp 1993; **Fellow:** Anatomic Pathology, Mass Genl Hosp 1994; Anatomic Pathology, Johns Hopkins Med Inst 1996

Sahin, Aysegul MD [Path] - **Spec Exp:** Breast Cancer; **Hospital:** UT MD Anderson Cancer Ctr; **Address:** 1515 Holcombe Blvd, Box 0085, Houston, TX 77030; **Phone:** 713-794-1500; **Board Cert:** Pathology 1987; **Med School:** Turkey 1980; **Resid:** Pathology, Oregon Hlth Sci Univ 1986; **Fellow:** Surgical Pathology, Univ Iowa Hosps & Clins 1987; **Fac Appt:** Prof Path, Univ Tex, Houston

Silva, Elvio G MD [Path] - **Spec Exp:** Gynecologic Pathology; Gynecologic Cancer; **Hospital:** UT MD Anderson Cancer Ctr, Cedars-Sinai Med Ctr; **Address:** MD Anderson Cancer Ctr, Dept Pathology, 1515 Holcombe Blvd, Unit 85, Houston, TX 77030; **Phone:** 713-792-3154; **Board Cert:** Anatomic Pathology 2007; **Med School:** Argentina 1969; **Resid:** Pathology, National Univ Med Ctr 1975; Anatomic Pathology, Univ Toronto 1978; **Fellow:** Surgical Pathology, MD Anderson Cancer Ctr 1979; **Fac Appt:** Prof Path

Wheeler, Thomas M MD [Path] - **Spec Exp:** Thyroid Disorders; Thyroid Cancer; **Hospital:** Ben Taub Genl Hosp; **Address:** Baylor Coll Med, Dept Pathology, One Baylor Plaza, rm T203, Houston, TX 77030; **Phone:** 713-798-4664; **Board Cert:** Anatomic & Clinical Pathology 1999; Cytopathology 1990; **Med School:** Baylor Coll Med 1977; **Resid:** Pathology, Baylor Coll Med 1981; **Fac Appt:** Prof Path, Baylor Coll Med

West Coast and Pacific

Amin, Mahul MD [Path] - **Spec Exp:** Genitourinary Pathology; Bladder Cancer; **Hospital:** Cedars-Sinai Med Ctr; **Address:** Cedars Sinai Hosp, 8700 Beverly Blvd, Ste 8728, Los Angeles, CA 90048; **Phone:** 310-423-6631; **Board Cert:** Anatomic & Clinical Pathology 1996; **Med School:** India 1983; **Resid:** Pathology, Henry Ford Hosp 1992; **Fellow:** Surgical Pathology, MD Anderson Cancer Ctr 1993; **Fac Appt:** Prof Path, Emory Univ

Arber, Daniel A MD [Path] - **Spec Exp:** Bone Marrow Pathology; Lymph Node Pathology; Spleen Pathology; **Hospital:** Stanford Univ Med Ctr, Lucile Packard Chldn's Hosp; **Address:** Clinic Laboratories, Stanford Univ Med Ctr, 300 Pasteur Drive, rm H1507, MC 5627, Stanford, CA 94305; **Phone:** 650-725-5604; **Board Cert:** Anatomic & Clinical Pathology 1991; Hematology 1993; **Med School:** Univ Tex, San Antonio 1986; **Resid:** Anatomic & Clinical Pathology, Scott & White Meml Hosp 1991; **Fellow:** Hematopathology, City of Hope Natl Med Ctr 1993; **Fac Appt:** Prof Path, Stanford Univ

Bastian, Boris C MD [Path] - **Spec Exp:** Melanoma; Skin Cancer; **Hospital:** UCSF Med Ctr; **Address:** UCSF Comprehensive Cancer Center, Box 0808, San Francisco, CA 94143; **Phone:** 415-476-5132; **Med School:** Germany 1988; **Resid:** Dermatology, University of Wurzburg 1994; **Fellow:** Hematology, Ludwig-Maximilian-University 1989; **Fac Appt:** Asst Prof D, UCSF

Bollen, Andrew W MD [Path] - **Spec Exp:** Neuro-Pathology; Brain Tumors; **Hospital:** UCSF Med Ctr, San Francisco Genl Hosp; **Address:** Dept Pathology/Neuropathology, 505 Parnassus Ave, M551, Box 0102, San Francisco, CA 94143-0511; **Phone:** 415-476-5236; **Board Cert:** Neuropathology 1992; Anatomic Pathology 1992; Clinical Pathology 1993; **Med School:** UCSD 1985; **Resid:** Anatomic Pathology, UCSF Med Ctr 1991; **Fellow:** Neuropathology, UCSF Med Ctr 1989; **Fac Appt:** Prof Path, UCSF

Pathology

Chandrasoma, Parakrama T MD [Path] - **Spec Exp:** Gastrointestinal Pathology; Gastrointestinal Cancer; Neuro-Pathology; **Hospital:** LAC & USC Med Ctr; **Address:** LAC-USC Med Ctr, Dept Path, Clinic Tower Fl 7 - rm A7A127, 1100 N State St, Los Angeles, CA 90033; **Phone:** 323-226-4600; **Board Cert:** Anatomic Pathology 1982; **Med School:** Sri Lanka 1971; **Resid:** Anatomic Pathology, Univ Sri Lanka 1978; Anatomic Pathology, LAC-USC Med Ctr 1982; **Fac Appt:** Prof Path, USC Sch Med

Chang, Karen L MD [Path] - **Spec Exp:** Leukemia; **Hospital:** City of Hope Natl Med Ctr & Beckman Rsch (page 69); **Address:** 1500 E Duarte Rd, Duarte, CA 91010-3012; **Phone:** 626-256-4673 x62456; **Board Cert:** Anatomic & Clinical Pathology 1992; **Med School:** Mount Sinai Sch Med 1985; **Resid:** Anatomic Pathology, Stanford Univ Med Ctr 1988; Clinical Pathology, Stanford Univ Med Ctr 1991; **Fellow:** Surgical Pathology, Stanford Univ Med Ctr 1989

Cochran, Alistair J MD [Path] - **Spec Exp:** Melanoma; Dermatopathology; **Hospital:** UCLA Ronald Reagan Med Ctr; **Address:** UCLA Med Ctr, Dept Path & Med, 10833 Le Conte Ave, rm 13145CHS, MC 173216, Los Angeles, CA 90095-1713; **Phone:** 310-825-2743; **Med School:** Scotland, UK 1959; **Resid:** Dermatopathology, Western Infirmary 1968; Pathology, Western Infirmary 1968; **Fellow:** Immunology, Karolinska Inst 1970; **Fac Appt:** Prof Path, UCLA

Dubeau, Louis MD/PhD [Path] - **Spec Exp:** Ovarian Cancer; Breast Cancer; **Hospital:** USC Norris Cancer Hosp; **Address:** USC Norris Cancer Ctr, Dept Pathology, 1441 Eastlake Ave, rm 6338, Los Angeles, CA 90033-1048; **Phone:** 323-865-0720; **Board Cert:** Anatomic Pathology 1984; **Med School:** McGill Univ 1979; **Resid:** Anatomic Pathology, McGill Univ Med Ctr 1984; **Fac Appt:** Prof Path, USC Sch Med

Hammar, Samuel P MD [Path] - **Spec Exp:** Lung Cancer; Pulmonary Pathology; **Hospital:** Harrison Meml Hosp; **Address:** Diagnostic Specialties Laboratory, 700 Lebo Blvd, Bremerton, WA 98310; **Phone:** 360-479-7707; **Board Cert:** Anatomic & Clinical Pathology 1975; **Med School:** Univ Wash 1970

Hendrickson, Michael MD [Path] - **Spec Exp:** Gynecologic Cancer; Gynecologic Pathology; **Hospital:** Stanford Univ Med Ctr; **Address:** Stanford Univ Med Ctr, Surg Path Lab, 300 Pasteur Drive, rm H2110, MC 5324, Stanford, CA 94305; **Phone:** 650-723-7211; **Board Cert:** Anatomic Pathology 1975; **Med School:** Stanford Univ 1971; **Resid:** Anatomic Pathology, Stanford Univ Med Sch 1974; **Fac Appt:** Prof Path, Stanford Univ

Koss, Michael N MD [Path] - **Spec Exp:** Pulmonary Pathology; Lung Cancer; Mediastinal Tumors; **Hospital:** USC Norris Cancer Hosp, USC Univ Hosp; **Address:** 2222 Ocean View Ave, Ste 212, 2011 Zonal Ave, Los Angeles, CA 90057; **Phone:** 323-226-6507; **Board Cert:** Anatomic Pathology 1979; **Med School:** Stanford Univ 1970; **Resid:** Pathology, Columbia Presby Med Ctr 1974; **Fellow:** Renal Pathology, Columbia Presby Med Ctr 1975; Pulmonary Pathology, Armed Forces Inst Path 1978; **Fac Appt:** Prof Path, USC Sch Med

Le Boit, Philip E MD [Path] - **Spec Exp:** Cutaneous Lymphoma; Skin Cancer; Dermatopathology; **Hospital:** UCSF Med Ctr; **Address:** UCSF - Dermatopathology Section, 1701 Divisadero St, rm 350, San Francisco, CA 94115; **Phone:** 415-353-7546; **Board Cert:** Anatomic Pathology 1983; Dermatopathology 1983; Clinical Pathology 1986; **Med School:** Albany Med Coll 1979; **Resid:** Anatomic Pathology, UCSF Med Ctr 1981; Clinical Pathology, Mt Sinai Hosp 1982; **Fellow:** Dermatopathology, New York Hosp-Cornell Med Ctr 1983; **Fac Appt:** Prof Path, UCSF

Ljung, Britt-Marie E MD [Path] - **Spec Exp:** Breast Cancer; Cytopathology; Fine Needle Aspiration Biopsy; **Hospital:** UCSF - Mt Zion Med Ctr; **Address:** UCSF - Dept Pathology, 1600 Divisadero St, Box 1785, rm r-200, San Francisco, CA 94143-1785; **Phone:** 415-353-7320; **Board Cert:** Anatomic Pathology 1985; Cytopathology 1989; **Med School:** Sweden 1975; **Resid:** Pathology, Karolinska Hosp 1979; Anatomic Pathology, UCLA Med Ctr 1983; **Fac Appt:** Prof Path, UCSF

Mischel, Paul S MD [Path] - **Spec Exp:** Neuro-Pathology; Brain Tumors; **Hospital:** UCLA Ronald Reagan Med Ctr; **Address:** UCLA Med Ctr, Div Neuropathology, 10833 Le Conte Ave, rm 13-317 CHS, Los Angeles, CA 90095-1732; **Phone:** 310-825-0377; **Board Cert:** Anatomic Pathology 1997; Neuropathology 1997; **Med School:** Cornell Univ-Weill Med Coll 1991; **Resid:** Anatomic & Clinical Pathology, UCLA Med Center 1996; **Fellow:** Neurological Pathology, UCLA 1995; Research, Howard Hughes Med Inst/UCSF 1998; **Fac Appt:** Prof Path, UCLA

Nathwani, Bharat N MD [Path] - **Spec Exp:** Hematopathology; Leukemia; Lymphoma; **Hospital:** LAC & USC Med Ctr; **Address:** LAC & USC Med Ctr, Dept Pathology, 1200 N State St, rm 2422, Los Angeles, CA 90033-4526; **Phone:** 323-226-7064; **Board Cert:** Anatomic Pathology 1977; **Med School:** India 1969; **Resid:** Pathology, JJ Group-Grant Med Ctr 1972; Pathology, Rush-Presby-St Lukes Med Ctr 1974; **Fellow:** Hematopathology, City Hope Natl Med Ctr 1975; **Fac Appt:** Prof Path, USC Sch Med

Rutgers, Joanne MD [Path] - **Spec Exp:** Gynecologic Cancer; Gastrointestinal Pathology; **Hospital:** Long Beach Meml Med Ctr; **Address:** 2801 Atlantic Ave, Dept of Pathology, Long Beach, CA 90806; **Phone:** 562-933-0717; **Board Cert:** Clinical Pathology 1992; Anatomic Pathology 1985; Cytopathology 1997; **Med School:** UCSD 1981; **Resid:** Pathology, Montefiore Med Ctr 1983; Pathology, NYU Med Ctr 1985; **Fellow:** Gynecologic Pathology, Mass Genl Hosp 1989; **Fac Appt:** Assoc Clin Prof Path, UCLA

Sibley, Richard K MD [Path] - **Spec Exp:** Kidney Pathology; Breast Pathology; Liver Pathology; **Hospital:** Stanford Univ Med Ctr; **Address:** Stanford Univ Med Ctr, Surg Path Lab, 300 Pasteur Drive, rm H2110, MC 5243, Stanford, CA 94305; **Phone:** 650-723-7211; **Board Cert:** Anatomic Pathology 1975; **Med School:** Univ Tex SW, Dallas 1971; **Resid:** Anatomic Pathology, Univ Chicago Hosps 1974; **Fellow:** Stanford Univ Med Ctr 1975; **Fac Appt:** Prof Path, Stanford Univ

Triche, Timothy J MD/PhD [Path] - **Spec Exp:** Pediatric Pathology; Pediatric Cancers; Sarcoma; **Hospital:** Chldns Hosp - Los Angeles; **Address:** Chldns Hosp of Los Angeles, Dept Path, 4650 Sunset Blvd, MS 43, Los Angeles, CA 90027; **Phone:** 323-361-4516; **Board Cert:** Anatomic Pathology 1975; **Med School:** Tulane Univ 1971; **Resid:** Anatomic Pathology, Barnes Hosp-Wash Univ 1973; Surgical Pathology, Barnes Hosp 1974; **Fellow:** Pathology, Natl Cancer Inst 1975; **Fac Appt:** Prof Path, USC Sch Med

True, Lawrence D MD [Path] - **Spec Exp:** Urologic Pathology; Prostate Cancer; Bladder Cancer; **Hospital:** Univ Wash Med Ctr; **Address:** Univ Wash Med Ctr, Dept Anatomic Path, 1959 NE Pacific St, rm NE110, Box 356100, Seattle, WA 98195-6100; **Phone:** 206-598-6400; **Board Cert:** Anatomic Pathology 1981; **Med School:** Tulane Univ 1971; **Resid:** Pathology, Univ Colo Hlth Sci Ctr 1980; **Fac Appt:** Prof Path, Univ Wash

Warnke, Roger A MD [Path] - **Spec Exp:** Lymphoma; Hematopathology; **Hospital:** Stanford Univ Med Ctr; **Address:** Stanford Hosp, 300 Pasteur Drive, Pathology, rm L235, Stanford, CA 94305-5324; **Phone:** 650-725-5167; **Board Cert:** Anatomic Pathology 1975; **Med School:** Washington Univ, St Louis 1971; **Resid:** Pathology, Stanford Univ Med Ctr 1974; **Fellow:** Surgical Pathology, Stanford Univ Med Ctr 1975; Immunology, Stanford Univ Med Ctr 1976; **Fac Appt:** Prof Path, Stanford Univ

Weiss, Lawrence M MD [Path] - **Spec Exp:** Lymphoma; Hematopathology; Adrenal Pathology; **Hospital:** City of Hope Natl Med Ctr & Beckman Rsch (page 69); **Address:** City of Hope Natl Med Ctr, Div Pathology, 1500 E Duarte Rd, Duarte, CA 91010-0269; **Phone:** 626-359-8111 x62456; **Board Cert:** Anatomic Pathology 1985; **Med School:** Univ MD Sch Med 1981; **Resid:** Pathology, Brigham & Women's Hosp 1983; **Fellow:** Surgical Pathology, Stanford Univ Hosp 1984

Pathology

Wilczynski, Sharon P MD/PhD [Path] - **Spec Exp:** Gynecologic Cancer; Breast Cancer; Ovarian Cancer; Clinical Trials; **Hospital:** City of Hope Natl Med Ctr & Beckman Rsch (page 69); **Address:** City Hope Natl Med Ctr-Dept of Pathology, 1500 E Duarte Blvd, Duarte, CA 91010; **Phone:** 626-256-4673 x62456; **Board Cert:** Anatomic & Clinical Pathology 1985; Cytopathology 1991; **Med School:** Med Coll PA Hahnemann 1981; **Resid:** Pathology, Hosp Univ Penn 1983; Anatomic & Clinical Pathology, Long Beach Meml Hosp 1985; **Fac Appt:** Prof Path, USC-Keck School of Medicine

Cancer Institute

NYU LANGONE MEDICAL CENTER

Pediatrics

A pediatrician is concerned with the physical, emotional and social health of children from birth to young adulthood. Care encompasses a broad spectrum of health services ranging from preventive healthcare to the diagnosis and treatment of acute and chronic diseases.

A pediatrician deals with biological, social and environmental influences on the developing child, and with the impact of disease and dysfunction on development.

Training Required: Three years. Certification in one or more of the following specialties requires additional training

Pediatric Hematology/Oncology: A pediatrician trained in the combination of pediatrics, hematology and oncology to recognize and manage pediatric blood disorders and cancerous diseases.

Pediatric Allergy and Immunology: An allergist-immunologist is trained in evaluation, physical and laboratory diagnosis and management of disorders involving the immune system. Selected examples of such conditions include asthma, anaphylaxis, rhinitis, eczema and adverse reactions to drugs, foods and insect stings as well as immune deficiency diseases (both acquired and congenital), defects in host defense and problems related to autoimmune disease, organ transplantation or malignancies of the immune system. As our understanding of the immune system develops, the scope of this specialty is widening.

Training programs are available at some medical centers to provide individuals with expertise in both allergy/immunology and pediatric pulmonology. Such individuals are candidates for dual certification.

Pediatric Endocrinology: A pediatrician who provides expert care to infants, children and adolescents who have diseases that result from an abnormality in the endocrine glands (glands which secrete hormones) These diseases include diabetes mellitus, growth failure, unusual size for age, early or late pubertal development, birth defects, the genital region and disorders of the thyroid, the adrenal and pituitary glands.

Pediatric Otolaryngology: A pediatric otolaryngologist has special expertise in the management of infants and children with disorders that include congenital and acquired conditions involving the aerodigestive tract, nose and paranasal sinuses, the ear and other areas of the head and neck. The pediatric otolaryngologist has special skills in the diagnosis, treatment and management of childhood disorders of voice, speech, language and hearing.

Pediatric Surgery: A surgeon with expertise in the management of surgical conditions in premature and newborn infants, children and adolescents.

Pediatric Hematology-Oncology

New England

Albritton, Karen H MD [PHO] - **Spec Exp:** Sarcoma; **Hospital:** Dana-Farber Cancer Inst; **Address:** Dana Farber Cancer Inst, 44 Binney St, Smith 338, Boston, MA 02115; **Phone:** 617-582-7976; **Board Cert:** Pediatric Hematology-Oncology 2002; Medical Oncology 2001; **Med School:** Univ Tex, San Antonio 1992; **Resid:** Internal Medicine & Pediatrics, Univ NC Hosps 1996; **Fellow:** Hematology & Oncology, Univ NC Hosps 2000

Altman, Arnold MD [PHO] - **Spec Exp:** Leukemia; **Hospital:** CT Chldns Med Ctr; **Address:** CT Childrens Med Ctr, Hematology/Oncology, 282 Washington St, Ste 2J, Hartford, CT 06106; **Phone:** 860-545-9630; **Board Cert:** Pediatrics 1971; Pediatric Hematology-Oncology 1974; **Med School:** Johns Hopkins Univ 1965; **Resid:** Pediatrics, Chldns Hosp Med Ctr 1970; **Fellow:** Pediatric Hematology-Oncology, Chldns Hosp Med Ctr 1972; **Fac Appt:** Prof Ped, Univ Conn

Diller, Lisa R MD [PHO] - **Spec Exp:** Neuroblastoma; Cancer Survivors-Late Effects of Therapy; **Hospital:** Dana-Farber Cancer Inst; **Address:** Dana-Farber Cancer Inst, 44 Binney St, Shields Warren 312, Boston, MA 02115; **Phone:** 617-632-5642; **Board Cert:** Pediatric Hematology-Oncology 2007; **Med School:** UCSD 1985; **Resid:** Pediatrics, Chldns Hosp 1988; **Fellow:** Pediatric Hematology-Oncology, Chldns Hosp-Dana Farber Cancer Inst 1991; **Fac Appt:** Assoc Prof Ped, Harvard Med Sch

Grier, Holcombe E MD [PHO] - **Spec Exp:** Bone Cancer; Ewing's Sarcoma; **Hospital:** Dana-Farber Cancer Inst, Children's Hospital - Boston; **Address:** Dana Farber Cancer Inst, 44 Binney St, SW350, Boston, MA 02115; **Phone:** 617-632-3971; **Board Cert:** Pediatrics 1983; Internal Medicine 1980; Pediatric Hematology-Oncology 2005; **Med School:** Univ Pennsylvania 1976; **Resid:** Pediatrics, NC Meml Hosp 1980; Internal Medicine, NC Meml Hosp 1980; **Fellow:** Pediatric Oncology, Dana Farber Chldn's Hosp 1984; **Fac Appt:** Assoc Prof Ped, Harvard Med Sch

Homans, Alan C MD [PHO] - **Spec Exp:** Leukemia; **Hospital:** Fletcher Allen Health Care-Med Ctr Campus; **Address:** Vermont Childrens Hosp, 111 Colchester Ave, Smith 5-rm 559, Burlington, VT 05401; **Phone:** 802 847 2850; **Board Cert:** Pediatrics 1985, Pediatric Hematology-Oncology 1987; **Med School:** Ohio State Univ 1979; **Resid:** Pediatrics, Med Ctr Hosp 1981; Pediatrics, Univ Mass Med Ctr 1982; **Fellow:** Pediatric Hematology-Oncology, Rhode Island Hosp 1985; **Fac Appt:** Prof Ped, Univ VT Coll Med

Kieran, Mark W MD/PhD [PHO] - **Spec Exp:** Brain Tumors; Neuro-Oncology; **Hospital:** Dana-Farber Cancer Inst, Children's Hospital - Boston; **Address:** Dana Farber Cancer Inst, 44 Binney St, Shields Warren Ste 331, Boston, MA 02115; **Phone:** 617-632-4386; **Board Cert:** Pediatric Hematology-Oncology 2004; **Med School:** Univ Calgary 1986; **Resid:** Pediatrics, Montreal Chldns Hosp 1992; **Fellow:** Pediatric Hematology-Oncology, Chldns Hosp 1995; **Fac Appt:** Asst Prof Ped, Harvard Med Sch

Kretschmar, Cynthia S MD [PHO] - **Spec Exp:** Brain Tumors; Neuroblastoma; Drug Discovery & Development; **Hospital:** Tufts Med Ctr; **Address:** Floating Hosp, Div Pediatric Hem/Onc, 750 Washington St, NEMC 14, Boston, MA 02111; **Phone:** 617-636-5535; **Board Cert:** Pediatrics 1984; Pediatric Hematology-Oncology 1987; **Med School:** Yale Univ 1978; **Resid:** Pediatrics, Yale-New Haven Hosp 1981; **Fellow:** Pediatric Hematology-Oncology, Dana Farber Cancer Inst 1984; **Fac Appt:** Prof Ped, Tufts Univ

Pediatric Hematology-Oncology

Sallan, Stephen MD [PHO] - **Spec Exp:** Pediatric Cancers; Leukemia; **Hospital:** Children's Hospital - Boston; **Address:** Dana Farber Cancer Inst, Dept Ped Oncology, 44 Binney St, Ste 1642, Boston, MA 02115; **Phone:** 617-632-3316; **Board Cert:** Pediatrics 1972; **Med School:** Wayne State Univ 1967; **Resid:** Pediatrics, Chldns Hosp 1969; Pediatrics, Hosp Sick Chldn 1970; **Fellow:** Pediatric Oncology, Chldns Hosp Med Ctr 1975; **Fac Appt:** Prof Ped, Harvard Med Sch

Schwartz, Cindy Lee MD [PHO] - **Spec Exp:** Hodgkin's Disease; Bone Cancer; Cancer Survivors-Late Effects of Therapy; **Hospital:** Rhode Island Hosp; **Address:** RI Hospital, Dept Ped-Div Ped Hem/Onc, 593 Eddy St, MPS, rm 117, Providence, RI 02903-4923; **Phone:** 401-444-5171; **Board Cert:** Pediatrics 1985; Pediatric Hematology-Oncology 2009; **Med School:** Brown Univ 1979; **Resid:** Pediatrics, Johns Hopkins Hosp 1982; **Fellow:** Pediatric Hematology-Oncology, Johns Hopkins Hosp 1985; **Fac Appt:** Prof Med, Brown Univ

van Hoff, Jack MD [PHO] - **Spec Exp:** Brain Tumors; Clinical Trials; **Hospital:** Dartmouth - Hitchcock Med Ctr; **Address:** DHMC, Dept Pediatric Hem/Onc, One Medical Center Drive, Lebanon, NH 03756; **Phone:** 603-650-5541; **Board Cert:** Pediatrics 1985; Pediatric Hematology-Oncology 1987; **Med School:** UMDNJ-NJ Med Sch, Newark 1981; **Resid:** Pediatrics, Yale New Haven Hosp 1984; **Fellow:** Pediatric Hematology-Oncology, Yale New Haven Hosp 1986

Weinstein, Howard J MD [PHO] - **Spec Exp:** Bone Marrow Transplant; Leukemia; Lymphoma; **Hospital:** Mass Genl Hosp, Dana-Farber Cancer Inst; **Address:** 55 Fruit St, Yawkey 8B-8893, Boston, MA 02114-2622; **Phone:** 617-724-3315; **Board Cert:** Pediatrics 1977; **Med School:** Univ MD Sch Med 1972; **Resid:** Pediatrics, Mass Genl Hosp 1974; **Fellow:** Pediatric Hematology-Oncology, Dana Farber Cancer Inst/Chldns Hosp 1977; **Fac Appt:** Prof Ped, Harvard Med Sch

Mid Atlantic

Adamson, Peter C MD [PHO] - **Spec Exp:** Drug Development; Clinical Trials; Rhabdomyosarcoma; Pediatric Cancers; **Hospital:** Chldns Hosp of Philadelphia, The; **Address:** Chldns Hosp of Philadelphia, 34th St & Civic Ctr Blvd Abramson Bldg, Philadelphia, PA 19104; **Phone:** 215-590-2299; **Board Cert:** Pediatric Hematology-Oncology 2005; **Med School:** Cornell Univ-Weill Med Coll 1984; **Resid:** Pediatrics, Chldns Hosp 1987; **Fellow:** Pediatric Hematology-Oncology, Natl Cancer Inst 1990; **Fac Appt:** Assoc Prof Pharm, Univ Pennsylvania

Aledo, Alexander MD [PHO] - **Spec Exp:** Leukemia; Lymphoma; Bone Tumors; **Hospital:** NY-Presby Hosp/Weill Cornell (page 79), NY Hosp Queens; **Address:** 525 E 68th St, rm P695, New York, NY 10021-4870; **Phone:** 212-746-3447; **Board Cert:** Pediatrics 2002; Pediatric Hematology-Oncology 2004; **Med School:** NYU Sch Med 1984; **Resid:** Pediatrics, NY Hosp 1987; **Fellow:** Pediatric Hematology-Oncology, Meml Sloan Kettering Cancer Ctr 1990; **Fac Appt:** Assoc Clin Prof Ped, Cornell Univ-Weill Med Coll

Arceci, Robert J MD/PhD [PHO] - **Spec Exp:** Leukemia; Histiocytoma; Bone Marrow Transplant; **Hospital:** Johns Hopkins Hosp; **Address:** Kimmel Cancer Ctr, Bunting-Blaustein Bldg, 1650 Orleans St, I-207, Baltimore, MD 21231-1000; **Phone:** 410-502-7519; **Board Cert:** Pediatrics 1987; Pediatric Hematology-Oncology 2005; **Med School:** Univ Rochester 1981; **Resid:** Pediatrics, Chldns Hosp 1983; **Fellow:** Pediatric Hematology-Oncology, Chldns Hosp/Dana Farber Cancer Ctr 1986; **Fac Appt:** Prof Ped, Johns Hopkins Univ

Brecher, Martin L MD [PHO] - **Spec Exp:** Brain Tumors; Lymphoma; Hodgkin's Disease; Leukemia; **Hospital:** Roswell Park Cancer Inst, Women's & Chldn's Hosp of Buffalo, The; **Address:** Roswell Park Cancer Inst, Dept Pediatrics, Elm & Carlton Sts, Buffalo, NY 14263; **Phone:** 716-845-2333; **Board Cert:** Pediatrics 1977; Pediatric Hematology-Oncology 1978; **Med School:** SUNY Buffalo 1972; **Resid:** Pediatrics, Buffalo Chldns Hosp 1975; **Fellow:** Hematology & Oncology, Buffalo Chldns Hosp/Roswell Park Cancer Inst 1977; **Fac Appt:** Prof Ped, SUNY Buffalo

Bussel, James MD [PHO] - **Spec Exp:** Autoimmune Disease; Bleeding/Coagulation Disorders; **Hospital:** NY-Presby Hosp/Weill Cornell (page 79), Lenox Hill Hosp; **Address:** 525 E 68th St, rm P-695, New York, NY 10021; **Phone:** 212-746-3474; **Board Cert:** Pediatrics 1979; Pediatric Hematology-Oncology 1981; **Med School:** Columbia P&S 1975; **Resid:** Pediatrics, Chldns Hosp 1978; **Fellow:** Pediatric Hematology-Oncology, NY Hosp 1981; **Fac Appt:** Prof Ped, Cornell Univ-Weill Med Coll

Cairo, Mitchell S MD [PHO] - **Spec Exp:** Bone Marrow Transplant; Leukemia; Lymphoma; **Hospital:** NYPresby-Morgan Stanley Children's Hosp (page 79); **Address:** Babies/Chldns Hosp-Presby Med Ctr, 3959 Broadway, CHN 10-03, New York, NY 10032; **Phone:** 212-305-8316; **Board Cert:** Pediatrics 1980; Pediatric Hematology-Oncology 1982; **Med School:** UCSF 1976; **Resid:** Pediatrics, UCLA Med Ctr 1979; **Fellow:** Pediatric Hematology-Oncology, Indiana Univ Med Ctr 1981; **Fac Appt:** Prof Ped, Columbia P&S

Carroll, William L MD [PHO] - **Spec Exp:** Leukemia; **Hospital:** NYU Langone Med Ctr (page 80); **Address:** NYU Med Ctr, Div Ped Hem/Onc, 160 E 32nd St Fl 2, New York, NY 10016; **Phone:** 212-263-9947; **Board Cert:** Pediatrics 1984; Pediatric Hematology-Oncology 1987; **Med School:** UC Irvine 1978; **Resid:** Pediatrics, Chldns Hosp Med Ctr 1981; **Fellow:** Pediatric Hematology-Oncology, Stanford Univ 1987; **Fac Appt:** Prof Ped, NYU Sch Med

Chen, Allen R MD/PhD [PHO] - **Spec Exp:** Bone Marrow Transplant; Hodgkin's Disease; Immunotherapy; Graft vs Host Disease; **Hospital:** Johns Hopkins Hosp; **Address:** Johns Hopkins Hosp, Div Peds Oncology, 1650 Orleans St, CRB 2M53, Baltimore, MD 21231; **Phone:** 410-955-7385; **Board Cert:** Pediatrics 2002; Pediatric Hematology-Oncology 2006; **Med School:** Duke Univ 1986; **Resid:** Pediatrics, Chldns Hosp Med Ctr 1989; **Fellow:** Pediatric Hematology-Oncology, Fred Hutchinson Canc Ctr 1993; Bone Marrow Transplant, Fred Hutchinson Canc Ctr 1994; **Fac Appt:** Assoc Prof Ped, Johns Hopkins Univ

Civin, Curt Ingraham MD [PHO] - **Spec Exp:** Pediatric Cancers; Leukemia; Bone Marrow Transplant; **Hospital:** Johns Hopkins Hosp; **Address:** Univ Maryland Office of Dean, 655 W Baltimore St, rm 14-023, Baltimore, MD 21201; **Phone:** 410-706-1181; **Board Cert:** Pediatrics 1979; Pediatric Hematology-Oncology 1980; **Med School:** Harvard Med Sch 1974; **Resid:** Pediatrics, Chldns Hosp 1976; **Fellow:** Pediatric Hematology-Oncology, Natl Cancer Inst 1979; **Fac Appt:** Prof Ped, Johns Hopkins Univ

Drachtman, Richard A MD [PHO] - **Spec Exp:** Pediatric Cancers; **Hospital:** Robert Wood Johnson Univ Hosp - New Brunswick, Jersey Shore Univ Med Ctr; **Address:** Cancer Inst of New Jersey, 195 Little Albany St, New Brunswick, NJ 08903-2681; **Phone:** 732-235-5437; **Board Cert:** Pediatric Hematology-Oncology 2007; **Med School:** Ros Franklin Univ/Chicago Med Sch 1984; **Resid:** Pediatrics, N Shore Univ Hosp 1988; **Fellow:** Pediatric Hematology-Oncology, Mount Sinai Hosp 1991; **Fac Appt:** Prof Ped, UMDNJ-RW Johnson Med Sch

Dunkel, Ira J MD [PHO] - **Spec Exp:** Retinoblastoma; Brain & Spinal Cord Tumors; Brain Tumors; Pediatric Cancers; **Hospital:** Meml Sloan-Kettering Cancer Ctr (page 76); **Address:** 1275 York Avenue, New York, NY 10065; **Phone:** 800-525-2225; **Board Cert:** Pediatric Hematology-Oncology 2007; **Med School:** Duke Univ 1985; **Resid:** Pediatrics, Duke Univ Med Ctr 1988; **Fellow:** Pediatric Hematology-Oncology, Memorial-Sloan Kettering 1992; **Fac Appt:** Asst Prof Ped, Cornell Univ-Weill Med Coll

Pediatric Hematology-Oncology

Felix, Carolyn A MD [PHO] - **Spec Exp:** Leukemia; Leukemia in Infants; **Hospital:** Chldns Hosp of Philadelphia, The; **Address:** Chldns Hosp of Philadelphia, 34th St & Civic Ctr Blvd Abramson Bldg, Philadelphia, PA 19104; **Phone:** 215-590-2831; **Board Cert:** Pediatrics 1987; Pediatric Hematology-Oncology 1987; **Med School:** Boston Univ 1981; **Resid:** Pediatrics, Chldns Hosp 1984; **Fellow:** Pediatric Hematology-Oncology, Natl Cancer Inst-Pediatric Br 1987; **Fac Appt:** Assoc Prof Ped, Univ Pennsylvania

Frantz, Christopher N MD [PHO] - **Spec Exp:** Solid Tumors; Neuroblastoma; Leukemia; **Hospital:** Alfred I duPont Hosp for Children, Christiana Care Hlth Svs; **Address:** Alfred I duPont Hosp for Chldn, 1600 Rockland Rd, Box 269, Wilmington, DE 19899; **Phone:** 302-651-5500; **Board Cert:** Pediatrics 1977; Pediatric Hematology-Oncology 2005; **Med School:** Albert Einstein Coll Med 1971; **Resid:** Pediatrics, Chldns Hosp 1976; **Fellow:** Pediatric Hematology-Oncology, Chldns Hosp/Dana Farber Cancer Inst 1979

Garvin, James H MD/PhD [PHO] - **Spec Exp:** Brain Tumors; Pediatric Cancers; Bone Marrow Transplant; **Hospital:** NYPresby-Morgan Stanley Children's Hosp (page 79); **Address:** 161 Fort Washington Ave Fl 7 - rm 708, New York, NY 10032-3729; **Phone:** 212-305-8685; **Board Cert:** Pediatrics 1982; Pediatric Hematology-Oncology 1984; **Med School:** Jefferson Med Coll 1976; **Resid:** Pediatrics, Chldns Hosp 1978; Pediatrics, Middlesex Hosp 1979; **Fellow:** Pediatric Hematology-Oncology, Dana Farber Cancer Inst/Childrens Hosp 1982; **Fac Appt:** Clin Prof Ped, Columbia P&S

Grupp, Stephan A MD [PHO] - **Spec Exp:** Stem Cell Transplant; Neuroblastoma; Bone Marrow Transplant; **Hospital:** Chldns Hosp of Philadelphia, The; **Address:** Childrens Hosp - Oncology, 34th St & Civic Ctr Blvd Abramson Bldg, Philadelphia, PA 19104; **Phone:** 215-590-2821; **Board Cert:** Pediatric Hematology-Oncology 2002; **Med School:** Univ Cincinnati 1987; **Resid:** Pediatrics, Chldns Hosp 1990; **Fellow:** Pediatric Hematology-Oncology, Dana Farber Cancer Inst/Chldns Hosp 1992; **Fac Appt:** Asst Prof Ped, Univ Pennsylvania

Guarini, Ludovico MD [PHO] - **Spec Exp:** Leukemia; Solid Tumors; **Hospital:** Maimonides Med Ctr (page 75); **Address:** 6300 8th Ave, Brooklyn, NY 11220; **Phone:** 718-765-2671; **Board Cert:** Pediatrics 1984; Pediatric Hematology-Oncology 2007; **Med School:** Italy 1974; **Resid:** Pediatrics, Beth Israel Hosp 1981; **Fellow:** Pediatric Hematology-Oncology, Columbia-Presby Med Ctr 1984; **Fac Appt:** Assoc Prof Ped, Mount Sinai Sch Med

Halligan, Gregory E MD [PHO] - **Spec Exp:** Clinical Trials; Solid Tumors; **Hospital:** St Christopher's Hosp for Chldn; **Address:** St Christophers Hosp for Children, Dept Oncology, Erie Ave at Front St, Philadelphia, PA 19134; **Phone:** 215-427-4447; **Board Cert:** Pediatrics 1982; Pediatric Hematology-Oncology 1984; **Med School:** Belgium 1977; **Resid:** Pediatrics, St Christophers Hosp for Chldn 1982; **Fellow:** Pediatric Hematology-Oncology, St Christophers Hosp for Chldn 1984; **Fac Appt:** Assoc Prof Ped, Drexel Univ Coll Med

Halpern, Steven MD [PHO] - **Spec Exp:** Leukemia & Lymphoma; Brain Tumors; Hodgkin's Disease; **Hospital:** Hackensack Univ Med Ctr (page 73); **Address:** 30 Prospect Ave, Ste TCI, Hackensack, NJ 07601; **Phone:** 201-996-5437; **Board Cert:** Pediatrics 1981; Pediatric Hematology-Oncology 1982; **Med School:** Ros Franklin Univ/Chicago Med Sch 1976; **Resid:** Pediatrics, St Christophers Hosp for Children 1979; **Fellow:** Pediatric Hematology-Oncology, Childrens Hosp 1982; **Fac Appt:** Asst Prof Ped, UMDNJ-NJ Med Sch, Newark

Harris, Michael B MD [PHO] - **Spec Exp:** Leukemia & Lymphoma; Bone Tumors; Cancer Survivors-Late Effects of Therapy; **Hospital:** Hackensack Univ Med Ctr (page 73); **Address:** Tomorrows Chldns Inst, JM Sanzari Chldns Hosp, 30 Prospect Ave, Imus 1-TCI, rm PC116, Hackensack, NJ 07601; **Phone:** 201-996-5437; **Board Cert:** Pediatrics 1974; Pediatric Hematology-Oncology 1974; **Med School:** Albert Einstein Coll Med 1969; **Resid:** Pediatrics, Chldns Hosp 1971; **Fellow:** Pediatric Hematology-Oncology, Chldns Hosp 1974; **Fac Appt:** Prof Ped, UMDNJ-NJ Med Sch, Newark

Helman, Lee Jay MD [PHO] - **Spec Exp:** Solid Tumors; **Hospital:** Natl Inst of Hlth - Clin Ctr; **Address:** National Cancer Inst, NIH, 31 Center Drive, rm 3A11, Bethesda, MD 20892-2440; **Phone:** 301-496-4257; **Board Cert:** Internal Medicine 1983; Medical Oncology 1985; **Med School:** Univ MD Sch Med 1980; **Resid:** Internal Medicine, Barnes Hosp 1983; **Fellow:** Oncology, Natl Inst Hlth 1986

Hinkle, Andrea S MD [PHO] - **Spec Exp:** Cancer Survivors-Late Effects of Therapy; **Hospital:** Univ of Rochester Strong Meml Hosp; **Address:** Golisano Childrens Hosp at Strong, 601 Elmwood Ave, Box 667, Rochester, NY 14642; **Phone:** 585-275-8138; **Board Cert:** Pediatrics 2006; Pediatric Hematology-Oncology 2008; **Med School:** Brown Univ 1987; **Resid:** Pediatrics, Boston City Hosp 1991; **Fellow:** Pediatric Hematology-Oncology, Chldns Natl Med Ctr 1994; **Fac Appt:** Asst Prof Ped, Univ Rochester

Jakacki, Regina I MD [PHO] - **Spec Exp:** Neuro-Oncology; Clinical Trials; Palliative Care; **Hospital:** Chldns Hosp of Pittsburgh - UPMC; **Address:** Children's Hospital Pittsburgh, 45th & Penn Drive, Pittsburgh, PA 15201; **Phone:** 412-692-7056; **Board Cert:** Pediatric Hematology-Oncology 2007; **Med School:** Univ Pennsylvania 1985; **Resid:** Pediatrics, Childrens Hosp 1988; **Fellow:** Pediatric Hematology-Oncology, Childrens Hosp 1991; **Fac Appt:** Assoc Prof Ped, Univ Pittsburgh

Jayabose, Somasundaram MD [PHO] - **Spec Exp:** Leukemia; Lymphoma; Wilms' Tumor; Neuroblastoma; **Hospital:** Westchester Med Ctr, Good Samaritan Hosp - Suffern; **Address:** 19 Bradhurst Ave, Hawthorne, NY 10532; **Phone:** 914-493-7997; **Board Cert:** Pediatrics 1975; Pediatric Hematology-Oncology 1976; **Med School:** India 1969; **Resid:** Pediatrics, Metropolitan Hosp Ctr 1974; **Fellow:** Pediatric Hematology-Oncology, LI Jewish Med Ctr 1976; **Fac Appt:** Prof Ped, NY Med Coll

Kamen, Barton A MD/PhD [PHO] **Spec Exp:** Drug Development; Leukemia; **Hospital:** Robert Wood Johnson Univ Hosp - New Brunswick; **Address:** Cancer Inst of New Jersey, 195 Little Albany St, rm 3507, New Brunswick, NJ 08903; **Phone:** 732 235 8864; **Board Cert:** Pediatrics 1981; Pediatric Hematology-Oncology 1987; **Med School:** Case West Res Univ 1976; **Resid:** Pediatrics, Yale-New Haven Hosp 1978; **Fellow:** Pediatric Hematology-Oncology, Yale-New Haven Hosp 1980; **Fac Appt:** Prof Ped, UMDNJ-RW Johnson Med Sch

Korones, David N MD [PHO] - **Spec Exp:** Brain Tumors; Palliative Care; Pediatric Cancers; **Hospital:** Univ of Rochester Strong Meml Hosp; **Address:** Golisano Childrens Hosp at Strong, 601 Elmwood Ave, Box 777, Rochester, NY 14642-8777; **Phone:** 585-275-2981; **Board Cert:** Pediatrics 1987; Pediatric Hematology-Oncology 2006; Hospice & Palliative Medicine 2002; **Med School:** Vanderbilt Univ 1983; **Resid:** Pediatrics, Strong Meml Hosp 1986; **Fellow:** Pediatrics, Yale Univ 1988; Pediatric Hematology-Oncology, Strong Meml Hosp 1991; **Fac Appt:** Assoc Prof Ped, Univ Rochester

Pediatric Hematology-Oncology

Kushner, Brian H MD [PHO] - **Spec Exp:** Neuroblastoma; Bone Marrow Transplant; Immunotherapy; **Hospital:** Meml Sloan-Kettering Cancer Ctr (page 76); **Address:** 1275 York Avenue, New York, NY 10065; **Phone:** 800-525-2225; **Board Cert:** Pediatrics 1983; Pediatric Hematology-Oncology 1987; **Med School:** Johns Hopkins Univ 1976; **Resid:** Pediatrics, Columbia-Presby Med Ctr 1978; Pediatrics, NY Hosp 1979; **Fellow:** Pediatric Hematology-Oncology, Boston Chldns Hosp 1980; Pediatric Hematology-Oncology, Meml Sloan Kettering Cancer Ctr 1986; **Fac Appt:** Prof Ped, Cornell Univ-Weill Med Coll

Lange, Beverly J MD [PHO] - **Spec Exp:** Leukemia; Brain & Spinal Cord Tumors; Cognitive Rehabilitation; **Hospital:** Chldns Hosp of Philadelphia, The; **Address:** Chldns Hosp Phila, Medical Oncology, 34th St & Civic Ctr Blvd, Wood Center, 4th Fl, Philadelphia, PA 19104; **Phone:** 215-590-2249; **Board Cert:** Pediatrics 1976; Pediatric Hematology-Oncology 1997; **Med School:** Temple Univ 1971; **Resid:** Pediatrics, Philadelphia Genl Hosp 1973; **Fellow:** Pediatric Oncology, Chldns Hosp; **Fac Appt:** Prof Ped, Univ Pennsylvania

Lipton, Jeffrey M MD/PhD [PHO] - **Spec Exp:** Bone Marrow Failure Disorders; Stem Cell Transplant; Bone Marrow Transplant; **Hospital:** Schneider Chldn's Hosp; **Address:** Div Hem-Onc & Stem Cell Transplant, 269-01 76th Ave, rm 255, MC-07670, New Hyde Park, NY 11040-1433; **Phone:** 718-470-3460; **Board Cert:** Pediatrics 1981; **Med School:** St Louis Univ 1975; **Resid:** Pediatrics, Boston Chldns Hosp 1977; **Fellow:** Pediatric Hematology-Oncology, Boston Chldns Hosp/Dana Farber Cancer Inst 1979; **Fac Appt:** Prof Ped, Albert Einstein Coll Med

Luchtman-Jones, Lori MD [PHO] - **Spec Exp:** Leukemia; Bleeding/Coagulation Disorders; **Hospital:** Chldns Natl Med Ctr; **Address:** Chldn's Natl Med Ctr, 111 Michigan Ave NW Fl 4 - Ste 4043, Washington, DC 20010; **Phone:** 202-476-2140; **Board Cert:** Pediatric Hematology-Oncology 2004; **Med School:** UCSD 1987; **Resid:** Pediatrics, UCSD School Med 1990; **Fellow:** Pediatric Hematology-Oncology, Washington Univ 1995; **Fac Appt:** Asst Prof Ped, Washington Univ, St Louis

Maris, John M MD [PHO] - **Spec Exp:** Neuroblastoma; Clinical Trials; **Hospital:** Chldns Hosp of Philadelphia, The; **Address:** Chldns Hosp Philadelphia - Oncology, 34th St & Civic Ctr Blvd Abramson Bldg, Philadelphia, PA 19104-4318; **Phone:** 215-590-5244; **Board Cert:** Pediatric Hematology-Oncology 2004; **Med School:** Univ Pennsylvania 1989; **Resid:** Pediatrics, Chldns Hosp 1992; **Fellow:** Pediatric Hematology-Oncology, Chldns Hosp 1996

Meek, Rita S MD [PHO] - **Hospital:** Alfred I duPont Hosp for Children, Christiana Care Hlth Svs; **Address:** Dupont Hosp for Chldn, Div Hem/Oncology, 1600 Rockland Rd, Wilmington, DE 19899; **Phone:** 302-651-5500; **Board Cert:** Pediatrics 1979; Pediatric Hematology-Oncology 1980; **Med School:** Geo Wash Univ 1974; **Resid:** Pediatrics, Childns Hosp Natl Med Ctr 1977; **Fellow:** Pediatric Hematology-Oncology, Chldns Hosp Natl Med Ctr 1979; **Fac Appt:** Assoc Clin Prof Ped, Jefferson Med Coll

Meyers, Paul A MD [PHO] - **Spec Exp:** Pediatric Cancers; Bone Tumors; Sarcoma; **Hospital:** Meml Sloan-Kettering Cancer Ctr (page 76), NY-Presby Hosp/Weill Cornell (page 79); **Address:** 1275 York Avenue, New York, NY 10065; **Phone:** 800-525-2225; **Board Cert:** Pediatrics 1978; Pediatric Hematology-Oncology 1978; **Med School:** Mount Sinai Sch Med 1973; **Resid:** Pediatrics, Mt Sinai Hosp 1976; **Fellow:** Pediatric Hematology-Oncology, NY Hosp-Cornell Med Ctr 1979; **Fac Appt:** Prof Ped, Cornell Univ-Weill Med Coll

O'Reilly, Richard MD [PHO] - **Spec Exp:** Bone Marrow Transplant; **Hospital:** Meml Sloan-Kettering Cancer Ctr (page 76), NY-Presby Hosp/Weill Cornell (page 79); **Address:** 1275 York Avenue, New York, NY 10065; **Phone:** 800-525-2225; **Board Cert:** Pediatrics 1974; **Med School:** Univ Rochester 1968; **Resid:** Pediatrics, Chldrns Hosp 1972; **Fellow:** Infectious Disease, Chldrns Hosp 1973; **Fac Appt:** Prof Ped, Cornell Univ-Weill Med Coll

Parker, Robert MD [PHO] - **Spec Exp:** Pediatric Cancers; Bleeding/Coagulation Disorders; Lymphoma; **Hospital:** Stony Brook Univ Med Ctr; **Address:** Stony Brook Univ Hosp, Dept Peds, HSC T-11, Rm 029, Stony Brook, NY 11794-8111; **Phone:** 631-444-7720; **Board Cert:** Pediatrics 1983; Pediatric Hematology-Oncology 1984; **Med School:** Brown Univ 1976; **Resid:** Internal Medicine, Roger Williams Med Ctr 1977; Pediatrics, Rhode Island Hosp 1979; **Fellow:** Pediatric Hematology-Oncology, Natl Cancer Inst 1981; Hematology, Natl Cancer Inst 1984; **Fac Appt:** Prof Ped, SUNY Stony Brook

Rausen, Aaron R MD [PHO] - **Spec Exp:** Leukemia & Lymphoma; Bone Tumors; Retinoblastoma; **Hospital:** NYU Langone Med Ctr (page 80), Lenox Hill Hosp; **Address:** NYU Medical Ctr, 160 E 32nd St Fl 2, New York, NY 10016; **Phone:** 212-263-7144; **Board Cert:** Pediatrics 1960; Pediatric Hematology-Oncology 1974; **Med School:** SUNY Downstate 1954; **Resid:** Pediatrics, Bellevue Hosp 1956; Pediatrics, Mount Sinai 1959; **Fellow:** Hematology, Chldns Hosp 1961; **Fac Appt:** Prof Ped, NYU Sch Med

Reaman, Gregory MD [PHO] - **Spec Exp:** Leukemia; Lymphoma; Cancer Survivors-Late Effects of Therapy; **Hospital:** Chldns Natl Med Ctr; **Address:** 111 Michigan Ave NW, Washington, DC 20010-2916; **Phone:** 202-476-2800; **Board Cert:** Pediatrics 1978; Pediatric Hematology-Oncology 1978; **Med School:** Loyola Univ-Stritch Sch Med 1973; **Resid:** Hematology, Montreal Chldns Hosp 1975; Pediatrics, Montreal Chldns Hosp 1976; **Fellow:** Pediatric Oncology, Natl Cancer Inst 1979; **Fac Appt:** Prof Ped, Geo Wash Univ

Rheingold, Susan R MD [PHO] - **Spec Exp:** Leukemia; Clinical Trials; **Hospital:** Chldns Hosp of Philadelphia, The; **Address:** Chldns Hosp Phila - Div Oncology, 34th & Civic Ctr Blvd, Philadelphia, PA 19104; **Phone:** 215-590-3025; **Board Cert:** Pediatrics 2003; Pediatric Hematology-Oncology 2008; **Med School:** Univ Pennsylvania 1992; **Resid:** Pediatrics, Johns Hopkins Hosp 1995; **Fellow:** Pediatric Hematology-Oncology, Chldns Hosp 1999; **Fac Appt:** Asst Prof Ped, Univ Pennsylvania

Ritchey, A Kim MD [PHO] - **Spec Exp:** Leukemia; **Hospital:** Chldns Hosp of Pittsburgh - UPMC; **Address:** Chldns Hosp, Div Hematology/Oncology, 3705 Fifth Ave, Desoto Wing 4B, Ste 385, Pittsburgh, PA 15213; **Phone:** 412-692-5055; **Board Cert:** Pediatrics 1977; Pediatric Hematology-Oncology 2007; **Med School:** Univ Cincinnati 1972; **Resid:** Pediatrics, Johns Hopkins Hosp 1975; **Fellow:** Pediatric Hematology-Oncology, Yale-New Haven Hosp 1980; **Fac Appt:** Prof Ped, Univ Pittsburgh

Steinherz, Peter G MD [PHO] - **Spec Exp:** Leukemia & Lymphoma; Pediatric Cancers; Wilms' Tumor; **Hospital:** Meml Sloan-Kettering Cancer Ctr (page 76), NY-Presby Hosp/Weill Cornell (page 79); **Address:** 1275 York Avenue, New York, NY 10065; **Phone:** 800-525-2225; **Board Cert:** Pediatrics 1973; Pediatric Hematology-Oncology 1978; **Med School:** Albert Einstein Coll Med 1968; **Resid:** Pediatrics, NY Hosp-Cornell 1971; **Fellow:** Pediatric Hematology-Oncology, NY Hosp-Cornell 1975; **Fac Appt:** Prof Ped, Cornell Univ-Weill Med Coll

Weinblatt, Mark E MD [PHO] - **Spec Exp:** Leukemia & Lymphoma; Bleeding/Coagulation Disorders; Solid Tumors; **Hospital:** Winthrop - Univ Hosp; **Address:** Winthrop Univ Hosp, 120 Mineola Blvd, Ste 460, Mineola, NY 11501; **Phone:** 516-663-9400; **Board Cert:** Pediatrics 1980; Pediatric Hematology-Oncology 1982; **Med School:** Albert Einstein Coll Med 1976; **Resid:** Pediatrics, Jacobi Med Ctr 1979; **Fellow:** Pediatric Hematology-Oncology, Children's Hosp 1981; **Fac Appt:** Prof Ped, SUNY Stony Brook

Pediatric Hematology-Oncology

Weiner, Michael MD [PHO] - **Spec Exp:** Hodgkin's Disease; Lymphoma; Leukemia; **Hospital:** NY-Presby Hosp/Columbia (page 79); **Address:** 161 Fort Washington Ave, Irving Pavilion-FL 7, New York, NY 10032-3710; **Phone:** 212-305-9770; **Board Cert:** Pediatrics 1980; Pediatric Hematology-Oncology 1980; **Med School:** SUNY Hlth Sci Ctr 1972; **Resid:** Pediatrics, Montefiore Med Ctr 1974; **Fellow:** Pediatric Hematology-Oncology, NYU Med Ctr 1976; Pediatric Hematology-Oncology, Johns Hopkins Hosp 1977; **Fac Appt:** Prof Ped, Columbia P&S

Wexler, Leonard MD [PHO] - **Spec Exp:** Rhabdomyosarcoma; Bone Cancer; Gastrointestinal Stromal Tumors; Sarcoma-Soft Tissue; **Hospital:** Meml Sloan-Kettering Cancer Ctr (page 76); **Address:** 1275 York Avenue, New York, NY 10065; **Phone:** 800-525-2225; **Board Cert:** Pediatrics 2000; Pediatric Hematology-Oncology 2000; **Med School:** Boston Univ 1985; **Resid:** Pediatrics, Montefiore Med Ctr 1988; **Fellow:** Pediatric Hematology-Oncology, National Cancer Inst 1991; **Fac Appt:** Assoc Prof Ped, Columbia P&S

Wolfe, Lawrence C MD [PHO] - **Spec Exp:** Leukemia; Neuro-Oncology; Cancer Survivors-Late Effects of Therapy; Pain Management-Pediatric; **Hospital:** Long Island Jewish Med Ctr; **Address:** LIJ Medical Ctr, Div Pediatric Hematology/Oncology, 269-01 76th Ave, New Hyde Park, NY 11040; **Phone:** 718-470-3460; **Board Cert:** Pediatrics 1981; Pediatric Hematology-Oncology 1987; **Med School:** Harvard Med Sch 1976; **Resid:** Pediatrics, Chldns Hosp 1978; **Fellow:** Pediatric Hematology-Oncology, Chldns Hosp 1991

Southeast

Barredo, Julio C MD [PHO] - **Spec Exp:** Cancer Survivors-Late Effects of Therapy; Clinical Trials; **Hospital:** Univ of Miami Hosp & Clins/Sylvester Comp Canc Ctr (page 82); **Address:** Dept Pediatrics, R131 PO Box 016960, Miami, FL 33136; **Phone:** 305-585-5635; **Board Cert:** Pediatric Hematology-Oncology 2007; **Med School:** Peru 1982; **Resid:** Pediatrics, Kings Co Hosp 1987; **Fellow:** Pediatric Hematology-Oncology, Chldns Hosp/USC 1988; **Fac Appt:** Prof Ped, Univ Miami Sch Med

Bertolone, Salvatore MD [PHO] - **Spec Exp:** Bone Marrow Transplant; Kasabach-Merritt Syndrome (KMS); **Hospital:** Kosair Chldn's Hosp, Norton Hosp; **Address:** Kosair Childrens Hosp, Dept Ped Hem/Onc, 601 Floyd St, rm 403, Louisville, KY 40202-3820; **Phone:** 502-629-7750; **Board Cert:** Pediatrics 1975; Pediatric Hematology-Oncology 1976; **Med School:** Univ Louisville Sch Med 1970; **Resid:** Pediatrics, Univ Louisville 1972; **Fellow:** Pediatric Hematology-Oncology, Univ Colorado 1974; **Fac Appt:** Prof Ped, Univ Louisville Sch Med

Blatt, Julie MD [PHO] - **Spec Exp:** Neuroblastoma; Cancer Survivors-Late Effects of Therapy; **Hospital:** Univ NC Hosps; **Address:** UNC, Dept Ped Hematology Oncology, CB 7236, Chapel Hill, NC 27599-7236; **Phone:** 919-966-1178; **Board Cert:** Pediatrics 1981; Pediatric Hematology-Oncology 1982; **Med School:** Johns Hopkins Univ 1976; **Resid:** Pediatrics, Columbia-Presby Hosp 1978; **Fellow:** Pediatric Oncology, Natl Cancer Inst 1982; **Fac Appt:** Prof Ped, Univ NC Sch Med

Castellino, Sharon M MD [PHO] - **Spec Exp:** Cancer Survivors-Late Effects of Therapy; Leukemia; Lymphoma; **Hospital:** Brenner Chldn's Hosp; **Address:** Wake Forest Univ Baptist Med Ctr, Div Pediatric Hematology/Oncology, Medical Center Blvd, Winston-Salem, NC 27157; **Phone:** 336-716-4324; **Board Cert:** Pediatrics 2003; Pediatric Hematology-Oncology 2006; **Med School:** Duke Univ 1992; **Resid:** Pediatrics, Childrens Hosp 1994; Pediatrics, Duke Univ Med Ctr 1995; **Fellow:** Pediatric Hematology-Oncology, Duke Univ 1997; **Fac Appt:** Asst Prof Ped, Wake Forest Univ

Frangoul, Haydar A MD [PHO] - **Spec Exp:** Stem Cell Transplant; **Hospital:** Vanderbilt Univ Med Ctr; **Address:** Ped Hem/Onc Clinic, 2200 Children's Way, Nashville, TN 37232-6310; **Phone:** 615-936-1762; **Board Cert:** Pediatric Hematology-Oncology 2008; **Med School:** Amer Univ Beirut 1990; **Resid:** Pediatrics, Duke Univ Med Ctr 1993; **Fellow:** Pediatric Hematology-Oncology, Duke Univ Med Ctr 1994; **Fac Appt:** Assoc Prof Ped, Vanderbilt Univ

Friedman, Debra L MD [PHO] - **Spec Exp:** Cancer Survivors-Late Effects of Therapy; Hodgkin's Disease; Retinoblastoma; **Hospital:** Vanderbilt Children's Hosp, Vanderbilt Univ Med Ctr; **Address:** Vanderbilt Univ Med Ctr, 2525 West End Ave Fl 6 - Ste 600, Nashville, TN 37232; **Phone:** 615-322-4708; **Board Cert:** Pediatric Hematology-Oncology 2006; **Med School:** UMDNJ-RW Johnson Med Sch 1991; **Resid:** Pediatrics, Chldns Hosp 1994; **Fellow:** Pediatric Hematology-Oncology, Chldns Hosp 1997; **Fac Appt:** Asst Prof Ped, Vanderbilt Univ

Friedman, Henry S MD [PHO] - **Spec Exp:** Neuro-Oncology; Brain & Spinal Cord Tumors; **Hospital:** Duke Univ Med Ctr; **Address:** Preston Robert Tisch, Brain Tumor Ctr at Duke, DUMC, Box 3624, Durham, NC 27710; **Phone:** 919-684-5301; **Board Cert:** Pediatrics 1982; Pediatric Hematology-Oncology 1982; **Med School:** SUNY Upstate Med Univ 1977; **Resid:** Pediatrics, SUNY Upstate Med Ctr 1980; **Fellow:** Pediatric Hematology-Oncology, Duke Univ Med Ctr 1983; **Fac Appt:** Prof Ped, Duke Univ

Furman, Wayne L MD [PHO] - **Spec Exp:** Neuroblastoma; Liver Cancer; Drug Development; **Hospital:** St Jude Children's Research Hosp; **Address:** St Jude Children's Research Hospital, 332 N Lauderdale St, MS 260, Memphis, TN 38105; **Phone:** 901-595-2800; **Board Cert:** Pediatrics 1985; Pediatric Hematology-Oncology 1987; **Med School:** Ohio State Univ 1979; **Resid:** Pediatrics, Children's Hosp 1983; **Fellow:** Pediatric Hematology-Oncology, St Jude Chldn's Rsch Hosp 1985; **Fac Appt:** Prof Ped, Univ Tenn Coll Med, Memphis

Gajjar, Amar J MD [PHO] - **Spec Exp:** Brain Tumors; Medulloblastoma; Neuro-Oncology; Drug Development; **Hospital:** St Jude Children's Research Hosp; **Address:** St Judes Children's Hosp, Dept Oncology, 262 Danny Thomas Pl, rm C6024, MS 260, Memphis, TN 38105-2794; **Phone:** 901-495-4599; **Board Cert:** Pediatric Hematology-Oncology 2007; **Med School:** India 1984; **Resid:** Pediatrics, All Chldns Hosp 1989; **Fellow:** Hematology & Oncology, St Jude Chldns Hosp 1990; **Fac Appt:** Prof Ped, Univ Tenn Coll Med, Memphis

Godder, Kamar MD/PhD [PHO] **Spec Exp:** Stem Cell Transplant, Leukemia, Palliative Care; **Hospital:** Med Coll of VA Hosp; **Address:** PO Box 980121, Richmond, VA 23219; **Phone:** 804-828-9605; **Board Cert:** Pediatric Hematology-Oncology 2005; **Med School:** Israel 1980; **Resid:** Pediatrics, Hadassah-Mt Scopus 1984; **Fellow:** Pediatric Hematology-Oncology, Meml Sloan Kettering Cancer Ctr 1988; **Fac Appt:** Prof Ped, Va Commonwealth Univ Sch Med

Gold, Stuart H MD [PHO] - **Spec Exp:** Leukemia; Brain Tumors; Cancer Survivors-Late Effects of Therapy; **Hospital:** Univ NC Hosps; **Address:** Univ of NC at Chapel Hill, Dept Ped Hem-Onc, CB# 7236 POB 1185A Bldg, Chapel Hill, NC 27599-7236; **Phone:** 919-966-1178; **Board Cert:** Pediatrics 1986; Pediatric Hematology-Oncology 1987; **Med School:** Vanderbilt Univ 1981; **Resid:** Pediatrics, Univ Colorado Hlth Sci Ctr 1984; **Fellow:** Pediatric Hematology-Oncology, Univ Colorado Hlth Sci Ctr 1989; **Fac Appt:** Prof Ped, Univ NC Sch Med

Green, Daniel M MD [PHO] - **Spec Exp:** Wilms' Tumor; Fertility in Cancer Survivors; Cancer Survivors-Late Effects of Therapy; **Hospital:** St Jude Children's Research Hosp; **Address:** Dept Epidemiology & Cancer Control, St Jude Chldn's Rsch Hosp, 332 N Lauderdale St, MS 735, Memphis, TN 38105-2794; **Phone:** 901-595-5915; **Board Cert:** Pediatrics 1986; Pediatric Hematology-Oncology 1997; **Med School:** St Louis Univ 1973; **Resid:** Pediatrics, Boston City Hosp 1975; **Fellow:** Pediatric Hematology-Oncology, Chldns Hosp Med Ctr 1978

Hudson, Melissa M MD [PHO] - **Spec Exp:** Cancer Survivors-Late Effects of Therapy; Hodgkin's Disease; **Hospital:** St Jude Children's Research Hosp; **Address:** St Jude Children's Research Hosp, 262 Danny Thomas Pl, MS 735, Memphis, TN 38105; **Phone:** 901-495-3384; **Board Cert:** Pediatrics 1988; Pediatric Hematology-Oncology 2006; **Med School:** Univ Tex SW, Dallas 1983; **Resid:** Pediatrics, Univ Texas Affil Hosps 1986; **Fellow:** Pediatric Hematology-Oncology, MD Anderson Cancer Ctr 1989

Johnston, J Martin MD [PHO] - **Spec Exp:** Leukemia; Lymphoma; **Hospital:** Meml Hlth Univ Med Ctr - Savannah; **Address:** Backus Children's Hosp Outpatient Ctr, 4700 Waters Ave, PO Box 23089, Savannah, GA 31403-3089; **Phone:** 912-350-8194; **Board Cert:** Pediatric Hematology-Oncology 2002; **Med School:** Duke Univ 1984; **Resid:** Pediatrics, Univ Utah Med Ctr 1988; **Fellow:** Pediatric Hematology-Oncology, Barnes Jewish Hosp 1991

Kane, Javier R MD [PHO] - **Spec Exp:** Palliative Care; **Hospital:** St Jude Children's Research Hosp; **Address:** St Jude Chldns Rsch Hosp, Dept Oncology, 262 Danny Thomas Pl, MS 260, Memphis, TN 38105-2794; **Phone:** 901-495-4152; **Board Cert:** Pediatrics 2007; Pediatric Hematology-Oncology 2004; **Med School:** Mexico 1986; **Resid:** Pediatrics, Austin Med Ed Prog 1992; **Fellow:** Pediatric Hematology-Oncology, Univ Tennessee

Keller Jr, Frank G MD [PHO] - **Spec Exp:** Leukemia; Hodgkin's Disease; **Hospital:** Chldns Hlthcare Atlanta @ Egleston; **Address:** Emory Childrens Ctr-Aflac Cancer Ctr, 2015 Uppergate Drive NE Fl 4, Atlanta, GA 30322; **Phone:** 404-785-1200; **Board Cert:** Pediatric Hematology-Oncology 2002; **Med School:** Univ NC Sch Med 1986; **Resid:** Pediatrics, Vanderbilt Univ Med Ctr 1990; **Fellow:** Pediatric Hematology-Oncology, Duke Univ Med Ctr 1993; **Fac Appt:** Assoc Prof Ped, Emory Univ

Kreissman, Susan G MD [PHO] - **Spec Exp:** Neuroblastoma; Clinical Trials; **Hospital:** Duke Univ Med Ctr; **Address:** Duke Univ Med Ctr, Box 2916, Durham, NC 27710; **Phone:** 919-684-3401; **Board Cert:** Pediatric Hematology-Oncology 2004; **Med School:** Mount Sinai Sch Med 1985; **Resid:** Pediatrics, Chldns Hosp 1988; **Fellow:** Pediatric Hematology-Oncology, Chldns Hosp/Dana Farber Cancer Inst 1991; **Fac Appt:** Assoc Prof Ped, Duke Univ

Kurtzberg, Joanne MD [PHO] - **Spec Exp:** Stem Cell Transplant; Bone Marrow Transplant; **Hospital:** Duke Univ Med Ctr; **Address:** Duke Univ Med Ctr, Box 3350, Durham, NC 27710; **Phone:** 919-668-1100; **Board Cert:** Pediatrics 1982; Pediatric Hematology-Oncology 1982; **Med School:** NY Med Coll 1976; **Resid:** Pediatrics, Dartmouth Med Ctr 1977; Pediatrics, Upstate Med Ctr 1979; **Fellow:** Pediatric Hematology-Oncology, Upstate Med Ctr 1980; Pediatric Hematology-Oncology, Duke Med Ctr 1983; **Fac Appt:** Prof Ped, Duke Univ

Kuttesch, John F MD [PHO] - **Spec Exp:** Brain Tumors; Brain Tumors-Recurrent; **Hospital:** Vanderbilt Children's Hosp; **Address:** Vanderbilt Pediatric Hem/Oncology, 2220 Pierce Ave, Rm 397 PRB, Nashville, TN 37232-6310; **Phone:** 615-936-1762; **Board Cert:** Pediatric Hematology-Oncology 2007; **Med School:** Univ Tex, Houston 1985; **Resid:** Pediatrics, Vanderbilt Univ Med Ctr 1988; **Fellow:** Pediatric Hematology-Oncology, St Judes Chldns Hosp 1992; **Fac Appt:** Assoc Prof Ped, Vanderbilt Univ

Moscow, Jeffrey A MD [PHO] - **Spec Exp:** Pediatric Cancers; **Hospital:** Univ of Kentucky Chandler Hosp; **Address:** Univ Kentucky - Kentucky Clinic, 740 S Limestone, rm J457, Lexington, KY 40536-0001; **Phone:** 859-257-4554; **Board Cert:** Pediatrics 1988; Pediatric Hematology-Oncology 2007; **Med School:** Dartmouth Med Sch 1982; **Resid:** Pediatrics, Univ Texas SW Med Ctr 1985; **Fellow:** Pediatric Hematology-Oncology, Natl Cancer Inst 1986; **Fac Appt:** Prof Ped, Univ KY Coll Med

Neuberg, Ronnie W MD [PHO] - **Spec Exp:** Pediatric Cancers; Gene Therapy; Clinical Trials; Brain Tumors; **Hospital:** Palmetto Richland Mem Hosp, MUSC Chldns Hosp; **Address:** Palmetto Health Richland, 7 Richland Medical Park Drive, Ste 7215, Columbia, SC 29203; **Phone:** 803-434-3533; **Board Cert:** Pediatrics 1982; Pediatric Hematology-Oncology 1982; **Med School:** SUNY Buffalo 1977; **Resid:** Pediatrics, Chldns Hosp 1980; **Fellow:** Pediatric Hematology-Oncology, SUNY Upstate Med Ctr 1982; **Fac Appt:** Assoc Prof Ped, Univ SC Sch Med

Nieder, Michael L MD [PHO] - **Spec Exp:** Bone Marrow Transplant; **Hospital:** All Children's Hosp; **Address:** 801 6th St S, Dept 7865, St Petersburg, FL 33701-4816; **Phone:** 727-767-6856; **Board Cert:** Pediatrics 1986; Pediatric Hematology-Oncology 1987; **Med School:** Univ IL Coll Med 1982; **Resid:** Pediatrics, Children's Meml Hosp 1985; **Fellow:** Pediatric Hematology-Oncology, Children's Meml Hosp 1988; **Fac Appt:** Prof Ped, Univ S Fla Coll Med

Olson, Thomas A MD [PHO] - **Spec Exp:** Sarcoma; Brain Tumors; **Hospital:** Chldns Hlthcare Atlanta @ Egleston; **Address:** Emory Childrens Ctr-Aflac Cancer Ctr, 2015 Uppergate Drive NE Fl 4, Atlanta, GA 30322; **Phone:** 404-785-1200; **Board Cert:** Pediatrics 1982; Pediatric Hematology-Oncology 1984; **Med School:** Loyola Univ-Stritch Sch Med 1978; **Resid:** Pediatrics, Walter Reed AMC 1981; **Fellow:** Pediatric Hematology-Oncology, Walter Reed AMC 1983; **Fac Appt:** Assoc Prof Ped, Emory Univ

Pui, Ching-Hon MD [PHO] - **Spec Exp:** Leukemia; Lymphoma; **Hospital:** St Jude Children's Research Hosp; **Address:** St Jude Chldns Rsch Hosp, 332 N Lauderdale St, Memphis, TN 38105; **Phone:** 901-495-3335; **Board Cert:** Pediatrics 1980; Pediatric Hematology-Oncology 1982; **Med School:** Taiwan 1976; **Resid:** Pediatrics, St Jude Chldns Rsch Hosp 1979; **Fellow:** Hematology & Oncology, St Jude Chldns Rsch Hosp 1981; **Fac Appt:** Prof Ped, Univ Tenn Coll Med, Memphis

Rosoff, Philip M MD [PHO] - **Spec Exp:** Cancer Survivors-Late Effects of Therapy; Leukemia; **Hospital:** Duke Univ Med Ctr; **Address:** Duke Univ Med Ctr, Box 2916, Durham, NC 27710-0001; **Phone:** 919-684-3401; **Board Cert:** Pediatrics 1984; Pediatric Hematology-Oncology 2002; **Med School:** Case West Res Univ 1978; **Resid:** Pediatrics, Chldns Hosp 1980; **Fellow:** Pediatric Hematology-Oncology, Chldns Hosp/Dana Farber Cancer Inst 1984; **Fac Appt:** Assoc Prof Ped, Duke Univ

Sandler, Eric MD [PHO] - **Spec Exp:** Bone Marrow Transplant; Leukemia; Clinical Trials; **Hospital:** Wolfson Chldns Hosp; **Address:** 807 Childrens Way, Jacksonville, FL 32207; **Phone:** 904-390-3793; **Board Cert:** Pediatric Hematology-Oncology 2007; Pediatrics 2008; **Med School:** Univ VT Coll Med 1985; **Resid:** Pediatrics, UCSF Med Ctr 1988; **Fellow:** Pediatric Hematology-Oncology, Univ Fla Med Sch 1991; **Fac Appt:** Assoc Prof Ped, Mayo Med Sch

Sandlund Jr, John T MD [PHO] - **Spec Exp:** Lymphoma, Non-Hodgkin's; Leukemia & Lymphoma; **Hospital:** St Jude Children's Research Hosp, Le Bonheur Chldns Med Ctr; **Address:** St Jude Children's Research Hosp, 262 Danny Thomas Pl, MS 260, Memphis, TN 38105; **Phone:** 901-595-2153; **Board Cert:** Pediatrics 1986; Pediatric Hematology-Oncology 1987; **Med School:** Ohio State Univ 1980; **Resid:** Pediatrics, Columbus Chldns Hosp 1983; **Fellow:** Hematology, Natl Cancer Inst 1986; Research, Natl Cancer Inst 1987

Santana, Victor M MD [PHO] - **Spec Exp:** Solid Tumors; **Hospital:** St Jude Children's Research Hosp; **Address:** St Jude Chldn's Rsch Hosp, Dept Oncology, 226 Danny Thomas Pl, rm C6041, MS 260, Memphis, TN 38105-2794; **Phone:** 901-495-2424; **Board Cert:** Pediatrics 1982; Pediatric Hematology-Oncology 1984; **Med School:** Puerto Rico 1978; **Resid:** Pediatrics, Johns Hopkins Hosp 1981; **Fellow:** Pediatric Hematology-Oncology, Johns Hopkins Hosp 1984

Pediatric Hematology-Oncology

Shearer, Patricia C MD [PHO] - **Spec Exp:** Wilms' Tumor; Cancer Survivors-Late Effects of Therapy; **Hospital:** Shands at Univ of FL; **Address:** Univ Florida HSC, Div Ped Hem/Oncology, PO Box 100296, Gainesville, FL 32610; **Phone:** 352-392-5633; **Board Cert:** Pediatric Hematology-Oncology 2007; **Med School:** Louisiana State U, New Orleans 1986; **Resid:** Pediatrics, Johns Hopkins Hosp 1989; **Fellow:** Hematology & Oncology, St Jude Chldns Rsch Hosp 1992

Tebbi, Cameron MD [PHO] - **Spec Exp:** Hemophilia; Leukemia; Sickle Cell Disease; **Hospital:** St Josephs Chldns Hosp, Tampa Genl Hosp; **Address:** 3001 W Martin Luther King Jr Blvd, Tampa, FL 33607; **Phone:** 813-870-4286; **Board Cert:** Pediatrics 1974; Pediatric Hematology-Oncology 1980; **Med School:** Iran 1968; **Resid:** Pediatrics, Cincinnati Chldns Hosp 1972; Pediatric Hematology-Oncology, MD Anderson Cancer Inst 1972; **Fellow:** Pediatric Hematology-Oncology, St Louis Chldns Hosp 1973; Medical Oncology, Ontario Cancer Inst 1974

Whitlock, James A MD [PHO] - **Spec Exp:** Leukemia; Drug Development; **Hospital:** Vanderbilt Children's Hosp, Vanderbilt Univ Med Ctr; **Address:** Vanderbilt Univ Med Ctr, Dept Peds, 2220 Pierce Ave, rm 397 PRB, Nashville, TN 37232-6310; **Phone:** 615-936-1762; **Board Cert:** Pediatric Hematology-Oncology 2007; **Med School:** Vanderbilt Univ 1984; **Resid:** Pediatrics, Vanderbilt Univ Med Ctr 1987; **Fellow:** Pediatric Hematology-Oncology, Vanderbilt Univ Med Ctr 1990; **Fac Appt:** Assoc Prof Ped, Vanderbilt Univ

Woods, William G MD [PHO] - **Spec Exp:** Leukemia; Neuroblastoma; **Hospital:** Chldns Hlthcare Atlanta @ Egleston, Chldns Hlthcare Atlanta - Scottish Rite; **Address:** AFLAC Cancer Ctr & Blood Disorders Svc, 2015 Uppergate Drive, rm 404, Atlanta, GA 30322; **Phone:** 404-785-6170; **Board Cert:** Pediatrics 1976; Pediatric Hematology-Oncology 1978; **Med School:** Univ Pennsylvania 1972; **Resid:** Pediatrics, Univ Minnesota Hosps 1975; **Fellow:** Hematology, Univ Minnesota Hosps 1977; **Fac Appt:** Prof Ped, Emory Univ

Midwest

Arndt, Carola A MD [PHO] - **Spec Exp:** Sarcoma; Brain Tumors; Stem Cell Transplant; **Hospital:** Mayo Med Ctr & Clin - Rochester; **Address:** Mayo Clinic, Dept Pediatrics, 200 1st St SW, Rochester, MN 55905; **Phone:** 507-284-2652; **Board Cert:** Pediatrics 1982; Pediatric Hematology-Oncology 1987; **Med School:** Boston Univ 1978; **Resid:** Pediatrics, Naval Reg Med Ctr 1981; **Fellow:** Pediatric Hematology-Oncology, Natl Inst Hlth 1984

Camitta, Bruce M MD [PHO] - **Spec Exp:** Leukemia; Anemia-Aplastic; Bone Marrow Transplant; **Hospital:** Chldns Hosp - Wisconsin; **Address:** Midwest Childrens Cancer Ctr, 8701 Watertown Plank Rd, Ste 3018, Milwaukee, WI 53226; **Phone:** 414-456-4170; **Board Cert:** Pediatrics 1971; Pediatric Hematology-Oncology 1976; **Med School:** Johns Hopkins Univ 1966; **Resid:** Pediatrics, Chldns Hosp 1968; Pediatrics, Johns Hopkins Hosp 1969; **Fellow:** Pediatric Hematology-Oncology, Chldns Hosp 1973; **Fac Appt:** Prof Ped, Med Coll Wisc

Castle, Valerie P MD [PHO] - **Spec Exp:** Neuroblastoma; Cancer Survivors-Late Effects of Therapy; **Hospital:** Univ Michigan Hlth Sys; **Address:** Univ Mich Comp Cancer Ctr, 1500 E Med Ctr Drive, Desk B1-358, Ann Arbor, MI 48109-0911; **Phone:** 734-936-9814; **Board Cert:** Pediatric Hematology-Oncology 2006; **Med School:** McMaster Univ 1983; **Resid:** Pediatrics, McMaster Univ Med Ctr 1986; **Fellow:** Pediatric Hematology-Oncology, Univ Mich Hosps 1989; **Fac Appt:** Prof Ped, Univ Mich Med Sch

Cohn, Susan L MD [PHO] - **Spec Exp:** Neuroblastoma; **Hospital:** Univ of Chicago Med Ctr; **Address:** Univ Chicago, 5841 S Maryland Ave, MC 4060, Chicago, IL 60637-1470; **Phone:** 773-702-2571; **Board Cert:** Pediatrics 1985; Pediatric Hematology-Oncology 1987; **Med School:** Univ IL Coll Med 1980; **Resid:** Pediatrics, Michael Reese Hosp 1984; **Fellow:** Hematology & Oncology, Chldns Meml Hosp 1985; **Fac Appt:** Prof Ped, Univ Chicago-Pritzker Sch Med

Corey, Seth J MD [PHO] - **Spec Exp:** Bone Marrow Failure Disorders; Leukemia; Myelodysplastic Syndromes; **Hospital:** Children's Mem Hosp; **Address:** Robert Lurie Comp Cancer Ctr, Lurie 5-107, 303 E Superior St, Chicago, IL 60611; **Phone:** 312-503-6694; **Board Cert:** Pediatrics 1986; Pediatric Hematology-Oncology 2004; **Med School:** Tulane Univ 1982; **Resid:** Pediatrics, St Louis Chldns Hosp 1985; **Fellow:** Hematology & Oncology, Tufts Med Sch 1992; Research, Boston Chldns-Dana Farber Ctr 1989; **Fac Appt:** Prof Ped, Northwestern Univ-Feinberg Sch Med

Croop, James M MD/PhD [PHO] - **Spec Exp:** Rhabdomyosarcoma; Clinical Trials; **Hospital:** Riley Hosp for Children (page 74); **Address:** Riley Hosp for Children, Hem/Onc, 702 Barnhill Drive, ROC 4340, Indianapolis, IN 46202; **Phone:** 317-274-8784; **Board Cert:** Pediatrics 1985; Pediatric Hematology-Oncology 2005; **Med School:** Univ Pennsylvania 1980; **Resid:** Pediatrics, Childrens Hosp 1983; **Fellow:** Pediatric Hematology-Oncology, Childrens Hosp 1985; **Fac Appt:** Prof Ped, Indiana Univ

Davies, Stella M MD/PhD [PHO] - **Spec Exp:** Leukemia; Bone Marrow Transplant; Stem Cell Transplant; **Hospital:** Cincinnati Chldns Hosp Med Ctr; **Address:** Cincinnati Chldns Hosp Med Ctr, 3333 Burnet Ave, MLC 7015, Cincinnati, OH 45229-3039; **Phone:** 513-636-2469; **Med School:** England, UK 1981; **Resid:** Pediatrics, Univ Newcastle Med Ctr 1985; **Fellow:** Pediatric Hematology-Oncology, Univ Minn Med Ctr 1993; **Fac Appt:** Prof Ped, Univ Cincinnati

Fallon, Robert J MD/PhD [PHO] - **Spec Exp:** Lymphoma; Hodgkin's Disease; Stem Cell Transplant; Adolescent/Young Adult Cancers; **Hospital:** Riley Hosp for Children (page 74); **Address:** Riley Childrens Hospital, 702 Barnhill Drive, rm Riley 4340, Indianapolis, IN 46202; **Phone:** 317-274-8784; **Board Cert:** Internal Medicine 1983; Medical Oncology 1985; **Med School:** NYU Sch Med 1980; **Resid:** Internal Medicine, Brigham & Womens Hosp 1983; **Fellow:** Hematology & Oncology, Brigham & Womens Hosp/Dana Farber Cancer Inst 1985; **Fac Appt:** Prof Ped, Indiana Univ

Ferrara, James MD [PHO] - **Spec Exp:** Bone Marrow Transplant; Graft vs Host Disease; **Hospital:** Univ Michigan Hlth Sys; **Address:** Univ Michigan Comprehensive Cancer Ctr, 1500 E Medical Center Drive, Ste 6308, Ann Arbor, MI 48109-0942; **Phone:** 734-615-1340; **Board Cert:** Pediatrics 2005; Pediatric Hematology-Oncology 2006; **Med School:** Georgetown Univ 1980; **Resid:** Pediatrics, Children's Hosp 1982; **Fellow:** Pediatric Hematology-Oncology, Children's Hosp 1985; **Fac Appt:** Prof Ped, Univ Mich Med Sch

Friebert, Sarah E MD [PHO] - **Spec Exp:** Palliative Care; Cancer Survivors-Late Effects of Therapy; **Hospital:** Children's Hosp & Med Ctr- Akron; **Address:** Children's Hosp Med Ctr of Akron, One Perkins Sq Fl 5, Akron, OH 44308; **Phone:** 330-543-3343; **Board Cert:** Pediatrics 2004; Pediatric Hematology-Oncology 2008; **Med School:** Case West Res Univ 1993; **Resid:** Pediatrics, Chldns Hosp 1996; **Fellow:** Pediatric Hematology-Oncology, Rainbow Babies-Chldns Hosp 1999; **Fac Appt:** Asst Prof Ped, NE Ohio Univ

Goldman, Stewart MD [PHO] - **Spec Exp:** Neuro-Oncology; Brain Tumors; Clinical Trials; **Hospital:** Children's Mem Hosp; **Address:** Childrens Meml Hosp, Div Hem/Onc, 2300 Childrens Plaza, Box 30, Chicago, IL 60614; **Phone:** 773-880-3004; **Board Cert:** Pediatric Hematology-Oncology 2004; **Med School:** Loyola Univ-Stritch Sch Med 1985; **Resid:** Pediatrics, Univ Chicago Hosps 1988; **Fellow:** Pediatric Hematology-Oncology, Univ Chicago Hosps 1991

Haut, Paul R MD [PHO] - **Spec Exp:** Stem Cell Transplant; Bone Marrow Transplant; Leukemia; **Hospital:** Riley Hosp for Children (page 74); **Address:** Riley Hospital for Children, 702 Barnhill Drive, rm 4340, Indianapolis, IN 46202; **Phone:** 317-274-2143; **Board Cert:** Pediatric Hematology-Oncology 2008; **Med School:** Univ Ark 1990; **Resid:** Pediatrics, Arkansas Children's Hosp 1994; **Fellow:** Pediatric Hematology-Oncology, Children's Meml Hosp 1997; **Fac Appt:** Assoc Prof Ped, Indiana Univ

Pediatric Hematology-Oncology

Hayani, Ammar MD [PHO] - **Spec Exp:** Leukemia; Solid Tumors; **Hospital:** Adv Christ Med Ctr, Central DuPage Hosp; **Address:** Hope Children's Hospital, 4440 W 95th St, Oak Lawn, IL 60453-2600; **Phone:** 708-684-4094; **Board Cert:** Pediatric Hematology-Oncology 2005; **Med School:** Syria 1982; **Resid:** Pediatrics, Louisiana State Univ Hosp 1987; **Fellow:** Pediatric Hematology-Oncology, Baylor Coll Med Affil Hosp 1991

Hayashi, Robert J MD [PHO] - **Spec Exp:** Bone Marrow Transplant; Cancer Survivors-Late Effects of Therapy; Leukemia; **Hospital:** St Louis Chldns Hosp; **Address:** St Louis Chldns Hosp, Div Ped Hem Onc, One Children's Pl, Ste 9 South, Campus Box 8116, St Louis, MO 63110; **Phone:** 314-454-6018; **Board Cert:** Pediatrics 2007; Pediatric Hematology-Oncology 2007; **Med School:** Washington Univ, St Louis 1986; **Resid:** Pediatrics, St Louis Childrens Hosp 1989; **Fellow:** Pediatric Hematology-Oncology, Johns Hopkins Hosp 1992; **Fac Appt:** Asst Prof Ped, Washington Univ, St Louis

Hetherington, Maxine MD [PHO] - **Spec Exp:** Brain Tumors; **Hospital:** Chldns Mercy Hosps & Clinics; **Address:** Childrens Mercy Hosptial, 2401 Gillham Rd, Kansas City, MO 64108; **Phone:** 816-234-3265; **Board Cert:** Pediatrics 1983; Pediatric Hematology-Oncology 1987; **Med School:** Univ Tenn Coll Med, Memphis 1978; **Resid:** Pediatrics, Childrens Med Ctr 1981; **Fellow:** Pediatric Hematology-Oncology, Univ Texas Hlth Sci Ctr 1987; **Fac Appt:** Assoc Prof Ped, Univ MO-Kansas City

Hilden, Joanne M MD [PHO] - **Spec Exp:** Brain Tumors; Leukemia & Lymphoma; Bone Tumors; Soft Tissue Tumors; **Hospital:** St Vincent Indianapolis Hosp; **Address:** Peyton Manning Children's Hospital, at St Vincent, 8402 Harcourt Rd, Ste 603, Indianapolis, IN 46260; **Phone:** 317-338-4673; **Board Cert:** Pediatrics 2006; Pediatric Hematology-Oncology 2002; Hospice & Palliative Medicine 2008; **Med School:** Univ Minn 1988; **Resid:** Pediatrics, Univ Minn Med Ctr 1991; **Fellow:** Pediatric Hematology-Oncology, Univ Minn Med Ctr 1994; **Fac Appt:** Assoc Prof Ped, Indiana Univ

Hord, Jeffrey D MD [PHO] - **Spec Exp:** Hematologic Malignancies; Bone Marrow Failure Disorders; Pediatric Cancers; **Hospital:** Children's Hosp & Med Ctr- Akron; **Address:** Akron Childrens Hosp, Hematology/Oncology, One Perkins Square, Akron, OH 44308; **Phone:** 330-543-8580; **Board Cert:** Pediatric Hematology-Oncology 2004; **Med School:** Univ KY Coll Med 1989; **Resid:** Pediatrics, Childrens Hosp 1992; **Fellow:** Pediatric Hematology-Oncology, Vanderbilt Univ Med Ctr 1995; **Fac Appt:** Prof Ped, NE Ohio Univ

Hutchinson, Raymond MD [PHO] - **Spec Exp:** Leukemia; Hodgkin's Disease; **Hospital:** Univ Michigan Hlth Sys; **Address:** Univ Michigan Hosp, 1500 E Med Ctr Drive, rm L2110, Flr 1-Recep B1, Ann Arbor, MI 48109-5238; **Phone:** 734-763-6336; **Board Cert:** Pediatrics 1979; Pediatric Hematology-Oncology 1980; **Med School:** Harvard Med Sch 1973; **Resid:** Pediatrics, New England Med Ctr 1975; **Fellow:** Pediatric Hematology-Oncology, Childrens Hosp 1978; **Fac Appt:** Prof Ped, Univ Mich Med Sch

Lusher, Jeanne M MD [PHO] - **Hospital:** Chldns Hosp of Michigan; **Address:** Children's Hospital Michigan, Div Hem/Onc, 3901 Beaubien Blvd, Detroit, MI 48201; **Phone:** 313-745-5515; **Board Cert:** Pediatrics 1986; Pediatric Hematology-Oncology 1986; **Med School:** Univ Cincinnati 1960; **Resid:** Pediatrics, Charity Hosp/Tulane Univ 1963; **Fellow:** Hematology & Oncology, Charity Hosp/Tulane Univ 1965; Hematology & Oncology, Saint Louis Children's Hosp 1966; **Fac Appt:** Prof Ped, Wayne State Univ

Manera, Ricarchito B MD [PHO] - **Spec Exp:** Leukemia; Brain Tumors; Lymphoma; **Hospital:** Loyola Univ Med Ctr; **Address:** Loyola University Med Ctr, 2160 S First Ave, Maywood, IL 60611; **Phone:** 708-327-9136; **Board Cert:** Pediatrics 2003; Pediatric Hematology-Oncology 2004; **Med School:** Philippines 1984; **Resid:** Pediatrics, Bronx-Lebanon Hosp Ctr 1995; **Fellow:** Pediatric Hematology-Oncology, MD Anderson Cancer Ctr 1994; Pediatric Hematology-Oncology, Columbia-Presby Med Ctr 1996; **Fac Appt:** Assoc Prof Ped, Loyola Univ-Stritch Sch Med

Morgan, Elaine MD [PHO] - **Spec Exp:** Leukemia; Palliative Care; Ethics; **Hospital:** Children's Mem Hosp; **Address:** Children's Meml Hosp, Div Hem/Onc, 2300 Children's Plaza, Box 30, Chicago, IL 60614; **Phone:** 773-880-4562; **Board Cert:** Pediatrics 1976; Pediatric Hematology-Oncology 1978; Hospice & Palliative Medicine 2005; **Med School:** Univ Pennsylvania 1971; **Resid:** Pediatrics, Chldns Hosp 1974; **Fellow:** Pediatric Hematology-Oncology, Chldns Hosp Med Ctr 1975; Pediatric Hematology-Oncology, Chldns Meml Med Ctr 1976; **Fac Appt:** Prof Ped, Northwestern Univ-Feinberg Sch Med

Nachman, James MD [PHO] - **Spec Exp:** Leukemia & Lymphoma; Bone Tumors; Hodgkin's Disease; **Hospital:** Univ of Chicago Med Ctr; **Address:** Univ Chicago Hosps, 5841 S Maryland Ave, rm C-429, MC 4060, Chicago, IL 60637; **Phone:** 773-702-6808; **Board Cert:** Pediatrics 1979; Pediatric Hematology-Oncology 1980; **Med School:** Johns Hopkins Univ 1974; **Resid:** Pediatrics, Chldns Meml Hosp 1977; Pediatrics, Fell-Wylers Chldns Hosp 1980; **Fellow:** Pediatric Hematology-Oncology, Chldns Meml Hosp 1979; **Fac Appt:** Prof Ped, Univ Chicago-Pritzker Sch Med

Neglia, Joseph MD [PHO] - **Spec Exp:** Cancer Survivors-Late Effects of Therapy; **Hospital:** Univ Minn Med Ctr, Fairview - Univ Campus; **Address:** Univ Minnesota-Div Ped Hem/Oncology, 420 Delaware St SE, MMC 484, Minneapolis, MN 55455; **Phone:** 612-626-2778; **Board Cert:** Pediatrics 1986; Pediatric Hematology-Oncology 1987; **Med School:** Loma Linda Univ 1981; **Resid:** Pediatrics, Baylor Coll Med 1984; **Fellow:** Pediatric Hematology-Oncology, Univ Minn Hosp 1987; **Fac Appt:** Prof Ped, Univ Minn

O'Dorisio, M Sue MD/PhD [PHO] - **Spec Exp:** Neuroblastoma; Medulloblastoma; Neuroendocrine Tumors; **Hospital:** Univ Iowa Hosp & Clinics; **Address:** UIHC Pediatrics Hema/Oncology, 200 Hawkins Drive, rm 2520 JCP, Iowa City, IA 52242; **Phone:** 319-356-7873; **Board Cert:** Pediatrics 2007; Pediatric Hematology-Oncology 2007; **Med School:** Ohio State Univ 1985; **Resid:** Pediatrics, Chldns Hosp 1988; **Fellow:** Pediatric Hematology-Oncology, Chldns Hosp 1992; **Fac Appt:** Prof Ped, Univ Iowa Coll Med

Plautz, Gregory E MD [PHO] - **Spec Exp:** Brain Tumors; Leukemia & Lymphoma; Wilms' Tumor; Cancer Survivors-Late Effects of Therapy; **Hospital:** Cleveland Clin Fdn (page 70); **Address:** Cleveland Clinic Fdn - Div Ped Hem Onc, 9500 Euclid Ave, MC S20, Cleveland, OH 44195; **Phone:** 216-445-3800; **Board Cert:** Pediatric Hematology-Oncology 2005; **Med School:** Indiana Univ 1984; **Resid:** Pediatrics, Johns Hopkins Hosp 1987; **Fellow:** Pediatric Hematology-Oncology, Univ Michigan Affil Hosp 1990; **Fac Appt:** Assoc Prof S, Case West Res Univ

Puccetti, Diane M MD [PHO] - **Spec Exp:** Brain Tumors; Neuro-Oncology; Cancer Survivors-Late Effects of Therapy; **Hospital:** Univ WI Hosp & Clins; **Address:** Univ Wisconsin Childrens Hosp, 600 Highland Ave, MC 4672, Madison, WI 53792; **Phone:** 608-263-6420; **Board Cert:** Pediatric Hematology-Oncology 2007; **Med School:** Med Coll OH 1985; **Resid:** Pediatrics, UC-Irvine Med Ctr 1986; Pediatrics, Med Coll Ohio 1988; **Fellow:** Pediatric Hematology-Oncology, Riley Hosp Chldn 1991; **Fac Appt:** Assoc Clin Prof Ped, Univ Wisc

Pediatric Hematology-Oncology

Razzouk, Bassem I MD [PHO] - **Spec Exp:** Leukemia; Clinical Trials; **Hospital:** St Vincent Indianapolis Hosp; **Address:** St Vincent Hosp & Hlth Services, Center for Cancer & Blood Diseases, 2001 W 86th St, Indianapolis, IN 46260; **Phone:** 317-338-4673; **Board Cert:** Pediatric Hematology-Oncology 2004; **Med School:** Lebanon 1987; **Resid:** Pediatrics, American Univ Med Ctr 1990; Pediatrics, SUNY Hlth Sci Ctr 1992; **Fellow:** Hematology & Oncology, St Jude Chldns Rsch Hosp 1995

Salvi, Sharad MD [PHO] - **Spec Exp:** Leukemia; **Hospital:** Adv Christ Med Ctr, Central DuPage Hosp; **Address:** Hope Chldns Hosp, 4440 W 95th St, Oak Lawn, IL 60453; **Phone:** 708-684-4094; **Board Cert:** Pediatrics 1982; Pediatric Hematology-Oncology 1982; **Med School:** India 1974; **Resid:** Pediatrics, Lincoln Meml Hosp 1979; **Fellow:** Pediatric Hematology-Oncology, Chldns Hosp/Roswell Park Meml Cancer Inst 1981

Sencer, Susan F MD [PHO] - **Spec Exp:** Pediatric Cancers; Complementary Medicine; **Hospital:** Chldns Hosp and Clinics - Minneapolis; **Address:** Chldns Specialty Clinic, Hem/Onc Clin, 2525 Chicago Ave S, Fl 4 - Ste 4150, Minneapolis, MN 55404; **Phone:** 612-813-5940; **Board Cert:** Pediatric Hematology-Oncology 2007; **Med School:** Univ Minn 1984; **Resid:** Pediatrics, Univ Minnesota Affil Hosp 1988; **Fellow:** Pediatric Hematology-Oncology, Univ Minnesota Affil Hosp 1991

Sondel, Paul M MD [PHO] - **Spec Exp:** Immunotherapy; Stem Cell Transplant; Pediatric Cancers; **Hospital:** Univ WI Hosp & Clins; **Address:** 600 Highland Ave, K4-448 Clin Sci Ctr, Madison, WI 53792-4672; **Phone:** 608-263-6200; **Board Cert:** Pediatrics 1981; **Med School:** Harvard Med Sch 1977; **Resid:** Pediatrics, Univ Wisconsin Hosp 1980; **Fellow:** Research, Sidney Farber Cancer Inst/Harvard 1977; **Fac Appt:** Prof Ped, Univ Wisc

Tannous, Raymond MD [PHO] - **Spec Exp:** Wilms' Tumor; Leukemia & Lymphoma; Pain-Cancer; **Hospital:** Univ Iowa Hosp & Clinics; **Address:** Univ Iowa Hosps & Clinics, Dept Peds, 200 Hawkins Drive, rm 2528 JCP, Iowa City, IA 52242; **Phone:** 319-356-1905; **Board Cert:** Pediatrics 1976; Pediatric Hematology-Oncology 1978; **Med School:** France 1972; **Resid:** Pediatrics, St Jude Chldns Rsch Hosp 1976; **Fellow:** Pediatric Hematology-Oncology, St Jude Chldns Rsch Hosp 1977; **Fac Appt:** Assoc Prof Ped, Univ Iowa Coll Med

Vik, Terry A MD [PHO] - **Spec Exp:** Neuroblastoma; Clinical Trials; Cancer Survivors-Late Effects of Therapy; Leukemia; **Hospital:** Riley Hosp for Children (page 74); **Address:** Riley Hosp Children, 702 Barnhill Drive, Riley 4340, Indianapolis, IN 46202; **Phone:** 317-274-2143; **Board Cert:** Pediatrics 1987; Pediatric Hematology-Oncology 2004; **Med School:** Johns Hopkins Univ 1983; **Resid:** Pediatrics, UCLA Med Ctr 1986; **Fellow:** Pediatric Hematology-Oncology, Chldns Hosp 1989; **Fac Appt:** Assoc Clin Prof Ped, Indiana Univ

Yaddanapudi, Ravindranath MD [PHO] - **Spec Exp:** Leukemia; **Hospital:** Chldns Hosp of Michigan; **Address:** Children's Hospital Michigan, Div Hem/Onc, 3901 Beaubien Blvd, Detroit, MI 48201; **Phone:** 313-745-5515; **Board Cert:** Pediatrics 1970; Pediatric Hematology-Oncology 1974; **Med School:** India 1964; **Resid:** Pathology, Western Penn Hosp 1967; Pediatrics, Children's Hosp 1969; **Fellow:** Pediatric Hematology-Oncology, Children's Hosp Michigan 1971; **Fac Appt:** Prof Ped, Wayne State Univ

Great Plains and Mountains

Abromowitch, Minnie MD [PHO] - **Hospital:** Children's Hosp - Omaha; **Address:** Children's Hosp-Dept Ped Hem Oncology, 8200 Dodge St, Omaha, NE 68114; **Phone:** 402-955-3950; **Board Cert:** Pediatrics 1980; Pediatric Hematology-Oncology 1982; **Med School:** Canada 1972; **Resid:** Pediatrics, Hospital for Sick Children 1976; **Fellow:** Pediatric Hematology-Oncology, Univ Manitoba 1978; Pediatric Hematology-Oncology, St Jude Chldns Research Hosp 1980; **Fac Appt:** Assoc Prof Ped, Univ Nebr Coll Med

Bruggers, Carol S MD [PHO] - **Spec Exp:** Brain Tumors; Clinical Trials; **Hospital:** Primary Children's Med Ctr; **Address:** Primary Children's Medical Ctr, 100 N Medical Drive, Salt Lake City, UT 84113; **Phone:** 801-662-4700; **Board Cert:** Pediatrics 2008; Pediatric Hematology-Oncology 2008; **Med School:** Mich State Univ 1984; **Resid:** Pediatrics, Univ Colorado Health Sci Ctr 1987; **Fellow:** Pediatric Hematology-Oncology, Duke Univ Med Ctr 1991; **Fac Appt:** Prof Ped, Univ Utah

Coccia, Peter F MD [PHO] - **Spec Exp:** Bone Marrow Transplant; Leukemia & Lymphoma; Solid Tumors; **Hospital:** Nebraska Med Ctr, Children's Hosp - Omaha; **Address:** Univ Nebr Med Ctr, Dept Pediatrics, 982168 Nebraska Med Ctr, Omaha, NE 68198-2168; **Phone:** 402-559-7257; **Board Cert:** Clinical Pathology 1972; Hematology 1975; Pediatrics 1976; Pediatric Hematology-Oncology 1976; **Med School:** SUNY Upstate Med Univ 1968; **Resid:** Pathology, Upstate Med Ctr 1970; Pediatrics, Univ Minn 1973; **Fellow:** Pediatric Hematology-Oncology, Univ Minn 1974; **Fac Appt:** Prof Ped, Univ Nebr Coll Med

Odom, Lorrie F MD [PHO] - **Spec Exp:** Leukemia; Solid Tumors; Cancer Survivors-Late Effects of Therapy; **Hospital:** Presby - St Luke's Med Ctr, Sky Ridge Med Ctr; **Address:** Rocky Mountain Ped Hem Onc, 1601 E 19th Ave, Ste 6600, Denver, CO 80218; **Phone:** 303-832-2344; **Board Cert:** Pediatrics 1974; Pediatric Hematology-Oncology 1976; **Med School:** Univ Colorado 1969; **Resid:** Pediatrics, Chldns Hosp 1972; **Fellow:** Pediatric Hematology-Oncology, Dana-Farber Cancer Inst 1974; Pediatric Hematology-Oncology, Univ Colorado Med Ctr 1975; **Fac Appt:** Clin Prof Ped, Univ Colorado

Southwest

Abella, Esteban MD [PHO] - **Spec Exp:** Leukemia; Anemia-Aplastic; Neuroblastoma; Bone Marrow Transplant; **Hospital:** Banner Desert Med Ctr, St Joseph's Hosp & Med Ctr - Phoenix; **Address:** 1432 S Dobson, Ste 107, Mesa, AZ 85202; **Phone:** 480-833-1123; **Board Cert:** Pediatric Hematology-Oncology 2009; **Med School:** Dominican Republic 1985; **Resid:** Pediatrics, Chldns Hosp Michigan 1988; **Fellow:** Pediatric Hematology-Oncology, Chldns Hosp Michigan/Wayne St Univ 1991

Berg, Stacey MD [PHO] - **Spec Exp:** Drug Discovery & Development; Brain Tumors; Solid Tumors; **Hospital:** Texas Chldns Hosp; **Address:** Texas Chldns Cancer Ctr, Ped Hem-Onc, 6621 Fannin St, MC 3-3320, Houston, TX 77030; **Phone:** 832-824-4240; **Board Cert:** Pediatrics 2007; Pediatric Hematology-Oncology 2007; **Med School:** Univ Pittsburgh 1985; **Resid:** Pediatrics, Chldns Hosp 1988; **Fellow:** Pediatric Hematology-Oncology, Natl Inst Hlth 1991; **Fac Appt:** Prof Ped, Baylor Coll Med

Blaney, Susan MD [PHO] - **Spec Exp:** Brain Tumors; Neuro-Oncology; Drug Development; Clinical Trials; **Hospital:** Texas Chldns Hosp; **Address:** 6621 Fannin St #CC 1410.00, Houston, TX 77030; **Phone:** 832-822-1482; **Board Cert:** Pediatric Hematology-Oncology 2005; **Med School:** Med Coll OH 1984; **Resid:** Pediatrics, Letterman AMC 1987; **Fellow:** Pediatric Oncology, Walter Reed AMC 1990; **Fac Appt:** Prof Ped, Baylor Coll Med

Dreyer, ZoAnn E MD [PHO] - **Spec Exp:** Cancer Survivors-Late Effects of Therapy; Leukemia in Infants; **Hospital:** Texas Chldns Hosp; **Address:** Texas Childrens Hosp, Clinical Care Ctr, 6701 Fannin Fl 14, MC CC1400, Houston, TX 77030; **Phone:** 832-822-4242; **Board Cert:** Pediatrics 1988; Pediatric Hematology-Oncology 2005; **Med School:** UC Davis 1982; **Resid:** Pediatrics, Baylor Affil Hosps 1985; **Fellow:** Pediatric Hematology-Oncology, Baylor Coll Med 1988; **Fac Appt:** Assoc Prof Ped, Baylor Coll Med

Pediatric Hematology-Oncology

Goldman, Stanton C MD [PHO] - **Spec Exp:** Leukemia; Lymphoma; Stem Cell Transplant; **Hospital:** Med City Dallas Hosp; **Address:** 7777 Forest Ln, Ste D400, Dallas, TX 75230; **Phone:** 972-566-6647; **Board Cert:** Pediatric Hematology-Oncology 2004; **Med School:** Boston Univ 1990; **Resid:** Pediatrics, Chldns Natl Med Ctr 1996; **Fellow:** Pediatric Hematology-Oncology, Johns Hopkins Hosp

Graham, Michael L MD [PHO] - **Spec Exp:** Bone Marrow Transplant; Leukemia; Stem Cell Transplant; **Hospital:** Univ Med Ctr - Tucson; **Address:** Univ Arizona Hlth Science Ctr, 1501 N Campbell Ave, rm 4341, Box 245073, Tucson, AZ 85724-5073; **Phone:** 520-626-6527; **Board Cert:** Pediatrics 1980; Pediatric Hematology-Oncology 1984; **Med School:** Brown Univ 1975; **Resid:** Pediatrics, Johns Hopkins Hosp 1978; Pediatric Hematology-Oncology, Johns Hopkins Hosp 1980; **Fellow:** Medical Oncology, Yale-New Haven Hosp 1982; **Fac Appt:** Assoc Prof Ped, Univ Ariz Coll Med

Meyer, William H MD [PHO] - **Spec Exp:** Sarcoma; Pediatric Cancers; **Hospital:** Chldns Hosp OU Med Ctr; **Address:** OU Childrens Physicians, 940 NE 13th St, J Everett Tower, Fl 3 (Rm MRI 3000), Oklahoma City, OK 73104; **Phone:** 405-271-4412; **Board Cert:** Pediatrics 1980; Pediatric Hematology-Oncology 1980; **Med School:** Jefferson Med Coll 1974; **Resid:** Pediatrics, Wilmington Med Ctr 1977; **Fellow:** Pediatric Hematology-Oncology, Johns Hopkins Hosp 1980; **Fac Appt:** Prof Ped, Univ Okla Coll Med

Scher, Charles D MD [PHO] - **Spec Exp:** Pediatric Cancers; Leukemia; **Hospital:** Tulane Univ Hosp & Clin; **Address:** Tulane Univ Hosp, Dept Pediatrics, 1430 Tulane Ave, Box SL-37, New Orleans, LA 70112; **Phone:** 504-988-5412; **Board Cert:** Pediatrics 1972; **Med School:** Univ Pennsylvania 1965; **Resid:** Pediatrics, Bronx Muni Hosp Ctr 1967; Pediatrics, Chldns Hosp Med Ctr 1972; **Fellow:** Pediatric Hematology-Oncology, Chldns Hosp Med Ctr 1974; **Fac Appt:** Prof Ped, Tulane Univ

Tomlinson, Gail E MD [PHO] - **Spec Exp:** Cancer Survivors-Late Effects of Therapy; Cancer Genetics; Liver Cancer; Kidney Cancer; **Hospital:** Christus Santa Rosa Children's Hosp, Univ Hlth Syst-San Antonio; **Address:** UT HSC at San Antonio, 7703 Floyd Curl Drive, San Antonio, TX 78229; **Phone:** 210-704-3405; **Board Cert:** Pediatrics 2008; Pediatric Hematology-Oncology 2002; **Med School:** Geo Wash Univ 1984; **Resid:** Pediatrics, Chldns Hosp Natl Med Ctr 1987; **Fellow:** Pediatric Hematology-Oncology, MD Anderson Cancer Ctr 1989; Pediatric Hematology-Oncology, Univ Texas SW Med Ctr 1992; **Fac Appt:** Prof Ped, Univ Tex, San Antonio

Winick, Naomi J MD [PHO] - **Spec Exp:** Leukemia; **Hospital:** Chldns Med Ctr of Dallas; **Address:** Ctr for Cancer & Blood Disorders, 1935 Motor St Brides Bldg Fl 3, Dallas, TX 75235-7794; **Phone:** 214-456-2382; **Board Cert:** Pediatrics 1984; Pediatric Hematology-Oncology 1987; **Med School:** Northwestern Univ 1978; **Resid:** Pediatrics, Babies Hosp-Columbia Presbyterian Med Ctr 1981; **Fellow:** Pediatric Hematology-Oncology, Sloan-Kettering Cancer Ctr 1983; **Fac Appt:** Prof Ped, Univ Tex SW, Dallas

West Coast and Pacific

Andrews, Robert G MD [PHO] - **Spec Exp:** Bone Marrow Transplant; Leukemia; Lymphoma; **Hospital:** Chldns Hosp and Regl Med Ctr - Seattle; **Address:** Fred Hutchinson Cancer Rsch Ctr, FHCRC, Box 358080, PO Box 19024, Seattle, WA 98109-1024; **Phone:** 206-667-5000; **Board Cert:** Pediatrics 1984; Pediatric Hematology-Oncology 1984; **Med School:** Univ Minn 1976; **Resid:** Pediatrics, New England Med Ctr 1979; **Fellow:** Pediatric Hematology-Oncology, Children's Hosp Med Ctr 1983; **Fac Appt:** Assoc Prof Ped, Univ Wash

America's Top Doctors® for Cancer 5th Edition

Ducore, Jonathan M MD [PHO] - **Spec Exp:** Brain Tumors; Bone & Soft Tissue Tumors; **Hospital:** UC Davis Med Ctr; **Address:** UC Davis Med Ctr, Dept Pediatrics, Div Pediatric Hematology/Oncology, 2516 Stockton Blvd, Sacramento, CA 95817; **Phone:** 916-734-2781; **Board Cert:** Pediatrics 1978; Pediatric Hematology-Oncology 1978; **Med School:** Duke Univ 1973; **Resid:** Pediatrics, Chldns Med Ctr 1975; **Fellow:** Pediatric Hematology-Oncology, Univ Colorado Med Ctr 1977; Cancer Research, Natl Cancer Inst 1980; **Fac Appt:** Assoc Prof Ped, UC Davis

Finklestein, Jerry Z MD [PHO] - **Spec Exp:** Cancer Survivors-Late Effects of Therapy; Anemias & Red Cell Disorders; **Hospital:** Long Beach Meml Med Ctr, LAC - Harbor - UCLA Med Ctr; **Address:** 2653 Elm Ave, Ste 200, Long Beach, CA 90806-1652; **Phone:** 562-492-1062; **Board Cert:** Pediatrics 1980; Pediatric Hematology-Oncology 1974; **Med School:** McGill Univ 1963; **Resid:** Pediatrics, Montreal Chldns Hosp 1966; **Fellow:** Pediatric Hematology-Oncology, LA Chldns Hosp 1968; **Fac Appt:** Clin Prof Ped, UCLA

Finlay, Jonathan MD [PHO] - **Spec Exp:** Brain Tumors; **Hospital:** Chldns Hosp - Los Angeles, Chldns Hosp - Oakland; **Address:** Chldns Hosp-LA, Ped Hematology/Oncology, 4650 Sunset Blvd, MS 54, Los Angeles, CA 90027-6016; **Phone:** 323-361-8147; **Board Cert:** Pediatrics 1984; Pediatric Hematology-Oncology 1987; **Med School:** England, UK 1973; **Resid:** Pediatrics, Univ Birmingham 1975; Pediatrics, Christie Hosp 1976; **Fellow:** Pediatric Allergy & Immunology, Univ Wisconsin Hosp 1978; Pediatric Hematology-Oncology, Univ Wisconsin Hosp 1980; **Fac Appt:** Prof Ped, USC-Keck School of Medicine

Geyer, J Russell MD [PHO] - **Spec Exp:** Brain Tumors; **Hospital:** Chldns Hosp and Regl Med Ctr - Seattle, Univ Wash Med Ctr; **Address:** Chldns Hosp & Reg Med Ctr - Div Hem/Onc, 4800 Sands Point Way NE, MS B-6553, Seattle, WA 98105; **Phone:** 206-987-2106; **Board Cert:** Pediatrics 1983; Pediatric Hematology-Oncology 1987; **Med School:** Wayne State Univ 1977; **Resid:** Pediatrics, Chldns Hosp Michigan 1980; **Fellow:** Pediatric Hematology-Oncology, Univ Michigan Med Ctr 1981; **Fac Appt:** Prof Ped, Univ Wash

Hawkins, Douglas MD [PHO] - **Spec Exp:** Bone Tumors; Ewing's Sarcoma; Leukemia; Rhabdomyosarcoma; **Hospital:** Chldns Hosp and Regl Med Ctr - Seattle; **Address:** Children's Hosp & Regl Med Ctr, 4800 Sand Point Way NE, Box 5371, MS B6553, Seattle, WA 98105; **Phone:** 206-987-2106; **Board Cert:** Pediatric Hematology-Oncology 2004; **Med School:** Harvard Med Sch 1990; **Resid:** Pediatrics, Univ Washington Med Ctr 1993; **Fellow:** Pediatric Hematology-Oncology, Fred Hutchinson Cancer Research Ctr 1996

Horn, Biljana N MD [PHO] - **Spec Exp:** Bone Marrow Transplant; Brain Tumors; Stem Cell Transplant; Immunotherapy; **Hospital:** UCSF Med Ctr; **Address:** UCSF Med Ctr, Pediatric BMT Program, 505 Parnassus Ave, rm M-659, San Francisco, CA 94143; **Phone:** 415-476-2188; **Board Cert:** Pediatrics 2006; Pediatric Hematology-Oncology 2004; **Med School:** Croatia 1983; **Resid:** Pediatrics, Rainbow Babies & Chldns Hosp 1991; **Fellow:** Pediatric Hematology-Oncology, Natl Cancer Inst 1994; Pediatric Neuro-Oncology, UCSF 1998; **Fac Appt:** Assoc Prof Ped, UCSF

Kadota, Richard P MD [PHO] - **Spec Exp:** Bone Marrow Transplant; Brain Tumors; Clinical Trials; **Hospital:** Rady Children's Hosp - San Diego; **Address:** Children's Hospital San Diego, 3020 Children's Way, MC 5035, San Diego, CA 92123; **Phone:** 858-966-5811; **Board Cert:** Pediatrics 1984; Pediatric Hematology-Oncology 1984; **Med School:** Northwestern Univ 1979; **Resid:** Pediatrics, Mayo Clinic 1983; **Fellow:** Pediatric Hematology-Oncology, Mayo Clinic 1985; **Fac Appt:** Clin Prof Ped, UCSD

Kapoor, Neena MD [PHO] - **Spec Exp:** Bone Marrow Transplant; **Hospital:** Chldns Hosp - Los Angeles; **Address:** Chlds Hosp LA-Rsch Immunology/BMT, 4650 Sunset Blvd, MS 62, Los Angeles, CA 90027; **Phone:** 323-361-2546; **Board Cert:** Pediatrics 1978; **Med School:** India 1972; **Resid:** Pediatrics, Rhode Island Hosp 1976; **Fellow:** Pediatric Hematology-Oncology, Meml Sloan-Kettering Cancer Ctr 1978; **Fac Appt:** Prof Ped, USC Sch Med

Pediatric Hematology-Oncology

Kung, Faith H MD [PHO] - **Spec Exp:** Leukemia & Lymphoma; Bleeding/Coagulation Disorders; Cancer Survivors-Late Effects of Therapy; **Hospital:** Rady Children's Hosp - San Diego; **Address:** UCSD Med Ctr, Div Ped Hem/Oncology, 200 W Arbor Drive, San Diego, CA 92103-8447; **Phone:** 619-543-6844; **Board Cert:** Pediatrics 1967; Pediatric Hematology-Oncology 1974; **Med School:** Univ VA Sch Med 1957; **Resid:** Pediatrics, NC Meml Hosp 1960; **Fellow:** Pediatric Hematology-Oncology, Chldns Hosp/Babies Hosp 1962; **Fac Appt:** Prof Ped, UCSD

Link, Michael P MD [PHO] - **Spec Exp:** Stem Cell Transplant; **Hospital:** Lucile Packard Chldn's Hosp, Stanford Univ Med Ctr; **Address:** 1000 Welch Rd, Ste 300, Palo Alto, CA 94304; **Phone:** 650-723-5535; **Board Cert:** Pediatrics 1979; Pediatric Hematology-Oncology 1980; **Med School:** Stanford Univ 1974; **Resid:** Pediatrics, Chldns Hosp Med Ctr 1976; **Fellow:** Hematology & Oncology, Dana Farber Cancer Inst 1979; **Fac Appt:** Prof Ped, Stanford Univ

Marina, Neyssa MD [PHO] - **Spec Exp:** Sarcoma; Cancer Survivors-Late Effects of Therapy; Germ Cell Tumors; **Hospital:** Lucile Packard Chldn's Hosp; **Address:** Pediatric Hematology & Oncology, 725 Walsh Rd-Clinic E, Palo Alto, CA 94304; **Phone:** 650-497-8953; **Board Cert:** Pediatrics 1987; Pediatric Hematology-Oncology 2005; **Med School:** Puerto Rico 1983; **Resid:** Pediatrics, Univ Pediatric Hosp 1986; **Fellow:** Pediatric Hematology-Oncology, St Jude Children's Hosp 1989; **Fac Appt:** Prof Ped, Stanford Univ

Matthay, Katherine K MD [PHO] - **Spec Exp:** Neuroblastoma; Bone Marrow & Stem Cell Transplant; **Hospital:** UCSF Med Ctr; **Address:** UCSF, Dept Ped Onc, 505 Parnassus Ave, Box 0106, San Francisco, CA 94143; **Phone:** 415-476-0603; **Board Cert:** Pediatrics 1979; Pediatric Hematology-Oncology 1980; **Med School:** Univ Pennsylvania 1973; **Resid:** Pediatrics, Univ Colorado 1976; **Fellow:** Pediatric Hematology-Oncology, UCSF 1979; **Fac Appt:** Prof Ped, UCSF

Nicholson, Henry Stacy MD [PHO] - **Spec Exp:** Brain Tumors; Cancer Survivors-Late Effects of Therapy; **Hospital:** Doernbecher Chldns Hosp/OHSU, OR Hlth & Sci Univ; **Address:** OR Hlth Scis Univ, 707 SW Gaines Rd, CDRCP, Portland, OR 97239; **Phone:** 503-494-4265; **Board Cert:** Pediatric Hematology-Oncology 2007; **Med School:** Med Coll GA 1985; **Resid:** Pediatrics, Chldns National Med Ctr 1988; **Fellow:** Pediatric Hematology-Oncology, Chldns National Med Ctr 1991; **Fac Appt:** Prof Ped, Oregon Hlth Sci Univ

Pendergrass, Thomas W MD [PHO] - **Spec Exp:** Sarcoma; Leukemia & Lymphoma; Retinoblastoma; **Hospital:** Chldns Hosp and Regl Med Ctr - Seattle, Univ Wash Med Ctr; **Address:** Children's Hosp Regional Med Ctr, 4800 Sandpoint Way NE, Box 5371, MS B6553, Seattle, WA 98105; **Phone:** 206-987-2106; **Board Cert:** Pediatrics 1978; **Med School:** Univ Tenn Coll Med, Memphis 1971; **Resid:** Pediatrics, Children's Memorial Hosp 1973; **Fellow:** Pediatric Hematology-Oncology, Children's Hosp Med Ctr 1977; **Fac Appt:** Prof Ped, Univ Wash

Rosenthal, Joseph MD [PHO] - **Spec Exp:** Bone Marrow Transplant; Clinical Trials; **Hospital:** City of Hope Natl Med Ctr & Beckman Rsch (page 69); **Address:** City of Hope Med Ctr, 1500 E Duarte Rd, Duarte, CA 91010; **Phone:** 626-256-4673 x68442; **Board Cert:** Pediatrics 2003; Pediatric Hematology-Oncology 2004; **Med School:** Israel 1984; **Resid:** Pediatrics, Soroka Med Ctr 1988; Pediatrics, Chldn Hosp 1995; **Fellow:** Pediatric Hematology-Oncology, Univ Colorado Affil Hosp 1991; Pediatric Hematology-Oncology, Chldn Hosp 1994; **Fac Appt:** Assoc Prof Ped, USC-Keck School of Medicine

Russo, Carolyn MD [PHO] - **Spec Exp:** Brain Tumors; Cancer Survivors-Late Effects of Therapy; Palliative Care; **Hospital:** Kaiser Permanente Santa Clara Med Ctr; **Address:** 710 Lawrence Expwy, Dept 160, Santa Clara, CA 95051; **Phone:** 408-554-9810; **Board Cert:** Pediatric Hematology-Oncology 2005; **Med School:** UCLA 1984; **Resid:** Pediatrics, Harbor-UCLA Med Ctr 1987; **Fellow:** Pediatric Hematology-Oncology, Stanford Med Ctr 1990

Sakamoto, Kathleen M MD [PHO] - **Spec Exp:** Leukemia; Pediatric Cancers; Bone Marrow Transplant; **Hospital:** Mattel Chldns Hosp at UCLA; **Address:** Mattel Chldns Hosp UCLA, Div Hem-Onc, 10833 Le Conte Ave, Los Angeles, CA 90095-1752; **Phone:** 310-825-6708; **Board Cert:** Pediatrics 2007; Pediatric Hematology-Oncology 2007; **Med School:** Univ Cincinnati 1985; **Resid:** Pediatrics, Children's Hosp 1988; **Fellow:** Pediatric Hematology-Oncology, Children's Hosp 1991; **Fac Appt:** Prof Ped, UCLA

Siegel, Stuart E MD [PHO] - **Spec Exp:** Leukemia & Lymphoma; Infections in Cancer Patients; Psychosocial Support in Childhood Cancer; Solid Tumors; **Hospital:** Chldns Hosp - Los Angeles, Ventura Cnty Med Ctr; **Address:** Childrens Hospital, 4650 Sunset Blvd, MS 54, Los Angeles, CA 90027-6062; **Phone:** 323-361-2205; **Board Cert:** Pediatrics 1973; Pediatric Hematology-Oncology 1976; **Med School:** Boston Univ 1967; **Resid:** Pediatrics, Univ Minnesota Hosps 1969; **Fellow:** Pediatric Hematology-Oncology, Natl Cancer Inst 1972; **Fac Appt:** Prof Ped, USC-Keck School of Medicine

Wilkinson, Robert W MD [PHO] - **Hospital:** Kapiolani Med Ctr for Women & Chldn; **Address:** Kapiolani Med Ctr for Women & Children, 1319 Punahou St, Ste 1050, Honolulu, HI 96826; **Phone:** 808-942-8144; **Board Cert:** Pediatrics 1986; Pediatric Hematology-Oncology 1986; **Med School:** Tulane Univ 1967; **Resid:** Pediatrics, LAC-USC Med Ctr 1971; **Fellow:** Pediatric Hematology-Oncology, LAC-USC Med Ctr 1972; **Fac Appt:** Assoc Prof Ped, Univ Hawaii JA Burns Sch Med

PEDIATRIC ALLERGY & IMMUNOLOGY

Mid Atlantic

Kamani, Naynesh R MD [PA&I] - **Spec Exp:** Stem Cell Transplant; Immunotherapy; Bone Marrow Transplant; **Hospital:** Chldns Natl Med Ctr; **Address:** Chldns Natl Med Ctr, Div Hematology, 111 Michigan Ave NW, Washington, DC 20010; **Phone:** 202-476-2800; **Board Cert:** Pediatrics 1983; Pediatric Allergy & Immunology 1983; Diagnostic Lab Immunology 1986; **Med School:** Ethiopia 1975; **Resid:** Pediatrics, Downstate Med Ctr-Kings Co Hosp 1981; **Fellow:** Pediatric Allergy & Immunology, Chldns Hosp 1983; **Fac Appt:** Prof Ped, Geo Wash Univ

West Coast and Pacific

Cowan, Morton J MD [PA&I] - **Spec Exp:** Bone Marrow Transplant; **Hospital:** UCSF Med Ctr; **Address:** UCSF Med Ctr, Peds BMT Program, 505 Parnassus Ave, rm M659, San Francisco, CA 94143-1278; **Phone:** 415-476-2188; **Board Cert:** Pediatrics 1981; Allergy & Immunology 1983; **Med School:** Univ Pennsylvania 1970; **Resid:** Surgery, Duke Univ Med Ctr 1972; Pediatrics, UCSF Med Ctr 1977; **Fellow:** Research, Natl Inst Hlth 1975; Immunology, UCSF Med Ctr 1979; **Fac Appt:** Prof Ped, UCSF

PEDIATRIC CARDIOLOGY

Mid Atlantic

Steinherz, Laurel MD [PCd] - **Spec Exp:** Cardiac Effects of Cancer/Cancer Therapy; **Hospital:** Meml Sloan-Kettering Cancer Ctr (page 76), NY-Presby Hosp/Weill Cornell (page 79); **Address:** 1275 York Avenue, New York, NY 10065; **Phone:** 212-639-8103; **Board Cert:** Pediatrics 1976; Pediatric Cardiology 1978; **Med School:** Albert Einstein Coll Med 1970; **Resid:** Pediatrics, Chldns Hosp 1972; **Fellow:** Pediatric Cardiology, NY Hosp-Cornell Med Ctr 1975; **Fac Appt:** Prof Ped, Cornell Univ-Weill Med Coll

PEDIATRIC ENDOCRINOLOGY

Mid Atlantic

Sklar, Charles A MD [PEn] - **Spec Exp:** Cancer Survivors-Late Effects of Therapy; Growth Disorders in Childhood Cancer; **Hospital:** Meml Sloan-Kettering Cancer Ctr (page 76); **Address:** 1275 York Avenue, New York, NY 10065; **Phone:** 800-525-2225; **Board Cert:** Pediatrics 1979; Pediatric Endocrinology 1980; **Med School:** USC Sch Med 1974; **Resid:** Pediatrics, Childrens Hosp 1976; **Fellow:** Pediatric Endocrinology, UCSF Med Ctr 1979; **Fac Appt:** Assoc Prof Ped, Cornell Univ-Weill Med Coll

Southeast

Meacham, Lillian R MD [PEn] - **Spec Exp:** Growth Disorders in Childhood Cancer; Cancer Survivors-Late Effects of Therapy; **Hospital:** Chldns Hlthcare Atlanta @ Egleston, Emory Univ Hosp; **Address:** Emory Childrens Ctr, 2015 Uppergate Drive, Atlanta, GA 30322; **Phone:** 404-778-2400; **Board Cert:** Pediatrics 2006; Pediatric Endocrinology 2006; **Med School:** Emory Univ 1984; **Resid:** Pediatrics, Emory Univ Hosp 1987; **Fellow:** Pediatric Endocrinology, Emory Univ Hosp 1990; **Fac Appt:** Assoc Prof Ped, Emory Univ

Midwest

Zimmerman, Donald MD [PEn] - **Spec Exp:** Growth Disorders in Childhood Cancer; Thyroid Cancer; Thyroid Disorders; **Hospital:** Children's Mem Hosp; **Address:** Children's Memorial Hosp, 2300 Children's Plaza, Div Endocrinology, Box 54, Chicago, IL 60614; **Phone:** 773-327-7740; **Board Cert:** Internal Medicine 1977; Endocrinology 1979; Pediatrics 1983; Pediatric Endocrinology 2001; **Med School:** Univ IL Coll Med 1974; **Resid:** Internal Medicine, Johns Hopkins Hosp 1977; Pediatrics, Mayo Clinic 1981; **Fellow:** Endocrinology, Diabetes & Metabolism, Mayo Clinic 1980; **Fac Appt:** Prof Ped, Northwestern Univ

PEDIATRIC OTOLARYNGOLOGY

New England

McGill, Trevor J MD [PO] - **Spec Exp:** Head & Neck Tumors; **Hospital:** Children's Hospital - Boston; **Address:** Childrens Hosp, Dept Otolaryngology, 300 Longwood Ave, MS LO-367, Boston, MA 02115; **Phone:** 617-355-8589; **Board Cert:** Otolaryngology 1988; **Med School:** Ireland 1967; **Resid:** Otolaryngology, Royal Natl Throat Nose & Ear Hosp 1974; **Fellow:** Otolaryngology, Mass Eye & Ear Infirm 1976; **Fac Appt:** Prof Oto, Harvard Med Sch

West Coast and Pacific

Crockett, Dennis M MD [PO] - **Spec Exp:** Head & Neck Cancer; **Hospital:** USC Univ Hosp; **Address:** 26726 Crown Valley Pkwy, Ste 200, Mission Viejo, CA 92691; **Phone:** 949-364-4361; **Board Cert:** Otolaryngology 1985; **Med School:** USC Sch Med 1979; **Resid:** Otolaryngology, LAC-USC Med Ctr 1984; **Fellow:** Pediatrics, Boston Chldns Hosp 1985; **Fac Appt:** Assoc Prof Oto, USC Sch Med

Geller, Kenneth Allen MD [PO] - **Spec Exp:** Head & Neck Cancer; Pediatric Airway Disorders; **Hospital:** Chldns Hosp - Los Angeles, Huntington Memorial Hosp; **Address:** Chldns Hosp, Div Otolaryngology, 4650 Sunset Blvd, MS 58, Los Angeles, CA 90027; **Phone:** 323-361-2145; **Board Cert:** Otolaryngology 1978; **Med School:** USC Sch Med 1972; **Resid:** Surgery, Wadsworth VA Hosp 1975; Otolaryngology, UCLA Hlth Scis Ctr 1978; **Fellow:** Pediatric Otolaryngology, Chldns Hosp 1979; **Fac Appt:** Assoc Clin Prof Oto, USC Sch Med

PEDIATRIC PULMONOLOGY

West Coast and Pacific

Cooper, Dan M MD [PPul] - **Hospital:** Chldns Hosp Orange Co; **Address:** 455 S Main St, Orange, CA 92868; **Phone:** 714-532-7983; **Board Cert:** Pediatrics 1980; Pediatric Pulmonology 2002; **Med School:** UCSF 1974; **Resid:** Internal Medicine, Hadassah Hosp; Pediatrics, Children's Hosp Med Ctr; **Fellow:** Pediatric Pulmonology, Babies' Hosp-Columbia Univ; **Fac Appt:** Prof Ped, UC Irvine

PEDIATRIC SURGERY

New England

Latchaw, Laurie MD [PS] - **Spec Exp:** Thoracic Surgery; Cancer Surgery; Neonatal Surgery; **Hospital:** Dartmouth - Hitchcock Med Ctr; **Address:** DHMC, Clinic 6M, One Medical Center Drive, Lebanon, NH 03756; **Phone:** 603-653-9883; **Board Cert:** Surgery 2001; Pediatric Surgery 2003; **Med School:** Rush Med Coll 1976; **Resid:** Surgery, Univ Texas 1981; **Fellow:** Pediatric Surgery, Montreal Chldns Hosp 1983; **Fac Appt:** Assoc Prof S, Dartmouth Med Sch

Shamberger, Robert C MD [PS] - **Spec Exp:** Cancer Surgery; **Hospital:** Children's Hospital - Boston; **Address:** Children's Hosp-Dept Surgery, 300 Longwood Ave, Fegan - 3, Boston, MA 02115; **Phone:** 617-355-8326; **Board Cert:** Surgery 2002; Surgical Critical Care 1999; Pediatric Surgery 2003; **Med School:** Harvard Med Sch 1975; **Resid:** Surgery, Massachusetts Genl Hosp 1978; Pediatric Surgery, Children's Hosp 1985; **Fellow:** Surgical Oncology, NCI-Surgical Branch 1980; **Fac Appt:** Prof S, Harvard Med Sch

Mid Atlantic

Alexander, Frederick MD [PS] - **Spec Exp:** Solid Tumors; **Hospital:** Hackensack Univ Med Ctr (page 73); **Address:** Joseph M Sanzari Chldns Hosp-HUMC, 30 Prospect Ave, Ste PC311, Hackensack, NJ 07601; **Phone:** 201-996-2921; **Board Cert:** Pediatric Surgery 1999; **Med School:** Columbia P&S 1977; **Resid:** Surgery, Brigham-Womens Hosp 1984; **Fellow:** Pediatric Surgery, Chldns Hosp 1986; **Fac Appt:** Clin Prof S

Colombani, Paul M MD [PS] - **Spec Exp:** Thoracic Surgery; Transplant-Kidney; Transplant-Liver; Cancer Surgery; **Hospital:** Johns Hopkins Hosp; **Address:** 600 N Wolfe St, Harvey 319, Baltimore, MD 21287; **Phone:** 410-955-2717; **Board Cert:** Surgery 2003; Pediatric Surgery 2003; **Med School:** Univ KY Coll Med 1976; **Resid:** Surgery, Geo Wash Univ Hosp 1981; **Fellow:** Pediatric Surgery, Johns Hopkins Hosp 1983; **Fac Appt:** Prof S, Johns Hopkins Univ

Pediatric Surgery

Ginsburg, Howard B MD [PS] - **Spec Exp:** Neonatal Surgery; Tumor Surgery; Pediatric Urology; Gastrointestinal Surgery; **Hospital:** NYU Langone Med Ctr (page 80), Bellevue Hosp Ctr; **Address:** NYU Medical Ctr, Div Pediatric Surgery, 530 1st Ave, Ste 10W, New York, NY 10016-6402; **Phone:** 212-263-7391; **Board Cert:** Pediatric Surgery 2001; **Med School:** Univ Cincinnati 1972; **Resid:** Surgery, NYU-Bellvue Hosp 1977; Pediatric Surgery, Columbia-Presby Med Ctr 1979; **Fellow:** Pediatric Surgery, Mass Genl Hosp 1980; **Fac Appt:** Assoc Prof S, NYU Sch Med

La Quaglia, Michael MD [PS] - **Spec Exp:** Cancer Surgery; Neuroblastoma; Liver Tumors; Colon & Rectal Cancer; **Hospital:** Meml Sloan-Kettering Cancer Ctr (page 76), NY-Presby Hosp/Weill Cornell (page 79); **Address:** 1275 York Ave, Ste H1315, New York, NY 10065; **Phone:** 212-639-7002; **Board Cert:** Surgery 2003; Pediatric Surgery 2007; **Med School:** UMDNJ-NJ Med Sch, Newark 1976; **Resid:** Surgery, Mass Genl Hosp 1983; **Fellow:** Cardiothoracic Surgery, Broadgreen Ctr 1984; Pediatric Surgery, Chldns Hosp 1985; **Fac Appt:** Prof S, Cornell Univ-Weill Med Coll

Stolar, Charles J H MD [PS] - **Spec Exp:** Pediatric Cancers; Neonatal Surgery; **Hospital:** NYPresby-Morgan Stanley Children's Hosp (page 79); **Address:** Morgan Stanley Chldns Hosp NY-Presby, 3959 Broadway, Fl 2 - rm 215 North, New York, NY 10032; **Phone:** 212-342-8586; **Board Cert:** Surgery 2001; Pediatric Surgery 2007; **Med School:** Georgetown Univ 1974; **Resid:** Surgery, Univ Illinois Hosp 1980; **Fellow:** Pediatric Surgery, Chldns Hosp Natl Med Ctr 1982; **Fac Appt:** Prof S, Columbia P&S

Southeast

Davidoff, Andrew M MD [PS] - **Spec Exp:** Neuroblastoma; Cancer Surgery; **Hospital:** St Jude Children's Research Hosp, Le Bonheur Chldns Med Ctr; **Address:** St Jude Chldns Rsch Hosp, Dept Surg, 262 Danny Thomas Pl, MS 133, Memphis, TN 38105; **Phone:** 901-495-4060; **Board Cert:** Surgery 2005; Pediatric Surgery 2007; **Med School:** Univ Pennsylvania 1987; **Resid:** Surgery, Duke Med Ctr 1994; **Fellow:** Pediatric Surgery, Chldns Hosp 1996; **Fac Appt:** Assoc Prof S, Univ Tenn Coll Med, Memphis

Morgan III, Walter M MD [PS] - **Spec Exp:** Germ Cell Tumors; Neuroblastoma; Bone Cancer; **Hospital:** Vanderbilt Children's Hosp, Vanderbilt Univ Med Ctr; **Address:** Vanderbilt Children's Hosp-Dept Ped Surgery, 2200 Children's Way, Ste 4150, Nashville, TN 37232-9780; **Phone:** 615-936-1050; **Board Cert:** Pediatric Surgery 2001; **Med School:** Vanderbilt Univ 1982; **Resid:** Surgery, Johns Hopkins Hosp 1988; **Fellow:** Pediatric Surgery, Johns Hopkins Hosp 1990; **Fac Appt:** Asst Prof S, Vanderbilt Univ

Paidas, Charles N MD [PS] - **Spec Exp:** Pediatric Cancers; **Hospital:** Tampa Genl Hosp, Univ of S FL - Tampa; **Address:** Tampa Genl Hosp, Div Ped Surgery, 1 Tampa General Cir, rm G-441, Tampa, FL 33606; **Phone:** 813-259-0929; **Board Cert:** Surgery 1999; Pediatric Surgery 2001; Surgical Critical Care 2002; **Med School:** NY Med Coll 1981; **Resid:** Surgery, NY Med Coll Affil Hosps 1987; **Fellow:** Pediatric Surgery, Johns Hopkins Hosp 1991; **Fac Appt:** Prof S, Univ S Fla Coll Med

Rice, Henry MD [PS] - **Spec Exp:** Neonatal Surgery; Cancer Surgery; **Hospital:** Duke Univ Med Ctr; **Address:** Duke Univ Med Ctr, Dept Ped Surg, DUMC, Box 3815, Durham, NC 27710; **Phone:** 919-681-5077; **Board Cert:** Surgery 2006; Pediatric Surgery 2000; **Med School:** Yale Univ 1988; **Resid:** Surgery, Univ Wash Affil Hosps 1996; **Fellow:** Pediatric Surgery, Chldns Hosp of Buffalo 1998; **Fac Appt:** Assoc Prof S, Duke Univ

Ricketts, Richard R MD [PS] - **Spec Exp:** Neonatal Surgery; Cancer Surgery; Gastrointestinal Surgery; **Hospital:** Chldns Hlthcare Atlanta @ Egleston; **Address:** 1975 Century Blvd, Ste 6, Atlanta, GA 30345; **Phone:** 404-982-9938; **Board Cert:** Surgery 2004; Pediatric Surgery 2001; **Med School:** Northwestern Univ 1973; **Resid:** Surgery, LAC-USC Med Ctr 1978; **Fellow:** Pediatric Surgery, Chldns Meml Hosp 1980; **Fac Appt:** Prof S, Emory Univ

Shochat, Stephen J MD [PS] - **Spec Exp:** Cancer Surgery; **Hospital:** St Jude Children's Research Hosp; **Address:** St Jude Childrens Research Hosp, Dept Surgery, 262 Danny Thomas Pl, Memphis, TN 38105; **Phone:** 901-495-4060; **Board Cert:** Surgery 1969; Thoracic Surgery 1975; Pediatric Surgery 2005; **Med School:** Med Coll VA 1963; **Resid:** Surgery, Barnes Hosp 1968; Pediatric Surgery, Boston Chldns Hosp 1970; **Fellow:** Thoracic Surgery, George Washington Univ Med Ctr 1974; **Fac Appt:** Prof S, Univ Tenn Coll Med, Memphis

Midwest

Aiken, John J MD [PS] - **Spec Exp:** Tumor Surgery; Solid Tumors; **Hospital:** Chldns Hosp - Wisconsin; **Address:** 999 N 92nd St, Ste C-320, Milwaukee, WI 53226; **Phone:** 414-266-6550; **Board Cert:** Surgery 2004; Pediatric Surgery 2000; **Med School:** Univ Cincinnati 1984; **Resid:** Surgery, Mass Genl Hosp 1991; **Fellow:** Pediatric Surgery, Chldns Hosp 1993; **Fac Appt:** Assoc Prof S, Med Coll Wisc

Ehrlich, Peter F MD [PS] - **Spec Exp:** Pediatric Cancers; Wilms' Tumor; Thyroid Cancer; **Hospital:** Mott Chldns Hosp, Mich State Univ-Hurley Med Ctr; **Address:** Mott Children's Hospital, 1500 E Medical Center Drive, rm F3970, Ann Arbor, MI 48109-0245; **Phone:** 734-764-4151; **Board Cert:** Surgery 1997; Pediatric Surgery 2000; **Med School:** Canada 1989; **Resid:** Surgery, Univ Toronto Med Ctr 1996; **Fellow:** Pediatric Surgery, Children's Natl Med Ctr 1998; **Fac Appt:** Assoc Clin Prof S, Univ Mich Med Sch

Rescorla, Frederick J MD [PS] - **Spec Exp:** Cancer Surgery; Head & Neck Cancer; Gastrointestinal Surgery; **Hospital:** Riley Hosp for Children (page 74); **Address:** 702 Barnhill Drive, Ste 2500, Indianapolis, IN 46202; **Phone:** 317-274-4681; **Board Cert:** Surgery 2004; Surgical Critical Care 1998; Pediatric Surgery 2007; **Med School:** Univ Wisc 1981; **Resid:** Surgery, Indiana Univ Med Ctr 1986; Pediatric Surgery, Indiana Univ Med Ctr 1988; **Fac Appt:** Prof S, Indiana Univ

Warner, Brad MD [PS] - **Spec Exp:** Gastrointestinal Surgery; Neonatal Surgery; Cancer Surgery; **Hospital:** St Louis Chldns Hosp; **Address:** 1 Children's Pl, Ste 5S40, St. Louis, MO 63110; **Phone:** 314-454-6066; **Board Cert:** Surgery 1998; Pediatric Surgery 2001; **Med School:** Univ MO-Kansas City 1982; **Resid:** Surgery, Univ Cincinnati Med Ctr 1989; **Fellow:** Pediatric Surgery, Chldns Hosp Med Ctr 1991; **Fac Appt:** Prof S, Univ Cincinnati

Great Plains and Mountains

Meyers, Rebecka L MD [PS] - **Spec Exp:** Transplant-Liver; Tumor Surgery; Biliary Surgery; Pancreatic Surgery; **Hospital:** Primary Children's Med Ctr, Univ Utah Hosps and Clins; **Address:** Primary Chlds Med Ctr, Dept Ped Surg, 100 N Mario Capecchi Drive, Ste 2600, Salt Lake City, UT 84113-1103; **Phone:** 801-662-2950; **Board Cert:** Surgery 2003; Pediatric Surgery 2005; **Med School:** Oregon Hlth Sci Univ 1985; **Resid:** Surgery, UCSF Med Ctr 1990; **Fellow:** Research, Cardio Rsch Inst-UCSF 1992; Pediatric Surgery, St Christophers Hosp for Chldn 1994; **Fac Appt:** Assoc Prof S, Univ Utah

Pediatric Surgery

Ziegler, Moritz M MD [PS] - **Spec Exp:** Gastrointestinal Surgery; Neuroblastoma; Tumor Surgery; **Hospital:** Chldn's Hosp - Aurora, The, Univ Colorado Hosp; **Address:** Chldns Hosp, Dept Surgery, 13123 E 16th Ave, Box 323, Aurora, CO 80045; **Phone:** 720-777-6524; **Board Cert:** Surgery 1975; Pediatric Surgery 2007; **Med School:** Univ Mich Med Sch 1968; **Resid:** Surgery, Univ Penn Hosp 1975; Pediatric Surgery, Chldns Hosp 1977; **Fellow:** Surgical Oncology, Amer Oncologic Hosp 1975; **Fac Appt:** Prof S, Univ Colorado

Southwest

Jackson, Richard J MD [PS] - **Spec Exp:** Pediatric Cancers; Neonatal Surgery; Robotic Surgery; **Hospital:** Cook Chldns Med Ctr; **Address:** 1433 W Humbolt, Fort Worth, TX 76104; **Phone:** 682-885-7080; **Board Cert:** Surgery 1997; Pediatric Surgery 2001; Surgical Critical Care 1998; **Med School:** W VA Univ 1983; **Resid:** Surgery, W Va Univ Hosps 1988; Pediatric Surgery, Chldns Hosp 1989; **Fellow:** Surgical Critical Care, Chldns Hosp-Univ Pittsburgh 1990; Pediatric Surgery, Chldns Hosp-Univ Pittsburgh 1992

Nuchtern, Jed MD [PS] - **Spec Exp:** Thoracic Surgery; Cancer Surgery; Laparoscopic Surgery; **Hospital:** Texas Chldns Hosp, Ben Taub Genl Hosp; **Address:** Texas Children's Hosp, 6621 Fannin St, MC CC650, Houston, TX 77030; **Phone:** 832-822-3135; **Board Cert:** Surgery 2003; Surgical Critical Care 2002; Pediatric Surgery 2007; **Med School:** Harvard Med Sch 1985; **Resid:** Surgery, Univ Washington 1992; Pediatric Surgery, Baylor Coll Med 1995; **Fellow:** Cellular Molecular Biology, Natl Inst Hlth 1990; **Fac Appt:** Prof S, Baylor Coll Med

Skinner, Michael A MD [PS] - **Spec Exp:** Endocrine Cancers; Thyroid Cancer; **Hospital:** UT Southwestern Med Ctr at Dallas; **Address:** UT Southwestern Med Ctr at Dallas, 1935 Medical District Drive, Ste B3250, Dallas, TX 75235; **Phone:** 214-456-6040; **Board Cert:** Surgery 2000; Pediatric Surgery 2003; **Med School:** Rush Med Coll 1984; **Resid:** Surgery, Duke Univ Med Ctr 1991; **Fellow:** Pediatric Surgery, Indiana Univ 1993; **Fac Appt:** Assoc Prof S, Univ Tex SW, Dallas

West Coast and Pacific

Farmer, Diana MD [PS] - **Spec Exp:** Pediatric Cancers; Pediatric Cancer Surgery; **Hospital:** CA Pacific Med Ctr - Pacific Campus, UCSF Med Ctr; **Address:** 400 Parnassus Ave, rm A123, San Francisco, CA 94143; **Phone:** 415-476-2538; **Board Cert:** Surgery 2001; Pediatric Surgery 2005; **Med School:** Univ Wash 1983; **Resid:** Surgery, UCSF 1993; **Fellow:** Pediatric Surgery, Chldn's Hosp 1995; **Fac Appt:** Assoc Prof S, UCSF

Sawin, Robert S MD [PS] - **Spec Exp:** Pediatric Cancers; Thoracic Surgery; **Hospital:** Chldns Hosp and Regl Med Ctr - Seattle; **Address:** Chldns Hosp & Regl Med Ctr, 4800 Sand Point Way NE, Box 5371, Seattle, WA 98105-0371; **Phone:** 206-987-2039; **Board Cert:** Surgery 1999; Surgical Critical Care 2001; Pediatric Surgery 1999; **Med School:** Univ Pittsburgh 1982; **Resid:** Surgery, Brigham Women's Hosp 1987; **Fellow:** Pediatric Surgery, Chldns Hosp 1989; **Fac Appt:** Prof S, Univ Wash

PEDIATRICS

Mid Atlantic

Oeffinger, Kevin MD [Ped] - **Spec Exp:** Cancer Survivors-Late Effects of Therapy; **Hospital:** Meml Sloan-Kettering Cancer Ctr (page 76); **Address:** 1275 York Ave, Box 396, New York, NY 10065; **Phone:** 800-525-2225; **Board Cert:** Family Medicine 2000; **Med School:** Univ Tex, San Antonio 1984; **Resid:** Family Medicine, Baylor Coll Med 1985; **Fellow:** Family Medicine, Fam Practice Faculty Dev Ctr 1999; Natl Cancer Inst 2000

Southwest

Kleinerman, Eugenie S MD [Ped] - **Spec Exp:** Ewing's Sarcoma; Cancer Survivors-Late Effects of Therapy; **Hospital:** UT MD Anderson Cancer Ctr; **Address:** MD Anderson Cancer Ctr, Dept Pediatrics, 1515 Holcombe Blvd, Unit 87, Houston, TX 77030; **Phone:** 713-792-8110; **Board Cert:** Pediatrics 1980; **Med School:** Duke Univ 1975; **Resid:** Pediatrics, Chldns Hosp-Natl Med Ctr 1978; **Fellow:** Immunology, Natl Cancer Inst 1981; **Fac Appt:** Prof Ped, Univ Tex, Houston

NYU Cancer Institute
NYU LANGONE MEDICAL CENTER

NYU Clinical Cancer Center
160 East 34th Street
New York, New York 10016
www.nyuci.org/atcd

NYU Langone Medical Center
550 First Avenue
(at 31st Street)
New York, New York 10016
www.nyumc.org/atcd

Stephen D. Hassenfeld
Children's Center
for Cancer and Blood
Disorders
160 East 32nd Street
New York, New York 10016
www.nyumc.org/hassenfeld

A Collaborative Approach
The NYU Cancer Institute, an NCI designated center, is a "matrix cancer center" without walls operating within the larger NYU Langone Medical Center. With over 175 members and a research funding base of over $81 million, this structure strengthens our capabilities to forge collaborations across medical and scientific disciplines, which translates to comprehensive care for our patients and discoveries that will influence the future of this disease.

Renowned Expertise
Team members' compassion and expertise help patients better manage the symptoms of their disease as well as their special needs. Our highly skilled Magnet™ nursing team not only plays a pivotal role in coordinating direct patient care, but is also a source of invaluable patient education.

A Patient-Focused Setting
The NYU Clinical Cancer Center, with over 70 faculty members from various disciplines at the New York University School of Medicine, is the principal outpatient facility of the Cancer Institute and serves as home for our patients and their caregivers. The center and its multidisciplinary team of experts provide access to the latest treatment options and clinical trials along with a variety of programs in cancer prevention, screening, diagnostics, genetic counseling, and supportive services. When it comes to kids and cancer, the Stephen D. Hassenfeld Children's Center for Cancer and Blood Disorders offers not just innovation but insight. As a leading member of the NCI-sponsored Children's Oncology Group, our physicians are known for developing new ways to treat childhood cancer. Our affiliation with Bellevue Hospital, the oldest public hospital in the country, affords clinically distinctive opportunities to learn and care for patients with cancer by observing its presentation and behavior in a variety of patient groups.

Cancer Institute
NYU LANGONE MEDICAL CENTER

Plastic Surgery

A plastic surgeon deals with the repair, reconstruction or replacement of physical defects of form or function involving the skin, musculoskeletal system, craniomaxillofacial structures, hand, extremities, breast and trunk and external genitalia. He/she uses aesthetic surgical principles not only to improve undesirable qualities of normal structures (commonly called "cosmetic surgery") but in all reconstructive procedures as well.

A plastic surgeon possesses special knowledge and skill in the design and surgery of grafts, flaps, free tissue transfer and replantation. Competence in the management of complex wounds, the use of implantable materials, and in tumor surgery is required.

Training Required: Five to seven years

Plastic Surgery within the Head and Neck: A plastic surgeon with additional training in plastic and reconstructive procedures within the head, face, neck and associated structures, including cutaneous head and neck oncology and reconstruction, management of maxillofacial trauma, soft tissue repair and neural surgery.

The field is diverse and involved a wide range of patients, from the newborn to the aged. While both cosmetic and reconstructive surgery are practiced, there are many additional procedures which interface with them.

Surgery of the Hand:
(See Hand Surgery under Orthopaedic Surgery)

PLASTIC SURGERY

New England

Collins, Dale MD [PlS] - **Spec Exp:** Breast Cancer; Breast Reconstruction; **Hospital:** Dartmouth - Hitchcock Med Ctr; **Address:** Div Plastic Surgery, 1 Medical Center Drive, Lebanon, NH 03756; **Phone:** 603-653-3500; **Board Cert:** Plastic Surgery 2007; **Med School:** Emory Univ 1989; **Resid:** Plastic Surgery, Washington Univ Med Ctr 1994; **Fellow:** Microsurgery, Washington Univ Med Ctr 1995; **Fac Appt:** Prof S, Dartmouth Med Sch

May Jr, James W MD [PlS] - **Spec Exp:** Breast Reconstruction; **Hospital:** Mass Genl Hosp; **Address:** Mass Genl Hosp, 15 Parkman St, WACC 435, Boston, MA 02114; **Phone:** 617-726-8220; **Board Cert:** Surgery 1975; Plastic Surgery 1977; **Med School:** Northwestern Univ 1969; **Resid:** Plastic Surgery, Mass Genl Hosp 1975; **Fellow:** Hand Surgery, Univ Louisville 1975; **Fac Appt:** Prof S, Harvard Med Sch

Stadelmann, Wayne K MD [PlS] - **Spec Exp:** Melanoma-Head & Neck; Breast Reconstruction; **Hospital:** Concord Hospital, Elliot Hosp; **Address:** 248 Pleasant St, Ste 201, Concord, NH 03301; **Phone:** 603-224-5200; **Board Cert:** Plastic Surgery 1999; **Med School:** Univ Chicago-Pritzker Sch Med 1990; **Resid:** Surgery, Univ Chicago Hosps 1994; Plastic Surgery, Univ S Florida/H Lee Moffit Cancer Ctr 1997

Stahl, Richard S MD [PlS] - **Spec Exp:** Breast Reconstruction; Chest Wall Reconstruction; Abdominal Wall Reconstruction; **Hospital:** Yale-New Haven Hosp, Hosp of St Raphael; **Address:** 5 Durham Rd, Guilford, CT 06437; **Phone:** 203-458-4440; **Board Cert:** Surgery 2001; Plastic Surgery 1984; **Med School:** Vanderbilt Univ 1976; **Resid:** Surgery, Yale New Haven Hosp 1981; **Fellow:** Plastic Surgery, Emory Univ Med Ctr 1983; **Fac Appt:** Clin Prof S, Yale Univ

Mid Atlantic

Cordeiro, Peter G MD [PlS] - **Spec Exp:** Reconstructive Surgery; Breast Reconstruction; Facial Plastic & Reconstructive Surgery; **Hospital:** Meml Sloan-Kettering Cancer Ctr (page 76), Lenox Hill Hosp (Manh Eye, Ear & Throat Hosp); **Address:** 1275 York Avenue, New York, NY 10065; **Phone:** 800-525-2225; **Board Cert:** Surgery 1998; Plastic Surgery 1994; **Med School:** Harvard Med Sch 1983; **Resid:** Surgery, New Eng Deaconess Hosp-Harvard 1989; Plastic Surgery, NYU Med Ctr 1991; **Fellow:** Microsurgery, Meml Sloan-Kettering Cancer Ctr. 1992; Craniofacial Surgery, Univ Miami 1992; **Fac Appt:** Prof S, Cornell Univ-Weill Med Coll

Hoffman, Lloyd MD [PlS] - **Spec Exp:** Breast Reconstruction; **Hospital:** NY-Presby Hosp/Columbia (page 79), Lenox Hill Hosp; **Address:** 12A E 68th St, New York, NY 10021; **Phone:** 212-861-1640; **Board Cert:** Plastic Surgery 1989; **Med School:** Northwestern Univ 1978; **Resid:** Surgery, New York Hosp 1983; Plastic Surgery, NYU Med Ctr 1986; **Fellow:** Hand Surgery, NYU Med Ctr 1987; **Fac Appt:** Assoc Prof PlS, Cornell Univ-Weill Med Coll

Loree, Thom R MD [PlS] - **Spec Exp:** Head & Neck Cancer; Thyroid Cancer; Reconstructive Surgery; **Hospital:** Roswell Park Cancer Inst, Millard Fillmore Gates Cir Hosp; **Address:** Roswell Park Cancer Inst, Dept Head & Neck Surgery, Elm & Carlton Sts, Buffalo, NY 14263; **Phone:** 716-845-3158; **Board Cert:** Surgery 1997; Plastic Surgery 2004; **Med School:** Geo Wash Univ 1982; **Resid:** Surgery, St Lukes-Roosevelt Hosp 1987; Plastic Surgery, St Lukes-Roosevelt Hosp 1989; **Fellow:** Head & Neck Surgical Oncology, Meml Sloan-Kettering Cancer Ctr 1990; **Fac Appt:** Assoc Prof S, SUNY Buffalo

Noone, R Barrett MD [PlS] - **Spec Exp:** Breast Reconstruction; **Hospital:** Bryn Mawr Hosp, Lankenau Hosp; **Address:** 888 Glenbrook Ave, Bryn Mawr, PA 19010-2506; **Phone:** 610-527-4833; **Board Cert:** Surgery 1972; Plastic Surgery 1974; **Med School:** Univ Pennsylvania 1965; **Resid:** Surgery, Hosp Univ Penn 1971; Plastic Surgery, Hosp Univ Penn 1973; **Fac Appt:** Clin Prof S, Univ Pennsylvania

Serletti, Joseph M MD [PlS] - **Spec Exp:** Breast Reconstruction; Reconstructive Surgery; **Hospital:** Hosp Univ Penn - UPHS (page 81); **Address:** Hosp Univ Penn, 3400 Spruce St, 10 Penn Tower, Philadelphia, PA 19104; **Phone:** 215-662-3743; **Board Cert:** Plastic Surgery 2003; **Med School:** Univ Rochester 1982; **Resid:** Surgery, U Rochester Med Ctr 1986; Plastic Surgery, U Rochester Med Ctr 1988; **Fellow:** Reconstructive Surgery, Johns Hopkins Hosp 1990; **Fac Appt:** Prof PlS, Univ Pennsylvania

Slezak, Sheri MD [PlS] - **Spec Exp:** Breast Reconstruction; **Hospital:** Univ of MD Med Ctr; **Address:** Univ Maryland, Dept Plastic Surgery, 22 S Greene St, rm S8D12, Baltimore, MD 21201; **Phone:** 410-328-2360; **Board Cert:** Plastic Surgery 1991; **Med School:** Harvard Med Sch 1980; **Resid:** Surgery, Columbia-Presby Med Ctr 1985; Plastic Surgery, Johns Hopkins Hosp 1989; **Fac Appt:** Assoc Prof PlS, Univ MD Sch Med

Sultan, Mark MD [PlS] - **Spec Exp:** Breast Reconstruction; **Hospital:** St Luke's - Roosevelt Hosp Ctr - Roosevelt Div (page 71); **Address:** 1100 Park Ave, New York, NY 10128; **Phone:** 212-360-0700; **Board Cert:** Plastic Surgery 1992; **Med School:** Columbia P&S 1982; **Resid:** Surgery, Columbia-Presby Hosp 1987; Plastic Surgery, Columbia-Presby Hosp 1990; **Fellow:** Head and Neck Surgery, Emory Univ Hosp 1989; **Fac Appt:** Assoc Prof S, Columbia P&S

Ting, Jess MD [PlS] - **Spec Exp:** Reconstructive Microvascular Surgery; Nerve Surgery & Transplantation; Breast Reconstruction; **Hospital:** Mount Sinai Med Ctr (page 77); **Address:** Dept of Surgery Mount Sinai Sch Med, 5 E 98th St, Box 1259, New York, NY 10029; **Phone:** 212-241-4410; **Board Cert:** Plastic Surgery 2002; Hand Surgery 2003; **Med School:** Columbia P&S 1995; **Resid:** Surgery, Columbia Presby Med Ctr 1998; Plastic Surgery, Univ Pittsburgh Med Ctr 2000; **Fellow:** Hand Surgery, Hosp Special Surgery 2001; **Fac Appt:** Asst Prof S, Mount Sinai Sch Med

Southeast

Allen, Robert J MD [PlS] - **Spec Exp:** Breast Reconstruction; **Hospital:** Roper Hosp, New York Eye & Ear Infirm (page 78); **Address:** 125 Doughty St, Ste 590, Charleston, SC 29403; **Phone:** 888-890-3437; **Board Cert:** Plastic Surgery 1985; **Med School:** Med Univ SC 1976; **Resid:** Surgery, LSU Med Ctr 1982; Plastic Surgery, LSU Med Ctr 1981; **Fellow:** Microsurgery, NYU Med Ctr 1983; **Fac Appt:** Assoc Clin Prof PlS, Louisiana State U, New Orleans

Fix, R Jobe MD [PlS] - **Spec Exp:** Breast Reconstruction; Microsurgery; **Hospital:** Univ of Ala Hosp at Birmingham, Children's Hospital - Birmingham; **Address:** Univ of Alabama Hosp, Div Plastic Surg, 510 S 20th St, FOT-Ste 1102, Birmingham, AL 35294; **Phone:** 205-934-3358; **Board Cert:** Surgery 1997; Plastic Surgery 1991; Hand Surgery 2001; **Med School:** Univ Nebr Coll Med 1982; **Resid:** Surgery, Valley Med Ctr 1987; Plastic Surgery, Univ Ala Hosp 1989; **Fac Appt:** Prof PlS, Univ Alabama

Georgiade, Gregory MD [PlS] - **Spec Exp:** Breast Reconstruction; **Hospital:** Duke Univ Med Ctr; **Address:** Duke Univ Med Ctr, Box 3960, Durham, NC 27710; **Phone:** 919-684-3039; **Board Cert:** Plastic Surgery 1981; Surgery 2001; **Med School:** Duke Univ 1973; **Resid:** Surgery, Duke Univ Med Ctr 1978; Plastic Surgery, Duke Univ Med Ctr 1980; **Fac Appt:** Prof S, Duke Univ

Plastic Surgery

Hester Jr, T Roderick MD [PlS] - **Spec Exp:** Breast Reconstruction; **Hospital:** Emory Univ Hosp; **Address:** Paces Plastic Surgery, 3200 Dunwood Circle, Ste 6340, Atlanta, GA 30327-1610; **Phone:** 404-351-0051; **Board Cert:** Plastic Surgery 1980; Surgery 1973; **Med School:** Emory Univ 1967; **Resid:** Surgery, Emory Affil Hosps 1972; Plastic Reconstructive Surgery, Emory Affil Hosps 1978; **Fac Appt:** Assoc Prof PlS, Emory Univ

Maxwell, G Patrick MD [PlS] - **Spec Exp:** Breast Reconstruction; **Hospital:** Baptist Hosp - Nashville, Centennial Med Ctr; **Address:** 2020 21st Ave S, Nashville, TN 37212; **Phone:** 615-932-7700; **Board Cert:** Plastic Surgery 1981; **Med School:** Vanderbilt Univ 1972; **Resid:** Surgery, Johns Hopkins Hosp 1976; Plastic Surgery, Johns Hopkins Hosp 1979; **Fellow:** Microsurgery, Davies Med Ctr 1975; **Fac Appt:** Asst Clin Prof PlS, Vanderbilt Univ

McCraw, John MD [PlS] - **Spec Exp:** Breast Reconstruction; **Hospital:** Univ Mississippi Med Ctr; **Address:** Univ Mississippi Med Ctr, Div Plastic Surg, 2500 N State St, Jackson, MS 39216; **Phone:** 601-815-1343; **Board Cert:** Surgery 1972; Plastic Surgery 1974; **Med School:** Univ MO-Columbia Sch Med 1966; **Resid:** Orthopaedic Surgery, Duke U Med Ctr 1969; Surgery, Univ Florida Med Ctr 1971; **Fellow:** Plastic Surgery, Univ Florida Med Ctr 1973; **Fac Appt:** Prof PlS, Univ Miss

Smith Jr, David J MD [PlS] - **Spec Exp:** Breast Reconstruction; **Hospital:** Univ of S FL - Tampa; **Address:** Div Plastic Surg, 2 Tampa General Circle Fl 7, Tampa, FL 33606; **Phone:** 813-259-0929; **Board Cert:** Plastic Surgery 1981; **Med School:** Indiana Univ 1973; **Resid:** Surgery, Emory Univ-Grady Hosp 1988; Plastic Surgery, Inidana Univ 1980; **Fellow:** Hand Surgery, Univ Louisville 1979; **Fac Appt:** Prof S, Univ S Fla Coll Med

Vasconez, Luis O MD [PlS] - **Spec Exp:** Breast Reconstruction; **Hospital:** Univ of Ala Hosp at Birmingham; **Address:** 510 20th St S, FOT 1102, Birmingham, AL 35294-3411; **Phone:** 205-934-3245; **Board Cert:** Surgery 1970; Plastic Surgery 1971; **Med School:** Washington Univ, St Louis 1962; **Resid:** Surgery, Strong Meml Hosp 1970; Plastic Surgery, Shands Hosp-Univ FL 1969; **Fac Appt:** Prof S, Univ Alabama

Midwest

Brandt, Keith Eric MD [PlS] - **Spec Exp:** Breast Reconstruction; Reconstructive Surgery; Microsurgery; **Hospital:** Barnes-Jewish Hosp, Barnes-Jewish West County Hosp; **Address:** 4921 Parkview Pl, Ste 6G, St Louis, MO 63110-1010; **Phone:** 314-362-7388; **Board Cert:** Surgery 1999; Plastic Surgery 2003; Hand Surgery 2005; **Med School:** Univ Tex, Houston 1983; **Resid:** Surgery, Univ Nebraska Med Ctr 1989; Plastic Surgery, Univ Tennessee 1991; **Fellow:** Hand Surgery, Wash Univ 1992; Microsurgery, Wash Univ 1993; **Fac Appt:** Prof S, Washington Univ, St Louis

Coleman, John J MD [PlS] - **Spec Exp:** Cancer Reconstruction; Breast Reconstruction; Head & Neck Surgery; Pediatric Plastic Surgery; **Hospital:** Indiana Univ Hosp (page 74), Riley Hosp for Children (page 74); **Address:** 545 Barnhill Dr, Emerson Hall, Ste 232, Indianapolis, IN 46202-5120; **Phone:** 317-274-8106; **Board Cert:** Surgery 1998; Plastic Surgery 1981; **Med School:** Harvard Med Sch 1973; **Resid:** Surgery, Emory Univ Affil Hosp 1978; Plastic Surgery, Emory Univ Affil Hosp 1979; **Fellow:** Surgical Oncology, Univ Maryland Med Ctr 1981; **Fac Appt:** Prof S, Indiana Univ

Ness, John A MD [PlS] - **Hospital:** Northern Meml Hlth Care; **Address:** Wayzata Plastic Surgery, 319 Barry Ave, Ste 300, Wayzata, MN 55391; **Phone:** 952-473-1111; **Board Cert:** Otolaryngology 1992; Plastic Surgery 2009; **Med School:** Univ Minn 1986; **Resid:** Otolaryngology, Loyola U- Stritch Sch Med 1991; **Fellow:** Facial Plastic & Reconstr Surgery, UC Davis 1993; Craniofacial Surgery, Australian Craniofacial Inst 1996; **Fac Appt:** Asst Prof PlS, Univ Minn

Walton Jr, Robert L MD [PlS] - **Spec Exp:** Nasal Reconstruction; Breast Reconstruction; **Hospital:** Univ of Chicago Med Ctr, Resurrection Hlth Care St Joseph Hosp; **Address:** 60 E Delaware, Ste 1430, Chicago, IL 60611-1495; **Phone:** 312-337-7795; **Board Cert:** Plastic Surgery 1980; **Med School:** Univ Kans 1972; **Resid:** Surgery, Johns Hopkins Hosp 1974; Plastic Surgery, Yale-New Haven Hosp 1978; **Fellow:** Hand Surgery, Hartford Hosp 1978

Wilkins, Edwin G MD [PlS] - **Spec Exp:** Breast Reconstruction; Microsurgery; **Hospital:** Univ Michigan Hlth Sys; **Address:** Univ Mich, Div Plastic Surg, 1500 E Med Ctr Drive, rm 2130 Taubman Ctr, Ann Arbor, MI 48109-5340; **Phone:** 734-998-6022; **Board Cert:** Plastic Surgery 1991; **Med School:** Wake Forest Univ 1981; **Resid:** Surgery, Charlotte Meml Hosp 1986; Plastic Surgery, Vanderbilt Univ Med Ctr 1988; **Fellow:** Reconstructive Microsurgery, Univ Louisville Sch Med 1989; **Fac Appt:** Assoc Prof PlS, Univ Mich Med Sch

Yetman, Randall MD [PlS] - **Spec Exp:** Breast Reconstruction; Melanoma; **Hospital:** Cleveland Clin Fdn (page 70); **Address:** 9500 Euclid Ave, Desk A60, Cleveland, OH 44195; **Phone:** 216-444-6908; **Board Cert:** Plastic Surgery 1984; **Med School:** Univ Miami Sch Med 1975; **Resid:** Surgery, Montefiore Med Ctr 1979; Plastic Surgery, NY Cornell Med Ctr 1981; **Fellow:** Plastic Surgery, Cleveland Clin Fdn 1982

Southwest

Menick, Frederick J MD [PlS] - **Spec Exp:** Reconstructive Surgery-Face; Nasal Reconstruction; Cancer Reconstruction; **Hospital:** St Joseph's Hosp - Tucson; **Address:** 1102 N Eldorado Pl, Tucson, AZ 85712; **Phone:** 520-881-4525; **Board Cert:** Plastic Surgery 1983; **Med School:** Yale Univ 1970; **Resid:** Surgery, Stanford Med Ctr; Surgery, Univ Ariz Med Ctr 1979; **Fellow:** Plastic Surgery, Queen Victoria Hosp/Univ Miami 1982; **Fac Appt:** Assoc Clin Prof S, Univ Ariz Coll Med

Robb, Geoffrey L MD [PlS] - **Spec Exp:** Breast Reconstruction; Head & Neck Cancer Reconstruction; Facial Plastic & Reconstructive Surgery; **Hospital:** UT MD Anderson Cancer Ctr, St Luke's Episcopal Hosp-Houston; **Address:** 1515 Holcombe Blvd, Unit 443, Houston, TX 77030; **Phone:** 713-794-1247; **Board Cert:** Otolaryngology 1979; Plastic Surgery 1986; **Med School:** Univ Miami Sch Med 1974; **Resid:** Otolaryngology, Naval Reg Med Ctr 1979; Plastic Surgery, Univ Pittsburgh 1985; **Fellow:** Microvascular Surgery, Univ Pittsburgh 1986; **Fac Appt:** Prof PlS, Univ Tex, Houston

Rohrich, Rod J MD [PlS] - **Spec Exp:** Breast Reconstruction; **Hospital:** UT Southwestern Med Ctr at Dallas, Baylor Univ Medical Ctr; **Address:** Univ Tex SW Med Ctr, Plastic Surgery, 1801 Inwood Rd, Dallas, TX 75390-9132; **Phone:** 214-645-3119; **Board Cert:** Plastic Surgery 1987; Hand Surgery 1990; **Med School:** Baylor Coll Med 1979; **Resid:** Plastic Surgery, Univ Mich Hosp 1985; Plastic Surgery, Radcliffe Infirm/Oxford 1983; **Fellow:** Hand Surgery, Mass Genl Hosp-Harvard 1987; **Fac Appt:** Prof PlS, Univ Tex SW, Dallas

Schusterman, Mark A MD [PlS] - **Spec Exp:** Breast Reconstruction; Cancer Reconstruction; **Hospital:** St Luke's Episcopal Hosp-Houston, Park Plaza Hosp; **Address:** 1200 Binz St, Ste 1200, Houston, TX 77030; **Phone:** 713-794-0368; **Board Cert:** Plastic Surgery 1989; **Med School:** Univ Louisville Sch Med 1980; **Resid:** Surgery, Univ Hosp 1985; Pediatric Surgery, Univ Pittsburgh Med Ctr 1987; **Fellow:** Microsurgery, Univ Pittsburgh Med Ctr 1988; **Fac Appt:** Clin Prof PlS, Baylor Coll Med

Plastic Surgery

Yuen, James C MD [PlS] - **Spec Exp:** Breast Reconstruction; Head & Neck Cancer Reconstruction; Chest Wall Reconstruction; Limb Sparing Surgery; **Hospital:** UAMS Med Ctr; **Address:** 4301 W Markham, Ste 720, Little Rock, AR 72205; **Phone:** 501-686-8711; **Board Cert:** Surgery 2001; Plastic Surgery 2004; **Med School:** Med Coll VA 1985; **Resid:** Surgery, West Va Med Ctr 1990; Plastic Reconstructive Surgery, Duke Univ Med Ctr 1993; **Fellow:** Hand & Microvascular Surgery, Kleinert Inst of Hand & Microsurgery 1991; **Fac Appt:** Assoc Prof S, Univ Ark

West Coast and Pacific

Andersen, James S MD [PlS] - **Spec Exp:** Breast Reconstruction; Head & Neck Reconstruction; Microsurgery; **Hospital:** City of Hope Natl Med Ctr & Beckman Rsch (page 69), Huntington Memorial Hosp; **Address:** City of Hope National Cancer Ctr, Div Plastic Surgery, 1500 E Duarte Rd, Duarte, CA 91010; **Phone:** 626-471-7100; **Board Cert:** Plastic Surgery 1994; **Med School:** Jefferson Med Coll 1983; **Resid:** Surgery, Hosp U Penn 1989; Plastic Surgery, Hosp U Penn 1991; **Fellow:** Microsurgery, USC Med Ctr 1992; **Fac Appt:** Assoc Clin Prof S, USC Sch Med

Hansen, Juliana MD [PlS] - **Spec Exp:** Breast Reconstruction; Cancer Reconstruction; **Hospital:** OR Hlth & Sci Univ; **Address:** 3303 SW Bond Ave, MC CH5P, Portland, OR 97239; **Phone:** 503-494-6687; **Board Cert:** Plastic Surgery 2008; **Med School:** Univ Wash 1988; **Resid:** Surgery, UCSF Med Ctr 1994; Plastic Surgery, UCSF Med Ctr 1996

Isik, Ferda Frank MD [PlS] - **Spec Exp:** Breast Reconstruction; **Hospital:** Swedish Med Ctr - Seattle; **Address:** The Polyclinic, 1145 Broadway, Seattle, WA 98122; **Phone:** 206-860-4566; **Board Cert:** Surgery 2001; Plastic Surgery 2007; **Med School:** Mount Sinai Sch Med 1985; **Resid:** Surgery, Boston Univ Hosps 1990; Plastic Surgery, Univ Wash Affil Hosp 1995; **Fellow:** Pathology, NIH / Univ Wash 1992

Jewell, Mark L MD [PlS] - **Spec Exp:** Breast Reconstruction; **Hospital:** Sacred Heart Med Ctr; **Address:** 10 Coburg Rd, Ste 300, Eugene, OR 97401; **Phone:** 541-683-3234; **Board Cert:** Plastic Surgery 1981; **Med School:** Univ Kans 1973; **Resid:** Surgery, LAC-Harbor Med Ctr 1976; Plastic Surgery, Erlanger Hosp 1979; **Fellow:** Burn Surgery, LAC-USC Med Ctr 1977; **Fac Appt:** Asst Clin Prof PlS, Oregon Hlth Sci Univ

Miller, Timothy A MD [PlS] - **Spec Exp:** Eyelid Cancer & Reconstruction; Skin Cancer; Nasal Reconstruction; **Hospital:** UCLA Ronald Reagan Med Ctr; **Address:** 200 UCLA Medical Plaza, Ste 465, Los Angeles, CA 90095-8344; **Phone:** 310-825-5644; **Board Cert:** Surgery 1971; Plastic Surgery 1973; **Med School:** UCLA 1963; **Resid:** Surgery, Johns Hopkins Hosp 1967; Thoracic Surgery, UCLA Med Ctr 1969; **Fellow:** Plastic Surgery, Univ Pittsburgh 1971; **Fac Appt:** Prof S, UCLA

Sherman, Randolph MD [PlS] - **Spec Exp:** Breast Reconstruction; **Hospital:** Cedars-Sinai Med Ctr; **Address:** 8635 W 3rd St, Ste 770W, Los Angeles, CA 90048; **Phone:** 310-423-2129; **Board Cert:** Surgery 2004; Plastic Surgery 1986; Hand Surgery 2000; **Med School:** Univ MO-Columbia Sch Med 1977; **Resid:** Surgery, UCSF Hosps 1981; Surgery, State Univ of New York 1983; **Fellow:** Plastic Surgery, USC Med Ctr 1985; **Fac Appt:** Prof S, USC Sch Med

Psychiatry

A psychiatrist specializes in the prevention, diagnosis and treatment of mental, addictive and emotional disorders such as schizophrenia and other psychotic disorders, mood disorders, anxiety disorders, substance-related disorders, sexual and gender identity disorders and adjustment disorders. The psychiatrist is able to understand the biologic, psychologic and social components of illness, and therefore is uniquely prepared to treat the whole person. A psychiatrist is qualified to order diagnostic laboratory tests and to prescribe medications, evaluate and treat psychologic and interpersonal problems and to intervene with families who are coping with stress, crises and other problems in living.

Training Required: Four years

Certification in one of the following subspecialties requires additional training and examination.

Addiction Psychiatry: A psychiatrist who focuses on the evaluation and treatment of individuals with alcohol, drug, or other substancerelated disorders and of individuals with the dual diagnosis of substance-related and other psychiatric disorders.

Child & Adolescent Psychiatry: A psychiatrist with additional training in the diagnosis and treatment of developmental, behavioral, emotional and mental disorders of childhood and adolescence

Geriatric Psychiatry: A psychiatrist with expertise in the prevention, evaluation, diagnosis and treatment of mental and emotional disorders in the elderly. The geriatric psychiatrist seeks to improve the psychiatric care of the elderly both in health and in disease.

PSYCHIATRY

New England

Block, Susan D MD [Psyc] - **Spec Exp:** Psychiatry in Cancer; Palliative Care; **Hospital:** Dana-Farber Cancer Inst, Brigham & Women's Hosp; **Address:** Dana Farber Cancer Inst, 44 Binney St, SW 411, Boston, MA 02115; **Phone:** 617-632-5788; **Board Cert:** Psychiatry 1984; Internal Medicine 1981; Hospice & Palliative Medicine 2003; **Med School:** Case West Res Univ 1977; **Resid:** Internal Medicine, Beth Israel Hosp 1980; Psychiatry, Beth Israel Hosp 1982; **Fac Appt:** Prof Psyc, Harvard Med Sch

Greenberg, Donna B MD [Psyc] - **Spec Exp:** Psychiatry in Cancer; **Hospital:** Mass Genl Hosp; **Address:** Mass General Hospital, Warren 605, 55 Fruit St, Boston, MA 02114-2696; **Phone:** 617-724-8400; **Board Cert:** Internal Medicine 1978; Psychiatry 1990; **Med School:** Univ Rochester 1975; **Resid:** Internal Medicine, Boston City Hosp 1978; Psychiatry, Mass Genl Hosp 1989; **Fellow:** Psychiatry, Mass Genl Hosp 1979; **Fac Appt:** Assoc Prof Psyc, Harvard Med Sch

Rauch, Paula K MD [Psyc] - **Spec Exp:** Psychiatry in Childhood Cancer; Children/Families with Severe Illness; Parent Guidance in Parental Cancer; **Hospital:** Mass Genl Hosp; **Address:** Mass General Hosp, Dept Child Psychiatry, 32 Fruit St, Yawkey 6, Boston, MA 02114; **Phone:** 617-724-5600; **Board Cert:** Psychiatry 1990; Child & Adolescent Psychiatry 1991; **Med School:** Univ Cincinnati 1981; **Resid:** Psychiatry, Mass Genl Hosp 1984; **Fac Appt:** Asst Prof Psyc, Harvard Med Sch

Mid Atlantic

Basch, Samuel MD [Psyc] - **Spec Exp:** Psychiatry in Physical Illness; Psychiatry in Cancer; **Hospital:** Mount Sinai Med Ctr (page 77); **Address:** 10 E 85th St, Ste 1B, New York, NY 10028-0412; **Phone:** 212-427-0344; **Board Cert:** Psychiatry 1970; **Med School:** Hahnemann Univ 1961; **Resid:** Psychiatry, Mount Sinai Hosp 1965; **Fellow:** Psychoanalysis, Columbia Presby Hosp 1976; **Fac Appt:** Clin Prof Psyc, Mount Sinai Sch Med

Breitbart, William MD [Psyc] - **Spec Exp:** Psychiatry in Cancer; AIDS Related Cancers; Pain-Cancer; Palliative Care; **Hospital:** Meml Sloan-Kettering Cancer Ctr (page 76); **Address:** 1275 York Avenue, New York, NY 10065; **Phone:** 646-888-0100; **Board Cert:** Internal Medicine 1982; Psychiatry 1986; Psychosomatic Medicine 2005; **Med School:** Albert Einstein Coll Med 1978; **Resid:** Internal Medicine, Bronx Muni Hosp Ctr 1982; Psychiatry, Bronx Muni Hosp Ctr 1984; **Fellow:** Psychiatric Oncology, Meml Sloan Kettering Cancer Ctr 1986; **Fac Appt:** Prof Psyc, Cornell Univ-Weill Med Coll

Klagsbrun, Samuel C MD [Psyc] - **Spec Exp:** Psychiatry in Cancer; Psychiatry in Terminal Illness; **Hospital:** Four Winds Hosp; **Address:** Four Winds Hospital, 800 Cross River Rd, Katonah, NY 10536; **Phone:** 914-763-8151 x2222; **Board Cert:** Psychiatry 1977; **Med School:** Ros Franklin Univ/Chicago Med Sch 1962; **Resid:** Psychiatry, Yale-New Haven Hosp 1966; **Fac Appt:** Clin Prof Psyc, Albert Einstein Coll Med

Kunkel, Elisabeth J MD [Psyc] - **Spec Exp:** Psychiatry in Cancer; Psychiatry in Physical Illness; **Hospital:** Thomas Jefferson Univ Hosp (page 83), Methodist Hosp; **Address:** Thomas Jefferson Univ, 1020 Samson St, Thompson Bldg, Ste 1652, Philadelphia, PA 19107; **Phone:** 215-955-9545; **Board Cert:** Psychiatry 1989; Addiction Psychiatry 1998; Psychosomatic Medicine 2005; **Med School:** McGill Univ 1983; **Resid:** Psychiatry, NYU Med Ctr 1987; **Fellow:** Liaison Psychiatry, Meml Sloan Kettering Cancer Ctr 1989; Consultation Psychiatry, Meml Sloan Kettering Cancer Ctr 1989; **Fac Appt:** Prof Psyc, Jefferson Med Coll

Roth, Andrew J MD [Psyc] - **Spec Exp:** Psychiatry of Prostate Cancer; Bereavement/Traumatic Grief; **Hospital:** Meml Sloan-Kettering Cancer Ctr (page 76); **Address:** 641 Lexington Ave Fl 7, New York, NY 10022; **Phone:** 646-888-0024; **Board Cert:** Psychiatry 1993; Geriatric Psychiatry 2005; Psychosomatic Medicine 2005; **Med School:** NY Med Coll 1988; **Resid:** Psychiatry, Mt Sinai Med Ctr 1992; **Fellow:** Liaison Psychiatry, Meml Sloan-Kettering Canc Ctr 1994

Midwest

Riba, Michelle B MD [Psyc] - **Spec Exp:** Psychiatry in Cancer; **Hospital:** Univ Michigan Hlth Sys; **Address:** Univ Mich Med Ctr, Dept Psychiatry, 1500 E Medical Center Dr, MCHC, rm F6236, Ann Arbor, MI 48109-0295; **Phone:** 734-764-6879; **Board Cert:** Psychiatry 1991; Psychosomatic Medicine 2005; **Med School:** Univ Conn 1985; **Resid:** Psychiatry, Univ Connecticut 1988; **Fac Appt:** Clin Prof Psyc, Univ Mich Med Sch

Great Plains and Mountains

Greiner, Carl B MD [Psyc] - **Spec Exp:** Psychiatry in Cancer; Psychiatry in Physical Illness; Palliative Care; Ethics; **Hospital:** Nebraska Med Ctr; **Address:** UNMC, dept Psychiatry, 985575 Nebraska Medical Ctr, Omaha, NE 68198-5575; **Phone:** 402-552-6002; **Board Cert:** Psychiatry 1984; Forensic Psychiatry 1999; **Med School:** Univ Cincinnati 1978; **Resid:** Psychiatry, Univ Cincinnati Med Ctr 1982; **Fac Appt:** Prof Psyc, Univ Nebr Coll Med

Southwest

Baile, Walter F MD [Psyc] - **Spec Exp:** Psychiatry in Cancer; **Hospital:** UT MD Anderson Cancer Ctr; **Address:** Brain & Spine Inst, MD Anderson, Main Bldg Fl 7, 1515 Holcombe Blvd, Texas, TX 77030; **Phone:** 713-563-1484; **Board Cert:** Psychiatry 1980; **Med School:** Italy 1973; **Resid:** Psychiatry, Johns Hopkins Hosp 1976; **Fellow:** Behavioral Medicine, Natl Inst Aging 1978; **Fac Appt:** Prof Psyc, Univ Tex, Houston

Valentine, Alan D MD [Psyc] - **Spec Exp:** Psychiatry in Cancer; Palliative Care; **Hospital:** UT MD Anderson Cancer Ctr; **Address:** MD Anderson Cancer Center, Dept Psychiatry Unit 453, PO Box 301402, Houston, TX 77230-1402; **Phone:** 713-745-3344; **Board Cert:** Psychiatry 1992; Geriatric Psychiatry 2006; Psychosomatic Medicine 2005; **Med School:** Univ Tex, Houston 1986; **Resid:** Psychiatry, Univ Texas Affil Hosps; **Fac Appt:** Assoc Prof Psyc, Univ Tex, Houston

Psychiatry

West Coast and Pacific

Fann, Jesse R MD [Psyc] - **Spec Exp:** Psychiatry in Physical Illness; Psychiatry in Cancer; Neuro-Psychiatry; **Hospital:** Univ Wash Med Ctr, Harborview Med Ctr; **Address:** Univ Washington Med Ctr, Psychiatry-Box 356560, 1959 NE Pacific St, Seattle, WA 98195-6560; **Phone:** 206-685-4280; **Board Cert:** Psychiatry 2005; **Med School:** Northwestern Univ 1989; **Resid:** Psychiatry, Univ Washington Med Ctr 1993; **Fellow:** Liaison Psychiatry, Univ Washington Med Ctr 1995; Epidemiology, Univ Washington 1996; **Fac Appt:** Assoc Prof Psyc, Univ Wash

Kerrihard, Thomas MD [Psyc] - **Spec Exp:** Psychiatry in Physical Illness; Psychiatry in Cancer; **Hospital:** Cedars-Sinai Med Ctr; **Address:** Cedars Sinai Medical Ctr, Dept Psychiatry, 8700 Beverly Blvd, Ste AC1004, Los Angeles, CA 90048; **Phone:** 310-423-8030; **Board Cert:** Psychiatry 1999; Pain Medicine 2005; **Med School:** Harvard Med Sch 1994; **Resid:** Psychiatry, Mass Genl Hosp 1998; **Fellow:** Liaison Psychiatry, Meml Sloan Kettering Cancer Ctr 1999

Spiegel, David MD [Psyc] - **Spec Exp:** Psychiatry in Cancer; **Hospital:** Stanford Univ Med Ctr; **Address:** Stanford Univ Sch Medicine, Dept Psychiatry & Behavioral Sciences, 401 Quarry Rd, rm 2325, Stanford, CA 94305-5718; **Phone:** 650-723-6421; **Board Cert:** Psychiatry 1976; **Med School:** Harvard Med Sch 1971; **Resid:** Psychiatry, Mass Mental Hlth Ctr 1974; Psychiatry, Cambridge Hosp-Harvard Med Sch 1974; **Fellow:** Community Psychiatry, Harvard Med Sch 1974; **Fac Appt:** Prof Psyc, Stanford Univ

Strouse, Thomas B MD [Psyc] - **Spec Exp:** Psychiatry in Cancer; Pain-Cancer; Psychiatry in Physical Illness; **Hospital:** UCLA Ronald Reagan Med Ctr, Cedars-Sinai Med Ctr; **Address:** Resnick Neuropsychiatric Hosp at UCLA, 150 Medical Plaza, Ste 4230B, Los Angeles, CA 90025; **Phone:** 310-267-9159; **Board Cert:** Psychiatry 1993; Pain Medicine 2000; **Med School:** Case West Res Univ 1987; **Resid:** Psychiatry, UCLA Med Ctr 1991; **Fac Appt:** Clin Prof Psyc, UCLA

Pulmonary Disease

a subspecialty of Internal Medicine

An internist who treats diseases of the lungs and airways. The pulmonologist diagnoses and treats cancer, pneumonia, pleurisy, asthma, occupational diseases, bronchitis, sleep disorders, emphysema and other complex disorders of the lungs.

Training Required: Three years in internal medicine plus additional training and examination for certification in pulmonary disease.

PULMONARY DISEASE

Mid Atlantic

King, Earl D MD [Pul] - **Spec Exp:** Lung Cancer; **Hospital:** Fox Chase Cancer Ctr (page 72); **Address:** Fox Chase Cancer Center, 333 Cottman Ave, Philadelphia, PA 19111; **Phone:** 215-728-5703; **Board Cert:** Internal Medicine 1989; Pulmonary Disease 2002; Critical Care Medicine 2003; **Med School:** Penn State Univ-Hershey Med Ctr 1986; **Resid:** Internal Medicine, Temple Univ Med Ctr 1989; **Fellow:** Pulmonary Disease, Johns Hopkins Hosp 1993; Sleep Medicine, Johns Hopkins Hosp 1993

Libby, Daniel M MD [Pul] - **Spec Exp:** Lung Cancer; **Hospital:** NY-Presby Hosp/Weill Cornell (page 79); **Address:** 635 Madison Ave, Ste 1101, New York, NY 10021; **Phone:** 212-628-6611; **Board Cert:** Internal Medicine 1977; Pulmonary Disease 1980; **Med School:** Baylor Coll Med 1974; **Resid:** Internal Medicine, NY Hosp 1977; **Fellow:** Pulmonary Disease, NY Hosp 1979; **Fac Appt:** Clin Prof Med, Cornell Univ-Weill Med Coll

Nelson, Judith E MD [Pul] - **Spec Exp:** Palliative Care; **Hospital:** Mount Sinai Med Ctr (page 77); **Address:** Mt Sinai Medical Ctr, One Gustave Levy Pl, Box 1232, New York, NY 10029; **Phone:** 212-241-2587; **Board Cert:** Internal Medicine 1989; Pulmonary Disease 2002; Critical Care Medicine 2003; Hospice & Palliative Medicine 2005; **Med School:** NYU Sch Med 1986; **Resid:** Internal Medicine, Mt Sinai Med Ctr 1989; **Fellow:** Pulmonary Critical Care Medicine, Mt Sinai Med Ctr 1992; **Fac Appt:** Assoc Prof Med, Mount Sinai Sch Med

Steinberg, Harry MD [Pul] - **Spec Exp:** Lung Cancer; **Hospital:** Long Island Jewish Med Ctr, N Shore Univ Hosp; **Address:** LI Jewish Med Ctr, Dept Med, 270-05 76th Ave, New Hyde Park, NY 11040-1433; **Phone:** 516-465-5400; **Med School:** Temple Univ 1966; **Resid:** Internal Medicine, LI Jewish Med Ctr 1969; Pulmonary Critical Care Medicine, LI Jewish Med Ctr 1970; **Fellow:** Pulmonary Disease, Hosp Univ Penn 1974; **Fac Appt:** Clin Prof Med, Albert Einstein Coll Med

Teirstein, Alvin S MD [Pul] - **Spec Exp:** Lung Cancer; **Hospital:** Mount Sinai Med Ctr (page 77), VA Med Ctr - Bronx; **Address:** Mount Sinai Med Ctr, 1 Gustave Levy Pl, Box 1232, New York, NY 10029; **Phone:** 212-241-5656; **Board Cert:** Internal Medicine 1961; Pulmonary Disease 1969; **Med School:** SUNY Downstate 1953; **Resid:** Internal Medicine, Mt Sinai Med Ctr 1957; **Fellow:** Pulmonary Disease, Mt Sinai Med Ctr 1954; Pulmonary Disease, VA Med Ctr 1956; **Fac Appt:** Prof Med, Mount Sinai Sch Med

Unger, Michael MD [Pul] - **Spec Exp:** Lung Cancer; Cancer Prevention; **Hospital:** Fox Chase Cancer Ctr (page 72); **Address:** Fox Chase Cancer Center, 7701 Burholme Ave, Philadelphia, PA 19111; **Phone:** 215-728-6900; **Board Cert:** Internal Medicine 1977; Pulmonary Disease 1978; **Med School:** France 1971; **Resid:** Internal Medicine, Mt Sinai Hosp 1974; **Fellow:** Pulmonary Disease, NY Hosp-Cornell 1976; **Fac Appt:** Clin Prof Med, Thomas Jefferson Univ

White, Dorothy MD [Pul] - **Spec Exp:** Lung Cancer; Lung Disease(Immunocompromised); **Hospital:** Meml Sloan-Kettering Cancer Ctr (page 76); **Address:** 1275 York Avenue, New York, NY 10065; **Phone:** 800-525-2225; **Board Cert:** Internal Medicine 1980; Pulmonary Disease 1984; **Med School:** SUNY Hlth Sci Ctr 1977; **Resid:** Internal Medicine, New York Hosp 1980; Internal Medicine, Meml Sloan Kettering Cancer Ctr 1981; **Fellow:** Pulmonary Disease, Yale-New Haven Hosp 1984; **Fac Appt:** Prof Med, Cornell Univ-Weill Med Coll

Southeast

Alberts, W Michael MD [Pul] - **Spec Exp:** Lung Cancer; **Hospital:** H Lee Moffitt Cancer Ctr & Research Inst; **Address:** H Lee Moffitt Cancer Ctr, Thoracic Onc, 12902 Magnolia Drive, Tampa, FL 33612; **Phone:** 813-979-3067; **Board Cert:** Internal Medicine 1980; Pulmonary Disease 1982; **Med School:** Univ IL Coll Med 1977; **Resid:** Internal Medicine, Ohio State Univ Hosp 1980; **Fellow:** Pulmonary Critical Care Medicine, UCSD Med Ctr 1983; **Fac Appt:** Prof Med, Univ S Fla Coll Med

Garver Jr, Robert MD [Pul] - **Spec Exp:** Lung Cancer; **Hospital:** Univ of Ala Hosp at Birmingham; **Address:** 1900 University Blvd, THT 215, Birmingham, AL 35294; **Phone:** 205-934-7556; **Board Cert:** Internal Medicine 1984; Pulmonary Disease 1986; **Med School:** Johns Hopkins Univ 1981; **Resid:** Internal Medicine, Johns Hopkins Hosp 1984; **Fellow:** Pulmonary Disease, NHLBI 1985; **Fac Appt:** Prof Med, Univ Alabama

Goldman, Allan L MD [Pul] - **Spec Exp:** Lung Cancer; **Hospital:** Tampa Genl Hosp, James A Haley VA Hosp; **Address:** USF Coll Med, Dept Internal Medicine, 12901 Bruce B Downs Blvd, Box MDC19, Tampa, FL 33612-4742; **Phone:** 813-974-2271; **Board Cert:** Internal Medicine 1972; Pulmonary Disease 1972; **Med School:** Univ Minn 1968; **Resid:** Internal Medicine, Brooke Army Hosp 1970; **Fellow:** Pulmonary Disease, Walter Reed Army Hosp 1972; **Fac Appt:** Prof Med, Univ S Fla Coll Med

Midwest

Jett, James R MD [Pul] - **Spec Exp:** Lung Cancer; Mesothelioma; Thymoma; **Hospital:** Mayo Med Ctr & Clin - Rochester; **Address:** Mayo Clinic, Thoracic Diseases, 200 First St SW, Rochester, MN 55905; **Phone:** 507-284-5398; **Board Cert:** Internal Medicine 1976; Pulmonary Disease 1978; **Med School:** Univ MO-Columbia Sch Med 1973; **Resid:** Internal Medicine, Mayo Clinic 1976; **Fellow:** Pulmonary Disease, Mayo Clinic 1978; **Fac Appt:** Prof Med, Mayo Med Sch

McLennan, Geoffrey MD/PhD [Pul] - **Spec Exp:** Lung Cancer; **Hospital:** Univ Iowa Hosp & Clinics; **Address:** Univ Iowa Hosp, 200 Hawkins Drive, Ste 4900JPP, Iowa City, IA 52242; **Phone:** 319-353-8201; **Med School:** Australia 1970; **Resid:** Internal Medicine, Royal Adelaide Medical Sch; **Fellow:** Pulmonary Disease, Queen Elizabeth Hosp; **Fac Appt:** Prof Med, Univ Iowa Coll Med

Silver, Michael R MD [Pul] - **Spec Exp:** Lung Cancer; **Hospital:** Rush Univ Med Ctr, Rush Oak Park Hosp; **Address:** Rush Univ Med Ctr, Professional Office Bldg 3, 1725 W Harrison St, Ste 054, Chicago, IL 60612; **Phone:** 312-942-6744; **Board Cert:** Internal Medicine 1984; Pulmonary Disease 1988; Critical Care Medicine 1999; **Med School:** Albany Med Coll 1981; **Resid:** Internal Medicine, Rush-Presby-St Luke's Med Ctr 1985; **Fellow:** Pulmonary Critical Care Medicine, Rush-Presby-St Luke's Med Ctr 1987; **Fac Appt:** Assoc Prof Med, Rush Med Coll

Radiology

A radiologist is a physician who utilizes imaging methodologies to diagnose and manage patients and provide therapeutic options. They specialize in Diagnostic Radiology or Radiation Oncology.

Radiation Oncology: A subspecialist in radiation oncology deals with the therapeutic applications of radiant energy and its modifiers and the study and management of disease, especially malignant tumors.

Diagnostic Radiology: A radiologist who utilizes X-ray, radionuclides, ultrasound and electromagnetic radiation to diagnose and treat disease.

Training Required: Four years. Subspecialties which include Interventional Radiology and Neuroradiology, require additional training and examination.

Interventional Radiology: A radiologist who diagnoses and treats diseases by various radiologic imaging modalities. These include fluoroscopy, digital radiography, computed tomography, sonography and magnetic resonance imaging.

Neuroradiology: A radiologist who diagnoses and treats diseases utilizing imaging procedures as they relate to the brain, spine and spinal cord, head, neck and organs of special sense in adults and children.

Additional certification in subspecialties such as Pediatric Radiology and Interventional Radiology require additional training and examination.

Nuclear Medicine: A nuclear medicine specialist employs the properties of radioactive atoms and molecules in the diagnosis and treatment of disease, and in research. Radiation detection and imaging instrument systems are used to detect disease as it changes the function and metabolism of normal cells, tissues and organs. A wide variety of diseases can be found in this way, usually before the structure of the organ involved by the disease can be seen to be abnormal by any other techniques. Early detection of coronary artery disease (including acute heart attack); early cancer detection and evaluation of the effect of tumor treatment; diagnosis of infection and inflammation anywhere in the body; and early detection of blood clot in the lungs, are all possible with these techniques. Unique forms or radioactive molecules can attack and kill cancer cells (e.g., lymphoma, thyroid cancer) or can relieve the severe pain of cancer that has spread to bone.

The nuclear medicine specialist has special knowledge in the biologic effects of radiation exposure, the fundamentals of the physical sciences and the principles and operation of radiation detection and imaging instrumentation systems.

Training Required: Three years

RADIATION ONCOLOGY

New England

Choi, Noah C MD [RadRO] - **Spec Exp:** Lung Cancer; Esophageal Cancer; Mesothelioma; **Hospital:** Mass Genl Hosp; **Address:** Mass Genl Hosp, Dept Rad Oncology, 100 Blossom St, Cox 307, Boston, MA 02114; **Phone:** 617-726-6050; **Board Cert:** Therapeutic Radiology 1970; **Med School:** South Korea 1963; **Resid:** Radiation Oncology, Princess Margaret Hosp 1970; **Fac Appt:** Prof RadRO, Harvard Med Sch

D'Amico, Anthony V MD/PhD [RadRO] - **Spec Exp:** Prostate Cancer; Brachytherapy; **Hospital:** Dana-Farber Cancer Inst, Brigham & Women's Hosp; **Address:** Brigham & Women's Hosp, Dept Rad Onc, 75 Francis St, Ste L2, Boston, MA 02115; **Phone:** 617-732-7936; **Board Cert:** Radiation Oncology 1999; **Med School:** Univ Pennsylvania 1990; **Resid:** Radiation Oncology, Hosp Univ Penn 1994; **Fac Appt:** Prof RadRO, Harvard Med Sch

DeLaney, Thomas Francis MD [RadRO] - **Spec Exp:** Sarcoma; Proton Beam Therapy; **Hospital:** Mass Genl Hosp; **Address:** Francis H. Burr Proton Therapy Ctr, 30 Fruit St, Bosont, MA 02114; **Phone:** 617-726-6876; **Board Cert:** Therapeutic Radiology 1986; Radiation Oncology 1999; **Med School:** Harvard Med Sch 1982; **Resid:** Therapeutic Radiology, Mass Genl Hosp 1986; **Fac Appt:** Assoc Prof RadRO, Harvard Med Sch

Harris, Jay R MD [RadRO] - **Spec Exp:** Breast Cancer; **Hospital:** Brigham & Women's Hosp, Dana-Farber Cancer Inst; **Address:** Dana Farber Cancer Inst, 44 Binney St, rm D1622, Boston, MA 02115; **Phone:** 617-632-2291; **Board Cert:** Therapeutic Radiology 1999; **Med School:** Stanford Univ 1970; **Resid:** Radiation Oncology, Joint Ctr Rad Ther 1976; **Fellow:** Radiation Therapy, Harvard Med Sch 1977; **Fac Appt:** Prof RadRO, Harvard Med Sch

Knisely, Jonathan MD [RadRO] - **Spec Exp:** Brain Tumors; Stereotactic Radiosurgery; Gastrointestinal Cancer; **Hospital:** Yale-New Haven Hosp; **Address:** Dept Therapeutic Radiology, 15 York St, Hunter Bldg-HRT 133, New Haven, CT 06520-8040; **Phone:** 203-785-2960; **Board Cert:** Internal Medicine 1989; Radiation Oncology 1993; **Med School:** Univ Pennsylvania 1986; **Resid:** Internal Medicine, Michael Reese Hosp 1989; Radiation Oncology, Univ Toronto Med Ctr 1992; **Fac Appt:** Assoc Prof RadRO, Yale Univ

Mauch, Peter M MD [RadRO] - **Spec Exp:** Lymphoma; Hodgkin's Disease; **Hospital:** Dana-Farber Cancer Inst; **Address:** Dana Farber Cancer Inst, 75 Francis St, Ste RadOnc L2, Boston, MA 02115; **Phone:** 617-632-4116; **Board Cert:** Therapeutic Radiology 1978; **Med School:** St Louis Univ 1974; **Resid:** Radiation Therapy, Harvard Joint Ctr 1978; **Fac Appt:** Prof, Harvard Med Sch

Peschel, Richard E MD [RadRO] - **Spec Exp:** Prostate Cancer; **Hospital:** Yale-New Haven Hosp, Bridgeport Hosp; **Address:** Yale-New Haven Hosp, Dept Therapeutic Radiology, 15 York St, rm HRT 142, New Haven, CT 06510; **Phone:** 203-785-2958; **Board Cert:** Therapeutic Radiology 1982; **Med School:** Yale Univ 1977; **Resid:** Radiation Oncology, Yale-New Haven Hosp 1981; **Fac Appt:** Prof RadRO, Yale Univ

Recht, Abram MD [RadRO] - **Spec Exp:** Breast Cancer; Gastrointestinal Cancer; Gynecologic Cancer; **Hospital:** Beth Israel Deaconess Med Ctr - Boston; **Address:** Beth Israel Deaconess Med Ctr, 330 Brookline Ave, Boston, MA 02215; **Phone:** 617-667-2345; **Board Cert:** Therapeutic Radiology 1984; **Med School:** Johns Hopkins Univ 1980; **Resid:** Radiation Oncology, Joint Ctr Radiation Therapy 1984; **Fac Appt:** Assoc Prof RadRO, Harvard Med Sch

Radiation Oncology

Roberts, Kenneth MD [RadRO] - **Spec Exp:** Pediatric Cancers; Lymphoma; Hodgkin's Disease; **Hospital:** Yale-New Haven Hosp, Backus Hosp, Norwich; **Address:** Yale Univ School of Medicine, Dept Radiation Therapy, 15 York St, New Haven, CT 06520-8040; **Phone:** 203-785-2957; **Board Cert:** Internal Medicine 1987; Medical Oncology 1989; Radiation Oncology 1995; **Med School:** Duke Univ 1984; **Resid:** Internal Medicine, Ohio State Univ Hosps 1987; Radiation Oncology, Duke Univ Med Ctr 1992; **Fellow:** Hematology & Oncology, Duke Univ Med Ctr 1989; **Fac Appt:** Assoc Prof Rad, Yale Univ

Shipley, William U MD [RadRO] - **Spec Exp:** Bladder Cancer; Prostate Cancer; **Hospital:** Mass Genl Hosp; **Address:** Mass Genl Hosp, Dept Rad Oncology, 100 Blossom St, Cox Bldg, rm 347, Boston, MA 02114; **Phone:** 617-726-8146; **Board Cert:** Therapeutic Radiology 1975; **Med School:** Harvard Med Sch 1966; **Resid:** Surgery, Mass Genl Hosp 1971; Radiation Therapy, Harvard Joint Ctr Rad Therapy 1973; **Fellow:** Radiation Therapy, Royal Marsden Hosp 1974; **Fac Appt:** Prof RadRO, Harvard Med Sch

Tarbell, Nancy MD [RadRO] - **Spec Exp:** Brain Tumors-Pediatric; Proton Beam Therapy; **Hospital:** Mass Genl Hosp; **Address:** Massachusetts Genl Hosp, Proton Ctr, Boston, MA 02114; **Phone:** 617-724-1836; **Board Cert:** Therapeutic Radiology 1983; **Med School:** SUNY Upstate Med Univ 1979; **Resid:** Radiation Therapy, Harvard Med School 1983; **Fac Appt:** Prof RadRO, Harvard Med Sch

Wazer, David E MD [RadRO] - **Spec Exp:** Breast Cancer; Melanoma; **Hospital:** Rhode Island Hosp, Tufts Med Ctr; **Address:** 593 Eddy St, Providence, RI 02903; **Phone:** 401-444-8311; **Board Cert:** Radiation Oncology 1988; **Med School:** NYU Sch Med 1982; **Resid:** Radiation Oncology, Tufts New Eng Med Ctr 1988; **Fellow:** Neurological Chemistry, NYU Med Ctr 1984; **Fac Appt:** Prof RadRO, Tufts Univ

Wilson, Lynn D MD [RadRO] - **Spec Exp:** Lymphoma, Cutaneous T Cell (CTCL); Lymphoma, Cutaneous B Cell (CBCL); Lung Cancer; Head & Neck Cancer; **Hospital:** Yale-New Haven Hosp; **Address:** Yale Univ Sch Med, Dept Therapeutic Rad, PO Box 208040, New Haven, CT 06520-8040; **Phone:** 203-688-1861; **Board Cert:** Radiation Oncology 2004; **Med School:** Geo Wash Univ 1990; **Resid:** Therapeutic Radiology, Yale-New Haven Hosp 1994; **Fac Appt:** Prof RadRO, Yale Univ

Zietman, Anthony L MD [RadRO] - **Spec Exp:** Prostate Cancer; Urologic Cancer; Proton Beam Therapy; **Hospital:** Mass Genl Hosp; **Address:** Mass Genl Hosp, 100 Blossom St Cox Bldg, rm 3, Boston, MA 02114; **Phone:** 617-724-4000; **Board Cert:** Radiation Oncology 1994; **Med School:** England, UK 1983; **Resid:** Internal Medicine, St Stephens & Westminster Hosp 1986; Radiation Oncology, Mass Genl Hosp 1989; **Fellow:** Radiation Oncology, Middlesex/Mt Vernon Hosps 1991; **Fac Appt:** Prof RadRO, Harvard Med Sch

Mid Atlantic

Berg, Christine D MD [RadRO] - **Spec Exp:** Breast Cancer-Early Detection; Breast Cancer-High Risk Women; **Hospital:** Natl Inst of Hlth - Clin Ctr; **Address:** 6130 Executive Blvd, Bethesda, MD 20892-7346; **Phone:** 301-496-8544; **Board Cert:** Internal Medicine 1980; Medical Oncology 1983; Therapeutic Radiology 1986; Radiation Oncology 1999; **Med School:** Northwestern Univ 1977; **Resid:** Internal Medicine, Northwestern Meml Hosp 1981; Radiation Oncology, Georgetown Univ Hosp 1986; **Fellow:** Medical Oncology, Natl Cancer Inst-NIH 1984

Bogart, Jeffrey A MD [RadRO] - **Spec Exp:** Lung Cancer; Thoracic Cancers; Clinical Trials; **Hospital:** Univ Hosp - SUNY Upstate; **Address:** SUNY Upstate Medical Ctr, Dept Radiation Oncology, 750 E Adams St, Syracuse, NY 13210; **Phone:** 315-464-5276; **Med School:** SUNY Upstate Med Univ 1989; **Resid:** Radiation Oncology, SUNY Hlth Sci Ctr 1993

Constine, Louis Sanders MD [RadRO] - **Spec Exp:** Pediatric Cancers; Lymphoma; Cancer Survivors-Late Effects of Therapy; Sarcoma; **Hospital:** Univ of Rochester Strong Meml Hosp; **Address:** 601 Elmwood Ave, Box 647, Rochester, NY 14642; **Phone:** 585-275-5622; **Board Cert:** Pediatrics 1978; Therapeutic Radiology 1981; Pediatric Hematology-Oncology 1978; **Med School:** Johns Hopkins Univ 1973; **Resid:** Pediatrics, Moffitt Hosp-UCSF Med Ctr 1975; Pediatrics, Stanford Hosp Med Ctr 1976; **Fellow:** Therapeutic Radiology, Stanford Hosp Med Ctr 1981; Pediatric Hematology-Oncology, Univ Wash/Chldns Ortho Hosp 1978; **Fac Appt:** Prof RadRO, Univ Rochester

Cooper, Jay MD [RadRO] - **Spec Exp:** Head & Neck Cancer; Skin Cancer; Chemo-Radiation Combined Therapy; **Hospital:** Maimonides Med Ctr (page 75); **Address:** Maimonides Cancer Ctr, 6300 8th Ave, Brooklyn, NY 11220; **Phone:** 718-765-2700; **Board Cert:** Therapeutic Radiology 1977; **Med School:** NYU Sch Med 1973; **Resid:** Radiation Oncology, NYU Med Ctr 1977; **Fac Appt:** Prof RadRO, Albert Einstein Coll Med

DeWeese, Theodore L MD [RadRO] - **Spec Exp:** Urologic Cancer; Prostate Cancer; Testicular Cancer; **Hospital:** Johns Hopkins Hosp; **Address:** Johns Hopkins Hosp, Weinberg Bldg, 401 N Broadway, rm 1363, Baltimore, MD 21231; **Phone:** 410-955-8893; **Board Cert:** Radiation Oncology 1995; **Med School:** Univ Colorado 1990; **Resid:** Radiation Oncology, Johns Hopkins Hosp 1994; **Fellow:** Urologic Oncology, Johns Hopkins Hosp 1995; **Fac Appt:** Prof RadRO, Johns Hopkins Univ

Dicker, Adam P MD/PhD [RadRO] - **Spec Exp:** Prostate Cancer; **Hospital:** Thomas Jefferson Univ Hosp (page 83); **Address:** Bodine Cancer Treatment Ctr, 111 South 11th St, Philadelphia, PA 19107-5097; **Phone:** 215-955-6527; **Board Cert:** Radiation Oncology 2000; **Med School:** Cornell Univ-Weill Med Coll 1992; **Resid:** Surgery, Lenox Hill Hosp 1994; Radiation Oncology, Meml Sloan Kettering Cancer Ctr 1997; **Fac Appt:** Assoc Prof RadRO, Thomas Jefferson Univ

Donahue, Bernadine R MD [RadRO] - **Spec Exp:** Brain Tumors; Gastrointestinal Cancer; Pediatric Cancers; Solid Tumors; **Hospital:** Maimonides Med Ctr (page 75); **Address:** Maimonides Med Ctr, Dept Radiation Oncology, 6300 8th Ave, Lower Level, Brooklyn, NY 11220; **Phone:** 718-765-2700; **Board Cert:** Internal Medicine 1987; Radiation Oncology 1991; **Med School:** Boston Univ 1984; **Resid:** Internal Medicine, Boston Univ Med Ctr 1987; **Fellow:** Radiation Oncology, NYU Med Ctr 1990

Dritschilo, Anatoly MD [RadRO] - **Spec Exp:** Prostate Cancer; **Hospital:** Georgetown Univ Hosp; **Address:** Georgetown Univ Hosp, Dept Radiation Medicine, LL-Bliss, 3800 Reservoir Rd NW, Washington, DC 20007; **Phone:** 202-687-2144; **Board Cert:** Therapeutic Radiology 1977; **Med School:** UMDNJ-NJ Med Sch, Newark 1973; **Resid:** Radiation Therapy, Harvard Joint Rad Ther Ctr 1977; **Fac Appt:** Prof Med, Georgetown Univ

Ennis, Ronald D MD [RadRO] - **Spec Exp:** Prostate Cancer; Brachytherapy; Gynecologic Cancer; **Hospital:** St Luke's - Roosevelt Hosp Ctr - Roosevelt Div (page 71), Beth Israel Med Ctr - Petrie Division (page 71); **Address:** St Luke's Roosevelt Hosp, Dept Rad Oncol, 1000 10th Ave, Lower Level, New York, NY 10019; **Phone:** 212-523-7165; **Board Cert:** Radiation Oncology 2005; **Med School:** Yale Univ 1990; **Resid:** Therapeutic Radiology, Yale-New Haven Hosp 1994

Flickinger, John C MD [RadRO] - **Spec Exp:** Neuro-Oncology; Brain & Spinal Tumors; **Hospital:** UPMC Presby, Pittsburgh; **Address:** UPMC Cancer Ctr, Radiation Oncology, 5230 Centre Ave, Pittsburgh, PA 15213; **Phone:** 412-647-3600; **Board Cert:** Therapeutic Radiology 1985; **Med School:** Univ Chicago-Pritzker Sch Med 1981; **Resid:** Radiation Therapy, Mass Genl Hosp 1985; **Fac Appt:** Prof RadRO, Univ Pittsburgh

Radiation Oncology

Formenti, Silvia C MD [RadRO] - **Spec Exp:** Breast Cancer; Chemo-Radiation Combined Therapy; **Hospital:** NYU Langone Med Ctr (page 80); **Address:** NYU Med Ctr, Dept Radiation Oncology, 160 E 34th St, New York, NY 10016; **Phone:** 212-263-2601; **Board Cert:** Radiation Oncology 1991; **Med School:** Italy 1980; **Resid:** Internal Medicine, San Carlo Borromeo Hosp 1983; Medical Oncology, Univ of Pavia Med Ctr 1985; **Fellow:** Radiation Oncology, USC Med Ctr 1990; **Fac Appt:** Asst Prof RadRO, NYU Sch Med

Freedman, Gary M MD [RadRO] - **Spec Exp:** Breast Cancer; **Hospital:** Fox Chase Cancer Ctr (page 72), Jeanes Hosp; **Address:** Fox Chase Cancer Ctr-Radiation Onc Dept, 333 Cottman Ave, Philadelphia, PA 19111; **Phone:** 215-728-3815; **Board Cert:** Radiation Oncology 2000; **Med School:** Temple Univ 1993; **Resid:** Radiation Oncology, Fox Chase Cancer Ctr 1998

Gejerman, Glen MD [RadRO] - **Spec Exp:** Prostate Cancer; Intensity Modulated Radiotherapy (IMRT); Breast Cancer; Brachytherapy; **Hospital:** Hackensack Univ Med Ctr (page 73); **Address:** Hackensack Univ Med Ctr, Radiation Onc, 30 Prospect Ave, Hackensack, NJ 07601; **Phone:** 201-996-2464; **Board Cert:** Radiation Oncology 2006; **Med School:** UMDNJ-NJ Med Sch, Newark 1990; **Resid:** Radiation Oncology, Montefiore Med Ctr 1995; **Fac Appt:** Asst Clin Prof RadRO, Albert Einstein Coll Med

Glassburn, John R MD [RadRO] - **Spec Exp:** Gynecologic Cancer; Prostate Cancer; Breast Cancer; **Hospital:** Pennsylvania Hosp (page 81), Hosp Univ Penn - UPHS (page 81); **Address:** Pennsylvania Hosp, Dept Radiation Oncology, 800 Spruce St, Philadelphia, PA 19107; **Phone:** 215-829-3873; **Board Cert:** Therapeutic Radiology 1973; **Med School:** Hahnemann Univ 1966; **Resid:** Radiation Oncology, Hahnemann Hosp 1972; **Fac Appt:** Clin Prof RadRO, Univ Pennsylvania

Glatstein, Eli MD [RadRO] - **Spec Exp:** Lymphoma; Lung Cancer; Photodynamic Therapy; Sarcoma; **Hospital:** Hosp Univ Penn - UPHS (page 81); **Address:** Hosp Univ Penn, Dept Rad Oncology, 3400 Spruce St, Donner Bldg Fl 2, Philadelphia, PA 19104; **Phone:** 215-662-3383; **Board Cert:** Therapeutic Radiology 1972; **Med School:** Stanford Univ 1964; **Resid:** Radiation Therapy, Stanford Med Ctr 1970; **Fellow:** Radiological Biology, Hammersmith Hosp 1972; **Fac Appt:** Prof RadRO, Univ Pennsylvania

Goodman, Robert L MD [RadRO] - **Spec Exp:** Breast Cancer; Lymphoma; Prostate Cancer; Brain Tumors; **Hospital:** St Barnabas Med Ctr; **Address:** St Barnabas Med Ctr, Dept Rad Oncology, 94 Old Short Hills Rd, Livingston, NJ 07039; **Phone:** 973-322-5133; **Board Cert:** Internal Medicine 1971; Therapeutic Radiology 1974; Medical Oncology 1975; **Med School:** Columbia P&S 1966; **Resid:** Internal Medicine, Beth Israel Hosp 1970; Radiation Therapy, Harvard Joint Ctr Rad Therapy 1974; **Fellow:** Hematology, NY-Presby Hosp 1969

Greenberger, Joel S MD [RadRO] - **Spec Exp:** Lung Cancer; Esophageal Cancer; **Hospital:** UPMC Presby, Pittsburgh; **Address:** UPMC Cancer Ctr, Radiation Oncology, 5230 Centre Ave, Pittsburgh, PA 15232; **Phone:** 412-647-3600; **Board Cert:** Therapeutic Radiology 1977; **Med School:** Harvard Med Sch 1971; **Resid:** Radiation Therapy, Mass General Hosp 1977; **Fac Appt:** Prof RadRO, Univ Pittsburgh

Haffty, Bruce MD [RadRO] - **Spec Exp:** Breast Cancer; Head & Neck Cancer; Lung Cancer; **Hospital:** Robert Wood Johnson Univ Hosp - New Brunswick, Robert Wood Johnson Univ Hosp Hamilton; **Address:** The Cancer Institute of New Jersey, 195 Little Albany St, rm 2038, New Brunswick, NJ 08903; **Phone:** 732-253-3939; **Board Cert:** Radiation Oncology 1988; **Med School:** Yale Univ 1984; **Resid:** Radiation Oncology, Yale-New Haven Hosp 1988; **Fac Appt:** Prof RadRO, Robert W Johnson Med Sch

Hahn, Stephen M MD [RadRO] - **Spec Exp:** Lung Cancer; Prostate Cancer; Sarcoma; Photodynamic Therapy; **Hospital:** Hosp Univ Penn - UPHS (page 81), Penn Presby Med Ctr - UPHS (page 81); **Address:** Hosp of the Univ of Penn, 3400 Spruce St 2 Donner Bldg, Philadelphia, PA 19104; **Phone:** 215-662-7296; **Board Cert:** Radiation Oncology 2004; Internal Medicine 1987; Medical Oncology 2001; **Med School:** Temple Univ 1984; **Resid:** Internal Medicine, UCSF Med Ctr 1988; Medical Oncology, Natl Inst Hlth 1991; **Fellow:** Radiation Oncology, Natl Inst Hlth 1994; **Fac Appt:** Prof RadRO, Univ Pennsylvania

Harrison, Louis B MD [RadRO] - **Spec Exp:** Brachytherapy; Head & Neck Cancer; Radiation Therapy-Intraoperative; **Hospital:** Beth Israel Med Ctr - Petrie Division (page 71), St Luke's - Roosevelt Hosp Ctr - Roosevelt Div (page 71); **Address:** Beth Israel Med Ctr, Dept Rad Onc, 10 Union Square East, Ste 4G, New York, NY 10003-3314; **Phone:** 212-844-8087; **Board Cert:** Therapeutic Radiology 1986; **Med School:** SUNY Downstate 1982; **Resid:** Therapeutic Radiology, Yale-New Haven Hosp 1986; **Fac Appt:** Prof RadRO, Albert Einstein Coll Med

Horwitz, Eric MD [RadRO] - **Spec Exp:** Prostate Cancer; Intensity Modulated Radiotherapy (IMRT); Brachytherapy; **Hospital:** Fox Chase Cancer Ctr (page 72); **Address:** Fox Chase Cancer Ctr, Dept Radiation Oncology, 333 Cottman Ave, Philadelphia, PA 19111; **Phone:** 215-728-2995; **Board Cert:** Radiation Oncology 1999; **Med School:** Albany Med Coll 1992; **Resid:** Radiation Oncology, William Beaumont Hosp 1997

Isaacson, Steven R MD [RadRO] - **Spec Exp:** Brain Tumors; Neuro-Oncology; Stereotactic Radiosurgery; Arteriovenous Malformations; **Hospital:** NY-Presby Hosp/Columbia (page 79); **Address:** Columbia Presby Med Ctr, Dept Radiation Oncology, 622 W 168th St BHN Bldg - rm B-11, New York, NY 10032-3720; **Phone:** 212-305-2611; **Board Cert:** Radiation Oncology 1988; Otolaryngology 1978; **Med School:** Jefferson Med Coll 1973; **Resid:** Otolaryngology, Hosp Univ Penn 1978; Radiation Oncology, SUNY Hlth Sci Ctr 1988; **Fac Appt:** Clin Prof RadRO, Columbia P&S

Kleinberg, Lawrence MD [RadRO] - **Spec Exp:** Brain & Spinal Cord Tumors; Brain Tumors-Metastatic; Stereotactic Radiosurgery; Esophageal Cancer; **Hospital:** Johns Hopkins Hosp; **Address:** Johns Hopkins Oncology Ctr Weinberg Bldg, 401 N Broadway, Ste 1440, Baltimore, MD 21231; **Phone:** 410-614-2597; **Board Cert:** Radiation Oncology 1994; **Med School:** Yale Univ 1989; **Resid:** Radiation Oncology, Meml Sloan-Kettering Canc Ctr 1993; **Fac Appt:** Assoc Prof RadRO, Johns Hopkins Univ

Kuettel, Michael MD/PhD [RadRO] - **Spec Exp:** Prostate Cancer; **Hospital:** Roswell Park Cancer Inst; **Address:** Roswell Park Cancer Inst, Radiation Med, Elm and Carlton St, Buffalo, NY 14263; **Phone:** 716-845-1562; **Board Cert:** Radiation Oncology 1992; **Med School:** Northwestern Univ-Feinberg Sch Med 1985; **Resid:** Internal Medicine, Northwestern Hosp 1986; Radiation Oncology, Johns Hopkins Hosp 1990; **Fac Appt:** Prof RadRO, SUNY Buffalo

Lepanto, Philip B MD [RadRO] - **Hospital:** St Mary's Med Ctr - Huntington, Cabell Huntington Hosp; **Address:** St Mary's Med Ctr, Dept Radiation Oncology, 2900 First Ave, Huntington, WV 25702; **Phone:** 304-526-1143; **Board Cert:** Therapeutic Radiology 1975; **Med School:** Univ Louisville Sch Med 1970; **Resid:** Diagnostic Radiology, Graduate Hosp 1972; Radiation Therapy, Hosp Univ Penn 1975; **Fac Appt:** Clin Prof Rad, Marshall Univ

Machtay, Mitchell MD [RadRO] - **Spec Exp:** Head & Neck Cancer; Skin Cancer; Skull Base Tumors; **Hospital:** Thomas Jefferson Univ Hosp (page 83); **Address:** Bodine Ctr for Cancer Treatment, Dept Rad Onc, 111 S 11 St, Bodine Ctr, Philadelphia, PA 19107-5097; **Phone:** 215-955-6706; **Board Cert:** Radiation Oncology 1994; **Med School:** NYU Sch Med 1989; **Resid:** Radiation Oncology, Hosp Univ Penn 1993; **Fac Appt:** Assoc Prof RadRO, Jefferson Med Coll

Radiation Oncology

McCormick, Beryl MD [RadRO] - **Spec Exp:** Breast Cancer; Eye Tumors/Cancer; **Hospital:** Meml Sloan-Kettering Cancer Ctr (page 76), NY-Presby Hosp/Weill Cornell (page 79); **Address:** 1275 York Avenue, New York, NY 10065; **Phone:** 800-525-2225; **Board Cert:** Therapeutic Radiology 1977; **Med School:** UMDNJ-NJ Med Sch, Newark 1973; **Resid:** Therapeutic Radiology, Meml Sloan Kettering Cancer Ctr 1977; **Fac Appt:** Prof RadRO, Cornell Univ-Weill Med Coll

Nicolaou, Nicos MD [RadRO] - **Spec Exp:** Lymphoma; Hodgkin's Disease; **Hospital:** Fox Chase Cancer Ctr (page 72); **Address:** 333 Cottman Avenue, Philadelphia, PA 19111-2497; **Phone:** 215-728-3058; **Board Cert:** Radiation Oncology 1999; **Med School:** Canada 1984; **Resid:** Radiation Oncology, British Columbia Cancer Agency 1989; **Fellow:** Radiation Oncology, Fox Chase Cancer Ctr 1990

Nori, Dattatreyudu MD [RadRO] - **Spec Exp:** Prostate Cancer; Brachytherapy; **Hospital:** NY-Presby Hosp/Weill Cornell (page 79), NY Hosp Queens; **Address:** 525 E 68th St, Box 575, New York, NY 10021-4870; **Phone:** 212-746-3679; **Board Cert:** Therapeutic Radiology 1979; **Med School:** India 1970; **Resid:** Radiation Oncology, Meml Sloan Kettering Cancer Ctr 1975; **Fellow:** Radiation Oncology, Meml Sloan Kettering Cancer Ctr 1978; **Fac Appt:** Prof RadRO, Cornell Univ-Weill Med Coll

Porrazzo, Michael S MD [RadRO] - **Spec Exp:** Prostate Cancer; Central Nervous System Cancer; Breast Cancer; Stereotactic Radiosurgery; **Hospital:** Washington Hosp Ctr; **Address:** Wash Hosp Ctr-Dept. Radiation Onc, 110 Irving St NW, Rm CG-107, Washington, DC 20010; **Phone:** 202-877-3925; **Board Cert:** Radiation Oncology 1990; **Med School:** Meharry Med Coll 1985; **Resid:** Radiation Oncology, Univ Hosp Brooklyn-SUNY Hlth 1989

Regine, William F MD [RadRO] - **Spec Exp:** Stereotactic Radiosurgery; Brain & Spinal Tumors; Gastrointestinal Cancer; **Hospital:** Univ of MD Med Ctr; **Address:** Univ MD Med System-Greenbaum Cancer Ctr, 22 S Green St Guldelsky Bldg, Baltimore, MD 21201; **Phone:** 410-328-6080; **Board Cert:** Radiation Oncology 1992; **Med School:** SUNY Upstate Med Univ 1987; **Resid:** Radiation Oncology, Thomas Jefferson Univ Hosp 1991; **Fellow:** Radiation Oncology, Thomas Jefferson Univ Hosp 1992; **Fac Appt:** Prof RadRO, Univ MD Sch Med

Rotman, Marvin MD [RadRO] - **Spec Exp:** Bladder Cancer; Gynecologic Cancer; Breast Cancer; Prostate Cancer; **Hospital:** SUNY Downstate Med Ctr, Long Island Coll Hosp (page 71); **Address:** 450 Clarkson Ave, Box 1211, Brooklyn, NY 11203-2056; **Phone:** 718-270-2181; **Board Cert:** Diagnostic Radiology 1966; Radiation Oncology 1999; **Med School:** Jefferson Med Coll 1958; **Resid:** Internal Medicine, Albert Einstein Med Ctr 1960; Radiation Oncology, Montefiore Hosp Med Ctr 1965; **Fac Appt:** Prof RadRO, SUNY Downstate

Schiff, Peter B MD/PhD [RadRO] - **Spec Exp:** Prostate Cancer; Gynecologic Cancer; Breast Cancer; **Hospital:** NYU Langone Med Ctr (page 80); **Address:** NYU Clinical Cancer Ctr, 160 E 34th St Fl 1, New York, NY 10016; **Phone:** 212-731-5003; **Board Cert:** Radiation Oncology 1990; **Med School:** Albert Einstein Coll Med 1984; **Resid:** Radiation Oncology, Meml Sloan Kettering Cancer Ctr 1988; **Fac Appt:** Prof RadRO, NYU Sch Med

Solin, Lawrence J MD [RadRO] - **Spec Exp:** Breast Cancer; Head & Neck Cancer; **Hospital:** Albert Einstein Med Ctr; **Address:** Albert Einstein Medical Ctr, Dept Radiation Oncology, 5501 Old York Rd, Philadelphia, PA 19141; **Phone:** 215-456-6280; **Board Cert:** Radiation Oncology 1999; Therapeutic Radiology 1984; **Med School:** Brown Univ 1978; **Resid:** Surgery, Thos Jefferson Univ Hosp 1981; Radiation Oncology, Thos Jefferson Univ Hosp 1984; **Fac Appt:** Prof RadRO, Univ Pennsylvania

Stock, Richard MD [RadRO] - **Spec Exp:** Prostate Cancer; **Hospital:** Mount Sinai Med Ctr (page 77); **Address:** Dept Radiation Oncology, Box 1236, New York, NY 10029; **Phone:** 212-241-7502; **Board Cert:** Radiation Oncology 1993; **Med School:** Mount Sinai Sch Med 1988; **Resid:** Radiation Oncology, Meml Sloan Kettering Cancer Ctr 1992; **Fac Appt:** Prof RadRO, Mount Sinai Sch Med

Streeter Jr, Oscar E MD [RadRO] - **Spec Exp:** Lung Cancer; Head & Neck Cancer; **Hospital:** Howard Univ Hosp; **Address:** Howard Univ Hosp, Dept Radiation Onc, 2041 Georgia Ave NW, Washington, DC 20060; **Phone:** 202-865-6100; **Board Cert:** Radiation Oncology 1989; **Med School:** Howard Univ 1982; **Resid:** Radiation Oncology, Howard Univ 1986; **Fac Appt:** Assoc Prof RadRO, USC Sch Med

Weiss, Marisa C MD [RadRO] - **Spec Exp:** Breast Cancer; **Hospital:** Lankenau Hosp; **Address:** Lankenau Hospital, Dept Rad Oncology, 100 Lancaster Ave, Wynnewood, PA 19096; **Phone:** 610-645-2433; **Board Cert:** Radiation Oncology 1988; **Med School:** Univ Pennsylvania 1984; **Resid:** Radiation Oncology, Hosp Univ Penn 1988; **Fellow:** Radiological Biology, Hosp Univ Penn 1990

Werner-Wasik, Maria MD [RadRO] - **Spec Exp:** Brain Tumors; Lung Cancer; Melanoma; Breast Cancer; **Hospital:** Thomas Jefferson Univ Hosp (page 83); **Address:** Bodine Ctr, Ste G-301, 111 S 11 St, Philadelphia, PA 19107; **Phone:** 215-955-6702; **Board Cert:** Radiation Oncology 1994; **Med School:** Poland 1979; **Resid:** Internal Medicine, Framingham Union Hosp 1990; Radiation Oncology, Tufts/New England Med Ctr 1993; **Fellow:** Radiation Oncology, Hosp Univ Penn 1994; **Fac Appt:** Assoc Prof RadRO, Thomas Jefferson Univ

Wharam Jr, Moody D MD [RadRO] - **Spec Exp:** Pediatric Cancers; Brain Tumors; Sarcoma-Soft Tissue; **Hospital:** Johns Hopkins Hosp; **Address:** Kimmel Cancer Ctr, Dept Rad Oncology, 401 N Broadway St, Ste 1440, Baltimore, MD 21231-1146; **Phone:** 410-955-7313; **Board Cert:** Therapeutic Radiology 1974; **Med School:** Univ VA Sch Med 1969; **Resid:** Radiation Oncology, UCSF Med Ctr 1973; **Fac Appt:** Prof RadRO, Johns Hopkins Univ

Yahalom, Joachim MD [RadRO] - **Spec Exp:** Lymphoma; Hodgkin's Disease; Multiple Myeloma; **Hospital:** Meml Sloan-Kettering Cancer Ctr (page 76); **Address:** 1275 York Ave, SM03, Dept Radiation Onc, New York, NY 10065; **Phone:** 212-639-5999; **Board Cert:** Radiation Oncology 1988; **Med School:** Israel 1976; **Resid:** Internal Medicine, Hadassah Hosp 1979; Radiation Oncology, Hadassah Hosp 1984; **Fellow:** Radiation Oncology, Meml Sloan Kettering Canc Ctr 1986; **Fac Appt:** Prof RadRO, Cornell Univ-Weill Med Coll

Zelefsky, Michael J MD [RadRO] - **Spec Exp:** Prostate Cancer; Brachytherapy; Head & Neck Cancer; **Hospital:** Meml Sloan-Kettering Cancer Ctr (page 76); **Address:** 1275 York Avenue, New York, NY 10065; **Phone:** 800-525-2225; **Board Cert:** Radiation Oncology 1991; **Med School:** Albert Einstein Coll Med 1986; **Resid:** Radiation Oncology, Meml Sloan Kettering Cancer Ctr 1990; **Fac Appt:** Prof RadRO, Cornell Univ-Weill Med Coll

Southeast

Anscher, Mitchell S MD [RadRO] - **Spec Exp:** Prostate Cancer; Brachytherapy; **Hospital:** Med Coll of VA Hosp, Henrico Doctors Hosp; **Address:** Virginia Commonwealth Univ, Department of Radiation Oncology, Box 980058, Richmond, VA 23298-0058; **Phone:** 804-828-7238; **Board Cert:** Internal Medicine 1984; Radiation Oncology 1987; **Med School:** Med Coll VA 1981; **Resid:** Internal Medicine, St Marys Hosp 1984; Radiation Oncology, Duke Univ Med Ctr 1987; **Fac Appt:** Prof RadRO, Va Commonwealth Univ Sch Med

Radiation Oncology

Blackstock, Arthur William MD [RadRO] - **Spec Exp:** Lung Cancer; Gastrointestinal Cancer; Clinical Trials; **Hospital:** Wake Forest Univ Baptist Med Ctr (page 84); **Address:** Wake Forest Univ Medical Ctr, Dept Radiation Oncology, Medical Center Blvd, Winston-Salem, NC 27157; **Phone:** 336-713-3600; **Board Cert:** Radiation Oncology 2006; **Med School:** E Carolina Univ 1989; **Resid:** Radiation Oncology, Univ NC Hosps 1994; **Fac Appt:** Prof RadRO, Wake Forest Univ

Bonner, James Alan MD [RadRO] - **Spec Exp:** Head & Neck Cancer; Lung Cancer; **Hospital:** Univ of Ala Hosp at Birmingham; **Address:** 1824 6th Ave S, WTI, rm 105, Birmingham, AL 35294; **Phone:** 205-934-2761; **Board Cert:** Radiation Oncology 1990; **Med School:** Wayne State Univ 1985; **Resid:** Radiation Oncology, Univ Michigan Med Ctr 1989; **Fac Appt:** Prof RadRO, Univ Alabama

Brizel, David M MD [RadRO] - **Spec Exp:** Head & Neck Cancer; Sarcoma; **Hospital:** Duke Univ Med Ctr; **Address:** Duke Univ Med Ctr, Dept Rad Onc, Box 3085, Durham, NC 27710-0001; **Phone:** 919-668-5637; **Board Cert:** Radiation Oncology 1987; **Med School:** Northwestern Univ 1983; **Resid:** Radiation Oncology, Harvard Joint Ctr Radiation Ther 1987; **Fac Appt:** Prof RadRO, Duke Univ

Chakravarthy, Anuradha MD [RadRO] - **Spec Exp:** Breast Cancer; Gastrointestinal Cancer; **Hospital:** Vanderbilt Univ Med Ctr; **Address:** Vanderbilt Univ Med Ctr, Dept Rad Onc, 1301 22nd Ave S, Preston Research Bldg, Ste 1003, Nashville, TN 37232; **Phone:** 615-322-2555; **Board Cert:** Radiation Oncology 1994; Internal Medicine 1986; Medical Oncology 1989; **Med School:** Geo Wash Univ 1983; **Resid:** Internal Medicine, Mayo Clinic 1986; Medical Oncology, Univ MD Cancer Ctr 1989; **Fellow:** Radiation Oncology, Johns Hopkins Hosp; **Fac Appt:** Asst Prof RadRO, Vanderbilt Univ

Crocker, Ian R MD [RadRO] - **Spec Exp:** Brain Tumors; Eye Tumors/Cancer; Vascular Brachytherapy; **Hospital:** Emory Univ Hosp, Emory Univ Hosp Midtown; **Address:** The Emory Clinic, Dept Radiation Onc, 1365 Clifton Rd NE, CT-104, Atlanta, GA 30322; **Phone:** 404-778-3473; **Board Cert:** Therapeutic Radiology 1999; Internal Medicine 1980; **Med School:** Univ Saskatchewan 1976; **Resid:** Internal Medicine, Univ Hosp-Univ West Ontario 1980; **Fellow:** Radiation Oncology, Princess Margaret Hosp-Univ Toronto 1983; **Fac Appt:** Prof RadRO, Emory Univ

Halle, Jan MD [RadRO] - **Spec Exp:** Breast Cancer; Lung Cancer; **Hospital:** Univ NC Hosps; **Address:** Univ North Carolina Sch Med, Dept Rad Onc, 101 Manning Drive, CB 7512, Gravely Bldg, Chapel Hill, NC 27599; **Phone:** 919-966-7700; **Board Cert:** Therapeutic Radiology 1982; **Med School:** Tufts Univ 1975; **Resid:** Radiation Oncology, North Carolina Meml Hosp 1981; **Fac Appt:** Assoc Prof RadRO, Univ NC Sch Med

Jose, Baby Oliapuram MD [RadRO] - **Spec Exp:** Head & Neck Cancer; Lung Cancer; Gynecologic Cancer; Prostate Cancer; **Hospital:** Univ of Louisville Hosp; **Address:** James G. Brown Cancer Center, 529 S Jackson St Fl 4, Louisville, KY 40202; **Phone:** 502-561-2700; **Board Cert:** Therapeutic Radiology 1978; **Med School:** India 1971; **Resid:** Surgery, CMC Hosp 1974; Radiation Oncology, CMC Hosp 1976; **Fellow:** Radiation Oncology, Brown Univ-RI Hosp 1979; **Fac Appt:** Prof RadRO, Univ Louisville Sch Med

Kiel, Krystyna D MD [RadRO] - **Spec Exp:** Breast Cancer; Sarcoma; Gastrointestinal Cancer; Colon & Rectal Cancer; **Hospital:** Meml Hlth Univ Med Ctr - Savannah; **Address:** Savannah Radiation Cancer Care, 4700 Waters Ave, Dept Radiation Onc, Savanna, GA 31404; **Phone:** 912-350-8490; **Board Cert:** Therapeutic Radiology 1983; Radiation Oncology 2000; **Med School:** Univ Mass Sch Med 1977; **Resid:** Radiation Oncology, Mass Genl Hosp 1982

Kun, Larry E MD [RadRO] - **Spec Exp:** Brain Tumors; Pediatric Cancers; **Hospital:** St Jude Children's Research Hosp, Le Bonheur Chldns Med Ctr; **Address:** St Jude Chldns Research Hosp-Dept Rad Onc, 262 Danny Thomas Pl, MS 220, Memphis, TN 38105; **Phone:** 901-495-3565; **Board Cert:** Therapeutic Radiology 1973; **Med School:** Jefferson Med Coll 1968; **Resid:** Therapeutic Radiology, Penrose Cancer Hosp 1972; **Fellow:** Radiation Oncology, Natl Cancer Inst 1974; Radiation Oncology, Rotterdam Radiotherapy Inst 1975; **Fac Appt:** Prof, Univ Tenn Coll Med, Memphis

Landry, Jerome C MD [RadRO] - **Spec Exp:** Gastrointestinal Cancer; Sarcoma-Soft Tissue; **Hospital:** Emory Univ Hosp, Grady Hlth Sys; **Address:** Emory Dept Rad Oncology, 1365 Clifton Rd NE, Ste A-1304, Atlanta, GA 30322; **Phone:** 404-778-3473; **Board Cert:** Radiation Oncology 1988; **Med School:** Harvard Med Sch 1983; **Resid:** Radiation Oncology, Mass Genl Hosp 1987; **Fac Appt:** Prof RadRO, Emory Univ

Larner, James M MD [RadRO] - **Spec Exp:** Neuro-Oncology; Brain Tumors; **Hospital:** Univ Virginia Med Ctr; **Address:** Univ Virginia Medical Ctr, Dept Radiation Oncology, PO Box 800383, Charlottesville, VA 22908; **Phone:** 434-924-5191; **Board Cert:** Internal Medicine 1983; Medical Oncology 1987; Hematology 1988; Radiation Oncology 1989; **Med School:** Univ VA Sch Med 1980; **Resid:** Internal Medicine, Thos Jefferson Univ Hosp 1983; Radiation Oncology, Montefiore-Einstein Med Ctr 1989; **Fellow:** Hematology & Oncology, Thos Jefferson Univ Hosp 1986; **Fac Appt:** Assoc Prof Med, Univ VA Sch Med

Lee, W Robert MD [RadRO] - **Spec Exp:** Prostate Cancer; Brachytherapy; Intensity Modulated Radiotherapy (IMRT); **Hospital:** Duke Univ Med Ctr; **Address:** Duke Univ Med Ctr, Div Radiation Oncology, Box 3085, Durham, NC 27710; **Phone:** 919-668-5640; **Board Cert:** Radiation Oncology 1994; **Med School:** Univ VA Sch Med 1989; **Resid:** Radiation Oncology, Univ Florida 1993; **Fac Appt:** Prof RadRO, Duke Univ

Lewin, Alan A MD [RadRO] - **Spec Exp:** Breast Cancer; Lung Cancer; Brain & Spinal Cord Tumors; **Hospital:** Baptist Hosp of Miami; **Address:** Baptist Hosp Miami, Dept Radiation Oncology, 8900 N Kendall Drive, Miami, FL 33176-2118; **Phone:** 786-596-6566; **Board Cert:** Therapeutic Radiology 1982; Internal Medicine 1976; Hematology 1978; Medical Oncology 1981; **Med School:** Geo Wash Univ 1973; **Resid:** Internal Medicine, Mt Sinai Hosp 1976; **Fellow:** Hematology & Oncology, Beth Israel Med Ctr 1978; Radiation Oncology, Joint Ctr Radiation Therapy 1980; **Fac Appt:** Clin Prof RadRO, Univ Miami Sch Med

Marcus Jr, Robert B MD [RadRO] - **Spec Exp:** Pediatric Cancers; Sarcoma; Bone Cancer; Brain/CNS Tumors; **Hospital:** Shands Jacksonville; **Address:** Univ Florida Proton Therapy Inst, 2015 N Jefferson St NE, Jacksonville, FL 32206; **Phone:** 904-588-1800; **Board Cert:** Therapeutic Radiology 1980; **Med School:** Univ Fla Coll Med 1975; **Resid:** Radiation Oncology, Shands Hosp 1979; **Fac Appt:** Prof RadRO, Univ Fla Coll Med

Markoe, Arnold M MD [RadRO] - **Spec Exp:** Eye Tumors/Cancer; Orbital Tumors/Cancer; Central Nervous System Cancer; Lymphoma; **Hospital:** Univ of Miami Hosp & Clins/Sylvester Comp Canc Ctr (page 82), Jackson Meml Hosp (page 82); **Address:** Univ of Miami Sylvester Comp Cancer Ctr, 1475 NW 12th Ave, Dept Radiation Onc-D31, Miami, FL 33136; **Phone:** 305-243-4319; **Board Cert:** Therapeutic Radiology 1983; **Med School:** Hahnemann Univ 1977; **Resid:** Radiation Oncology, Hahnemann Hosp 1981; **Fac Appt:** Prof RadRO, Univ Miami Sch Med

Marks, Lawrence MD [RadRO] - **Spec Exp:** Breast Cancer; Lung Cancer; **Hospital:** Univ NC Hosps; **Address:** UNC Dept Rad Onc, Campus Box 7512, Chapel Hill, NC 27599-7512; **Phone:** 919-966-0400; **Board Cert:** Radiation Oncology 1989; **Med School:** Univ Rochester 1985; **Resid:** Radiation Oncology, Mass Genl Hosp 1989; **Fac Appt:** Prof RadRO, Univ NC Sch Med

Radiation Oncology

McGarry, Ronald C MD/PhD [RadRO] - **Spec Exp:** Lung Cancer; Lymphoma; Clinical Trials; Stereotactic Radiosurgery; **Hospital:** Univ of Kentucky Chandler Hosp; **Address:** Chandler Medical Ctr, Radiation Medicine, 800 Rose St, rm C1, Lexington, KY 40536; **Phone:** 859-323-6486; **Board Cert:** Radiation Oncology 1999; **Med School:** Canada 1992; **Resid:** Radiation Oncology, Univ W Ontario Regl Cancer Ctr 1997; **Fac Appt:** Prof RadRO, Univ KY Coll Med

Mendenhall, Nancy P MD [RadRO] - **Spec Exp:** Breast Cancer; Lymphoma; Hodgkin's Disease; **Hospital:** Shands at Univ of FL; **Address:** Univ Florida, Dept Radiation Oncology, Box 100385, Gainesville, FL 32610-0385; **Phone:** 352-265-0287; **Board Cert:** Therapeutic Radiology 1985; **Med School:** Univ Fla Coll Med 1980; **Resid:** Diagnostic Radiology, Shands-Univ of Florida 1984; **Fac Appt:** Prof RadRO, Univ Fla Coll Med

Mendenhall, William M MD [RadRO] - **Spec Exp:** Head & Neck Cancer; Stereotactic Radiosurgery; Colon Cancer; **Hospital:** Shands at Univ of FL; **Address:** Univ Florida, Dept Radiation Oncology, Box 100385, Gainesville, FL 32610-0385; **Phone:** 352-265-0287; **Board Cert:** Therapeutic Radiology 1983; **Med School:** Univ S Fla Coll Med 1978; **Resid:** Radiation Oncology, Univ Fla 1983; **Fac Appt:** Prof RadRO, Univ Fla Coll Med

Merchant, Thomas E DO [RadRO] - **Spec Exp:** Brain Tumors-Pediatric; **Hospital:** St Jude Children's Research Hosp; **Address:** St Jude Children's Research Hosp, 262 Danny Thomas Pl, MS 220, Memphis, TN 38105; **Phone:** 901-495-3604; **Board Cert:** Radiation Oncology 2004; **Med School:** Chicago Coll Osteo Med 1989; **Resid:** Radiation Oncology, Meml Sloan Kettering Cancer Ctr 1994

Meredith, Ruby F MD [RadRO] - **Spec Exp:** Multiple Myeloma; Breast Cancer; Radionuclide Therapy; Bone Tumors-Metastatic; **Hospital:** Univ of Ala Hosp at Birmingham; **Address:** Univ Alabama Hosps-Radiation Oncology, 619 19th St S, Birmingham, AL 35233; **Phone:** 205-934-2763; **Board Cert:** Radiation Oncology 1987; **Med School:** Ohio State Univ 1983; **Resid:** Radiation Oncology, Med College Va Hosps 1987; **Fac Appt:** Prof RadRO, Univ Alabama

Pollack, Alan MD/PhD [RadRO] - **Spec Exp:** Prostate Cancer; Genitourinary Cancer; Sarcoma; **Hospital:** Univ of Miami Hosp & Clins/Sylvester Comp Canc Ctr (page 82); **Address:** 1475 NW 12th Ave, Miami, FL 33136; **Phone:** 305-243-4200; **Board Cert:** Radiation Oncology 1993; **Med School:** Univ Miami Sch Med 1987; **Resid:** Radiation Oncology, MD Anderson Cancer Ctr 1992; **Fac Appt:** Prof RadRO, Univ Miami Sch Med

Prosnitz, Leonard MD [RadRO] - **Spec Exp:** Lymphoma; Breast Cancer; Hyperthermia Treatment of Cancer; Sarcoma; **Hospital:** Duke Univ Med Ctr; **Address:** Duke Univ Med Ctr, Dept Rad Onc, Box 3085, Durham, NC 27710; **Phone:** 919-668-5637; **Board Cert:** Therapeutic Radiology 1970; **Med School:** SUNY Downstate 1961; **Resid:** Internal Medicine, Dartmouth Affil Hosps 1963; Radiation Oncology, Yale-New Haven Hosp 1969; **Fellow:** Hematology & Oncology, Yale-New Haven Hosp 1967; **Fac Appt:** Prof RadRO, Duke Univ

Randall, Marcus MD [RadRO] - **Spec Exp:** Gynecologic Cancer; Stereotactic Radiosurgery; **Hospital:** Univ of Kentucky Chandler Hosp; **Address:** Univ Kentucky Medical Ctr, 800 Rose St, rm C11-14D, Office of Radiation Med, Lexington, KY 40536-0001; **Phone:** 859-323-6487; **Board Cert:** Therapeutic Radiology 1986; **Med School:** Univ NC Sch Med 1982; **Resid:** Radiation Oncology, Univ Va Med Ctr 1986; **Fellow:** Radiation Oncology, Univ Va Med Ctr 1986; **Fac Appt:** Prof RadRO, Univ KY Coll Med

Rich, Tyvin Andrew MD [RadRO] - **Spec Exp:** Colon & Rectal Cancer; Chemo-Radiation Combined Therapy; Esophageal Cancer; Gallbladder & Biliary Cancer; **Hospital:** Univ Virginia Med Ctr; **Address:** Univ Va Hlth Sys, Dept Rad Onc, Box 800383, Charlottesville, VA 22908-0383; **Phone:** 434-924-5191; **Board Cert:** Radiation Oncology 1978; **Med School:** Univ VA Sch Med 1973; **Resid:** Mass Genl Hosp 1978; **Fellow:** Radiation Oncology, Mt Vernon Hosp/Gray Lab 1978; **Fac Appt:** Prof RadRO, Univ VA Sch Med

Rosenman, Julian MD/PhD [RadRO] - **Spec Exp:** Lung Cancer; Breast Cancer; Prostate Cancer; **Hospital:** Univ NC Hosps; **Address:** Univ North Carolina, Dept Rad Onc, 101 Manning Drive, CB 7512, Gravely Bldg, Chapel Hill, NC 27599-7512; **Phone:** 919-966-7700; **Board Cert:** Therapeutic Radiology 1981; **Med School:** Univ Tex SW, Dallas 1977; **Resid:** Therapeutic Radiology, Mass Genl Hosp 1981; **Fac Appt:** Prof RadRO, Univ NC Sch Med

Sailer, Scott MD [RadRO] - **Spec Exp:** Head & Neck Cancer; Genitourinary Cancer; Pediatric Cancers; **Hospital:** WakeMed Cary, WakeMed New Bern; **Address:** 300 Ashville Ave, Ste 110, Cary, NC 27518; **Phone:** 919-854-4588; **Board Cert:** Radiation Oncology 1988; **Med School:** Harvard Med Sch 1984; **Resid:** Radiation Therapy, Mass Genl Hosp 1988

Shaw, Edward G MD [RadRO] - **Spec Exp:** Stereotactic Radiosurgery; Brain Tumors; **Hospital:** Wake Forest Univ Baptist Med Ctr (page 84); **Address:** Wake Forest Med Ctr, Dept Rad Onc, Medical Center Blvd, Comp Cancer Ctr, Winston-Salem, NC 27157-1029; **Phone:** 336-713-6506; **Board Cert:** Radiation Oncology 1987; **Med School:** Rush Med Coll 1983; **Resid:** Radiation Oncology, Mayo Grad Sch Med 1987; **Fac Appt:** Prof RadRO, Wake Forest Univ

Tepper, Joel E MD [RadRO] - **Spec Exp:** Gastrointestinal Cancer; Sarcoma; Rectal Cancer; **Hospital:** Univ NC Hosps; **Address:** North Carolina Clin Cancer Ctr, Dept Rad Onc - CB#7512, Chapel Hill, NC 27599-7512; **Phone:** 919-966-0400; **Board Cert:** Therapeutic Radiology 1976; **Med School:** Washington Univ, St Louis 1972; **Resid:** Therapeutic Radiology, Mass Genl Hosp 1976; **Fellow:** Therapeutic Radiology, Mass Genl Hosp 1977; **Fac Appt:** Prof RadRO, Univ NC Sch Med

Toonkel, Leonard M MD [RadRO] - **Spec Exp:** Prostate Cancer; Breast Cancer; Brachytherapy; **Hospital:** Mount Sinai Med Ctr - Miami; **Address:** Dept Radiation Oncology, 4300 Alton Rd, Miami Beach, FL 33140; **Phone:** 305-535-3400; **Board Cert:** Therapeutic Radiology 1979; **Med School:** Univ Miami Sch Med 1975; **Resid:** Radiation Therapy, Jackson Meml Hosp 1977; Diagnostic Radiology, MD Anderson Hosp 1978; **Fellow:** Radiation Oncology, MD Anderson Hosp 1979; **Fac Appt:** Assoc Clin Prof Rad, Univ Miami Sch Med

Trotti, Andrea MD [RadRO] - **Spec Exp:** Head & Neck Cancer; Gastrointestinal Cancer; Skin Cancer; **Hospital:** H Lee Moffitt Cancer Ctr & Research Inst; **Address:** H Lee Moffitt Cancer Ctr, Dept Rad Onc, 12902 Magnolia Drive, Tampa, FL 33612-9416; **Phone:** 813-745-8424; **Board Cert:** Radiation Oncology 1988; **Med School:** Univ Fla Coll Med 1984; **Resid:** Radiation Oncology, Univ Alabama 1988; **Fac Appt:** Prof RadRO, Univ S Fla Coll Med

Vijayakumar, Srinivasan MD [RadRO] - **Spec Exp:** Brachytherapy; Prostate Cancer; **Hospital:** Univ Mississippi Med Ctr; **Address:** 2500 N State St, Jackson, MS 39216; **Phone:** 601-815-2005; **Board Cert:** Therapeutic Radiology 1986; **Med School:** India 1978; **Resid:** Radiation Oncology, Madras Univ Med Ctr 1981; Radiation Oncology, Michael Reese Hosp 1984; **Fellow:** Brachytherapy, Univ Chicago Hosps 1985; **Fac Appt:** Prof RadRO, Univ Miss

Willett, Christopher MD [RadRO] - **Spec Exp:** Gastrointestinal Cancer; Clinical Trials; **Hospital:** Duke Univ Med Ctr; **Address:** Duke Univ Med Ctr, PO Box 3085, Durham, NC 27710; **Phone:** 919-668-5640; **Board Cert:** Therapeutic Radiology 1985; **Med School:** Tufts Univ 1981; **Resid:** Radiation Oncology, Mass Genl Hosp 1986; **Fac Appt:** Prof RadRO, Duke Univ

Radiation Oncology

Wolfson, Aaron H MD [RadRO] - **Spec Exp:** Bone Tumors; Sarcoma-Soft Tissue; **Hospital:** Univ of Miami Hosp & Clins/Sylvester Comp Canc Ctr (page 82); **Address:** Univ of Miami Sylvester Comp Cancer Ctr, 1475 NW 12th Ave, Box D31, Miami, FL 33101; **Phone:** 305-243-4319; **Board Cert:** Radiation Oncology 1999; **Med School:** Univ Fla Coll Med 1982; **Resid:** Radiation Oncology, Med Coll of Virginia 1989; **Fac Appt:** Prof RadRO, Univ Miami Sch Med

Midwest

Abrams, Ross A MD [RadRO] - **Spec Exp:** Gastrointestinal Cancer; Lymphoma; **Hospital:** Rush Univ Med Ctr; **Address:** Women's Center for Radiation Therapy, 500 S Paulina, Ground Floor Atrium, Chicago, IL 60612; **Phone:** 312-942-5751; **Board Cert:** Internal Medicine 1976; Medical Oncology 1979; Hematology 1982; Radiation Oncology 1987; **Med School:** Univ Pennsylvania 1973; **Resid:** Internal Medicine, Pennsylvania Hosp 1975; Hematology & Oncology, Hosp Univ Penn 1976; **Fellow:** Hematology & Oncology, Natl Cancer Inst 1978; Radiation Oncology, Med Coll Wisconsin 1987; **Fac Appt:** Prof RadRO, Rush Med Coll

Ben-Josef, Edgar MD [RadRO] - **Spec Exp:** Bone Cancer; Gastrointestinal Cancer; Pancreatic Cancer; Intensity Modulated Radiotherapy (IMRT); **Hospital:** Univ Michigan Hlth Sys; **Address:** Univ of Mich Hosp, 1500 E Medical Ctr Drive, rm UH B2C490, Ann Arbor, MI 48109-0010; **Phone:** 734-936-8207; **Board Cert:** Radiation Oncology 1994; **Med School:** Israel 1986; **Resid:** Radiation Oncology, Wayne State Univ Hosp 1994; **Fellow:** Cancer Biology, Wayne State Univ Hosp 1995; **Fac Appt:** Assoc Prof RadRO, Univ Mich Med Sch

Bradley, Jeffrey D MD [RadRO] - **Spec Exp:** Lung Cancer; Esophageal Cancer; Thoracic Cancers; Clinical Trials; **Hospital:** Barnes-Jewish Hosp; **Address:** Siteman Cancer Ctr, 4921 Parkview Pl Fl LL, St Louis, MO 63110; **Phone:** 314-747-7236; **Board Cert:** Radiation Oncology 1998; **Med School:** Univ Ark 1993; **Resid:** Radiation Oncology, Univ Chicago 1998; **Fac Appt:** Assoc Prof RadRO, Washington Univ, St Louis

Buatti, John M MD [RadRO] - **Spec Exp:** Central Nervous System Cancer; **Hospital:** Univ Iowa Hosp & Clinics; **Address:** 200 Hawkins Drive, rm 01626, Iowa City, IA 52242; **Phone:** 319-356-2699; **Board Cert:** Radiation Oncology 1994; **Med School:** Georgetown Univ 1986; **Resid:** Internal Medicine, Georgetown Univ 1989; **Fellow:** Radiation Oncology, Univ Arizona 1993; **Fac Appt:** Prof RadRO, Univ Iowa Coll Med

Charboneau, J William MD [RadRO] - **Spec Exp:** Radiofrequency Tumor Ablation; Liver Cancer; Thyroid Cancer; **Hospital:** Mayo Med Ctr & Clin - Rochester; **Address:** Mayo Clinic Dept of Radiology, 200 First St SW, Rochester, MN 55905-0002; **Phone:** 507-284-2097; **Board Cert:** Diagnostic Radiology 1980; **Med School:** Univ Wisc 1976; **Resid:** Diagnostic Radiology, Mayo Clinic 1980; **Fac Appt:** Prof, Mayo Med Sch

Ciezki, Jay P MD [RadRO] - **Spec Exp:** Brachytherapy; Prostate Cancer; Genitourinary Cancer; **Hospital:** Cleveland Clin Fdn (page 70); **Address:** Cleveland Clinic Fdn, 9500 Euclid Ave, MC T28, Cleveland, OH 44195; **Phone:** 216-445-9465; **Board Cert:** Radiation Oncology 2005; **Med School:** Med Coll Wisc 1991; **Resid:** Radiation Oncology, Cleveland Clinic 1995; **Fellow:** Brachytherapy, Cleveland Clinic 1996

Emami, Bahman MD [RadRO] - **Spec Exp:** Head & Neck Cancer; Lung Cancer; **Hospital:** Loyola Univ Med Ctr, Hines VA Hosp; **Address:** Loyola Univ Med Ctr, Dept Rad Onc, 2160 S First Ave Bldg 105 - rm 2932, Maywood, IL 60153-3328; **Phone:** 708-216-2729; **Board Cert:** Therapeutic Radiology 1976; **Med School:** Iran 1968; **Resid:** Radiation Therapy, St Vincents Hosp 1973; Radiation Therapy, New England Med Ctr 1977; **Fac Appt:** Prof RadRO, Loyola Univ-Stritch Sch Med

Forman, Jeffrey D MD [RadRO] - **Spec Exp:** Neutron Therapy for Advanced Cancer; Genitourinary Cancer; Prostate Cancer; **Address:** 70 Fulton St, Pontiac, MI 48341; **Phone:** 248-338-0300; **Board Cert:** Radiation Oncology 1986; **Med School:** NYU Sch Med 1982; **Resid:** Radiation Oncology, Johns Hopkins Hosp 1986; **Fellow:** Therapeutic Radiology, Johns Hopkins Hosp 1987; **Fac Appt:** Prof RadRO, Wayne State Univ

Grigsby, Perry W MD [RadRO] - **Spec Exp:** Gynecologic Cancer; Thyroid Cancer; **Hospital:** Barnes-Jewish Hosp, St Louis Chldns Hosp; **Address:** Washington Univ School Med, Dept Rad Onc, 4921 Parkview Pl, Box 8224, St Louis, MO 63110; **Phone:** 314-747-7236; **Board Cert:** Radiation Oncology 1987; **Med School:** Univ KY Coll Med 1982; **Resid:** Radiation Oncology, Barnes Jewish Hosp 1985; **Fac Appt:** Prof, Washington Univ, St Louis

Halpern, Howard MD/PhD [RadRO] - **Spec Exp:** Breast Cancer; Esophageal Cancer; Gynecologic Cancer; **Hospital:** Univ of Chicago Med Ctr, Univ of IL Med Ctr at Chicago; **Address:** 1801 W Taylor St, rm C400, MC-933, Chicago, IL 60612; **Phone:** 773-702-0817; **Board Cert:** Therapeutic Radiology 1984; **Med School:** Univ Miami Sch Med 1980; **Resid:** Therapeutic Radiology, Jnt Ctr Rad Ther Harvard 1984; **Fellow:** Therapeutic Radiology, Jnt Ctr Rad Ther Harvard 1985; **Fac Appt:** Prof Rad, Univ Chicago-Pritzker Sch Med

Haraf, Daniel J MD [RadRO] - **Spec Exp:** Head & Neck Cancer; Lung Cancer; Prostate Cancer; **Hospital:** Univ of Chicago Med Ctr; **Address:** Univ Chicago Hosps, Dept Rad Oncology, 5758 S Maryland, MS 9006, Chicago, IL 60637; **Phone:** 773-702-6870; **Board Cert:** Internal Medicine 1985; Radiation Oncology 1990; **Med School:** Ros Franklin Univ/Chicago Med Sch 1982; **Resid:** Internal Medicine, Michael Reese Hosp 1985; **Fellow:** Radiation Oncology, Michael Reese Hosp 1988; **Fac Appt:** Prof RadRO, Univ Chicago-Pritzker Sch Med

Harari, Paul M MD [RadRO] - **Spec Exp:** Head & Neck Cancer; **Hospital:** Univ WI Hosp & Clins; **Address:** Dept of Human Oncology, 600 Highland Ave, Ste K4/336, Madison, WI 53792; **Phone:** 608-263-5009; **Board Cert:** Radiation Oncology 1990; **Med School:** Univ VA Sch Med 1984; **Resid:** Radiation Oncology, Univ Arizona Med Ctr 1990; **Fac Appt:** Prof RadRO, Univ Wisc

Hayman, James A MD [RadRO] - **Spec Exp:** Breast Cancer; Stomach Cancer; Lung Cancer; Brain Tumors; **Hospital:** Univ Michigan Hlth Sys; **Address:** Univ Michigan Hosp, 1500 E Medical Ctr Drive, rm UH B2C490, Ann Arbor, MI 48109-0010; **Phone:** 734-647-9956; **Board Cert:** Radiation Oncology 2004; **Med School:** Univ Chicago-Pritzker Sch Med 1991; **Resid:** Radiation Therapy, Joint Ctr for Radiation Therapy 1996; **Fac Appt:** Assoc Prof RadRO, Univ Mich Med Sch

Kim, Jae Ho MD [RadRO] - **Spec Exp:** Brain Tumors; Spinal Cord Tumors; Breast Cancer; Lymphoma; **Hospital:** Henry Ford Hosp; **Address:** Radiation Oncology, 2799 W Grand Blvd, Detroit, MI 48202; **Phone:** 313-916-1029; **Board Cert:** Therapeutic Radiology 1973; **Med School:** Korea 1959; **Resid:** Therapeutic Radiology, Meml-Sloan-Kettering 1972; **Fellow:** Diagnostic Radiology, Meml-Sloan-Kettering 1968; **Fac Appt:** Prof RadRO, Wayne State Univ

Konski, Andre MD [RadRO] - **Spec Exp:** Esophageal Cancer; Rectal Cancer; Pancreatic Cancer; Gastrointestinal Cancer; **Hospital:** Karmanos Cancer Inst; **Address:** Dept Radiation Oncology, 4100 John R, Detroit, MI 48201; **Phone:** 313-745-2560; **Board Cert:** Radiation Oncology 2000; **Med School:** NY Med Coll 1984; **Resid:** Radiation Oncology, Stong Meml/Genesee Hosps 1988; **Fac Appt:** Prof RadRO, Wayne State Univ

Radiation Oncology

Lawrence, Theodore S MD/PhD [RadRO] - **Spec Exp:** Gastrointestinal Cancer; Liver Cancer; Pancreatic Cancer; **Hospital:** Univ Michigan Hlth Sys; **Address:** Univ of Mich Hosp, Dept Rad Onc, 1500 E Med Ctr Dr, SPC5010, Box 5010, UH-B2-C502, Ann Arbor, MI 48109-5010; **Phone:** 734-936-4300; **Board Cert:** Internal Medicine 1983; Medical Oncology 1985; Radiation Oncology 1987; **Med School:** Cornell Univ-Weill Med Coll 1980; **Resid:** Internal Medicine, Stanford Univ Hosp 1983; Radiation Oncology, Natl Cancer Inst 1987; **Fellow:** Medical Oncology, Natl Cancer Inst 1986; **Fac Appt:** Prof RadRO, Univ Mich Med Sch

Lee, Chung K MD [RadRO] - **Spec Exp:** Head & Neck Cancer; Breast Cancer; Lymphoma; Gastrointestinal Cancer; **Hospital:** Univ Minn Med Ctr, Fairview - Univ Campus; **Address:** Dept of Radiation Oncology, 420 Delaware St SE, MMC 400, Minneapolis, MN 55455; **Phone:** 612-273-6700; **Board Cert:** Therapeutic Radiology 1976; **Med School:** Korea 1965; **Resid:** Therapeutic Radiology, Univ of Minn Hosp 1976; Diagnostic Radiology, Yonsei Univ Hosp 1971; **Fac Appt:** Prof, Univ Minn

Macklis, Roger M MD [RadRO] - **Spec Exp:** Radioimmunotherapy of Cancer; Breast Cancer; Lymphoma; **Hospital:** Cleveland Clin Fdn (page 70); **Address:** Cleveland Cin Fdn, Dept Rad Onc, 9500 Euclid Ave, Desk T28, Cleveland, OH 44195; **Phone:** 216-444-5576; **Board Cert:** Radiation Oncology 1989; **Med School:** Harvard Med Sch 1983; **Resid:** Radiation Oncology, Joint Ctr Radiotherapy Inst 1987; **Fellow:** Research, Dana Farber Cancer Inst 1987; **Fac Appt:** Prof RadRO, Case West Res Univ

Martenson Jr, James A MD [RadRO] - **Spec Exp:** Mucositis; Esophageal Cancer; **Hospital:** Mayo Med Ctr & Clin - Rochester; **Address:** Mayo Clinic, Dept Rad/Onc, 200 First St SW, Rochester, MN 55905; **Phone:** 507-284-4561; **Board Cert:** Therapeutic Radiology 1985; **Med School:** Univ Wash 1981; **Resid:** Radiation Oncology, Mayo Clinic 1985; **Fac Appt:** Assoc Prof, Mayo Med Sch

Mehta, Minesh P MD [RadRO] - **Spec Exp:** Brain Tumors; Lung Cancer; Pediatric Cancers; **Hospital:** Univ WI Hosp & Clins; **Address:** Univ Wisconsin, Dept Rad Oncology, 600 Highland Ave, K4B-100, Madison, WI 53792; **Phone:** 608-263-8500; **Board Cert:** Radiation Oncology 1988; **Med School:** Zambia 1981; **Resid:** Internal Medicine, Ndola Central Hosp 1983; Radiation Oncology, Univ WI Hosps 1988; **Fac Appt:** Prof RadRO, Univ Wisc

Michalski, Jeff M MD [RadRO] - **Spec Exp:** Prostate Cancer; Sarcoma; Pediatric Cancers; **Hospital:** Barnes-Jewish Hosp, St Louis Chldns Hosp; **Address:** Washington Univ Sch Med, Dept Rad Oncology, 4921 Parkview Place, Lower Level, Box 8224, St Louis, MO 63110; **Phone:** 314-747-7236; **Board Cert:** Radiation Oncology 1991; **Med School:** Med Coll Wisc 1986; **Resid:** Radiation Oncology, Columbia Presby Med Ctr 1988; Radiation Oncology, Mallinckrodt Inst of Radiology 1990; **Fellow:** Radiation Oncology, Mallinckrodt Inst of Radiology 1991; **Fac Appt:** Assoc Prof RadRO, Washington Univ, St Louis

Mittal, Bharat B MD [RadRO] - **Spec Exp:** Head & Neck Cancer; Lymphoma; Skin Cancer; **Hospital:** Northwestern Meml Hosp; **Address:** 251 E Huron St, Bldg LC-178, Chicago, IL 60611; **Phone:** 312-926-2520; **Board Cert:** Radiation Oncology 1981; **Med School:** India 1975; **Resid:** Internal Medicine, Christian Med Coll 1976; Radiation Oncology, Northwestern Meml Hosp 1980; **Fellow:** Radiation Oncology, Mallinckrodt Inst 1981; **Fac Appt:** Prof RadRO, Northwestern Univ

Movsas, Benjamin MD [RadRO] - **Spec Exp:** Lung Cancer; Brain Tumors; Prostate Cancer; Stereotactic Radiosurgery; **Hospital:** Henry Ford Hosp; **Address:** Henry Ford Health Sys, Rad Oncology, 2799 W Grand Blvd, Detroit, MI 48202-2608; **Phone:** 313-916-5188; **Board Cert:** Radiation Oncology 1999; **Med School:** Washington Univ, St Louis 1990; **Resid:** Radiation Oncology, National Cancer Inst 1995

Myerson, Robert J MD [RadRO] - **Spec Exp:** Gastrointestinal Cancer; Breast Cancer; Hyperthermia Treatment of Cancer; **Hospital:** Barnes-Jewish Hosp; **Address:** Ctr for Advanced Med-Siteman Cancer Ctr, 4921 Parkview Pl, Box 9038635, St Louis, MO 63110; **Phone:** 314-747-7236; **Board Cert:** Therapeutic Radiology 1985; **Med School:** Univ Miami Sch Med 1980; **Resid:** Radiation Therapy, Hosp Univ Penn 1984; **Fac Appt:** Prof RadRO, Washington Univ, St Louis

Pierce, Lori J MD [RadRO] - **Spec Exp:** Breast Cancer; **Hospital:** Univ Michigan Hlth Sys; **Address:** Univ Hosp, Dept Rad Onc, 1500 E Med Ctr, rm B2C440, Box 5010, Ann Arbor, MI 48109-5099; **Phone:** 734-936-4300; **Board Cert:** Radiation Oncology 1989; **Med School:** Duke Univ 1985; **Resid:** Radiation Oncology, Hosp Univ Penn 1989; **Fac Appt:** Prof RadRO, Univ Mich Med Sch

Schomberg, Paula J MD [RadRO] - **Spec Exp:** Brain Tumors; Pediatric Cancers; **Hospital:** Mayo Med Ctr & Clin - Rochester; **Address:** Mayo Clinic - Charlton Bldg, Desk R, 200 1st St SW, Rochester, MN 55905; **Phone:** 507-284-3551; **Board Cert:** Therapeutic Radiology 1984; **Med School:** Med Coll Wisc 1979; **Resid:** Radiation Therapy, Mayo Clinic 1983; **Fac Appt:** Prof RadRO, Mayo Med Sch

Small Jr, William MD [RadRO] - **Spec Exp:** Gynecologic Cancer; Gastrointestinal Cancer; Breast Cancer; Pancreatic Cancer; **Hospital:** Northwestern Meml Hosp; **Address:** Northwestern Meml Hosp, Rad Oncology, 250 E Huron St Galter Bldg - Ste L178, Chicago, IL 60611; **Phone:** 312-472-3650; **Board Cert:** Radiation Oncology 2004; **Med School:** Northwestern Univ 1990; **Resid:** Radiation Oncology, Northwestern Univ 1994; **Fac Appt:** Prof RadRO, Northwestern Univ

Suh, John H MD [RadRO] - **Spec Exp:** Brain Tumors-Adult & Pediatric; Stereotactic Radiosurgery; Stereotactic Body Radiation Therapy; **Hospital:** Cleveland Clin Fdn (page 70); **Address:** Cleveland Clinic, Dept Rad/Onc, 9500 Euclid Ave, Desk T28, Cleveland, OH 44195-0001; **Phone:** 216-444-5574; **Board Cert:** Radiation Oncology 2000; **Med School:** Univ Miami Sch Med 1990; **Resid:** Radiation Oncology, Cleveland Clinic 1994; **Fellow:** Radiation Oncology, Cleveland Clinic 1995

Taylor, Marie E MD [RadRO] - **Spec Exp:** Breast Cancer; **Hospital:** Barnes-Jewish Hosp, Barnes-Jewish West County Hosp; **Address:** Center for Advanced Med-Siteman Cancer Ctr, 4921 Parkview Pl, Box 8224, St Louis, MO 63110; **Phone:** 314-747-7236; **Board Cert:** Radiation Oncology 1997; **Med School:** Univ Wash 1992; **Resid:** Radiation Oncology, Univ Wash Med Ctr 1996

Thornton Jr, Allan F MD [RadRO] - **Spec Exp:** Proton Beam Therapy; **Address:** Midwest Proton Radiotherapy Inst, 2425 N Milo B Sampson Lane, Bloomington, IN 47408; **Phone:** 812-349-5074; **Board Cert:** Radiation Oncology 1999; **Med School:** Univ VA Sch Med 1981; **Resid:** Radiation Oncology, Princess Margaret Hosp 1986

Vicini, Frank A MD [RadRO] - **Spec Exp:** Breast Cancer; Prostate Cancer; Brachytherapy; **Hospital:** William Beaumont Hosp; **Address:** William Beaumont Hospital, 3601 W 13 Mile Rd, Royal Oak, MI 48073; **Phone:** 248-551-1219; **Board Cert:** Radiation Oncology 1999; **Med School:** Wayne State Univ 1985; **Resid:** Radiation Oncology, William Beaumont Hosp 1989; **Fellow:** Radiation Oncology, Harvard Med Sch/Joint Ctr for Rad Ther 1990; **Fac Appt:** Clin Prof RadRO, Univ Mich Med Sch

Videtic, Gregory M MD [RadRO] - **Spec Exp:** Lung Cancer; Mesothelioma; Esophageal Cancer; Thymoma; **Hospital:** Cleveland Clin Fdn (page 70); **Address:** Cleveland Clinic, Radiation Oncology, 9500 Euclid Ave, MC T28, Cleveland, OH 44195; **Phone:** 216-444-9797; **Board Cert:** Radiation Oncology 1998; **Med School:** McGill Univ 1986; **Resid:** Radiation Oncology, Dalhousie Univ 1988; Radiation Oncology, London Regl Cancer Ctr 1997; **Fellow:** Radiation Oncology, Wayne State Univ 1998; **Fac Appt:** Assoc Prof Rad, Cleveland Cl Coll Med/Case West Res

Radiation Oncology

Weichselbaum, Ralph R MD [RadRO] - **Spec Exp:** Gene Targeted Radiotherapy; Head & Neck Cancer; Esophageal Cancer; **Hospital:** Univ of Chicago Med Ctr; **Address:** Univ Chicago, Dept Rad Onc, 5758 S Maryland Ave, MC-9006-DCAM-1D, Chicago, IL 60637; **Phone:** 773-702-0817; **Board Cert:** Therapeutic Radiology 1975; **Med School:** Univ IL Coll Med 1971; **Resid:** Therapeutic Radiology, Harvard Jt Ctr Rad Therapy 1975; **Fellow:** Diagnostic Radiology, Harvard Med Sch 1976; **Fac Appt:** Prof Rad, Univ Chicago-Pritzker Sch Med

Wilson, J Frank MD [RadRO] - **Spec Exp:** Breast Cancer; Skin Cancer; **Hospital:** Froedtert Meml Lutheran Hosp; **Address:** Dept Radiation Oncology, 9200 W Wisconsin Ave, Milwaukee, WI 53226; **Phone:** 414-805-4400; **Board Cert:** Therapeutic Radiology 1971; **Med School:** Univ MO-Columbia Sch Med 1965; **Resid:** Radiation Therapy, Penrose Cancer Hosp 1969; **Fellow:** Radiation Therapy, Natl Cancer Inst/NIH 1971; **Fac Appt:** Prof RadRO, Med Coll Wisc

Great Plains and Mountains

Gaffney, David K MD/PhD [RadRO] - **Spec Exp:** Breast Cancer; Gynecologic Cancer; **Hospital:** Univ Utah Hosps and Clins; **Address:** Huntsman Cancer Hosp, Dept Rad Oncology, 1950 Circle of Hope, rm 1440, Salt Lake City, UT 84112-5560; **Phone:** 801-581-2396; **Board Cert:** Radiation Oncology 2007; **Med School:** Med Coll Wisc 1992; **Resid:** Radiation Oncology, Univ Utah Hosps 1996; **Fac Appt:** Assoc Prof, Univ Utah

Rabinovitch, Rachel A MD [RadRO] - **Spec Exp:** Breast Cancer; Lymphoma; **Hospital:** Univ Colorado Hosp; **Address:** Anschutz Cancer Pavilion, Dept Rad Oncology, 1665 Aurora Court, Ste 1032, MS F-706, Aurora, CO 80045; **Phone:** 720-848-0156; **Board Cert:** Radiation Oncology 1994; **Med School:** Albert Einstein Coll Med 1989; **Resid:** Radiation Oncology, Meml Sloan Kettering Cancer Ctr 1993; **Fac Appt:** Assoc Prof RadRO, Univ Colorado

Shrieve, Dennis C MD [RadRO] - **Spec Exp:** Brain Tumors-Adult & Pediatric; Genitourinary Cancer; Gastrointestinal Cancer; **Hospital:** Univ Utah Hosps and Clins, Primary Children's Med Ctr; **Address:** Huntsman Cancer Inst, Dept Rad Oncology, 1950 Circle of Hope, rm 1440, Salt Lake City, UT 84112; **Phone:** 801-581-2396; **Board Cert:** Radiation Oncology 1993; **Med School:** Univ Miami Sch Med 1989; **Resid:** Radiation Oncology, UCSF Med Ctr; **Fac Appt:** Prof RadRO, Univ Utah

Smalley, Stephen R MD [RadRO] - **Spec Exp:** Colon Cancer; Gastrointestinal Cancer; **Hospital:** Olathe Med Ctr; **Address:** Olathe Med Ctr, 20375 W 151st St, Doctors Bldg - Ste 180, Olathe, KS 66061-4575; **Phone:** 913-768-7200; **Board Cert:** Internal Medicine 1982; Radiation Oncology 1987; Medical Oncology 1985; **Med School:** Univ MO-Kansas City 1979; **Resid:** Internal Medicine, Mayo Clinic 1982; Radiation Oncology, Mayo Clinic 1986; **Fellow:** Medical Oncology, Mayo Clinic 1984; **Fac Appt:** Prof RadRO, Univ Kans

Southwest

Ang, Kie-Kian MD/PhD [RadRO] - **Spec Exp:** Head & Neck Cancer; **Hospital:** UT MD Anderson Cancer Ctr; **Address:** UT MD Anderson Cancer Ctr, 1515 Holcombe Blvd, Box 97, Houston, TX 77030; **Phone:** 713-563-8400; **Board Cert:** Radiation Oncology 1987; **Med School:** Belgium 1975; **Resid:** Radiation Oncology, Univ Hosp Louvian 1980; **Fac Appt:** Prof, Univ Tex, Houston

Buchholz, Thomas A MD [RadRO] - **Spec Exp:** Breast Cancer; **Hospital:** UT MD Anderson Cancer Ctr; **Address:** Univ Texas MD Anderson Cancer Ctr, 1515 Holcombe Blvd, Unit 97, Houston, TX 77030-4000; **Phone:** 713-794-4892; **Board Cert:** Radiation Oncology 1993; **Med School:** Tufts Univ 1988; **Resid:** Radiation Oncology, Univ Washington Med Ctr 1993; **Fellow:** Research, Univ Washington Med Ctr 1994; **Fac Appt:** Prof RadRO, Univ Tex, Houston

Choy, Hak MD [RadRO] - **Spec Exp:** Lung Cancer; **Hospital:** UT Southwestern Med Ctr at Dallas; **Address:** UT SW Med Ctr - Dallas, Dept Rad-Onc, 5801 Forest Park Rd, Dallas, TX 75390-9183; **Phone:** 214-645-7600; **Board Cert:** Radiation Oncology 1993; **Med School:** Univ Tex Med Br, Galveston 1987; **Resid:** Radiation Oncology, Ohio State Univ Hosp 1989; Radiation Oncology, Univ Texas Hlth Sci Ctr 1991; **Fac Appt:** Prof RadRO, Univ Tex SW, Dallas

Cox, James D MD [RadRO] - **Spec Exp:** Lung Cancer; Esophageal Cancer; Thymoma; Thoracic Cancers; **Hospital:** UT MD Anderson Cancer Ctr; **Address:** Univ Tex MD Anderson Cancer Ctr, 1515 Holcombe Blvd, Unit 97, Houston, TX 77030; **Phone:** 713-563-2316; **Board Cert:** Radiation Oncology 1999; **Med School:** Univ Rochester 1965; **Resid:** Diagnostic Radiology, Penrose Cancer Hosp 1969; **Fellow:** Therapeutic Radiology, Inst Gustave-Roussy 1970; **Fac Appt:** Prof RadRO, Univ Tex, Houston

Eifel, Patricia J MD [RadRO] - **Spec Exp:** Cervical Cancer; Uterine Cancer; Vulvar Disease/Cancer; Vaginal Cancer; **Hospital:** UT MD Anderson Cancer Ctr; **Address:** MD Anderson Cancer Ctr, Dept Rad Onc, 1515 Holcombe Blvd, Unit 1202, Houston, TX 77030; **Phone:** 713-563-6830; **Board Cert:** Therapeutic Radiology 1983; **Med School:** Stanford Univ 1977; **Resid:** Radiation Oncology, Stanford Univ Med Ctr 1981; **Fellow:** Therapeutic Radiology, Stanford Univ Med Ctr 1982

Grado, Gordon L MD [RadRO] - **Spec Exp:** Prostate Cancer; Brachytherapy; **Hospital:** Scottsdale Hlthcare - Shea, Univ Minn Med Ctr, Fairview - Univ Campus; **Address:** 2926 N Civic Center Plaza, Scottsdale, AZ 85251; **Phone:** 480-614-6300; **Board Cert:** Therapeutic Radiology 1981; Radiation Oncology 1999; **Med School:** Southern IL Univ 1977; **Resid:** Therapeutic Radiology, Mayo Clinic 1981; **Fac Appt:** Assoc Prof RadRO, Univ Minn

Gunderson, Leonard MD [RadRO] - **Spec Exp:** Gastrointestinal Cancer; Brachytherapy; Sarcoma; **Hospital:** Mayo Clinic - Scottsdale; **Address:** Mayo Clinic, Dept Radiation Onc, 5777 E Mayo Blvd, Phoenix, AZ 85054; **Phone:** 480-342-1262; **Board Cert:** Therapeutic Radiology 1975; **Med School:** Univ KY Coll Med 1969; **Resid:** Radiation Oncology, Latter Day Saints Hosp 1974; **Fac Appt:** Prof RadRO, Mayo Med Sch

Herman, Terence S MD [RadRO] - **Spec Exp:** Breast Cancer; Sarcoma; Brain Tumors; **Hospital:** OU Med Ctr; **Address:** Oklahoma Univ Health Sci Ctr, 825 NE 10th St, OUPB 1430, Oklahoma City, OK 73104-5417; **Phone:** 405-271-5641; **Board Cert:** Internal Medicine 1975; Medical Oncology 1977; Therapeutic Radiology 1985; **Med School:** Univ Conn 1972; **Resid:** Internal Medicine, Univ Arizona Med Ctr 1975; Radiation Oncology, Stanford Univ Med Ctr 1985; **Fellow:** Medical Oncology, Univ Arizona 1977; **Fac Appt:** Prof RadRO, Univ Okla Coll Med

Jhingran, Anuja MD [RadRO] - **Spec Exp:** Gynecologic Cancer; Brachytherapy; **Hospital:** UT MD Anderson Cancer Ctr; **Address:** MD Anderson Cancer Ctr, 1515 Holcombe Ave, Box 1202, Houston, TX 77030; **Phone:** 713-563-6900; **Board Cert:** Radiation Oncology 1993; **Med School:** Texas Tech Univ 1988; **Resid:** Radiation Oncology, Baylor College Med 1993; **Fac Appt:** Assoc Prof RadRO, Univ Tex, Houston

Komaki, Ritsuko U MD [RadRO] - **Spec Exp:** Lung Cancer; Thymoma; Esophageal Cancer; **Hospital:** UT MD Anderson Cancer Ctr; **Address:** UT-MD Anderson Cancer Ctr, Dept Rad Onc, 1515 Holcombe Blvd, Unit 97, Houston, TX 77030; **Phone:** 713-563-2300; **Board Cert:** Therapeutic Radiology 1977; Radiation Oncology 2001; **Med School:** Japan 1969; **Resid:** Radiation Oncology, Med Coll Wisc 1978; **Fac Appt:** Prof RadRO, Univ Tex, Houston

Kuske, Robert R MD [RadRO] - **Spec Exp:** Breast Cancer; **Hospital:** Scottsdale Hlthcare - Shea; **Address:** 9055 E Del Camino Drive, Ste 200, Scottsdale, AZ 85258; **Phone:** 480-922-4600; **Board Cert:** Therapeutic Radiology 1985; **Med School:** Univ Cincinnati 1980; **Resid:** Radiation Oncology, Univ Cincinnati Med Ctr 1984

Radiation Oncology

Lee, Andrew K MD [RadRO] - **Spec Exp:** Prostate Cancer; Proton Beam Therapy; Genitourinary Cancer; **Hospital:** UT MD Anderson Cancer Ctr; **Address:** MD Anderson Cancer Ctr, 1515 Holcombe Blvd, Unit 1202, Houston, TX 77030; **Phone:** 713-563-2443; **Board Cert:** Radiation Oncology 2001; **Med School:** Univ Minn 1996; **Resid:** Radiation Oncology, Joint Ctr for Radiation Therapy/Harvard 2001; **Fac Appt:** Assoc Prof RadRO, Univ Tex, Houston

Medbery, Clinton A MD [RadRO] - **Spec Exp:** Breast Cancer; Prostate Cancer; Brachytherapy; Stereotactic Radiosurgery; **Hospital:** St Anthony Hosp -Oklahoma City; **Address:** Southwest Radiation Oncology, 1011 N Dewey Ave, Ste 101, Oklahoma City, OK 73101; **Phone:** 405-272-7311; **Board Cert:** Internal Medicine 1980; Medical Oncology 1983; Radiation Oncology 1987; **Med School:** Med Univ SC 1976; **Resid:** Internal Medicine, Naval Hosp 1980; Radiation Oncology, Natl Cancer Inst 1987; **Fellow:** Medical Oncology, Naval Hosp 1982

Schild, Steven E MD [RadRO] - **Spec Exp:** Lung Cancer; Brain Cancer; Gastrointestinal Cancer; Clinical Trials; **Hospital:** Mayo Clinic - Scottsdale; **Address:** Mayo Clinic, Dept Radiation Oncology, 13400 E Shea Blvd, Scottsdale, AZ 85259; **Phone:** 480-342-1262; **Board Cert:** Radiation Oncology 1989; **Med School:** Creighton Univ 1985; **Resid:** Radiation Oncology, Mayo Clinic 1989; **Fac Appt:** Prof RadRO, Mayo Med Sch

Senzer, Neil N MD [RadRO] - **Spec Exp:** Clinical Trials; Gene Targeted Radiotherapy; Gene Therapy; **Hospital:** Med City Dallas Hosp, Baylor Univ Medical Ctr; **Address:** Mary Crowley Cancer Research Ctr, 7777 Forest Ln C Bldg - Ste 707, Dallas, TX 75230; **Phone:** 214-370-1870; **Board Cert:** Pediatrics 1976; Pediatric Hematology-Oncology 1978; Therapeutic Radiology 1985; **Med School:** SUNY Buffalo 1971; **Resid:** Pediatrics, Johns Hopkins Hosp 1974; Radiation Oncology, St Barnabas Med Ctr 1985; **Fellow:** Pediatric Hematology-Oncology, St Jude Chldns Rsch Hosp 1978

Shina, Donald C MD [RadRO] - **Spec Exp:** Breast Cancer; **Hospital:** St Vincent Hosp - Santa Fe; **Address:** Santa Fe Cancer Ctr at St Vincent Hosp, 455 Saint Michael's Drive, Santa Fe, NM 87505; **Phone:** 505-820-5233; **Board Cert:** Internal Medicine 1977; Medical Oncology 1979; Therapeutic Radiology 1981; **Med School:** Case West Res Univ 1974; **Resid:** Internal Medicine, Univ Hosps 1977; **Fellow:** Radiation Oncology, Univ Hosps 1980; Medical Oncology, Univ Hosps 1980

Stea, Baldassarre MD/PhD [RadRO] - **Spec Exp:** Brain Tumors; Stereotactic Radiosurgery; Pediatric Cancers; **Hospital:** Univ Med Ctr - Tucson, Tucson Med Ctr; **Address:** Univ Hlth Scis Ctr, Dept Rad Onc, 1501 N Campbell Ave, Tucson, AZ 85724-0001; **Phone:** 520-626-6724; **Board Cert:** Radiation Oncology 1987; **Med School:** Geo Wash Univ 1983; **Resid:** Radiation Oncology, Natl Cancer Inst 1987; **Fac Appt:** Prof RadRO, Univ Ariz Coll Med

Woo, Shiao Y MD [RadRO] - **Spec Exp:** Brain Tumors-Adult & Pediatric; Proton Beam Therapy; Stereotactic Radiosurgery; Pediatric Cancers; **Hospital:** UT MD Anderson Cancer Ctr, Texas Chldns Hosp; **Address:** UT-MD Anderson Cancer Ctr, 1515 Holcombe, Box 1150, Unit 97, Houston, TX 77030; **Phone:** 713-563-2324; **Board Cert:** Radiation Oncology 1988; Pediatrics 1980; **Med School:** Malaysia 1972; **Resid:** Pediatrics, Georgetown Univ Hosp 1978; **Fellow:** Pediatric Hematology-Oncology, Georgetown Univ Hosp 1980; Radiation Oncology, Georgetown Univ Hosp 1988; **Fac Appt:** Prof RadRO, Baylor Coll Med

West Coast and Pacific

Bahn, Duke K MD [RadRO] - **Spec Exp:** Prostate Cancer-Cryosurgery; **Hospital:** Comm Meml Hosp - Ventura; **Address:** Prostate Inst of America, 168 N Brent St, Ste 402, Ventura, CA 93003; **Phone:** 805-585-3082; **Board Cert:** Diagnostic Radiology 1978; **Med School:** Korea 1970; **Resid:** Diagnostic Radiology, Wayne State Univ Med Ctr 1978

Donaldson, Sarah S MD [RadRO] - **Spec Exp:** Pediatric Cancers; Hodgkin's Disease; **Hospital:** Stanford Univ Med Ctr; **Address:** 875 Blake Wilbur Drive, CC Bldg Fl G - rm 226, MC 5847, Stanford, CA 94305-5847; **Phone:** 650-723-6195; **Board Cert:** Therapeutic Radiology 1974; **Med School:** Harvard Med Sch 1968; **Resid:** Radiation Oncology, Stanford Univ Med Ctr 1972; **Fellow:** Pediatric Hematology-Oncology, Inst Gustave-Roussy 1973; Pediatric Hematology-Oncology, MD Anderson Cancer Ctr 1971; **Fac Appt:** Prof RadRO, Stanford Univ

Douglas, James G MD [RadRO] - **Spec Exp:** Pediatric Cancers; Head & Neck Cancer; Brain Tumors; **Hospital:** Univ Wash Med Ctr, Chldns Hosp and Regl Med Ctr - Seattle; **Address:** Univ Washington Med Ctr, Dept Radiation Onc, 1959 NE Pacific St, Box 356043, Seattle, WA 98195-6043; **Phone:** 206-598-4100; **Board Cert:** Pediatrics 1986; Radiation Oncology 2007; **Med School:** Case West Res Univ 1980; **Resid:** Pediatrics, Children's Hosp Med Ctr 1983; Radiation Oncology, Univ Washington Med Ctr 1996; **Fellow:** Pediatric Hematology-Oncology, Natl Inst Hlth 1986; **Fac Appt:** Assoc Prof RadRO, Univ Wash

Fowble, Barbara MD [RadRO] - **Spec Exp:** Breast Cancer; **Hospital:** UCSF Med Ctr; **Address:** 1600 Divisiadero St, Ste H1031, 7701 Burholme Ave, San Francisco, CA 94143-1708; **Phone:** 415-353-9819; **Board Cert:** Therapeutic Radiology 1976; **Med School:** Jefferson Med Coll 1972; **Resid:** Therapeutic Radiology, Bellevue Hosp Ctr-NYU 1975; Therapeutic Radiology, Hahnemann 1976; **Fellow:** Radiation Therapy, Jefferson Hosp 1977; **Fac Appt:** Prof RadRO, UCSF

Halberg, Francine MD [RadRO] - **Spec Exp:** Breast Cancer; **Hospital:** Marin Genl Hosp, UCSF Med Ctr; **Address:** Marin Cancer Inst-Dept of Rad.Oncology, 1350 S Eliseo Drive, Ste 100, Greenbrae, CA 94904; **Phone:** 415-925-7326; **Board Cert:** Internal Medicine 1981; Therapeutic Radiology 1984; **Med School:** Cornell Univ-Weill Med Coll 1978; **Resid:** Internal Medicine, USPHS Hosp 1981; **Fellow:** Radiation Oncology, Stanford Univ Med Ctr 1984; **Fac Appt:** Assoc Prof RadRO, UCSF

Hancock, Steven MD [RadRO] - **Spec Exp:** Prostate Cancer; Breast Cancer; Cancer Survivors-Late Effects of Therapy; **Hospital:** Stanford Univ Med Ctr; **Address:** Stanford Cancer Center-Dept Rad Onc, 875 Blake Wilbur Drive, MC 5847, Stanford, CA 94305; **Phone:** 650-723-6440; **Board Cert:** Internal Medicine 1980; Therapeutic Radiology 1982; **Med School:** Stanford Univ 1976; **Resid:** Radiation Therapy, Stanford Univ Med Ctr 1981; Internal Medicine, Stanford Univ Med Ctr 1979; **Fac Appt:** Prof RadRO, Stanford Univ

Hoppe, Richard T MD [RadRO] - **Spec Exp:** Lymphoma; Hodgkin's Disease; **Hospital:** Stanford Univ Med Ctr; **Address:** Stanford Cancer Ctr, Dept Rad Onc, 875 Blake Wilbur, MC 5847, Stanford, CA 94305-5847; **Phone:** 650-723-5510; **Board Cert:** Therapeutic Radiology 1976; **Med School:** Cornell Univ-Weill Med Coll 1971; **Resid:** Radiation Therapy, Stanford Univ Med Ctr 1976; **Fac Appt:** Prof, Stanford Univ

Koh, Wui-Jin MD [RadRO] - **Spec Exp:** Gynecologic Cancer; Brachytherapy; Clinical Trials; **Hospital:** Univ Wash Med Ctr; **Address:** Univ Washington Med Ctr, Dept of Radiation Oncology, Box 356043, Seattle, WA 98195; **Phone:** 206-598-4121; **Board Cert:** Radiation Oncology 1988; **Med School:** Loma Linda Univ 1984; **Resid:** Radiation Oncology, Univ Washington Med Ctr 1988; **Fellow:** Tumor Imaging, Univ Washington Med Ctr 1988; **Fac Appt:** Prof RadRO, Univ Wash

Laramore, George E MD/PhD [RadRO] - **Spec Exp:** Neutron Therapy for Advanced Cancer; Salivary Gland Tumors; Head & Neck Cancer; Skin Cancer; **Hospital:** Univ Wash Med Ctr; **Address:** Univ Washington Med Ctr, Dept Rad Onc Box 356043, Seattle, WA 98195; **Phone:** 206-598-4110; **Board Cert:** Therapeutic Radiology 1980; Radiation Oncology 2000; **Med School:** Univ Miami Sch Med 1976; **Resid:** Radiation Oncology, Univ Washington 1980; **Fac Appt:** Prof RadRO, Univ Wash

Radiation Oncology

Larson, David A MD/PhD [RadRO] - **Spec Exp:** Neuro-Oncology; Brain Tumors; Stereotactic Radiosurgery; **Hospital:** UCSF Med Ctr; **Address:** UCSF Med Ctr, Dept Rad Onc, 505 Parnassus Ave, rm L-75, San Francisco, CA 94143-0226; **Phone:** 415-353-8900; **Board Cert:** Therapeutic Radiology 1986; **Med School:** Univ Miami Sch Med 1981; **Resid:** Radiation Therapy, Joint Ctr RadTherapy 1985; **Fac Appt:** Prof RadRO, UCSF

Le, Quynh-Thu Xuan MD [RadRO] - **Spec Exp:** Head & Neck Cancer; Lung Cancer; Thoracic Cancers; Clinical Trials; **Hospital:** Stanford Univ Med Ctr; **Address:** Stanford Univ, Dept Rad Oncology, 875 Blake Wilbur Drive, MC 5847, Ground Flr, Stanford, CA 94305; **Phone:** 650-498-5032; **Board Cert:** Radiation Oncology 1998; **Med School:** UCSF 1993; **Resid:** Radiation Oncology, UCSF Med Ctr 1997; **Fac Appt:** Prof RadRO, Stanford Univ

Mundt, Arno J MD [RadRO] - **Spec Exp:** Gynecologic Cancer; Intensity Modulated Radiotherapy (IMRT); **Hospital:** UCSD Med Ctr; **Address:** Moores UCSD Cancer Ctr, Radiation Oncology Dept, 3855 Health Sciences Drive, MC 0843, La Jolla, CA 92093-0843; **Phone:** 858-822-6046; **Board Cert:** Radiation Oncology 1994; **Med School:** Univ Mich Med Sch 1987; **Resid:** Physical Medicine & Rehabilitation, George Washington Univ Hosp 1990; Radiation Oncology, Univ Chicago Hosps 1993; **Fellow:** Physical Medicine & Rehabilitation, Univ Chicago Hosps 1994; **Fac Appt:** Assoc Prof RadRO, Univ Chicago-Pritzker Sch Med

Park, Catherine C MD [RadRO] - **Spec Exp:** Breast Cancer; Lymphoma; **Hospital:** UCSF Med Ctr; **Address:** 1600 Divisadero St, Ste H1031, Box 1708, San Francisco, CA 94115; **Phone:** 415-353-7175; **Board Cert:** Radiation Oncology 2000; **Med School:** UCLA 1995; **Resid:** Radiation Oncology, Mass Genl Hosp 2000; **Fac Appt:** Assoc Prof RadRO, UCSF

Pezner, Richard D MD [RadRO] - **Spec Exp:** Sarcoma-Soft Tissue; Breast Cancer; Stereotactic Radiosurgery; **Hospital:** City of Hope Natl Med Ctr & Beckman Rsch (page 69); **Address:** City of Hope Med Ctr-Div Radiation Onc, 1500 E Duarte Rd, Duarte, CA 91010-3000; **Phone:** 626-301-8247; **Board Cert:** Therapeutic Radiology 1979; **Med School:** Northwestern Univ 1975; **Resid:** Radiation Oncology, Oregon Health Sci Ctr 1979; **Fac Appt:** Clin Prof RadRO, UC Irvine

Quivey, Jeanne M MD [RadRO] - **Spec Exp:** Head & Neck Cancer; Breast Cancer; Eye Tumors/Cancer; Intensity Modulated Radiotherapy (IMRT); **Hospital:** UCSF Med Ctr; **Address:** UCSF Med Ctr @ Mt Zion, Radiation Oncology Dept, 1600 Divisadero St, Ste H1031, San Francisco, CA 94115-3010; **Phone:** 415-353-7175; **Board Cert:** Therapeutic Radiology 1974; **Med School:** UCSF 1970; **Resid:** Radiation Therapy, UCSF Med Ctr 1974; **Fac Appt:** Prof RadRO, UCSF

Roach III, Mack MD [RadRO] - **Spec Exp:** Prostate Cancer; Genitourinary Cancer; Lung Cancer; **Hospital:** UCSF - Mt Zion Med Ctr, UCSF Med Ctr; **Address:** UCSF Radiation Oncology, 1600 Divisadero St, Ste H1031, San Francisco, CA 94143-1708; **Phone:** 415-353-7181; **Board Cert:** Internal Medicine 1984; Medical Oncology 1985; Radiation Oncology 1987; **Med School:** Stanford Univ 1979; **Resid:** Internal Medicine, ML King Genl Hosp 1981; Radiation Oncology, Stanford Univ Med Ctr 1987; **Fellow:** Medical Oncology, UCSF Med Ctr 1983; **Fac Appt:** Prof RadRO, UCSF

Rose, Christopher M MD [RadRO] - **Spec Exp:** Prostate Cancer; Breast Cancer; Intensity Modulated Radiotherapy (IMRT); **Hospital:** Providence St Joseph Med Ctr; **Address:** Valley Radiotherapy Assocs, The Ctr for Radiation Therapy, 9229 Wilshire Blvd, Beverly Hills, CA 90210; **Phone:** 310-205-5777; **Board Cert:** Radiation Oncology 1999; **Med School:** Harvard Med Sch 1974; **Resid:** Internal Medicine, Beth Israel Deaconess 1976; Radiation Oncology, Joint Ctr Rad Therapy 1979; **Fellow:** Cancer Research, British Inst Cancer Rsch 1979; **Fac Appt:** Assoc Clin Prof RadRO, UCLA

Rossi, Carl John MD [RadRO] - **Spec Exp:** Prostate Cancer; Proton Beam Therapy; **Hospital:** Loma Linda Univ Med Ctr; **Address:** Loma Linda Univ Med Ctr, 11234 Anderson St, rm B124, Loma Linda, CA 92354; **Phone:** 909-558-4280; **Board Cert:** Radiation Oncology 1994; **Med School:** Loyola Univ-Stritch Sch Med 1988; **Resid:** Radiation Oncology, Loma Linda Univ Med Ctr 1992; **Fac Appt:** Asst Prof RadRO, Loma Linda Univ

Russell, Kenneth J MD [RadRO] - **Spec Exp:** Prostate Cancer; Lymphoma; Genitourinary Cancer; **Hospital:** Univ Wash Med Ctr; **Address:** Seattle Cancer Care Alliance, G1101, 825 East-lake Ave E, Seattle, WA 98109; **Phone:** 206-288-7318; **Board Cert:** Therapeutic Radiology 1984; **Med School:** Harvard Med Sch 1979; **Resid:** Radiation Therapy, Stanford Univ Med Ctr 1983; **Fellow:** Radiological Biology, Stanford Univ Med Ctr 1985; **Fac Appt:** Prof Rad, Univ Wash

Sandler, Howard M MD [RadRO] - **Spec Exp:** Prostate Cancer; Genitourinary Cancer; Brain Tumors; **Hospital:** Cedars-Sinai Med Ctr; **Address:** S Oschin Comprehensive Cancer Inst, Cedars-Sinai Med Ctr, 8700 Beverly Blvd, Los Angeles, CA 90048; **Phone:** 310-423-4234; **Board Cert:** Radiation Oncology 1989; **Med School:** Univ Conn 1985; **Resid:** Radiation Oncology, Hosp Univ Penn 1989

Seung, Steven K MD/PhD [RadRO] - **Spec Exp:** Stereotactic Radiosurgery; Brain Tumors; Esophageal Cancer; Lung Cancer; **Hospital:** Providence Portland Med Ctr; **Address:** 4805 NE Glisan St, Garden Level, Portland, OR 97213; **Phone:** 503-215-6029; **Board Cert:** Radiation Oncology 1999; **Med School:** Univ Chicago-Pritzker Sch Med 1994; **Resid:** Radiation Oncology, UCSF Med Ctr 1998

Thomas, Charles R MD [RadRO] - **Hospital:** OR Hlth & Sci Univ; **Address:** 3181 SW Sam Jackson Park Rd, MC KPV4, Portland, OR 97239; **Phone:** 503-494-8756; **Board Cert:** Internal Medicine 1989; Radiation Oncology 1999; **Med School:** Univ IL Coll Med 1985; **Resid:** Internal Medicine, Baylor Coll Med 1988; Radiation Oncology, Univ Wash Med Ctr 1997; **Fellow:** Medical Oncology, Rush Univ Med Ctr 1999; **Fac Appt:** Prof RadRO, Oregon Hlth Sci Univ

Tripuraneni, Prabhakar MD [RadRO] - **Spec Exp:** Prostate Cancer; Head & Neck Cancer; Lymphoma; **Hospital:** Scripps Green Hosp, Scripps Meml Hosp - La Jolla; **Address:** Scripps Clinic, Div Radiation Oncology, 10666 N Torrey Pines Rd, MSB 1, La Jolla, CA 92037; **Phone:** 858-554-2000; **Board Cert:** Therapeutic Radiology 1983; **Med School:** India 1976; **Resid:** Radiation Oncology, Univ Alberta 1981; Radiation Oncology, UCSF Med Ctr 1983; **Fac Appt:** Clin Prof RadRO, UCSD

Wara, William M MD [RadRO] - **Spec Exp:** Brain & Spinal Tumors; Sarcoma; Pediatric Cancers; **Hospital:** Kaiser Permanente S San Francisco Med Ctr; **Address:** Cancer Treatment Ctr, 220 Oyster Pt Blvd, San Francisco, CA 94080; **Phone:** 650-827-6500; **Board Cert:** Therapeutic Radiology 1974; **Med School:** UC Irvine 1969; **Resid:** Therapeutic Radiology, UCSF Medical Ctr 1973; **Fac Appt:** Prof RadRO, UCSF

Wong, Jeffrey Y C MD [RadRO] - **Spec Exp:** Radioimmunotherapy of Cancer; Prostate Cancer; Intensity Modulated Radiotherapy (IMRT); Multiple Myeloma; **Hospital:** City of Hope Natl Med Ctr & Beckman Rsch (page 69); **Address:** City of Hope Med Ctr-Dept Radiation Onc, 1500 E Duarte Rd, Duarte, CA 91768-3012; **Phone:** 626-359-8111 x62969; **Board Cert:** Therapeutic Radiology 1985; **Med School:** Johns Hopkins Univ 1981; **Resid:** Radiation Oncology, UCSF Med Ctr 1985; **Fac Appt:** Clin Prof RadRO, UC Irvine

DIAGNOSTIC RADIOLOGY

New England

Kopans, Daniel B MD [DR] - **Spec Exp:** Breast Imaging; Breast Cancer; **Hospital:** Mass Genl Hosp; **Address:** Mass Genl Hosp, Avon Comprehensive Breast Ctr, 15 Parkman St, WAC 240, Boston, MA 02114-3117; **Phone:** 617-726-3093; **Board Cert:** Diagnostic Radiology 1977; **Med School:** Harvard Med Sch 1973; **Resid:** Diagnostic Radiology, Mass Genl Hosp 1977; **Fac Appt:** Prof Rad, Harvard Med Sch

McCarthy, Shirley M MD/PhD [DR] - **Spec Exp:** Gynecologic Cancer; Pelvic Imaging; **Hospital:** Yale-New Haven Hosp; **Address:** Yale-New Haven Hosp, 333 Cedar St, Ste TE2, New Haven, CT 06520-3206; **Phone:** 203-785-2384; **Board Cert:** Diagnostic Radiology 1983; **Med School:** Yale Univ 1979; **Resid:** Diagnostic Radiology, Yale-New Haven Hosp 1983; **Fellow:** Cross Sectional Imaging, UCSF Med Ctr 1984; **Fac Appt:** Prof Rad, Yale Univ

Weinreb, Jeffrey C MD [DR] - **Spec Exp:** Breast Cancer; Abdominal Imaging; **Hospital:** Yale-New Haven Hosp; **Address:** Yale Univ Sch Medicine, Dept Radiology, 333 Cedar St, rm MRC147, Box 208042, New Haven, CT 06520-8042; **Phone:** 203-785-5913; **Board Cert:** Diagnostic Radiology 1983; **Med School:** Mount Sinai Sch Med 1978; **Resid:** Diagnostic Radiology, LI Jewish Med Ctr 1982; **Fellow:** Ultrasound/CT, Hosp Univ Penn 1983; **Fac Appt:** Prof Rad, Yale Univ

Mid Atlantic

Austin, John H M MD [DR] - **Spec Exp:** Lung Cancer; Thoracic Radiology; **Hospital:** NY-Presby Hosp/Columbia (page 79); **Address:** Columbia Presby Hosp, Dept Radiology, 622 W 168th St, HP 3-305, New York, NY 10032-3784; **Phone:** 212-305-2986; **Board Cert:** Diagnostic Radiology 1970; **Med School:** Yale Univ 1965; **Resid:** Diagnostic Radiology, UCSF Med Ctr 1968; **Fellow:** Diagnostic Radiology, UCSF Med Ctr 1970; **Fac Appt:** Prof Rad, Columbia P&S

Berg, Wendie A MD/PhD [DR] - **Spec Exp:** Breast Imaging; Breast Cancer; **Hospital:** Johns Hopkins Hosp; **Address:** Johns Hopkins, Greenspring Station Breast Ctr, 10755 Falls Rd, Ste 440, Lutherville, MD 21093; **Phone:** 410-583-2700; **Board Cert:** Diagnostic Radiology 1992; **Med School:** Johns Hopkins Univ 1987; **Resid:** Diagnostic Radiology, Johns Hopkins Hosp 1992; **Fellow:** Abdominal Imaging, Johns Hopkins Univ 1992

Brem, Rachel F MD [DR] - **Spec Exp:** Breast Imaging; Breast Cancer; **Hospital:** G Washington Univ Hosp; **Address:** GW Medical Faculty Assocs, 2150 Pennsylvania Ave NW, DC Level, Washington, DC 20037; **Phone:** 202-741-3036; **Board Cert:** Diagnostic Radiology 1990; **Med School:** Columbia P&S 1984; **Resid:** Diagnostic Radiology, Johns Hopkins Hosp 1989; **Fellow:** Mammography, Johns Hopkins Hosp 1990; **Fac Appt:** Prof Rad, Geo Wash Univ

Conant, Emily F MD [DR] - **Spec Exp:** Breast Cancer; Breast Imaging; **Hospital:** Hosp Univ Penn - UPHS (page 81); **Address:** Dept Radiology (Breast Imaging), 3400 Spruce St, 1 Silverstein, Philadelphia, PA 19104; **Phone:** 215-662-4032; **Board Cert:** Diagnostic Radiology 1989; **Med School:** Univ Pennsylvania 1983; **Resid:** Diagnostic Radiology, Hosp Univ Penn 1986; **Fellow:** Breast Imaging, Hosp Univ Penn 1989; **Fac Appt:** Prof Rad, Univ Pennsylvania

Dershaw, D David MD [DR] - **Spec Exp:** Breast Imaging; Breast Cancer; Mammography; **Hospital:** Meml Sloan-Kettering Cancer Ctr (page 76); **Address:** 1275 York Avenue, New York, NY 10065; **Phone:** 800-525-2225; **Board Cert:** Diagnostic Radiology 1978; **Med School:** Jefferson Med Coll 1974; **Resid:** Diagnostic Radiology, New York Hosp 1978; **Fellow:** Ultrasound, Thos Jefferson Univ Hosp 1979; **Fac Appt:** Prof Rad, Cornell Univ-Weill Med Coll

Edelstein, Barbara A MD [DR] - **Spec Exp:** Breast Cancer; **Address:** 1045 Park Ave, New York, NY 10028; **Phone:** 212-860-7700; **Board Cert:** Diagnostic Radiology 1983; **Med School:** NY Med Coll 1977; **Resid:** Diagnostic Radiology, Montefiore Hosp 1982

Evers, Kathryn A MD [DR] - **Spec Exp:** Breast Cancer; Mammography; **Hospital:** Fox Chase Cancer Ctr (page 72); **Address:** Fox Chase Cancer Ctr, Diagnostic Imaging, 333 Cottman Ave, Philadelphia, PA 19111; **Phone:** 215-728-4316; **Board Cert:** Diagnostic Radiology 1980; **Med School:** NYU Sch Med 1975; **Resid:** Diagnostic Radiology, Hosp Univ Penn 1980; **Fellow:** Diagnostic Radiology, Hosp Univ Penn 1981; **Fac Appt:** Assoc Clin Prof Rad, Temple Univ

Fishman, Elliot MD [DR] - **Spec Exp:** CT Body Scan; Abdominal Imaging; Cardiac Imaging; Cancer Imaging; **Hospital:** Johns Hopkins Hosp; **Address:** Johns Hopkins Hosp, Dept Radiology, 601 N Caroline St, JHOC 3254, Baltimore, MD 21287-0006; **Phone:** 410-955-5173; **Board Cert:** Diagnostic Radiology 1981; **Med School:** Univ MD Sch Med 1977; **Resid:** Diagnostic Radiology, Sinai Hosp 1980; **Fellow:** Computerized Tomography, Johns Hopkins Hosp 1981; **Fac Appt:** Prof Rad, Johns Hopkins Univ

Hann, Lucy MD [DR] - **Spec Exp:** Liver & Biliary Cancer Ultrasound; Ovarian Cancer Ultrasound Diagnosis; Thyroid Ultrasound; **Hospital:** Meml Sloan-Kettering Cancer Ctr (page 76); **Address:** 1275 York Avenue, New York, NY 10065; **Phone:** 800-525-2225; **Board Cert:** Diagnostic Radiology 1977; **Med School:** Harvard Med Sch 1971; **Resid:** Diagnostic Radiology, Hosp Univ Penn 1974; Diagnostic Radiology, Mass Genl Hosp 1977; **Fellow:** Body Imaging, Mass Genl Hosp 1978; **Fac Appt:** Prof Rad, Cornell Univ-Weill Med Coll

Henschke, Claudia L MD/PhD [DR] - **Spec Exp:** Lung Cancer; Lung Disease; Thoracic Radiology; **Hospital:** NY-Presby Hosp/Weill Cornell (page 79); **Address:** NY Weill Medical College, Dept Radiology, 525 E 68th St, Box 586, New York, NY 10021; **Phone:** 212-746-1325; **Board Cert:** Diagnostic Radiology 1981; **Med School:** Howard Univ 1977; **Resid:** Diagnostic Radiology, Brigham & Womens Hosp 1983; **Fac Appt:** Prof Rad, Cornell Univ-Weill Med Coll

Hricak, Hedvig MD/PhD [DR] - **Spec Exp:** Prostate Cancer-MR Spectroscopy (MRSI); Breast Imaging; Breast Cancer; **Hospital:** Meml Sloan-Kettering Cancer Ctr (page 76); **Address:** 1275 York Avenue, New York, NY 10065; **Phone:** 800-525-2225; **Board Cert:** Diagnostic Radiology 1978; **Med School:** Yugoslavia 1970; **Resid:** Diagnostic Radiology, St Joseph Mercy Hosp 1977; **Fellow:** Ultrasound/CT, Henry Ford Hosp 1978; **Fac Appt:** Prof Rad, Cornell Univ-Weill Med Coll

Levy, Angela D MD [DR] - **Spec Exp:** Abdominal Imaging; **Hospital:** Unif Serv Univ of the Hlth Sci, Armed Forces Inst of Path; **Address:** Uniformed Services Univ of the Hlth Scis, Dept Radiology, 4301 Jones Bridge Rd, rm C1071, Bethesda, MD 20814; **Phone:** 301-295-3145; **Board Cert:** Diagnostic Radiology 1993; **Med School:** Uniformed Srvs Univ, Bethesda 1988; **Resid:** Diagnostic Radiology, Walter Reed Army Hosp 1992; **Fac Appt:** Assoc Prof Rad, Uniformed Srvs Univ, Bethesda

Mitnick, Julie MD [DR] - **Spec Exp:** Mammography; Breast Cancer; **Address:** 650 1st Ave, New York, NY 10016; **Phone:** 212-686-4440; **Board Cert:** Diagnostic Radiology 1977; **Med School:** NYU Sch Med 1973; **Resid:** Diagnostic Radiology, NYU Med Ctr 1977; **Fellow:** Pediatric Radiology, NYU Med Ctr 1978; **Fac Appt:** Assoc Clin Prof Rad, NYU Sch Med

Diagnostic Radiology

Panicek, David M MD [DR] - **Spec Exp:** Bone Cancer; Soft Tissue Tumors; Musculoskeletal Tumor Imaging; **Hospital:** Meml Sloan-Kettering Cancer Ctr (page 76); **Address:** 1275 York Avenue, New York, NY 10065; **Phone:** 800-525-2225; **Board Cert:** Diagnostic Radiology 1984; **Med School:** Cornell Univ-Weill Med Coll 1980; **Resid:** Diagnostic Radiology, NY Hosp-Cornell Med Ctr 1984; **Fac Appt:** Prof Rad, Cornell Univ-Weill Med Coll

Parsons, Rosaleen B MD [DR] - **Spec Exp:** CT Body Scan; Gynecologic Cancer; Prostate Cancer; **Hospital:** Fox Chase Cancer Ctr (page 72); **Address:** Fox Chase Cancer Ctr, Dept of Diagnostic Imaging, 333 Cottman Ave, Philadelphia, PA 19111; **Phone:** 215-728-3024; **Board Cert:** Diagnostic Radiology 1991; **Med School:** Med Coll PA Hahnemann 1986; **Resid:** Diagnostic Radiology, Med Coll Penn Affil Hosp 1991; **Fac Appt:** Prof Rad, Temple Univ

Rao, Vijay M MD [DR] - **Spec Exp:** Head & Neck Tumors Imaging; **Hospital:** Thomas Jefferson Univ Hosp (page 83); **Address:** 132 S 10th St, 1087, Main Bldg, Philadelphia, PA 19107-4824; **Phone:** 215-955-4804; **Board Cert:** Diagnostic Radiology 1978; Neuroradiology 1997; **Med School:** India 1973; **Resid:** Diagnostic Radiology, Thomas Jefferson Univ Hosp 1978; **Fac Appt:** Prof Rad, Thomas Jefferson Univ

Roth, Susan G MD [DR] - **Spec Exp:** Breast Imaging; Breast Cancer; **Hospital:** Hosp Univ Penn - UPHS (page 81); **Address:** Hosp Univ Penn, Dept Radiology, 3400 Physics Ctr Blvd Fl Ground, Philadelphia, PA 19104; **Phone:** 215-614-0124; **Board Cert:** Diagnostic Radiology 1989; **Med School:** Univ Pennsylvania 1986; **Resid:** Diagnostic Radiology, Johns Hopkins Hosp 1989; **Fac Appt:** Prof Rad, Univ Pennsylvania

Yankelevitz, David MD [DR] - **Spec Exp:** Lung Cancer; Thoracic Radiology; **Hospital:** NY-Presby Hosp/Weill Cornell (page 79); **Address:** 520 E 70th St, Weill Cornell Starr Bldg, New York, NY 10021; **Phone:** 212-746-9729; **Board Cert:** Diagnostic Radiology 1987; Nuclear Medicine 1987; **Med School:** SUNY Hlth Sci Ctr 1981; **Resid:** Diagnostic Radiology, Long Island Coll Hosp 1984; Nuclear Medicine, NY-Cornell Med Ctr 1987; **Fellow:** Diagnostic Radiology, NY-Cornell Med Ctr 1987; **Fac Appt:** Prof Rad, Cornell Univ-Weill Med Coll

Southeast

Abbitt, Patricia L MD [DR] - **Spec Exp:** Breast Imaging; Breast Cancer; **Hospital:** Shands at Univ of FL; **Address:** Shands Healthcare, Dept Radiology, 1600 SW Archer Rd, PO Box 100374, Gainesville, FL 32610; **Phone:** 352-265-0291; **Board Cert:** Diagnostic Radiology 1986; **Med School:** Tufts Univ 1981; **Resid:** Diagnostic Radiology, Univ VA Med Ctr 1986; **Fellow:** Breast Imaging, Univ VA Med Ctr 1987; **Fac Appt:** Prof Rad, Univ Fla Coll Med

Cardenosa, Gilda MD [DR] - **Spec Exp:** Breast Imaging; **Hospital:** Med Coll of VA Hosp; **Address:** VCU Med Ctr at Stony Point, Dept Radiology, 9000 Stony Point Pkwy, Richmond, VA 23235; **Phone:** 804-560-8906 x7862; **Board Cert:** Diagnostic Radiology 1989; **Med School:** Columbia P&S 1984; **Resid:** Diagnostic Radiology, Mass Genl Hosp 1989; **Fac Appt:** Prof Rad, Med Coll VA

Patz, Edward F MD [DR] - **Spec Exp:** Thoracic Radiology; PET Imaging; Lung Cancer; **Hospital:** Duke Univ Med Ctr; **Address:** Duke Univ Med Ctr, Dept Radiology, Box 3808, Durham, NC 27710; **Phone:** 919-684-7367; **Board Cert:** Diagnostic Radiology 1990; **Med School:** Univ MD Sch Med 1985; **Resid:** Diagnostic Radiology, Brigham & Womens Hosp 1990; **Fellow:** Thoracic Radiology, Brigham & Womens Hosp 1990; **Fac Appt:** Prof, Duke Univ

Midwest

Helvie, Mark A MD [DR] - **Spec Exp:** Breast Imaging; Breast Cancer; Mammography; **Hospital:** Univ Michigan Hlth Sys; **Address:** 2910N Taubman Univ Michigan Health Ctr, 1500 E Medical Ctr Drive, Ann Arbor, MI 48109-0326; **Phone:** 734-936-4367; **Board Cert:** Internal Medicine 1983; Diagnostic Radiology 1986; **Med School:** Univ NC Sch Med 1980; **Resid:** Internal Medicine, Univ Michigan Hosps 1983; Diagnostic Radiology, Univ Michigan Hosps 1986; **Fellow:** Breast Imaging, Univ Michigan Hosps 1987; **Fac Appt:** Prof, Univ Mich Med Sch

Jackson, Valerie P MD [DR] - **Spec Exp:** Breast Imaging; **Hospital:** Indiana Univ Hosp (page 74), Wishard Hlth Srvs; **Address:** Indiana Univ Hosp, Dept Radiology, 550 N University Blvd, #0663, Indianapolis, IN 46202; **Phone:** 317-274-1866; **Board Cert:** Diagnostic Radiology 1982; **Med School:** Indiana Univ 1978; **Resid:** Diagnostic Radiology, Indiana Univ Med Ctr 1982; **Fac Appt:** Prof Rad, Indiana Univ

Monsees, Barbara MD [DR] - **Spec Exp:** Mammography; Breast Cancer; **Hospital:** Barnes-Jewish Hosp; **Address:** Ctr for Advanced Med, Campus Box 8131, 510 S Kingshighway Blvd, St Louis, MO 63110; **Phone:** 314-454-7500; **Board Cert:** Diagnostic Radiology 1980; **Med School:** Washington Univ, St Louis 1975; **Resid:** Pediatrics, St Louis Chldns Hosp 1977; Diagnostic Radiology, Mallinckrodt Inst Radiology 1980; **Fac Appt:** Prof, Washington Univ, St Louis

Sagel, Stuart S MD [DR] - **Spec Exp:** Lung Cancer; **Hospital:** Barnes-Jewish Hosp; **Address:** Mallinckrodt Inst Rad-Barnes Hosp, 510 S Kingshighway Blvd, Box 8131, St Louis, MO 63110-1016; **Phone:** 314-362-2927; **Board Cert:** Diagnostic Radiology 1970; **Med School:** Temple Univ 1965; **Resid:** Diagnostic Radiology, Yale New Haven Hosp 1968; Diagnostic Radiology, UCSF Med Ctr 1970; **Fac Appt:** Prof Rad, Washington Univ, St Louis

Swensen, Stephen J MD [DR] - **Spec Exp:** Lung Cancer; Lung Disease; **Hospital:** Mayo Med Ctr & Clin - Rochester; **Address:** Mayo Clinic - Diagnostic Radiology, 200 1st St SW, Rochester, MN 55905; **Phone:** 507-284-8550; **Board Cert:** Diagnostic Radiology 1986; **Med School:** Univ Wisc 1981; **Resid:** Diagnostic Radiology, Mayo Clinic 1986; **Fellow:** Pulmonary Radiology, Brigham & Womens Hosp 1987; **Fac Appt:** Prof Rad, Mayo Med Sch

Southwest

Erasmus, Jeremy J MD [DR] - **Spec Exp:** Lung Cancer; CT Body Scan; PET Imaging; **Hospital:** UT MD Anderson Cancer Ctr; **Address:** MD Anderson Cancer Ctr, Dept of Rad, 1515 Holcombe Blvd, Unit 0371, Houston, TX 77030; **Phone:** 713-792-5878; **Board Cert:** Diagnostic Radiology 1993; **Med School:** South Africa 1982; **Resid:** Diagnostic Radiology, Queens Univ 1993; **Fac Appt:** Prof Rad, Univ Tex, Houston

Huynh, Phan Tuong MD [DR] - **Spec Exp:** Mammography; Breast Cancer; **Hospital:** St Luke's Episcopal Hosp-Houston; **Address:** 6624 Fannin St, St Luke's Tower, Womens Ctr Fl 10, Houston, TX 77030; **Phone:** 832-355-8130; **Board Cert:** Diagnostic Radiology 1994; **Med School:** Univ VA Sch Med 1989; **Resid:** Diagnostic Radiology, Univ Virginia Med Ctr 1994; **Fellow:** Mammography, Univ Virginia 1995; **Fac Appt:** Assoc Clin Prof Rad, Baylor Coll Med

Otto, Pamela MD [DR] - **Spec Exp:** Breast Imaging; Breast Cancer; **Hospital:** Univ Hlth Syst-San Antonio, Audie L Murphy Meml Vets Hosp; **Address:** 7703 Floyd Curl Drive, MC 7800, San Antonio, TX 78229-3900; **Phone:** 210-567-3448; **Board Cert:** Diagnostic Radiology 1993; **Med School:** Univ MO-Columbia Sch Med 1988; **Resid:** Diagnostic Radiology, Univ Texas Hlth Sci Ctr 1993; **Fellow:** Breast Imaging, Univ Texas Hlth Sci Ctr 1993; **Fac Appt:** Assoc Prof Rad, Univ Tex, San Antonio

Diagnostic Radiology

West Coast and Pacific

Bassett, Lawrence W MD [DR] - **Spec Exp:** Breast Imaging; **Hospital:** UCLA Ronald Reagan Med Ctr; **Address:** 200 UCLA Med Plaza, rm 165-47, Los Angeles, CA 90095; **Phone:** 310-206-9608; **Board Cert:** Diagnostic Radiology 1975; **Med School:** UC Irvine 1968; **Resid:** Diagnostic Radiology, UCLA Med Ctr 1972; **Fac Appt:** Prof, UCLA

Feig, Stephen A MD [DR] - **Spec Exp:** Breast Imaging; Breast Cancer; **Hospital:** UC Irvine Med Ctr; **Address:** UCI Medical Ctr, 101 City Drive South Route 140, Orange, CA 92868-3298; **Phone:** 714-456-6905; **Board Cert:** Diagnostic Radiology 1972; **Med School:** NYU Sch Med 1967; **Resid:** Radiology, Bronx Muni Hosp-Einstein 1971; **Fac Appt:** Prof Rad, UC Irvine

Lehman, Constance D MD/PhD [DR] - **Spec Exp:** Breast Imaging; **Hospital:** Univ Wash Med Ctr; **Address:** Seattle Cancer Care Alliance, 825 Eastlake Ave E, rm G2600, Seattle, WA 98109-1023; **Phone:** 206-288-2046; **Board Cert:** Diagnostic Radiology 1995; **Med School:** Yale Univ 1990; **Resid:** Diagnostic Radiology, Univ Wash Med Ctr 1995; **Fellow:** Diagnostic Radiology, Univ Wash Med Ctr 1996; **Fac Appt:** Prof Rad, Univ Wash

NEURORADIOLOGY

Mid Atlantic

Loevner, Laurie A MD [NRad] - **Spec Exp:** Head & Neck Cancer; Thyroid Cancer; Brain Tumor Imaging; Spinal Tumor Imaging; **Hospital:** Hosp Univ Penn - UPHS (page 81), Pennsylvania Hosp (page 81); **Address:** Univ Penn Med Ctr-Dept Rad, 3400 Spruce St, Philadelphia, PA 19104; **Phone:** 215-662-3020; **Board Cert:** Diagnostic Radiology 1993; Neuroradiology 2006; **Med School:** Univ Pennsylvania 1988; **Resid:** Diagnostic Radiology, Univ Michigan Hosps 1993; **Fellow:** Neuroradiology, Hosp Univ Penn 1995; **Fac Appt:** Prof Rad, Univ Pennsylvania

Vezina, L Gilbert MD [NRad] - **Spec Exp:** Pediatric Neuroradiology; Brain Tumors; **Hospital:** Chldns Natl Med Ctr; **Address:** Chldns Natl Med Ctr, Dept Radiology, 111 Michigan Ave NW, Washington, DC 20010-2970; **Phone:** 202-476-3651; **Board Cert:** Diagnostic Radiology 1987; Neuroradiology 1998; **Med School:** McGill Univ 1983; **Resid:** Diagnostic Radiology, Mass Genl Hosp 1987; **Fellow:** Neurological Radiology, Mass Genl Hosp 1989; Pediatric Neuroradiology, Chldns Natl Med Ctr 1991; **Fac Appt:** Prof, Geo Wash Univ

Southeast

Murtagh, F Reed MD [NRad] - **Spec Exp:** Neuro-Oncology; Brain Tumor Imaging; Spinal Tumor Imaging; **Hospital:** H Lee Moffitt Cancer Ctr & Research Inst; **Address:** Univ Diagnostic Institute-USF, 3301 Alumni Drive, Tampa, FL 33612; **Phone:** 813-975-0725; **Board Cert:** Diagnostic Radiology 1978; Neuroradiology 2004; **Med School:** Temple Univ 1971; **Resid:** Diagnostic Radiology, Jackson Meml Hosp 1978; **Fellow:** Neurological Radiology, Univ Miami 1979; **Fac Appt:** Prof Rad, Univ S Fla Coll Med

Provenzale, James M MD [NRad] - **Spec Exp:** Brain Tumor Imaging; **Hospital:** Duke Univ Med Ctr; **Address:** Duke University Medical Ctr, Dept Radiology, Box 3808, Durham, NC 27710; **Phone:** 919-684-7218; **Board Cert:** Neurology 1988; Diagnostic Radiology 1991; Neuroradiology 2001; **Med School:** Albany Med Coll 1983; **Resid:** Neurology, NC Memorial Hosp 1987; Diagnostic Radiology, Mass Genl Hosp 1991; **Fellow:** Neuroradiology, Mass Genl Hosp 1992; **Fac Appt:** Prof, Duke Univ

Midwest

Koeller, Kelly K MD [NRad] - **Spec Exp:** Brain Tumor Imaging; Head & Neck Tumors; Spinal Tumor Imaging; **Hospital:** Mayo Med Ctr & Clin - Rochester; **Address:** Mayo Clinic, 200 First St SW Charlton Bldg - rm 2-290, Rochester, MN 55905; **Phone:** 507-266-3412; **Board Cert:** Diagnostic Radiology 1990; Neuroradiology 2004; **Med School:** Univ Tenn Coll Med, Memphis 1982; **Resid:** Diagnostic Radiology, Naval Hosp 1990; **Fellow:** Neuroradiology, UCSF Med Ctr 1992

West Coast and Pacific

Atlas, Scott W MD [NRad] - **Spec Exp:** Brain Tumors; **Hospital:** Stanford Univ Med Ctr; **Address:** Stanford Univ Med Ctr, Dept Rad, 300 Pasteur Drive, rm S-047, Stanford, CA 94304-2204; **Phone:** 650-498-7152; **Board Cert:** Diagnostic Radiology 1985; Neuroradiology 2005; **Med School:** Univ Chicago-Pritzker Sch Med 1981; **Resid:** Diagnostic Radiology, Northwestern Univ Med Ctr 1985; **Fellow:** Neuroradiology, Hosp Univ Pennsylvania 1987; **Fac Appt:** Prof, Stanford Univ

Cha, Soonmee MD [NRad] - **Spec Exp:** Brain Tumors; **Hospital:** UCSF Med Ctr; **Address:** 505 Parnassus Ave, Ste L-358, Neuroradiology Section, San Francisco, CA 94143-0628; **Phone:** 415-353-8913; **Board Cert:** Diagnostic Radiology 1996; Neuroradiology 1998; **Med School:** Georgetown Univ 1991; **Resid:** Diagnostic Radiology, North Shore Univ Hosp 1996; **Fellow:** Neuroradiology, NYU Med Ctr 1998; **Fac Appt:** Assoc Prof Rad, UCSF

Dillon, William P MD [NRad] - **Spec Exp:** Brain Tumors; **Hospital:** UCSF Med Ctr; **Address:** 505 Parnassus Ave, rm L-371, San Francisco, CA 94143-0628; **Phone:** 415-353-1668; **Board Cert:** Diagnostic Radiology 1982; Neuroradiology 2006; **Med School:** Loyola Univ-Stritch Sch Med 1978; **Resid:** Diagnostic Radiology, Univ Utah Hosp 1982; **Fellow:** Neuroradiology, UCSF Med Ctr 1983; **Fac Appt:** Prof, UCSF

VASCULAR & INTERVENTIONAL RADIOLOGY

New England

Hallisey, Michael J MD [VIR] - **Spec Exp:** Liver Cancer/Chemoembolization; **Hospital:** Hartford Hosp; **Address:** 399 Farmington Ave, Farmington, CT 06032; **Phone:** 860-246-6589; **Board Cert:** Diagnostic Radiology 1991; Vascular & Interventional Radiology 1998; **Med School:** Univ Conn 1986; **Resid:** Diagnostic Radiology, Hospital of St Raphael 1991

Mid Atlantic

Geschwind, Jean-Francois H MD [VIR] - **Spec Exp:** Liver Cancer/Chemoembolization; Cancer Chemoembolization; Cancer Radiotherapy; **Hospital:** Johns Hopkins Hosp; **Address:** Interventional Radiology, 600 N Wolfe St Blalock Bldg - rm 545, Baltimore, MD 21287; **Phone:** 410-955-6358; **Board Cert:** Diagnostic Radiology 1998; **Med School:** Boston Univ 1991; **Resid:** Diagnostic Radiology, UCSF Med Ctr 1996; **Fellow:** Interventional Radiology, Johns Hopkins Hosp 1998; **Fac Appt:** Assoc Prof, Johns Hopkins Univ

Haskal, Ziv MD [VIR] - **Spec Exp:** Liver Cancer/Chemoembolization; **Hospital:** Univ of MD Med Ctr; **Address:** 22 S Greene St, rm G2K14, Baltimore, MD 21201; **Phone:** 410-328-7467; **Board Cert:** Diagnostic Radiology 1991; Vascular & Interventional Radiology 1999; **Med School:** Boston Univ 1986; **Resid:** Diagnostic Radiology, UCSF Med Ctr 1991; **Fellow:** Vascular & Interventional Radiology, UCSF Med Ctr 1992; **Fac Appt:** Prof Rad, Univ MD Sch Med

Vascular & Interventional Radiology

Soulen, Michael C MD [VIR] - **Spec Exp:** Liver Cancer/Chemoembolization; Kidney Cancer; Radiofrequency Tumor Ablation; **Hospital:** Hosp Univ Penn - UPHS (page 81); **Address:** Hosp U Penn, Interventional Radiology, 3400 Spruce St, Philadelphia, PA 19104; **Phone:** 215-662-6839; **Board Cert:** Diagnostic Radiology 1989; Vascular & Interventional Radiology 1995; **Med School:** Univ Pennsylvania 1984; **Resid:** Diagnostic Radiology, Johns Hopkins Med Inst 1989; **Fellow:** Vascular & Interventional Radiology, Thomas Jefferson Univ Hosp 1991; **Fac Appt:** Prof Rad, Univ Pennsylvania

Wood, Bradford J MD [VIR] - **Spec Exp:** Radiofrequency Tumor Ablation; Liver Cancer; Kidney Cancer; Gene Therapy Delivery Systems; **Hospital:** Natl Inst of Hlth - Clin Ctr; **Address:** National Inst Health, Bldg 10, 9000 Rockville Pike, msc 1182, Bethesda, MD 20892; **Phone:** 301-594-4511; **Board Cert:** Diagnostic Radiology 1996; Vascular & Interventional Radiology 2000; **Med School:** Univ VA Sch Med 1991; **Resid:** Diagnostic Radiology, Georgetown Univ Med Ctr 1996; **Fellow:** Abdominal/Interventional Radiology, Mass General Hosp 1997; **Fac Appt:** Asst Clin Prof Rad, Georgetown Univ

Southeast

Mauro, Matthew MD [VIR] - **Spec Exp:** Cancer Chemoembolization; Cancer Radiotherapy; Gastrointestinal Cancer; **Hospital:** Univ NC Hosps; **Address:** University NC Hosps, Dept Radiology, CB 7510, 2006 Old Clinic Bldg, Chapel Hill, NC 27514; **Phone:** 919-966-4238; **Board Cert:** Diagnostic Radiology 1981; Vascular & Interventional Radiology 2003; **Med School:** Cornell Univ-Weill Med Coll 1977; **Resid:** Diagnostic Radiology, Univ NC Hosps 1981; **Fellow:** Interventional Radiology, Mallinckrodt Inst 1982; **Fac Appt:** Prof Rad, Univ NC Sch Med

Midwest

Rilling, William S MD [VIR] - **Spec Exp:** Liver Cancer/Chemoembolization; **Hospital:** Froedtert Meml Lutheran Hosp; **Address:** Froedtert Hosp, Dept Radiology, 9200 W Wisconsin Ave, Milwaukee, WI 53226; **Phone:** 414-805-3028; **Board Cert:** Diagnostic Radiology 1995; Vascular & Interventional Radiology 2007; **Med School:** Univ Wisc 1990; **Resid:** Diagnostic Radiology, Univ Wisc Affil Hosps 1995; **Fellow:** Vascular & Interventional Radiology, Northwestern Meml Hosp 1996; **Fac Appt:** Assoc Prof Rad, Univ Wisc

Salem, Riad MD [VIR] - **Spec Exp:** Cancer Radiotherapy; Cancer Chemoembolization; Liver Cancer/Chemoembolization; **Hospital:** Northwestern Meml Hosp; **Address:** Northwestern Univ Med Sch, Dept Radiology, 676 N St Clair St, Ste 800, Chicago, IL 60611; **Phone:** 312-695-5753; **Board Cert:** Diagnostic Radiology 1997; Vascular & Interventional Radiology 1999; **Med School:** McGill Univ 1993; **Resid:** Diagnostic Radiology, Geo Washington Univ Hosp 1997; **Fellow:** Interventional Radiology, Chldns Hosp 1998; Interventional Radiology, Hosp Univ Penn 1998; **Fac Appt:** Asst Prof Rad, Northwestern Univ

West Coast and Pacific

Goodwin, Scott C MD [VIR] - **Spec Exp:** Liver Cancer/Chemoembolization; **Hospital:** UC Irvine Med Ctr; **Address:** 101 S City Drive, MC 5005, Route 140, Orange, CA 92868; **Phone:** 714-456-5033; **Board Cert:** Diagnostic Radiology 1989; Vascular & Interventional Radiology 2007; **Med School:** Harvard Med Sch 1984; **Resid:** Diagnostic Radiology, UCLA Medical Ctr 1988; **Fellow:** Vascular & Interventional Radiology, UCLA Medical Ctr 1989; **Fac Appt:** Prof, UCLA

McGahan, John P MD [VIR] - **Spec Exp:** Radiofrequency Tumor Ablation; Liver Cancer; Kidney Cancer; **Hospital:** UC Davis Med Ctr; **Address:** UC Davis Medical Ctr, Dept Radiology, 4860 Y St, Ste 3100, Sacramento, CA 95817; **Phone:** 916-734-3606; **Board Cert:** Diagnostic Radiology 1979; **Med School:** Oregon Hlth Sci Univ 1974; **Resid:** Surgery, UC Davis Med Ctr 1976; Diagnostic Radiology, UC Davis Med Ctr 1979; **Fac Appt:** Prof Rad, UC Davis

NUCLEAR MEDICINE

Mid Atlantic

Alavi, Abass MD [NuM] - **Spec Exp:** Brain Tumors; Neurologic Imaging; PET Imaging-Brain; **Hospital:** Hosp Univ Penn - UPHS (page 81), Chldns Hosp of Philadelphia, The; **Address:** Hosp Univ Penn, Div Nuclear Med, 3400 Spruce St, Donner Bldg rm 110, Philadelphia, PA 19104; **Phone:** 215-662-3014; **Board Cert:** Nuclear Medicine 1973; Internal Medicine 1972; **Med School:** Iran 1964; **Resid:** Internal Medicine, Albert Einstein Med Ctr/Phila VA Hosp 1969; Hematology, Hosp Univ Penn 1970; **Fellow:** Nuclear Medicine, Hosp Univ Penn 1973; **Fac Appt:** Prof Rad, Univ Pennsylvania

Carrasquillo, Jorge A MD [NuM] - **Spec Exp:** Radioimmunotherapy of Cancer; PET Imaging; **Hospital:** Meml Sloan-Kettering Cancer Ctr (page 76); **Address:** 1275 York Avenue, Nuclear Medicine Svc, Box 77, New York, NY 10065; **Phone:** 212-639-2459; **Board Cert:** Internal Medicine 1977; Nuclear Medicine 1982; **Med School:** Univ Puerto Rico 1974; **Resid:** Internal Medicine, Univ Dist Hosp 1977; Nuclear Medicine, Univ Wash Hosp 1982

Goldsmith, Stanley J MD [NuM] - **Spec Exp:** Thyroid Cancer; Neuroendocrine Tumors; PET Imaging; Lymphoma; **Hospital:** NY-Presby Hosp/Weill Cornell (page 79); **Address:** 525 E 68th St Starr Bldg - rm 2-21, New York, NY 10021-9800; **Phone:** 212-746-4588; **Board Cert:** Internal Medicine 1969; Nuclear Medicine 1972; Endocrinology 1972; **Med School:** SUNY Downstate 1962; **Resid:** Internal Medicine, Kings Co Hosp 1967; **Fellow:** Endocrinology, Diabetes & Metabolism, Mt Sinai Hosp 1968; Nuclear Medicine, Bronx VA Hosp 1969; **Fac Appt:** Prof Rad, Cornell Univ-Weill Med Coll

Lamonica, Dominick M MD [NuM] - **Spec Exp:** Thyroid Cancer; **Hospital:** Roswell Park Cancer Inst; **Address:** Roswell Park Cancer Inst, Elm & Carlton St, Dept of Nuclear Medicine, Buffalo, NY 14263; **Phone:** 716-845-3282; **Board Cert:** Internal Medicine 2005; Nuclear Medicine 2006; **Med School:** Mount Sinai Sch Med 1987; **Resid:** Internal Medicine, Univ Hosp-SUNY Stony Brook 1991; Diagnostic Radiology, Nassau City Med Ctr 1992; **Fellow:** Nuclear Medicine, DVAMC North Port-SUNY Stony Brook 1994; Nuclear Medicine, SUNY Buffalo-RPCI 1995; **Fac Appt:** Asst Prof, SUNY Buffalo

Larson, Steven M MD [NuM] - **Spec Exp:** Thyroid Cancer; PET Imaging; **Hospital:** Meml Sloan-Kettering Cancer Ctr (page 76); **Address:** 1275 York Avenue, New York, NY 10065; **Phone:** 800-525-2225; **Board Cert:** Nuclear Medicine 1972; Internal Medicine 1973; **Med School:** Univ Wash 1965; **Resid:** Internal Medicine, Virginia Mason Hosp 1970; Nuclear Medicine, Natl Inst Hlth 1972; **Fac Appt:** Prof NuM, Cornell Univ-Weill Med Coll

Strauss, H William MD [NuM] - **Spec Exp:** Cardiac Imaging in Cancer Therapy; Thyroid Disorders; **Hospital:** Meml Sloan-Kettering Cancer Ctr (page 76); **Address:** 1275 York Avenue, New York, NY 10065; **Phone:** 212-639-7238; **Board Cert:** Nuclear Medicine 1988; **Med School:** SUNY Downstate 1965; **Resid:** Internal Medicine, Downstate Med Ctr 1967; Internal Medicine, Bellevue Hosp 1968; **Fellow:** Nuclear Medicine, Johns Hopkins Hosp 1970; **Fac Appt:** Prof NuM, Cornell Univ-Weill Med Coll

Nuclear Medicine

Wahl, Richard L MD [NuM] - **Spec Exp:** Radioimmunotherapy of Cancer; PET Imaging; PET Imaging-Breast; **Hospital:** Johns Hopkins Hosp; **Address:** Johns Hopkins Hosp, Radiology Dept, Nuclear Medicine Fl 3, 601 N Caroline St, JHOC-3223, Baltimore, MD 21287; **Phone:** 410-955-5465; **Board Cert:** Diagnostic Radiology 1982; Nuclear Radiology 1983; Nuclear Medicine 1985; **Med School:** Washington Univ, St Louis 1978; **Resid:** Diagnostic Radiology, Mallinckrodt Inst 1982; **Fellow:** Nuclear Radiology, Mallinckrodt Inst 1983; **Fac Appt:** Prof Rad, Johns Hopkins Univ

Southeast

Alazraki, Naomi P MD [NuM] - **Spec Exp:** Nuclear Oncology; **Hospital:** VA Med Ctr - Atlanta, Emory Univ Hosp; **Address:** VA Medical Ctr - Atlanta, 1670 Clairmont Rd, MC 115, Decatur, GA 30033; **Phone:** 404-728-7629; **Board Cert:** Nuclear Medicine 1972; Diagnostic Radiology 1972; **Med School:** Albert Einstein Coll Med 1966; **Resid:** Diagnostic Radiology, Univ Hospital 1971; **Fac Appt:** Prof, Emory Univ

Coleman, R Edward MD [NuM] - **Spec Exp:** PET Imaging; SPECT Imaging; Tumor Imaging; **Hospital:** Duke Univ Med Ctr; **Address:** Duke Univ Med Ctr, Erwin Rd, Box 3949, Durham, NC 27710-0001; **Phone:** 919-684-7244; **Board Cert:** Internal Medicine 1973; Nuclear Medicine 1973; **Resid:** Internal Medicine, Royal Victoria Hosp 1970; **Fellow:** Nuclear Medicine, Mallinckrodt Inst Radiology 1974; **Fac Appt:** Prof Rad

Midwest

Dillehay, Gary MD [NuM] - **Spec Exp:** Lymphoma; PET Imaging; **Hospital:** Northwestern Meml Hosp; **Address:** Northwestern Meml Hosp, Dept Nuclear Medicine, 675 N St Clair St, Galter 8-110, Chicago, IL 60611; **Phone:** 312-926-5119; **Board Cert:** Nuclear Medicine 1985; Nuclear Radiology 1987; **Med School:** Mayo Med Sch 1979; **Resid:** Diagnostic Radiology, Northwestern Meml Hosp 1983; Nuclear Medicine, Northwestern Meml Hosp 1984

Neumann, Donald R MD [NuM] - **Spec Exp:** Nuclear Oncology; Parathyroid Disease; **Hospital:** Cleveland Clin Fdn (page 70); **Address:** Cleveland Clinic, Dept Nuclear Medicine, 9500 Euclid Ave, MS Jb3, Cleveland, OH 44195; **Phone:** 216-444-2193; **Board Cert:** Diagnostic Radiology 1987; Nuclear Radiology 1990; **Med School:** Wright State Univ 1980; **Resid:** Diagnostic Radiology, Mount Sinai Med Ctr 1987; **Fellow:** Magnetic Resonance Imaging, Mount Sinai Med Ctr 1987

Siegel, Barry A MD [NuM] - **Spec Exp:** Cancer Detection & Staging; PET Imaging; **Hospital:** Barnes-Jewish Hosp, St Louis Chldns Hosp; **Address:** Mallinckrodt Inst of Radiology, 510 S Kingshighway Blvd, St Louis, MO 63110-1016; **Phone:** 314-362-2809; **Board Cert:** Nuclear Medicine 1973; Diagnostic Radiology 1977; Nuclear Radiology 1981; **Med School:** Washington Univ, St Louis 1969; **Resid:** Diagnostic Radiology, Mallinckrodt Inst Radiology 1973; **Fellow:** Nuclear Medicine, Mallinckrodt Inst Radiology 1973; **Fac Appt:** Prof Rad, Washington Univ, St Louis

Wiseman, Gregory MD [NuM] - **Spec Exp:** Lymphoma, Non-Hodgkin's; Multiple Myeloma; Radioimmunotherapy of Cancer; **Hospital:** Mayo Med Ctr & Clin - Rochester; **Address:** Mayo Clinic, Dept Nuc Med, 200 First St SW, Charlton Bldg, Rochester, MN 55905; **Phone:** 507-284-9599; **Board Cert:** Internal Medicine 1986; Hematology 1988; Nuclear Medicine 2002; **Med School:** Univ Utah 1983; **Resid:** Internal Medicine, Mayo Clinic 1986; Nuclear Medicine, Univ Washington Med Ctr 1992; **Fellow:** Hematology, Mayo Clinic 1989; Medical Oncology, Univ Washington 1991; **Fac Appt:** Asst Prof, Mayo Med Sch

Southwest

Podoloff, Donald MD [NuM] - **Spec Exp:** Prostate Cancer; Breast Cancer; Lymphoma; **Hospital:** UT MD Anderson Cancer Ctr; **Address:** UT MD Anderson Cancer Ctr, 1515 Holcombe Blvd, Box 57, Houston, TX 77030; **Phone:** 713-745-1160; **Board Cert:** Diagnostic Radiology 1973; Nuclear Medicine 1975; Nuclear Radiology 1975; **Med School:** SUNY Downstate 1964; **Resid:** Internal Medicine, Beth Israel Med Ctr 1968; Diagnostic Radiology, Wilford Hall USAF Med Ctr 1973; **Fac Appt:** Prof Rad, Univ Tex, Houston

West Coast and Pacific

Scheff, Alice M MD [NuM] - **Spec Exp:** PET Imaging; Thyroid Disorders; **Hospital:** Santa Clara Vly Med Ctr; **Address:** 751 S Bascom Ave, San Jose, CA 95128; **Phone:** 408-885-6970; **Board Cert:** Nuclear Medicine 1982; Nuclear Radiology 1983; **Med School:** Penn State Univ-Hershey Med Ctr 1978; **Resid:** Diagnostic Radiology, Penn State-Hershey Med Ctr 1982; Nuclear Medicine, Penn State-Hershey Med Ctr 1982; **Fellow:** Magnetic Resonance Imaging, Long Beach Meml Med Ctr 1993

Waxman, Alan D MD [NuM] - **Spec Exp:** PET Imaging-Brain; Thyroid Cancer; Cancer Detection & Staging; **Hospital:** Cedars-Sinai Med Ctr, USC Univ Hosp; **Address:** Cedars-Sinai Med Ctr, Taper Imaging, 8700 Beverly Blvd, rm 1251, Los Angeles, CA 90048-1804; **Phone:** 310-423-4216; **Board Cert:** Nuclear Medicine 1972; **Med School:** USC Sch Med 1963; **Resid:** Nuclear Medicine, Wadsworth VA Hosp 1965; **Fellow:** Internal Medicine, Natl Inst Hlth 1967; **Fac Appt:** Clin Prof, USC Sch Med

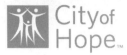

1500 East Duarte Road
Duarte, CA 91010
800-826-HOPE cityofhope.org

City of Hope is a recognized worldwide leader for its compassionate patient care, innovative science and translational research, which rapidly turn laboratory breakthroughs into promising new therapies. One of only 40 National Cancer Institute-designated Comprehensive Cancer Centers nationwide and a founding member of the National Comprehensive Cancer Network, City of Hope is ranked as one of "America's Best Hospitals" in cancer and urology by *U.S.News & World Report*.

ACADEMIC AND CLINICAL AFFILIATIONS

As an independent academic institution, City of Hope enables its researchers to pursue all avenues of scientific inquiry while encouraging collaboration with other researchers and institutions around the world. This helps to speed the development of novel cancer therapies. City of Hope's Graduate School of Biological Sciences also provides a fertile academic environment to prepare future scientists for careers in academia, medical and industrial fields.

MEDICAL STAFF

Guided by a humanistic approach to medicine, nationally recognized physicians and nurses lead collaborative treatment teams that address the whole patient, not just the disease, including emotional, psychological, spiritual and nutritional needs.

PIONEERING, COMPREHENSIVE MEDICAL CARE

City of Hope's Helford Clinical Research Hospital integrates the best of science and human caring in one state-of-the-art facility. There, lifesaving research and superior clinical care join forces as multidisciplinary teams of medical professionals pool their knowledge to bring promising new therapies to patients quickly, safely and effectively.

PHYSICIAN REFERRAL

City of Hope welcomes patient referrals from physicians throughout the world. Referring physicians are encouraged to contact our specialists directly or call 800-826-HOPE.

CENTER OF EXCELLENCE: RADIATION ONCOLOGY

Advances in radiation therapy technology are making a difference for cancer patients. TomoTherapy represents the next-generation radiation therapy and provides City of Hope oncologists with the unprecedented ability to deliver, with surgical precision, radiation to cancers. This means more effective treatment for the tumor and less radiation to normal organs, resulting in significantly reduced side effects.

To learn more, visit cityofhope.org/radonc

NYU Cancer Institute
NYU LANGONE MEDICAL CENTER

A Collaborative Approach

The NYU Cancer Institute, an NCI designated center, is a "matrix cancer center" without walls operating within the larger NYU Langone Medical Center. With over 175 members and a research funding base of over $81 million, this structure strengthens our capabilities to forge collaborations across medical and scientific disciplines, which translates to comprehensive care for our patients and discoveries that will influence the future of this disease.

Renowned Expertise

Team members' compassion and expertise help patients better manage the symptoms of their disease as well as their special needs. Our highly skilled Magnet™ nursing team not only plays a pivotal role in coordinating direct patient care, but is also a source of invaluable patient education.

A Patient-Focused Setting

The NYU Clinical Cancer Center, with over 70 faculty members from various disciplines at the New York University School of Medicine, is the principal outpatient facility of the Cancer Institute and serves as home for our patients and their caregivers. The center and its multidisciplinary team of experts provide access to the latest treatment options and clinical trials along with a variety of programs in cancer prevention, screening, diagnostics, genetic counseling, and supportive services. When it comes to kids and cancer, the Stephen D. Hassenfeld Children's Center for Cancer and Blood Disorders offers not just innovation but insight. As a leading member of the NCI-sponsored Children's Oncology Group, our physicians are known for developing new ways to treat childhood cancer. Our affiliation with Bellevue Hospital, the oldest public hospital in the country, affords clinically distinctive opportunities to learn and care for patients with cancer by observing its presentation and behavior in a variety of patient groups.

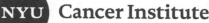

NYU Cancer Institute
NYU LANGONE MEDICAL CENTER

NYU Clinical Cancer Center
160 East 34th Street
New York, New York 10016
www.nyuci.org/atcd

NYU Langone Medical Center
550 First Avenue
(at 31st Street)
New York, New York 10016
www.nyumc.org/atcd

Stephen D. Hassenfeld Children's Center for Cancer and Blood Disorders
160 East 32nd Street
New York, New York 10016
www.nyumc.org/hassenfeld

A Collaborative Approach
The NYU Cancer Institute, an NCI designated center, is a "matrix cancer center" without walls operating within the larger NYU Langone Medical Center. With over 175 members and a research funding base of over $81 million, this structure strengthens our capabilities to forge collaborations across medical and scientific disciplines, which translates to comprehensive care for our patients and discoveries that will influence the future of this disease.

Renowned Expertise
Team members' compassion and expertise help patients better manage the symptoms of their disease as well as their special needs. Our highly skilled Magnet™ nursing team not only plays a pivotal role in coordinating direct patient care, but is also a source of invaluable patient education.

A Patient-Focused Setting
The NYU Clinical Cancer Center, with over 70 faculty members from various disciplines at the New York University School of Medicine, is the principal outpatient facility of the Cancer Institute and serves as home for our patients and their caregivers. The center and its multidisciplinary team of experts provide access to the latest treatment options and clinical trials along with a variety of programs in cancer prevention, screening, diagnostics, genetic counseling, and supportive services. When it comes to kids and cancer, the Stephen D. Hassenfeld Children's Center for Cancer and Blood Disorders offers not just innovation but insight. As a leading member of the NCI-sponsored Children's Oncology Group, our physicians are known for developing new ways to treat childhood cancer. Our affiliation with Bellevue Hospital, the oldest public hospital in the country, affords clinically distinctive opportunities to learn and care for patients with cancer by observing its presentation and behavior in a variety of patient groups.

NYU Cancer Institute

NYU LANGONE MEDICAL CENTER

NYU Clinical Cancer Center
160 East 34th Street
New York, New York 10016
www.nyuci.org/atcd

NYU Langone Medical Center
550 First Avenue
(at 31st Street)
New York, New York 10016
www.nyumc.org/atcd

Stephen D. Hassenfeld Children's Center for Cancer and Blood Disorders
160 East 32nd Street
New York, New York 10016
www.nyumc.org/hassenfeld

A Collaborative Approach

The NYU Cancer Institute, an NCI designated center, is a "matrix cancer center" without walls operating within the larger NYU Langone Medical Center. With over 175 members and a research funding base of over $81 million, this structure strengthens our capabilities to forge collaborations across medical and scientific disciplines, which translates to comprehensive care for our patients and discoveries that will influence the future of this disease.

Renowned Expertise

Team members' compassion and expertise help patients better manage the symptoms of their disease as well as their special needs. Our highly skilled Magnet™ nursing team not only plays a pivotal role in coordinating direct patient care, but is also a source of invaluable patient education.

A Patient-Focused Setting

The NYU Clinical Cancer Center, with over 70 faculty members from various disciplines at the New York University School of Medicine, is the principal outpatient facility of the Cancer Institute and serves as home for our patients and their caregivers. The center and its multidisciplinary team of experts provide access to the latest treatment options and clinical trials along with a variety of programs in cancer prevention, screening, diagnostics, genetic counseling, and supportive services. When it comes to kids and cancer, the Stephen D. Hassenfeld Children's Center for Cancer and Blood Disorders offers not just innovation but insight. As a leading member of the NCI-sponsored Children's Oncology Group, our physicians are known for developing new ways to treat childhood cancer. Our affiliation with Bellevue Hospital, the oldest public hospital in the country, affords clinically distinctive opportunities to learn and care for patients with cancer by observing its presentation and behavior in a variety of patient groups.

Cancer Institute

NYU LANGONE MEDICAL CENTER

FIGHTING **CANCER**
JUST GOT **EASIER.**

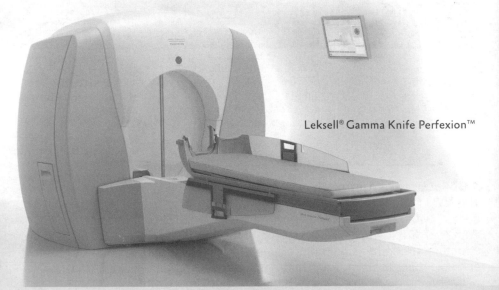

Leksell® Gamma Knife Perfexion™

IN THE FIGHT AGAINST CANCER,
NEW TECHNOLOGY REPRESENTS NEW HOPE.

So it is with genuine excitement that we announce the acquisition of two "next generation" tools that allow for treatment of tumors, from head to toe.

The Stereotactic Radiosurgery (SRS) Team at Wake Forest University Baptist Medical Center now offers **Leksell® Gamma Knife Perfexion™** and the **Axesse™** linear accelerator — the fastest, most accurate stereotactic radiosurgery/radiotherapy treatments available. For our patients, that means a faster return to daily life, with virtually no discomfort and no hospital stay.

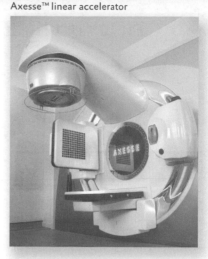
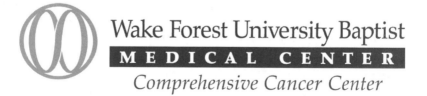

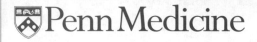

Philadelphia, PA 19104
800.789.PENN (7366)
PennMedicine.org

PENN RADIATION ONCOLOGY

Advancing Cancer Care

At Penn Medicine, the Department of Radiation Oncology is a national leader in clinical care, research, and education and has one of the largest and most respected clinical services in the Philadelphia region.

Excellence and Expertise

At Penn, our patient care is backed by a nationally recognized research and teaching program. The department conducts basic research to better understand tumor response to radiation and to increase that response, enabling us to develop new treatment approaches.

The department offers a wide range of services, including many that combine radiation therapy with chemotherapy and/or surgery. Penn provides complete evaluation, treatment and follow-up care for patients whose cancer can be effectively treated with radiation and also sees patients with benign (non-cancerous) diseases that can be treated with radiation.

Imaging procedures for treatment planning include X-ray filming and fluoroscopy, and CT linkage with computerized dosimetry. Treatment options include Intensity-Modulated Radiation Therapy (IMRT), Positron Emission Therapy (PET) and Conformal Radiation Therapy. Symptom management and access to innovative treatments, such as photodynamic and proton therapy, further differentiates Penn Radiation Oncology from other radiation oncology centers.

Leaders in Research

Our radiation oncologists are experts in cancer treatment and research, and have contributed many important advances in the field. This means that when you are treated by Penn physicians, you will benefit from their expertise in treating your type of cancer.

Penn Radiation Oncology also conducts a wide range of clinical trials involving the innovative use of radiation therapy in combination with other therapies in order to find better ways to treat patients with different types of cancer. This means that our patients have access to the latest research and advances, often before the research findings are published in medical journals. And, because we understand the emotional implications of cancer, we also provide support services to help patients and their families throughout their cancer experience.

Penn Radiation Oncology Network

Because we understand the needs of our patients, the Penn Radiation Oncology Network offers several convenient locations throughout Southeastern Pennsylvania and New Jersey. At each facility, full-time, board certified Penn radiation oncologists provide outstanding clinical and patient-focused care.

The Roberts Proton Therapy Center

Opening in 2009, the Roberts Proton Therapy Center will be the largest proton therapy center in the world and one of only eight such centers in the country. As the world's most comprehensive proton therapy center, it will offer the unique ability to fully integrate conventional radiation treatment with proton radiation for certain types of cancer. In addition, the Center will be connected to the Ruth and Raymond Perelman Center for Advanced Medicine, home of Penn's Abramson Cancer Center.

Because of its proximity to the Abramson Cancer Center, all cancer diagnostic and treatment services are available in one location. This allows patients to receive comprehensive care in one location, easily navigating from one service to the next, ensuring exceptional and timely care.

The Center will be the:

- first and only facility in the mid-Atlantic region

- first in the world to be fully integrated with a renowned cancer center, the Abramson Cancer Center of the University of Pennsylvania

- first proton therapy center to be located on the campus of an academic medical center

For more information or to schedule an appointment with Penn's Department of Radiation Oncology, call 800.789.PENN (7366) or visit PennMedicine.org.

Surgery

A surgeon manages a broad spectrum of surgical conditions affecting almost any area of the body. The surgeon establishes the diagnosis and provides the preoperative, operative and postoperative care to surgical patients and is usually responsible for the comprehensive management of the trauma victim and the critically ill surgical patient.

The surgeon uses a variety of diagnostic techniques, including endoscopy, for observing internal structures and may use specialized instruments during operative procedures. A general surgeon is expected to be familiar with the salient features of other surgical specialties in order to recognize problems in those areas and to know when to refer a patient to another specialist.

Training Required: Five years

SURGERY

New England

Becker, James M MD [S] - **Spec Exp:** Gastrointestinal Cancer; Gastrointestinal Surgery; **Hospital:** Boston Med Ctr, Qunicy Med Ctr; **Address:** Boston Med Ctr, Dept Surg, 88 E Newton St, rm C500, Boston, MA 02118-2393; **Phone:** 617-638-8600; **Board Cert:** Surgery 1999; **Med School:** Case West Res Univ 1975; **Resid:** Surgery, Univ Utah Med Ctr 1980; **Fellow:** Research, Mayo Clinic 1982; **Fac Appt:** Prof S, Boston Univ

Cioffi, William G MD [S] - **Spec Exp:** Cancer Surgery; **Hospital:** Rhode Island Hosp; **Address:** Rhode Island Hosp, Dept Surg, 2 Dudley St, Ste 470, Providence, RI 02905; **Phone:** 401-553-8348; **Board Cert:** Surgery 2007; Surgical Critical Care 1997; **Med School:** Univ VT Coll Med 1981; **Resid:** Surgery, Med Ctr Hosp 1986; **Fac Appt:** Prof S, Brown Univ

Eisenberg, Burton L MD [S] - **Spec Exp:** Breast Cancer; Melanoma; Sarcoma; **Hospital:** Dartmouth - Hitchcock Med Ctr; **Address:** DHMC, Dept General Surgery, One Medical Center Drive, Lebanon, NH 03756; **Phone:** 603-650-9479; **Board Cert:** Surgery 1999; **Med School:** Univ Tenn Coll Med, Memphis 1974; **Resid:** Surgery, Wilford Hall USAF Med Ctr 1979; **Fellow:** Surgical Oncology, Meml Sloan-Kettering Cancer Ctr 1981; **Fac Appt:** Prof S, Dartmouth Med Sch

Hughes, Kevin S MD [S] - **Spec Exp:** Breast Cancer; Ovarian Cancer; **Hospital:** Mass Genl Hosp; **Address:** Mass Genl Hosp, Dept Surgery, 55 Fruit St, Yawkey Center Fl 9 - Ste A, Boston, MA 02114; **Phone:** 617-724-4800; **Board Cert:** Surgery 2006; **Med School:** Dartmouth Med Sch 1979; **Resid:** Surgery, Mercy Hosp 1984; **Fellow:** Surgical Oncology, National Cancer Inst 1986; **Fac Appt:** Assoc Prof S, Harvard Med Sch

Iglehart, J Dirk MD [S] - **Spec Exp:** Breast Cancer; **Hospital:** Brigham & Women's Hosp, Dana-Farber Cancer Inst; **Address:** Dana-Farber Cancer Inst, 44 binney, Smith Bldg, Boston, MA 02115; **Phone:** 617-632-5178 x1; **Board Cert:** Surgery 2005; **Med School:** Harvard Med Sch 1975; **Resid:** Surgery, Duke Univ Med Ctr 1981; Thoracic Surgery, Duke Univ Med Ctr 1984; **Fac Appt:** Prof S, Harvard Med Sch

Jenkins, Roger L MD [S] - **Spec Exp:** Transplant-Liver; Liver & Biliary Cancer; Pancreatic Cancer; **Hospital:** Lahey Clin, Children's Hospital - Boston; **Address:** Lahey Clin, Dept Hepatobiliary Surg, 41 Mall Rd, Burlington, MA 01805; **Phone:** 781-744-2500; **Board Cert:** Surgery 2005; **Med School:** Univ VT Coll Med 1977; **Resid:** Surgery, New Eng Deaconess Hosp 1982; **Fellow:** Cardiac Surgery, New Eng Deaconess Hosp 1983; Transplant Surgery, Univ Pittsburgh Hosp 1983; **Fac Appt:** Prof S, Tufts Univ

Kavanah, Maureen MD [S] - **Spec Exp:** Breast Cancer; Gynecologic Cancer; Melanoma; **Hospital:** Boston Med Ctr; **Address:** Boston Medical Ctr, 820 Harrison Ave, rm 5009, Bldg FGH, Boston, MA 02118; **Phone:** 617-638-8473; **Board Cert:** Surgery 1999; **Med School:** Tufts Univ 1975; **Resid:** Surgery, St Elizabeths Hosp 1979; **Fellow:** Surgical Oncology, Boston Univ Med Ctr 1981; **Fac Appt:** Assoc Prof S, Boston Univ

Krag, David N MD [S] - **Spec Exp:** Sentinel Node Surgery; Breast Cancer; Cancer Surgery; Melanoma; **Hospital:** Fletcher Allen Health Care- Med Ctr Campus; **Address:** Univ Vermont Coll Med, Dept Surgery, 89 Beaumont Ave, Given Bldg - E309C, Burlington, VT 05405; **Phone:** 802-656-5830; **Board Cert:** Surgery 2006; **Med School:** Loyola Univ-Stritch Sch Med 1980; **Resid:** Surgery, UC Davis Med Ctr 1983; **Fellow:** Surgical Oncology, UCLA Med Ctr 1984; **Fac Appt:** Assoc Prof S, Univ VT Coll Med

Ponn, Teresa MD [S] - **Spec Exp:** Breast Cancer; **Hospital:** Elliot Hosp; **Address:** Elliot Breast Health Center, 275 Mammoth Rd, Ste 1, Manchester, NH 03109; **Phone:** 603-668-3067; **Board Cert:** Surgery 2000; **Med School:** Univ Fla Coll Med 1976; **Resid:** Surgery, Stanford Univ Med Ctr 1982

Salem, Ronald R MD [S] - **Spec Exp:** Cancer Surgery; Liver & Biliary Surgery; Gastrointestinal Cancer; **Hospital:** Yale-New Haven Hosp; **Address:** Dept Surgery, 333 Cedar St, TMP 202, New Haven, CT 06520-8062; **Phone:** 203-785-3577; **Board Cert:** Surgery 2000; **Med School:** Zimbabwe 1978; **Resid:** Surgery, Hammersmith Hosp 1985; Surgery, New England Deaconess Hosp 1989; **Fac Appt:** Assoc Prof S, Yale Univ

Smith, Barbara Lynn MD/PhD [S] - **Spec Exp:** Breast Cancer; **Hospital:** Mass Genl Hosp; **Address:** Mass Genl Hosp, Dept Surgery, 55 Fruit St, Yawkey Center Fl 9 - Ste A, Boston, MA 02114; **Phone:** 617-724-4800; **Board Cert:** Surgery 2000; **Med School:** Harvard Med Sch 1983; **Resid:** Surgery, Brigham & Women's Hosp 1989; **Fac Appt:** Asst Prof S, Harvard Med Sch

Sutton, John E MD [S] - **Spec Exp:** Esophageal Cancer; Liver & Biliary Surgery; Pancreatic Cancer; **Hospital:** Dartmouth - Hitchcock Med Ctr; **Address:** One Medical Center Drive, Lebanon, NH 03756; **Phone:** 603-650-8022; **Board Cert:** Surgery 2001; Surgical Critical Care 2007; **Med School:** Georgetown Univ 1974; **Resid:** Surgery, Dartmouth-Hitchcock Med Ctr 1981; **Fellow:** Surgical Critical Care, Dartmouth-Hitchcock Med Ctr 1983; **Fac Appt:** Prof S, Dartmouth Med Sch

Tanabe, Kenneth K MD [S] - **Spec Exp:** Liver Cancer; Colon & Rectal Cancer; Melanoma; **Hospital:** Mass Genl Hosp, Newton - Wellesley Hosp; **Address:** Mass General Hosp, Div Surgical Oncology, 55 Fruit St, Yawkey 7.924, Boston, MA 02114; **Phone:** 617-724-3868; **Board Cert:** Surgery 2000, **Med School:** UCSD 1985; **Resid:** Surgery, New York Hosp-Cornell 1990; **Fellow:** Surgical Oncology, MD Anderson Cancer Ctr 1993; **Fac Appt:** Assoc Prof S, Harvard Med Sch

Udelsman, Robert MD [S] - **Spec Exp:** Parathyroid Cancer; Adrenal Tumors; Thyroid Cancer; **Hospital:** Yale-New Haven Hosp; **Address:** Yale School Medicine, Dept Surgery, 330 Cedar St, FMB 102, New Haven, CT 06511; **Phone:** 203-785-2697; **Board Cert:** Surgery 1999; **Med School:** Geo Wash Univ 1981; **Resid:** Surgery, Natl Inst Hlth 1986; Surgery, Johns Hopkins Hosp 1989; **Fellow:** Gastrointestinal Surgery, Johns Hopkins Hosp 1990; **Fac Appt:** Prof S, Yale Univ

Ward, Barbara MD [S] - **Spec Exp:** Breast Cancer; **Hospital:** Greenwich Hosp; **Address:** 77 Lafayette Pl, Ste 302, Greenwich, CT 06830-5426; **Phone:** 203-863-4250; **Board Cert:** Surgery 2002; **Med School:** Temple Univ 1983; **Resid:** Surgery, Yale-New Haven Hosp 1990; **Fellow:** Surgical Oncology, Natl Cancer Inst 1987; **Fac Appt:** Assoc Clin Prof S, Yale Univ

Warshaw, Andrew L MD [S] - **Spec Exp:** Pancreatic Cancer; Pancreatic Surgery; **Hospital:** Mass Genl Hosp; **Address:** Mass Genl Hosp, Dept Surg, 55 Fruit St, WHT 506, Boston, MA 02114-2696; **Phone:** 617-726-8254; **Board Cert:** Surgery 1971; **Med School:** Harvard Med Sch 1963; **Resid:** Surgery, Mass Genl Hosp 1971; **Fellow:** Internal Medicine, Mass Genl Hosp 1970; **Fac Appt:** Prof S, Harvard Med Sch

Zinner, Michael MD [S] - **Spec Exp:** Colon & Rectal Cancer; Gastrointestinal Surgery; Pancreatic Cancer; **Hospital:** Brigham & Women's Hosp, Dana-Farber Cancer Inst; **Address:** Brigham & Women's Hosp, Dept Surg, 75 Francis St, Twr 1, Ste 220, Boston, MA 02115; **Phone:** 617-732-8181; **Board Cert:** Surgery 2000; **Med School:** Univ Fla Coll Med 1971; **Resid:** Surgery, Johns Hopkins Hosp 1974; Surgery, Johns Hopkins Hosp 1979; **Fac Appt:** Prof S, Harvard Med Sch

Surgery

Mid Atlantic

Alfonso, Antonio MD [S] - **Spec Exp:** Breast Cancer; Head & Neck Surgery; Thyroid Cancer; **Hospital:** Long Island Coll Hosp (page 71), SUNY Downstate Med Ctr; **Address:** Long Island Coll Hosp, 339 Hicks St, Brooklyn, NY 11201; **Phone:** 718-875-3244; **Board Cert:** Surgery 1973; **Med School:** Philippines 1968; **Resid:** Surgery, Temple Univ Hosp 1972; **Fellow:** Surgical Oncology, Meml Sloan Kettering Cancer Ctr 1974; **Fac Appt:** Prof S, SUNY Downstate

August, David MD [S] - **Spec Exp:** Pancreatic Cancer; Esophageal Cancer; Stomach Cancer; Sarcoma-Soft Tissue; **Hospital:** Robert Wood Johnson Univ Hosp - New Brunswick; **Address:** Canc Inst NJ, 195 Little Albany St, New Brunswick, NJ 08903-1914; **Phone:** 732-235-7701; **Board Cert:** Surgery 2005; **Med School:** Yale Univ 1980; **Resid:** Surgery, Yale-New Haven Hosp 1986; **Fellow:** Surgical Oncology, Natl Cancer Inst 1984; **Fac Appt:** Prof S, UMDNJ-RW Johnson Med Sch

Axelrod, Deborah MD [S] - **Spec Exp:** Breast Cancer; **Hospital:** NYU Langone Med Ctr (page 80), St Vincent Cath Med Ctrs - Manhattan; **Address:** NYU Clinical Cancer Ctr, 160 E 34th St, New York, NY 10016; **Phone:** 212-731-5366; **Board Cert:** Surgery 1997; **Med School:** Israel 1982; **Resid:** Surgery, Beth Israel Med Ctr 1988; **Fellow:** Surgical Oncology, Meml Sloan Kettering Cancer Ctr 1986; **Fac Appt:** Assoc Prof S, NYU Sch Med

Balch, Charles M MD [S] - **Spec Exp:** Sentinel Node Surgery; Melanoma; Cancer Surgery; **Hospital:** Johns Hopkins Hosp; **Address:** 600 N Wolfe St Osler Bldg - Ste 624, Baltimore, MD 21287; **Phone:** 410-502-5977; **Board Cert:** Surgery 1997; **Med School:** Columbia P&S 1967; **Resid:** Surgery, Univ Alabama Med Ctr 1971; Surgery, Univ Alabama Med Ctr 1975; **Fellow:** Immunology, Scripps Clin-Rsch Fdn 1973; **Fac Appt:** Prof Surg & Onc, Johns Hopkins Univ

Ballantyne, Garth H MD [S] - **Spec Exp:** Laparoscopic Surgery; Colon Cancer; **Hospital:** Hackensack Univ Med Ctr (page 73); **Address:** 20 Prospect Ave, Ste 901, Hackensack, NJ 07601-1974; **Phone:** 201-996-2959; **Board Cert:** Surgery 2006; Colon & Rectal Surgery 1985; **Med School:** Columbia P&S 1977; **Resid:** Surgery, UCLA Med Ctr 1980; Surgery, Northwestern Univ 1982; **Fellow:** Colon & Rectal Surgery, Mayo Clinic 1984; **Fac Appt:** Prof S, UMDNJ-NJ Med Sch, Newark

Bartlett, David L MD [S] - **Spec Exp:** Peritoneal Carcinomatosis; Pancreatic Cancer; Liver Cancer; Appendix Cancer; **Hospital:** UPMC Shadyside; **Address:** UPMC Cancer Ctr, 5150 Centre Ave Fl 4 - rm 415, Pittsburgh, PA 15232; **Phone:** 412-692-2852; **Board Cert:** Surgery 2004; **Med School:** Univ Tex, Houston 1987; **Resid:** Surgery, Hosp Univ Penn 1993; **Fellow:** Surgical Oncology, Meml Sloan-Kettering Cancer Ctr 1995; **Fac Appt:** Assoc Prof S, Univ Pittsburgh

Borgen, Patrick I MD [S] - **Spec Exp:** Breast Cancer; **Hospital:** Maimonides Med Ctr (page 75); **Address:** Maimonides Breast Ctr, 6300 8th Ave, Brooklyn, NY 11220; **Phone:** 718-765-2570; **Board Cert:** Surgery 2002; **Med School:** Louisiana State U, New Orleans 1984; **Resid:** Surgery, Ochsner Fdn Hosp 1989; **Fellow:** Surgical Oncology, Meml Sloan Kettering Canc Ctr 1990; **Fac Appt:** Prof S, Cornell Univ-Weill Med Coll

Brennan, Murray MD [S] - **Spec Exp:** Sarcoma; Pancreatic Cancer; Stomach Cancer; Endocrine Cancers; **Hospital:** Meml Sloan-Kettering Cancer Ctr (page 76); **Address:** 1275 York Avenue, New York, NY 10065; **Phone:** 800-525-2225; **Board Cert:** Surgery 1975; **Med School:** New Zealand 1964; **Resid:** Surgery, Univ Otago Hosp 1969; **Fellow:** Surgery, Harvard Med Sch 1972; Surgery, Peter Bent Brigham Hosp 1975; **Fac Appt:** Prof S, Cornell Univ-Weill Med Coll

Brooks, Ari D MD [S] - **Spec Exp:** Breast Cancer; **Hospital:** Hahnemann Univ Hosp; **Address:** Drexel Surgical Assocs, 219 N Broad St Fl 8, Philadelphia, PA 19107; **Phone:** 215-762-2295; **Board Cert:** Surgery 2000; **Med School:** Hahnemann Univ 1992; **Resid:** Surgery, NYU Med Ctr 1999; **Fellow:** Surgical Oncology, Meml Sloan-Kettering Cancer Ctr 2001; **Fac Appt:** Assoc Prof S, Drexel Univ Coll Med

Cance, William George MD [S] - **Spec Exp:** Pancreatic Cancer; Colon & Rectal Cancer; Endocrine Cancers; **Hospital:** Roswell Park Cancer Inst; **Address:** Roswell Park Cancer Inst, Dept Surgery, Elm & Carlton Sts, Buffalo, NY 14263; **Phone:** 716-845-8204; **Board Cert:** Surgery 1998; **Med School:** Duke Univ 1982; **Resid:** Surgery, Barnes Jewish Hosp 1988; **Fellow:** Surgical Oncology, Meml Sloan Kettering Canc Ctr 1990; **Fac Appt:** Prof S, SUNY Buffalo

Carty, Sally E MD [S] - **Spec Exp:** Endocrine Tumors; Parathyroid Surgery; **Hospital:** UPMC Montefiore; **Address:** 3471 Fifth Ave, Ste 101, Pittsburgh, PA 15213; **Phone:** 412-647-0467; **Board Cert:** Surgery 1999; **Med School:** Penn State Univ-Hershey Med Ctr 1984; **Resid:** Surgery, Penn State Hershey Med Ctr 1989; **Fellow:** Surgical Oncology, Natl Cancer Inst 1991; **Fac Appt:** Prof S, Univ Pittsburgh

Chabot, John A MD [S] - **Spec Exp:** Liver & Biliary Surgery; Pancreatic Cancer; Pancreatic Surgery; Thyroid & Parathyroid Surgery; **Hospital:** NY-Presby Hosp/Columbia (page 79); **Address:** NY Presby-Columbia Medical Ctr, 161 Ft Washington Ave Fl 8 - Ste 819, New York, NY 10032; **Phone:** 212-305-9468; **Board Cert:** Surgery 2000; **Med School:** Dartmouth Med Sch 1983; **Resid:** Surgery, Columbia-Presby Med Ctr 1990; **Fac Appt:** Prof S, Columbia P&S

Choti, Michael A MD [S] - **Spec Exp:** Pancreatic Cancer; Liver Cancer-Metastatic; Carcinoid Tumors; **Hospital:** Johns Hopkins Hosp; **Address:** Johns Hopkins Hosp, 600 N Wolfe St Blalock Bldg - rm 665, Baltimore, MD 21287; **Phone:** 410-955-7113; **Board Cert:** Surgery 2002; **Med School:** Yale Univ 1983; **Resid:** Surgery, Hosp Univ Penn 1990; **Fellow:** Surgical Oncology, Meml Sloan-Kettering Canc Ctr 1992; **Fac Appt:** Prof S, Johns Hopkins Univ

Coit, Daniel G MD [S] - **Spec Exp:** Melanoma; Pancreatic Cancer; Stomach Cancer; **Hospital:** Meml Sloan-Kettering Cancer Ctr (page 76); **Address:** 1275 York Avenue, New York, NY 10065; **Phone:** 800-525-2225; **Board Cert:** Surgery 2004; **Med School:** Univ Cincinnati 1976; **Resid:** Internal Medicine, New Eng Deaconess Hosp 1978; Surgery, New Eng Deaconess Hosp 1983; **Fellow:** Surgical Oncology, Meml Sloan Kettering Canc Ctr 1985; **Fac Appt:** Assoc Prof S, Cornell Univ-Weill Med Coll

Drebin, Jeffrey A MD/PhD [S] - **Spec Exp:** Pancreatic Cancer; Liver Cancer; Biliary Cancer; Gastrointestinal Cancer; **Hospital:** Hosp Univ Penn - UPHS (page 81); **Address:** Hosp Univ of Pennsylvania, 3400 Spruce St, 4 Silverstein Pavilion, Fl 4, Philadelphia, PA 19104; **Phone:** 215-662-2165; **Board Cert:** Surgery 2004; **Med School:** Harvard Med Sch 1987; **Resid:** Surgery, Johns Hopkins Hosp 1994; **Fellow:** Surgical Oncology, Johns Hopkins Hosp 1995

Edge, Stephen B MD [S] - **Spec Exp:** Breast Cancer; **Hospital:** Roswell Park Cancer Inst; **Address:** Roswell Park Cancer Inst, Dept Surg Onc, Elm & Carlton Streets, Buffalo, NY 14263; **Phone:** 716-845-3152; **Board Cert:** Surgery 2006; **Med School:** Case West Res Univ 1979; **Resid:** Surgery, Univ Hosp 1986; **Fellow:** Surgical Oncology, Natl Cancer Inst 1984; **Fac Appt:** Prof S, SUNY Buffalo

Edington, Howard D MD [S] - **Spec Exp:** Melanoma; Breast Reconstruction; Reconstructive Surgery; **Hospital:** Magee-Womens Hosp - UPMC; **Address:** Magee-Women's Hospital, Dept Surgery, 300 Halket St, rm 2502, Pittsburgh, PA 15213; **Phone:** 412-641-1342; **Board Cert:** Surgery 1998; Plastic Surgery 1993; **Med School:** Temple Univ 1983; **Resid:** Surgery, Univ Pittsburgh Med Ctr 1989; Plastic Surgery, Univ Pittsburgh Med Ctr 1990; **Fellow:** Hand Surgery, Univ Pittsburgh Med Ctr 1991; Surgical Oncology, National Cancer Inst 1993; **Fac Appt:** Assoc Prof S, Univ Pittsburgh

Surgery

Emond, Jean C MD [S] - **Spec Exp:** Transplant-Liver; Liver Cancer; Liver & Biliary Cancer; Hepatobiliary Surgery; **Hospital:** NY-Presby Hosp/Columbia (page 79), Holy Name Hosp; **Address:** 622 W 168th St, PH - Fl 14, New York, NY 10032; **Phone:** 212-305-9691; **Board Cert:** Surgery 2006; **Med School:** Univ Chicago-Pritzker Sch Med 1979; **Resid:** Surgery, Cook Cty Hosp 1984; **Fellow:** Surgery, Hopital P Brousse/Univ de Paris Sud 1985; Transplant Surgery, Univ Chicago Hosps 1987; **Fac Appt:** Prof S, Columbia P&S

Eng, Kenneth MD [S] - **Spec Exp:** Colon & Rectal Cancer & Surgery; Pancreatic Cancer; **Hospital:** NYU Langone Med Ctr (page 80); **Address:** 530 1st Ave, Ste 6B, New York, NY 10016-6402; **Phone:** 212-263-7301; **Board Cert:** Surgery 1982; **Med School:** NYU Sch Med 1967; **Resid:** Surgery, NYU Med Ctr 1972; **Fac Appt:** Prof S, NYU Sch Med

Estabrook, Alison MD [S] - **Spec Exp:** Breast Cancer; Breast Cancer-High Risk Women; **Hospital:** St Luke's - Roosevelt Hosp Ctr - Roosevelt Div (page 71); **Address:** 425 W 59th St, Ste 7A, New York, NY 10019-1104; **Phone:** 212-523-7500; **Board Cert:** Surgery 2004; **Med School:** NYU Sch Med 1978; **Resid:** Surgery, Columbia Presby Med Ctr 1984; **Fellow:** Surgical Oncology, Columbia Presby Med Ctr 1982; **Fac Appt:** Prof S, Columbia P&S

Fahey III, Thomas J MD [S] - **Spec Exp:** Endocrine Surgery; Pheochromocytoma; Pancreatic Cancer; **Hospital:** NY-Presby Hosp/Weill Cornell (page 79); **Address:** NY Presby Cornell Med Ctr, Dept Surgery, 525 E 68 St, rm F2024, Box 249, New York, NY 10065; **Phone:** 212-746-5130; **Board Cert:** Surgery 2002; **Med School:** Cornell Univ-Weill Med Coll 1986; **Resid:** Surgery, New York Hosp 1992; **Fellow:** Endocrine Surgery, Royal North Shore Hosp 1993; **Fac Appt:** Prof S, Cornell Univ-Weill Med Coll

Fong, Yuman MD [S] - **Spec Exp:** Pancreatic Cancer; Liver & Biliary Cancer; Stomach Cancer; **Hospital:** Meml Sloan-Kettering Cancer Ctr (page 76), NY-Presby Hosp/Weill Cornell (page 79); **Address:** 1275 York Avenue, New York, NY 10065; **Phone:** 800-525-2225; **Board Cert:** Surgery 2002; **Med School:** Cornell Univ-Weill Med Coll 1984; **Resid:** Surgery, NY Hosp-Cornell Med Ctr 1992; **Fellow:** Surgical Oncology, Meml Sloan-Kettering Cancer Ctr 1994; **Fac Appt:** Prof S, Cornell Univ-Weill Med Coll

Fraker, Douglas L MD [S] - **Spec Exp:** Melanoma; Endocrine Tumors; Liver Cancer; Sarcoma; **Hospital:** Hosp Univ Penn - UPHS (page 81); **Address:** Hosp Univ Penn, Dept Surgery, 3400 Spruce St, 4 Silverstein Pavilion, Philadelphia, PA 19104; **Phone:** 215-662-7866; **Board Cert:** Surgery 2002; **Med School:** Harvard Med Sch 1983; **Resid:** Surgery, UCSF Med Ctr 1986; Surgery, UCSF Med Ctr 1991; **Fellow:** Surgical Oncology, National Cancer Inst 1989; **Fac Appt:** Prof S, Univ Pennsylvania

Frazier, Thomas G MD [S] - **Spec Exp:** Breast Cancer; **Hospital:** Bryn Mawr Hosp; **Address:** 101 S Bryn Mawr Ave, Ste 201, Bryn Mawr, PA 19010; **Phone:** 610-520-0700; **Board Cert:** Surgery 2004; **Med School:** Univ Pennsylvania 1968; **Resid:** Surgery, Hosp Univ Penn 1975; **Fellow:** Surgical Oncology, MD Anderson Cancer Ctr 1976; **Fac Appt:** Clin Prof S, Drexel Univ Coll Med

Gibbs, John F MD [S] - **Spec Exp:** Liver Cancer; Liver & Biliary Surgery; Pancreatic Cancer; **Hospital:** Roswell Park Cancer Inst; **Address:** Roswell Park Cancer Inst, Dept Surg Onc, Elm & Carlton Streets, Buffalo, NY 14263-0001; **Phone:** 716-845-5807; **Board Cert:** Surgery 2000; **Med School:** UCSD 1985; **Resid:** Surgery, Rush Presby-St Luke's Med Ctr 1990; **Fellow:** Transplant Surgery, Baylor Univ Med Ctr 1992; Surgical Oncology, Roswell Park Cancer Inst 1996; **Fac Appt:** Assoc Prof S, SUNY Buffalo

Hanna, Nader N MD [S] - **Spec Exp:** Pancreatic Cancer; Adrenal Tumors; Peritoneal Carcino-matosis; Sarcoma-Soft Tissue; **Hospital:** Univ of MD Med Ctr; **Address:** Univ MD Med Sys, 22 S Greene St, Ste S4B-12, Baltimore, MD 21201; **Phone:** 410-328-7320; **Board Cert:** Surgery 2005; **Med School:** Egypt 1985; **Resid:** Surgery, St. Elizabeth's Med Ctr-Tuft's Univ 1994; **Fellow:** Surgical Oncology, Univ Chicago 1997; Research, Univ Chicago; **Fac Appt:** Assoc Prof Surg & Onc, Univ MD Sch Med

Hoffman, John P MD [S] - **Spec Exp:** Pancreatic Cancer; Gastrointestinal Cancer; Hepatobiliary Surgery; Liver Cancer; **Hospital:** Fox Chase Cancer Ctr (page 72); **Address:** Fox Chase Cancer Ctr, 333 Cottman Ave, Philadelphia, PA 19111-2497; **Phone:** 215-728-3518; **Board Cert:** Surgery 1998; **Med School:** Case West Res Univ 1970; **Resid:** Surgery, Virginia Mason Hosp 1977; **Fellow:** Surgical Oncology, Meml Sloan Kettering Cancer Ctr 1980; **Fac Appt:** Prof S, Temple Univ

Jarnagin, William MD [S] - **Spec Exp:** Hepatobiliary Surgery; Liver Cancer; Pancreatic Cancer; **Hospital:** Meml Sloan-Kettering Cancer Ctr (page 76); **Address:** 1275 York Ave, New York, NY 10065; **Phone:** 212-639-7601; **Board Cert:** Surgery 2006; **Med School:** Rush Med Coll 1988; **Resid:** Surgery, Univ Calif San Francisco 1996; **Fellow:** Hepatopancreatobiliary Surgery, Meml Sloan-Kettering Cancer Ctr 1997

Johnson, Ronald R MD [S] - **Spec Exp:** Breast Cancer; **Hospital:** Magee-Womens Hosp - UPMC; **Address:** Magee-Womens Hosp - UPMC, 300 Halket St, Ste 2601, Pittsburgh, PA 15213; **Phone:** 412-641-1225; **Board Cert:** Surgery 1999; **Med School:** Univ Pittsburgh 1983; **Resid:** Surgery, Univ Pittsburgh Med Ctr 1989; **Fac Appt:** Asst Prof S, Univ Pittsburgh

Julian, Thomas B MD [S] - **Spec Exp:** Breast Cancer & Surgery; Clinical Trials; **Hospital:** Allegheny General Hosp; **Address:** Allegheny Cancer Center, 320 E North Ave Fl 5, Pittsburgh, PA 15212; **Phone:** 412-359-8229; **Board Cert:** Surgery 2001; **Med School:** Univ Pittsburgh 1976; **Resid:** Surgery, Univ Pittsburgh Med Ctr 1982; **Fac Appt:** Assoc Prof S, Drexel Univ Coll Med

Karpeh Jr, Martin S MD [S] - **Spec Exp:** Gastrointestinal Cancer; Esophageal Cancer; Colon & Rectal Cancer; **Hospital:** Beth Israel Med Ctr - Petrie Division (page 71); **Address:** Beth Israel Med Ctr, Philips Ambulatory Ctr, 10 Union Square E, Ste 4C, New York, NY 10003; **Phone:** 212-420-4041; **Board Cert:** Surgery 1998; **Med School:** Penn State Univ-Hershey Med Ctr 1983; **Resid:** Surgery, Hosp Univ Penn 1989; **Fellow:** Surgical Oncology, Meml Sloan Kettering Cancer Ctr 1991; **Fac Appt:** Prof S, Mount Sinai Sch Med

Kaufman, Howard L MD [S] - **Spec Exp:** Cancer Surgery; Vaccine Therapy; Melanoma; Immunotherapy; **Hospital:** Mount Sinai Med Ctr (page 77); **Address:** Mount Sinai Med Ctr, Dept Surgery, 5 E 98th St, Box 1259, New York, NY 10029; **Phone:** 212-241-4757; **Board Cert:** Surgery 2007; **Med School:** Loyola Univ-Stritch Sch Med 1986; **Resid:** Surgery, Boston Univ Hosp 1995; **Fellow:** Surgical Oncology, Natl Cancer Inst 1996; **Fac Appt:** Prof S, Mount Sinai Sch Med

Lee, Kenneth K W MD [S] - **Spec Exp:** Pancreatic Cancer; Gastrointestinal Cancer & Surgery; **Hospital:** UPMC Presby, Pittsburgh, UPMC Shadyside; **Address:** UPMC Presbyterian, 200 Lothrop St, Ste 497, Scaife Hall, Pittsburgh, PA 15261; **Phone:** 412-647-0457; **Board Cert:** Surgery 1998; **Med School:** Univ Chicago-Pritzker Sch Med 1981; **Resid:** Surgery, Univ Chicago Hosps 1988; **Fac Appt:** Assoc Prof S, Univ Pittsburgh

Libutti, Steven K MD [S] - **Spec Exp:** Liver Cancer; Pancreatic Cancer; Endocrine Tumors; Gastrointestinal Cancer; **Hospital:** Montefiore Med Ctr - Div. Moses, Montefiore Med Ctr - Div. Weiler; **Address:** 3400 Bainbridge Ave Fl 4th, Bronx, NY 10467; **Phone:** 718-920-4231; **Board Cert:** Surgery 2004; **Med School:** Columbia P&S 1990; **Resid:** Surgery, Columbia Presby Med Ctr 1995; **Fellow:** Surgical Oncology, Natl Cancer Inst 1996; **Fac Appt:** Prof S, Albert Einstein Coll Med

Marsh Jr, James W MD [S] - **Spec Exp:** Transplant-Liver; Liver Cancer; Pancreatic Cancer; **Hospital:** UPMC Presby, Pittsburgh; **Address:** UPMC, Starzl Transplant Inst, 3459 Fifth Ave 7 South, Pittsburgh, PA 15213; **Phone:** 412-647-5800; **Board Cert:** Surgery 2003; **Med School:** Univ Ark 1979; **Resid:** Surgery, St Paul Hosp 1984; **Fellow:** Transplant Surgery, Mayo Clin 1985; Transplant Surgery, Univ Pittsburgh Hosps 1986; **Fac Appt:** Prof S, Univ Pittsburgh

Michelassi, Fabrizio MD [S] - **Spec Exp:** Gastrointestinal Cancer; Colon Cancer; **Hospital:** NY-Presby Hosp/Weill Cornell (page 79); **Address:** Weill Cornell Med College, Surg Dept, 525 E 68th St, rm F-739, New York, NY 10021; **Phone:** 212-746-6006; **Board Cert:** Surgery 2002; **Med School:** Italy 1975; **Resid:** Surgery, NYU Med Ctr 1981; **Fellow:** Research, Mass Genl Hosp 1983; **Fac Appt:** Prof S, Cornell Univ-Weill Med Coll

Morrow, Monica MD [S] - **Spec Exp:** Breast Cancer; **Hospital:** Meml Sloan-Kettering Cancer Ctr (page 76); **Address:** 1275 York Avenue, New York, NY 10065; **Phone:** 800-525-2225; **Board Cert:** Surgery 2001; **Med School:** Jefferson Med Coll 1976; **Resid:** Surgery, Med Ctr Hosp Vermont 1981; **Fellow:** Surgical Oncology, Meml Sloan Kettering Cancer Ctr 1983; **Fac Appt:** Prof S, Cornell Univ-Weill Med Coll

Nava-Villarreal, Hector MD [S] - **Spec Exp:** Esophageal Cancer; Stomach Cancer; Barrett's Esophagus; **Hospital:** Roswell Park Cancer Inst; **Address:** Roswell Park Cancer Inst, Elm & Carlton Sts, Buffalo, NY 14263; **Phone:** 716-845-5915; **Board Cert:** Surgery 2001; **Med School:** Mexico 1967; **Resid:** Surgery, Buffalo Genl Hosp 1974; **Fellow:** Surgical Oncology, Roswell Park Cancer Inst 1976; **Fac Appt:** Assoc Prof S, SUNY Buffalo

Nowak, Eugene MD [S] - **Spec Exp:** Breast Cancer; Gastrointestinal Surgery; Sentinel Node Surgery; **Hospital:** NY-Presby Hosp/Weill Cornell (page 79); **Address:** 325 E 79th St, New York, NY 10021-0954; **Phone:** 212-517-6693; **Board Cert:** Surgery 2002; **Med School:** UMDNJ-NJ Med Sch, Newark 1975; **Resid:** Surgery, NY Hosp-Cornell Med Ctr 1980; **Fac Appt:** Assoc Prof S, Cornell Univ-Weill Med Coll

O'Hea, Brian J MD [S] - **Spec Exp:** Breast Cancer; Sentinel Node Surgery; **Hospital:** Stony Brook Univ Med Ctr; **Address:** SUNY Stony Brook, Dept Surgery, HSC T-18, Rm 060, Stony Brook, NY 11794-8191; **Phone:** 631-444-1795; **Board Cert:** Surgery 2002; **Med School:** Georgetown Univ 1986; **Resid:** Surgery, St Vincent's Hosp 1991; **Fellow:** Breast Disease, Meml Sloan-Kettering Cancer Ctr 1996; **Fac Appt:** Asst Prof S, SUNY Stony Brook

Olthoff, Kim M MD [S] - **Spec Exp:** Transplant-Liver-Adult & Pediatric; Liver & Biliary Surgery; Liver Cancer; **Hospital:** Hosp Univ Penn - UPHS (page 81), Chldns Hosp of Philadelphia, The; **Address:** Hosp Univ Penn - Dept Surgery, 3400 Spruce St Dulles Bldg Fl 2, Philadelphia, PA 19104; **Phone:** 215-662-6136; **Board Cert:** Surgery 2003; **Med School:** Univ Chicago-Pritzker Sch Med 1986; **Resid:** Surgery, UCLA Med Ctr 1990; **Fellow:** Transplant Surgery, UCLA Med Ctr; **Fac Appt:** Prof S, Univ Pennsylvania

Osborne, Michael P MD [S] - **Spec Exp:** Breast Cancer; Breast Cancer-High Risk Women; **Hospital:** Beth Israel Med Ctr - Petrie Division (page 71); **Address:** Philip Ambulatory Care Ctr, 10 Union Square E, Ste 4E, New York, NY 10003; **Phone:** 212-844-8770; **Med School:** England, UK 1970; **Resid:** Surgery, Charing Cross Hosp 1977; Surgery, Royal Marsden Hosp 1980; **Fellow:** Surgical Oncology, Meml Sloan-Kettering Canc Ctr 1981; **Fac Appt:** Prof S, Cornell Univ-Weill Med Coll

Paty, Philip B MD [S] - **Spec Exp:** Colon & Rectal Cancer; Pelvic Tumors; Appendix Cancer; **Hospital:** Meml Sloan-Kettering Cancer Ctr (page 76); **Address:** 1275 York Avenue, New York, NY 10065; **Phone:** 800-525-2225; **Board Cert:** Surgery 2001; **Med School:** Stanford Univ 1983; **Resid:** Surgery, UCSF Med Ctr 1990; **Fellow:** Surgical Oncology, Meml Sloan Kettering Cancer Ctr 1992; **Fac Appt:** Prof S, Cornell Univ-Weill Med Coll

Petrelli, Nicholas J MD [S] - **Spec Exp:** Cancer Surgery; Gastrointestinal Cancer; Colon & Rectal Cancer; **Hospital:** Christiana Care Hlth Svs; **Address:** Helen F Graham Cancer Ctr, 4701 Ogletown-Stanton Rd, Ste 1213, Newark, DE 19713; **Phone:** 302-623-4550; **Board Cert:** Surgery 1997; **Med School:** Tulane Univ 1973; **Resid:** Surgery, St Mary's Hosp-Med Ctr 1978; **Fellow:** Surgical Oncology, Roswell Park Cancer Inst 1980; **Fac Appt:** Prof S, Thomas Jefferson Univ

Reich, David MD [S] - **Spec Exp:** Transplant-Liver; Hepatobiliary Surgery; Liver Cancer; **Hospital:** Hahnemann Univ Hosp; **Address:** 216 N Broad St Fl 5, Philadelphia, PA 19102; **Phone:** 215-762-8153; **Board Cert:** Surgery 2003; **Med School:** McGill Univ 1989; **Resid:** Surgery, Beth Israel Med Ctr 1994; **Fellow:** Hepatobiliary Surgery, Mt Sinai Med Ctr 1996

Ridge, John Andrew MD/PhD [S] - **Spec Exp:** Head & Neck Cancer & Surgery; Thyroid Cancer & Surgery; Laryngeal Cancer; **Hospital:** Fox Chase Cancer Ctr (page 72); **Address:** Fox Chase Cancer Ctr, Dept Surgical Oncology, 333 Cottman Ave, Philadelphia, PA 19111; **Phone:** 215-728-3517; **Board Cert:** Surgery 2006; **Med School:** Stanford Univ 1981; **Resid:** Surgery, Univ Colorado Med Ctr 1987; **Fellow:** Surgical Oncology, Meml Sloan-Kettering Cancer Ctr 1989

Roh, Mark S MD [S] - **Spec Exp:** Liver Cancer; Cancer Surgery; **Hospital:** Allegheny General Hosp; **Address:** Allegheny General Hospital, Dept Surgery, 320 E North Ave, Pittsburgh, PA 15212; **Phone:** 412-359-6738; **Board Cert:** Surgery 2006; **Med School:** Ohio State Univ 1979; **Resid:** Surgery, Univ Pittsburgh Med Ctr 1982; Surgery, Univ Pittsburgh Med Ctr 1986; **Fellow:** Surgical Oncology, Meml Sloan-Kettering Cancer Ctr 1984; Surgical Oncology, Meml Sloan-Kettering Cancer Ctr 1987; **Fac Appt:** Prof S, Drexel Univ Coll Med

Rosato, Ernest F MD [S] - **Spec Exp:** Gastrointestinal Cancer & Surgery; Esophageal Cancer; Pancreatic Cancer; **Hospital:** Hosp Univ Penn - UPHS (page 81); **Address:** Hosp Univ Penn, Dept Surg, 3400 Spruce St, 4 Silverstein, Philadelphia, PA 19104; **Phone:** 215-662-2033; **Board Cert:** Surgery 1969; **Med School:** Univ Pennsylvania 1962; **Resid:** Surgery, Hosp Univ Penn 1968; **Fac Appt:** Prof S, Univ Pennsylvania

Rosenberg, Steven A MD [S] - **Spec Exp:** Melanoma; Kidney Cancer; **Hospital:** Natl Inst of Hlth - Clin Ctr; **Address:** National Cancer Institute, 9000 Rockville Pike CRC Bldg, rm 3W-3940, Bethesda, MD 20892; **Phone:** 301-496-4164; **Board Cert:** Surgery 1975; **Med School:** Johns Hopkins Univ 1964; **Resid:** Surgery, Peter Bent Brigham Hosp 1974

Roses, Daniel F MD [S] - **Spec Exp:** Breast Cancer; Melanoma; Thyroid Cancer; Parathyroid Surgery; **Hospital:** NYU Langone Med Ctr (page 80); **Address:** 530 First Ave, Ste 6B, New York, NY 10016-6402; **Phone:** 212-263-7329; **Board Cert:** Surgery 1975; **Med School:** NYU Sch Med 1969; **Resid:** Surgery, NYU-Bellevue Hosp 1974; **Fellow:** Surgical Oncology, NYU-Bellevue Hosp 1978; **Fac Appt:** Prof Surg & Onc, NYU Sch Med

Schnabel, Freya MD [S] - **Spec Exp:** Breast Cancer; Breast Cancer-High Risk Women; **Hospital:** NYU Langone Med Ctr (page 80); **Address:** 160 E 34th St Fl 3, New York, NY 10016; **Phone:** 212-731-5367; **Board Cert:** Surgery 1998; **Med School:** NYU Sch Med 1982; **Resid:** Surgery, NYU Med Ctr 1987; **Fellow:** Research, SUNY Hlth Sci Ctr 1988; **Fac Appt:** Prof S, NYU Sch Med

Schraut, Wolfgang H MD [S] - **Spec Exp:** Gastrointestinal Surgery; Colon & Rectal Cancer & Surgery; Laparoscopic Surgery; **Hospital:** UPMC Presby, Pittsburgh, Magee-Womens Hosp - UPMC; **Address:** Univ Pittsburgh Med Ctr, Dept Surgery, 200 Lothrop St, Ste 497, Scaife Hall, Pittsburgh, PA 15261; **Phone:** 412-647-0457; **Board Cert:** Surgery 1999; **Med School:** Germany 1970; **Resid:** Surgery, Univ Chicago Hosps 1978; **Fac Appt:** Prof S, Univ Pittsburgh

Surgery

Shah, Jatin P MD/PhD [S] - **Spec Exp:** Head & Neck Cancer & Surgery; Thyroid Cancer & Surgery; Skull Base Tumors; Salivary Gland Tumors & Surgery; **Hospital:** Meml Sloan-Kettering Cancer Ctr (page 76); **Address:** 1275 York Avenue, New York, NY 10065; **Phone:** 800-525-2225; **Board Cert:** Surgery 1975; **Med School:** India 1964; **Resid:** Surgery, SSG Hosp 1967; Surgery, NY Eye & Ear Infirm 1974; **Fellow:** Head & Neck Surgical Oncology, Meml Sloan-Kettering Hosp 1972; **Fac Appt:** Prof S, Cornell Univ-Weill Med Coll

Sigurdson, Elin R MD [S] - **Spec Exp:** Breast Cancer; Colon & Rectal Cancer; Melanoma; Gastrointestinal Cancer; **Hospital:** Fox Chase Cancer Ctr (page 72); **Address:** 333 Cottman Ave, Philadelphia, PA 19111-2412; **Phone:** 215-728-3519; **Board Cert:** Surgery 2006; **Med School:** Canada 1980; **Resid:** Surgery, Univ Toronto Med Ctr 1984; **Fellow:** Surgical Oncology, Meml Sloan-Kettering Cancer Ctr 1987; **Fac Appt:** Assoc Prof S

Singer, Samuel MD [S] - **Spec Exp:** Sarcoma-Soft Tissue; **Hospital:** Meml Sloan-Kettering Cancer Ctr (page 76); **Address:** 1275 York Avenue, New York, NY 10065; **Phone:** 800-525-2225; **Board Cert:** Surgery 1998; **Med School:** Harvard Med Sch 1982; **Resid:** Surgery, Brigham & Women's Hosp 1988; **Fellow:** Surgical Oncology, Dana Farber Cancer Inst 1990; **Fac Appt:** Assoc Prof S, Cornell Univ-Weill Med Coll

Skinner, Kristin A MD [S] - **Spec Exp:** Breast Cancer; Gastrointestinal Cancer; Melanoma; **Hospital:** Univ of Rochester Strong Meml Hosp; **Address:** Univ Rochester Med Ctr, 601 Elmwood Ave, Box SURG, Rochester, NY 14642; **Phone:** 585-276-3332; **Board Cert:** Surgery 2005; **Med School:** Johns Hopkins Univ 1988; **Resid:** Surgery, UCLA Med Ctr 1995; **Fellow:** Surgical Oncology, UCLA Med Ctr 1994; **Fac Appt:** Assoc Prof S, Univ Rochester

Sugarbaker, Paul H MD [S] - **Spec Exp:** Appendix Cancer; Peritoneal Carcinomatosis; Cystadenocarcinoma; Ovarian Cancer; **Hospital:** Washington Hosp Ctr; **Address:** Washington Hosp Ctr, 106 Irving St NW, Ste 3900N, Washington, DC 20010; **Phone:** 202-877-3908; **Board Cert:** Surgery 1973; **Med School:** Cornell Univ-Weill Med Coll 1967; **Resid:** Surgery, Peter Bent Brigham Hosp 1973; **Fellow:** Surgical Oncology, Mass Genl Hosp 1976; **Fac Appt:** Prof S, Univ Wash

Sundaram, Magesh MD [S] - **Spec Exp:** Gastrointestinal Cancer & Surgery; Pancreatic Cancer; Stomach Cancer; Liver & Biliary Cancer; **Hospital:** WV Univ Hosp - Ruby Memorial; **Address:** WV Univ Hosp-Dept Surgery, P.O. BOX 9238, 6309 HSC, Morgantown, WV 26506; **Phone:** 304 293-7095; **Board Cert:** Surgery 2006; **Med School:** Univ MD Sch Med 1990; **Resid:** Surgery, Delaware Med Ctr 1995; **Fellow:** Surgical Oncology, Jackson Meml Hosp 1997; **Fac Appt:** Assoc Prof Surg & Onc, W VA Univ

Swistel, Alexander J MD [S] - **Spec Exp:** Breast Cancer; Sentinel Node Surgery; **Hospital:** NY-Presby Hosp/Weill Cornell (page 79), St Luke's - Roosevelt Hosp Ctr - Roosevelt Div (page 71); **Address:** 425 E 61st St Fl 10, New York, NY 10021; **Phone:** 212-821-0602; **Board Cert:** Surgery 2005; **Med School:** Brown Univ 1975; **Resid:** Surgery, St Luke's Roosevelt Hosp Ctr 1981; **Fellow:** Surgical Oncology, Meml Sloan Kettering Canc Ctr 1983; **Fac Appt:** Asst Prof S, Cornell Univ-Weill Med Coll

Tafra, Lorraine MD [S] - **Spec Exp:** Breast Cancer; **Hospital:** Anne Arundel Med Ctr; **Address:** 2002 Medical Parkway, Ste 120, Annapolis, MD 21401; **Phone:** 443-481-5300; **Board Cert:** Surgery 2005; **Med School:** Case West Res Univ 1986; **Resid:** Surgery, Rhode Island Hosp 1988; Surgery, Hosp Univ Penn 1992; **Fellow:** Surgical Oncology, John Wayne Cancer Inst 1994

Tartter, Paul MD [S] - **Spec Exp:** Breast Cancer; Breast Cancer in Elderly; Sentinel Node Surgery; **Hospital:** St Luke's - Roosevelt Hosp Ctr - Roosevelt Div (page 71), Mount Sinai Med Ctr (page 77); **Address:** 425 W 59th St, Ste 7A, New York, NY 10019-1104; **Phone:** 212-523-7500; **Board Cert:** Surgery 2003; **Med School:** Brown Univ 1977; **Resid:** Surgery, Mt Sinai Hosp 1982; **Fac Appt:** Assoc Prof S, Columbia P&S

Teperman, Lewis W MD [S] - **Spec Exp:** Transplant-Liver; Transplant-Kidney; Liver Tumors; **Hospital:** NYU Langone Med Ctr (page 80); **Address:** 403 E 34th St Fl 3, Transplant Assocs, New York, NY 10016; **Phone:** 212-263-8134; **Board Cert:** Surgery 1997; **Med School:** Mount Sinai Sch Med 1981; **Resid:** Surgery, Columbia Presby Med Ctr 1984; Surgery, LI Jewish Med Ctr 1986; **Fellow:** Transplant Surgery, Univ Pittsburgh 1988; **Fac Appt:** Assoc Prof S, NYU Sch Med

Tsangaris, Theodore N MD [S] - **Spec Exp:** Breast Cancer; **Hospital:** Johns Hopkins Hosp; **Address:** Johns Hopkins Hospital, 600 N Wolfe St, Carnegie 686, Baltimore, MD 21287; **Phone:** 410-955-2615; **Board Cert:** Surgery 2005; **Med School:** Geo Wash Univ 1983; **Resid:** Surgery, Geo Washington Univ Med Ctr 1989; **Fellow:** Surgical Oncology, Baylor Univ Med Ctr 1990; **Fac Appt:** Assoc Prof S, Johns Hopkins Univ

Willey, Shawna C MD [S] - **Spec Exp:** Breast Cancer; Clinical Trials; **Hospital:** Georgetown Univ Hosp; **Address:** 3800 Reservoir Rd NW, PHC Bldg Fl 4, Washington, DC 20007; **Phone:** 202-444-0241; **Board Cert:** Surgery 1998; **Med School:** Univ Iowa Coll Med 1982; **Resid:** Surgery, George Washington Univ Med Ctr 1988; **Fac Appt:** Asst Prof S, Georgetown Univ

Yang, James C MD [S] - **Spec Exp:** Kidney Cancer; Kidney Cancer Clinical Trials; Clinical Trials; Immunotherapy; **Hospital:** Natl Inst of Hlth - Clin Ctr; **Address:** National Cancer Institute, 9000 Rockville Pike CRC Bldg - rm 3-5952, Bethesda, MD 20892; **Phone:** 301-496-1574; **Board Cert:** Surgery 2005; **Med School:** UCSD 1978; **Resid:** Surgery, UCSD Med Ctr 1984; **Fellow:** Surgical Oncology, Natl Cancer Inst 1986

Yeo, Charles J MD [S] - **Spec Exp:** Pancreatic Cancer; Biliary Cancer; **Hospital:** Thomas Jefferson Univ Hosp (page 83); **Address:** 1015 Walnut St, Ste 620, Philadelphia, PA 19107; **Phone:** 215-955-9402; **Board Cert:** Surgery 2005; **Med School:** Johns Hopkins Univ 1979; **Resid:** Surgery, Johns Hopkins Hosp 1985; **Fellow:** Research, SUNY Downstate 1982; **Fac Appt:** Prof S, Thomas Jefferson Univ

Southeast

Adams, Reid B MD [S] - **Spec Exp:** Hepatobiliary Surgery; Liver Cancer; Pancreatic & Biliary Surgery; **Hospital:** Univ Virginia Med Ctr; **Address:** UVA Health System, Dept Surgery, PO Box 800709, Charlottesville, VA 22908; **Phone:** 434-924-2839; **Board Cert:** Surgery 2003; **Med School:** Univ VA Sch Med 1987; **Resid:** Surgery, Univ Va Hlth Sci Ctr 1994; **Fellow:** Hepatopancreatobiliary Surgery, Univ Toronto Med Ctr 1995; **Fac Appt:** Assoc Prof S, Univ VA Sch Med

Bear, Harry D MD/PhD [S] - **Spec Exp:** Breast Cancer; Melanoma; Gastrointestinal Cancer; **Hospital:** Med Coll of VA Hosp; **Address:** Med Coll Virginia - VCU, PO Box 980011, Richmond, VA 23298; **Phone:** 804-828-9325; **Board Cert:** Surgery 2003; **Med School:** Med Coll VA 1975; **Resid:** Surgery, Brigham & Women's Hosp 1983; **Fellow:** Surgical Oncology, Med Coll Virgina 1984; **Fac Appt:** Prof Surg & Onc, Med Coll VA

Beauchamp, Robert D MD [S] - **Spec Exp:** Breast Cancer; Colon & Rectal Cancer; Pancreatic Cancer; **Hospital:** Vanderbilt Univ Med Ctr; **Address:** Medical Center North, rm D4316, 1161 21st Ave S, Nashville, TN 37232; **Phone:** 615-322-2363; **Board Cert:** Surgery 2007; **Med School:** Univ Tex Med Br, Galveston 1982; **Resid:** Surgery, Univ Tex Med Br 1987; **Fellow:** Cellular Molecular Biology, Vanderbilt Univ 1989; **Fac Appt:** Prof S, Vanderbilt Univ

Behrns, Kevin E MD [S] - **Spec Exp:** Pancreatic Cancer; Gastrointestinal Cancer & Surgery; **Hospital:** Shands at Univ of FL; **Address:** Shands Healthcare at Univ Florida, PO Box 100286, Gainesville, FL 32610-0286; **Phone:** 352-265-0761; **Board Cert:** Surgery 2005; **Med School:** Mayo Med Sch 1988; **Resid:** Surgery, Mayo Clinic 1995; **Fac Appt:** Prof S, Univ Fla Coll Med

Bland, Kirby MD [S] - **Spec Exp:** Breast Cancer; Colon Cancer; Thyroid & Parathyroid Cancer & Surgery; **Hospital:** Univ of Ala Hosp at Birmingham; **Address:** UAB, Dept Surgery, 1530 3rd Ave S, BDB 502, Birmingham, AL 35294-0002; **Phone:** 205-975-2193; **Board Cert:** Surgery 2000; **Med School:** Univ Alabama 1968; **Resid:** Surgery, Univ Fla Hosp 1970; Surgery, Univ Fla Hosp 1976; **Fellow:** Surgical Oncology, MD Anderson Cancer Ctr 1977; **Fac Appt:** Prof S, Univ Alabama

Calvo, Benjamin MD [S] - **Spec Exp:** Colon Cancer; Endocrine Cancers; Breast Cancer; **Hospital:** Univ NC Hosps; **Address:** Dept Surg CB 7213, Chapel Hill, NC 27599; **Phone:** 919-966-5221; **Board Cert:** Surgery 1999; **Med School:** Univ MD Sch Med 1981; **Resid:** Surgery, G Washington Univ Hosp 1988; Surgery, Natl Inst Hlth 1991; **Fellow:** Surgery, Meml Sloan Kettering Cancer Ctr 1993; **Fac Appt:** Assoc Prof S, Univ NC Sch Med

Chari, Ravi S MD [S] - **Spec Exp:** Liver Cancer; Biliary Cancer; Transplant-Liver; **Hospital:** Centennial Med Ctr, Vanderbilt Univ Med Ctr; **Address:** Centennial Med Ctr, 2300 Patterson St, Nashville, TN 37203; **Phone:** 615-936-2573; **Board Cert:** Surgery 2005; **Med School:** Canada 1989; **Resid:** Surgery, Duke Univ Med Ctr 1996; **Fellow:** Transplant Surgery, Univ Toronto-Toronto Hosp 1998; **Fac Appt:** Prof S, Vanderbilt Univ

Cole, David J MD [S] - **Spec Exp:** Breast Brachytherapy; Gastrointestinal Cancer; Vaccine Therapy; Gene Therapy; **Hospital:** MUSC Med Ctr; **Address:** 96 Jonathan Lucas St, PO BOX 250613, Charleston, SC 29425; **Phone:** 843-792-4638; **Board Cert:** Surgery 2000; **Med School:** Cornell Univ-Weill Med Coll 1986; **Resid:** Surgery, Emory Univ Affil Hosp 1991; **Fellow:** Surgical Oncology, Natl Cancer Institute 1994; **Fac Appt:** Prof S, Med Univ SC

Dilawari, Raza A MD [S] - **Spec Exp:** Liver & Biliary Cancer; Melanoma; Skin Cancer; Breast Cancer; **Hospital:** Methodist Univ Hosp - Memphis, St Francis Hosp - Memphis; **Address:** Methodist Univ Hosp, 1325 Eastmoreland Ave, Ste 410, Memphis, TN 38104; **Phone:** 901-725-1921; **Board Cert:** Surgery 1975; **Med School:** Pakistan 1968; **Resid:** Surgery, SUNY-Upstate Med Ctr 1974; **Fellow:** Surgical Oncology, Roswell Park Meml Hosp 1976; **Fac Appt:** Prof S, Univ Tenn Coll Med, Memphis

Eason, James MD [S] - **Spec Exp:** Transplant-Kidney; Transplant-Pancreas & Liver; Liver Cancer; **Hospital:** Methodist Univ Hosp - Memphis; **Address:** Transplant Inst, 1265 Union Ave, rm S1011, Memphis, TN 38104; **Phone:** 866-805-7710; **Board Cert:** Surgery 2002; **Med School:** Univ Tenn Coll Med, Memphis 1987; **Resid:** Surgery, Wilford Hall USAF Med Ctr 1992; **Fellow:** Transplant Surgery, Mass Genl Hosp 1994; **Fac Appt:** Prof S, Univ Tenn Coll Med, Memphis

Flynn, Michael B MD [S] - **Spec Exp:** Head & Neck Cancer; Head & Neck Surgery; **Hospital:** Univ of Louisville Hosp, Norton Hosp; **Address:** 401 E Chestnut St, Ste 710, Louisville, KY 40202; **Phone:** 502-583-8303; **Board Cert:** Surgery 1972; **Med School:** Ireland 1962; **Resid:** Surgery, Univ Maryland Hosp 1969; **Fellow:** Surgical Oncology, MD Anderson Hosp 1971; **Fac Appt:** Prof S, Univ Louisville Sch Med

Gabram, Sheryl G A MD [S] - **Spec Exp:** Breast Cancer; Breast Cancer-High Risk Women; **Hospital:** Emory Univ Hosp, Grady Hlth Sys; **Address:** Winship Cancer Institute, 1365 Clifton Rd NE C Bldg Fl 2, Atlanta, GA 30322; **Phone:** 404-778-1230; **Board Cert:** Surgery 2006; **Med School:** Georgetown Univ 1982; **Resid:** Surgery, Washington Hosp Ctr 1987; **Fellow:** Trauma, Hartford Hosp 1988; **Fac Appt:** Prof S, Emory Univ

Goldstein, Richard E MD/PhD [S] - **Spec Exp:** Endocrine Tumors; Thyroid Cancer & Surgery; Parathyroid Cancer; Parathyroid Surgery; **Hospital:** Univ of Louisville Hosp; **Address:** University Surgical Assocs, 401 E Chestnut St, Ste 710, Louisville, KY 40202; **Phone:** 502-583-8303; **Board Cert:** Surgery 1999; **Med School:** Jefferson Med Coll 1982; **Resid:** Surgery, Vanderbilt Univ Hosp 1990; **Fac Appt:** Prof S, Univ Louisville Sch Med

Greene, Frederick L MD [S] - **Spec Exp:** Gastrointestinal Surgery; Gastrointestinal Cancer; **Hospital:** Carolinas Med Ctr; **Address:** Carolinas Medical Ctr, 1025 Morehead Medical Drive, Ste 275, Charlotte, NC 28203; **Phone:** 704-355-1813; **Board Cert:** Surgery 1998; **Med School:** Univ VA Sch Med 1970; **Resid:** Surgery, Yale-New Haven Hosp 1976; **Fellow:** Surgical Oncology, Yale-New Haven Hosp 1973; **Fac Appt:** Prof S, Univ NC Sch Med

Hanks, John B MD [S] - **Spec Exp:** Endocrine Cancers; Breast Cancer; Thyroid Cancer & Surgery; **Hospital:** Univ Virginia Med Ctr; **Address:** Univ VA Hlth Sys, Dept Surgery, PO Box 800709, Charlottesville, VA 22908-0709; **Phone:** 434-924-0376; **Board Cert:** Surgery 2001; **Med School:** Univ Rochester 1973; **Resid:** Surgery, Duke Univ Med Ctr 1982; **Fac Appt:** Prof S, Univ VA Sch Med

Hemming, Alan W MD [S] - **Spec Exp:** Liver Cancer; Transplant-Liver; Hepatobiliary Surgery; Pancreatic Cancer; **Hospital:** Shands at Univ of FL; **Address:** Univ Florida, Dept Surgery, 1600 SW Archer Rd, rm 6142, Gainesville, FL 32610; **Phone:** 352-265-0606; **Board Cert:** Surgery 2004; **Med School:** Canada 1987; **Resid:** Surgery, Univ British Columbia Med Ctr 1993; **Fellow:** Transplant Surgery, Univ Toronto/Hosp for Sick Children 1995; Hepatobiliary Surgery, Univ Toronto 1996; **Fac Appt:** Prof S, Univ Fla Coll Med

Herrmann, Virginia M MD [S] - **Spec Exp:** Breast Cancer; Nutrition & Cancer Prevention/Control; **Hospital:** Hilton Head Reg Med Ctr, MUSC Med Ctr; **Address:** Hilton Head Reg Med Ctr, 25 Hospital Center Drive, Ste 300, Hilton Head Isl, SC 29926; **Phone:** 843-682-7377; **Board Cert:** Surgery 2000; **Med School:** St Louis Univ 1974; **Resid:** Surgery, St Louis Univ Hosps 1979; **Fellow:** Surgery, Brigham & Women's Hosp 1980; **Fac Appt:** Prof S, Med Univ SC

Heslin, Martin J MD [S] - **Spec Exp:** Gastrointestinal Cancer; Pancreatic Cancer; Biliary Cancer; Sarcoma-Soft Tissue; **Hospital:** Univ of Ala Hosp at Birmingham; **Address:** Univ Alabama, 1922 7th Ave S, Ste 321, Birmingham, AL 35294-0016; **Phone:** 205-934-3064; **Board Cert:** Surgery 2006; **Med School:** SUNY Upstate Med Univ 1987; **Resid:** Surgery, NYU Med Ctr 1994; Surgery, Meml Sloan-Kettering Canc Ctr 1991; **Fellow:** Surgical Oncology, Meml Sloan-Kettering Cancer Ctr 1996; **Fac Appt:** Prof S, Univ Alabama

Kelley, Mark C MD [S] - **Spec Exp:** Breast Cancer; Melanoma; **Hospital:** Vanderbilt Univ Med Ctr; **Address:** Div Surgical Oncology, 2220 Pierce Ave, 597 Preston Rsch Bldg, Nashville, TN 37232; **Phone:** 615-322-2391; **Board Cert:** Surgery 2005, **Med School:** Univ Fla Coll Med 1989; **Resid:** Surgery, Univ Fla-Shands Hosp 1995; **Fellow:** Surgical Oncology, John Wayne Cancer Inst-St Johns Hosp 1997; **Fac Appt:** Asst Prof Surg & Onc, Vanderbilt Univ

Levi, Joe U MD [S] - **Spec Exp:** Pancreatic Cancer; Liver Tumors; Biliary Surgery; **Hospital:** Jackson Meml Hosp (page 82), Univ of Miami Hosp & Clins/Sylvester Comp Canc Ctr (page 82); **Address:** 1475 NW 12th Ave, Ste 3524, Miami, FL 33136; **Phone:** 305-243-4211; **Board Cert:** Surgery 1975; **Med School:** Univ Fla Coll Med 1967; **Resid:** Surgery, Johns Hopkins Hosp 1969; Surgery, Jackson Meml Hosp 1974; **Fac Appt:** Prof S, Univ Miami Sch Med

Levine, Edward A MD [S] - **Spec Exp:** Breast Cancer; Esophageal Cancer; Peritoneal Carcinomatosis; **Hospital:** Wake Forest Univ Baptist Med Ctr (page 84); **Address:** Wake Forest Univ Baptist Med Ctr, Dept Surgery, Medical Center Blvd, Winston-Salem, NC 27157; **Phone:** 336-716-4276; **Board Cert:** Surgery 1999; **Med School:** Ros Franklin Univ/Chicago Med Sch 1985; **Resid:** Surgery, Michael Reese Hosp 1990; **Fellow:** Surgical Oncology, Univ Illinois 1992; **Fac Appt:** Prof S, Wake Forest Univ

Lind, David Scott MD [S] - **Spec Exp:** Breast Cancer; Melanoma; Sarcoma; **Hospital:** Med Coll of GA Hosp and Clin (MCG Health Inc); **Address:** MCG Health-Comp Cancer Center, Div Surgical Oncology, 1120 15th St, Augusta, GA 30912; **Phone:** 706-721-6744; **Board Cert:** Surgery 2000; **Med School:** Eastern VA Med Sch 1984; **Resid:** Surgery, Univ Texas Affil Hosp 1989; **Fellow:** Medical Oncology, Med Coll Virginia 1992; **Fac Appt:** Prof Surg & Onc, Med Coll GA

Livingstone, Alan S MD [S] - **Spec Exp:** Liver & Biliary Cancer; Stomach Cancer; Esophageal Cancer; Pancreatic Cancer; **Hospital:** Jackson Meml Hosp (page 82), Univ of Miami Hosp & Clins/Sylvester Comp Canc Ctr (page 82); **Address:** Sylvester Comp Cancer Ctr, Dept Surgery (310T), 1475 NW 12th Ave, rm 3550, Miami, FL 33136-1002; **Phone:** 305-243-4902; **Board Cert:** Surgery 2007; **Med School:** McGill Univ 1971; **Resid:** Surgery, Montreal Genl Hosp 1976; Surgery, Jackson Meml Hosp 1975; **Fac Appt:** Prof S, Univ Miami Sch Med

Lyerly, H Kim MD [S] - **Spec Exp:** Breast Cancer; Immunotherapy; **Hospital:** Duke Univ Med Ctr, Durham Regional Hosp; **Address:** Duke Comprehensive Cancer Center, DUMC Box 2714, Durham, NC 27710; **Phone:** 919-684-5613; **Board Cert:** Surgery 2001; **Med School:** UCLA 1983; **Resid:** Surgery, Duke Univ Med Ctr 1990; **Fac Appt:** Prof S, Duke Univ

McGrath, Patrick C MD [S] - **Spec Exp:** Breast Cancer; Cancer Surgery; **Hospital:** Univ of Kentucky Chandler Hosp; **Address:** Univ Kentucky Med Ctr, Dept Genl Surgery, 800 Rose St, rm C224, Lexington, KY 40536-0293; **Phone:** 859-323-6346 x233; **Med School:** Univ IL Coll Med 1980; **Resid:** Surgery, Med Coll Virginia Hosp 1986; **Fellow:** Surgical Oncology, Med Coll Virginia Hosp 1988; **Fac Appt:** Prof S, Univ KY Coll Med

McMasters, Kelly M MD [S] - **Spec Exp:** Melanoma; Breast Cancer; Liver Cancer; **Hospital:** Univ of Louisville Hosp; **Address:** 401 S Chestnut St, Ste 710, Louisville, KY 40202; **Phone:** 502-583-8303; **Board Cert:** Surgery 2005; **Med School:** UMDNJ-RW Johnson Med Sch 1989; **Resid:** Surgery, Univ Louisville Sch Med 1994; **Fellow:** Surgical Oncology, Texas-MD Anderson Cancer Ctr 1995; **Fac Appt:** Prof S, Univ Louisville Sch Med

Neifeld, James P MD [S] - **Spec Exp:** Melanoma; Head & Neck Cancer; Gastrointestinal Cancer; **Hospital:** Med Coll of VA Hosp; **Address:** Medical College Virginia Hosp, PO Box 980645, Richmond, VA 23298-0645; **Phone:** 804-828-9324; **Board Cert:** Surgery 2009; **Med School:** Med Coll VA 1972; **Resid:** Surgery, Med Coll Va Hosps 1978; **Fac Appt:** Prof S, Va Commonwealth Univ Sch Med

Pappas, Theodore N MD [S] - **Spec Exp:** Pancreatic Surgery; Laparoscopic Surgery; **Hospital:** Duke Univ Med Ctr; **Address:** Duke Univ Med Ctr, Dept Surgery, DUMC Box 3479, Durham, NC 27710-0001; **Phone:** 919-681-3442; **Board Cert:** Surgery 1997; **Med School:** Ohio State Univ 1981; **Resid:** Surgery, Brigham & Womens Hosp 1988; **Fellow:** Research, Wadworth VA Med Ctr 1985; **Fac Appt:** Prof S, Duke Univ

Pinson, C Wright MD [S] - **Spec Exp:** Transplant-Liver; Liver & Biliary Cancer; Pancreatic Cancer; **Hospital:** Vanderbilt Univ Med Ctr; **Address:** Vanderbilt Univ Med Ctr, TVC 3810A, 1301 Med Center Drive, Nashville, TN 37232-5545; **Phone:** 615-343-9324; **Board Cert:** Surgery 2007; Surgical Critical Care 2007; **Med School:** Vanderbilt Univ 1980; **Resid:** Surgery, Oregon Health Sci Ctr 1986; **Fellow:** Gastrointestinal Surgery, Lahey Clinic 1987; Transplant Surgery, Deaconess Hosp 1988; **Fac Appt:** Prof S, Vanderbilt Univ

Rosemurgy, Alexander S MD [S] - **Spec Exp:** Pancreatic Cancer; Gastrointestinal Surgery; Minimally Invasive Surgery; **Hospital:** Tampa Genl Hosp; **Address:** Digestive Disorders Ctr, Tampa General Hospital, 2 Columbia Drive, rm F145, Tampa, FL 33601; **Phone:** 813-844-7393; **Board Cert:** Surgery 2005; **Med School:** Univ Mich Med Sch 1979; **Resid:** Surgery, Univ Chicago Hosps 1984; **Fac Appt:** Prof S, Univ S Fla Coll Med

Salo, Jonathan C MD [S] - **Spec Exp:** Gastrointestinal Cancer; Esophageal Cancer; **Hospital:** Carolinas Med Ctr; **Address:** Blumenthal Cancer Center, 1025 Morehead Medical Drive, Ste 600, Charlotte, NC 28204; **Phone:** 704-355-2884; **Board Cert:** Surgery 2005; **Med School:** UCSF 1981; **Resid:** Surgery, UCSF Med Ctr 1993; **Fellow:** Surgical Oncology, Natl Cancer Inst 1991; Surgical Oncology, Meml Sloan-Kettering Cancer Ctr 1998; **Fac Appt:** Asst Prof S, Univ NC Sch Med

Shen, Perry MD [S] - **Spec Exp:** Liver & Biliary Cancer; Pancreatic Cancer; Gastrointestinal Cancer; Melanoma; **Hospital:** Wake Forest Univ Baptist Med Ctr (page 84); **Address:** Wake Forest Univ Baptist Med Ctr, Dept Surgery, Medical Center Blvd, Winston-Salem, NC 27157; **Phone:** 336-716-4276; **Board Cert:** Surgery 1999; **Med School:** USC Sch Med 1992; **Resid:** Surgery, LAC-USC Med Ctr 1998; **Fellow:** Surgical Oncology, John Wayne Cancer Inst 2000; **Fac Appt:** Assoc Prof S, Wake Forest Univ

Slingluff Jr, Craig L MD [S] - **Spec Exp:** Melanoma; Immunotherapy; **Hospital:** Univ Virginia Med Ctr; **Address:** UVA Health System, Dept Surgery, PO Box 800709, Charlottesville, VA 22908; **Phone:** 434-924-1730; **Board Cert:** Surgery 2002; **Med School:** Univ VA Sch Med 1984; **Resid:** Surgery, Duke Univ Med Ctr 1991; **Fellow:** Surgical Research, Duke Univ Med Ctr 1992; **Fac Appt:** Prof S, Univ VA Sch Med

Sondak, Vernon K MD [S] - **Spec Exp:** Cancer Surgery; Melanoma; Sarcoma; **Hospital:** H Lee Moffitt Cancer Ctr & Research Inst; **Address:** H Lee Moffitt Cancer Ctr, Cutaneous Program, 12902 Magnolia Drive, Tampa, FL 33612; **Phone:** 813-745-1968; **Board Cert:** Surgery 1996; **Med School:** Boston Univ 1980; **Resid:** Surgery, UCLA Med Ctr 1987; **Fellow:** Surgical Oncology, UCLA Med Ctr 1984; **Fac Appt:** Prof S, Univ S Fla Coll Med

Tyler, Douglas S MD [S] - **Spec Exp:** Pancreatic Cancer; Colon & Rectal Cancer; Rectal Cancer/Sphincter Preservation; Melanoma; **Hospital:** Duke Univ Med Ctr; **Address:** Duke University Med Ctr, Box 3118, Durham, NC 27710; **Phone:** 919-684-6858; **Board Cert:** Surgery 2000; **Med School:** Dartmouth Med Sch 1985; **Resid:** Surgery, Duke Univ Med Ctr 1992; **Fellow:** Surgical Oncology, MD Anderson Cancer Ctr 1994; **Fac Appt:** Prof S, Duke Univ

Urist, Marshall M MD [S] - **Spec Exp:** Cancer Surgery; Breast Cancer; Melanoma; **Hospital:** Univ of Ala Hosp at Birmingham; **Address:** Univ Alabama Sch Med, Dept Surgery, 1922 7th Ave S, Kracke Bldg, Ste 321, Birmingham, AL 35294; **Phone:** 205-934-3065; **Board Cert:** Surgery 2000; **Med School:** Univ Chicago-Pritzker Sch Med 1971; **Resid:** Surgery, Johns Hopkins Hosp 1978; **Fellow:** Surgical Oncology, UCLA Med Ctr 1976; **Fac Appt:** Prof S, Univ Alabama

White Jr, Richard L MD [S] - **Spec Exp:** Breast Cancer; Melanoma; Sarcoma; Immunotherapy; **Hospital:** Carolinas Med Ctr; **Address:** Carolinas Medical Center, 1000 Blythe Blvd, Box 32861, Charlotte, NC 28203; **Phone:** 704-355-2884; **Board Cert:** Surgery 2002; **Med School:** Columbia P&S 1986; **Resid:** Surgery, Georgetown Univ Hosp 1992; **Fellow:** Surgical Oncology, NIH-Natl Cancer Inst 1995; **Fac Appt:** Assoc Clin Prof S, Univ NC Sch Med

Whitworth, Pat W MD [S] - **Spec Exp:** Breast Cancer; **Hospital:** Baptist Hosp - Nashville, Centennial Med Ctr; **Address:** 300 20th Ave N, Ste 401, Nashville, TN 37203; **Phone:** 615-620-5535; **Board Cert:** Surgery 1999; **Med School:** Univ Tenn Coll Med, Memphis 1983; **Resid:** Surgery, Univ Louisville Med Ctr 1988; **Fellow:** Surgical Oncology, MD Anderson Cancer Ctr 1991; **Fac Appt:** Assoc Clin Prof S, Vanderbilt Univ

Willis, Irvin MD [S] - **Spec Exp:** Pancreatic Surgery; Cancer Surgery; Laparoscopic Surgery; **Hospital:** Mount Sinai Med Ctr - Miami; **Address:** 4302 Alton Rd, Ste 630, Miami Beach, FL 33140-2876; **Phone:** 305-534-6050; **Board Cert:** Surgery 1970; **Med School:** Univ Cincinnati 1964; **Resid:** Surgery, Univ Miami-Jackson Meml 1969

Surgery

Wood, William C MD [S] - **Spec Exp:** Breast Cancer; **Hospital:** Emory Univ Hosp; **Address:** Emory Univ Hosp, Dept Surgery, 1364 Clifton Rd NE, Ste B206, Atlanta, GA 30322; **Phone:** 404-778-4720; **Board Cert:** Surgery 1974; **Med School:** Harvard Med Sch 1966; **Resid:** Surgery, Mass Genl Hosp 1968; Surgery, Mass Genl Hosp 1974; **Fac Appt:** Prof S, Emory Univ

Yeatman, Timothy J MD [S] - **Spec Exp:** Liver Cancer; **Hospital:** H Lee Moffitt Cancer Ctr & Research Inst; **Address:** H Lee Moffitt Cancer Ctr, 12902 Magnolia Drive, Tampa, FL 33612-9497; **Phone:** 813-979-7292; **Board Cert:** Surgery 2000; **Med School:** Emory Univ 1984; **Resid:** Surgery, Univ Florida 1990; **Fellow:** Surgical Oncology, MD Anderson Cancer Ctr 1992; **Fac Appt:** Prof S, Univ S Fla Coll Med

Midwest

Angelos, Peter MD/PhD [S] - **Spec Exp:** Endocrine Tumors; Thyroid Surgery; Parathyroid Surgery; Adrenal Tumors; **Hospital:** Univ of Chicago Med Ctr; **Address:** 5841 S Maryland Ave, MC 4052, Chicago, IL 60637; **Phone:** 773-702-4429; **Board Cert:** Surgery 2004; **Med School:** Boston Univ 1989; **Resid:** Surgery, Northwestern Univ 1995; **Fellow:** Medical Ethics, Univ of Chicago Hosps 1992; Endocrine Surgery, Univ of Michigan Med Sch 1996; **Fac Appt:** Prof S, Univ Chicago-Pritzker Sch Med

Aranha, Gerard V MD [S] - **Spec Exp:** Pancreatic & Biliary Surgery; Stomach Cancer; Esophageal Cancer; **Hospital:** Loyola Univ Med Ctr, Hines VA Hosp; **Address:** Loyola Univ Med Ctr, Dept Surg, 2160 S First Ave Bldg 110 - rm 3236, Maywood, IL 60153-3328; **Phone:** 708-327-3430; **Board Cert:** Surgery 2006; **Med School:** India 1969; **Resid:** Surgery, Loyola Univ Med Ctr 1975; **Fellow:** Surgical Oncology, Univ Minn Hosp 1977; **Fac Appt:** Prof S, Loyola Univ-Stritch Sch Med

Averbook, Bruce J MD [S] - **Spec Exp:** Melanoma; Clinical Trials; **Hospital:** MetroHealth Med Ctr; **Address:** Metrohealth Medical Ctr, Surgical Oncology, 2500 Metrohealth Drive, rm C2110, Cleveland, OH 44109; **Phone:** 216-778-4795; **Board Cert:** Surgery 2000; **Med School:** Geo Wash Univ 1983; **Resid:** Surgery, UC Irvine Med Ctr 1990; **Fellow:** Surgical Oncology, NCI, NIH Surg Br 1993; **Fac Appt:** Assoc Prof S, Case West Res Univ

Brems, John J MD [S] - **Spec Exp:** Pancreatic Cancer; Liver Cancer; Transplant-Liver; Liver & Biliary Surgery; **Hospital:** Loyola Univ Med Ctr; **Address:** 2160 S 1st Ave, MC-EMS-3268, Maywood, IL 60153-3328; **Phone:** 708-327-2539; **Board Cert:** Surgery 2004; Surgical Critical Care 2000; **Med School:** St Louis Univ 1981; **Resid:** Surgery, St Louis Univ 1986; **Fellow:** Transplant Surgery, UCLA Med Ctr 1987; **Fac Appt:** Prof S, Loyola Univ-Stritch Sch Med

Brunt, L Michael MD [S] - **Spec Exp:** Minimally Invasive Surgery; Adrenal Tumors; **Hospital:** Barnes-Jewish Hosp; **Address:** Washington Univ Sch Medicine, Dept Surg, 660 S Euclid Ave, Box 8109, St Louis, MO 63110; **Phone:** 314-454-7194; **Board Cert:** Surgery 2006; **Med School:** Johns Hopkins Univ 1980; **Resid:** Surgery, Barnes Jewish Hosp 1987; **Fellow:** Surgery, Barnes Jewish Hosp 1984; **Fac Appt:** Prof S, Washington Univ, St Louis

Chang, Alfred E MD [S] - **Spec Exp:** Breast Cancer; Gastrointestinal Cancer; Melanoma; Sarcoma; **Hospital:** Univ Michigan Hlth Sys; **Address:** Univ Mich Comp Cancer Ctr, 1500 E Med Ctr Dr 3302 CGC, Ann Arbor, MI 48109-5932; **Phone:** 734-936-6000; **Board Cert:** Surgery 2001; **Med School:** Harvard Med Sch 1974; **Resid:** Surgery, Duke Univ Med Ctr 1976; Surgery, Hosp Univ Penn 1982; **Fellow:** Surgical Oncology, Natl Cancer Inst 1979; **Fac Appt:** Prof S, Univ Mich Med Sch

Chapman, William C MD [S] - **Spec Exp:** Transplant-Liver-Adult & Pediatric; Liver Cancer; Liver & Biliary Surgery; **Hospital:** Barnes-Jewish Hosp, St Louis Chldns Hosp; **Address:** Washington Univ Sch Med, 660 S Euclid Ave, Box 8109, St Louis, MO 63110; **Phone:** 314-362-7792; **Board Cert:** Surgery 2001; Surgical Critical Care 2001; **Med School:** Med Univ SC 1984; **Resid:** Surgery, Vanderbilt Univ Med Ctr 1991; **Fellow:** Hepatobiliary Surgery, Kings College Hosp 1992; **Fac Appt:** Prof S, Washington Univ, St Louis

Crowe Jr, Joseph P MD [S] - **Spec Exp:** Breast Cancer; Tumor Surgery; **Hospital:** Cleveland Clin Fdn (page 70); **Address:** Cleveland Clinic Fdn, Dept Surg, 9500 Euclid Ave, Desk A10, Cleveland, OH 44195; **Phone:** 216-444-3024; **Board Cert:** Surgery 2004; **Med School:** Case West Res Univ 1978; **Resid:** Surgery, Univ Hosp-Case West Reserve 1983; **Fellow:** Surgical Oncology, Meml Sloan Kettering Cancer Ctr 1985

Donohue, John H MD [S] - **Spec Exp:** Gastrointestinal Cancer; Breast Cancer; Stomach Cancer; **Hospital:** Mayo Med Ctr & Clin - Rochester; **Address:** Mayo Clinic, Dept General Surgery, 200 First St SW, Rochester, MN 55905; **Phone:** 507-284-0362; **Board Cert:** Surgery 2005; **Med School:** Harvard Med Sch 1978; **Resid:** Surgery, UCSF Med Ctr 1981; Surgery, UCSF Med Ctr 1985; **Fellow:** Surgery, Natl Inst Hlth 1983; Surgical Oncology, Meml Sloan-Kettering Canc Ctr 1987; **Fac Appt:** Prof S, Mayo Med Sch

Eberlein, Timothy J MD [S] - **Spec Exp:** Breast Cancer; Melanoma; Immunotherapy; **Hospital:** Barnes-Jewish Hosp, St Louis Chldns Hosp; **Address:** Wash Univ School Med, Dept Surgery, 660 S Euclid Ave, Box 8109, St Louis, MO 63110-1093; **Phone:** 314-362-8020; **Board Cert:** Surgery 2006; **Med School:** Univ Pittsburgh 1977; **Resid:** Surgery, Peter Bent Brigham Hosp 1979; Surgery, Brigham-Womens Hosp 1985; **Fellow:** Allergy & Immunology, Natl Inst Hlth 1982; **Fac Appt:** Prof S, Washington Univ, St Louis

Edwards, Michael J MD [S] - **Spec Exp:** Breast Cancer; Melanoma; **Hospital:** Univ Hosp - Cincinnati; **Address:** 234 Goodman St, ML 0772, Cincinnati, OH 45219; **Phone:** 513-584-8900; **Board Cert:** Surgery 2005; **Med School:** Emory Univ 1981; **Resid:** Surgery, Univ Louisville Hosp 1986; **Fellow:** Surgical Oncology, MD Anderson Cancer Ctr 1987; **Fac Appt:** Prof S, Univ Ark

Ellison, E Christopher MD [S] - **Spec Exp:** Biliary Cancer; Pancreatic Cancer; **Hospital:** Ohio St Univ Med Ctr; **Address:** 1654 Upham Drive, Ste 327 Means Hall, Columbus, OH 43210-1236; **Phone:** 614-293-9722; **Board Cert:** Surgery 2001; **Med School:** Univ Wisc 1975; **Resid:** Surgery, Ohio State Univ 1981; **Fac Appt:** Prof S, Ohio State Univ

Evans, Douglas B MD [S] - **Spec Exp:** Pancreatic Cancer; Thyroid Cancer; Endocrine Cancers; **Hospital:** Froedtert Meml Lutheran Hosp, Clement J Zablocki VA Med Ctr; **Address:** Medical Coll Wisconsin, Dept Surgery, 9200 W Wisconsin Ave, Ste 3510, Milwaukee, WI 53226-6533; **Phone:** 414-805-5706; **Board Cert:** Surgery 1996; **Med School:** Boston Univ 1983; **Resid:** Surgery, Dartmouth-Hitchcock Med Ctr 1988; **Fellow:** Surgical Oncology, MD Anderson Cancer Ctr 1990; **Fac Appt:** Prof S, Med Coll Wisc

Farrar, William B MD [S] - **Spec Exp:** Breast Cancer; Thyroid Cancer; **Hospital:** Arthur G James Cancer Hosp & Research Inst, Ohio St Univ Med Ctr; **Address:** 410 W 10th Ave, N924 Doan Hall, Columbus, OH 43210-1240; **Phone:** 614-293-8890; **Board Cert:** Surgery 2000; **Med School:** Univ VA Sch Med 1975; **Resid:** Surgery, Ohio State Univ Hosps 1980; **Fellow:** Surgical Oncology, Meml Sloan-Kettering Cancer Ctr 1982; **Fac Appt:** Prof S, Ohio State Univ

Surgery

Fung, John J MD/PhD [S] - **Spec Exp:** Transplant-Liver; Transplant-Kidney; Liver & Biliary Cancer; **Hospital:** Cleveland Clin Fdn (page 70), Euclid Hosp; **Address:** Cleveland Clinic, Dept Surgery, 9500 Euclid Ave, Desk A80, Cleveland, OH 44195-0001; **Phone:** 216-444-3776; **Board Cert:** Surgery 2008; **Med School:** Univ Chicago-Pritzker Sch Med 1982; **Resid:** Surgery, Strong Memorial Hosp 1988; **Fellow:** Transplant Surgery, Univ Pittsburgh 1986; **Fac Appt:** Prof S, Cleveland Cl Coll Med/Case West Res

Goulet Jr, Robert J MD [S] - **Spec Exp:** Breast Cancer; Breast Surgery; **Hospital:** Indiana Univ Hosp (page 74); **Address:** Indiana Cancer Pavilion, 535 Barnhill Drive, Ste 253, Indianapolis, IN 46202-5112; **Phone:** 317-274-9800; **Board Cert:** Surgery 2006; **Med School:** SUNY Downstate 1979; **Resid:** Surgery, SUNY-Downstate Med Ctr 1986; **Fellow:** Surgical Research, SUNY-Downstate Med Ctr 1983; **Fac Appt:** Assoc Prof S, Indiana Univ

Grant, Clive S MD [S] - **Spec Exp:** Thyroid & Parathyroid Cancer & Surgery; Adrenal Tumors; Breast Cancer; **Hospital:** Mayo Med Ctr & Clin - Rochester; **Address:** Mayo Clinic, Dept Surgery, 200 First St SW, Rochester, MN 55905-0001; **Phone:** 507-284-2644; **Board Cert:** Surgery 2001; **Med School:** Univ Colorado 1975; **Resid:** Surgery, Mayo Clinic 1980; **Fac Appt:** Prof S, Mayo Med Sch

Hansen, Nora M MD [S] - **Spec Exp:** Sentinel Node Surgery; Breast Cancer-High Risk Women; Breast Cancer Risk Assessment; **Hospital:** Northwestern Meml Hosp; **Address:** Lynn Sage Breast Surgery Ctr, 250 E Superior St Fl 4 - Ste 420, Chicago, IL 60611; **Phone:** 312-472-4720; **Board Cert:** Surgery 2006; **Med School:** NY Med Coll 1988; **Resid:** Surgery, Univ Chicago Hosps 1995; **Fellow:** Surgical Oncology, Univ Chicago Hosps 1996; **Fac Appt:** Assoc Prof S, Northwestern Univ

Hinshaw, Daniel B MD [S] - **Spec Exp:** Palliative Care; **Hospital:** VA Med Ctr - Ann Arbor, Univ Michigan Hlth Sys; **Address:** VA Medical Ctr, 2215 Fuller Rd, rm 530, MS 112, Ann Arbor, MI 48105; **Phone:** 734-769-7100 x5939; **Board Cert:** Surgery 2003; **Med School:** Loma Linda Univ 1978; **Resid:** Surgery, Loma Linda U Med Ctr 1983; **Fellow:** Immunology, Scripps Clinic Rsch Fdn 1985; Cleveland Clinic 2001; **Fac Appt:** Clin Prof S, Univ Mich Med Sch

Howe, James MD [S] - **Spec Exp:** Endocrine Surgery; Gastrointestinal Cancer; Colon & Rectal Cancer; **Hospital:** Univ Iowa Hosp & Clinics; **Address:** Univ Iowa, Dept Surgery, 200 Hawkins Drive, 4645 JCP, Iowa City, IA 52242-1086; **Phone:** 319-356-1727; **Board Cert:** Surgery 2006; **Med School:** Univ VT Coll Med 1987; **Resid:** Surgery, Barnes Hosp-Wash Univ 1994; **Fellow:** Research, Wash Univ-NCI 1991; Surgical Oncology, Meml Sloan Kettering Cancer Ctr 1996; **Fac Appt:** Prof S, Univ Iowa Coll Med

Kim, Julian A MD [S] - **Spec Exp:** Melanoma; Breast Cancer; Gastrointestinal Cancer; Immunotherapy; **Hospital:** Univ Hosps Case Med Ctr; **Address:** Univ Hosps of Cleveland, LKS 5047, 11100 Euclid Ave, Cleveland, OH 44106-1716; **Phone:** 216-844-8247; **Board Cert:** Surgery 2002; **Med School:** Med Univ Ohio at Toledo 1986; **Resid:** Surgery, Univ Maryland Hosps 1991; **Fellow:** Surgical Oncology, Arthur James Cancer Hosp & Rsch Inst 1993; Immunotherapy, Ohio State Univ Comp Cancer Ctr 1994; **Fac Appt:** Assoc Prof S, Case West Res Univ

Leeming, Rosemary A MD [S] - **Spec Exp:** Breast Cancer & Surgery; Clinical Trials; **Hospital:** Univ Hosps Case Med Ctr; **Address:** 3909 Orange Pl, Beechwood, OH 44122; **Phone:** 216-591-1909; **Board Cert:** Surgery 2000; **Med School:** Hahnemann Univ 1983; **Resid:** Surgery, Mt Sinai Med Ctr 1989; **Fellow:** Breast Disease, Univ Pitts-Shadyside Hosp 1989; **Fac Appt:** Asst Prof S, Case West Res Univ

Lillemoe, Keith D MD [S] - **Spec Exp:** Pancreatic Cancer; Colon Cancer; Pancreatic & Biliary Surgery; Gastrointestinal Cancer; **Hospital:** Indiana Univ Hosp (page 74); **Address:** Indiana Univ, Dept Surgery, 545 Barnhill Drive, EH 203, Indianapolis, IN 46202-5112; **Phone:** 317-274-5707; **Board Cert:** Surgery 2007; **Med School:** Johns Hopkins Univ 1978; **Resid:** Surgery, Johns Hopkins Hosp 1985; **Fac Appt:** Prof S, Indiana Univ

Mamounas, Eleftherios P MD [S] - **Spec Exp:** Breast Cancer; **Hospital:** Aultman Hosp; **Address:** Aultman Cancer Ctr, 2600 6th St SW, Main 1, Clinical Trials Dept, Canton, OH 44710; **Phone:** 330-363-6281; **Board Cert:** Surgery 1999; **Med School:** Greece 1983; **Resid:** Surgery, McKeesport Hosp 1989; **Fellow:** Clinical Oncology, Univ Pittsburgh 1991; Surgical Oncology, Roswell Park Cancer Inst 1992; **Fac Appt:** Prof S, NE Ohio Univ

Melvin, W Scott MD [S] - **Spec Exp:** Liver & Biliary Surgery; Pancreatic Cancer; Laparoscopic Surgery; **Hospital:** Ohio St Univ Med Ctr; **Address:** 410 W 10th Ave, Ste N729 Doan, Columbus, OH 43210; **Phone:** 614-293-4499; **Board Cert:** Surgery 2002; **Med School:** Med Coll OH 1987; **Resid:** Surgery, Univ Maryland 1992; **Fellow:** Gastrointestinal Surgery, Grant Med Ctr 1993; **Fac Appt:** Prof S, Ohio State Univ

Merrick III, Hollis W MD [S] - **Spec Exp:** Cancer Surgery; **Hospital:** Univ of Toledo Med Ctr; **Address:** 3065 Arlington Ave, Toledo, OH 43614-2570; **Phone:** 419-383-3759; **Board Cert:** Surgery 1997; **Med School:** McGill Univ 1964; **Resid:** Surgery, Royal Victoria Hosp 1972; **Fac Appt:** Prof S, Med Coll OH

Millis, J Michael MD [S] - **Spec Exp:** Transplant-Liver-Adult & Pediatric; Liver Cancer; Transplant-Pancreas; **Hospital:** Univ of Chicago Med Ctr; **Address:** Univ Chicago, Dept Surgery, 5841 S Maryland Ave, MC 5027, Chicago, IL 60637; **Phone:** 773-702-6319; **Board Cert:** Surgery 2001; Surgical Critical Care 2001; **Med School:** Univ Tenn Coll Med, Memphis 1985; **Resid:** Surgery, UCLA Med Ctr 1992; **Fellow:** Transplant Surgery, UCLA Med Ctr 1994; **Fac Appt:** Prof S, Univ Chicago-Pritzker Sch Med

Moley, Jeffrey F MD [S] - **Spec Exp:** Thyroid Cancer & Surgery; Endocrine Cancers; Melanoma; **Hospital:** Barnes-Jewish Hosp; **Address:** Washington Univ School Med, Dept Surgery, 660 S Euclid Ave, Box 8109, St Louis, MO 63110; **Phone:** 314-362-2280; **Board Cert:** Surgery 2005; **Med School:** Columbia P&S 1980; **Resid:** Surgery, Yale-New Haven Hosp 1985; **Fellow:** Surgical Oncology, National Cancer Inst 1987; **Fac Appt:** Prof S, Washington Univ, St Louis

Nagorney, David M MD [S] - **Spec Exp:** Pancreatic Cancer; Hepatobiliary Surgery; Gastrointestinal Cancer; **Hospital:** Mayo Med Ctr & Clin - Rochester; **Address:** Mayo Clin, Dept Surgery, 200 1st St SW, Mayo E12, Rochester, MN 55905; **Phone:** 507-284-2644; **Board Cert:** Surgery 2001; **Med School:** Univ Kans 1975; **Resid:** Surgery, Mayo Clin 1982; **Fellow:** Hepatobiliary Surgery, Hammersmith Hosp 1985; **Fac Appt:** Prof S, Mayo Med Sch

Nathanson, S David MD [S] - **Spec Exp:** Breast Cancer; Breast Cancer Risk Assessment; Melanoma; Sarcoma; **Hospital:** Henry Ford Hosp; **Address:** 2799 W Grand Blvd, Detroit, MI 48202; **Phone:** 313-916-2917; **Board Cert:** Surgery 2002; **Med School:** South Africa 1966; **Resid:** Surgery, Univ Witwaterstrand 1974; Surgical Oncology, UCLA Med Ctr 1980; **Fellow:** Surgery, UC Davis 1982; **Fac Appt:** Prof S, Case West Res Univ

Newman, Lisa A MD [S] - **Spec Exp:** Breast Cancer; **Hospital:** Univ Michigan Hlth Sys; **Address:** Univ Michigan Cancer Center, 1500 E Medical Center Drive, rm 3308-CGC, Ann Arbor, MI 48109-5932; **Phone:** 734-936-8771; **Board Cert:** Surgery 2001; **Med School:** SUNY Downstate 1985; **Resid:** Surgery, Downstate Med Ctr 1990; **Fac Appt:** Assoc Prof S, Univ Mich Med Sch

Surgery

Onders, Raymond P MD [S] - **Spec Exp:** Laparoscopic Surgery; Gastrointestinal Cancer; **Hospital:** Univ Hosps Case Med Ctr; **Address:** University Hosps Cleveland, 11100 Euclid Ave, LKS 5047, Cleveland, OH 44106; **Phone:** 216-844-5797; **Board Cert:** Surgery 2001; **Med School:** NE Ohio Univ 1988; **Resid:** Surgery, Case Western Reserve Univ 1993; **Fac Appt:** Asst Prof S, Case West Res Univ

Posner, Mitchell C MD [S] - **Spec Exp:** Pancreatic Cancer; Gastrointestinal Cancer; Esophageal Cancer; **Hospital:** Univ of Chicago Med Ctr; **Address:** Univ Chicago Hospitals, 5841 S Maryland Ave, Ste G209, MC 9045, Chicago, IL 60637-1447; **Phone:** 773-834-0156; **Board Cert:** Surgery 2006; **Med School:** SUNY Buffalo 1981; **Resid:** Surgery, Univ Colorado Med Ctr 1986; **Fellow:** Surgical Oncology, Meml Sloan Kettering Cancer Ctr 1988; **Fac Appt:** Prof S, Univ Chicago-Pritzker Sch Med

Rikkers, Layton F MD [S] - **Spec Exp:** Pancreatic Cancer; Liver & Biliary Cancer; **Hospital:** Univ WI Hosp & Clins; **Address:** 600 Highland Ave, rm K4/761, Madison, WI 53705-2275; **Phone:** 608-263-1383; **Board Cert:** Surgery 2007; **Med School:** Stanford Univ 1970; **Resid:** Surgery, Univ Utah Hosp 1973; Surgery, Univ Utah Hosp 1976; **Fellow:** Hepatology, Royal Free Hosp 1974; **Fac Appt:** Prof S, Univ Wisc

Saha, Sukamal MD [S] - **Spec Exp:** Sentinel Node Surgery; Colon Cancer; Head & Neck Cancer & Surgery; **Hospital:** McLaren Reg Med Ctr, Genesys Reg Med Ctr - St Joseph Campus; **Address:** 3500 Calkins Rd, Ste A, Flint, MI 48532; **Phone:** 810-230-9600 x500; **Board Cert:** Surgery 2000; **Med School:** India 1977; **Resid:** Surgery, Hahnemann Univ Hosp 1985; Surgery, Easton Hosp 1987; **Fellow:** Surgical Oncology, Tulane Univ Med Ctr 1989; Head and Neck Surgery, Roswell Park Meml Hosp; **Fac Appt:** Asst Prof S, Mich State Univ

Sarr, Michael G MD [S] - **Spec Exp:** Pancreatic Cancer; Gastrointestinal Cancer; **Hospital:** Mayo Med Ctr & Clin - Rochester; **Address:** Mayo Clinic, Dept Surg, Desk West 12A, Rochester, MN 55905; **Phone:** 507-284-2863; **Board Cert:** Surgery 2001; **Med School:** Johns Hopkins Univ 1976; **Resid:** Surgery, Johns Hopkins Hosp 1982; **Fellow:** Surgery, Mayo Clinic 1984; Surgery, Johns Hopkins Hosp 1985; **Fac Appt:** Prof S, Mayo Med Sch

Schwartzentruber, Douglas J MD [S] - **Spec Exp:** Cancer Surgery; Melanoma; Kidney Cancer; Cancer Surgery; **Hospital:** Goshen Genl Hosp; **Address:** Cancer Ctr at Goshen Health System, 200 High Park Ave, Goshen, IN 46526; **Phone:** 574-535-2888; **Board Cert:** Surgery 1997; **Med School:** Indiana Univ 1982; **Resid:** Surgery, Indiana Univ Med Ctr 1987; **Fellow:** Surgical Oncology, Natl Cancer Inst 1990; **Fac Appt:** Assoc Clin Prof S, Indiana Univ

Scott-Conner, Carol E H MD/PhD [S] - **Spec Exp:** Breast Cancer; Cancer Surgery; Laparoscopic Surgery; **Hospital:** Univ Iowa Hosp & Clinics, VA Med Ctr - Iowa City; **Address:** Univ Iowa, Dept Surg, 200 Hawkins Drive, 4622-JCP, Iowa City, IA 52242-1086; **Phone:** 319-356-0330; **Board Cert:** Surgery 2000; Surgical Critical Care 1998; **Med School:** NYU Sch Med 1976; **Resid:** Surgery, NYU Med Ctr 1981; **Fac Appt:** Prof S, Univ Iowa Coll Med

Sener, Stephen F MD [S] - **Spec Exp:** Breast Cancer; Pancreatic Cancer; Lymphedema; Gastrointestinal Cancer & Surgery; **Hospital:** Evanston/Northshore Univ Hlth Syst; **Address:** Evanston Hospital, Dept Surgery, 2650 Ridge Ave, rm 2507, Evanston, IL 60201-1718; **Phone:** 847-570-1328; **Board Cert:** Surgery 2001; **Med School:** Northwestern Univ 1977; **Resid:** Surgery, Northwestern Univ 1982; **Fellow:** Surgery, Meml Sloan Kettering Cancer Ctr 1984; **Fac Appt:** Prof S, Northwestern Univ

America's Top Doctors® for Cancer 5th Edition

Shenk, Robert R MD [S] - **Spec Exp:** Breast Cancer; Melanoma; Pancreatic Cancer; Stomach Cancer; **Hospital:** Univ Hosps Case Med Ctr; **Address:** Univ Hosp Case Med Ctr, 11100 Euclid Ave, Dept General Surgery, Cleveland, OH 44106; **Phone:** 216-844-3026; **Board Cert:** Surgery 2004; **Med School:** Case West Res Univ 1978; **Resid:** Surgery, Univ Hosp 1985; Immunology, Natl Cancer Inst 1982; **Fellow:** Surgical Oncology, Anderson Hosp 1987; **Fac Appt:** Assoc Prof S, Case West Res Univ

Sielaff, Timothy D MD/PhD [S] - **Spec Exp:** Liver Cancer; Pancreatic Cancer; Gallbladder & Biliary Cancer; **Hospital:** Abbott - Northwestern Hosp; **Address:** Virginia Piper Cancer Inst, Liver and Pancreas Clinic, 800 E 28th St, Minneapolis, MN 55407; **Phone:** 612-863-7553; **Board Cert:** Surgery 1998; **Med School:** Med Coll VA 1989; **Resid:** Surgery, Univ Minn Hosps 1997; **Fellow:** Transplant Surgery, Univ Toronto Affil Hosp 1998; **Fac Appt:** Assoc Prof S, Univ Minn

Simeone, Diane M MD [S] - **Spec Exp:** Pancreatic Cancer; Cancer Surgery; **Hospital:** Univ Michigan Hlth Sys; **Address:** Univ Michigan Hlth Sys, 1500 E Med Ctr Drive, 2210B Taubman Center SPC 5343, Ann Arbor, MI 48109-5331; **Phone:** 734-936-5738; **Board Cert:** Surgery 2005; **Med School:** Duke Univ 1988; **Resid:** Surgery, Univ Mich Med Ctr 1995; **Fac Appt:** Prof S, Univ Mich Med Sch

Siperstein, Allan E MD [S] - **Spec Exp:** Laparoscopic Surgery; Endocrine Tumors; Thyroid & Parathyroid Cancer & Surgery; **Hospital:** Cleveland Clin Fdn (page 70); **Address:** Cleveland Clinic Fdn, Dept Genl Surg, 9500 Euclid Ave, Desk A80, Cleveland, OH 44195; **Phone:** 216-444-5664; **Board Cert:** Surgery 1997; **Med School:** Univ Tex SW, Dallas 1983; **Resid:** Surgery, UCSF Med Ctr 1990; **Fellow:** Research, UCSF Med Ctr 1988

Stahl, Donna L MD [S] - **Spec Exp:** Breast Cancer; Breast Surgery; **Hospital:** Jewish Hosp - Kenwood - Cincinnati; **Address:** 4750 E Galbraith Rd, Ste 112, Cincinnati, OH 45236; **Phone:** 513-686-3109; **Board Cert:** Surgery 2000; **Med School:** Univ Iowa Coll Med 1971; **Resid:** Surgery, Univ Cincinnati Hosps 1978

Staren, Edgar MD/PhD [S] - **Spec Exp:** Breast Cancer; Endocrine Cancers; Liver Cancer; **Hospital:** Midwest Reg Med Ctr; **Address:** Cancer Treatment Centers of America, 2610 Sheridan Rd, Zion, IL 60099; **Phone:** 847-731-5805; **Board Cert:** Surgery 2006; **Med School:** Loyola Univ-Stritch Sch Med 1982; **Resid:** Surgery, Rush-Presby-St Lukes Med Ctr 1987; **Fellow:** Surgical Oncology, Rush-Presby-St Lukes Med Ctr 1988

Talamonti, Mark S MD [S] - **Spec Exp:** Pancreatic Cancer; Liver Cancer; Gastrointestinal Cancer & Surgery; Melanoma; **Hospital:** Evanston/Northshore Univ Hlth Syst, Highland Park/North Shore Univ Hlth Syst; **Address:** North Shore Univ Health System, 2560 Ridge Ave, Evanston, IL 60201; **Phone:** 847-570-1700; **Board Cert:** Surgery 1999; **Med School:** Northwestern Univ 1983; **Resid:** Surgery, Northwestern Meml Hosp 1989; **Fellow:** Surgical Oncology, MD Anderson Cancer Ctr 1991; **Fac Appt:** Prof S, Northwestern Univ

Tuttle, Todd M MD [S] - **Spec Exp:** Breast Cancer; Minimally Invasive Surgery; Cancer Surgery; **Hospital:** Univ Minn Med Ctr, Fairview - Univ Campus; **Address:** Univ Minn, Dept Surgery, 420 Delaware St SE, MMC 195, Minneapolis, MN 55455; **Phone:** 612-625-2991; **Board Cert:** Surgery 2004; **Med School:** Johns Hopkins Univ 1988; **Resid:** Surgery, Med Coll Virginia Hosps 1994; **Fellow:** Surgical Oncology, MD Anderson Cancer Ctr 1996; **Fac Appt:** Assoc Prof S

Vickers, Selwyn M MD [S] - **Spec Exp:** Pancreatic Cancer; Liver Tumors; Gastrointestinal Surgery; **Hospital:** Univ Minn Med Ctr, Fairview - Univ Campus; **Address:** University of Minnesota, 420 Delaware St SE, Phillips Wangensteen Bldg, MMC 88, Minneapolis, MN 55455; **Phone:** 612-625-5411; **Board Cert:** Surgery 2003; **Med School:** Johns Hopkins Univ 1986; **Resid:** Surgery, Johns Hopkins Hosp 1992; **Fac Appt:** Prof S, Johns Hopkins Univ

Surgery

Walker, Alonzo P MD [S] - **Spec Exp:** Breast Cancer; **Hospital:** Froedtert Meml Lutheran Hosp; **Address:** Dept Surgery, 9200 W Wisconsin Ave, Milwaukee, WI 53226-3522; **Phone:** 414-805-5737; **Board Cert:** Surgery 2004; **Med School:** Univ Fla Coll Med 1976; **Resid:** Surgery, Univ Maryland Hosps 1983; **Fac Appt:** Prof S, Med Coll Wisc

Walsh, R Matthew MD [S] - **Spec Exp:** Pancreatic Cancer; Gastrointestinal Surgery; Hepatobiliary Surgery; **Hospital:** Cleveland Clin Fdn (page 70); **Address:** Cleveland Clin Dept Surgery, Desk A110, 9500 Euclid Ave, Cleveland, OH 44195; **Phone:** 216-445-7576; **Board Cert:** Surgery 1999; **Med School:** Med Coll Wisc 1985; **Resid:** Surgery, Loyola Univ Hosp 1990; **Fellow:** Endoscopy, Mass General Hosp 1991; Hepatopancreatobiliary Surgery, Cleveland Clinic; **Fac Appt:** Assoc Prof S, Cleveland Cl Coll Med/Case West Res

Weigel, Ronald J MD/PhD [S] - **Spec Exp:** Breast Cancer; Endocrine Surgery; **Hospital:** Univ Iowa Hosp & Clinics; **Address:** Univ Iowa Carver Coll Med-Dept Surgery, 200 Hawkins Drive, 1516 JCP, Iowa City, IA 52242-1086; **Phone:** 319-356-4200; **Board Cert:** Surgery 2001; **Med School:** Yale Univ 1986; **Resid:** Surgery, Duke Univ Med Ctr 1992; **Fellow:** Immunology, Duke Univ Med Ctr; **Fac Appt:** Prof S, Univ Iowa Coll Med

Wiebke, Eric A MD [S] - **Spec Exp:** Gastrointestinal Cancer & Surgery; Laparoscopic Surgery; Gastrointestinal Motility Disorders; **Hospital:** Indiana Univ Hosp (page 74); **Address:** Indiana Univ Med Ctr-Emerson Hall 244, 545 Barnhill Drive, Indianapolis, IN 46202; **Phone:** 317-274-4990; **Board Cert:** Surgery 1998; Surgical Critical Care 2002; **Med School:** Vanderbilt Univ 1983; **Resid:** Surgery, Johns Hopkins Hosp 1989; **Fellow:** Surgical Oncology, Natl Cancer Inst/NIH 1987; **Fac Appt:** Prof S, Indiana Univ

Witt, Thomas R MD [S] - **Spec Exp:** Breast Cancer; **Hospital:** Rush Univ Med Ctr, Glenbrook/NorthShore Univ Hlth Syst; **Address:** 1725 W Harrison St, Ste 409, Chicago, IL 60612-3828; **Phone:** 312-942-2302; **Board Cert:** Surgery 2000; **Med School:** Northwestern Univ 1975; **Resid:** Surgery, Rush Presby-St Lukes Med Ctr 1980; **Fellow:** Surgical Oncology, Meml Sloan Kettering Cancer Ctr 1982; **Fac Appt:** Assoc Prof S, Rush Med Coll

Great Plains and Mountains

Edney, James A MD [S] - **Spec Exp:** Breast Cancer; Thyroid & Parathyroid Cancer & Surgery; Cancer Surgery; **Hospital:** Nebraska Med Ctr; **Address:** Univ Nebraska Med Ctr, Dept Surgery, 984030 Nebraska Medical Ctr, Omaha, NE 68198-4030; **Phone:** 402-559-7272; **Board Cert:** Surgery 2000; **Med School:** Univ Nebr Coll Med 1975; **Resid:** Surgery, Univ Nebraska Med Ctr 1980; **Fellow:** Surgical Oncology, Univ Colorado Med Ctr 1981; **Fac Appt:** Prof S, Univ Nebr Coll Med

Finlayson, Christina A MD [S] - **Spec Exp:** Breast Cancer; Breast Disease; **Hospital:** Univ Colorado Hosp; **Address:** Univ Colorado Hlth Sci Ctr, Dept Surgery, GI Tumor C313 Academic Office 1, rm 6001, 12631 E 17th Ave, PO Box 6511, Aurora, CO 80045; **Phone:** 720-848-1030; **Board Cert:** Surgery 1995; **Med School:** Univ Utah 1989; **Resid:** Surgery, Univ Colorado Hlth Sci Ctr 1994; **Fellow:** Surgical Oncology, Fox Chase Cancer Ctr 1996; **Fac Appt:** Assoc Prof S, Univ Colorado

Mulvihill, Sean J MD [S] - **Spec Exp:** Gastrointestinal Surgery; Liver & Biliary Cancer; Pancreatic Cancer; **Hospital:** Univ Utah Hosps and Clins; **Address:** Univ Utah, Dept Surgery, 30 N 1900 E, rm 3B110, Salt Lake City, UT 84132; **Phone:** 801-581-7304; **Board Cert:** Surgery 1999; **Med School:** USC Sch Med 1981; **Resid:** Surgery, UCLA Med Ctr 1987; **Fac Appt:** Prof S, Univ Utah

America's Top Doctors® for Cancer 5th Edition

Nelson, Edward W MD [S] - **Spec Exp:** Breast Cancer; **Hospital:** Univ Utah Hosps and Clins; **Address:** University Utah Medical Ctr, Div Genl Surgery, 30 N 1900 E, rm 3B322, Salt Lake City, UT 84132; **Phone:** 801-581-7738; **Board Cert:** Surgery 1999; **Med School:** Univ Utah 1974; **Resid:** Surgery, Univ Utah Med Ctr 1979; **Fac Appt:** Prof S, Univ Utah

Pearlman, Nathan W MD [S] - **Spec Exp:** Gastrointestinal Cancer; Melanoma; Head & Neck Cancer; **Hospital:** Univ Colorado Hosp; **Address:** 12631 E 17th Ave, MS C-313, Aurora, CO 80045; **Phone:** 303-724-2728; **Board Cert:** Surgery 1974; **Med School:** Univ IL Coll Med 1966; **Resid:** Surgery, Univ Colorado Med Ctr 1973; **Fellow:** Surgical Oncology, Sloan-Kettering Cancer Ctr 1975; **Fac Appt:** Prof S, Univ Colorado

Sasson, Aaron R MD [S] - **Spec Exp:** Gastrointestinal Cancer; Pancreatic Cancer; Liver Cancer; Neuroendocrine Tumors; **Hospital:** Nebraska Med Ctr; **Address:** Univ Nebraska Med Ctr, Box 984030, Omaha, NE 68198-0001; **Phone:** 402-559-8941; **Board Cert:** Surgery 2000; **Med School:** UMDNJ-NJ Med Sch, Newark 1993; **Resid:** Surgery, UCSD Med Ctr 1999; **Fellow:** Surgical Oncology, Fox Chase Cancer Ctr 2001; **Fac Appt:** Assoc Prof S, Univ Nebr Coll Med

Southwest

Ames, Frederick C MD [S] - **Spec Exp:** Breast Cancer; **Hospital:** UT MD Anderson Cancer Ctr; **Address:** MD Anderson Cancer Ctr, Dept Surgery, 1515 Holcombe Blvd, Unit 444, Houston, TX 77030-4009; **Phone:** 713-792-6929; **Board Cert:** Surgery 1975; **Med School:** Univ Tex Med Br, Galveston 1969; **Resid:** Surgery, Univ Texas Med Branch 1971; Surgery, St Joseph Hosp 1974; **Fellow:** Surgical Oncology, MD Anderson Cancer Ctr 1975; **Fac Appt:** Prof S, Univ Tex, Houston

Babiera, Gildy V MD [S] - **Spec Exp:** Breast Cancer; **Hospital:** UT MD Anderson Cancer Ctr; **Address:** MD Anderson Cancer Ctr, 1515 Holcombe Blvd., Unit 444, Houston, TX 77030-4009; **Phone:** 713-792-6937; **Board Cert:** Surgery 2007; **Med School:** NY Med Coll 1991; **Resid:** Surgery, NYU Med Ctr 1995; Surgery, NYU Med Ctr 1997; **Fellow:** Surgical Oncology, MD Anderson Cancer Ctr 1996; **Fac Appt:** Assoc Prof Surg & Onc, Univ Tex, Houston

Beitsch, Peter D MD [S] - **Spec Exp:** Breast Cancer; **Hospital:** Med City Dallas Hosp, Presby Hosp of Dallas; **Address:** 7777 Forrest Ln C Bldg - Ste 760, Dallas, TX 75230; **Phone:** 972-566-8039; **Board Cert:** Surgery 2002; **Med School:** Univ Tex SW, Dallas 1986; **Resid:** Surgery, Univ TX SW Med Ctr 1993; **Fellow:** Surgical Oncology, MD Anderson Cancer Ctr 1990; Surgical Oncology, John Wayne Cancer Inst 1994

Bolton, John MD [S] - **Spec Exp:** Cancer Surgery; Esophageal Cancer; Pancreatic Cancer; Liver Cancer; **Hospital:** Ochsner Fdn Hosp; **Address:** Ochsner Clin, Dept Surg, 1514 Jefferson Hwy, New Orleans, LA 70121; **Phone:** 504-842-4072; **Board Cert:** Surgery 2002; **Med School:** Louisiana State U, New Orleans 1976; **Resid:** Surgery, Charity Hosp 1981; **Fellow:** Hepatopancreatobiliary Surgery, Lahey Clinic 1980; Surgical Oncology, Meml Sloan Kettering Cancer Ctr 1982; **Fac Appt:** Asst Clin Prof S, Louisiana State U, New Orleans

Brunicardi, F Charles MD [S] - **Spec Exp:** Pancreatic Cancer; **Hospital:** St Luke's Episcopal Hosp-Houston; **Address:** 6620 Main St, Ste 1475, Houston, TX 77030; **Phone:** 713-798-8070; **Board Cert:** Surgery 1998; **Med School:** UMDNJ-Rutgers Med Sch 1980; **Resid:** Surgery, SUNY Brooklyn Hlth Sci Ctr 1989; **Fellow:** Pancreatic Physiology, SUNY Brooklyn Hlth Sci Ctr 1986; **Fac Appt:** Prof S, Baylor Coll Med

Curley, Steven A MD [S] - **Spec Exp:** Colon & Rectal Cancer; Liver Cancer; Hepatobiliary Surgery; **Hospital:** UT MD Anderson Cancer Ctr; **Address:** MD Anderson Cancer Ctr, Dept Surg Oncology, Unit 444, PO Box 301402, Houston, TX 77230-1402; **Phone:** 713-792-6937; **Board Cert:** Surgery 1997; **Med School:** Univ Tex, Houston 1982; **Resid:** Surgery, Univ New Mexico Hosps 1988; **Fellow:** Surgical Oncology, MD Anderson Cancer Ctr 1990; **Fac Appt:** Prof S, Univ Tex, Houston

Dooley, William C MD [S] - **Spec Exp:** Breast Cancer; Tumors-Rare & Multiple; **Hospital:** OU Med Ctr, VA Med Ctr - Oklahoma City; **Address:** 825 NE 10th St, Ste 4500, Oklahoma City, OK 73104; **Phone:** 405-271-7867; **Board Cert:** Surgery 1997; **Med School:** Vanderbilt Univ 1982; **Resid:** Surgery, Johns Hopkins Hosp 1987; Surgical Oncology, Oxford Univ 1986; **Fellow:** Surgical Oncology, Johns Hopkins 1988; **Fac Appt:** Prof S, Univ Okla Coll Med

Ellis, Lee M MD [S] - **Spec Exp:** Liver Cancer; Colon & Rectal Cancer; Metastatic Cancer; Peritoneal Carcinomatosis; **Hospital:** UT MD Anderson Cancer Ctr; **Address:** MD Anderson Cancer Ctr, Dept Surgery, 1515 Holcombe Blvd, Box 444, Houston, TX 77030; **Phone:** 713-792-6937; **Board Cert:** Surgery 1999; **Med School:** Univ VA Sch Med 1983; **Resid:** Surgery, Univ Fla-Shands Hosp 1990; **Fellow:** Surgical Oncology, MD Anderson Cancer Ctr 1992; **Fac Appt:** Prof S, Univ Tex, Houston

Euhus, David M MD [S] - **Spec Exp:** Breast Cancer; **Hospital:** UT Southwestern Med Ctr at Dallas; **Address:** Univ Texas SW Med Ctr - Div Surg Oncology, 5323 Harry Hines Blvd, MC 9155, Dallas, TX 75390-9155; **Phone:** 214-648-6467; **Board Cert:** Surgery 2001; **Med School:** St Louis Univ 1984; **Resid:** Surgery, UCLA Med Ctr 1991; **Fellow:** Surgical Oncology, UCLA Med Ctr 1988; Breast Disease, Queens Med Ctr 1990; **Fac Appt:** Prof S, Univ Tex SW, Dallas

Feig, Barry W MD [S] - **Spec Exp:** Gastrointestinal Cancer; Sarcoma; Breast Cancer; **Hospital:** UT MD Anderson Cancer Ctr; **Address:** UT MD Anderson Cancer Ctr, Dept Surg Onc, Unit 444, PO Box 301402, Houston, TX 77230-1402; **Phone:** 713-792-6937; **Board Cert:** Surgery 1998; **Med School:** SUNY Upstate Med Univ 1984; **Resid:** Surgery, Northwestern Univ Med Ctr 1990; **Fellow:** Trauma, Univ Minnesota Affil Hosp 1991; Surgical Oncology, UT MD Anderson Cancer Ctr 1994; **Fac Appt:** Prof S, Univ Tex, Houston

Fisher, William E MD [S] - **Spec Exp:** Pancreatic Cancer; **Hospital:** St Luke's Episcopal Hosp-Houston; **Address:** 6620 Main St, Ste 1475, Houston, TX 77030; **Phone:** 713-798-8070; **Board Cert:** Surgery 2006; **Med School:** Univ Cincinnati 1990; **Resid:** Surgery, Ohio State U Hosps 1996; **Fellow:** Cancer Research, Ohio State U Hosps 1998; **Fac Appt:** Asst Prof S, Baylor Coll Med

Grant, Michael D MD [S] - **Spec Exp:** Breast Cancer; Breast Surgery; **Hospital:** Baylor Univ Medical Ctr; **Address:** 3900 Junius, Ste 220, Baylor Medical Pavillion, Dallas, TX 75246; **Phone:** 214-826-7300; **Board Cert:** Surgery 2001; **Med School:** Univ Tex, Houston 1987; **Resid:** Surgery, Baylor Univ Med Ctr 1992; **Fellow:** Breast Cancer, Baylor Univ Med Ctr 1993

Gray, Richard J MD [S] - **Spec Exp:** Breast Cancer; Melanoma; **Hospital:** Mayo Clinic - Phoenix, Mayo Clinic - Scottsdale; **Address:** Mayo Clinic, 5777 E Mayo Blvd, Phoenix, AZ 85054; **Phone:** 480-342-2849; **Board Cert:** Surgery 2001; **Med School:** Mich State Univ 1995; **Resid:** Surgery, Mayo Clinic 2000; **Fellow:** Surgical Oncology, H Lee Moffitt Cancer Ctr 2001; **Fac Appt:** Assoc Prof S, Mayo Med Sch

Hunt, Kelly K MD [S] - **Spec Exp:** Breast Cancer; Sarcoma-Soft Tissue; Gene Therapy; **Hospital:** UT MD Anderson Cancer Ctr; **Address:** MD Anderson Cancer Ctr, 1515 Holcombe Blvd, Box 444, Houston, TX 77030-4000; **Phone:** 713-792-7216; **Board Cert:** Surgery 2001; **Med School:** Univ Tenn Coll Med, Memphis 1986; **Resid:** Surgery, UCLA Med Ctr 1993; **Fellow:** Surgical Oncology, MD Anderson Cancer Ctr 1996; **Fac Appt:** Prof S, Univ Tex, Houston

Jackson, Gilchrist MD [S] - **Spec Exp:** Thyroid & Parathyroid Surgery; Head & Neck Cancer & Surgery; Endocrine Tumors; Gastrointestinal Cancer & Surgery; **Hospital:** St Luke's Episcopal Hosp-Houston, Woman's Hosp TX; **Address:** 2727 W Holcombe Blvd Fl 3 A, Houston, TX 77027; **Phone:** 713-442-1132; **Board Cert:** Surgery 1998; **Med School:** Univ Louisville Sch Med 1974; **Resid:** Surgery, Parkland Hosp 1979; **Fellow:** Surgical Oncology, MD Anderson Hosp 1980; **Fac Appt:** Assoc Clin Prof S, Baylor Coll Med

Klimberg, Vicki S MD [S] - **Spec Exp:** Breast Cancer; Radiofrequency Tumor Ablation; Sentinel Node Surgery; **Hospital:** UAMS Med Ctr; **Address:** Univ Arkansas Medical Sciences, 4301 W Markham, MS 725, Little Rock, AR 72205-7199; **Phone:** 501-686-5669; **Board Cert:** Surgery 1999; **Med School:** Univ Fla Coll Med 1984; **Resid:** Surgery, Univ Fla Med Ctr 1989; **Fellow:** Clinical Oncology, Univ Fla 1990; Breast Disease, Univ Arkansas for Med Scis 1991; **Fac Appt:** Prof S, Univ Ark

Krouse, Robert S MD [S] - **Spec Exp:** Cancer Surgery; Gastrointestinal Cancer; Palliative Care; **Hospital:** VA Medical Center - Tucson; **Address:** Southern AZ VA Hosp Care System, Surg Care Line, 2-112, 3601 S 6th Ave, Tucson, AZ 85723; **Phone:** 520-792-1450 x6145; **Board Cert:** Surgery 2007; **Med School:** Hahnemann Univ 1991; **Resid:** Surgery, Univ Hawaii Integrated Surg Prog 1993; Immunotherapy, Natl Cancer Inst 1994; **Fellow:** Surgery, W Virginia Univ Sch Med 1997; Surgical Oncology, City of Hope Natl Med Ctr 2000; **Fac Appt:** Asst Prof S, Univ Ariz Coll Med

Kuhn, Joseph A MD [S] - **Spec Exp:** Liver Cancer; Peritoneal Carcinomatosis; Melanoma; Thyroid Cancer; **Hospital:** Baylor Univ Medical Ctr; **Address:** 7777 Forest Lane St, Ste C-410, Dallas, TX 75230; **Phone:** 214-823-5000; **Board Cert:** Surgery 1999; Surgical Critical Care 2003; **Med School:** Univ Tex Med Br, Galveston 1984; **Resid:** Surgery, Baylor Univ Med Ctr 1989; **Fellow:** Surgical Oncology, City Hosp Natl Med Ctr 1992

Lee, Jeffrey E MD [S] - **Spec Exp:** Melanoma; Pancreatic Cancer; Endocrine Tumors; **Hospital:** UT MD Anderson Cancer Ctr; **Address:** UT MD Anderson Cancer Ctr, 1400 Holcombe Blvd, Unit 444 Fl 12, Houston, TX 77030-4009; **Phone:** 713-792-7218; **Board Cert:** Surgery 1999; **Med School:** Stanford Univ 1984; **Resid:** Surgery, Stanford Univ Hosp 1987; Surgery, Stanford Univ Hosp 1991; **Fellow:** Immunology, Stanford Univ Sch Med 1989; Surgical Oncology, Univ Tex-MD Anderson Cancer Ctr 1993; **Fac Appt:** Prof S, Univ Tex, Houston

Leitch, A Marilyn MD [S] - **Spec Exp:** Breast Cancer & Surgery; Melanoma; Sarcoma; **Hospital:** UT Southwestern Med Ctr at Dallas; **Address:** UT Southwestern Med Ctr - Dept Surgery, 5323 Harry Hines Blvd, MC 9155, Dallas, TX 75390-9155; **Phone:** 214-648-3039; **Board Cert:** Surgery 2003; **Med School:** Univ Tex SW, Dallas 1978; **Resid:** Surgery, UCLA Med Ctr 1984; **Fellow:** Surgical Oncology, MD Anderson Cancer Ctr 1985; **Fac Appt:** Prof S, Univ Tex SW, Dallas

Li, Benjamin D L MD [S] - **Spec Exp:** Gastrointestinal Cancer; Sarcoma; Breast Cancer; **Hospital:** Louisiana State Univ Hosp, Willis Knighton Hlth Sys; **Address:** LSU Hlth Scis Ctr, Dept Surgery, 1501 Kings Hwy, Shreveport, LA 71130; **Phone:** 318-675-6100; **Board Cert:** Surgery 2002; **Med School:** Yale Univ 1986; **Resid:** Surgery, Northwestern Univ-McGraw Med Ctr 1992; **Fellow:** Surgical Oncology, Roswell Park Cancer Inst 1995; **Fac Appt:** Prof S, Louisiana State U, New Orleans

Mansfield, Paul F MD [S] - **Spec Exp:** Appendix Cancer; Stomach Cancer; Colon Cancer; Melanoma; **Hospital:** UT MD Anderson Cancer Ctr; **Address:** UT MD Anderson Cancer Ctr, 1515 Holcombe Blvd, rm 444, Houston, TX 77030; **Phone:** 713-794-5499; **Board Cert:** Surgery 2006; **Med School:** Jefferson Med Coll 1983; **Resid:** Surgery, Pennsylvania Hosp 1988; **Fellow:** Surgical Oncology, MD Anderson Cancer Ctr 1991; **Fac Appt:** Prof Surg & Onc, Univ Tex, Houston

Surgery

Pisters, Peter MD [S] - **Spec Exp:** Pancreatic Cancer; Sarcoma-Soft Tissue; Gastrointestinal Cancer; **Hospital:** UT MD Anderson Cancer Ctr; **Address:** MD Anderson Cancer Ctr, PO Box 301402, Unit 444, Houston, TX 77230-1402; **Phone:** 713-792-6397; **Board Cert:** Surgery 2001; **Med School:** Univ Western Ontario 1985; **Resid:** Surgery, NYU/Bellevue Hosp 1992; **Fellow:** Surgical Research, Meml Sloan-Kettering Cancer Ctr 1989; Surgical Oncology, Meml Sloan-Kettering Cancer Ctr 1994; **Fac Appt:** Prof S, Univ Tex, Houston

Pockaj, Barbara A MD [S] - **Spec Exp:** Melanoma; Breast Cancer; Stomach Cancer; Clinical Trials; **Hospital:** Mayo Clinic - Scottsdale; **Address:** Mayo Clinic, Dept Surgery, 5779 E Mayo Blvd, Phoenix, AZ 85054; **Phone:** 480-342-1051; **Board Cert:** Surgery 2005; **Med School:** Vanderbilt Univ 1987; **Resid:** Surgery, Case Western Res Univ Affil Hosps 1995; **Fellow:** Surgical Oncology, Natl Inst Hlth 1992; **Fac Appt:** Assoc Prof S, Mayo Med Sch

Pollock, Raphael E MD/PhD [S] - **Spec Exp:** Sarcoma; **Hospital:** UT MD Anderson Cancer Ctr; **Address:** MD Anderson Cancer Ctr, Dept Surg Oncology, 1515 Holcombe Blvd, Unit 444, Houston, TX 77030; **Phone:** 713-792-6928; **Board Cert:** Surgery 2003; **Med School:** St Louis Univ 1977; **Resid:** Surgery, Univ Chicago 1979; Surgery, Rush Presby-St Lukes Hosp 1982; **Fellow:** Surgical Oncology, MD Anderson Cancer Ctr 1984; **Fac Appt:** Prof S, Univ Tex, Houston

Postier, Russell G MD [S] - **Spec Exp:** Pancreatic Cancer; Biliary Surgery; **Hospital:** OU Med Ctr; **Address:** OU Physicians, Dept Surgery, 825 NE 10th St, Ste 4500, Oklahoma City, OK 73104; **Phone:** 405-271-1400; **Board Cert:** Surgery 2000; **Med School:** Univ Okla Coll Med 1975; **Resid:** Surgery, Johns Hopkins Hosp 1981; **Fac Appt:** Prof S, Univ Okla Coll Med

Ross, Merrick I MD [S] - **Spec Exp:** Sentinel Node Surgery; Breast Cancer; Melanoma; **Hospital:** UT MD Anderson Cancer Ctr; **Address:** UT MD Anderson Cancer Ctr, Dept Surg Onc, PO Box 301402, Unit 444, Houston, TX 77230-1402; **Phone:** 713-792-6937; **Board Cert:** Surgery 2007; **Med School:** Univ IL Coll Med 1980; **Resid:** Surgery, Univ Illinois Hosp & Clin 1982; Surgery, Univ Illinois Hosp & Clin 1987; **Fellow:** Research, Scripps Clin & Rsch 1984; Surgical Oncology, Univ TX-MD Anderson Cancer Ctr 1989; **Fac Appt:** Prof S, Univ Tex, Houston

Singletary, S Eva MD [S] - **Spec Exp:** Breast Cancer; **Hospital:** UT MD Anderson Cancer Ctr; **Address:** Univ Tex MD Anderson Cancer Ctr, 1515 Holcombe Blvd, Box 444, Houston, TX 77030-4009; **Phone:** 713-792-6937; **Board Cert:** Surgery 2003; **Med School:** Med Univ SC 1977; **Resid:** Surgery, Shands Hosp-Univ Florida 1983; **Fellow:** Surgery, UT MD Anderson Hosp 1985; **Fac Appt:** Prof S, Univ Tex, Houston

Skibber, John M MD [S] - **Spec Exp:** Rectal Cancer/Sphincter Preservation; Colon & Rectal Cancer-Familial Polyposis; **Hospital:** UT MD Anderson Cancer Ctr; **Address:** Unit 444 PO Box 301402, Houston, TX 77230-1402; **Phone:** 713-792-5165; **Board Cert:** Surgery 1998; **Med School:** Jefferson Med Coll 1981; **Resid:** Surgery, NYU Med Ctr 1989; **Fellow:** Surgical Oncology, Univ Texas-MD Anderson 1991; **Fac Appt:** Prof S, Univ Tex, Houston

Stolier, Alan J MD [S] - **Spec Exp:** Breast Cancer; **Hospital:** Ochsner Baptist Med Ctr, Louisiana State Univ Hosp; **Address:** 2525 Severn Ave, Metairie, LA 70002; **Phone:** 504-832-4200; **Board Cert:** Surgery 2006; **Med School:** Louisiana State U, New Orleans 1970; **Resid:** Surgery, Charity Hosp 1974; **Fellow:** Surgical Oncology, MD Anderson Hosp 1976

Vauthey, Jean Nicholas MD [S] - **Spec Exp:** Hepatobiliary Surgery; Liver Cancer; Gallbladder & Biliary Cancer; **Hospital:** UT MD Anderson Cancer Ctr; **Address:** UT MD Anderson Cancer Ctr -Surg Oncology, 1515 Holcombe Blvd, Unit 444, Houston, TX 77030; **Phone:** 713-792-6937; **Board Cert:** Surgery 2000; **Med School:** Switzerland 1979; **Resid:** Surgery, Ochsner Med Fdn 1989; **Fellow:** Hepatobiliary Surgery, Med Fac Univ Bern 1991; Surgical Oncology, Meml Sloan-Kettering Cancer Ctr 1993; **Fac Appt:** Prof S, Univ Tex, Houston

Woltering, Eugene MD [S] - **Spec Exp:** Carcinoid Tumors; **Hospital:** Ochsner Fdn Hosp; **Address:** 200 W Esplanade, Ste 200, Kenner, LA 70062; **Phone:** 504-464-8500; **Board Cert:** Surgery 2002; **Med School:** Ohio State Univ 1975; **Resid:** Surgery, Vanderbilt Med Ctr 1982; Surgical Oncology, Natl Inst Hlth 1979; **Fellow:** Surgical Oncology, Ohio State Univ 1984; **Fac Appt:** Prof S, Louisiana State U, New Orleans

Wood, R Patrick MD [S] - **Spec Exp:** Liver Cancer; **Hospital:** St Luke's Episcopal Hosp-Houston; **Address:** 6624 Fannin St, Ste 1200, Houston, TX 77030; **Phone:** 713-795-8994; **Board Cert:** Surgery 2004; **Med School:** Univ Rochester 1979; **Resid:** Surgery, NYU/Bellevue Hosp Ctr 1984; **Fellow:** Transplant Surgery, Univ Pittsburgh 1985; **Fac Appt:** Clin Prof S, Univ Tex, Houston

Zannis, Victor J MD [S] - **Spec Exp:** Breast Cancer; **Hospital:** Phoenix Baptist Hosp & Med Ctr, J C Lincoln Hosp - North Mountain; **Address:** 2525 W Greenway Rd, Ste 130, Phoenix, AZ 85023; **Phone:** 602-942-8000; **Board Cert:** Surgery 2000; **Med School:** UCLA 1976; **Resid:** Surgery, Maricopa Med Ctr 1982

West Coast and Pacific

Anderson, Benjamin O MD [S] - **Spec Exp:** Breast Cancer & Surgery; **Hospital:** Univ Wash Med Ctr; **Address:** Univ Washington Dept Surgery, 1959 NE Pacific St, Box 356410, Seattle, WA 98195-6410; **Phone:** 206-288-6487; **Board Cert:** Surgery 2002; **Med School:** Albert Einstein Coll Med 1985; **Resid:** Surgery, Univ Colorado 1992; **Fellow:** Surgical Oncology, Meml Sloan Kettering Cancer Ctr 1994; **Fac Appt:** Prof S, Univ Wash

Bilchik, Anton J MD/PhD [S] - **Spec Exp:** Gastrointestinal Cancer; Laparoscopic Surgery; **Hospital:** St John's Hlth Ctr, Santa Monica, Cedars-Sinai Med Ctr; **Address:** John Wayne Cancer Institute, 2336 Santa Monica Blvd, Ste 206, Santa Monica, CA 90404; **Phone:** 310-696-0716; **Board Cert:** Surgery 2004; **Med School:** South Africa 1985; **Resid:** Surgery, UCLA Med Ctr 1996; **Fellow:** John Wayne Cancer Inst. 1998; **Fac Appt:** Asst Clin Prof S, UCLA

Busuttil, Ronald W MD/PhD [S] - **Spec Exp:** Transplant-Liver; Liver Cancer; **Hospital:** UCLA Ronald Reagan Med Ctr; **Address:** UCLA Dept Surg, Transplant, 77-120 CHS Box 957054, Los Angeles, CA 90095-7054; **Phone:** 310-825-5318; **Board Cert:** Surgery 2007; **Med School:** Tulane Univ 1971; **Resid:** Surgery, UCLA Med Ctr 1976; **Fellow:** Surgery, UCLA Med Ctr 1975; **Fac Appt:** Prof S, UCLA

Butler, John A MD [S] - **Spec Exp:** Breast Cancer; Thyroid Cancer; Adrenal Tumors; Small Bowel Cancer; **Hospital:** UC Irvine Med Ctr; **Address:** UC-Irvine Medical Ctr, 101 City Drive S, Bldg 56 Office 252 Rt 81, Orange, CA 92868-3298; **Phone:** 714-456-8030; **Board Cert:** Surgery 2003; **Med School:** Loyola Univ-Stritch Sch Med 1976; **Resid:** Surgery, LAC-USC Med Ctr 1982; Surgery, Harbor-UCLA Med Ctr 1982; **Fellow:** Surgical Oncology, Meml Sloan-Kettering Cancer Ctr 1984; **Fac Appt:** Prof S, UC Irvine

Byrd, David MD [S] - **Spec Exp:** Tumor Surgery; Breast Cancer; Melanoma; **Hospital:** Univ Wash Med Ctr; **Address:** Univ Washington Med Ctr, Dept Surgical Specialites Center, 1959 NE Pacific St, Box 356165, Seattle, WA 98195; **Phone:** 206-598-4477; **Board Cert:** Surgery 1998; **Med School:** Tulane Univ 1982; **Resid:** Surgery, Univ Wash Med Ctr 1987; **Fellow:** Surgical Oncology, Univ Tex-MD Anderson Cancer Ctr 1992; **Fac Appt:** Assoc Prof S, Univ Wash

Chang, Helena MD [S] - **Spec Exp:** Breast Cancer; Cancer Surgery; **Hospital:** UCLA Ronald Reagan Med Ctr; **Address:** 200 Westwood Plaza Drive, Ste B265, Revlon Breast Clinic, Los Angeles, CA 90095-7028; **Phone:** 310-825-2144; **Board Cert:** Surgery 1997; **Med School:** Temple Univ 1981; **Resid:** Surgery, Episcopal Hosp 1986; **Fellow:** Cellular Molecular Biology, Temple Univ 1977; Surgical Oncology, Meml Sloan-Kettering Cancer Ctr 1988; **Fac Appt:** Prof S, UCLA

Clark, Orlo H MD [S] - **Spec Exp:** Thyroid Cancer & Surgery; Neuroendocrine Tumors; Parathyroid Cancer; **Hospital:** UCSF - Mt Zion Med Ctr, UCSF Med Ctr; **Address:** UCSF Mt Zion Med Ctr, 1600 Divisadero St Fl 3, Box 1674, San Francisco, CA 94115-1926; **Phone:** 415-353-7687; **Board Cert:** Surgery 1974; **Med School:** Cornell Univ-Weill Med Coll 1967; **Resid:** Surgery, UCSF Med Ctr 1970; Surgery, UCSF Med Ctr 1973; **Fellow:** Surgery, Royal Med Sch London 1971; **Fac Appt:** Prof S, UCSF

Colquhoun, Steven D MD [S] - **Spec Exp:** Liver Cancer; Transplant-Liver; Pancreatic Cancer; Hepatobiliary Surgery; **Hospital:** Cedars-Sinai Med Ctr; **Address:** Cedars-Sinai Med Center, 8635 W 3rd St, Ste 590-W, Los Angeles, CA 90048; **Phone:** 310-423-2641; **Board Cert:** Surgery 2003; Surgical Critical Care 2008; **Med School:** Loyola Univ-Stritch Sch Med 1984; **Resid:** Surgery, UCLA Med Ctr 1990; **Fellow:** Surgical Oncology, UCLA Med Ctr 1993; Transplant Surgery, UCLA Med Ctr 1994; **Fac Appt:** Assoc Clin Prof S, UCLA

Duh, Quan-Yang MD [S] - **Spec Exp:** Endocrine Surgery; Thyroid & Parathyroid Cancer & Surgery; Adrenal Tumors; Minimally Invasive Surgery; **Hospital:** UCSF Med Ctr, VA Med Ctr - San Francisco; **Address:** UCSF Medical Ctr, Box 1926, San Francisco, CA 94143-1926; **Phone:** 415-353-7687; **Board Cert:** Surgery 2007; **Med School:** UCSF 1981; **Resid:** Surgery, UCSF Med Ctr 1988; **Fellow:** Endocrine Surgery, UCSF Med Ctr 1987; **Fac Appt:** Prof S, UCSF

Eilber, Frederick R MD [S] - **Spec Exp:** Tumor Surgery; Sarcoma; **Hospital:** UCLA Ronald Reagan Med Ctr; **Address:** 200 UCLA Medical Plaza, Ste 120, Los Angeles, CA 90095-1718; **Phone:** 310-825-7086; **Board Cert:** Surgery 1973; **Med School:** Univ Mich Med Sch 1965; **Resid:** Surgery, Univ Maryland Hosp 1972; **Fellow:** Surgery, Univ Tex-MD Anderson Hosp 1973; **Fac Appt:** Prof S, UCLA

Ellenhorn, Joshua DI MD [S] - **Spec Exp:** Gastrointestinal Cancer; Pancreatic Surgery; Cancer Surgery; **Hospital:** City of Hope Natl Med Ctr & Beckman Rsch (page 69), Huntington Memorial Hosp; **Address:** City of Hope Med Ctr, 1500 E Duarte Rd, Duarte, CA 91010; **Phone:** 626-471-7100; **Board Cert:** Surgery 2000; **Med School:** Boston Univ 1984; **Resid:** Surgery, Univ Cincinnati Hosp 1991; **Fellow:** Surgical Oncology, Meml Sloan-Kettering Cancer Ctr 1993

Esserman, Laura J MD [S] - **Spec Exp:** Breast Cancer; **Hospital:** UCSF - Mt Zion Med Ctr, UCSF Med Ctr; **Address:** UCSF-Helen Diller Family Comp Cancer Ctr, 1600 Divisadero St Fl 2, Box 1710, San Francisco, CA 94115; **Phone:** 415-353-7070; **Board Cert:** Surgery 2001; **Med School:** Stanford Univ 1983; **Resid:** Surgery, Stanford Univ Med Ctr 1991; **Fellow:** Oncology, Stanford Univ Med Ctr 1988; **Fac Appt:** Assoc Prof S, UCSF

Essner, Richard MD [S] - **Spec Exp:** Sentinel Node Surgery; Melanoma; Gastrointestinal Surgery; **Hospital:** St John's Hlth Ctr, Santa Monica, Century City Hosp; **Address:** John Wayne Cancer Inst, 2336 Santa Monica Blvd, Ste 206, Santa Monica, CA 90404-2302; **Phone:** 310-696-0716; **Board Cert:** Surgery 2002; **Med School:** Emory Univ 1985; **Resid:** Surgery, Univ NC Hosps 1992; **Fac Appt:** Asst Clin Prof S, USC Sch Med

Giuliano, Armando E MD [S] - **Spec Exp:** Breast Cancer; Thyroid & Parathyroid Surgery; **Hospital:** St John's Hlth Ctr, Santa Monica, UCLA Ronald Reagan Med Ctr; **Address:** John Wayne Cancer Inst, 2200 Santa Monica Blvd, Santa Monica, CA 90404; **Phone:** 310-829-8089; **Board Cert:** Surgery 1999; **Med School:** Univ Chicago-Pritzker Sch Med 1973; **Resid:** Surgery, UCSF Med Ctr 1980; **Fellow:** Surgical Oncology, UCLA Med Ctr 1978; **Fac Appt:** Prof S, UCLA

Goodnight, James E MD [S] - **Spec Exp:** Melanoma; Breast Cancer; Bone & Soft Tissue Tumors; **Hospital:** UC Davis Med Ctr; **Address:** 4610 X St, Ste 3101, Sacramento, CA 95817; **Phone:** 916-703-5569; **Board Cert:** Surgery 2007; **Med School:** Baylor Coll Med 1968; **Resid:** Surgery, Univ Utah Hosp 1976; **Fellow:** Surgical Oncology, UCLA Med Ctr 1978; **Fac Appt:** Prof S, UC Davis

Goodson III, William H MD [S] - **Spec Exp:** Breast Cancer; **Hospital:** CA Pacific Med Ctr - Pacific Campus, UCSF - Mt Zion Med Ctr; **Address:** 2100 Webster St, Ste 401, San Francisco, CA 94115-2378; **Phone:** 415-923-3925; **Board Cert:** Surgery 2006; **Med School:** Harvard Med Sch 1971; **Resid:** Surgery, Univ Hosps 1976; Surgery, Childrens Hosp 1977

Johnson, Denise L MD [S] - **Spec Exp:** Melanoma; Breast Cancer; **Hospital:** Stanford Univ Med Ctr; **Address:** Stanford Univ Med Ctr-Dept Surgery, 300 Pasteur Drive, Ste H3680, MC 5655, Stanford, CA 94305; **Phone:** 650-723-5672; **Board Cert:** Surgery 2001; **Med School:** Washington Univ, St Louis 1978; **Resid:** Surgery, Univ Illinois Med Ctr 1986; Immunology, Univ Texas SW Med Ctr 1982; **Fellow:** Surgical Oncology, City of Hope Med Ctr 1989; **Fac Appt:** Assoc Prof S, Stanford Univ

Karlan, Scott R MD [S] - **Spec Exp:** Breast Cancer & Surgery; **Hospital:** Cedars-Sinai Med Ctr; **Address:** 310 N San Vicente Blvd Fl 3, Los Angeles, CA 90048; **Phone:** 310-423-9331; **Board Cert:** Surgery 2005; **Med School:** Harvard Med Sch 1982; **Resid:** Surgery, Yale-New Haven Hosp 1987; **Fac Appt:** Clin Prof S, UCLA

Kaufman, Cary S MD [S] - **Spec Exp:** Breast Cancer; **Hospital:** St Joseph Hosp - Bellingham; **Address:** 2940 Squalicum Pkwy, Ste 101, Bellingham, WA 98225; **Phone:** 360-671-9877; **Board Cert:** Surgery 2000; **Med School:** UCLA 1973; **Resid:** Surgery, Univ Wash Med Ctr 1975; Surgery, Harbor-UCLA Med Ctr 1979; **Fac Appt:** Asst Clin Prof S, Univ Wash

Klein, Andrew S MD [S] - **Spec Exp:** Transplant-Liver; Liver Cancer; **Hospital:** Cedars-Sinai Med Ctr; **Address:** Liver & Transplant Ctr at Cedars-Sinai, 8635 W Third St, Ste 590W, Los Angeles, CA 90048; **Phone:** 310-423-2641; **Board Cert:** Surgery 2007; **Med School:** Johns Hopkins Univ 1979; **Resid:** Surgery, Johns Hopkins Hosp 1982; Surgery, Johns Hopkins Hosp 1986; **Fellow:** Transplant Surgery, UCLA-CHS 1988; **Fac Appt:** Clin Prof S, UCLA

Knudson, Mary Margaret MD [S] - **Spec Exp:** Breast Cancer; **Hospital:** UCSF Med Ctr, San Francisco Genl Hosp; **Address:** 1001 Potrero Ave, Ste 3A, San Francisco, CA 94110; **Phone:** 415-206-4623; **Board Cert:** Surgery 2002; Surgical Critical Care 1998; **Med School:** Univ Mich Med Sch 1976; **Resid:** Surgery, Beth Israel Hosp 1979; Surgery, Univ Mich Med Ctr 1982; **Fellow:** Pediatric Surgery, Stanford Univ Hosps 1983; **Fac Appt:** Assoc Prof S, UCSF

Moossa, AR MD [S] - **Spec Exp:** Pancreatic Cancer; Gastrointestinal Cancer; Hepatobiliary Surgery; **Hospital:** UCSD Med Ctr; **Address:** 9300 Campus Point Drive, MC 7212, La Jolla, CA 92037; **Phone:** 858-657-6113; **Med School:** England, UK 1965; **Resid:** Surgery, Liverpool Univ Hosps 1970; **Fellow:** Surgical Oncology, Johns Hopkins Hosp 1972; **Fac Appt:** Prof S, UCSD

Nakakura, Eric MD/PhD [S] - **Spec Exp:** Pancreatic Cancer; Liver Cancer; Gastrointestinal Cancer; Sarcoma; **Hospital:** UCSF Med Ctr; **Address:** 1600 Divisadero St Fl 4 - rm 4202, San Francisco, CA 94115; **Phone:** 415-353-9888; **Board Cert:** Surgery 2004; **Med School:** Stanford Univ 1995; **Resid:** Surgery, Johns Hopkins Hosp 2000; **Fellow:** Surgical Oncology, Johns Hopkins Hosp 2004; **Fac Appt:** Asst Prof S, UCSF

Nissen, Nicholas N MD [S] - **Spec Exp:** Liver Cancer; Transplant-Liver; Pancreatic Cancer; Minimally Invasive Surgery; **Hospital:** Cedars-Sinai Med Ctr; **Address:** Cedars-Sinai Medical Center, 8635 W 3rd St, Ste 590-W, Los Angeles, CA 90048; **Phone:** 310-423-2641; **Board Cert:** Surgery 1999; Surgical Critical Care 1999; **Med School:** Univ Minn 1991; **Resid:** Surgery, Loyola Univ Med Ctr 1998; **Fellow:** Surgical Critical Care, Univ Pittsburgh Med Ctr 1999; Hepatobiliary Surgery, UCLA Med Ctr 2001

Surgery

Norton, Jeffrey A MD [S] - **Spec Exp:** Pancreatic Cancer; Gastrointestinal Cancer & Surgery; Endocrine Surgery; **Hospital:** Stanford Univ Med Ctr; **Address:** 875 Blake Wilbur Drive, Clinic F, Stanford, CA 94305; **Phone:** 650-723-5461; **Board Cert:** Surgery 2001; **Med School:** SUNY Upstate Med Univ 1973; **Resid:** Surgery, Duke Univ Med Ctr 1982; **Fellow:** Research, Natl Cancer Inst 1989; **Fac Appt:** Prof S, Stanford Univ

Paz, Isaac Benjamin MD [S] - **Spec Exp:** Breast Cancer; Esophageal Cancer; **Hospital:** City of Hope Natl Med Ctr & Beckman Rsch (page 69); **Address:** 209 S Fair Oaks Ave, South Pasadena, CA 91030; **Phone:** 626-256-4673 x67100; **Board Cert:** Surgery 2000; **Med School:** Chile 1981; **Resid:** Surgery, Univ Catolica de Chile 1985; Surgery, Univ Arizona 1990; **Fellow:** Surgical Oncology, City of Hope Med Ctr 1993

Pellegrini, Carlos MD [S] - **Spec Exp:** Esophageal Cancer; Esophageal Surgery; Gastrointestinal Cancer & Surgery; Minimally Invasive Surgery; **Hospital:** Univ Wash Med Ctr; **Address:** Univ Washington Medical Ctr, Dept Surgery, 1959 NE Pacific St, Box 356165, Seattle, WA 98195; **Phone:** 206-598-4477; **Board Cert:** Surgery 1998; **Med School:** Argentina 1971; **Resid:** Surgery, Granadero Hosp 1975; Surgery, Univ Chicago Hosps 1979; **Fac Appt:** Prof S, Univ Wash

Peterson, Laura D MD [S] - **Spec Exp:** Breast Cancer; **Hospital:** Kapiolani Med Ctr for Women & Chldn; **Address:** Kapi'olani Womens Ctr, 1907 S Beretania St, Ste 501, Honolulu, HI 96826; **Phone:** 808-949-3444; **Board Cert:** Surgery 2004; **Med School:** UCSD 1998; **Resid:** Surgery, UCSD Med Ctr 2004

Reber, Howard A MD [S] - **Spec Exp:** Pancreatic Cancer; Gastrointestinal Cancer; **Hospital:** UCLA Ronald Reagan Med Ctr; **Address:** UCLA General Surgery, Box 956904, Los Angeles, CA 90095-6904; **Phone:** 310-825-4976; **Board Cert:** Surgery 1971; **Med School:** Univ Pennsylvania 1964; **Resid:** Surgery, Hosp Univ Penn 1970; **Fac Appt:** Prof S, UCLA

Silverstein, Melvin J MD [S] - **Spec Exp:** Breast Cancer; **Hospital:** Hoag Meml Hosp Presby; **Address:** 1 Hoag Drive, Breast Care Ctr, Newport Beach, CA 92658; **Phone:** 949-764-8281; **Board Cert:** Surgery 1971; **Med School:** Albany Med Coll 1965; **Resid:** Surgery, Boston City Hosp-Tufts Univ 1970; **Fellow:** Surgical Oncology, UCLA Med Ctr 1975

Sinanan, Mika N MD [S] - **Spec Exp:** Gastrointestinal Surgery; Gastrointestinal Cancer; Liver & Biliary Cancer; Laparoscopic Surgery; **Hospital:** Univ Wash Med Ctr; **Address:** Univ Washington, Dept Surgery, 1959 NE Pacific St, Box 356165, Seattle, WA 98195-6410; **Phone:** 206-598-7915; **Board Cert:** Surgery 1998; **Med School:** Johns Hopkins Univ 1980; **Resid:** Surgery, Univ Washington Hosp 1988; **Fellow:** Gastrointestinal Surgery, Univ Brit Columbia Med Ctr 1986; **Fac Appt:** Prof S, Univ Wash

Traverso, L William MD [S] - **Spec Exp:** Pancreatic Cancer; Laparoscopic Surgery; **Hospital:** Virginia Mason Med Ctr; **Address:** Virginia Mason Med Ctr, Dept Surg, 1100 9th Ave, Seattle, WA 98101; **Phone:** 206-223-8855; **Board Cert:** Surgery 1998; **Med School:** UCLA 1973; **Resid:** Surgery, UCLA Med Ctr 1978; **Fac Appt:** Clin Prof S, Univ Wash

Trisal, Vijay MD [S] - **Spec Exp:** Skin Cancer; **Hospital:** City of Hope Natl Med Ctr & Beckman Rsch (page 69); **Address:** 1500 E Duarte Rd, Duarte, CA 91010; **Phone:** 626-256-4673 x67100; **Board Cert:** Surgery 2003; **Med School:** India 1993; **Resid:** Surgery, Providence Hosp & Med Ctrs 2002; **Fellow:** Surgical Oncology, City of Hope Natl Med Ctr 2004

Vetto, John MD [S] - **Spec Exp:** Cancer Surgery; **Hospital:** OR Hlth & Sci Univ; **Address:** 3181 SW Sam Jackson Park Rd, MC L619, Portland, OR 97239; **Phone:** 503-494-5501; **Board Cert:** Surgery 2000; **Med School:** Oregon Hlth Sci Univ 1982; **Resid:** Surgery, Brigham & Women's Hosp 1984; Surgery, UCLA Med Ctr 1989; **Fellow:** Surgical Oncology, Natl Cancer Inst 1986; Surgical Oncology, Meml Sloan Kettering Cancer Ctr 1991; **Fac Appt:** Assoc Prof S, Oregon Hlth Sci Univ

Wagman, Lawrence D MD [S] - **Spec Exp:** Liver Cancer; Gastrointestinal Cancer; Breast Cancer; **Hospital:** St Joseph's Hosp - Orange, City of Hope Natl Med Ctr & Beckman Rsch (page 69); **Address:** Ctr for Cancer Prevention & Treatment, 1000 W La Veta Ave, Orange, CA 92868; **Phone:** 714-734-6215; **Board Cert:** Surgery 2004; **Med School:** Columbia P&S 1978; **Resid:** Surgery, Med Coll Virginia Hosp 1985; **Fellow:** Surgical Oncology, NIH/NCI 1982; **Fac Appt:** Assoc Clin Prof S, UCSD

Wallace, Anne Marie MD [S] - **Spec Exp:** Breast Cancer; Breast Reconstruction; Melanoma; **Hospital:** UCSD Med Ctr; **Address:** UCSD Moores Cancer Ctr, 3855 Health Sciences Drive, La Jolla, CA 92093; **Phone:** 858-822-6193; **Board Cert:** Surgery 2001; Plastic Surgery 2005; **Med School:** Creighton Univ 1987; **Resid:** Surgery, Washington Hosp Ctr 1992; Plastic Surgery, UCSD Med Ctr 1994; **Fellow:** Surgical Breast Oncology, MD Anderson Cancer Ctr 1995; **Fac Appt:** Clin Prof S, UCSD

Warren, Robert Samuel MD [S] - **Spec Exp:** Liver Cancer; **Hospital:** UCSF Med Ctr; **Address:** UCSF Comprehensive Cancer Center, 1600 Divisadero St Fl 4, San Francisco, CA 94115; **Phone:** 415-353-9846; **Board Cert:** Surgery 1998; **Med School:** Univ Minn 1980; **Resid:** Surgery, Univ Minn Hosps 1988; **Fellow:** Surgical Oncology, Meml Sloan-Kettering Cancer Ctr 1986; **Fac Appt:** Prof S, UCSF

Yeung, Raymond S W MD [S] - **Spec Exp:** Liver & Biliary Cancer; Liver Cancer; Melanoma; Breast Cancer; **Hospital:** Univ Wash Med Ctr; **Address:** Univ of Washington, Dept Surgery, 1959 NE Pacific St, Box 356165, Seattle, WA 98195; **Phone:** 202-598-4477; **Board Cert:** Surgery 1999; **Med School:** Univ Toronto 1982; **Resid:** Surgery, University of Toronto 1987; **Fellow:** Surgical Oncology, Fox Chase Cancer Ctr 1992; **Fac Appt:** Prof S, Univ Wash

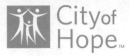

City of Hope

1500 East Duarte Road
Duarte, CA 91010
800-826-HOPE cityofhope.org

City of Hope is a recognized worldwide leader for its compassionate patient care, innovative science and translational research, which rapidly turn laboratory breakthroughs into promising new therapies. One of only 40 National Cancer Institute-designated Comprehensive Cancer Centers nationwide and a founding member of the National Comprehensive Cancer Network, City of Hope is ranked as one of "America's Best Hospitals" in cancer and urology by *U.S.News & World Report*.

ACADEMIC AND CLINICAL AFFILIATIONS

As an independent academic institution, City of Hope enables its researchers to pursue all avenues of scientific inquiry while encouraging collaboration with other researchers and institutions around the world. This helps to speed the development of novel cancer therapies. City of Hope's Graduate School of Biological Sciences also provides a fertile academic environment to prepare future scientists for careers in academia, medical and industrial fields.

MEDICAL STAFF

Guided by a humanistic approach to medicine, nationally recognized physicians and nurses lead collaborative treatment teams that address the whole patient, not just the disease, including emotional, psychological, spiritual and nutritional needs.

PIONEERING, COMPREHENSIVE MEDICAL CARE

City of Hope's Helford Clinical Research Hospital integrates the best of science and human caring in one state-of-the-art facility. There, lifesaving research and superior clinical care join forces as multidisciplinary teams of medical professionals pool their knowledge to bring promising new therapies to patients quickly, safely and effectively.

PHYSICIAN REFERRAL

City of Hope welcomes patient referrals from physicians throughout the world. Referring physicians are encouraged to contact our specialists directly or call 800-826-HOPE.

CENTER OF EXCELLENCE: SURGERY

As a recognized leader in the field of laparoscopic and robotic-assisted surgery, City of Hope uses the most advanced *da Vinci*® robotic system. Guided by skilled surgeons, da Vinci goes beyond the reach of humans and performs with greater precision, removing tumors without disturbing the healthy tissue around them. The result is less blood loss, minimal discomfort and faster recovery times. Robotic-assisted surgery is used for many cancers, including colon, kidney, liver, lung and prostate cancer.

To learn more, visit cityofhope.org/davinci

Cleveland Clinic

Recognized Leader in Breast Health

At Cleveland Clinic Taussig Cancer Institute, more than 250 cancer specialists, researchers, nurses and technicians are dedicated to developing and applying the latest and most effective medical techniques to achieve the long-term survival and improve the quality of life for 7,500 new cancer patients every year. Because of our patient-centered care, leading-edge treatments, innovative research, 350 clinical trials and state-of-the-art medical technologies, *U.S.News & World Report* has ranked Cleveland Clinic's cancer program one of the top cancer centers in the nation.

Working in multidisciplinary teams, Taussig Cancer Institute specialists and Cleveland Clinic Breast Center physicians use innovative therapies for breast cancer, including treatments that may reduce the risk of onset or progression of the disease. **To schedule an appointment or get a second opinion, call 866.223.8100 today or visit clevelandclinic.org/breastTCD.**

Treatment with Image-Guided Radiation Therapy and Hyperthermia

Patients undergoing radiation treatment for early-stage breast cancer treatment may benefit from more accurate targeting of the treatment area with Clarity (TM) Breast System, an image guided radiation therapy (IRGT) system that more accurately locates the treatment area for potentially fewer side effects and no additional risks to patients.

For recurrent breast cancer, hyperthermia, a non-invasive method of increasing tumor temperature to stimulate blood flow, increase oxygenation and render tumor cells more sensitive to radiation, is an option to treat tumors located within a few centimeters of the surface of the body.

Detection and Diagnosis

Patients have access to the latest breast imaging capabilities, including digital mammography, expert interpretation by dedicated breast imaging physicians and special care for high-risk patients.

Breast Center specialists use breast magnetic resonance imaging to complement existing screening, diagnostic and surgical strategies. Breast MRI is used to stage newly diagnosed patients, particularly those with dense breast tissue; to evaluate women with a history of breast cancer, especially those who have had breast conservation surgery; and to assess patients when diagnostic results are inconclusive.

Treatment and Reconstruction

The Breast Center offers patients the latest treatments for breast cancer, including the latest state-of-the-art techniques and reconstructive surgery performed alone or together with therapeutic cancer surgery; including a nipple-sparing procedure that allows for a more natural looking breast reconstruction and DIEP (Deep Inferior Epigastric Perforator) that allows the patient to use their own tissue for reconstruction. Patients who undergo radiation therapy are fitted with a unique device developed at Cleveland Clinic that shields the opposite breast from scatter radiation.

Additional treatments include partial breast irradiation and neo-adjuvant chemotherapy. What's more, we have been leaders in developing circulating tumor cell assays to treat breast cancer and we offer comprehensive genetic counseling for breast cancer patients. For patients with more advanced breast cancer, our physicians and scientists are at the forefront of clinical trials and anti-cancer drug development.

To schedule an appointment or for more information about the Cleveland Clinic Taussig Cancer Institute, call 866.223.8100 or visit clevelandclinic.org/breastTCD.

Cleveland Clinic Taussig Cancer Institute | Cleveland, OH

FOX CHASE
CANCER CENTER

333 Cottman Avenue
Philadelphia, PA 19111-2497
Phone: 1-888-FOX CHASE
www.fccc.edu

SURGICAL ONCOLOGY

The most experienced surgical oncologists have the best treatment outcomes. At Fox Chase, our surgeons are fellowship-trained, meaning they have one to three years of additional training in the highly complex techniques of cancer surgery. They focus entirely on cancer care, including a wide variety of options from minimally invasive approaches to complex plastic and reconstructive surgery.

Breast Cancer: We offer the most advanced diagnostic techniques, including digital mammography, stereotactic breast biopsy and sentinel lymph-node surgery. Treatment options include breast-preserving surgery with radiation therapy as well as skin-sparing mastectomy with cosmetic reconstructive surgery.

Gastrointestinal Cancers: Our gastrointestinal surgeons have extensive expertise with colorectal, pancreatic, gallbladder, liver and other bowel cancers and are the most experienced laparoscopic and robotic experts in the region. We also offer the most advanced endoscopic and minimally invasive techniques to avoid major surgery.

Genitourinary Cancers: Our urologic surgical oncologists have extensive expertise in the treatment of prostate, bladder, kidney, ureteral, adrenal, testicular and penile cancers. Our urologists emphasize organ preservation, quality of life and minimally invasive/robotic approaches to cancer surgery.

Gynecologic Cancers: Our gynecologic surgeons offer the most advanced laparoscopic and robotic techniques as well as complex open surgery for women with cancers of the uterus, ovary and cervix.

Head and Neck Cancers: The head and neck cancer center at Fox Chase provides patients with one-stop consultations with surgical, radiation and medical oncologists. Expertise includes otolaryngology, transoral laser surgery, plastic and microvascular reconstruction as well as robotic surgery.

Lung and Esophageal Cancers: Our thoracic surgeons offer a variety of minimally invasive techniques for patients with lung and esophageal cancers, including video-assisted thoracic surgery (VATS) and laparoscopic esophageal surgery. Fox Chase is one of only a few centers in the country offering these options.

Minimally Invasive Surgery

At Fox Chase, we offer the broadest range of minimally invasive treatment options for your cancer. Our highly skilled surgeons specialize in da Vinci robot-assisted surgery for more types of cancers than other hospitals across the country. This includes prostate, gynecologic, kidney, bladder, colon, lung, and head and neck cancers. In addition, Fox Chase is one of only a few places in the nation to offer advanced laparoscopic and minimally invasive techniques for patients with cancers of the liver, pancreas, bile ducts, and gallbladder.

For more about Fox Chase physicians and services, visit our web site, www.fccc.edu, or call 1-888-FOX CHASE.

442

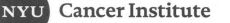

NYU Cancer Institute

NYU LANGONE MEDICAL CENTER

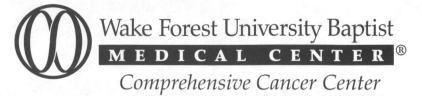

Wake Forest University Baptist
MEDICAL CENTER ®
Comprehensive Cancer Center
Breast Cancer Center of Excellence

Medical Center Boulevard • Winston-Salem, NC 27157
PAL® (Physician-to-physician calls) 1-800-277-7654
Health On-Call® (Patient access) 1-800-446-2255
www.wfubmc.edu/cancer/

OVERVIEW

In 1996, the cross-programmatic nature of breast cancer research at Wake Forest Baptist was formally recognized, and the Breast Cancer Center of Excellence was established to facilitate collaboration among the Cancer Center's four programs.

RESEARCH

The Breast Cancer Center of Excellence takes a multidisciplinary, comprehensive approach involving basic scientists, public health scientists and clinicians. Areas of emphasis at the Center include breast carcinogenesis (what causes cells to mutate into cancer cells), breast cancer risk assessment and prevention, novel modes of breast imaging and quality of life issues for breast cancer patients. The clinical arm is mediated via the Breast Care Center, which has enabled us to initiate a variety of translational research projects.

MULTIDISCIPLINARY CARE

Breast Care Center — As the area's only truly multidisciplinary breast care program, the Center consolidates the services of a multidisciplinary team in a central location so the patient can be seen by multiple specialists during a single visit. With a pathology laboratory located in the clinic, they can provide "on the spot" diagnosis.

The team includes surgical oncologists, radiologists, medical and radiation oncologists, plastic surgeons, pathologists, specialty nurses and genetic counselors.

In most cases, by the end of the day the patient leaves with a ***comprehensive*** treatment plan in place, thus reducing the stressful period between the diagnosis of breast cancer and the beginning of treatment. This also decreases the number of visits to the medical center required to set up complex multimodality care.

In addition to receiving the latest advances in treatment such as sentinel lymph node mapping, breast conserving surgery, immediate breast reconstruction and radiation implants, patients have access to the latest clinical trials on breast cancer treatment and prevention.

The Center's extensive laboratory research programs in breast cancer allow for rapid translation of research from the lab to the clinic. Patients benefit from clinical trials assessing the most up-to-date approaches in the prevention, diagnosis, treatment, and follow-up of breast cancer, so both doctors and their patients make informed decisions.

Genetic screening is available for those who are concerned about hereditary risk factors. Patients who are at high risk may elect to participate in breast cancer prevention trials.

To make an appointment or find a specialist at Wake Forest University Baptist Medical Center, call Health On-Call® 1-800-446-2255.

KNOWLEDGE MAKES ALL THE DIFFERENCE.

Thoracic Surgery

A thoracic surgeon provides the operative, perioperative care and critical care of patients with pathologic conditions within the chest. Included is the surgical care of coronary artery disease, cancers of the lung, esophagus and chest wall, abnormalities of the trachea, abnormalities of the great vessels and heart valves, congenital anomalies, tumors of the mediastinum and diseases of the diaphragm. The management of the airway and injuries of the chest is within the scope of the specialty.

Thoracic surgeons have the knowledge, experience and technical skills to accurately diagnose, operate upon safely and effectively manage patients with thoracic diseases of the chest. This requires substantial knowledge of cardiorespiratory physiology and oncology, as well as capability in the use of heart assist devices, management of abnormal heart rhythms and drainage of the chest cavity, respiratory support systems, endoscopy and invasive and noninvasive diagnostic techniques.

Training Required: Six to eight years

THORACIC SURGERY

New England

Bueno, Raphael MD [TS] - **Spec Exp:** Lung Cancer; **Hospital:** Brigham & Women's Hosp, Dana-Farber Cancer Inst; **Address:** Brigham and Women's Hospital, 75 Francis St, Division of Thoracic Surgery Clin, Boston, MA 02115; **Phone:** 617-732-6824; **Board Cert:** Thoracic Surgery 2006; Surgery 2002; Surgical Critical Care 2003; **Med School:** Harvard Med Sch 1985; **Resid:** Surgery, Brigham & Women's Hosp 1992; **Fellow:** Surgical Critical Care, Brigham & Women's Hosp 1993; Cardiothoracic Surgery, Mass Genl Hosp 1997; **Fac Appt:** Assoc Prof S, Harvard Med Sch

Gaissert, Henning A MD [TS] - **Spec Exp:** Esophageal Cancer; Tracheal Surgery; Lung Cancer; **Hospital:** Mass Genl Hosp; **Address:** Division of Thoracic Surgery, 55 Fruit St, BLK 1570, Boston, MA 02114; **Phone:** 617-726-5341; **Board Cert:** Surgery 2001; Thoracic Surgery 2004; **Med School:** Germany 1984; **Resid:** Surgery, Mass Genl Hosp 1989; Surgery, Barnes Jewish Hosp 1991; **Fellow:** Research, Harvard Med Sch 1993; Cardiothoracic Surgery, Barnes Jewish Hosp 1996; **Fac Appt:** Assoc Prof S, Harvard Med Sch

Mathisen, Douglas MD [TS] - **Spec Exp:** Tracheal Surgery; Lung Cancer; Esophageal Cancer; **Hospital:** Mass Genl Hosp, Newton - Wellesley Hosp; **Address:** Mass Genl Hosp, Dept Thor Surg, 55 Fruit St, Blake 1570, Boston, MA 02114; **Phone:** 617-726-6826; **Board Cert:** Thoracic Surgery 2002; **Med School:** Univ IL Coll Med 1974; **Resid:** Surgery, Mass Genl Hosp 1981; Thoracic Surgery, Mass Genl Hosp 1982; **Fellow:** Surgical Oncology, Natl Cancer Inst 1979; **Fac Appt:** Prof S, Harvard Med Sch

Nugent, William C MD [TS] - **Spec Exp:** Thoracic Cancers; **Hospital:** Dartmouth - Hitchcock Med Ctr; **Address:** Dartmouth-Hitchcock Med Ctr, Dept Cardiothoracic Surgery, 1 Medical Center Drive, Lebanon, NH 03756-1000; **Phone:** 603-650-8572; **Board Cert:** Thoracic Surgery 2002; **Med School:** Albany Med Coll 1975; **Resid:** Surgery, Beth Israel Hosp 1980; Thoracic Surgery, Univ Michigan Med Ctr 1983; **Fellow:** Cardiothoracic Surgery, Mass Genl Hosp 1981; **Fac Appt:** Prof S, Dartmouth Med Sch

Sugarbaker, David J MD [TS] - **Spec Exp:** Mesothelioma; Transplant-Lung; Esophageal Cancer; **Hospital:** Brigham & Women's Hosp, Dana-Farber Cancer Inst; **Address:** Brigham & Women's Hosp, 75 Francis St, Division of Thoracic Surgery, Boston, MA 02115-6110; **Phone:** 617-732-6824; **Board Cert:** Thoracic Surgery 1999; **Med School:** Cornell Univ-Weill Med Coll 1979; **Resid:** Surgery, Brigham & Women's Hosp 1982; Surgery, Brigham & Women's Hosp 1986; **Fellow:** Thoracic Surgery, Toronto Genl Hosp 1988; **Fac Appt:** Prof S, Harvard Med Sch

Swanson, Scott J MD [TS] - **Spec Exp:** Lung Cancer; Video Assisted Thoracic Surgery (VATS); Esophageal Cancer; **Hospital:** Brigham & Women's Hosp, Dana-Farber Cancer Inst; **Address:** Div Thoracic Surgery, Brigham & Women's Hosp, 75 Francis St, Boston, MA 02115; **Phone:** 617-525-7532; **Board Cert:** Surgery 2003; Thoracic Surgery 2006; **Med School:** Harvard Med Sch 1985; **Resid:** Surgery, Brigham & Womens Hosp 1990; **Fellow:** Cardiothoracic Surgery, Brigham & Womens Hosp 1994

Wain, John MD [TS] - **Spec Exp:** Lung Cancer; Esophageal Cancer; **Hospital:** Mass Genl Hosp; **Address:** Mass Genl Hosp, Dept Thoracic Surg, 55 Fruit St, Blake 1570, Boston, MA 02114; **Phone:** 617-726-5200; **Board Cert:** Thoracic Surgery 2000; **Med School:** Jefferson Med Coll 1980; **Resid:** Surgery, Mass Genl Hosp 1985; **Fellow:** Cardiothoracic Surgery, Mass Genl Hosp 1988; **Fac Appt:** Asst Prof TS, Harvard Med Sch

Wright, Cameron D MD [TS] - **Spec Exp:** Lung Cancer; Esophageal Cancer; Tracheal Surgery; **Hospital:** Mass Genl Hosp; **Address:** Mass Genl Hosp, Div Thoracic Surg, 55 Fruit St, Blake 1570, Boston, MA 02114-2696; **Phone:** 617-726-5801; **Board Cert:** Surgery 2006; Thoracic Surgery 2007; **Med School:** Univ Mich Med Sch 1980; **Resid:** Surgery, Mass Genl Hosp 1986; Thoracic Surgery, Mass Genl Hosp 1988; **Fac Appt:** Assoc Prof S, Harvard Med Sch

Mid Atlantic

Altorki, Nasser MD [TS] - **Spec Exp:** Esophageal Cancer; Lung Cancer; Thoracic Cancers; Vaccine Therapy; **Hospital:** NY-Presby Hosp/Weill Cornell (page 79); **Address:** 525 E 68th St, New York, NY 10021-4870; **Phone:** 212-746-5156; **Board Cert:** Surgery 2006; Thoracic Surgery 1998; **Med School:** Egypt 1978; **Resid:** Surgery, Univ Chicago Hosps 1985; **Fellow:** Cardiothoracic Surgery, Univ Chicago Hosps 1987; **Fac Appt:** Prof S, Cornell Univ-Weill Med Coll

Bains, Manjit MD [TS] - **Spec Exp:** Esophageal Cancer; Lung Cancer; **Hospital:** Meml Sloan-Kettering Cancer Ctr (page 76); **Address:** 1275 York Avenue, New York, NY 10065; **Phone:** 800-525-2225; **Board Cert:** Surgery 1971; Thoracic Surgery 1972; **Med School:** India 1963; **Resid:** Surgery, Rochester Genl Hosp 1970; **Fellow:** Thoracic Surgery, Sloan Kettering Cancer Ctr 1972; **Fac Appt:** Clin Prof S, Cornell Univ-Weill Med Coll

Battafarano, Richard J MD [TS] - **Spec Exp:** Lung Cancer; Barrett's Esophagus; Esophageal Surgery; Mesothelioma; **Hospital:** Barnes-Jewish Hosp; **Address:** Univ MD Med Ctr, Greenebaum Cancer Ctr-Dept Thoracic Surgery, 22 S Greeene St, Baltimore, MD 21210; **Phone:** 410-328-6366; **Board Cert:** Surgery 1998; Thoracic Surgery 2000; **Med School:** Hahnemann Univ 1988; **Resid:** Surgery, Univ Minn Hosp & Clin 1997; **Fellow:** Thoracic Surgery, Meml Sloan Kettering Cancer Ctr 1999; **Fac Appt:** Assoc Prof S, Univ MD Sch Med

Demmy, Todd L MD [TS] - **Spec Exp:** Lung Cancer; Thoracic Cancers; Esophageal Cancer; **Hospital:** Roswell Park Cancer Inst, Buffalo General Hosp; **Address:** Roswell Park Cancer Inst, Dept Thoracic Surgery, Elm & Carlton Sts, Buffalo, NY 14263; **Phone:** 716-845-5873; **Board Cert:** Surgery 1997; Thoracic Surgery 2000; Surgical Critical Care 2001; **Med School:** Jefferson Med Coll 1983; **Resid:** Surgery, Baylor Univ Medical Ctr 1988; Thoracic Surgery, Allegheny Genl Hosp 1991; **Fac Appt:** Assoc Prof S, SUNY Buffalo

Friedberg, Joseph MD [TS] - **Spec Exp:** Lung Cancer; Mesothelioma; Photodynamic Therapy; Thoracic Cancers; **Hospital:** Penn Presby Med Ctr - UPHS (page 81), Hosp Univ Penn - UPHS (page 81); **Address:** Penn-Presbyterian Medical Ctr, 51 N 39th St, rm W250, Philadelphia, PA 19104; **Phone:** 215-662-9195; **Board Cert:** Surgery 2006; Thoracic Surgery 2006; **Med School:** Harvard Med Sch 1986; **Resid:** Surgery, Mass General Hosp 1994; **Fellow:** Cardiothoracic Surgery, Brigham & Womens Hosp 1996

Gharagozloo, Farid MD [TS] - **Spec Exp:** Video Assisted Thoracic Surgery (VATS); Lung Cancer; **Hospital:** G Washington Univ Hosp, Harbor Hosp Ctr; **Address:** 2175 K St NW, Ste 300, Washington, DC 20037; **Phone:** 202-775-8600; **Board Cert:** Thoracic Surgery 2001; **Med School:** Johns Hopkins Univ 1983; **Resid:** Surgery, Mayo Clinic 1989; Research, Harvard Med Sch 1986; **Fellow:** Cardiothoracic Surgery, Mayo Clinic 1992; **Fac Appt:** Prof S, Geo Wash Univ

Heitmiller, Richard F MD [TS] - **Spec Exp:** Esophageal Surgery; Esophageal Cancer; Lung Cancer; **Hospital:** Union Meml Hosp-Baltimore; **Address:** 3333 N Calvert St, Ste 610, Baltimore, MD 21218; **Phone:** 410-554-2063; **Board Cert:** Surgery 1997; Thoracic Surgery 1999; **Med School:** Johns Hopkins Univ 1979; **Resid:** Surgery, Mass Genl Hosp 1985; **Fellow:** Thoracic Surgery, Mass Genl Hosp 1987; **Fac Appt:** Assoc Prof Surg & Onc, Johns Hopkins Univ

Thoracic Surgery

Keenan, Robert J MD [TS] - **Spec Exp:** Lung Cancer; Esophageal Cancer; Mediastinal Tumors; **Hospital:** Allegheny General Hosp, Westmoreland Hosp; **Address:** Allegheny Genl Hosp, 14th Fl, 320 E North Ave, Pittsburgh, PA 15212; **Phone:** 412-359-6137; **Board Cert:** Surgery 2000; **Med School:** Canada 1984; **Resid:** Surgery, Univ Toronto Med Ctr 1989; **Fellow:** Thoracic Surgery, Univ Pittsburgh Med Ctr 1990; Thoracic Surgery, Univ Toronto Med Ctr 1991; **Fac Appt:** Prof TS, Drexel Univ Coll Med

Keller, Steven M MD [TS] - **Spec Exp:** Lung Cancer; Esophageal Cancer; **Hospital:** Montefiore Med Ctr - Div. Moses, Montefiore Med Ctr - Div. Weiler; **Address:** Montefiore-Moses Medical Ctr, 3400 Bainbridge Ave Fl 5 - Ste A, Bronx, NY 10467-2404; **Phone:** 718-920-7580; **Board Cert:** Thoracic Surgery 2008; **Med School:** Albany Med Coll 1977; **Resid:** Surgery, Mount Sinai Hosp 1985; Thoracic Surgery, Mem Sloan Kettering Cancer Ctr 1987; **Fellow:** Surgical Oncology, NIH/National Cancer Inst 1983; **Fac Appt:** Prof TS, Albert Einstein Coll Med

Kiev, Jonathan MD [TS] - **Spec Exp:** Chest Wall Tumors; Esophageal Cancer; Lung Cancer; **Hospital:** Anne Arundel Med Ctr; **Address:** Annapolis Thoracic Surgery, 2001 Medical Pkwy, Donner Pavilion, 2nd Fl, Annapolis, MD 21401; **Phone:** 443-481-3300; **Board Cert:** Surgery 2005; Thoracic Surgery 2002; **Med School:** Tulane Univ 1989; **Resid:** Surgery, Hahnemann Univ Hosp 1996; Cardiothoracic Surgery, Loma Linda Univ 2000; **Fellow:** Thoracic Surgery, Univ Pittsburgh 2001; Thoracic Surgery, Mayo Clinic 2001

Krasna, Mark MD [TS] - **Spec Exp:** Esophageal Cancer; Lung Cancer; Mesothelioma; **Hospital:** St Joseph Med Ctr, Univ of MD Med Ctr; **Address:** 7501 Osler Drive Odea Bldg - Ste 204, Towson, MD 21204; **Phone:** 410-427-2220; **Board Cert:** Thoracic Surgery 2000; **Med School:** Israel 1982; **Resid:** Surgery, CMDNJ-Rutgers Med Sch 1988; **Fellow:** Cardiothoracic Surgery, New England Deaconess-Harvard 1990; **Fac Appt:** Prof S, Univ MD Sch Med

Krellenstein, Daniel J MD [TS] - **Spec Exp:** Lung Cancer; Minimally Invasive Thoracic Surgery; **Hospital:** Mount Sinai Med Ctr (page 77), Lenox Hill Hosp; **Address:** 16 E 98th St, Ste 1F, New York, NY 10029-6545; **Phone:** 212-423-9311; **Board Cert:** Surgery 1974; Thoracic Surgery 2006; **Med School:** SUNY Buffalo 1964; **Resid:** Surgery, SUNY Downstate Med Ctr 1972; **Fac Appt:** Assoc Clin Prof TS, Mount Sinai Sch Med

Marshall, Margaret Blair MD [TS] - **Spec Exp:** Lung Cancer; Esophageal Cancer; Thymoma; Chest Wall Tumors; **Hospital:** Georgetown Univ Hosp, Sibley Mem Hosp; **Address:** Georgetown Univ Hosp, 3800 Reservoir Rd NW, 4PHC, Washington, DC 20007; **Phone:** 202-444-5045; **Board Cert:** Surgery 2000; Thoracic Surgery 2002; **Med School:** Georgetown Univ 1991; **Resid:** Surgery, Georgetown Univ Med Ctr 1995; Cardiothoracic Surgery, Hosp Univ Penn 2001; **Fellow:** Research, Chldn's Hosp 1998; **Fac Appt:** Assoc Prof S, Georgetown Univ

Pass, Harvey MD [TS] - **Spec Exp:** Lung Cancer; Mesothelioma; Clinical Trials; **Hospital:** NYU Langone Med Ctr (page 80); **Address:** NYU Cancer Ctr, 160 E 34th St Fl 8, New York, NY 10016; **Phone:** 212-731-5414; **Board Cert:** Thoracic Surgery 2001; **Med School:** Duke Univ 1973; **Resid:** Surgery, Duke Univ Med Ctr 1975; Surgery, Univ Miss Med Ctr 1980; **Fellow:** Cardiothoracic Surgery, MUSC Med Ctr 1982; **Fac Appt:** Prof S, NYU Sch Med

Pierson III, Richard N MD [TS] - **Spec Exp:** Transplant-Lung; Lung Cancer; **Hospital:** Univ of MD Med Ctr; **Address:** Univ Md Med Ctr, Dept Cardiothoracic Surg, 22 S Greene St, rm N4W94, Baltimore, MD 21201; **Phone:** 410-328-5842; **Board Cert:** Surgery 2000; Thoracic Surgery 2002; **Med School:** Columbia P&S 1983; **Resid:** Surgery, Univ Mich Med Ctr 1990; **Fellow:** Cardiothoracic Surgery, Mass General Hosp 1992; **Fac Appt:** Assoc Prof TS, Univ MD Sch Med

Scott, Walter J MD [TS] - **Spec Exp:** Lung Cancer; Esophageal Cancer; Mediastinal Tumors; Minimally Invasive Surgery; **Hospital:** Fox Chase Cancer Ctr (page 72); **Address:** Fox Chase Cancer Ctr, 333 Cottman Ave, rm C308, Philadelphia, PA 19111; **Phone:** 215-214-1427; **Board Cert:** Thoracic Surgery 1998; **Med School:** Univ Chicago-Pritzker Sch Med 1981; **Resid:** Surgery, Univ Chicago Med Ctr 1987; **Fellow:** Cardiothoracic Surgery, Univ Chicago Med Ctr 1989; **Fac Appt:** Assoc Prof TS, Temple Univ

Sonett, Joshua R MD [TS] - **Spec Exp:** Minimally Invasive Thoracic Surgery; Transplant-Lung; Thoracic Cancers; **Hospital:** NY-Presby Hosp/Columbia (page 79); **Address:** 161 Fort Washington Ave, Ste 301, New York, NY 10032; **Phone:** 212-305-8086; **Board Cert:** Surgery 1994; Thoracic Surgery 1997; **Med School:** E Carolina Univ 1988; **Resid:** Surgery, Univ Mass Med Ctr 1993; **Fellow:** Cardiothoracic Surgery, Univ Pittsburgh Med Ctr 1994; Thoracic Surgery, Meml Sloan Kettering Cancer Ctr; **Fac Appt:** Assoc Prof S, Columbia P&S

Watson, Thomas J MD [TS] - **Spec Exp:** Esophageal Cancer; Lung Cancer; **Hospital:** Univ of Rochester Strong Meml Hosp, Highland Hosp of Rochester; **Address:** 601 Elmwood Ave, Box SURG, Rochester, NY 14642; **Phone:** 585-275-1509; **Board Cert:** Thoracic Surgery 2007; Surgery 2003; **Med School:** Univ SC Sch Med 1988; **Resid:** Surgery, LAC-USC Med Ctr 1993; Cardiothoracic Surgery, LAC-USC Med Ctr 1996; **Fellow:** Esophageal Surgery, LAC-USC Med Ctr 1994; **Fac Appt:** Assoc Prof S, Univ Rochester

Weksler, Benny MD [TS] - **Spec Exp:** Thoracic Cancers; Cancer Surgery; Esophageal Cancer; Minimally Invasive Thoracic Surgery; **Hospital:** Thomas Jefferson Univ Hosp (page 83); **Address:** 1025 Walnut St, 607 College, Philadelphia, PA 19107; **Phone:** 215-955-6996; **Board Cert:** Surgery 2007; Thoracic Surgery 2007; **Med School:** Brazil 1987; **Resid:** Surgery, NY Med Coll/ Lincoln Med Ctr 1991; Surgery, NY Med Coll/Lincoln Med Ctr 1995; **Fellow:** Cardiothoracic Surgery, Meml Sloan Kettering Cancer Ctr 1997; Minimally Invasive Surgery, Univ Pittsburgh Med Ctr 2008; **Fac Appt:** Assoc Prof S, Thomas Jefferson Univ

Yang, Stephen C MD [TS] - **Spec Exp:** Mesothelioma; Lung Cancer; Esophageal Cancer; **Hospital:** Johns Hopkins Hosp, Johns Hopkins Bayview Med Ctr; **Address:** Johns Hopkins Hosp, 600 N Wolfe St Blalock Bldg - rm 240, Baltimore, MD 21287-5674; **Phone:** 410-614-3891; **Board Cert:** Surgery 2003; Thoracic Surgery 2005; **Med School:** Med Coll VA 1984; **Resid:** Surgery, Univ Tex Hlth Sci Ctr 1990; **Fellow:** Thoracic Surgery, MD Anderson Cancer Ctr 1992; Cardiothoracic Surgery, Med Coll Virginia 1994; **Fac Appt:** Assoc Prof TS, Johns Hopkins Univ

Southeast

Cerfolio, Robert J MD [TS] - **Spec Exp:** Lung Cancer; Tracheal Surgery; Chest Wall Tumors; Esophageal Cancer; **Hospital:** Univ of Ala Hosp at Birmingham; **Address:** 703 19th St S, Ste 739, Zigler Rsch Bldg, Birmingham, AL 35294-0007; **Phone:** 205-934-5937; **Board Cert:** Surgery 2003; Thoracic Surgery 2006; **Med School:** Univ Rochester 1988; **Resid:** Surgery, Cornell-NY Hosp 1990; Surgery, Mayo Clinic 1993; **Fellow:** Cardiothoracic Surgery, Mayo Clinic 1996; **Fac Appt:** Prof TS, Univ Alabama

D'Amico, Thomas MD [TS] - **Spec Exp:** Lung Cancer; Esophageal Cancer; **Hospital:** Duke Univ Med Ctr; **Address:** Duke Univ Med Ctr, Dept Thoracic Surg, Box 3496, Durham, NC 27710; **Phone:** 919-684-4891; **Board Cert:** Surgery 2004; Thoracic Surgery 2006; **Med School:** Columbia P&S 1987; **Resid:** Surgery, Duke Univ Med Ctr 1989; Cardiothoracic Surgery, Duke Univ Med Ctr 1996; **Fellow:** Thoracic Oncology, Meml Sloan Kettering Cancer Ctr; **Fac Appt:** Assoc Prof S, Duke Univ

Harpole Jr, David H MD [TS] - **Spec Exp:** Lung Cancer; Mesothelioma; Esophageal Cancer; **Hospital:** Duke Univ Med Ctr; **Address:** Duke Univ Med Ctr-Thoracic Surgery, 2424 Erwin Rd, Ste 403 - rm 4071, Durham, NC 27705; **Phone:** 919-668-8413; **Board Cert:** Surgery 2002; Thoracic Surgery 2003; **Med School:** Univ VA Sch Med 1984; **Resid:** Surgery, Duke Univ Med Ctr 1991; **Fellow:** Thoracic Surgery, Duke Univ Med Ctr 1993; **Fac Appt:** Prof S, Duke Univ

Jones, David R MD [TS] - **Spec Exp:** Lung Cancer; Esophageal Cancer; Minimally Invasive Thoracic Surgery; **Hospital:** Univ Virginia Med Ctr; **Address:** Department of Surgery, Box 800679, Charlottesville, VA 22901; **Phone:** 434-243-6443; **Board Cert:** Surgery 2005; Thoracic Surgery 2007; **Med School:** W VA Univ 1989; **Resid:** Surgery, West Va Univ 1995; **Fellow:** Thoracic Surgery, Univ North Carolina 1998; **Fac Appt:** Assoc Prof S, Univ VA Sch Med

Kiernan, Paul D MD [TS] - **Spec Exp:** Lung Cancer; Esophageal Cancer; Mediastinal Tumors; **Hospital:** Inova Fairfax Hosp, Inova Alexandria Hosp; **Address:** 2921 Telestar Court, Falls Church, VA 22042; **Phone:** 703-280-5858; **Board Cert:** Thoracic Surgery 2002; **Med School:** Georgetown Univ 1974; **Resid:** Surgery, Mayo Clinic 1979; Cardiothoracic Surgery, Mayo Clinic 1981; **Fellow:** Vascular Surgery, Mayo Clinic 1982; **Fac Appt:** Assoc Clin Prof S, Georgetown Univ

Miller, Daniel L MD [TS] - **Spec Exp:** Esophageal Cancer; Lung Cancer; Mesothelioma; **Hospital:** Emory Univ Hosp; **Address:** The Emory Clinic, 1365A Clifton Rd NE, Ste 2219, Atlanta, GA 30322; **Phone:** 404-778-3755; **Board Cert:** Thoracic Surgery 2005; Surgery 2001; **Med School:** Univ KY Coll Med 1985; **Resid:** Surgery, Georgetown Univ Hosp 1991; **Fellow:** Cardiothoracic Surgery, Mayo Clinic 1994; **Fac Appt:** Assoc Prof S, Emory Univ

Miller, Joseph I MD [TS] - **Spec Exp:** Lung Cancer; **Hospital:** Emory Univ Hosp, Emory Univ Hosp Midtown; **Address:** 550 Peachtree St NE, MOT-6th Fl, Atlanta, GA 30308; **Phone:** 404-686-2515; **Board Cert:** Surgery 1973; Thoracic Surgery 1975; **Med School:** Emory Univ 1965; **Resid:** Surgery, Mayo Clin 1972; Thoracic Surgery, Emory Univ Hosp 1974; **Fac Appt:** Prof S, Emory Univ

Mullett, Timothy W MD [TS] - **Spec Exp:** Lung Cancer; Esophageal Surgery; **Hospital:** Univ of Kentucky Chandler Hosp; **Address:** 800 Rose St Fl 4th, Lexington, KY 40536; **Phone:** 859-323-1691; **Board Cert:** Thoracic Surgery 1997; Surgery 2005; **Med School:** Univ Fla Coll Med 1987; **Resid:** Surgery, Shands/Univ of FL 1993; **Fellow:** Pediatric Surgery, Shands/Univ of FL 1994; Cardiothoracic Surgery, Shands/Univ of FL 1995; **Fac Appt:** Assoc Prof S, Univ KY Coll Med

Nesbitt, Jonathan C MD [TS] - **Spec Exp:** Lung Cancer; Esophageal Cancer; **Hospital:** Vanderbilt Univ Med Ctr, Saint Thomas Hosp - Nashville; **Address:** The Vanderbilt Clinic, 609 Oxford House, 1313 21st Ave S, Nashville, TN 37232-4682; **Phone:** 615-322-0064; **Board Cert:** Surgery 1998; Thoracic Surgery 1998; **Med School:** Georgetown Univ 1981; **Resid:** Surgery, Vanderbilt Univ Med Ctr 1987; Thoracic Surgery, Albany Med Ctr 1989; **Fac Appt:** Asst Clin Prof S, Vanderbilt Univ

Ninan, Mathews MD [TS] - **Spec Exp:** Lung Cancer; Transplant-Lung; Esophageal Cancer; **Hospital:** Baptist Memorial Hospital - Memphis, Methodist Univ Hosp - Memphis; **Address:** 7945 Wolf River Blvd, Ste 280, Germantown, TN 38138; **Phone:** 901-347-8270; **Med School:** India 1988; **Resid:** Surgery, Univ London Affil Hosp 1994; **Fellow:** Cardiothoracic Surgery, Univ Pittsburgh Affil Hosp 1998; **Fac Appt:** Assoc Prof TS, Vanderbilt Univ

Putnam Jr, Joe B MD [TS] - **Spec Exp:** Lung Cancer; Esophageal Cancer; Sarcoma-Soft Tissue; **Hospital:** Vanderbilt Univ Med Ctr, VA Med Ctr - Nashville; **Address:** Vanderbilt Univ Med Ctr - Thoracic Surgery, 609 Oxford House, 1313 21st Ave S, Nashville, TN 37232-4682; **Phone:** 615-343-9202; **Board Cert:** Thoracic Surgery 2007; **Med School:** Univ NC Sch Med 1979; **Resid:** Surgery, Univ Rochester 1986; Thoracic Surgery, Univ Mich Med Ctr 1988; **Fellow:** Surgical Oncology, NCI/NIH-Surg Branch 1984; **Fac Appt:** Prof TS, Vanderbilt Univ

Reed, Carolyn E MD [TS] - **Spec Exp:** Esophageal Cancer; Lung Cancer; **Hospital:** MUSC Med Ctr; **Address:** Med Univ S Carolina, 25 Courtenay Drive, Ste 7018, Charleston, SC 29425; **Phone:** 843-876-4845; **Board Cert:** Thoracic Surgery 2006; **Med School:** Univ Rochester 1977; **Resid:** Surgery, NY Hosp 1982; Thoracic Surgery, NY Hosp 1985; **Fellow:** Surgical Oncology, Meml Sloan Kettering Cancer Ctr 1983; **Fac Appt:** Prof S, Med Univ SC

Robinson, Lary A MD [TS] - **Spec Exp:** Lung Cancer; Mesothelioma; **Hospital:** H Lee Moffitt Cancer Ctr & Research Inst, Tampa Genl Hosp; **Address:** H Lee Moffitt Cancer Ctr, Div Thoracic Oncology, 12902 Magnolia Drive, Tampa, FL 33612-9497; **Phone:** 813-745-7282; **Board Cert:** Thoracic Surgery 2003; Surgery 2002; Surgical Critical Care 2000; **Med School:** Washington Univ, St Louis 1972; **Resid:** Surgery, Duke Univ Med Ctr 1974; Thoracic Surgery, Duke Univ Med Ctr 1981; **Fellow:** Cardiothoracic Surgery, St Thomas Hosp 1982; Cardiothoracic Surgery, Duke Univ Med Ctr 1983; **Fac Appt:** Prof S, Univ S Fla Coll Med

Zwischenberger, Joseph B MD [TS] - **Spec Exp:** Thoracic Cancers; Lung Cancer; Esophageal Cancer; **Hospital:** Univ of Kentucky Chandler Hosp; **Address:** MN264 A B Chandler Med Ctr, 800 Rose St, Lexington, KY 40536; **Phone:** 859-323-6013; **Board Cert:** Surgery 2002; Thoracic Surgery 2005; Surgical Critical Care 1996; **Med School:** Univ KY Coll Med 1977; **Resid:** Surgery, Univ Michigan Hosp 1984; Cardiothoracic Surgery, Univ Michigan Hosp 1985; **Fellow:** Cardiac Surgery, Natl Inst Hlth 1981; **Fac Appt:** Prof S, Univ KY Coll Med

Midwest

Deschamps, Claude MD [TS] - **Spec Exp:** Esophageal Cancer; Lung Cancer; **Hospital:** St Mary's Hosp - Rochester; **Address:** Mayo Clinic, Div Thoracic Surgery, 200 First St SW, Rochester, MN 55905; **Phone:** 507-284-8462; **Board Cert:** Surgery 2004; **Med School:** Univ Montreal 1979; **Resid:** Surgery, Univ Montreal Hosps 1984; Thoracic Surgery, Univ Montreal Hosps 1985; **Fellow:** Thoracic Surgery, Mayo Clinic 1987; **Fac Appt:** Prof S, Mayo Med Sch

Ferguson, Mark K MD [TS] - **Spec Exp:** Barrett's Esophagus; Esophageal Cancer; Lung Cancer; **Hospital:** Univ of Chicago Med Ctr; **Address:** 5841 S Maryland Ave, MC 5035, Univ Chicago Hosps, Chicago, IL 60637-1470; **Phone:** 773-702-3551; **Board Cert:** Thoracic Surgery 2003; **Med School:** Univ Chicago-Pritzker Sch Med 1977; **Resid:** Surgery, Univ Chicago Hosps 1982; **Fellow:** Cardiothoracic Surgery, Univ Chicago Hosps 1984; **Fac Appt:** Prof S, Univ Chicago-Pritzker Sch Med

Howington, John A MD [TS] - **Spec Exp:** Lung Cancer; Esophageal Cancer; Thymoma; Minimally Invasive Thoracic Surgery; **Hospital:** NorthShore Univ HlthSys, Highland Park/North Shore Univ Hlth Syst; **Address:** Evanston Northwestern Hosp, 2650 Ridge Ave, Walgreen Bldg - Ste 3507, Evanston, IL 60201; **Phone:** 847-570-2868; **Board Cert:** Thoracic Surgery 2006; Surgery 2004; **Med School:** Univ Tenn Coll Med, Memphis 1989; **Resid:** Surgery, Truman Med Ctr/U Missouri 1994; Cardiothoracic Surgery, Vanderbilt Univ Med Ctr 1997; **Fac Appt:** Assoc Prof S, Northwestern Univ

Iannettoni, Mark D MD [TS] - **Spec Exp:** Transplant-Lung; Lung Cancer; Esophageal Surgery; **Hospital:** Univ Iowa Hosp & Clinics; **Address:** Univ Iowa Hosp & Clinics, 200 Hawkins Drive, rm SE514GH, Iowa City, IA 52242; **Phone:** 319-356-1133; **Board Cert:** Surgery 2002; Thoracic Surgery 2002; **Med School:** SUNY Upstate Med Univ 1985; **Resid:** Surgery, SUNY Upstate Med Ctr 1991; Thoracic Surgery, Univ Mich Med Ctr 1993; **Fellow:** Thoracic Surgery, Univ Mich Med Sch 1994

Thoracic Surgery

Maddaus, Michael A MD [TS] - **Spec Exp:** Esophageal Cancer; Lung Cancer; Minimally Invasive Thoracic Surgery; **Hospital:** Univ Minn Med Ctr, Fairview - Univ Campus, Abbott - Northwestern Hosp; **Address:** Div General Thoracic Surgery, 420 Delaware St SE, MMC 207, Minneapolis, MN 55455; **Phone:** 612-624-9461; **Board Cert:** Surgery 2000; Thoracic Surgery 2003; **Med School:** Univ Minn 1982; **Resid:** Surgery, Univ Minn Affil Hosp 1990; Thoracic Surgery, Univ Toronto Affil Hosp 1991; **Fellow:** Cardiac Surgery, St Michael's Hosp/Hosp Sick Chldn 1992; Thoracic Oncology, Meml Sloan Kettering Cancer Ctr 1992; **Fac Appt:** Prof S, Univ Minn

Meyers, Bryan MD [TS] - **Spec Exp:** Lung Cancer; Esophageal Cancer; Transplant-Lung; **Hospital:** Barnes-Jewish Hosp, Barnes-Jewish West County Hosp; **Address:** 4921 Parkview Pl, Ste 8B, St Louis, MO 63110; **Phone:** 314-362-8598; **Board Cert:** Surgery 1998; Thoracic Surgery 1999; **Med School:** Univ Chicago-Pritzker Sch Med 1986; **Resid:** Surgery, Mass Genl Hosp 1996; **Fellow:** Cardiothoracic Surgery, Barnes Hosp-Wash Univ 1998; **Fac Appt:** Assoc Prof S, Washington Univ, St Louis

Naunheim, Keith S MD [TS] - **Spec Exp:** Lung Cancer; Esophageal Cancer; Chest Wall Tumors; Video Assisted Thoracic Surgery (VATS); **Hospital:** St Louis Univ Hosp, SSM St Mary's Hlth Ctr - St Louis; **Address:** St Louis Univ Med Ctr, Dept Surgery, 3635 Vista Ave, St Louis, MO 63110-0250; **Phone:** 314-577-8360; **Board Cert:** Thoracic Surgery 2004; **Med School:** Univ Chicago-Pritzker Sch Med 1978; **Resid:** Surgery, Univ Chicago Hosp 1983; **Fellow:** Cardiothoracic Surgery, Univ Chicago Hosp 1985; **Fac Appt:** Prof S, St Louis Univ

Orringer, Mark B MD [TS] - **Spec Exp:** Esophageal Cancer; Lung Cancer; Mediastinal Tumors; Lung Cancer; **Hospital:** Univ Michigan Hlth Sys; **Address:** Univ Mich, Taubman Ctr, 1500 E Med Ctr Drive, rm TC 2120, Box 0344, Ann Arbor, MI 48109-0344; **Phone:** 734-936-4975; **Board Cert:** Surgery 1973; Thoracic Surgery 1974; **Med School:** Univ Pittsburgh 1967; **Resid:** Thoracic Surgery, Johns Hopkins Hosp 1973; **Fac Appt:** Prof S, Univ Mich Med Sch

Patterson, G Alexander MD [TS] - **Spec Exp:** Lung Cancer; Esophageal Cancer; Transplant-Lung; **Hospital:** Barnes-Jewish Hosp; **Address:** 660 S Euclid Ave, Box 8234, St Louis, MO 63110; **Phone:** 314-362-6025; **Board Cert:** Surgery 1978; Thoracic Surgery 1981; Vascular Surgery 1982; **Med School:** Canada 1974; **Resid:** Surgery, Queens Univ Med Ctr 1978; Vascular Surgery, Univ Toronto Med Ctr 1979; **Fellow:** Research, Toronto Genl Hosp 1981; Surgical Critical Care, Johns Hopkins Hosp 1982; **Fac Appt:** Prof S, Washington Univ, St Louis

Rice, Thomas W MD [TS] - **Spec Exp:** Esophageal Surgery; Minimally Invasive Thoracic Surgery; Lung Cancer; **Hospital:** Cleveland Clin Fdn (page 70); **Address:** Cleveland Clinic, 9500 Euclid Ave, Desk J4-1, Cleveland, OH 44195; **Phone:** 216-444-1921; **Board Cert:** Surgery 2004; Thoracic Surgery 2005; **Med School:** Univ Toronto 1978; **Resid:** Surgery, Univ Toronto Med Ctr 1983; Thoracic Surgery, Univ Toronto Med Ctr 1986; **Fellow:** Pulmonary Disease, UCSF Med Ctr 1984; **Fac Appt:** Prof S, Cleveland Cl Coll Med/Case West Res

Great Plains and Mountains

Bull, David A MD [TS] - **Spec Exp:** Esophageal Cancer; **Hospital:** Univ Utah Hosps and Clins; **Address:** Univ Utah, Dept Cardiothoracic Surgery, 30 N 1900 East, rm 3C127, Salt Lake City, UT 84132; **Phone:** 801-581-5311; **Board Cert:** Thoracic Surgery 2004; Vascular Surgery 2003; Surgery 1999; Surgical Critical Care 1999; **Med School:** UCSF 1985; **Resid:** Surgery, UCSF Medical Ctr 1987; Surgery, Univ Arizona Hosps 1990; **Fellow:** Vascular Surgery, Univ Arizona Hosps 1992; Cardiothoracic Surgery, Univ Arizona Hosps 1994; **Fac Appt:** Assoc Prof TS, Univ Utah

Karwande, Shreekanth V MD [TS] - **Spec Exp:** Thoracic Cancers; Lung Cancer; **Hospital:** St Mark's Hosp - Salt Lake City; **Address:** St Mark's Hosp, 1160 E 3900 St, Ste 3500, Salt Lake City, UT 84124; **Phone:** 801-743-4750; **Board Cert:** Thoracic Surgery 2003; **Med School:** India 1973; **Resid:** Surgery, Erie Co Med Ctr 1981; Cardiothoracic Surgery, NY Hosp 1985; **Fellow:** Cardiothoracic Surgery, Meml Sloan Kettering Cancer Ctr

Southwest

Lanza, Louis MD [TS] - **Spec Exp:** Lung Cancer; **Hospital:** Mayo Clinic - Scottsdale; **Address:** Mayo Clinic Hosp, 5779 E Mayo Blvd MCSB Bldg Fl 1, Phoenix, AZ 85054; **Phone:** 480-342-2270; **Board Cert:** Thoracic Surgery 2002; **Med School:** Loyola Univ-Stritch Sch Med 1981; **Resid:** Surgery, Univ Michigan Med Ctr 1988; Cardiovascular Surgery, Texas Heart Inst 1991; **Fellow:** Surgical Oncology, Natl Cancer Inst 1986; Thoracic Oncology, MD Anderson Cancer Ctr 1989

Reardon, Michael J MD [TS] - **Spec Exp:** Cardiac Tumors/Cancer; **Hospital:** Methodist Hosp - Houston, UT MD Anderson Cancer Ctr; **Address:** 6560 Fannin St, Ste 1401, Houston, TX 77030; **Phone:** 713-441-5200; **Board Cert:** Thoracic Surgery 2006; **Med School:** Baylor Coll Med 1978; **Resid:** Surgery, Baylor Affil Hosps 1983; Thoracic Surgery, Texas Heart Inst 1985; **Fac Appt:** Clin Prof S, Baylor Coll Med

Roth, Jack MD [TS] - **Spec Exp:** Esophageal Cancer; Lung Cancer; Gene Therapy; **Hospital:** UT MD Anderson Cancer Ctr; **Address:** Dept Thoracic & Cardiovasc Surg Unit 445, 1515 Holcombe Blvd, Houston, TX 77030-4000; **Phone:** 713-792-7664; **Board Cert:** Thoracic Surgery 2002; **Med School:** Johns Hopkins Univ 1971; **Resid:** Surgery, Johns Hopkins Hosp 1973; Thoracic Surgery, UCLA Ctr Hlth Sci 1979; **Fellow:** Surgical Oncology, UCLA 1975; **Fac Appt:** Prof TS, Univ Tex, Houston

Smythe, W Roy MD [TS] - **Spec Exp:** Lung Cancer; Mesothelioma; **Hospital:** Scott & White Mem Hosp; **Address:** 2401 S 31st St, Temple, TX 76508; **Phone:** 254-724-2334; **Board Cert:** Surgery 1998; Thoracic Surgery 2000; **Med School:** Texas A&M Univ 1989; **Resid:** Surgery, Hosp Univ Penn 1996; **Fellow:** Cardiothoracic Surgery, Hosp Univ Penn 1998; Surgical Oncology, Am Cancer Soc 1996; **Fac Appt:** Asst Prof S, Univ Tex, Houston

Swisher, Stephen G MD [TS] - **Spec Exp:** Esophageal Cancer; Lung Cancer; Mesothelioma; Thoracic Cancers; **Hospital:** UT MD Anderson Cancer Ctr; **Address:** Dept of Thoracic & Cardiovasc Surg, 1515 Holcombe Blvd, Unit 445, Houston, TX 77030; **Phone:** 713-792-8659; **Board Cert:** Surgery 2002; Thoracic Surgery 2006; **Med School:** UCSD 1986; **Resid:** Surgery, UCLA Med Ctr 1993; **Fellow:** Surgical Oncology, UCLA Med Ctr 1990; Cardiothoracic Surgery, MD Anderson Canc Ctr 1996; **Fac Appt:** Prof TS, Univ Tex, Houston

West Coast and Pacific

De Meester, Tom R MD [TS] - **Spec Exp:** Stomach Cancer; Esophageal Cancer; Lung Cancer; Tracheal Surgery; **Hospital:** USC Univ Hosp; **Address:** 1510 San Pablo St, Ste 514, Los Angeles, CA 90033; **Phone:** 323-442-5925; **Board Cert:** Surgery 1971; Thoracic Surgery 1971; **Med School:** Univ Mich Med Sch 1963; **Resid:** Surgery, Johns Hopkins Hosp 1966; **Fellow:** Thoracic Surgery, Johns Hopkins Hosp 1968; **Fac Appt:** Prof S, USC Sch Med

Thoracic Surgery

Grannis Jr, Frederic W MD [TS] - **Spec Exp:** Lung Cancer; Thoracic Cancers; Palliative Care; Mediastinal Tumors; **Hospital:** City of Hope Natl Med Ctr & Beckman Rsch (page 69), Methodist Hosp - Southern California; **Address:** Thor Surg-City of Hope Natl Med Ctr, 1500 E Duarte Rd, Duarte, CA 91010; **Phone:** 626-359-8111 x62669; **Board Cert:** Surgery 1975; Thoracic Surgery 2000; **Med School:** NY Med Coll 1969; **Resid:** Surgery, Mayo Clinic 1974; Thoracic Surgery, Mayo Clinic 1977; **Fac Appt:** Assoc Prof TS, UCSD

Handy Jr, John R MD [TS] - **Spec Exp:** Lung Cancer; Esophageal Cancer; Mesothelioma; Chest Wall Tumors; **Hospital:** Providence Portland Med Ctr; **Address:** Oregon Clinic-Cardiothoracic Surgery, 1111 NE 99th Ave, Ste 201, Portland, OR 97220; **Phone:** 503-963-3030; **Board Cert:** Thoracic Surgery 2001; Surgery 1999; **Med School:** Duke Univ 1983; **Resid:** Surgery, Brown Univ Hosp 1990; **Fellow:** Cardiothoracic Surgery, MUSC Med Ctr 1993

Jablons, David M MD [TS] - **Spec Exp:** Lung Cancer; Mesothelioma; Esophageal Surgery; **Hospital:** UCSF - Mt Zion Med Ctr; **Address:** UCSF Thoracic Surgery, 1600 Divisadero St Fl 4, San Francisco, CA 94115; **Phone:** 415-885-3882; **Board Cert:** Thoracic Surgery 2002; **Med School:** Albany Med Coll 1984; **Resid:** Surgery, New Eng Med Ctr-Tufts Univ 1986; Surgery, New Eng Med Ctr-Tufts Univ 1991; **Fellow:** Surgical Oncology, Natl Cancer Inst-NIH 1989; Cardiothoracic Surgery, New York Hosp-Cornell 1993; **Fac Appt:** Prof S, UCSF

Kernstine, Kemp H MD/PhD [TS] - **Spec Exp:** Lung Cancer; Esophageal Cancer; Tracheal Surgery; Esophageal Surgery; **Hospital:** City of Hope Natl Med Ctr & Beckman Rsch (page 69); **Address:** City of Hope Comprehensive Cancer Ctr, 1500 E Duarte Rd, Duarte, CA 91010; **Phone:** 626-359-8111 x68845; **Board Cert:** Thoracic Surgery 2004; Surgery 2001; **Med School:** Duke Univ 1982; **Resid:** Surgery, Univ Minn Med Ctr 1988; **Fellow:** Cardiothoracic Surgery, Brigham & Women's Hosp 1994; **Fac Appt:** Prof S, Univ Iowa Coll Med

Shrager, Joseph B MD [TS] - **Spec Exp:** Lung Cancer; Thymoma; Mediastinal Tumors; Chest Wall Tumors; **Hospital:** Stanford Univ Med Ctr, VA Hlth Care Sys - Palo Alto; **Address:** Stanford Univ Medical Ctr, Falk Bldg, 300 Pasteur Drive Fl 2 - rm CV207, Stanford, CA 94305-5407; **Phone:** 650-721-2086; **Board Cert:** Thoracic Surgery 1999; **Med School:** Harvard Med Sch 1988; **Resid:** Surgery, Hosp Univ Penn 1995; Thoracic Surgery, Mass Genl Hosp 1997; **Fac Appt:** Prof TS, Stanford Univ

Vallieres, Eric MD [TS] - **Spec Exp:** Lung Cancer; Mesothelioma; Mediastinal Tumors; Thoracic Cancers; **Hospital:** Swedish Med Ctr - Seattle; **Address:** 1101 Madison St, Ste 850, Seattle, WA 98104; **Phone:** 206-215-6800; **Board Cert:** Surgery 1988; Thoracic Surgery 1990; **Med School:** Canada 1982; **Resid:** Surgery, Univ Toronto Affil Hosp 1988; Thoracic Surgery, Univ Toronto Affil Hosp 1989; **Fellow:** Cardiovascular Surgery, Univ Montreal 1990

Whyte, Richard MD [TS] - **Spec Exp:** Lung Cancer; Esophageal Cancer; Chest Wall Tumors; **Hospital:** Stanford Univ Med Ctr; **Address:** Stanford Univ Sch Med, Div Thor Surg, 300 Pasteur Dr, Bldg CVRB - rm 205, Stanford, CA 94305-5407; **Phone:** 650-723-6649; **Board Cert:** Surgery 2001; Thoracic Surgery 2003; **Med School:** Univ Pittsburgh 1983; **Resid:** Surgery, Mass Genl Hosp 1990; Thoracic Surgery, Univ Michigan Hosp 1992; **Fac Appt:** Prof TS, Stanford Univ

Wood, Douglas E MD [TS] - **Spec Exp:** Lung Cancer; Esophageal Cancer; Mesothelioma; **Hospital:** Univ Wash Med Ctr, Northwest Hosp; **Address:** Univ Washington, Div Cardiothoracic Surg, 1959 NE Pacific St, AA Bldg - rm 115, Box 356310, Seattle, WA 98195-6310; **Phone:** 206-685-3228; **Board Cert:** Surgery 1999; Thoracic Surgery 2001; **Med School:** Harvard Med Sch 1983; **Resid:** Surgery, Mass Genl Hosp 1989; Thoracic Surgery, Mass Genl Hosp 1991; **Fellow:** Surgical Critical Care, Mass Genl Hosp 1991; **Fac Appt:** Prof S, Univ Wash

Cleveland Clinic

Taussig Cancer Institute Focus on Lung Cancer

At Cleveland Clinic Taussig Cancer Institute, more than 250 cancer specialists, researchers, nurses and technicians are dedicated to developing and applying the latest and most effective medical techniques to achieve the long-term survival and improve the quality of life for 7,500 new cancer patients every year. Because of our patient-centered care, leading-edge treatments, innovative research, 350 clinical trials and state-of-the-art medical technologies, *U.S.News & World Report* has ranked Cleveland Clinic's cancer program one of the top cancer centers in the nation.

The Cleveland Clinic Taussig Cancer Institute's Lung Cancer Clinic brings together multidisciplinary teams of medical and radiation oncologists, thoracic surgeons, pulmonologists, radiologists, palliative medicine physicians and clinical nurse specialists to provide patients with the latest therapies, reduce treatment complications and improve quality of life. **To schedule an appointment or get a second opinion, call 866.223.8100 today or visit clevelandclinic.org/lungTCD.**

Treatment Advances

Gamma Knife radiosurgery may improve quality of life when lung cancer metastasizes to the brain. The Gamma Knife may also provide extended control of multiple metastatic tumors and even increase survival in some patients.

Novel experimental drugs and radiation protocols are available to Taussig Cancer Institute lung cancer patients through many clinical trials.

The colorimetric sensor array system uses a novel optical chemical sensor to detect and identify odor-producing chemicals or patterns. A color fingerprint demonstrates changes in color due to exposure to exhaled breath generated from a colorimetric sensor array.

The use of implantable intrathecal pumps for the long-term delivery of medications such as narcotics can provide superior pain relief.

Combined PET-CT imaging for lung cancer staging offers major clinical advantages by providing more accurate tumor detection and localization.

Video-assisted thoracoscopy benefits lung cancer patients who develop dangerous fluid levels in the pleural space. For patients with early-stage lung cancer, surgical resection offers the best chance of survival. In addition to advanced surgical and palliative procedures, patients may benefit from treatment with targeted drug therapy or novel technologies.

To schedule an appointment, or for more information about Cleveland Clinic Taussig Cancer Institute, call 866.223.8100 or visit clevelandclinic.org/lungTCD.

Cleveland Clinic Taussig Cancer Institute | Cleveland, OH

NYU Cancer Institute
NYU LANGONE MEDICAL CENTER

NYU Clinical Cancer Center
160 East 34th Street
New York, New York 10016
www.nyuci.org/atcd

NYU Langone Medical Center
550 First Avenue
(at 31st Street)
New York, New York 10016
www.nyumc.org/atcd

Stephen D. Hassenfeld Children's Center for Cancer and Blood Disorders
160 East 32nd Street
New York, New York 10016
www.nyumc.org/hassenfeld

A Collaborative Approach

The NYU Cancer Institute, an NCI designated center, is a "matrix cancer center" without walls operating within the larger NYU Langone Medical Center. With over 175 members and a research funding base of over $81 million, this structure strengthens our capabilities to forge collaborations across medical and scientific disciplines, which translates to comprehensive care for our patients and discoveries that will influence the future of this disease.

Renowned Expertise

Team members' compassion and expertise help patients better manage the symptoms of their disease as well as their special needs. Our highly skilled Magnet™ nursing team not only plays a pivotal role in coordinating direct patient care, but is also a source of invaluable patient education.

A Patient-Focused Setting

The NYU Clinical Cancer Center, with over 70 faculty members from various disciplines at the New York University School of Medicine, is the principal outpatient facility of the Cancer Institute and serves as home for our patients and their caregivers. The center and its multidisciplinary team of experts provide access to the latest treatment options and clinical trials along with a variety of programs in cancer prevention, screening, diagnostics, genetic counseling, and supportive services. When it comes to kids and cancer, the Stephen D. Hassenfeld Children's Center for Cancer and Blood Disorders offers not just innovation but insight. As a leading member of the NCI-sponsored Children's Oncology Group, our physicians are known for developing new ways to treat childhood cancer. Our affiliation with Bellevue Hospital, the oldest public hospital in the country, affords clinically distinctive opportunities to learn and care for patients with cancer by observing its presentation and behavior in a variety of patient groups.

Urology

A urologist manages benign and malignant medical and surgical disorders of the genitourinary system and the adrenal gland. This specialist has comprehensive knowledge of, and skills in, endoscopic, percutaneous and open surgery of congenital and acquired conditions of the urinary and reproductive systems and their contiguous structures.

Training Required: Five years

UROLOGY

New England

Heney, Niall M MD [U] - **Spec Exp:** Urologic Cancer; **Hospital:** Mass Genl Hosp; **Address:** Mass Genl Hosp, Dept Urol, 55 Fruit St Fl 5th, 528 rm, Boston, MA 02114; **Phone:** 617-726-3011; **Board Cert:** Urology 1977; **Med School:** Ireland 1965; **Resid:** Urology, Regional Hosp 1972; Urology, Mass Genl Hosp 1976; **Fac Appt:** Prof U, Harvard Med Sch

Janeiro Jr, John J MD [U] - **Spec Exp:** Urologic Cancer; **Hospital:** Southern NH Med Ctr, St Joseph Hosp; **Address:** Urology Center Southern New Hampshire, 17 Riverside St, Ste 201, Nashua, NH 03062; **Phone:** 603-883-1550; **Board Cert:** Urology 2008; **Med School:** Univ Mass Sch Med 1982; **Resid:** Urology, Lahey Clinic 1987; **Fellow:** Pediatric Urology, Childrens Hosp 1989

Libertino, John A MD [U] - **Spec Exp:** Kidney Cancer; Prostate Cancer; Adrenal Tumors; **Hospital:** Lahey Clin; **Address:** Lahey Clinic, Dept Urology, 41 Mall Rd, Burlington, MA 01805-0001; **Phone:** 781-744-2750; **Board Cert:** Urology 1973; **Med School:** Georgetown Univ 1965; **Resid:** Urology, Univ Rochester-Strong Meml Hosp 1967; Urology, Yale-New Haven Hosp 1970; **Fellow:** Surgery, Yale-New Haven Hosp 1968; **Fac Appt:** Assoc Clin Prof S, Harvard Med Sch

Loughlin, Kevin R MD [U] - **Spec Exp:** Prostate Cancer; Bladder Cancer; Penile Cancer; Incontinence-Female; **Hospital:** Brigham & Women's Hosp, Dana-Farber Cancer Inst; **Address:** Brigham & Women's Hosp, Div Urology, 45 Francis St, ASBII-3, Boston, MA 02115; **Phone:** 617-732-6325; **Board Cert:** Urology 2004; **Med School:** NY Med Coll 1975; **Resid:** Pediatrics, New York Hosp-Cornell 1978; Surgery, Bellevue Hosp Ctr-NYU 1979; **Fellow:** Urology, Brigham & Women's Hosp 1983; Urologic Oncology, Meml Sloan Kettering Cancer Ctr 1983; **Fac Appt:** Prof S, Harvard Med Sch

McDougal, W Scott MD [U] - **Spec Exp:** Penile Cancer; Prostate Cancer; Bladder Cancer; Urologic Cancer; **Hospital:** Mass Genl Hosp; **Address:** Mass Genl Hosp, 55 Fruit St, Bldg GRB - rm 1102, Boston, MA 02114; **Phone:** 617-726-3010; **Board Cert:** Surgery 1975; Urology 1978; **Med School:** Cornell Univ-Weill Med Coll 1968; **Resid:** Surgery, Univ Hosps Cleveland 1975; Urology, Univ Hosps Cleveland 1975; **Fellow:** Physiology, Yale Med Sch 1972; **Fac Appt:** Prof U, Harvard Med Sch

McGovern, Francis MD [U] - **Spec Exp:** Prostate Cancer; **Hospital:** Mass Genl Hosp; **Address:** One Hawthorne Pl, Ste 109, Boston, MA 02114; **Phone:** 617-726-3560; **Board Cert:** Urology 1999; **Med School:** Case West Res Univ 1983; **Resid:** Urology, Mass Genl Hosp 1989

Richie, Jerome MD [U] - **Spec Exp:** Prostate Cancer; Testicular Cancer; Kidney Cancer; **Hospital:** Brigham & Women's Hosp, Dana-Farber Cancer Inst; **Address:** Brigham & Womens Hosp, 75 Francis St, Ste ASB2, Boston, MA 02115; **Phone:** 617-732-6325; **Board Cert:** Urology 1992; **Med School:** Univ Tex Med Br, Galveston 1969; **Resid:** Surgery, UCLA Med Ctr 1971; Urology, UCLA Med Ctr 1975; **Fac Appt:** Prof U, Harvard Med Sch

Sanda, Martin G MD [U] - **Spec Exp:** Prostate Cancer; Bladder Cancer; Kidney Cancer; Urologic Cancer; **Hospital:** Beth Israel Deaconess Med Ctr - Boston; **Address:** Beth Israel Deaconess Medical Ctr, 330 Brookline Ave, Rabb 440, Boston, MA 02115; **Phone:** 617-735-2100; **Board Cert:** Urology 2007; **Med School:** Columbia P&S 1987; **Resid:** Surgery, Med Coll Virginia 1989; Urology, Johns Hopkins Hosp 1994; **Fellow:** Surgical Oncology, Natl Cancer Inst 1991; **Fac Appt:** Assoc Prof U, Harvard Med Sch

Mid Atlantic

Alexander, Richard B MD [U] - **Spec Exp:** Prostate Cancer; **Hospital:** Univ of MD Med Ctr; **Address:** 29 SE Greene St, Ste 500, Baltimore, MD 21201; **Phone:** 410-328-5109; **Board Cert:** Urology 1999; **Med School:** Johns Hopkins Univ 1981; **Resid:** Surgery, Vanderbilt Univ Affl Hosps 1983; Urology, Johns Hopkins Hosp 1988; **Fellow:** Cancer Immunology, Natl Cancer Inst 1989; **Fac Appt:** Prof U, Univ MD Sch Med

Bagley, Demetrius H MD [U] - **Spec Exp:** Kidney Cancer; Ureter & Renal Pelvis Cancer; Minimally Invasive Urologic Surgery; **Hospital:** Thomas Jefferson Univ Hosp (page 83); **Address:** 833 Chestnut St E, Ste 703, Philadelphia, PA 19107; **Phone:** 215-955-1000; **Board Cert:** Urology 1981; **Med School:** Johns Hopkins Univ 1970; **Resid:** Surgery, Yale-New Haven Hosp 1972; Urology, Yale-New Haven Hosp 1979; **Fellow:** Surgery, NCI-USPHS 1975; **Fac Appt:** Prof U, Thomas Jefferson Univ

Benson, Mitchell C MD [U] - **Spec Exp:** Prostate Cancer/Robotic Surgery; Bladder Cancer; Kidney Cancer; Continent Urinary Diversions; **Hospital:** NY-Presby Hosp/Columbia (page 79); **Address:** NY Presby Hosp-Columbia, Dept Urology, 161 Ft Washington Ave Fl 11 - rm 1102, New York, NY 10032-3713; **Phone:** 212-305-5201; **Board Cert:** Urology 1984; **Med School:** Columbia P&S 1977; **Resid:** Surgery, Mount Sinai Med Ctr 1979; Urology, Columbia-Presby Hosp 1982; **Fellow:** Oncology, Johns Hopkins Hosp 1984; **Fac Appt:** Prof U, Columbia P&S

Burnett II, Arthur L MD [U] - **Spec Exp:** Prostate Cancer; Erectile Dysfunction; **Hospital:** Johns Hopkins Hosp; **Address:** 600 N Wolfe St, Marburg Bldg, Ste 407, Baltimore, MD 21287; **Phone:** 410-614-3986; **Board Cert:** Urology 2007; **Med School:** Johns Hopkins Univ 1988; **Resid:** Surgery, Johns Hopkins Hosp 1990; Urology, Johns Hopkins Hosp 1994; **Fac Appt:** Prof U, Johns Hopkins Univ

Carter, H Ballentine MD [U] - **Spec Exp:** Prostate Cancer; **Hospital:** Johns Hopkins Hosp; **Address:** Brady Urological Inst, Johns Hopkins Hosp, 600 N Wolfe St Marburg Bldg - rm 145, Baltimore, MD 21287-2101; **Phone:** 410-955-0833; **Board Cert:** Urology 1999; **Med School:** Med Univ SC 1981; **Resid:** Surgery, New York Hosp 1983; Urology, New York Hosp 1987; **Fellow:** Research, Johns Hopkins Hosp 1989; **Fac Appt:** Prof U, Johns Hopkins Univ

Droller, Michael J MD [U] - **Spec Exp:** Urologic Cancer; Bladder Cancer; Prostate Cancer; Kidney Cancer; **Hospital:** Mount Sinai Med Ctr (page 77); **Address:** 5 E 98th St Fl 6, Box 1272, New York, NY 10029-6501; **Phone:** 212-241-3868; **Board Cert:** Urology 2001; **Med School:** Harvard Med Sch 1968; **Resid:** Surgery, Peter Bent Brigham Hosp 1970; Urology, Stanford Univ Med Ctr 1976; **Fellow:** Immunology, Univ Stockholm 1977; **Fac Appt:** Prof U, Mount Sinai Sch Med

Gomella, Leonard G MD [U] - **Spec Exp:** Prostate Cancer; Minimally Invasive Urologic Surgery; Urologic Cancer; **Hospital:** Thomas Jefferson Univ Hosp (page 83); **Address:** Thomas Jefferson Univ, 1015 Walnut St Fl 11 - Ste 1112, Philadelphia, PA 19107-5001; **Phone:** 215-955-1000; **Board Cert:** Urology 1998; **Med School:** Univ KY Coll Med 1980; **Resid:** Surgery, Univ Kentucky Med Ctr 1982; Urology, Univ Kentucky Med Ctr 1986; **Fellow:** Urologic Oncology, Natl Cancer Inst 1988; **Fac Appt:** Prof U, Jefferson Med Coll

Grasso, Michael MD [U] - **Spec Exp:** Urologic Cancer; Laparoscopic Surgery; Testicular Cancer; **Hospital:** St Vincent Cath Med Ctrs - Manhattan; **Address:** 170 W 12th St, Dept Urology - Cronin 205, New York, NY 10011; **Phone:** 212-604-1270; **Board Cert:** Urology 2002; **Med School:** Jefferson Med Coll 1986; **Resid:** Surgery, Jefferson Univ Hosp 1988; Urology, Jefferson Univ Hosp 1992; **Fac Appt:** Prof U, NY Med Coll

Urology

Greenberg, Richard E MD [U] - **Spec Exp:** Prostate Cancer; Bladder Cancer; Kidney Cancer; Prostate Cancer/Robotic Surgery; **Hospital:** Fox Chase Cancer Ctr (page 72), Abington Mem Hosp; **Address:** Fox Chase Cancer Ctr, Div Urol-Dept Surg, 333 Cottman Ave, Ste H3 - rm H3-116, Philadelphia, PA 19111; **Phone:** 215-728-5341; **Board Cert:** Urology 2005; **Med School:** Cornell Univ-Weill Med Coll 1976; **Resid:** Surgery, New York Hosp 1979; Urology, New York Hosp 1983; **Fac Appt:** Prof U, Temple Univ

Hall, Simon J MD [U] - **Spec Exp:** Urologic Cancer; Minimally Invasive Urologic Surgery; Continent Urinary Diversions; Prostate Cancer; **Hospital:** Mount Sinai Med Ctr (page 77); **Address:** Mount Sinai Medical Ctr, 5 98th St, Box 1272, New York, NY 10029; **Phone:** 212-241-4812; **Board Cert:** Urology 2009; **Med School:** Columbia P&S 1988; **Resid:** Surgery, Mt Sinai Med Ctr 1990; Urology, Boston Univ 1994; **Fellow:** Urology, Baylor Coll Med 1996; **Fac Appt:** Assoc Prof U, Mount Sinai Sch Med

Herr, Harry W MD [U] - **Spec Exp:** Bladder Cancer; Prostate Cancer; Testicular Cancer; **Hospital:** Meml Sloan-Kettering Cancer Ctr (page 76), NY-Presby Hosp/Weill Cornell (page 79); **Address:** 1275 York Avenue, New York, NY 10065; **Phone:** 800-525-2225; **Board Cert:** Urology 1976; **Med School:** UCSF 1969; **Resid:** Urology, UC Irvine Med Ctr 1974; **Fellow:** Urology, Meml Sloan Kettering Cancer Ctr 1976; **Fac Appt:** Assoc Prof S, Cornell Univ-Weill Med Coll

Hrebinko Jr, Ronald L MD [U] - **Spec Exp:** Urologic Cancer; Kidney Cancer; Bladder Cancer; Testicular Cancer; **Hospital:** UPMC Presby, Pittsburgh; **Address:** Univ Pittsburgh Dept of Urology, Shadyside Medical Bldg, Ste 209, 5200 Centre Ave, Pittsburgh, PA 15232; **Phone:** 412-605-3022; **Board Cert:** Urology 2004; **Med School:** Univ Pittsburgh 1986; **Resid:** Urology, Univ Pittsburgh Med Ctr 1992; **Fellow:** Urologic Oncology, Roswell Park Cancer Ctr 1993; **Fac Appt:** Assoc Prof U, Univ Pittsburgh

Huben, Robert P MD [U] - **Spec Exp:** Prostate Cancer; Kidney Cancer; Urologic Cancer; **Hospital:** Roswell Park Cancer Inst; **Address:** Roswell Park Cancer Inst, Elm & Carlton Sts, Buffalo, NY 14263-0001; **Phone:** 716-845-3389; **Board Cert:** Urology 1983; **Med School:** Cornell Univ-Weill Med Coll 1976; **Resid:** Urology, East Virginia Med Ctr 1981; **Fellow:** Urologic Oncology, Roswell Park Meml Inst 1982

Jackman, Stephen V MD [U] - **Spec Exp:** Prostate Cancer/Robotic Surgery; Laparoscopic Surgery; **Hospital:** UPMC Shadyside, UPMC Presby, Pittsburgh; **Address:** UPMC, Kaufman Bldg, 3471 Fifth Ave, Ste 700, Pittsburgh, PA 15213; **Phone:** 412-692-4095; **Board Cert:** Urology 2002; **Med School:** Yale Univ 1994; **Resid:** Urology, Johns Hopkins Hosp 1999; **Fac Appt:** Assoc Prof U, Univ Pittsburgh

Jarow, Jonathan P MD [U] - **Spec Exp:** Prostate Cancer; Erectile Dysfunction; Incontinence after Prostate Cancer; **Hospital:** Johns Hopkins Hosp; **Address:** Johns Hopkins Outpatient Ctr-Urology, 601 N Caroline St, Fl 4, Baltimore, MD 21287; **Phone:** 410-955-3617; **Board Cert:** Urology 2007; **Med School:** Northwestern Univ 1980; **Resid:** Surgery, Johns Hopkins Hosp 1982; Urology, Johns Hopkins Hosp 1986; **Fellow:** Andrology, Baylor Univ 1989; **Fac Appt:** Assoc Prof U, Johns Hopkins Univ

Kaplan, Steven A MD [U] - **Spec Exp:** Incontinence after Prostate Cancer; **Hospital:** NY-Presby Hosp/Weill Cornell (page 79); **Address:** NY Presbyterian-Weill Cornell Med Ctr, 525 E 68th St, rm F9West, New York, NY 10021-4870; **Phone:** 212-746-4811; **Board Cert:** Urology 2001; **Med School:** Mount Sinai Sch Med 1982; **Resid:** Surgery, Mount Sinai Hosp 1984; Urology, Columbia Presby Med Ctr 1988; **Fellow:** Urology, Columbia Presby Med Ctr 1990; **Fac Appt:** Prof U, Cornell Univ-Weill Med Coll

Katz, Aaron E MD [U] - **Spec Exp:** Prostate Cancer-Cryosurgery; Kidney Cancer-Cryosurgery; Complementary Medicine; Nutrition & Cancer Prevention; **Hospital:** NY-Presby Hosp/Columbia (page 79); **Address:** NY Presby Med Ctr, Herbert Irving Pav, 161 Ft Washington Ave Fl 11, New York, NY 10032; **Phone:** 212-305-6408; **Board Cert:** Urology 2006; **Med School:** NY Med Coll 1986; **Resid:** Urology, Maimonides Med Ctr 1992; **Fellow:** Urologic Oncology, Columbia Presby Med Ctr 1993; **Fac Appt:** Assoc Clin Prof U, Columbia P&S

Kavoussi, Louis R MD [U] - **Spec Exp:** Laparoscopic Surgery; Urologic Cancer; Prostate Cancer; **Hospital:** Long Island Jewish Med Ctr, N Shore Univ Hosp; **Address:** 450 Lakeville Rd, Ste M-41, New Hyde Park, NY 11040; **Phone:** 516-734-8558; **Board Cert:** Urology 1999; **Med School:** SUNY Buffalo 1983; **Resid:** Surgery, Barnes Jewish Hosp 1985; Urology, Barnes Jewish Hosp 1989; **Fac Appt:** Prof U, NYU Sch Med

Kirschenbaum, Alexander M MD [U] - **Spec Exp:** Prostate Cancer; Bladder Cancer; Kidney Cancer; **Hospital:** Mount Sinai Med Ctr (page 77); **Address:** 58A E 79th St, New York, NY 10021; **Phone:** 646-422-0926; **Board Cert:** Urology 2006; **Med School:** Mount Sinai Sch Med 1980; **Resid:** Surgery, Mt Sinai Hosp 1982; Urology, Mt Sinai Hosp 1985; **Fellow:** Urologic Oncology, Mt Sinai Hosp 1987; **Fac Appt:** Assoc Prof U, Mount Sinai Sch Med

Lanteri, Vincent J MD [U] - **Spec Exp:** Prostate Cancer/Robotic Surgery; Urologic Cancer; Minimally Invasive Urologic Surgery; **Hospital:** Hackensack Univ Med Ctr (page 73), Monmouth Med Ctr; **Address:** 255 W Spring Valley Ave, Ste 101, Maywood, NJ 07607; **Phone:** 201-487-8866; **Board Cert:** Urology 1982; **Med School:** Mexico 1974; **Resid:** Surgery, UMDNJ Med Ctr 1977; Urology, UMDNJ Med Ctr 1980; **Fellow:** Urologic Oncology, Roswell Park Cancer Inst 1981

Lepor, Herbert MD [U] - **Spec Exp:** Prostate Cancer; **Hospital:** NYU Langone Med Ctr (page 80); **Address:** 150 E 32nd St Fl 2, New York, NY 10016; **Phone:** 646-825-6327; **Board Cert:** Urology 2006; **Med School:** Johns Hopkins Univ 1975; **Resid:** Urology, Johns Hopkins Hosp 1986; **Fac Appt:** Prof U, NYU Sch Med

Lowe, Franklin MD [U] - **Spec Exp:** Complementary Medicine; Prostate Cancer; **Hospital:** St Luke's - Roosevelt Hosp Ctr - Roosevelt Div (page 71), NY-Presby Hosp/Columbia (page 79); **Address:** 425 W 59th St, Ste 3A, New York, NY 10019-1104; **Phone:** 212-523-7790; **Board Cert:** Urology 2006; **Med School:** Columbia P&S 1979; **Resid:** Surgery, Johns Hopkins Hosp 1981; Urology, Johns Hopkins Hosp 1984; **Fac Appt:** Clin Prof U, Columbia P&S

Malkowicz, S Bruce MD [U] - **Spec Exp:** Prostate Cancer; Bladder Cancer; Kidney Cancer; Gene Therapy; **Hospital:** Hosp Univ Penn - UPHS (page 81); **Address:** Hosp Univ Penn, Dept Urology, 3400 Spruce St, 9 Penn Tower, Philadelphia, PA 19104; **Phone:** 215-662-2891; **Board Cert:** Urology 2000; **Med School:** Univ Pennsylvania 1981; **Resid:** Surgery, Hosp Univ Penn 1983; Urology, Hosp Univ Penn 1987; **Fellow:** Urologic Oncology, USC Med Ctr 1998; Urologic Oncology, Hosp Univ Penn/Wistar Inst 1990; **Fac Appt:** Assoc Prof U, Univ Pennsylvania

Mostwin, Jacek L MD/PhD [U] - **Spec Exp:** Prostate Cancer; **Hospital:** Johns Hopkins Hosp; **Address:** Johns Hopkins Hosp, 600 N Wolfe St Park 207 Bldg, Baltimore, MD 21287; **Phone:** 410-955-4461; **Board Cert:** Urology 2007; **Med School:** Univ MD Sch Med 1975; **Resid:** Surgery, Univ Michigan Med Ctr 1978; Urology, Johns Hopkins Hosp 1983; **Fac Appt:** Prof U, Johns Hopkins Univ

Naslund, Michael MD [U] - **Spec Exp:** Prostate Cancer; **Hospital:** Univ of MD Med Ctr; **Address:** Maryland Prostate Ctr, 419 W Redwood St, Ste 320, Baltimore, MD 21201; **Phone:** 410-328-0800; **Board Cert:** Urology 2008; **Med School:** Johns Hopkins Univ 1981; **Resid:** Surgery, Johns Hopkins Hosp 1983; Urology, Johns Hopkins Hosp 1987; **Fac Appt:** Prof U, Univ MD Sch Med

Nelson, Joel B MD [U] - **Spec Exp:** Prostate Cancer; **Hospital:** UPMC Shadyside; **Address:** UPMC Shadyside Med Ctr, 5200 Centre Ave, Ste 209, Pittsburgh, PA 15232-1312; **Phone:** 412-605-3013; **Board Cert:** Urology 2008; **Med School:** Northwestern Univ 1988; **Resid:** Surgery, Northwestern Meml Hosp 1990; Urology, Northwestern Meml Hosp 1994; **Fellow:** Urology, Johns Hopkins Hosp; **Fac Appt:** Prof U, Univ Pittsburgh

Partin, Alan W MD/PhD [U] - **Spec Exp:** Prostate Cancer; **Hospital:** Johns Hopkins Hosp; **Address:** Johns Hopkins Hosp, 600 N Wolfe St Marburg Bldg - rm 134, Baltimore, MD 21287; **Phone:** 410-614-4876; **Board Cert:** Urology 2007; **Med School:** Johns Hopkins Univ 1989; **Resid:** Surgery, Johns Hopkins Hosp 1991; Urology, Johns Hopkins Hosp 1996; **Fac Appt:** Prof U, Johns Hopkins Univ

Samadi, David B MD [U] - **Spec Exp:** Prostate Cancer/Robotic Surgery; Kidney Cancer; Bladder Cancer; Robotic Surgery; **Hospital:** Mount Sinai Med Ctr (page 77), N Genl Hosp; **Address:** 625 Madison Ave Fl 2 - Ste 230, New York, NY 10029; **Phone:** 212-241-8779; **Board Cert:** Urology 2004; **Med School:** SUNY Stony Brook 1994; **Resid:** Surgery, Montefiore Med Ctr 2000; Urology, Montefiore Med Ctr 2002; **Fellow:** Urologic Oncology, Meml Sloan Kettering Cancer Ctr 2003; Laparoscopic Surgery, Henri Mondor Hosp; **Fac Appt:** Asst Prof U, Mount Sinai Sch Med

Sawczuk, Ihor S MD [U] - **Spec Exp:** Kidney Cancer; Bladder Cancer; Prostate Cancer/Robotic Surgery; Bladder Reconstruction; **Hospital:** Hackensack Univ Med Ctr (page 73), NY-Presby Hosp/Columbia (page 79); **Address:** Hackensack Univ Med Ctr, 360 Essex St, Ste 403, Hackensack, NJ 07601; **Phone:** 201-336-8090; **Board Cert:** Urology 2005; **Med School:** Med Coll PA Hahnemann 1979; **Resid:** Surgery, St Vincents Hosp 1981; Urology, Columbia-Presby Med Ctr 1984; **Fellow:** Urologic Oncology, Columbia-Presby Med Ctr 1986; **Fac Appt:** Prof U, Columbia P&S

Scardino, Peter T MD [U] - **Spec Exp:** Prostate Cancer; Bladder Cancer; Urologic Cancer; Urinary Reconstruction; **Hospital:** Meml Sloan-Kettering Cancer Ctr (page 76); **Address:** 1275 York Avenue, New York, NY 10065; **Phone:** 646-422-4329; **Board Cert:** Urology 1981; **Med School:** Duke Univ 1971; **Resid:** Surgery, Mass Genl Hosp 1973; Urology, UCLA Med Ctr 1979; **Fellow:** Urology, Natl Cancer Inst 1976; **Fac Appt:** Prof U, Cornell Univ-Weill Med Coll

Scherr, Douglas S MD [U] - **Spec Exp:** Prostate Cancer/Robotic Surgery; Bladder Cancer; Robotic Surgery; Testicular Cancer; **Hospital:** NY-Presby Hosp/Weill Cornell (page 79); **Address:** NY Cornell Medical Ctr, Dept Urology, 525 E 68th St Starr 900, New York, NY 10021; **Phone:** 212-746-5788; **Board Cert:** Urology 2003; **Med School:** Geo Wash Univ 1994; **Resid:** Urology, NY Hosp-Cornell Med Ctr 1999; **Fellow:** Urologic Oncology, Meml Sloan-Kettering Canc Ctr 2002; **Fac Appt:** Assoc Prof U, Cornell Univ-Weill Med Coll

Schlegel, Peter N MD [U] - **Spec Exp:** Prostate Cancer; **Hospital:** NY-Presby Hosp/Weill Cornell (page 79); **Address:** 525 E 68th St, Starr 900, New York, NY 10021-4870; **Phone:** 212-746-5491; **Board Cert:** Urology 2001; **Med School:** Univ Mass Sch Med 1983; **Resid:** Surgery, Johns Hopkins Hosp 1985; Urology, Johns Hopkins Hosp 1989; **Fellow:** Medical Oncology, Johns Hopkins Hosp 1987; Male Reproduction, NY Hosp-Cornell Med Ctr 1991; **Fac Appt:** Prof U, Cornell Univ-Weill Med Coll

Schoenberg, Mark P MD [U] - **Spec Exp:** Bladder Cancer; Urinary Reconstruction; **Hospital:** Johns Hopkins Hosp; **Address:** Johns Hopkins Hospital, 150 Marburg Bldg, 600 N Wolfe St, Baltimore, MD 21287-2101; **Phone:** 410-502-3803; **Board Cert:** Urology 2005; **Med School:** Univ Tex, Houston 1986; **Resid:** Surgery, Hosp U Penn 1988; Urologic Surgery, Hosp U Penn 1992; **Fellow:** Urologic Oncology, Brady Inst/Johns Hopkins 1994; **Fac Appt:** Prof U, Johns Hopkins Univ

Sheinfeld, Joel MD [U] - **Spec Exp:** Testicular Cancer; Bladder Cancer; Fertility Preservation in Cancer; **Hospital:** Meml Sloan-Kettering Cancer Ctr (page 76); **Address:** 1275 York Avenue, New York, NY 10065; **Phone:** 800-525-2225; **Board Cert:** Urology 2000; **Med School:** Univ Fla Coll Med 1981; **Resid:** Urology, Strong Meml Hosp 1986; **Fellow:** Urologic Oncology, Meml Sloan Kettering Cancer Ctr 1989; **Fac Appt:** Assoc Prof U, Cornell Univ-Weill Med Coll

Taneja, Samir S MD [U] - **Spec Exp:** Kidney Cancer; Prostate Cancer; Bladder Cancer; **Hospital:** NYU Langone Med Ctr (page 80); **Address:** NYU Urology Assocs, 150 E 32nd St Fl 2, New York, NY 10016-6024; **Phone:** 646-825-6321; **Board Cert:** Urology 1999; **Med School:** Northwestern Univ 1990; **Resid:** Urology, UCLA Med Ctr 1996; **Fellow:** Urologic Oncology, NYU Med Ctr 1998; **Fac Appt:** Assoc Prof U, NYU Sch Med

Tewari, Ashutosh MD [U] - **Spec Exp:** Prostate Cancer/Robotic Surgery; **Hospital:** NY-Presby Hosp/Weill Cornell (page 79); **Address:** Weill Cornell Brady Urologic Health Ct, 525 E 68th St, Starr 916, New York, NY 10065; **Phone:** 212-746-5638; **Board Cert:** Urology 2006; **Med School:** India 1984; **Resid:** Surgery, GSVM Medical College 1990; Urology, Henry Ford Hosp 2003; **Fellow:** Transplant Surgery, Liverpool Univ Med Ctr 1993; Urologic Oncology, Shands Healthcare 1995; **Fac Appt:** Assoc Prof U, Cornell Univ-Weill Med Coll

Uzzo, Robert MD [U] - **Spec Exp:** Bladder Cancer; Prostate Cancer; Robotic Surgery; Minimally Invasive Urologic Surgery; **Hospital:** Fox Chase Cancer Ctr (page 72); **Address:** 333 Cottman Ave, rm H3116, Philadelphia, PA 19111; **Phone:** 215-728-3501; **Board Cert:** Urology 2001; **Med School:** Cornell Univ-Weill Med Coll 1991; **Resid:** Surgery, New York Hosp-Cornell Med Ctr 1993; Urology, New York Hosp-Cornell Med Ctr 1997; **Fellow:** Urologic Oncology, Cleveland Clinic 1999; Renal Transplant, Cleveland Clinic 2000; **Fac Appt:** Assoc Prof S, Temple Univ

Van Arsdalen, Keith N MD [U] - **Spec Exp:** Urologic Cancer; **Hospital:** Hosp Univ Penn - UPHS (page 81), Chldns Hosp of Philadelphia, The; **Address:** Hosp Univ Penn, Div Urology, 3400 Spruce St, 9 Penn Tower, Philadelphia, PA 19104-4283; **Phone:** 215-662-2891; **Board Cert:** Urology 1984; **Med School:** Med Coll VA 1977; **Resid:** Surgery, Univ Maryland Hosp 1979; Urology, Med Coll Virginia 1982; **Fellow:** Urodynamics, Hosp Univ Penn 1983; **Fac Appt:** Prof U, Univ Pennsylvania

Vaughan, Edwin D MD [U] - **Spec Exp:** Urologic Cancer; Adrenal Tumors; **Hospital:** NY-Presby Hosp/Weill Cornell (page 79); **Address:** New York Presby Hosp, Dept Urology, 525 E 68th St, Starr 900, Box 94, New York, NY 10021-4870; **Phone:** 212-746-5480; **Board Cert:** Urology 1986; **Med School:** Univ VA Sch Med 1965; **Resid:** Surgery, Vanderbilt Univ Med Ctr 1967; Urology, Univ Virginia Hosp 1971; **Fellow:** Internal Medicine, Columbia Univ 1973; **Fac Appt:** Prof U, Cornell Univ-Weill Med Coll

Walsh, Patrick MD [U] - **Spec Exp:** Prostate Cancer; **Hospital:** Johns Hopkins Hosp; **Address:** Brady Urological Inst, 600 N Wolfe St, Park 224, Baltimore, MD 21287-2101; **Phone:** 410-955-6100; **Board Cert:** Urology 1975; **Med School:** Case West Res Univ 1964; **Resid:** Surgery, Peter Bent Brigham Hosp/Childrens Hosp 1967; Urology, UCLA Med Ctr 1971; **Fellow:** Endocrinology, Harbor Genl Hosp 1970; **Fac Appt:** Prof U, Johns Hopkins Univ

Wein, Alan J MD [U] - **Spec Exp:** Prostate Cancer; Testicular Cancer; Bladder Cancer; Kidney Cancer; **Hospital:** Hosp Univ Penn - UPHS (page 81), Pennsylvania Hosp (page 81); **Address:** Univ Penn Hlth System, Div Urology, 34th & Civic Center Blvd, 9 Penn Tower, Philadelphia, PA 19104-4283; **Phone:** 215-662-6755; **Board Cert:** Urology 1995; **Med School:** Univ Pennsylvania 1966; **Resid:** Surgery, Hosp Univ Penn 1968; Urology, Hosp Univ Penn 1972; **Fellow:** Urology, Hosp Univ Penn 1969; **Fac Appt:** Prof U, Univ Pennsylvania

Urology

Weiss, Robert E MD [U] - **Spec Exp:** Bladder Cancer; Kidney Cancer; Testicular Cancer; **Hospital:** Robert Wood Johnson Univ Hosp - New Brunswick, Univ Med Ctr - Princeton; **Address:** 1 Robert Wood Johnson Pl Ste MB588, New Brunswick, NJ 08901-1928; **Phone:** 732-235-7775; **Board Cert:** Urology 2004; **Med School:** NYU Sch Med 1985; **Resid:** Surgery, Mount Sinai Med Ctr 1987; Urology, Mount Sinai Med Ctr 1991; **Fellow:** Urologic Oncology, Meml Sloan Kettering Cancer Ctr 1994; **Fac Appt:** Assoc Prof U, UMDNJ-RW Johnson Med Sch

Yu, George W MD [U] - **Spec Exp:** Nutrition & Disease Prevention/Control; Nutrition & Cancer Prevention/Control; **Hospital:** G Washington Univ Hosp, Anne Arundel Med Ctr; **Address:** 122 Defense Hwy, Ste 224, Annapolis, MD 21401; **Phone:** 410-897-0540; **Board Cert:** Urology 1981; **Med School:** Tufts Univ 1973; **Resid:** Surgery, Brigham & Women's Hosp 1976; Urology, Johns Hopkins Hosp 1981; **Fac Appt:** Prof U, Geo Wash Univ

Southeast

Beall, Michael E MD [U] - **Spec Exp:** Prostate Cancer; Testicular Cancer; **Hospital:** Inova Fairfax Hosp, Reston Hosp Ctr; **Address:** 8503 Arlington Blvd, Ste 310, Fairfax, VA 22031; **Phone:** 703-208-4200; **Board Cert:** Urology 1979; **Med School:** Geo Wash Univ 1972; **Resid:** Urology, Geo Wash Univ Hosp 1977; **Fac Appt:** Assoc Clin Prof U, Geo Wash Univ

Chang, Sam S MD [U] - **Spec Exp:** Urologic Cancer; Prostate Cancer; Prostate Cancer-HIFU Therapy; High Intensity Focused Ultrasound(HIFU); **Hospital:** Vanderbilt Univ Med Ctr; **Address:** Vanderbilt University Med Ctr, A-1302 MCN, Nashville, TN 37232-2765; **Phone:** 615-322-2880; **Board Cert:** Urology 2002; **Med School:** Vanderbilt Univ 1992; **Resid:** Surgery, Vanderbilt Univ 1998; **Fellow:** Urologic Oncology, Meml Sloan Kettering Cancer Ctr 1999; **Fac Appt:** Assoc Prof U, Vanderbilt Univ

Cookson, Michael MD [U] - **Spec Exp:** Bladder Cancer; Testicular Cancer; Prostate Cancer; **Hospital:** Vanderbilt Univ Med Ctr, Saint Thomas Hosp - Nashville; **Address:** Vanderbilt Univ Med Ctr, Urol Surg A1302 MCN, Nashville, TN 37232-0001; **Phone:** 615-322-2101; **Board Cert:** Urology 2006; **Med School:** Univ Okla Coll Med 1988; **Resid:** Urology, Univ Tex San Antonio-Univ Hosp 1994; **Fellow:** Urologic Oncology, Meml Sloan-Kettering Cancer Ctr 1996; **Fac Appt:** Prof U, Vanderbilt Univ

El-Galley, Rizk MD [U] - **Spec Exp:** Urologic Cancer; Laparoscopic Surgery; Bladder Cancer; **Hospital:** Univ of Ala Hosp at Birmingham; **Address:** UAB Hosp FOT-1105, 1530 3rd Ave S, Birmingham, AL 35294-3411; **Phone:** 205-996-8765; **Board Cert:** Urology 2003; **Med School:** Egypt 1983; **Resid:** Urology, Emory Univ Hosp 1999; **Fac Appt:** Asst Prof U, Univ Alabama

Fraser, Lionel B MD [U] - **Spec Exp:** Prostate Cancer; Incontinence after Prostate Cancer; Erectile Dysfunction; **Hospital:** Baptist Hosp - Jackson; **Address:** Metropolitan Urology, St Dominics West Med Tower, 971 Lakeland Drive, Ste 360, Jackson, MS 39216; **Phone:** 601-982-0982; **Board Cert:** Urology 2005; **Med School:** Univ Mich Med Sch 1977; **Resid:** Surgery, New England Deaconness Hosp 1979; **Fellow:** Urology, Brigham & Womens Hosp 1983

Harty, James MD [U] - **Spec Exp:** Urologic Cancer; **Hospital:** Norton Hosp, Jewish Hosp HlthCre Svcs Inc; **Address:** Allied Urology, 250 E Liberty St, Ste 500, Louisville, KY 40202; **Phone:** 502-584-0651; **Board Cert:** Urology 1979; **Med School:** Ireland 1969; **Resid:** Surgery, Johns Hopkins Hosp 1973; Urology, Johns Hopkins Hosp 1977; **Fac Appt:** Prof S, Univ Louisville Sch Med

Hemal, Ashok K MD [U] - **Spec Exp:** Urologic Cancer; Robotic Urologic Surgery; Reconstructive Urologic Surgery; Laparoscopic Surgery; **Hospital:** Wake Forest Univ Baptist Med Ctr (page 84); **Address:** Wake Forest Sch Med, Dept Urology, 140 Charlois Blvd, Winston-Salem, NC 27103; **Phone:** 336-716-4131; **Med School:** India 1981; **Resid:** Surgery, G R Med College 1985; Urology, Post Grad Inst Med Ed & Rsch 1988; **Fellow:** Robotic Surgery, Henry Ford Hosp; **Fac Appt:** Prof U, Wake Forest Univ

Jordan, Gerald H MD [U] - **Spec Exp:** Urinary Reconstruction; Prostate Cancer; **Hospital:** Sentara Norfolk Genl Hosp; **Address:** 400 W Brambleton Ave, Ste 100, Norfolk, VA 23510; **Phone:** 757-457-5100; **Board Cert:** Urology 2008; **Med School:** Univ Tex, San Antonio 1977; **Resid:** Urology, Naval Reg Med Ctr 1978; **Fellow:** Reconstructive Surgery, Eastern Va Med Sch 1984; **Fac Appt:** Prof U, Eastern VA Med Sch

Keane, Thomas E MD [U] - **Spec Exp:** Urologic Cancer; Genitourinary Cancer; Prostate Cancer; Clinical Trials; **Hospital:** MUSC Med Ctr; **Address:** MUSC-Urology Dept, 96 Jonathan Lucas St, Ste CSB644, Charleston, SC 29425; **Phone:** 843-792-1666; **Board Cert:** Urology 2003; **Med School:** Ireland 1981; **Resid:** Urology, St Vincents Hosp 1986; Urology, N Tees Gen Hosp 1988; **Fellow:** Urology, Duke Univ Med Ctr 1993; **Fac Appt:** Prof U, Univ SC Sch Med

Kim, Edward D MD [U] - **Spec Exp:** Prostate Cancer; Bladder Cancer; **Hospital:** Univ of Tennesee Mem Hosp; **Address:** University Urology, 1928 Alcoa Hwy, Med Office B Bldg - Ste 222, Knoxville, TN 37920; **Phone:** 865-305-9254; **Board Cert:** Urology 2007; **Med School:** Northwestern Univ 1989; **Resid:** Urology, Northwestern Meml Hosp 1995; **Fellow:** Baylor Coll Med 1996; **Fac Appt:** Assoc Prof U, Univ Tenn Coll Med, Memphis

Lockhart, Jorge L MD [U] - **Spec Exp:** Bladder Cancer; Incontinence; Urinary Reconstruction; Pelvic Reconstruction; **Hospital:** Tampa Genl Hosp, H Lee Moffitt Cancer Ctr & Research Inst; **Address:** USF College of Medicine, Div Urology, 2 Tampa General Circle Fl 7, Tampa, FL 33606; **Phone:** 813-259-8702; **Board Cert:** Urology 1980; **Med School:** Uruguay 1973; **Resid:** Urology, Duke Univ Med Ctr 1977; **Fellow:** Urodynamics, Duke Univ Med Ctr 1978; **Fac Appt:** Prof S, Univ S Fla Coll Med

Marshall, Fray F MD [U] - **Spec Exp:** Prostate Cancer; **Hospital:** Emory Univ Hosp; **Address:** Emory Urology, 1365 Clifton Rd NE B Bldg - Ste 1400, Atlanta, GA 30322; **Phone:** 404-778-4898; **Board Cert:** Urology 1977; **Med School:** Univ VA Sch Med 1969; **Resid:** Surgery, Univ Mich Hosps 1972; Urology, Mass Genl Hosp 1975; **Fac Appt:** Prof U, Emory Univ

McConnell, John D MD [U] - **Spec Exp:** Prostate Cancer; **Hospital:** Wake Forest Univ Baptist Med Ctr (page 84); **Address:** Wake Forest Univ Baptist Med Ctr, Medical Center Blvd, Winston-Salem, NC 27157; **Phone:** 336-716-3408; **Board Cert:** Urology 2004; **Med School:** Loyola Univ-Stritch Sch Med 1978; **Resid:** Surgery, Parkland Hosp 1980; Urology, Parkland Hosp 1984; **Fac Appt:** Prof U, Wake Forest Univ

Moul, Judd W MD [U] - **Spec Exp:** Prostate Cancer; Testicular Cancer; Minimally Invasive Urologic Surgery; Clinical Trials; **Hospital:** Duke Univ Med Ctr, VA Med Ctr - Durham; **Address:** Duke Univ Med Ctr, Div Urologic Surgery, Box 3707, Durham, NC 27710; **Phone:** 919-668-8180; **Board Cert:** Urology 2007; **Med School:** Jefferson Med Coll 1982; **Resid:** Urology, Walter Reed Army Med Ctr 1987; **Fellow:** Urologic Oncology, Duke Univ Med Ctr 1989; **Fac Appt:** Prof S, Duke Univ

Patel, Vipul R MD [U] - **Spec Exp:** Prostate Cancer/Robotic Surgery; Kidney Cancer; **Hospital:** Florida Hosp Celebration Hlth; **Address:** 410 Celebration Pl, Ste 200, Celebration, FL 34747; **Phone:** 407-303-4673; **Board Cert:** Urology 2004; **Med School:** Baylor Coll Med 1995; **Resid:** Urology, Univ Miami; **Fellow:** Urologic Laparoscopic Surgery-Endourology, Univ Miami

Urology

Pow-Sang, Julio M MD [U] - **Spec Exp:** Prostate Cancer; **Hospital:** H Lee Moffitt Cancer Ctr & Research Inst; **Address:** H Lee Moffitt Cancer Ctr, GU Clinic, 12902 Magnolia Drive, Tampa, FL 33612-9416; **Phone:** 813-972-8418; **Board Cert:** Urology 1999; **Med School:** Mexico 1978; **Resid:** Surgery, Univ Miami Sch Med 1983; Urology, Univ Miami Sch Med 1986; **Fellow:** Urologic Oncology, Univ Fla Coll Med 1987; **Fac Appt:** Prof S, Univ S Fla Coll Med

Robertson, Cary N MD [U] - **Spec Exp:** Prostate Cancer; Kidney Cancer; Testicular Cancer; **Hospital:** Duke Univ Med Ctr; **Address:** Duke Univ Med Ctr, Trent Drive, Box 3833, Durham, NC 27710; **Phone:** 919-681-6768; **Board Cert:** Urology 2006; **Med School:** Tulane Univ 1977; **Resid:** Urology, Duke Univ Med Ctr 1985; **Fellow:** Urologic Oncology, Natl Inst Hlth 1987; **Fac Appt:** Assoc Prof U, Duke Univ

Rowland, Randall MD [U] - **Spec Exp:** Urologic Cancer; **Hospital:** Univ of Kentucky Chandler Hosp; **Address:** Univ Kentucky Med Ctr, Div Urology, 800 Rose St, rm MS283, Lexington, KY 40536-0001; **Phone:** 859-323-6677; **Board Cert:** Urology 1980; **Med School:** Northwestern Univ 1972; **Resid:** Urology, Northwestern Meml Hosp 1978; **Fellow:** Urology, Northwestern Meml Hosp 1977; **Fac Appt:** Prof U, Univ KY Coll Med

Sanders, William H MD [U] - **Spec Exp:** Prostate Cancer; Kidney Cancer; **Hospital:** St Joseph's Hosp - Atlanta, Northside Hosp; **Address:** 980 Johnson Ferry Rd, Ste 490, Atlanta, GA 30342-1767; **Phone:** 404-257-0133; **Board Cert:** Urology 2006; **Med School:** Emory Univ 1988; **Resid:** Urology, Yale-New Haven Hosp 1993

Smith, Joseph A MD [U] - **Spec Exp:** Prostate Cancer/Robotic Surgery; Bladder Cancer; Kidney Cancer; **Hospital:** Vanderbilt Univ Med Ctr; **Address:** Vanderbilt Univ Med Ctr, Dept Urology, A-1302 MCN, Nashville, TN 37232-2765; **Phone:** 615-343-0234; **Board Cert:** Urology 2000; **Med School:** Univ Tenn Coll Med, Memphis 1974; **Resid:** Surgery, Parkland Meml Hosp 1976; Urology, Univ Utah 1979; **Fellow:** Urologic Oncology, Meml Sloan Kettering Cancer Ctr 1980; **Fac Appt:** Prof U, Vanderbilt Univ

Soloway, Mark S MD [U] - **Spec Exp:** Bladder Cancer; Kidney Cancer; Prostate Cancer; Urologic Pathology; **Hospital:** Jackson Meml Hosp (page 82), Univ of Miami Hosp & Clins/Sylvester Comp Canc Ctr (page 82); **Address:** 1150 NW 14th St, Ste 309, Miami, FL 33136; **Phone:** 305-243-6596; **Board Cert:** Urology 1977; **Med School:** Case West Res Univ 1968; **Resid:** Surgery, Univ Hosps 1970; Urology, Univ Hosps 1975; **Fellow:** Surgery, Natl Cancer Inst 1972; **Fac Appt:** Prof U, Univ Miami Sch Med

Strup, Stephen E MD [U] - **Spec Exp:** Urologic Cancer; Minimally Invasive Urologic Surgery; Robotic Surgery; **Hospital:** Univ of Kentucky Chandler Hosp; **Address:** MS-283 Chandler Medical Ctr, 800 Rose St, Lexington, KY 40536; **Phone:** 859-323-6679; **Board Cert:** Urology 2007; **Med School:** Indiana Univ 1988; **Resid:** Urology, Thomas Jefferson Univ Hosp 1994; **Fellow:** Urologic Oncology, National Cancer Inst 1996; **Fac Appt:** Prof S, Univ KY Coll Med

Teigland, Chris M MD [U] - **Spec Exp:** Prostate Cancer/Robotic Surgery; Kidney Cancer; **Hospital:** Carolinas Med Ctr; **Address:** Mckay Urology, 1023 Edgehill Rd S, Charlotte, NC 28207; **Phone:** 704-355-8686; **Board Cert:** Urology 2007; **Med School:** Duke Univ 1980; **Resid:** Surgery, Univ Utah Affil Hosps 1982; Urology, Univ Texas SW Med Ctr 1987; **Fac Appt:** Clin Prof S, Univ NC Sch Med

Terris, Martha K MD [U] - **Spec Exp:** Prostate Cancer; Brachytherapy; Urologic Cancer; Bladder Cancer; **Hospital:** VA Medical Ctr - Augusta, Med Coll of GA Hosp and Clin (MCG Health Inc); **Address:** Charlie Norwood VA Medical Center, 1 Freedom Way, Augusta, GA 30904; **Phone:** 706-733-0188; **Board Cert:** Urology 2007; **Med School:** Univ Miss 1986; **Resid:** Surgery, Duke Univ Med Ctr 1988; Urology, Stanford Univ Med Ctr 1995; **Fellow:** Ultrasound, Stanford Univ 1991; **Fac Appt:** Prof S, Med Coll GA

Theodorescu, Dan MD/PhD [U] - **Spec Exp:** Prostate Cancer; Clinical Trials; Bladder Cancer; Kidney Cancer; **Hospital:** Univ Virginia Med Ctr; **Address:** UVA Health System, Dept Urology, PO Box 800422, Charlottesville, VA 22908; **Phone:** 434-924-0042; **Board Cert:** Urology 2007; **Med School:** Canada 1986; **Resid:** Urology, Univ Toronto Med Ctr 1993; **Fellow:** Urologic Oncology, Meml Sloan Kettering Cancer Ctr 1995; **Fac Appt:** Prof U, Univ VA Sch Med

Midwest

Andriole, Gerald L MD [U] - **Spec Exp:** Urologic Cancer; Prostate Cancer; Laparoscopic Surgery; **Hospital:** Barnes-Jewish Hosp; **Address:** 4960 Children's Place, Campus Box 8242, St Louis, MO 63110; **Phone:** 314-362-8212; **Board Cert:** Urology 2003; **Med School:** Jefferson Med Coll 1978; **Resid:** Surgery, Strong Meml Hosp 1980; Urology, Brigham & Womens Hosp 1983; **Fellow:** Urologic Oncology, NCI/NIH 1985; **Fac Appt:** Prof U, Washington Univ, St Louis

Bahnson, Robert MD [U] - **Spec Exp:** Prostate Cancer; Bladder Cancer; Continent Urinary Diversions; **Hospital:** Ohio St Univ Med Ctr, Arthur G James Cancer Hosp & Research Inst; **Address:** 456 West 10th Avenue, Dept of Urology, 4960 Cramblett Med Ctr, Columbus, OH 43210-1228; **Phone:** 614-293-3646; **Board Cert:** Urology 2006; **Med School:** Tufts Univ 1979; **Resid:** Surgery, Northwestern Univ 1981; Urology, Northwestern Univ 1985; **Fellow:** Urology, Northwestern Univ 1984; Research, Univ Pittsburgh 1991; **Fac Appt:** Prof U, Ohio State Univ

Brendler, Charles B MD [U] - **Spec Exp:** Prostate Cancer; **Hospital:** NorthShore Univ HlthSys; **Address:** Evanston Northwestern Hosp, 2650 Ridge Ave Walgreen Bldg - Ste 2507, Evanston, IL 60201; **Phone:** 847-657-5730; **Board Cert:** Urology 1981; **Med School:** Univ VA Sch Med 1974; **Resid:** Surgery, Duke Univ Med Ctr 1976; Urology, Duke Univ Med Ctr 1979; **Fellow:** Urologic Oncology, Univ Hosp Wales 1980; Urologic Oncology, Johns Hopkins Hosp 1982; **Fac Appt:** Prof U, Northwestern Univ-Feinberg Sch Med

Campbell, Steven C MD/PhD [U] - **Spec Exp:** Kidney Cancer; Prostate Cancer; Bladder Cancer; **Hospital:** Cleveland Clin Fdn (page 70); **Address:** Cleveland Clinic, Glickman Urological Inst, 9500 Euclid Ave, MS Q10-1, Cleveland, OH 44195; **Phone:** 216-444-5595; **Board Cert:** Urology 1999; **Med School:** Univ Chicago-Pritzker Sch Med 1989; **Resid:** Urology, Cleveland Clinic 1995; **Fellow:** Urology, Meml Sloan Kettering Cancer Ctr 1996; **Fac Appt:** Prof S, Cleveland Cl Coll Med/Case West Res

Catalona, William J MD [U] - **Spec Exp:** Prostate Cancer; **Hospital:** Northwestern Meml Hosp; **Address:** Northwestern Med Faculty Foundation, 675 N St Clair St, Ste 20-150, Chicago, IL 60611; **Phone:** 312-695-6126; **Board Cert:** Urology 1978; **Med School:** Yale Univ 1968; **Resid:** Surgery, UCSF Med Ctr 1970; Urology, Johns Hopkins Hosp 1976; **Fellow:** Surgical Oncology, Natl Cancer Inst 1972; **Fac Appt:** Prof U, Northwestern Univ

Coplen, Douglas E MD [U] - **Spec Exp:** Pediatric Urology; Urologic Cancer-Pediatric; Testicular Cancer-Pediatric; **Hospital:** St Louis Chldns Hosp; **Address:** St Louis Children's Hosp, 4990 Children's Pl, Northwest Tower, Ste 1120, St Louis, MO 63110; **Phone:** 314-454-6034; **Board Cert:** Urology 2005; Pediatric Urology 2008; **Med School:** Indiana Univ 1985; **Resid:** Urology, Barnes Jewish Hosp 1992; **Fellow:** Pediatric Urology, Childrens Hosp 1994; **Fac Appt:** Asst Prof S, Washington Univ, St Louis

Donovan Jr, James F MD [U] - **Spec Exp:** Prostate Cancer/Robotic Surgery; Kidney Cancer; Adrenal Tumors; Laparoscopic Surgery; **Hospital:** Univ Hosp - Cincinnati, Christ Hospital; **Address:** Univ Cincinnati Med Ctr, Medical Arts Bldg, 222 Piedmont Ave, Ste 7000, Cincinnati, OH 45219; **Phone:** 513-475-8787; **Board Cert:** Surgery 1997; Urology 1999; **Med School:** Northwestern Univ 1978; **Resid:** Surgery, Northwestern Meml Hosp 1982; Urology, Northwestern Meml Hosp 1986; **Fellow:** Male Infertility, Baylor Coll Med 1986; **Fac Appt:** Prof U, Univ Cincinnati

Urology

Flanigan, Robert C MD [U] - **Spec Exp:** Prostate Cancer; Bladder Cancer; Kidney Cancer; **Hospital:** Loyola Univ Med Ctr; **Address:** Loyola Univ Med-Fahey Bldg 54, 2160 S First Ave, rm 267, Maywood, IL 60153; **Phone:** 708-216-5100; **Board Cert:** Surgery 1998; Urology 2001; **Med School:** Case West Res Univ 1972; **Resid:** Surgery, Case West Univ Med Ctr 1978; Urology, Case West Univ Med Ctr 1978; **Fac Appt:** Prof U, Loyola Univ-Stritch Sch Med

Foster, Richard S MD [U] - **Spec Exp:** Testicular Cancer; Reconstructive Surgery; **Hospital:** Indiana Univ Hosp (page 74); **Address:** 535 N Barnhill Drive, Ste 420, Indianapolis, IN 46202; **Phone:** 317-274-3458; **Board Cert:** Urology 2008; **Med School:** Indiana Univ 1980; **Resid:** Urology, Indiana Univ Hosp 1986; **Fac Appt:** Prof U, Indiana Univ

Gluckman, Gordon R MD [U] - **Spec Exp:** Prostate Cancer; Kidney Cancer; Minimally Invasive Urologic Surgery; Bladder Cancer; **Hospital:** Adv Luth Genl Hosp, Resurrection Med Ctr; **Address:** 900 Grand Rd, Ste 120, Des Plaines, IL 60016; **Phone:** 847-823-3185; **Board Cert:** Urology 2006; **Med School:** Northwestern Univ 1989; **Resid:** Surgery, UCSF Med Ctr 1991; Urology, UCSF Med Ctr 1995

Kaouk, Jihad MD [U] - **Spec Exp:** Minimally Invasive Urologic Surgery; Robotic Surgery; Kidney Cancer; Bladder Cancer; **Hospital:** Cleveland Clin Fdn (page 70); **Address:** Cleveland Clinic main campus, 9500 Euclid Ave, MC Q10-1, Cleveland, OH 44195; **Phone:** 216-444-2976; **Med School:** Lebanon 1993; **Resid:** Urology, Amer Univ of Beirut Med Ctr; Surgery, Amer Univ of Beitut Med Ctr; **Fellow:** Minimally Invasive Surgery, Cleveland Clinic; Research, Cleveland Clinic; **Fac Appt:** Assoc Prof S, Cleveland Cl Coll Med/Case West Res

Kibel, Adam S MD [U] - **Spec Exp:** Prostate Cancer; Bladder Cancer; Kidney Cancer; **Hospital:** Barnes-Jewish Hosp; **Address:** Director Urologic Oncology, Washington Univ School of Medicine, 4960 Children's Place, Box 8242, St Louis, MO 63105-1000; **Phone:** 314-362-8295; **Board Cert:** Urology 2001; **Med School:** Cornell Univ-Weill Med Coll 1991; **Resid:** Urology, Brigham & Women's Hosp 1996; **Fellow:** Urologic Oncology, Johns Hopkins Hosp 1999; **Fac Appt:** Prof U, Washington Univ, St Louis

Klein, Eric A MD [U] - **Spec Exp:** Prostate Cancer; Testicular Cancer; Urologic Cancer; **Hospital:** Cleveland Clin Fdn (page 70); **Address:** Cleveland Clinic Fdn, Dept Urol, Sect Urol-Onc, 9500 Euclid Ave, Desk A100, Cleveland, OH 44195-0001; **Phone:** 216-444-5591; **Board Cert:** Urology 2008; **Med School:** Univ Pittsburgh 1981; **Resid:** Urology, Cleveland Clinic Fdn 1986; **Fellow:** Urologic Oncology, Meml Sloan Kettering Canc Ctr 1989; **Fac Appt:** Prof S, Cleveland Cl Coll Med/Case West Res

Kozlowski, James M MD [U] - **Spec Exp:** Prostate Cancer; Continent Urinary Diversions; Laparoscopic Surgery; **Hospital:** Northwestern Meml Hosp, Jesse A Brown VA Med Ctr; **Address:** 675 N St Clair St, Galter Bldg Fl 20 - Ste 150, Chicago, IL 60611; **Phone:** 312-695-8146; **Board Cert:** Surgery 2004; Urology 1983; **Med School:** Northwestern Univ 1975; **Resid:** Surgery, Northwestern Univ-McGaw 1979; Urology, Northwestern Univ-McGaw 1981; **Fellow:** Research, NCI-Frederick Cancer Rsch 1984; **Fac Appt:** Assoc Prof U, Northwestern Univ

Lee, Cheryl T MD [U] - **Spec Exp:** Urologic Cancer; Bladder Cancer; **Hospital:** Univ Michigan Hlth Sys; **Address:** Univ of Michigan Cancer Ctr, 1500 E Medical Ctr Drive, Reception D LB1-229, Ann Arbor, MI 48109-5913; **Phone:** 734-647-8903; **Board Cert:** Urology 2002; **Med School:** Albany Med Coll 1991; **Resid:** Urology, Albany Med Ctr; **Fellow:** Urologic Oncology, Meml Sloan Kettering Cancer Ctr 2000; **Fac Appt:** Assoc Prof U, Univ Mich Med Sch

McVary, Kevin MD [U] - **Spec Exp:** Prostate Cancer; Erectile Dysfunction; **Hospital:** Northwestern Meml Hosp; **Address:** 675 N St Clair St, Galter Bldg Fl 20 - Ste 150, Chicago, IL 60611-4813; **Phone:** 312-695-8146; **Board Cert:** Urology 2000; **Med School:** Northwestern Univ 1983; **Resid:** Surgery, Northwestern Meml Hosp 1985; Urology, Northwestern Meml Hosp 1988; **Fellow:** Research, Northwestern Meml Hosp; **Fac Appt:** Prof U, Northwestern Univ

Menon, Mani MD [U] - **Spec Exp:** Prostate Cancer/Robotic Surgery; Transplant-Kidney; Urologic Cancer; **Hospital:** Henry Ford Hosp; **Address:** Henry Ford Hosp - Vattikuti Urology Inst, 2799 W Grand Bvd, Clinic Bldg - #K-9, Detroit, MI 48202; **Phone:** 888-881-1117; **Board Cert:** Urology 1982; **Med School:** India 1969; **Resid:** Urology, Bryn Mawr Hosp 1974; Urology, Johns Hopkins Hosp 1980; **Fellow:** Transplant Surgery, Johns Hopkins Univ 1977; **Fac Appt:** Prof S, Univ Mass Sch Med

Montie, James MD [U] - **Spec Exp:** Bladder Cancer; Prostate Cancer; Genitourinary Cancer; **Hospital:** Univ Michigan Hlth Sys; **Address:** UMH Cancer Ctr, Team 3, Reception D, Level B1-229, 1500 E Med Ctr Drive, Ann Arbor, MI 48109-5913; **Phone:** 734-647-8903; **Board Cert:** Urology 1978; **Med School:** Univ Mich Med Sch 1971; **Resid:** Urology, Cleveland Clinic Fdn 1976; **Fellow:** Urologic Oncology, Meml Sloan-Kettering Cancer Ctr 1979; **Fac Appt:** Prof U, Univ Mich Med Sch

Myers, Robert P MD [U] - **Spec Exp:** Prostate Cancer; **Hospital:** Mayo Med Ctr & Clin - Rochester, Rochester Methodist Hosp; **Address:** Mayo Clinic, Dept Urology, 200 First St SW, Rochester, MN 55905; **Phone:** 507-284-3077; **Board Cert:** Urology 1976; **Med School:** Columbia P&S 1967; **Resid:** Urology, Mayo Clinic 1972; **Fac Appt:** Prof U, Mayo Med Sch

O'Donnell, Michael A MD [U] - **Spec Exp:** Bladder Cancer; Immunotherapy; Urologic Cancer; **Hospital:** Univ Iowa Hosp & Clinics; **Address:** Univ Iowa Hosp & Clins, Dept Urology, 200 Hawkins Drive, 3RCP, Iowa City, IA 52242-1089; **Phone:** 319-384-6040; **Board Cert:** Urology 2005; **Med School:** Duke Univ 1984; **Resid:** Surgery, Brigham & Womens Hosp 1987; Urology, Brigham & Womens Hosp 1991; **Fellow:** Urology, Brigham & Womens Hosp 1993; **Fac Appt:** Prof U, Univ Iowa Coll Med

Schaeffer, Anthony MD [U] - **Spec Exp:** Incontinence after Prostate Cancer; **Hospital:** Northwestern Meml Hosp; **Address:** 675 N St Clair, Galter Bldg Fl 20 - Ste 150, Chicago, IL 60611; **Phone:** 312-695-8146; **Board Cert:** Urology 1978; **Med School:** Northwestern Univ 1968; **Resid:** Surgery, Northwestern Meml Hosp 1970; Urology, Stanford Med Ctr 1976; **Fac Appt:** Prof U, Northwestern Univ

See, William A MD [U] - **Spec Exp:** Prostate Cancer; Bladder Cancer; Testicular Cancer; **Hospital:** Froedtert Meml Lutheran Hosp; **Address:** Med Coll Wisconsin, Dept Urology, 9200 W Wisconsin Ave, Milwaukee, WI 53226; **Phone:** 414-805-0805; **Board Cert:** Urology 2008; **Med School:** Univ Chicago-Pritzker Sch Med 1982; **Resid:** Urology, Univ Washington 1988; **Fellow:** Research, Natl Kidney Fdn/Univ Wash 1986; Research, Amer Fdn for Urol Dis/Univ Iowa 1990; **Fac Appt:** Prof U, Med Coll Wisc

Steinberg, Gary D MD [U] - **Spec Exp:** Bladder Cancer; Kidney Cancer; Prostate Cancer; **Hospital:** Univ of Chicago Med Ctr; **Address:** 5841 S Maryland Ave, rm J653, MC 6038, Chicago, IL 60637-1447; **Phone:** 773-702-3080; **Board Cert:** Urology 2003; **Med School:** Univ Chicago-Pritzker Sch Med 1985; **Resid:** Surgery, Johns Hopkins Hosp 1987; Urology, Brady Urol Inst/Johns Hopkins 1991; **Fellow:** Oncology, Johns Hopkins Hosp 1989; **Fac Appt:** Prof U, Univ Chicago-Pritzker Sch Med

Urology

Williams, Richard D MD [U] - **Spec Exp:** Kidney Cancer; Bladder Cancer; Prostate Cancer; **Hospital:** Univ Iowa Hosp & Clinics; **Address:** Univ Iowa Hosp, Dept Urology, 200 Hawkins Dr, rm 3251 RCP, Iowa City, IA 52242-1089; **Phone:** 319-356-0760; **Board Cert:** Urology 1979; **Med School:** Univ Kans 1970; **Resid:** Surgery, Univ Minn Hosp 1972; Urology, Univ Minn Hosp 1976; **Fellow:** Urologic Oncology, Univ Minn Hosp 1979; **Fac Appt:** Prof U, Univ Iowa Coll Med

Wood, David P MD [U] - **Spec Exp:** Genitourinary Cancer; Bladder Cancer; Prostate Cancer; Robotic Surgery; **Hospital:** Univ Michigan Hlth Sys; **Address:** UMH Cancer Ctr, Team 3, Reception D, Level B1-229, 1500 E Medical Center Drive, Ann Arbor, MI 48109-5913; **Phone:** 734-647-8903; **Board Cert:** Urology 2002; **Med School:** Univ Mich Med Sch 1983; **Resid:** Urology, Cleveland Clinic 1988; **Fellow:** Urologic Oncology, Meml Sloan-Kettering Cancer Ctr 1991; **Fac Appt:** Prof U, Univ Mich Med Sch

Zippe, Craig D MD [U] - **Spec Exp:** Prostate Cancer; Bladder Cancer; Incontinence after Prostate Cancer; **Hospital:** Univ Hosps Case Med Ctr; **Address:** 88 Center Rd, Ste 360, Bedford, OH 44146; **Phone:** 440-232-8955; **Board Cert:** Urology 2007; **Med School:** Rush Med Coll 1980; **Resid:** Urology, Columbia Presby Med Ctr 1989; **Fellow:** Urologic Oncology, Meml Sloan Kettering Cancer Ctr 1992

Great Plains and Mountains

Childs, Stacy J MD [U] - **Spec Exp:** Prostate Cancer; Bladder Cancer; Incontinence after Prostate Cancer; **Hospital:** Yampa Valley Med Ctr, Memorial Hosp - Craig; **Address:** 501 Anglers Drive, Ste 202, Steamboat Springs, CO 80487-8841; **Phone:** 970-871-9710; **Board Cert:** Urology 1979; **Med School:** Louisiana State U, New Orleans 1972; **Resid:** Urology, Carraway Meth Med Ctr 1977; **Fac Appt:** Clin Prof U, Univ Colorado

Crawford, E David MD [U] - **Spec Exp:** Prostate Cancer; Testicular Cancer; Bladder Cancer; **Hospital:** Univ Colorado Hosp; **Address:** Urologic Oncology, MS F710, 1665 Aurora Ct, rm 1004, Box 6510, Aurora, CO 80045; **Phone:** 720-848-0170; **Board Cert:** Urology 1980; **Med School:** Univ Cincinnati 1973; **Resid:** Urology, Good Samaritan Hosp 1977; **Fellow:** Genitourinary Surgery, UCLA Med Ctr 1978; **Fac Appt:** Prof U, Univ Colorado

Davis, Bradley E MD [U] - **Spec Exp:** Urologic Cancer; Bladder Cancer; Reconstructive Surgery; Prostate Cancer; **Hospital:** Overland Pk Regl Med Ctr, St Luke's Hosp of Kansas City; **Address:** Urologic Surgical Associates, 10550 Quivira Rd, Ste 105, Overland Park, KS 66215; **Phone:** 913-438-3833; **Board Cert:** Urology 2004; **Med School:** Univ Kans 1986; **Resid:** Surgery, St Lukes Hosp 1991; Urology, Univ Kansas Med Ctr 1991; **Fellow:** Urologic Oncology, Meml Sloan-Kettering Cancer Ctr 1993; **Fac Appt:** Asst Clin Prof U, Univ Kans

Lugg, James A MD [U] - **Spec Exp:** Prostate Cancer; Laparoscopic Surgery; Incontinence after Prostate Cancer; **Hospital:** Cheyenne Regl Med Ctr, Univ Colorado Hosp; **Address:** 2301 House Ave, Ste 502, Cheyenne, WY 82001; **Phone:** 307-635-4131; **Board Cert:** Urology 2008; **Med School:** Northwestern Univ 1990; **Resid:** Urology, UCLA Med Ctr 1995; **Fac Appt:** Asst Prof U, Univ Colorado

Southwest

Bans, Larry L MD [U] - **Spec Exp:** Prostate Cancer; **Hospital:** Banner Good Samaritan Regl Med Ctr - Phoenix; **Address:** Prostate Solutions of Arizona, 2525 E Arizona Biltmore Cir, Ste C236, Phoenix, AZ 85016; **Phone:** 602-426-9772; **Board Cert:** Urology 2004; **Med School:** Cornell Univ-Weill Med Coll 1978; **Resid:** Urology, Ind Univ Med Ctr 1983

Bardot, Stephen F MD [U] - **Spec Exp:** Urologic Cancer; Prostate Cancer; **Hospital:** Ochsner Fdn Hosp; **Address:** Ochsner Clinic, 1514 Jefferson Hwy Fl 4, Atrium 4 West, Dept of Urology, New Orleans, LA 70121-2483; **Phone:** 504-842-4083; **Board Cert:** Urology 2002; **Med School:** Univ Kans 1985; **Resid:** Surgery, St Luke's Hosp 1987; Urology, Kansas City Univ Med Ctr 1990; **Fellow:** Urologic Oncology, Cleveland Clinic 1991

Basler, Joseph W MD [U] - **Spec Exp:** Prostate Cancer; Urologic Cancer; **Hospital:** Audie L Murphy Meml Vets Hosp; **Address:** 7703 Floyd Curl Dr, MC-7845, San Antonio, TX 78229-3900; **Phone:** 210-567-5640; **Board Cert:** Urology 2001; **Med School:** Univ MO-Columbia Sch Med 1984; **Resid:** Surgery, Univ Missouri Affil Hosp 1986; Urology, Barnes Hosp/Wash Univ 1990; **Fac Appt:** Prof U, Univ Tex, San Antonio

Culkin, Daniel J MD [U] - **Spec Exp:** Urologic Cancer; Laparoscopic Surgery; **Hospital:** OU Med Ctr, VA Med Ctr - Oklahoma City; **Address:** Oklahoma Univ Med Ctr, Div Urology, 920 Stanton L Young Blvd, Ste WP 3150, Oklahoma City, OK 73104; **Phone:** 405-271-8156; **Board Cert:** Urology 2006; **Med School:** Creighton Univ 1979; **Resid:** Surgery, Loyola Univ Med Ctr 1981; Urology, Loyola Univ Med Ctr 1983; **Fellow:** Neurourology, Loyola Univ Med Ctr 1984; **Fac Appt:** Prof U, Univ Okla Coll Med

Ellis, David S MD [U] - **Spec Exp:** Prostate Cancer-Cryosurgery; **Hospital:** Arlington Meml Hosp; **Address:** Urology Assocs of N Texas (UANT), Arlington-North, 1001 Waldrop Drive, Ste 708, Arlington, TX 76012; **Phone:** 817-465-0373; **Board Cert:** Urology 2000; **Med School:** Univ Tex, Houston 1982; **Resid:** Urology, Univ Texas Med Ctr 1988

Greene, Graham MD [U] - **Spec Exp:** Urologic Cancer; **Hospital:** UAMS Med Ctr, Arkansas Chldns Hosp; **Address:** 4301 W Markham, Slot 774, Little Rock, AR 72205; **Phone:** 501-296-1545; **Board Cert:** Urology 2007; **Med School:** Dalhousie Univ 1989; **Resid:** Urology, Victoria Genl 1994; **Fellow:** Urologic Oncology, M.D. Anderson Cancer Ctr 1997; **Fac Appt:** Assoc Prof U, Univ Ark

Grossman, H Barton MD [U] - **Spec Exp:** Bladder Cancer; Bladder Reconstruction; Urinary Reconstruction; **Hospital:** UT MD Anderson Cancer Ctr; **Address:** MD Anderson Cancer Ctr, Dept Urology, 1373, 1515 Holcombe Blvd, Houston, TX 77030; **Phone:** 713-792-3250; **Board Cert:** Urology 1979; **Med School:** Temple Univ 1972; **Resid:** Surgery, St Joseph Mercy Hosp 1974; Urology, Univ Michigan Med Ctr 1977; **Fellow:** Research, Meml Sloan Kettering Cancer Ctr 1979; **Fac Appt:** Prof U, Univ Tex, Houston

Kadmon, Dov MD [U] - **Spec Exp:** Prostate Cancer; **Hospital:** St Luke's Episcopal Hosp-Houston, Methodist Hosp - Houston; **Address:** Baylor Dept Urology, 6620 Main St, Ste 1325, Houston, TX 77030; **Phone:** 713-798-4001; **Board Cert:** Urology 1984; **Med School:** Israel 1970; **Resid:** Surgery, Barnes Jewish Hosp 1977; Urology, Barnes Jewish Hosp 1980; **Fellow:** Urology, Barnes Jewish Hosp 1982; **Fac Appt:** Prof U, Baylor Coll Med

Lerner, Seth P MD [U] - **Spec Exp:** Bladder Cancer; Testicular Cancer; Urinary Reconstruction; **Hospital:** St Luke's Episcopal Hosp-Houston, Methodist Hosp - Houston; **Address:** 6620 Main St, Ste 1325, Houston, TX 77030; **Phone:** 713-798-6841; **Board Cert:** Urology 2002; **Med School:** Baylor Coll Med 1984; **Resid:** Surgery, Virginia Mason Hosp 1986; Urology, Baylor Coll Med 1990; **Fellow:** Urologic Oncology, LAC-USC Med Ctr 1992; **Fac Appt:** Prof U, Baylor Coll Med

Miles, Brian J MD [U] - **Spec Exp:** Prostate Cancer; Urologic Cancer; Gene Therapy; **Hospital:** Methodist Hosp - Houston, St Luke's Episcopal Hosp-Houston; **Address:** 6624 Fannin St, Ste 2280, Houston, TX 77030-2769; **Phone:** 713-799-8896; **Board Cert:** Urology 1984; **Med School:** Univ Mich Med Sch 1974; **Resid:** Urology, Walter Reed Army Med Ctr 1982; **Fac Appt:** Clin Prof U, Baylor Coll Med

Urology

Pisters, Louis L MD [U] - **Spec Exp:** Prostate Cancer; Bladder Cancer; Genitourinary Cancer; Prostate Cancer/Robotic Surgery; **Hospital:** UT MD Anderson Cancer Ctr; **Address:** MD Anderson Cancer Ctr, 1515 Holcombe Blvd, Unit 1373, Houston, TX 77030; **Phone:** 713-792-3250; **Board Cert:** Urology 2003; **Med School:** Univ Western Ontario 1986; **Resid:** Urology, Shands Hosp/UNIV Florida 1991; **Fellow:** Urologic Oncology, MD Anderson Cancer Ctr 1993; **Fac Appt:** Assoc Prof U, Univ Tex, Houston

Sagalowsky, Arthur I MD [U] - **Spec Exp:** Urologic Cancer; Transplant-Kidney; Testicular Cancer; **Hospital:** UT Southwestern Med Ctr at Dallas; **Address:** UT SW Med Ctr, Dept Urology, 5323 Harry Hines Blvd, J8.114, Dallas, TX 75390-9110; **Phone:** 214-648-3976; **Board Cert:** Urology 1980; **Med School:** Indiana Univ 1973; **Resid:** Surgery, Indiana Univ Hosps 1975; Urology, Indiana Univ Hosps 1978; **Fellow:** Clinical Pharmacology, Univ Tex SW Med Ctr 1980; **Fac Appt:** Prof U, Univ Tex SW, Dallas

Slawin, Kevin Mark MD [U] - **Spec Exp:** Prostate Cancer; Prostate Cancer/Robotic Surgery; **Hospital:** Meml Hermann Hosp - Texas Med Ctr, Methodist Hosp - Houston; **Address:** Vanguard Urologic Inst, Memorial Hermann Medical Plaza, 6400 Fannin, Ste 2300, Houston, TX 77030; **Phone:** 713-366-7848; **Board Cert:** Urology 2005; **Med School:** Columbia P&S 1986; **Resid:** Surgery, Mt Sinai Med Ctr 1988; Urology, Columbia-Presby Hosp 1992; **Fellow:** Urologic Oncology, Am Fdn Urol Dis/Baylor Coll Med 1994; **Fac Appt:** Clin Prof U, Baylor Coll Med

Swanson, David A MD [U] - **Spec Exp:** Kidney Cancer; Prostate Cancer; Testicular Cancer; **Hospital:** UT MD Anderson Cancer Ctr; **Address:** UT MD Anderson Canc Ctr, Dept Urol, 1515 Holcombe Blvd , Unit 1373, Houston, TX 77030-4009; **Phone:** 713-792-3250; **Board Cert:** Urology 1977; **Med School:** Univ Pennsylvania 1967; **Resid:** Surgery, Harbor Genl Hosp 1969; Urology, UC Davis Med Ctr 1975; **Fellow:** Urologic Oncology, Univ Tex-MD Anderson Hosp 1978

Thompson Jr, Ian M MD [U] - **Spec Exp:** Prostate Cancer; **Hospital:** Univ Hlth Syst-San Antonio; **Address:** Univ Tex Hlth Scis Ctr, Dept Urol, 7703 Floyd Curl Drive, rm 306L, MC 7845, San Antonio, TX 78229-3900; **Phone:** 210-567-5643; **Board Cert:** Urology 2005; **Med School:** Tulane Univ 1980; **Resid:** Urology, Brooke Army Med Ctr 1985; **Fellow:** Medical Oncology, Meml Sloan-Kettering Canc Ctr 1988; **Fac Appt:** Prof S, Univ Tex, San Antonio

West Coast and Pacific

Ahlering, Thomas E MD [U] - **Spec Exp:** Prostate Cancer/Robotic Surgery; **Hospital:** UC Irvine Med Ctr, VA Med Ctr - Long Beach, CA; **Address:** UC Irvine Med Ctr, 333 City Blvd W, Ste 2100, Orange, CA 92868; **Phone:** 714-456-6068; **Board Cert:** Urology 2005; **Med School:** St Louis Univ 1979; **Resid:** Urology, LAC-USC Med Ctr 1984; **Fellow:** Urologic Oncology, USC-Norris Comp Cancer Ctr 1986; **Fac Appt:** Prof U, UC Irvine

Amling, Christopher L MD [U] - **Spec Exp:** Prostate Cancer/Robotic Surgery; Kidney Cancer; Bladder Cancer; Testicular Cancer; **Hospital:** OR Hlth & Sci Univ; **Address:** 3303 SW Bond Ave, MC CC10U, Portland, OR 97239; **Phone:** 503-494-4779; **Board Cert:** Urology 1999; **Med School:** Oregon Hlth Sci Univ 1985; **Resid:** Urology, Duke Univ Med Ctr 1996; **Fellow:** Urologic Oncology, Mayo Clinic 1997; **Fac Appt:** Prof U, Univ Alabama

Belldegrun, Arie S MD [U] - **Spec Exp:** Urologic Cancer; Gene Therapy; **Hospital:** UCLA Ronald Reagan Med Ctr; **Address:** UCLA-Geffen Sch Med, Dep Urology, 108-33 Leconte Ave, rm 66-118, Los Angeles, CA 90095; **Phone:** 310-206-1434; **Board Cert:** Urology 1999; **Med School:** Israel 1974; **Resid:** Urology, Brigham and Women's Hosp 1985; **Fellow:** Urologic Oncology, Natl Cancer Inst, NIH 1988; **Fac Appt:** Prof U, UCLA

Boyd, Stuart D MD [U] - **Spec Exp:** Urologic Cancer; **Hospital:** USC Norris Cancer Hosp, USC Univ Hosp; **Address:** 1441 Eastlake Ave, Ste 7416, Los Angeles, CA 90089-9178; **Phone:** 323-865-3704; **Board Cert:** Urology 1984; **Med School:** UCLA 1975; **Resid:** Urology, UCLA Med Ctr 1982; **Fac Appt:** Prof U, USC Sch Med

Carroll, Peter R MD [U] - **Spec Exp:** Testicular Cancer; Prostate Cancer; Bladder Cancer; Bladder Reconstruction; **Hospital:** UCSF - Mt Zion Med Ctr; **Address:** UCSF Urologic Oncology Practice, Fl 3, Box 1711, 1600 Divisadero St, San Francisco, CA 94115-1711; **Phone:** 415-353-7171; **Board Cert:** Urology 2006; **Med School:** Georgetown Univ 1979; **Resid:** Surgery, UCSF Med Ctr 1984; **Fellow:** Urology, Meml Sloan Kettering Cancer Ctr 1986; **Fac Appt:** Prof U, UCSF

Daneshmand, Siamak MD [U] - **Spec Exp:** Bladder Cancer; Prostate Cancer; Kidney Cancer; Testicular Cancer; **Hospital:** OR Hlth & Sci Univ; **Address:** Division of Urology, 10th FL, Center for Health & Healing, 3303 SW Bond Ave, Ste CH10U, Portland, OR 97239; **Phone:** 503-346-1500; **Board Cert:** Urology 2006; **Med School:** UC Davis 1996; **Resid:** Surgery, UC Med Ctr 1998; Urology, UC Med Ctr 2002; **Fellow:** Urologic Oncology, UC Med Ctr 2004; **Fac Appt:** Assoc Prof S, Oregon Hlth Sci Univ

Danoff, Dudley S MD [U] - **Spec Exp:** Prostate Cancer; Bladder Cancer; **Hospital:** Cedars-Sinai Med Ctr; **Address:** 8635 W 3rd St, Ste 1 West, Los Angeles, CA 90048; **Phone:** 310-854-9898; **Board Cert:** Urology 1974; **Med School:** Yale Univ 1963; **Resid:** Urology, Yale-New Haven Hosp 1965; Urology, Columbia-Presby Med Ctr 1969

de Kernion, Jean B MD [U] - **Spec Exp:** Urologic Cancer; Kidney Cancer; Prostate Cancer; **Hospital:** UCLA Ronald Reagan Med Ctr; **Address:** UCLA-Geffen Sch Med, Dept Urology, rm 66-133CHS, Box 951738, Los Angeles, CA 90095-1738; **Phone:** 310-206-6453; **Board Cert:** Surgery 1973; Urology 1975; **Med School:** Louisiana State U, New Orleans 1965; **Resid:** Surgery, Univ Hosps-Case West Res 1967; Urology, Univ Hosps-Case West Res 1973; **Fellow:** Urologic Oncology, Natl Cancer Inst 1969; **Fac Appt:** Prof U, UCLA

Ellis, William J MD [U] - **Spec Exp:** Prostate Cancer; Kidney Cancer; **Hospital:** Univ Wash Med Ctr; **Address:** Univ Wash Med Ctr, Dept Urology, 1959 NE Pacific St, Box 356158, Seattle, WA 98195; **Phone:** 206-598-4294; **Board Cert:** Urology 2001; **Med School:** Johns Hopkins Univ 1985; **Resid:** Surgery, Northwestern Meml Hosp 1987; Urology, Northwestern Meml Hosp 1991; **Fac Appt:** Assoc Prof U, Univ Wash

Gill, Harcharan Singh MD [U] - **Spec Exp:** Urologic Cancer; Prostate Cancer; **Hospital:** Stanford Univ Med Ctr; **Address:** 875 Blake Wilbur Drive, rm 2216, Stanford, CA 94305-5826; **Phone:** 650-725-5544; **Board Cert:** Urology 2004; **Med School:** Kenya 1977; **Resid:** Urology, Inst of Urol; Urology, Univ Penn 1991; **Fellow:** Urology, Univ Penn 1986; **Fac Appt:** Prof U, Stanford Univ

Gill, Inderbir Singh MD [U] - **Spec Exp:** Prostate Cancer; Kidney Cancer; Urologic Cancer; Minimally Invasive Urologic Surgery; **Hospital:** USC Norris Cancer Hosp; **Address:** USC/Norris Cancer Ctr, Dept Urology, 1441 Eastlake Ave, Ste 7416, Los Angeles, CA 90089; **Phone:** 323-865-3700; **Board Cert:** Urology 2008; **Med School:** India 1980; **Resid:** Surgery, Dayanand Med Coll & Hosp; Urology, Univ Kentucky Hosp 1993; **Fac Appt:** Prof U, Univ SC Sch Med

Holden, Stuart MD [U] - **Spec Exp:** Kidney Cancer; **Hospital:** Cedars-Sinai Med Ctr; **Address:** 8635 W 3rd St, Ste 1 West, Los Angeles, CA 90048; **Phone:** 310-854-9898; **Board Cert:** Urology 1977; **Med School:** Cornell Univ-Weill Med Coll 1968; **Resid:** Surgery, NY Hosp-Cornell 1970; Urology, Emory Univ Hosp 1975; **Fellow:** Urology, Meml Sloan Kettering Cancer Ctr 1978

Urology

Kawachi, Mark H MD [U] - **Spec Exp:** Prostate Cancer/Robotic Surgery; Minimally Invasive Urologic Surgery; **Hospital:** City of Hope Natl Med Ctr & Beckman Rsch (page 69); **Address:** Div Urologic Oncology, 1500 E Duarte Rd, Duarte, CA 91010-3012; **Phone:** 626-359-8111 x62655; **Board Cert:** Urology 2004; **Med School:** USC Sch Med 1979; **Resid:** Urology, USC Med Ctr 1984

Lange, Paul H MD [U] - **Spec Exp:** Prostate Cancer; **Hospital:** Univ Wash Med Ctr; **Address:** Univ Wash Med Ctr, Dept Urology, 1959 NE Pacific St, Box 356158, Seattle, WA 98195; **Phone:** 206-598-4294; **Board Cert:** Urology 2006; **Med School:** Washington Univ, St Louis 1967; **Resid:** Surgery, Duke Univ Med Ctr 1972; Urology, Univ Minn Med Ctr 1975; **Fellow:** Immunology, Univ Minn 1973; Research, Natl Inst Hlth 1970; **Fac Appt:** Prof U, Univ Wash

Lieskovsky, Gary MD [U] - **Spec Exp:** Prostate Cancer; **Hospital:** USC Norris Cancer Hosp, USC Univ Hosp; **Address:** 1441 Eastlake Ave, Ste 7416, Los Angeles, CA 90089-0112; **Phone:** 323-865-3702; **Board Cert:** Urology 1980; **Med School:** Canada 1973; **Resid:** Urology, Univ Alberta Hosp 1978; **Fellow:** Urology, UCLA Med Ctr 1980; **Fac Appt:** Prof U, USC Sch Med

Penson, David F MD [U] - **Spec Exp:** Urologic Cancer; Bladder Cancer; Erectile Dysfunction; **Hospital:** USC Univ Hosp, Good Sam Hosp; **Address:** 1441 Eastlake Ave, Ste 7416, Los Angeles, CA 90089; **Phone:** 323-865-3716; **Board Cert:** Urology 2001; **Med School:** Boston Univ 1991; **Resid:** Urology, UCLA Med Ctr 1997; **Fellow:** Urologic Oncology, Yale-New Haven Hosp 1999; **Fac Appt:** Assoc Prof U, USC-Keck School of Medicine

Presti Jr, Joseph C MD [U] - **Spec Exp:** Prostate Cancer; Bladder Cancer; Kidney Cancer; **Hospital:** Stanford Univ Med Ctr; **Address:** Stanford Cancer Ctr, 875 Blake Wilbur Dr MC 5826, Stanford, CA 94305; **Phone:** 650-725-5544; **Board Cert:** Urology 2002; **Med School:** UC Irvine 1984; **Resid:** Surgery, UCSF Med Ctr 1986; Urology, UCSF Med Ctr 1989; **Fellow:** Urologic Oncology, Meml Sloan-Kettering Cancer Ctr 1992; **Fac Appt:** Prof U, Stanford Univ

Skinner, Eila C MD [U] - **Spec Exp:** Urologic Cancer; Urinary Reconstruction; **Hospital:** USC Norris Cancer Hosp, USC Univ Hosp; **Address:** USC-Keck Sch Med, Dept Urology, 1441 Eastlake Ave, Ste 7416, Los Angeles, CA 90089; **Phone:** 323-865-3707; **Board Cert:** Urology 2001; **Med School:** USC Sch Med 1983; **Resid:** Urology, LAC-USC Med Ctr 1988; **Fellow:** Urologic Oncology, LAC-USC Med Ctr 1990; **Fac Appt:** Assoc Prof U, USC Sch Med

Wilson, Timothy G MD [U] - **Spec Exp:** Prostate Cancer/Robotic Surgery; Urinary Reconstruction; **Hospital:** City of Hope Natl Med Ctr & Beckman Rsch (page 69); **Address:** Div Urologic Oncology, 1500 E Duarte Rd, Duarte, CA 91010; **Phone:** 626-359-8111 x62655; **Board Cert:** Urology 2001; **Med School:** Oregon Hlth Sci Univ 1984; **Resid:** Urology, USC Med Ctr 1990; **Fellow:** Urologic Oncology, City Hosp Natl Med Ctr 1991; **Fac Appt:** Assoc Clin Prof U, USC Sch Med

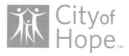

City of Hope™

1500 East Duarte Road
Duarte, CA 91010
800-826-HOPE cityofhope.org

City of Hope is a recognized worldwide leader for its compassionate patient care, innovative science and translational research, which rapidly turn laboratory breakthroughs into promising new therapies. One of only 40 National Cancer Institute-designated Comprehensive Cancer Centers nationwide and a founding member of the National Comprehensive Cancer Network, City of Hope is ranked as one of "America's Best Hospitals" in cancer and urology by *U.S.News & World Report*.

ACADEMIC AND CLINICAL AFFILIATIONS

As an independent academic institution, City of Hope enables its researchers to pursue all avenues of scientific inquiry while encouraging collaboration with other researchers and institutions around the world. This helps to speed the development of novel cancer therapies. City of Hope's Graduate School of Biological Sciences also provides a fertile academic environment to prepare future scientists for careers in academia, medical and industrial fields.

MEDICAL STAFF

Guided by a humanistic approach to medicine, nationally recognized physicians and nurses lead collaborative treatment teams that address the whole patient, not just the disease, including emotional, psychological, spiritual and nutritional needs.

PIONEERING, COMPREHENSIVE MEDICAL CARE

City of Hope's Helford Clinical Research Hospital integrates the best of science and human caring in one state-of-the-art facility. There, lifesaving research and superior clinical care join forces as multidisciplinary teams of medical professionals pool their knowledge to bring promising new therapies to patients quickly, safely and effectively.

PHYSICIAN REFERRAL

City of Hope welcomes patient referrals from physicians throughout the world. Referring physicians are encouraged to contact our specialists directly or call 800-826-HOPE.

CENTER OF EXCELLENCE: UROLOGY/ PROSTATE

Among the top in the nation, and the largest in California, City of Hope's program for prostate cancer delivers superior care to men diagnosed with this serious and increasingly common disease. City of Hope aggressively pursues and uses the newest, most innovative treatments known, including novel research therapies not available elsewhere. Integrating the skills of an extensive team of specialists, the hospital seamlessly coordinates all aspects of care. From diagnosis and treatment to recovery, prostate cancer patients at City of Hope have every advantage to beat this disease.

To learn more, visit cityofhope.org/prostate

Cancer Institute
NYU LANGONE MEDICAL CENTER

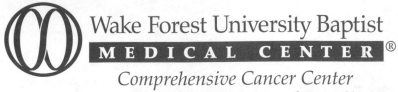

478   Sponsored Page

Other Specialties

Cardiology
(a subspecialty of INTERNAL MEDICINE)

Cardiovascular Disease: A cardiologist specializes in diseases of the heart, lungs and blood vessels and manages complex cardiac conditions such a heart attacks and life-threatening, abnormal heartbeat rhythms.

Cardiac Electrophysiology: A field of special interest within the subspecialty of cardiovascular disease which involves intricate technical procedures to evaluate heart rhythms and determine appropriate treatment for them.

Interventional Cardiology: An area of medicine within the subspecialty of cardiology which uses specialized imaging and other diagnostic techniques to evaluate blood flow and pressure in the coronary arteries and chambers of the heart, and uses technical procedures and medications to treat abnormalities that impair the function of the heart.

Training Required: Three years in internal medicine plus additional training and examination for certification in cardiovascular disease, clinical electrophysiology or interventional cardiology.

Clinical Genetics: A specialist trained in diagnostic and

therapeutic procedures for patients with genetically linked diseases. This specialist uses modern cytogenetics, radiologic and biochemical testing to assist in specialized genetic counseling, implements needed therapeutic interventions and provides prevention through prenatal diagnosis. A clinical geneticist demonstrates competence in providing comprehensive diagnostic, management and counseling services for genetic disorders. A medical geneticist plans and coordinates large scale screening programs for inborn errors of metabolism, hemoglobinopathies, chromosome abnormalities and neural tube defects.

Training Required: Two or four years

Infectious Disease:
(a subspecialty of INTERNAL MEDICINE)

An internist who deals with infectious diseases of all types and in all organs. Conditions requiring selective use of antibodies call for this special skill. This physician often diagnoses and treats AIDS patients and patients with fevers which have not been explained. Infectious disease specialists may also have expertise in preventive

medicine and conditions associated with travel.

Training Required: Three years in internal medicine plus additional training and examination for certification in infectious disease.

Internal Medicine: An internist is a personal physician who provides long-term, comprehensive care in the office and the hospital, managing both common and complex illness of adolescents, adults and the elderly. Internists are trained in the diagnosis and treatment of cancer, infections and diseases affecting the heart, blood, kidneys, joints and digestive, respiratory and vascular systems. They are also trained in the essentials of primary care internal medicine, which incorporates an understanding of disease prevention, wellness, substance abuse, mental health and effective treatment of common problems of the eyes, ears, skin, nervous system and reproductive organs.

Note: Internal Medicine normally includes many primary care physicians. However; for the purpose of this directory, no primary care physicians are included.

Training Required: Three years

Physical Medicine & Rehabilitation:

Physical medicine and rehabilitation, also referred to as rehabilitation medicine, is the medical specialty concerned with diagnosing, evaluations and treating patients with physical disabilities. these disabilities may arise from conditions affecting the musculoskeletal system such as neck and back pain, sports injuries, or other painful conditions affecting the limbs, for example carpal tunnel syndrome. Alternatively, the disabilities may result from neurological trauma or disease such as spinal cord injury, head injury or stroke.

A physician certified in physical medicine and rehabilitation is often called a physiatrist. The primary goal of the physiatrist is to achieve maximal comprehensive rehabilitation. Pain management is often an important part of the role of the physiatrist. for diagnosis and evaluation, a physiatrist may include the techniques of electromyography to supplement the standard history, physical, Xray and laboratory examinations. the physiatrist has expertise in orthotics and mechanical and electrical devices.

Training Required: Four years plus one year clinical practice.

Preventive Medicine: A preventative medicine specialist

focuses on the health of individuals and defined populations in order to protect, promote and maintain health and well-bing and prevent disease, disability and premature death. a preventive medicine physician may be a specialist in general preventive medicine, public health, occupational medicine, or aerospace medicine. this specialist works with large population groups as well as with individual patients to promote health and understand the resks of disease, injury, disability and death, seeking to modify and eliminate these risks.

Training Required: Three years

CARDIOVASCULAR DISEASE

Mid Atlantic

Steingart, Richard MD [Cv] - **Spec Exp:** Heart Disease in Cancer Patients; Cardiac Effects of Cancer/Cancer Therapy; **Hospital:** Meml Sloan-Kettering Cancer Ctr (page 76); **Address:** 1275 York Avenue, New York, NY 10065; **Phone:** 800-525-2225; **Board Cert:** Internal Medicine 1977; Cardiovascular Disease 1979; **Med School:** Mount Sinai Sch Med 1974; **Resid:** Internal Medicine, Yale-New Haven Hosp 1977; **Fellow:** Cardiovascular Disease, Mt Sinai Med Ctr 1979; **Fac Appt:** Prof Med, Cornell Univ-Weill Med Coll

CLINICAL GENETICS

New England

Bale, Allen E MD [CG] - **Spec Exp:** Cancer Genetics; **Hospital:** Yale-New Haven Hosp; **Address:** 333 Cedar St, SHM Bldg - rm 1321, New Haven, CT 06519; **Phone:** 203-785-5745; **Board Cert:** Internal Medicine 1983; Clinical Genetics 1987; Clinical Molecular Genetics 2006; **Med School:** Univ Mass Sch Med 1979; **Resid:** Internal Medicine, Western Penn Hosp 1983; **Fellow:** Medical Genetics, NIH 1987; **Fac Appt:** Assoc Prof CG, Yale Univ

Mid Atlantic

Ostrer, Harry MD [CG] - **Spec Exp:** Genetic Disorders; Hereditary Cancer; **Hospital:** NYU Langone Med Ctr (page 80); **Address:** NYU Medical Ctr, 550 1st Ave, rm MSB136, New York, NY 10016; **Phone:** 212-263-5746; **Board Cert:** Clinical Genetics 1984; Pediatrics 1985; Clinical Cytogenetics 1990; Clinical Molecular Genetics 2006; **Med School:** Columbia P&S 1976; **Resid:** Pediatrics, Johns Hopkins Hosp 1978; Clinical Genetics, Natl Inst Health 1981; **Fellow:** Molecular Genetics, Johns Hopkins Hosp 1983; **Fac Appt:** Prof Ped, NYU Sch Med

Shapiro, Lawrence R MD [CG] - **Spec Exp:** Hereditary Cancer; **Hospital:** Westchester Med Ctr; **Address:** Regional Med Genetics Ctr, Children/Women's Physicians of Westchester, 503 Grasslands Ave, Ste 200, Valhalla, NY 10595; **Phone:** 914-304-5300; **Board Cert:** Pediatrics 1967; Clinical Genetics 1982; Clinical Cytogenetics 1982; **Med School:** NYU Sch Med 1962; **Resid:** Pediatrics, Chldns Hosp 1964; Pediatrics, Bellevue Hosp 1965; **Fellow:** Clinical Genetics, Mount Sinai Med Ctr 1968; **Fac Appt:** Prof Ped, NY Med Coll

Southeast

Sutphen, Rebecca MD [CG] - **Spec Exp:** Genetic Disorders; Hereditary Cancer; Cancer Risk Assessment; **Hospital:** H Lee Moffitt Cancer Ctr & Research Inst; **Address:** H Lee Moffitt Cancer Ctr, 12902 Magnolia Drive, Tampa, FL 33612; **Phone:** 800-456-3434; **Board Cert:** Clinical Molecular Genetics 2007; Clinical Cytogenetics 2007; Clinical Genetics 2007; **Med School:** Temple Univ 1990; **Resid:** Pediatrics, All Children's Hosp 1993; **Fellow:** Clinical Genetics, Univ S Fla Coll Med 1995; **Fac Appt:** Assoc Prof CG, Univ S Fla Coll Med

Clinical Genetics

Midwest

Rubinstein, Wendy S MD/PhD [CG] - **Spec Exp:** Breast Cancer; Colon Cancer; Pancreatic Cancer; **Hospital:** Evanston/Northshore Univ Hlth Syst; **Address:** Ctr for Medical Genetics, 1000 Central St, Ste 620, Evanston, IL 60201; **Phone:** 847-570-1029; **Board Cert:** Internal Medicine 2003; Clinical Genetics 2007; Clinical Molecular Genetics 2007; **Med School:** Mount Sinai Sch Med 1989; **Resid:** Internal Medicine, Strong Meml Hosp 1992; **Fellow:** Clinical Genetics, Univ Pittsburgh 1996; Clinical Molecular Genetics, Univ Pittsburgh 1996; **Fac Appt:** Asst Prof Med, Northwestern Univ

Whelan, Alison MD [CG] - **Spec Exp:** Gynecologic Cancer Risk; Colon & Rectal Cancer Risk; Hereditary Cancer; **Hospital:** Barnes-Jewish Hosp, St Louis Chldns Hosp; **Address:** Washington Univ Sch Med, 660 S Euclid Ave, Campus Box 8116, St Louis, MO 63110; **Phone:** 314-454-6093; **Board Cert:** Internal Medicine 1989; Clinical Genetics 2007; **Med School:** Washington Univ, St Louis 1986; **Resid:** Internal Medicine, Barnes Hosp 1989; Pediatrics, Wash Univ Sch Med 1994; **Fellow:** Research, Wash Univ Sch Med 1991; Clinical Genetics, Wash Univ Sch Med 1994; **Fac Appt:** Prof Med, Washington Univ, St Louis

Southwest

Mulvihill, John J MD [CG] - **Spec Exp:** Genetic Disorders; Fertility in Cancer Survivors; **Hospital:** Chldns Hosp OU Med Ctr; **Address:** Childrens Hosp, 940 NE 13th St, rm 2B2418, Oklahoma City, OK 73104; **Phone:** 405-271-8685; **Board Cert:** Pediatrics 1975; Clinical Genetics 1982; **Med School:** Univ Wash 1969; **Resid:** Pediatrics, Johns Hopkins Hosp 1974; **Fellow:** Research, NCI-Natl Inst Hlth 1972; **Fac Appt:** Prof CG, Univ Okla Coll Med

Plon, Sharon E MD/PhD [CG] - **Spec Exp:** Hereditary Cancer; Cancer Risk Assessment; Breast Cancer Risk Assessment; Ovarian Cancer Genetics; **Hospital:** Texas Chldns Hosp, St Luke's Episcopal Hosp-Houston; **Address:** Kleberg Genetics Ctr, Texas Chldn's Hosp, 6621 Fannin St, MC 3-3320, Houston, TX 77030; **Phone:** 832-824-4251; **Board Cert:** Clinical Genetics 2006; **Med School:** Harvard Med Sch 1987; **Resid:** Internal Medicine, Univ Washington Affil Hosp 1988; **Fellow:** Molecular Genetics, National Cancer Inst 1990; Medical Genetics, Fred Hutchinson Cancer Research Ctr 1993; **Fac Appt:** Prof CG, Baylor Coll Med

West Coast and Pacific

Grody, Wayne W MD/PhD [CG] - **Spec Exp:** Genetic Disorders; Hereditary Cancer; **Address:** UCLA School Medicine, Div, Med Genetic & Molecular Pathology, 10833 Le Conte Ave, Los Angeles, CA 90095-1732; **Phone:** 310-825-5648; **Board Cert:** Clinical Genetics 1990; Anatomic & Clinical Pathology 1987; Clinical Biochemical Genetics 1990; Molecular Genetic Pathology 2001; **Med School:** Baylor Coll Med 1977; **Resid:** Pathology, UCLA Med Ctr 1986; **Fellow:** Clinical Genetics, UCLA Med Ctr 1987; **Fac Appt:** Prof CG, UCLA

Weitzel, Jeffrey N MD [CG] - **Spec Exp:** Breast Cancer; Ovarian Cancer; Hereditary Cancer; **Hospital:** City of Hope Natl Med Ctr & Beckman Rsch (page 69); **Address:** City of Hope Cancer Ctr, 1500 E Duarte Rd, Duarte, CA 91010; **Phone:** 626-256-8662; **Board Cert:** Internal Medicine 1986; Medical Oncology 1989; Clinical Genetics 1996; **Med School:** Univ Minn 1983; **Resid:** Internal Medicine, Univ Minn Hosps 1986; Hematology, Hammersmith Hosp 1987; **Fellow:** Hematology & Oncology, Tufts -New England Med Ctr 1992; Clinical Genetics, Tufts-New England Med Ctr 1996; **Fac Appt:** Assoc Clin Prof Med, USC Sch Med

INFECTIOUS DISEASE

Mid Atlantic

Polsky, Bruce W MD [Inf] - **Spec Exp:** Infections in Cancer Patients; AIDS Related Cancers; **Hospital:** St Luke's - Roosevelt Hosp Ctr - Roosevelt Div (page 71); **Address:** 1111 Amsterdam Ave, New York, NY 10025; **Phone:** 212-523-2525; **Board Cert:** Internal Medicine 1983; Infectious Disease 1986; **Med School:** Wayne State Univ 1980; **Resid:** Internal Medicine, Montefiore Hosp 1983; **Fellow:** Infectious Disease, Meml Sloan Kettering Cancer Ctr 1986; **Fac Appt:** Prof Med, Columbia P&S

Segal, Brahm H MD [Inf] - **Spec Exp:** Infections in Cancer Patients; Immune Deficiencies-Primary; **Hospital:** Roswell Park Cancer Inst; **Address:** Elm and Carlton Streets, Buffalo, NY 14263; **Phone:** 716-845-5721; **Board Cert:** Infectious Disease 1997; **Med School:** Albert Einstein Coll Med 1992; **Resid:** Internal Medicine, New England Med Ctr 1995; **Fellow:** Infectious Disease, Natl Inst Allergy/Inf Dis 1997; **Fac Appt:** Assoc Prof Med, SUNY Buffalo

Sepkowitz, Kent MD [Inf] - **Spec Exp:** Infections in Cancer Patients; **Hospital:** Meml Sloan-Kettering Cancer Ctr (page 76); **Address:** 1275 York Avenue, New York, NY 10065; **Phone:** 800-525-2225; **Board Cert:** Internal Medicine 1983; Infectious Disease 2000; **Med School:** Univ Okla Coll Med 1980; **Resid:** Internal Medicine, Roosevelt Hosp 1984; **Fellow:** Infectious Disease, Meml Sloan Kettering Cancer Ctr 1991; **Fac Appt:** Prof Med, Cornell Univ-Weill Med Coll

Great Plains and Mountains

Freifeld, Alison G MD [Inf] - **Spec Exp:** Infectious Disease during Chemotherapy; Infections in Cancer Patients; **Hospital:** Nebraska Med Ctr; **Address:** Univ Nebraska, 985400 Nebraska Medical Center, Omaha, NE 68198-5400; **Phone:** 402-559-8650; **Board Cert:** Internal Medicine 1985; Infectious Disease 1988; **Med School:** Johns Hopkins Univ 1982; **Resid:** Internal Medicine, Johns Hopkins Univ Med Ctr 1985

West Coast and Pacific

Palefsky, Joel M MD [Inf] - **Spec Exp:** AIDS Related Cancers; **Hospital:** UCSF - Mt Zion Med Ctr; **Address:** UCSF Med Ctr, Div Infectious Disease, 505 Parnassus Ave, Box 0162, San Francisco, CA 94143-0126; **Phone:** 415-476-1574; **Board Cert:** Internal Medicine 1984; Infectious Disease 1988; **Med School:** McGill Univ 1980; **Resid:** Internal Medicine, Royal Victoria Hosp 1984; **Fellow:** Infectious Disease, Stanford Univ 1989

INTERNAL MEDICINE

Mid Atlantic

Quill, Timothy E MD [IM] - **Spec Exp:** Palliative Care; **Hospital:** Univ of Rochester Strong Meml Hosp; **Address:** University of Rochester Medical Ctr, 601 Elmwood Ave, Box 687, Rochester, NY 14642; **Phone:** 585-273-1154; **Board Cert:** Internal Medicine 1979; Hospice & Palliative Medicine 1990; **Med School:** Univ Rochester 1976; **Resid:** Internal Medicine, U Rochester/Strong Meml Hosp 1979; **Fellow:** Liaison Psychiatry, U Rochester Med Psych Liason Program 1980; **Fac Appt:** Prof Med, Univ Rochester

Internal Medicine

Rivlin, Richard S MD [IM] - **Spec Exp:** Nutrition & Cancer Prevention/Control; Breast Cancer; Prostate Cancer; Colon Cancer; **Hospital:** NY-Presby Hosp/Weill Cornell (page 79); **Address:** 428 E 72nd St, Ste 600, New York, NY 10021; **Phone:** 646-898-2749; **Board Cert:** Internal Medicine 1969; **Med School:** Harvard Med Sch 1959; **Resid:** Internal Medicine, Johns Hopkins Hosp 1961; Internal Medicine, Johns Hopkins Hosp 1964; **Fellow:** Endocrinology, Diabetes & Metabolism, Natl Inst Hlth 1963; Biochemistry, Johns Hopkins Hosp 1966; **Fac Appt:** Prof Med, Cornell Univ-Weill Med Coll

Southeast

Heimburger, Douglas C MD [IM] - **Spec Exp:** Nutrition & Disease Prevention/Control; Nutrition & Cancer Prevention; **Hospital:** Univ of Ala Hosp at Birmingham, VA Med Ctr; **Address:** UAB, Dept Nutrition Sci & Med, 1675 University Blvd Webb Bldg - rm 439, Birmingham, AL 35294-3360; **Phone:** 205-996-5400; **Board Cert:** Internal Medicine 1981; **Med School:** Vanderbilt Univ 1978; **Resid:** Internal Medicine, Washington Univ Hosps 1981; **Fellow:** Nutrition, Univ Alabama Med Ctr 1982

Tucker, Rodney O MD [IM] - **Spec Exp:** Palliative Care; **Hospital:** Univ of Ala Hosp at Birmingham; **Address:** UAB Center for Palliative Care, CH19 219U, 1530 3rd Ave S, Birmingham, AL 35294-2041; **Phone:** 205-975-8197; **Board Cert:** Internal Medicine 2002; **Med School:** Univ Alabama 1989; **Resid:** Internal Medicine, Carraway Methodist Med Ctr 1993; **Fac Appt:** Asst Prof Med, Univ Alabama

Tulsky, James A MD [IM] - **Spec Exp:** Palliative Care; **Hospital:** Duke Univ Med Ctr; **Address:** Ctr for Palliative Care, Hock Plaza, 2424 Erwin Rd, Ste 1105, Durham, NC 27705; **Phone:** 919-668-7215; **Board Cert:** Internal Medicine 2000; Hospice & Palliative Medicine 2006; **Med School:** Univ IL Coll Med 1987; **Resid:** Internal Medicine, UCSF Med Ctr 1990; **Fellow:** Pain & Palliative Care, UCSF Med Ctr 1993; **Fac Appt:** Prof Med, Duke Univ

Southwest

Fine, Robert L MD [IM] - **Spec Exp:** Palliative Care; **Hospital:** Baylor Univ Medical Ctr; **Address:** 3434 Swiss Ave, Dallas, TX 75204; **Phone:** 214-828-5090; **Board Cert:** Internal Medicine 1981; Hospice & Palliative Medicine 1993; **Med School:** Univ Tex SW, Dallas 1978; **Resid:** Internal Medicine, Baylor Univ Med Ctr 1981

Wolff, Robert A MD [IM] - **Spec Exp:** Gastrointestinal Cancer; Pancreatic Cancer; Colon & Rectal Cancer; Clinical Trials; **Hospital:** UT MD Anderson Cancer Ctr; **Address:** 1515 Holcombe Blvd, Unit 421, Houston, TX 77030; **Phone:** 713-745-5476; **Board Cert:** Internal Medicine 1989; **Med School:** Albany Med Coll 1986; **Resid:** Internal Medicine, Duke Univ Med Ctr 1989; **Fellow:** Hematology & Oncology, Duke Univ Med Ctr 1992

West Coast and Pacific

Ferris, Frank D MD [IM] - **Spec Exp:** Palliative Care; **Hospital:** San Diego Hospice; **Address:** 4311 3rd Ave, San Diego, CA 92103-1407; **Phone:** 619-688-1600; **Board Cert:** Hospice & Palliative Medicine 1998; **Med School:** Canada 1981; **Resid:** Internal Medicine, Univ Toronto; Radiation Oncology, Univ Toronto; **Fellow:** Pain Management, Toronto-Sunnybrook Reg Cancer Ctr

Pantilat, Steven MD [IM] - **Spec Exp:** Palliative Care; **Hospital:** UCSF Med Ctr; **Address:** 521 Parnassus Ave, Box 0903, San Francisco, CA 94143-0903; **Phone:** 415-502-1414; **Board Cert:** Internal Medicine 2003; Hospice & Palliative Medicine 2001; **Med School:** UCSF 1989; **Resid:** Internal Medicine, UCSF Med Ctr 1992; **Fac Appt:** Asst Clin Prof Med, UCSF

Rabow, Michael W MD [IM] - **Spec Exp:** Palliative Care; **Hospital:** UCSF - Mt Zion Med Ctr; **Address:** 1701 Divisadero St, Ste 500, UCSF, San Francisco, CA 94143; **Phone:** 415-353-7300; **Board Cert:** Internal Medicine 1996; Hospice & Palliative Medicine 2002; **Med School:** UCSF 1993; **Resid:** Internal Medicine, UCSF Med Ctr 1996; **Fellow:** Gastroenterology, UCSF Med Ctr 1997; **Fac Appt:** Assoc Clin Prof Med, UCSF

PHYSICAL MEDICINE & REHABILITATION

Mid Atlantic

Francis, Kathleen D MD [PMR] - **Spec Exp:** Lymphedema; **Address:** Lymphedema Physician Services, 200 S Orange Ave, Livingston, NJ 07039; **Phone:** 973-322-7366; **Board Cert:** Physical Medicine & Rehabilitation 2004; **Med School:** UMDNJ-NJ Med Sch, Newark 1989; **Resid:** Physical Medicine & Rehabilitation, UMDNJ-Kessler Inst Rehab 1993; **Fac Appt:** Asst Clin Prof PMR, UMDNJ-NJ Med Sch, Newark

Schwartz, L Matthew MD [PMR] - **Spec Exp:** Lymphedema; Pain-Cancer; Cancer Rehabilitation; **Hospital:** Montgomery Rehab Hosp; **Address:** Montgomery Rehab Hosp, Medical Office, 8601 Stenton Ave, Wyndmoor, PA 19038; **Phone:** 215-233-6226; **Board Cert:** Physical Medicine & Rehabilitation 1992; Pain Medicine 2003; **Med School:** UMDNJ-NJ Med Sch, Newark 1987; **Resid:** Physical Medicine & Rehabilitation, Hosp U Penn 1989; Physical Medicine & Rehabilitation, Thos Jefferson Univ Hosp 1991; **Fac Appt:** Clin Prof PMR, Univ Pennsylvania

Stubblefield, Michael MD [PMR] - **Spec Exp:** Cancer Rehabilitation; Pain-Cancer; Radiation Fibrosis Syndrome; **Hospital:** Meml Sloan-Kettering Cancer Ctr (page 76); **Address:** 1275 York Avenue, New York, NY 10065; **Phone:** 212-639-7834; **Board Cert:** Internal Medicine 2001; Physical Medicine & Rehabilitation 2002; Electrodiagnostic Medicine 2003; **Med School:** Columbia P&S 1996; **Resid:** Internal Medicine, Columbia Presby Med Ctr 2001; Physical Medicine & Rehabilitation, Columbia Presby Med Ctr 2001; **Fac Appt:** Asst Prof PMR, Cornell Univ-Weill Med Coll

Southeast

King Jr, Richard W MD [PMR] - **Spec Exp:** Cancer Rehabilitation; Lymphedema; Soft Tissue Radiation Necrosis; Soft Tissue Radiation Necrosis-Breast; **Hospital:** WellStar Windy Hill Hosp, WellStar Cobb Hosp; **Address:** HyOx Medical Treatment Ctr, 2550 Windy Hill Rd, Ste 110, Marietta, GA 30067; **Phone:** 678-303-3200; **Board Cert:** Physical Medicine & Rehabilitation 1988; Undersea & Hyperbaric Medicine 2002; **Med School:** Emory Univ 1979; **Resid:** Physical Medicine & Rehabilitation, Emory Univ Hosp 1987; **Fac Appt:** Asst Clin Prof PMR, Emory Univ

Stewart, Paula JB MD [PMR] - **Spec Exp:** Lymphedema; Brain Tumors; Spinal Cord Tumors; Cancer Rehabilitation; **Hospital:** Healthsouth Lakeshore Rehab Hosp; **Address:** Healthsouth Lakeshore Rehab Hosp, 3800 Ridgeway Drive, Birmingham, AL 35209; **Phone:** 205-868-2347; **Board Cert:** Physical Medicine & Rehabilitation 1996; Spinal Cord Injury Medicine 2000; **Med School:** Univ Minn 1987; **Resid:** Physical Medicine & Rehabilitation, Mayo Clinic 1991

Physical Medicine & Rehabilitation

Midwest

Cheville, Andrea L MD [PMR] - **Spec Exp:** Lymphedema; Cancer Rehabilitation; Pain-Cancer; **Hospital:** Mayo Med Ctr & Clin - Rochester; **Address:** Mayo Clinic, Dept Physical Med & Rehab, 200 1st St SW, Rochester, MN 55905; **Phone:** 507-284-2747; **Board Cert:** Physical Medicine & Rehabilitation 2008; Pain Medicine 2004; **Med School:** Harvard Med Sch 1993; **Resid:** Physical Medicine & Rehabilitation, UMDNJ Med Ctr 1997; **Fellow:** Pain & Palliative Care, Meml Sloan Kettering Cancer Ctr 1999; **Fac Appt:** Asst Prof PMR, Mayo Med Sch

DePompolo, Robert W MD [PMR] - **Spec Exp:** Cancer Rehabilitation; Lymphedema; **Hospital:** St Mary's Hosp - Rochester, Mayo Med Ctr & Clin - Rochester; **Address:** Mayo Clinic, Dept Phys Med & Rehab, 200 1st St SW, Rochester, MN 55905; **Phone:** 507-255-8972; **Board Cert:** Physical Medicine & Rehabilitation 1981; **Med School:** Wayne State Univ 1977; **Resid:** Physical Medicine & Rehabilitation, Univ Minnesota Affil Hosp 1980

Feldman, Joseph L MD [PMR] - **Spec Exp:** Lymphedema; **Hospital:** Evanston/Northshore Univ Hlth Syst; **Address:** 2650 Ridge Ave, rm 2204, Evanston, IL 60201-1718; **Phone:** 847-570-2066; **Board Cert:** Physical Medicine & Rehabilitation 1971; **Med School:** Univ IL Coll Med 1965; **Resid:** Physical Medicine & Rehabilitation, Univ of Ilinois Med Ctr 1969; **Fac Appt:** Asst Prof PMR, Northwestern Univ

Gamble, Gail L MD [PMR] - **Spec Exp:** Lymphedema; Head & Neck Cancer; Bone Tumors-Metastatic; **Hospital:** Rehab Inst of Chicago; **Address:** Rehab Inst of Chicago, 345 E Superior St, Chicago, IL 60611; **Phone:** 312-238-7670; **Board Cert:** Physical Medicine & Rehabilitation 1985; **Med School:** Mayo Med Sch 1979; **Resid:** Physical Medicine & Rehabilitation, Mayo Clinic 1983

PREVENTIVE MEDICINE

Mid Atlantic

Lane, Dorothy S MD [PrM] - **Spec Exp:** Cancer Prevention; Health Promotion & Disease Prevention; **Hospital:** Stony Brook Univ Med Ctr; **Address:** Stony Brook Univ Sch Med, HSC L2, rm 142, Stony Brook, NY 11794-8222; **Phone:** 631-444-2094; **Board Cert:** Public Health & Genl Preventive Med 1970; **Med School:** Columbia P&S 1965; **Resid:** Public Health & Genl Preventive Med, NY Health Dept 1968; **Fac Appt:** Prof PrM, SUNY Stony Brook

Weiss, Stanley H MD [PrM] - **Spec Exp:** Cancer Epidemiology & Control; Infections in Cancer Patients; **Hospital:** UMDNJ-Univ Hosp-Newark; **Address:** NJ Medical School-UMDNJ, 30 Bergen St, ADMC16, Ste 1614, Newark, NJ 07107-3000; **Phone:** 973-972-4623; **Board Cert:** Internal Medicine 1981; Medical Oncology 1985; **Med School:** Harvard Med Sch 1978; **Resid:** Internal Medicine, Montefiore Med Ctr 1981; **Fellow:** Medical Oncology, National Cancer Inst 1985; Epidemiology, National Cancer Inst 1987; **Fac Appt:** Prof PrM, UMDNJ-NJ Med Sch, Newark

FOX CHASE
CANCER CENTER

333 Cottman Avenue
Philadelphia, PA 19111-2497
Phone: 1-888-FOX CHASE
www.fccc.edu

RISK ASSESSMENT

Unique programs for individuals at increased risk of cancer provide screening, education and early detection for people with a personal or family history of certain cancers or other special risk factors. The staff includes medical oncologists, gynecologists, gastroenterologists, dermatologists, radiation oncologists, nurses and nurse practitioners, genetic counselors, radiologists, pathologists and health educators trained in cancer prevention. Participants may also have the opportunity for genetic testing and counseling when appropriate and the option of enrolling in available prevention trials.

Fox Chase opened the region's first risk-assessment program in 1991. A memorial to Margaret M. Dyson, who died of ovarian cancer in 1990, the Margaret Dyson Family Risk Assessment Program was developed by Mary B. Daly, M.D., Ph.D., of Fox Chase and established with funds from the National Cancer Institute and the Dyson Foundation. The program became a model for additional Fox Chase risk-assessment programs focused on other cancers.

- **Margaret Dyson Family Risk Assessment Program:**

  1-800-325-4145 For women with a family history of breast and/or ovarian cancer

- **Melanoma Family Risk Assessment Program:**

  215-214-1448 For people with a family history of melanoma, a potentially fatal form of skin cancer

- **Gastrointestinal Tumor Risk Assessment Program:**

  215-728-7041 For people with increased risk of gastrointestinal cancers, including a family or personal history of colorectal polyps or inflammatory bowel disease

- **Prostate Cancer Risk Assessment Program:**

  215-728-2406 For men with increased risk of prostate cancer, including family history or being African American

- **Benign Breast Registry to Assess Valid Endpoints**

  (BeBrave): 1-800-325-4145 For women with a diagnosis of benign breast disease based on breast biopsy

CANCER PREVENTION

Our Research Institute for Cancer Prevention, the first comprehensive program of its kind in the nation, began in 2000, highlighting a decade of leadership in cancer prevention research. The research covers a broad spectrum from basic laboratory studies to clinical prevention trials and behavioral studies.

Fox Chase started its chemoprevention program in 1991—a laboratory program to develop and test natural or synthetic substances to prevent cancer. Director Margie L. Clapper, Ph.D., is collaborating with colleagues in preclinical studies of various agents aimed at preventing colitis-associated colorectal cancer. Fox Chase also participates in large nationwide clinical chemoprevention trials for people at increased cancer risk.

In addition, Fox Chase's behavioral research program conducts a wide range of studies to make cancer prevention and control programs more effective.

For more about Fox Chase physicians and services, visit our web site, www.fccc.edu, or call 1-888-FOX CHASE.

NYU Cancer Institute
NYU LANGONE MEDICAL CENTER

NYU Clinical Cancer Center
160 East 34th Street
New York, New York 10016
www.nyuci.org/atcd

NYU Langone Medical Center
550 First Avenue
(at 31st Street)
New York, New York 10016
www.nyumc.org/atcd

**Stephen D. Hassenfeld
Children's Center
for Cancer and Blood
Disorders**
160 East 32nd Street
New York, New York 10016
www.nyumc.org/hassenfeld

A Collaborative Approach
The NYU Cancer Institute, an NCI designated center, is a "matrix cancer center" without walls operating within the larger NYU Langone Medical Center. With over 175 members and a research funding base of over $81 million, this structure strengthens our capabilities to forge collaborations across medical and scientific disciplines, which translates to comprehensive care for our patients and discoveries that will influence the future of this disease.

Renowned Expertise
Team members' compassion and expertise help patients better manage the symptoms of their disease as well as their special needs. Our highly skilled Magnet™ nursing team not only plays a pivotal role in coordinating direct patient care, but is also a source of invaluable patient education.

A Patient-Focused Setting
The NYU Clinical Cancer Center, with over 70 faculty members from various disciplines at the New York University School of Medicine, is the principal outpatient facility of the Cancer Institute and serves as home for our patients and their caregivers. The center and its multidisciplinary team of experts provide access to the latest treatment options and clinical trials along with a variety of programs in cancer prevention, screening, diagnostics, genetic counseling, and supportive services. When it comes to kids and cancer, the Stephen D. Hassenfeld Children's Center for Cancer and Blood Disorders offers not just innovation but insight. As a leading member of the NCI-sponsored Children's Oncology Group, our physicians are known for developing new ways to treat childhood cancer. Our affiliation with Bellevue Hospital, the oldest public hospital in the country, affords clinically distinctive opportunities to learn and care for patients with cancer by observing its presentation and behavior in a variety of patient groups.

Section IV
Appendices

Appendix A:
Medical Boards

Intro to ABMS and Osteopathic Specialties

The following pages contain descriptions of the "official" medical specialties, approved by the American Board of Medical Specialists (for M.D.s) or by the American Osteopathic Association (for D.O.s). These are important because they are the only specialties recognized by the official governing boards. There may be physicians who call themselves one kind of specialist or another, but they may not be certified by the "official" boards. There are, in fact, over 100 such "self-designated" boards, some simply groups of physicians interested in a given area of medicine with no qualifications for membership to other groups with very specific qualifications for membership.

It is important for the medical consumer to seek out physicians certified by the ABMS or AOA to assure their doctor has had the appropriate training and passed the board certification exam.

ABMS

The ABMS is an organization of ABMS approved medical specialty boards. The mission of the ABMS is to maintain and improve the quality of medical care by assisting the Member Boards in their efforts to develop and utilize professional and educational standards for the evaluation and certification of physician specialists. The intent of certification of physicians is to provide assurance to the public that a physician specialist certified by a Member Board of the ABMS has successfully completed an approved educational program and evaluation process which includes an examination designed to assess the knowledge, skills, and experience required to provide quality patient care in that specialty. The ABMS serves to coordinate the activities of its Member Boards and to provide information to the public, the government, the profession and its Members concerning issues involving specialization and certification in medicine.

Following is a list of the addresses of the various medical specialty boards approved by the ABMS. Note that there are 24 board organizations for 25 medical specialties. Psychiatry and Neurology share the same board.

Appendix A: Medical Boards

To find out if a physician is certified, consumers can call the individual boards which may charge a fee for the information, or they can contact the ABMS at 866-275-2267 (no fee) or www.abms.org.

American Board of Allergy and Immunology
111 S. Independence Mall East, Suite 701
Philadelphia, PA 19106-3699
(215) 592-9466, (866) 264-5568

General Certification in Allergy and Immunology. Certifications awarded since 1989 are valid for 10 years. For those certified prior to 1989 there is no recertification requirement.

American Board of Anesthesiology
4101 Lake Boone Trail, Ste 510
Raleigh, NC 27607-7506
(919) 881-2570

General Certification in Anesthesiology; with Special and Added Qualifications in Critical Care Medicine and Pain Management. Certifications awarded since 2000 are valid for 10 years.

American Board of Colon and Rectal Surgery
20600 Eureka Road, Suite 600
Taylor, MI 48180
(734) 282-9400

General Certification in Colon and Rectal Surgery. Certifications awarded since 1990 are valid for 10 years.

American Board of Dermatology
Henry Ford Health System
1 Ford Place
Detriot, MI 48202-3450
(313) 874-1088

General Certification in Dermatology; with Special Qualifications in Clinical and Laboratory Dermatological Immunology, Dermatopathology, and Pediatric Dermatology. Certifications awarded since 1991 are valid for 10 years.

American Board of Emergency Medicine
3000 Coolidge Road
East Lansing, MI 48823-6319
(517) 332-4800

General Certification in Emergency Medicine; with Special and Added Qualifications in Medical Toxicology, Pediatric Emergency Medicine, Sports Medicine and Undersea and Hyperbaric Medicine. Certifications awarded since 1980 are valid for 10 years.

American Board of Family Practice
1648 McGrathiana Parkway, Suite 550
Lexington, KY 40505-4294
(859) 269-5626, (888) 995-5700

General Certification in Family Practice; with Added Qualifications in Adolescent Medicine, Geriatric Medicine and Sports Medicine. Certifications awarded since 1970 are valid for 7 years.

American Board of Internal Medicine
510 Walnut Street, Suite 1700
Philadelphia, PA 19106-3699
(215) 446-3500, (800) 2246

General Certification in Internal Medicine; with Special Qualifications in Cardiovascular Disease, Endocrinology, Diabetes and Metabolism, Gastroenterology, Hematology, Infectious Disease, Medical Oncology, Nephrology, Pulmonary Disease, and Rheumatology; and Added Qualifications in Adolescent Medicine, Clinical Cardiac Electrophysiology, Critical Care Medicine, Geriatric Medicine, Interventional Cardiology, Sleep Medicine, Sports Medicine and Transplant Hepatology. Certifications awarded since 1990 are valid for 10 years.

American Board of Medical Genetics
9650 Rockville Pike
Bethesda, MD 20814-3998
(301) 634-7315

General Certification in Clinical Genetics (MD), PhD Medical Genetics, Clinical Biochemical Genetics, Clinical Cytogenetics and Clinical Molecular Genetics; with Added Qualifications in Molecular Genetic Pathology. Certifications awarded since 2002 are valid for 2 years.

Appendix A: Medical Boards

American Board of Neurological Surgery
6550 Fannin Street, Suite 2139
Houston, TX 77030-2701
(713) 441-6015

General Certification in Neurological Surgery. Certifications awarded since 1999 are valid for 10 years.

American Board of Nuclear Medicine
4555 Forest Park Boulevard, Suite 119
St. Louis, MO 63108
(314) 367-2225

General Certification in Nuclear Medicine. Certifications awarded since 1992 are valid for 10 years.

American Board of Obstetrics and Gynecology
2915 Vine Street
Dallas, TX 75204
(214) 871-1619

General Certification in Obstetrics and Gynecology; with Special Qualifications in Gynecologic Oncology, Maternal and Fetal Medicine, Reproductive Endocrinology; and Added Qualifications in Critical Care Medicine. Certifications awarded since 1986 are valid for 6 years.

American Board of Ophthalmology
111 Presidential Boulevard, Suite 241
Bala Cynwyd, PA 19004-1075
(610) 664-1175

General Certification in Orthopaedic Surgery; with Added Qualifications in Hand Surgery and Orthopaedic Sports Medicine. Certifications awarded since 1986 are valid for 10 years.

American Board of Orthopaedic Surgery
400 Silver Cedar Court
Chapel Hill, NC 27514
(919) 929-7103

General Certification in Orthopaedic Surgery; with Added Qualification in Hand Surgery.

American Board of Otolaryngology
  5615 Kirby Drive, Suite 600
  Houston, TX 77005
  (713) 850-0399

General Certification in Otolaryngology; with Added Qualifications in Neurotology, Pediatric Otolaryngology and Plastic Surgery within the Head and Neck. Certifications awarded since 2002 are valid for 10 years.

American Board of Pathology
  P.O. Box 25915
  Tampa, FL 33622-5915
  (813) 286-2444

General Certification in Anatomic and Clinical Pathology, Anatomic Pathology and Clinical Pathology; with Special Qualifications in Blood Banking/Transfusion Medicine, Chemical Pathology, Dermatopathology, Forensic Pathology, Hematology, Medical Microbiology, Molecular Genetic Pathology, Neuropathology and Pediatric Pathology; and Added Qualifications in Cytopathology. Certifications awarded since 1997 are valid for 10 years.

American Board of Pediatrics
  111 Silver Cedar Court
  Chapel Hill, NC 27514-1651
  (919) 929-0461

General Certification in Pediatrics; with Special Qualifications in Adolescent Medicine, Developmental-Behavioral Pediatrics, Neonatal-Perinatal Medicine, Pediatric Cardiology, Pediatric Critical Care Medicine, Pediatric Emergency Medicine, Pediatric Endocrinology, Pediatric Gastroenterology, Pediatric Hematology-Oncology, Pediatric Infectious Diseases, Pediatric Nephrology, Pediatric Pulmonology, and Pediatric Rheumatology; and Added Qualifications in Medical Toxicology, Neurodevelopmental Disabilities, Pediatric Transplant Hepatology and Sports Medicine. Certifications awarded since 1988 valid for 7 years.

American Board of Physical Medicine and Rehabilitation
  3015 Allegro Park Lane, S.W.
  Rochester, MN 55902-4139
  (507) 282-1776

General Certification in Physical Medicine and Rehabilitation; with Special Qualifications in Pain Medicine, Pediatric Rehabilitation Medicine, and Spinal Cord Injury Medicine. Certifications awarded since 1993 are valid for 10 years.

American Board of Plastic Surgery
  Seven Penn Center, Suite 400
  1635 Market Street
  Philadelphia, PA 19103-2204
  (215) 587-9322

General Certification in Plastic Surgery; with Added Qualifications in Hand Surgery. Certifications awarded since 1995 are valid for 10-years.

American Board of Preventive Medicine
  111 West Jackson Boulevard, Suite 1110
  Chicago, IL 60604
  (312) 939-2276

General Certification in Aerospace Medicine, Occupational Medicine and Public Health and General Preventive Medicine; with Added Qualifications in Undersea and Hyperbaric Medicine and Medical Toxicology. Certifications awarded since 1997 are valid for 10 years.

American Board of Psychiatry and Neurology
  2150 E. Lake Cook Road, Suite 900
  Buffalo Grove, IL 60089
  (847) 229-6500

General Certification in Psychiatry, Neurology and Neurology with Special Qualification in Child Neurology; with Special Qualifications in Child and Adolescent Psychiatry, Pain Medicine and Sleep Medicine; and Added Qualifications in Addiction Psychiatry, Clinical Neurophysiology, Forensic Psychiatry, Geriatric Psychiatry, Neurodevelopmental Disabilities, Psychosomatic Medicine and Vascular Neurology . Certifications awarded since 1994 are valid for 10 years.

American Board of Radiology
  5441 E. Williams Boulevard, Suite 200
  Tucson, AZ 85711
  (520) 790-2900

General Certification in Diagnostic Radiology or Radiation Oncology; with Special Competency in Nuclear Radiology; and Added Qualifications in Neuroradiology, Pediatric Radiology and Vascular and Interventional Radiology. Radiological Physics is a non-clinical certification. Certificates are valid for 10 years.

American Board of Surgery
1617 John F. Kennedy Boulevard, Suite 860
Philadelphia, PA 19103-1847
(215) 568-4000

General Certification in Surgery and Vascular Surgery; with Special Qualifications in Pediatric Surgery and Surgery of the Hand; and Added Qualifications in Surgical Critical Care. Certifications awarded since 1976 are valid for 10 years.

American Board of Thoracic Surgery
633 North St. Clair Street, Suite 2320
Chicago, IL 60611
(312) 202-5900

General Certification in Thoracic Surgery. Certifications awarded since 1976 are valid for 10 years.

American Board of Urology
2216 Ivy Road, Suite 210
Charlottesville, VA 22903
(434) 979-0059

General Certification in Urology. Certifications awarded as of 1985 are valid for 10 years.

Osteopathic

The American Osteopathic Association (AOA) is a member association representing more than 56,000 osteopathic physicians (D.O.s). The AOA serves as the primary certifying body for D.O.s, and is the accrediting agency for all osetopathic medical colleges and healthcare facilities. The AOA's mission is to advance the philosophy and practice of osteopathic medicine by promoting excellence in education, research, and the delivery of quality, cost-effective healthcare within a distinct, unified profession.

American Osteopathic Association
142 E Ontario Street
Chicago, IL 60611

Consumers may call the American Osteopathic Association at (800) 621-1773 or visit the website, www.osteopathic.org, for general certification information.

Appendix A: Medical Boards

American Osteopathic Board of Anesthesiology

General certification in Anesthesiology; with Added Qualifications in Addiction Medicine, Critical Care Medicine, and Pain Management. Certifications awarded since 2004 are valid for 10 years. For those certified prior to 2004 there is no recertification requirement.

American Osteopathic Board of Dermatology

General certification in Dermatology; with Added Qualifications in Dermatopathology and Mohs'-Micrographic Surgery. Certifications awarded since 2004 are valid for 10 years.

American Osteopathic Board of Emergency Medicine

General certification in Emergency Medicine; with Added Qualifications in Emergency Medical Services, Medical Toxicology, and Sports Medicine. Certifications awarded since 1994 are valid for 10 years.

American Osteopathic Board of Family Physicians

General certification in Family Practice and Osteopathic Manipulative Treatment (OMT); with Added Qualifications in Geriatric Medicine and Sports Medicine. Certifications awarded since March 1,1997 are valid for 8 years.

American Osteopathic Board of Internal Medicine

General certification in Internal Medicine; with Special Qualifications in Allergy/Immunology, Cardiology, Endocrinology, Gastroenterology, Hematology, Infectious Disease, Nephrology, Oncology, Pulmonary Disease, Rheumatology; with Added Qualifications in Addiction Medicine, Critical Care Medicine, Clinical Cardiac Electrophysiology, Geriatric Medicine, Interventional Cardiology and Sports Medicine. Certifications awarded since 1993 are valid for 10 years.

American Osteopathic Board of Neurology and Psychiatry

General certification in Neurology and Psychiatry; with Special Qualifications in Child/Adolescent Psychiatry and Child/Adolescent Neurology; with Added Qualifications in Addiction Medicine, Neurophysiology, and Sports Medicine. Certifications awarded since 1995 are valid for 10 years.

American Osteopathic Board of Neuromusculoskeletal Medicine

(Formerly American Osteopathic Board of Special Proficiency in Osteopathic Manipulative Medicine)

American Osteopathic Board of Nuclear Medicine

General certification in Nuclear Medicine. Certifications awarded since 1995 are valid for 10 years.

American Osteopathic Board of Obstetrics and Gynecology

General certification in Obstetrics and Gynecology; with Special Qualifications in Gynecologic Oncology; Maternal and Fetal Medicine and Reproductive Endocrinology. Certifications awarded since June 2002 are valid for 6 years.

American Osteopathic Board of Ophthalmology and Otolaryngology/Head and Neck Surgery

General certification in Ophthalmology, Otolaryngology, Facial Plastic Surgery and Otolaryngology/Facial Plastic Surgery; with Added Qualifications in Otolaryngic Allergy. Certifications awarded in Ophthalmology since 2000 are valid for 10 years. For those certified prior to 2000 there is no recertification requirement. Certifications awarded in Otolaryngology and/or Otolaryngology/Facial Plastic Surgery since 2002 are valid for 10 years.

American Osteopathic Board of Orthopaedic Surgery

General certification in Orthopaedic Surgery; with Added Qualifications in Hand Surgery. Certifications awarded since 1994 are valid for 10 years.

American Osteopathic Board of Pathology

General certification in Laboratory Medicine, Anatomic Pathology and Anatomic Pathology and Laboratory Medicine; with Special Qualifications in Forensic Pathology; and with Added Qualifications in Dermatopathology. Certifications awarded since 1995 are valid for 10 years.

American Osteopathic Board of Pediatrics

General certification in Pediatrics with Special Qualifications in Adolescent and Young Adult Medicine, Neonatology, Pediatric Allergy/Immunology and Pediatric Endocrinology; with Added Qualifications in Sports Medicine. Certifications awarded since 1995 are valid for 7 years.

American Osteopathic Board of Physical Medicine and Rehabilitation Medicine

General certification in Physical Medicine and Rehabilitation; with Added Qualifications in Sports Medicine. Certifications awarded since 2004 are valid for 10 years.

Appendix A: Medical Boards

American Osteopathic Board of Preventive Medicine

General certification in Preventive Medicine/Aerospace Medicine, Preventive Medicine/Occupational-Environmental Medicine and Preventive Medicine/Public Health; with Added Qualifications in Occupational Medicine and Sports Medicine. Certifications awarded since 1994 are valid for 10 years.

American Osteopathic Board of Proctology

General certification in Proctology. Certifications awarded since 2004 are valid for 10 years.

American Osteopathic Board of Radiology

General certification in Diagnostic Radiology and Radiation Oncology; with Added Qualifications in Body Imaging, Diagnostic Ultrasound, Neuroradiology, Pediatric Radiology and Vascular and Interventional Radiology. Certifications awarded since 2002 are valid for 10 years.

American Osteopathic Board of Surgery

General certification in Surgery, Neurological Surgery, Plastic and Reconstructive Surgery, Cardiothoracic Surgery, Urological Surgery and General Vascular Surgery; with Added Qualifications in Surgical Critical Care. Certifications awarded since 1997 are valid for 10 years.

APPENDIX B:
Hospital Listings

The following is an alphabetical listing of all hospitals that have at least one Castle Connolly Top Doctor in this guide. Institutions listed in **Bold** are profiled in this Guide in association with Castle Connolly's Partnership for Excellence program. The abbreviations as they appear in the listings are in italics below. Due to the many changes taking place in the hospital industry, the names on this list may have changed subsequent to publication of this guide.

Abbott - Northwestern Hospital		(612) 863-4000
Abbott - Northwestern Hosp		
800 E 28th St	Minneapolis, MN 55407	MIDWEST
Advocate Christ Medical Center		(708) 684-8000
Adv Christ Med Ctr		
4440 W 95th St	Oak Lawn, IL 60453	MIDWEST
Advocate Lutheran General Hospital		(847) 723-2210
Adv Luth Genl Hosp		
1775 West Dempster St	Park Ridge, IL 60068	MIDWEST
Albany Medical Center		(518) 262-3125
Albany Med Ctr		
43 New Scotland Ave	Albany, NY 12208	MID ATLANTIC
Albert Einstein Medical Center		(215) 456-7890
Albert Einstein Med Ctr		
5501 Old York Rd	Philadelphia, PA 19141	MID ATLANTIC
Alfred I duPont Hospital for Children		(302) 651-4000
Alfred I duPont Hosp for Children		
1600 Rockland Rd	Wilmington, DE 19803	MID ATLANTIC
All Children's Hospital		(727) 767-7451
All Children's Hosp		
801 Sixth Street South	St. Petersburg, FL 33701	SOUTHEAST
Allegheny General Hospital		(412) 359-3131
Allegheny General Hosp		
320 E. North Avenue	Pittsburgh, PA 15212	MID ATLANTIC
Allenmore Hospital		(206) 552-5000
Allenmore Hosp		
S 19th & Union, Box 11414	Tacoma, WA 98405	WEST COAST AND PACIFIC

Alta Bates Summit Medical Center-Alta Bates Campus   (510) 204-4444
Alta Bates Summit Med Ctr-Alta Bates Campus
2450 Ashby Avenue   Berkeley, CA 94705   WEST COAST AND PACIFIC

Anne Arundel Medical Center   (443) 481-1000
Anne Arundel Med Ctr
64 Franklin Street   Annapolis, MD 21401   MID ATLANTIC

Arlington Memorial Hospital   (817) 548-6100
Arlington Meml Hosp
800 W Randol Mill Rd   Arlington, TX 76012-2503   SOUTHWEST

Arthur G. James Cancer Hospital & Research Institute   (614) 293-3300
Arthur G James Cancer Hosp & Research Inst
300 West 10th Avenue   Columbus, OH 43210   MIDWEST

Audie L Murphy Memorial Veterans Hospital   (210) 617-5300
Audie L Murphy Meml Vets Hosp
7400 Merton Minter Blvd   San Antonio, TX 78229   SOUTHWEST

Aultman Hospital   (330) 452-9911
Aultman Hosp
2600 6th St SW   Canton, OH 44710-1799   MIDWEST

Banner Desert Medical Center   (480) 512-3000
Banner Desert Med Ctr
1400 S Dobson Rd   Mesa, AZ 85202   SOUTHWEST

Banner Good Samaritan Regional Medical Center - Phoenix   (602) 239-2000
Banner Good Samaritan Regl Med Ctr - Phoenix
1111 E McDowell Rd   Phoenix, AZ 85060   SOUTHWEST

Baptist Hospital - Jackson   (601) 968-1000
Baptist Hosp - Jackson
1225 N State St   Jackson, MS 39202   SOUTHEAST

Baptist Hospital - Nashville   (615) 284-5555
Baptist Hosp - Nashville
2000 Church St   Nashville, TN 37236   SOUTHEAST

Baptist Hospital of Miami   (786) 596-1960
Baptist Hosp of Miami
8900 N Kendall Dr   Miami, FL 33176   SOUTHEAST

Baptist Memorial Hospital - Memphis   (901) 226-5000
Baptist Memorial Hospital - Memphis
6019 Walnut Grove Rd   Memphis, TN 38120   SOUTHEAST

Barnes-Jewish Hospital		(314) 362-5000
Barnes-Jewish Hosp		
One Barnes-Jewish Hospital Plaza	St. Louis, MO 63110	MIDWEST
Bascom Palmer Eye Institute		(305) 326-6000
Bascom Palmer Eye Inst		
900 NW 17 St	Miami, FL 33136	SOUTHEAST
Baylor University Medical Center		(214) 820-0111
Baylor Univ Medical Ctr		
3500 Gaston Avenue	Dallas, TX 75246	SOUTHWEST
Ben Taub General Hospital		(713) 873-2000
Ben Taub Genl Hosp		
1504 Taub Loop	Houston, TX 77001	SOUTHWEST
Beth Israel Deaconess Medical Center - Boston		(617) 667-7000
Beth Israel Deaconess Med Ctr - Boston		
330 Brookline Ave	Boston, MA 02215	NEW ENGLAND
Beth Israel Medical Center - Milton & Caroll Petrie Division		(212) 420-2000
Beth Israel Med Ctr - Petrie Division		
First Avenue @ 16th Street	New York, NY 10003	MID ATLANTIC
Boca Raton Community Hospital		(561) 395-7100
Boca Raton Comm Hosp		
800 Meadows Road	Boca Raton, FL 33486	SOUTHEAST
Boston Medical Center		(617) 638-8000
Boston Med Ctr		
1 Boston Medical Center Pl	Boston, MA 02118	NEW ENGLAND
Brenner Children's Hospital		(336) 716-2011
Brenner Chldrn's Hosp		
Medical Center Blvd	Winston-Salem, NC 27157-1015	SOUTHEAST
Brigham & Women's Hospital		(617) 732-5500
Brigham & Women's Hosp		
75 Francis St	Boston, MA 02115	NEW ENGLAND
Bryn Mawr Hospital		(610) 526-3000
Bryn Mawr Hosp		
130 S Bryn Mawr Ave	Bryn Mawr, PA 19010-3143	MID ATLANTIC
California Pacific Medical Center		(415) 600-6000
CA Pacific Med Ctr		
PO Box 7999	San Francisco, CA 94120	WEST COAST AND PACIFIC

California Pacific Medical Center - Pacific Campus   (415) 600-6000
CA Pacific Med Ctr - Pacific Campus
2333 Buchanan St   San Francisco, CA 94115   WEST COAST AND PACIFIC

Carolinas Medical Center   (704) 355-2000
Carolinas Med Ctr
1000 Blythe Blvd   Charlotte, NC 28203-5871   SOUTHEAST

Cedars-Sinai Medical Center   (310) 423-3277
Cedars-Sinai Med Ctr
8700 Beverly Boulevard   Los Angeles, CA 90048   WEST COAST AND PACIFIC

Centennial Medical Center   (615) 342-1000
Centennial Med Ctr
2300 Patterson Street   Nashville, TN 37203   SOUTHEAST

Cheyenne Regional Medical Center   (307) 634-2273
Cheyenne Regl Med Ctr
214 E 23rd St   Cheyenne, WY 82001   GREAT PLAINS AND MOUNTAINS

Children's Healthcare of Atlanta at Egleston   (404) 325-6000
Chldns Hlthcare Atlanta @ Egleston
1405 Clifton Rd NE   Atlanta, GA 30322   SOUTHEAST

Children's Hospital - Aurora, The   (720) 777-1234
Chldn's Hosp - Aurora, The
13123 E 16th Ave   Aurora, CO 80045   GREAT PLAINS AND MOUNTAINS

Children's Hospital - Boston   (617) 355-6000
Children's Hospital - Boston
300 Longwood Avenue   Boston, MA 02115   NEW ENGLAND

Children's Hospital - Los Angeles   (323) 660-2450
Chldns Hosp - Los Angeles
4650 Sunset Blvd   Los Angeles, CA 90027   WEST COAST AND PACIFIC

Children's Hospital - Oakland   (510) 428-3000
Chldns Hosp - Oakland
747 52nd St   Oakland, CA 94609   WEST COAST AND PACIFIC

Children's Hospital - Omaha   (402) 955-5400
Children's Hosp - Omaha
8200 Dodge St   Omaha, NE 68114   GREAT PLAINS AND MOUNTAINS

Children's Hospital and Clinics - Minneapolis   (612) 813-6111
Chldns Hosp and Clinics - Minneapolis
2525 Chicago Ave S   Minneapolis, MN 55404   MIDWEST

Children's Hospital and Regional Medical Center - Seattle   (206) 987-2000
Chldns Hosp and Regl Med Ctr - Seattle
4800 Sand Point Way NE   Seattle, WA 98145   WEST COAST AND PACIFIC

Children's Hospital at OU Medical Center   (405) 271-5437
Chldns Hosp OU Med Ctr
940 Northeast 13th St   Oklahoma City, OK 73104   SOUTHWEST

Children's Hospital Medical Center - Akron   (330) 379-8200
Children's Hosp & Med Ctr- Akron
One Perkins Square   Akron, OH 44308   MIDWEST

Children's Hospital of Michigan   (313) 745-5437
Chldns Hosp of Michigan
3901 Beaubian Blvd   Detroit, MI 48201   MIDWEST

Children's Hospital of Orange County   (714) 997-3000
Chldns Hosp Orange Co
455 South Main Street   Orange, CA 92868   WEST COAST AND PACIFIC

Children's Hospital of Philadelphia, The   (215) 590-1000
Chldns Hosp of Philadelphia, The
34th St & Civic Center Blvd   Philadelphia, PA 19104   MID ATLANTIC

Children's Hospital of Pittsburgh - UPMC   (412) 692-5325
Chldns Hosp of Pittsburgh - UPMC
3705 Fifth Avenue   Pittsburgh, PA 15213   MID ATLANTIC

Children's Hospital of Wisconsin   (414) 266-2000
Chldns Hosp - Wisconsin
9000 W Wisconsin Ave   Milwaukee, WI 53201   MIDWEST

Children's Medical Center of Dallas   (214) 456-7000
Chldns Med Ctr of Dallas
1935 Motor St   Dallas, TX 75235   SOUTHWEST

Children's Memorial Hospital   (773) 880-4000
Children's Mem Hosp
2300 Children's Plaza   Chicago, IL 60614   MIDWEST

Children's Mercy Hospitals & Clinics   (816) 234-3000
Chldns Mercy Hosps & Clinics
2401 Gilham Rd   Kansas City, MO 64108   MIDWEST

Children's National Medical Center - DC   (202) 884-5000
Chldns Natl Med Ctr
111 Michigan Ave NW   Washington, DC 20010   MID ATLANTIC

Christiana Care Health Services   (302) 428-2229
Christiana Care Hlth Svs
501 W 14th St   Wilmington, DE 19899-1038   MID ATLANTIC

Christiana Hospital   (302) 733-1000
Christiana Hospital
4755 Ogletown-Stanton Rd   Newark, DE 19718-0001   MID ATLANTIC

Christus Santa Rosa Children's Hospital   (512) 228-2011
Christus Santa Rosa Children's Hosp
333 N Santa Rosa St   San Antonio, TX 78207   SOUTHWEST

Cincinnati Children's Hospital Medical Center   (800) 344-2462
Cincinnati Chldns Hosp Med Ctr
3333 Burnet Ave   Cincinnati, OH 45229-3039   MIDWEST

City of Hope National Medical Center & Beckman Research   (626) 359-8111
City of Hope Natl Med Ctr & Beckman Rsch
1500 E Duarte Rd   Duarte, CA 91010   WEST COAST AND PACIFIC

Cleveland Clinic Florida - Weston   (954) 659-5000
Cleveland Clin - Weston
2950 Cleveland Clinic Blvd   Weston, FL 33331   SOUTHEAST

Cleveland Clinic Foundation   (800) 223-2273
Cleveland Clin Fdn
9500 Euclid Avenue   Cleveland, OH 44195   MIDWEST

Community Memorial Hospital - Ventura   (805) 652-5011
Comm Meml Hosp - Ventura
147 N Brent St   Ventura, CA 93003   WEST COAST AND PACIFIC

Concord Hospital   (603) 225-2711
Concord Hospital
250 Pleasant St   Concord, NH 03301-2598   NEW ENGLAND

Connecticut Children's Medical Center   (860) 545-9000
CT Chldns Med Ctr
282 Washington St   Hartford, CT 06106   NEW ENGLAND

Cook Children's Medical Center   (682) 885-4000
Cook Chldns Med Ctr
801 7th Ave   Fort Worth, TX 76104-2796   SOUTHWEST

Cooper University Hospital   (856) 342-2000
Cooper Univ Hosp
1 Cooper Plaza   Camden, NJ 08103-1489   MID ATLANTIC

Covenant Medical Center   (319) 272-8000
Covenant Med Ctr
3421 W 9th St   Waterloo, IA 50702-5499   MIDWEST

Dana-Farber Cancer Institute   (617) 632-3000
Dana-Farber Cancer Inst
44 Binney St   Boston, MA 02115   NEW ENGLAND

Dartmouth - Hitchcock Medical Center   (603) 650-5000
Dartmouth - Hitchcock Med Ctr
1 Medical Center Dr   Lebanon, NH 03756-0002   NEW ENGLAND

Detroit Medical Center   (313) 578-3930
Detroit Med Ctr
3663 Woodward Ave, Ste 200   Detroit, MI 48201-2403   MIDWEST

Doctors' Hospital   (305) 666-2111
Doctors' Hosp
5000 University Dr   Coral Gables, FL 33146   SOUTHEAST

Doernbecher Children's Hospital/Oregon Health Science University   (503) 494-8811
Doernbecher Chldns Hosp/OHSU
3181 SW Sam Jackson Park Rd   Portland, OR 97201-3098   WEST COAST AND PACIFIC

Duke University Medical Center   (919) 684-8111
Duke Univ Med Ctr
DUMC, Box 3708   Durham, NC 27710   SOUTHEAST

El Camino Hospital   (650) 940-7000
El Camino Hosp
2500 Grant Road   Mountain View, CA 94039   WEST COAST AND PACIFIC

Elliot Hospital   (603) 669-5300
Elliot Hosp
1 Elliot Way   Manchester, NH 03103   NEW ENGLAND

Emory University Hospital   (404) 712-2000
Emory Univ Hosp
1364 Clifton Rd NE   Atlanta, GA 30322   SOUTHEAST

Englewood Hospital & Medical Center   (201) 894-3000
Englewood Hosp & Med Ctr
350 Engle Street   Englewood, NJ 07631   MID ATLANTIC

Evanston/Northshore University Health System   (847) 570-2000
Evanston/Northshore Univ Hlth Syst
2650 Ridge Ave   Evanston, IL 60201   MIDWEST

Fletcher Allen Health Care-Medical Center Campus   (802) 658-4310
Fletcher Allen Health Care- Med Ctr Campus
111 Colchester Ave   Burlington, VT 05401   NEW ENGLAND

Florida Hospital - Celebration Health   (407) 764-4000
Florida Hosp Celebration Hlth
400 Celebration Pl   Celebration, FL 34747   SOUTHEAST

Forsyth Medical Center   (336) 718-5000
Forsyth Med Ctr
3333 Silas Creek Pkwy   Winston-Salem, NC 27103   SOUTHEAST

Four Winds Hospital   (914) 763-8151
Four Winds Hosp
800 Cross River Road   Katonah, NY 10536   MID ATLANTIC

Fox Chase Cancer Center   (215) 728-6900
Fox Chase Cancer Ctr
333 Cottman Avenue   Philadelphia, PA 19111   MID ATLANTIC

Franklin Square Hospital   (443) 777-7000
Franklin Square Hosp
9000 Franklin Square Drive   Baltimore, MD 21237   MID ATLANTIC

Froedtert Memorial Lutheran Hospital   (414) 805-6644
Froedtert Meml Lutheran Hosp
9200 W Wisconsin Ave   Milwaukee, WI 53226   MIDWEST

Geisinger Medical Center   (570) 271-6211
Geisinger Med Ctr
100 N Academy Ave   Danville, PA 17822   MID ATLANTIC

George Washington University Hospital   (202) 715-4000
G Washington Univ Hosp
900 23rd St NW   Washington, DC 20037   MID ATLANTIC

Georgetown University Hospital   (202) 444-2000
Georgetown Univ Hosp
3800 Reservoir Rd NW   Washington, DC 20007   MID ATLANTIC

Goshen General Hospital   (574) 533-2141
Goshen Genl Hosp
200 High Park Ave   Goshen, IN 46526   MIDWEST

Grady Health System   (404) 616-4307
Grady Hlth Sys
80 Jesse Hill Jr Dr   Atlanta, GA 30303   SOUTHEAST

Greater Baltimore Medical Center — (443) 849-2000
Greater Baltimore Med Ctr
6701 N Charles St — Baltimore, MD 21204 — MID ATLANTIC

Greenwich Hospital — (203) 863-3000
Greenwich Hosp
Five Perryridge Road — Greenwich, CT 06830 — NEW ENGLAND

H Lee Moffitt Cancer Center & Research Institute — (813) 972-4673
H Lee Moffitt Cancer Ctr & Research Inst
12902 Magnolia Drive — Tampa, FL 33612-9497 — SOUTHEAST

Hackensack University Medical Center — (201) 996-2000
Hackensack Univ Med Ctr
30 Prospect Avenue — Hackensack, NJ 07601 — MID ATLANTIC

Hahnemann University Hospital — (215) 762-7000
Hahnemann Univ Hosp
Broad & Vine St — Philadelphia, PA 19102 — MID ATLANTIC

Harborview Medical Center — (206) 731-3000
Harborview Med Ctr
325 9th Ave, Box 359717 — Seattle, WA 98104 — WEST COAST AND PACIFIC

Harper University Hospital — (313) 745-8040
Harper Univ Hosp
3990 John R St — Detroit, MI 48201-2097 — MIDWEST

Harrison Memorial Hospital — (360) 377-3911
Harrison Meml Hosp
2520 Cherry Ave — Bremerton, WA 98310-4270 — WEST COAST AND PACIFIC

Hartford Hospital — (860) 545-5000
Hartford Hosp
80 Seymour St, Box 5037 — Hartford, CT 06102-5037 — NEW ENGLAND

Healthsouth Lakeshore Rehabilitation Hospital — (205) 868-2000
Healthsouth Lakeshore Rehab Hosp
3800 Ridgeway — Birmingham, AL 35209 — SOUTHEAST

Henry Ford Hospital — (313) 916-2600
Henry Ford Hosp
2799 W Grand Blvd — Detroit, MI 48202 — MIDWEST

Hilton Head Regional Medical Center — (843) 681-6122
Hilton Head Reg Med Ctr
25 Hospital Ctr Blvd, PO Box 21117 — Hartsville, SC 29925-1117 — SOUTHEAST

Hoag Memorial Hospital Presbyterian   (949) 645-8600
Hoag Meml Hosp Presby
One Hoag Drive   Newport Beach, CA 92663   WEST COAST AND PACIFIC

Holy Cross Hospital - Silver Spring   (301) 754-7000
Holy Cross Hospital - Silver Spring
1500 Forest Glen Road   Silver Spring, MD 20910   MID ATLANTIC

Hospital for Joint Diseases   (212) 598-6000
Hosp For Joint Diseases
301 East 17th Street   New York, NY 10003   MID ATLANTIC

Hospital for Special Surgery   (212) 606-1000
Hosp For Special Surgery
535 East 70th Street   New York, NY 10021   MID ATLANTIC

Hospital of the University of Pennsylvania - UPHS   (215) 662-4000
Hosp Univ Penn - UPHS
3400 Spruce Street   Philadelphia, PA 19104   MID ATLANTIC

Howard University Hospital   (202) 865-6100
Howard Univ Hosp
2041 Georgia Ave NW   Washington, DC 20060   MID ATLANTIC

Indiana University Hospital   (317) 274-5000
Indiana Univ Hosp
550 N University Blvd   Indianapolis, IN 46202   MIDWEST

Inova Fairfax Hospital   (703) 698-1110
Inova Fairfax Hosp
3300 Gallows Road   Falls Church, VA 22042   SOUTHEAST

Inova Fairfax Hospital for Children   (703) 204-6777
Inova Fairfax Hosp for Chldn
3300 Gallows Rd   Fairfax, VA 22042   SOUTHEAST

Jackson Memorial Hospital   (305) 585-1111
Jackson Meml Hosp
1611 NW 12th Ave   Miami, FL 33136   SOUTHEAST

Jewish Hospital - Kenwood - Cincinnati   (513) 686-3000
Jewish Hosp - Kenwood - Cincinnati
4777 E Galbraith Rd   Cincinnati, OH 45236-2891   MIDWEST

Johns Hopkins Hospital   (410) 955-5000
Johns Hopkins Hosp
600 N Wolfe St   Baltimore, MD 21287   MID ATLANTIC

Kaiser Permanente Santa Clara Medical Center   (408) 236-6400
Kaiser Permanente Santa Clara Med Ctr
700 Lawrence Expy   Santa Clara, CA 95051   WEST COAST AND PACIFIC

Kaiser Permanente South San Francisco Medical Center   (650) 742-2000
Kaiser Permanente S San Francisco Med Ctr
1200 El Camino Real   South San Francisco, CA 94080   WEST COAST AND PACIFIC

Kapiolani Medical Center for Women & Children   (808) 983-6000
Kapiolani Med Ctr for Women & Chldn
1319 Punahou St   Honolulu, HI 96826   WEST COAST AND PACIFIC

Karmanos Cancer Institute   (800) 527-6266
Karmanos Cancer Inst
4100 John R   Detroit, MI 48201   MIDWEST

Kootenai Medical Center   (208) 666-2000
Kootenai Med Ctr
2003 Lincoln Way   Coeur d'Alene, ID 83814-2677   GREAT PLAINS AND MOUNTAINS

Kosair Children's Hospital   (502) 629-6000
Kosair Chldn's Hosp
231 E Chestnut St   Louisville, KY 40202   SOUTHEAST

LAC & USC Medical Center   (323) 226-2622
LAC & USC Med Ctr
1200 N State St   Los Angeles, CA 90033-4525   WEST COAST AND PACIFIC

LAC - Harbor - UCLA Medical Center   (310) 222-2345
LAC - Harbor - UCLA Med Ctr
1000 W Carson St   Torrance, CA 90509-2059   WEST COAST AND PACIFIC

Lahey Clinic   (781) 744-5100
Lahey Clin
41 Mall Road   Burlington, MA 01805   NEW ENGLAND

Lankenau Hospital   (610) 645-2000
Lankenau Hosp
100 Lancaster Ave   Wynnewood, PA 19096-3498   MID ATLANTIC

LDS Hospital   (801) 408-1100
LDS Hosp
8th Ave & C St   Salt Lake City, UT 84143   GREAT PLAINS AND MOUNTAINS

Le Bonheur Children's Medical Center   (901) 572-3000
Le Bonheur Chldns Med Ctr
50 N Dunlap   Memphis, TN 38103-2893   SOUTHEAST

Lenox Hill Hospital   (212) 434-2000
Lenox Hill Hosp
100 East 77th Street   New York, NY 10021   MID ATLANTIC

Loma Linda University Medical Center   (909) 558-4000
Loma Linda Univ Med Ctr
11234 Anderson St   Loma Linda, CA 92354   WEST COAST AND PACIFIC

Long Beach Memorial Medical Center   (562) 933-2000
Long Beach Meml Med Ctr
2801 Atlantic Ave   Long Beach, CA 90801   WEST COAST AND PACIFIC

Long Island College Hospital   (718) 780-1000
Long Island Coll Hosp
339 Hicks Street   Brooklyn, NY 11201   MID ATLANTIC

Long Island Jewish Medical Center   (516) 470-7000
Long Island Jewish Med Ctr
270-05 76th Avenue   New Hyde Park, NY 11040   MID ATLANTIC

Louisiana State University Hospital   (318) 675-4239
Louisiana State Univ Hosp
1501 Kings Highway P.O. Box 33932   Shreveport, LA 71130   SOUTHWEST

Loyola University Medical Center   (708) 216-9000
Loyola Univ Med Ctr
2160 S 1st Ave   Maywood, IL 60153   MIDWEST

LSU Interim Public Hospital   (504) 903-3000
LSU Interim Public Hosp
2021 Perdido St   New Orleans, LA 70112   SOUTHWEST

Lucile Packard Children's Hospital   (650) 497-8000
Lucile Packard Chldn's Hosp
725 Welch Rd   Palo Alto, CA 94304   WEST COAST AND PACIFIC

Magee-Womens Hospital - UPMC   (412) 641-1000
Magee-Womens Hosp - UPMC
300 Halket Street   Pittsburgh, PA 15213   MID ATLANTIC

Maimonides Medical Center   (718) 283-6000
Maimonides Med Ctr
4802 Tenth Avenue   Brooklyn, NY 11219   MID ATLANTIC

Maine Medical Center   (207) 871-0111
Maine Med Ctr
22 Bramhall St   Portland, ME 04102   NEW ENGLAND

Marin General Hospital		(415) 925-7000
Marin Genl Hosp		
250 Bon Air Rd	Greenbrae, CA 94904	WEST COAST AND PACIFIC

Massachusetts Eye and Ear Infirmary		(617) 523-7900
Mass Eye & Ear Infirmary		
243 Charles Street	Boston, MA 02114	NEW ENGLAND

Massachusetts General Hospital		(617) 726-2000
Mass Genl Hosp		
55 Fruit St	Boston, MA 02114	NEW ENGLAND

Mattel Children's Hospital at UCLA		(310) 825-9111
Mattel Chldns Hosp at UCLA		
10833 Le Conte Ave	Los Angeles, CA 90095-1752	WEST COAST AND PACIFIC

Mayo Clinic - Jacksonville, FL		(904) 953-2000
Mayo - Jacksonville		
4500 San Pablo Road	Jacksonville, FL 32224	SOUTHEAST

Mayo Clinic - Phoenix		(480) 515-6296
Mayo Clinic - Phoenix		
5777 E Mayo Blvd	Phoenix, AZ 85054	SOUTHWEST

Mayo Clinic - Rochester, MN		(507) 284-2511
Mayo Med Ctr & Clin - Rochester		
200 First St SW	Rochester, MN 55905	MIDWEST

Mayo Clinic - Scottsdale		(480) 301-8000
Mayo Clinic - Scottsdale		
13400 E Shea Blvd	Scottsdale, AZ 85259	SOUTHWEST

McLaren Regional Medical Center		(810) 342-2000
McLaren Reg Med Ctr		
401 S. Ballenger Highway	Flint, MI 48532	MIDWEST

Medical City Dallas Hospital		(972) 566-7000
Med City Dallas Hosp		
7777 Forest Ln	Dallas, TX 75230-2594	SOUTHWEST

Medical College of Georgia Hospital & Clinic (MCG Health Inc)		(706) 721-6569
Med Coll of GA Hosp and Clin (MCG Health Inc)		
1120 15th Street	Augusta, GA 30912	SOUTHEAST

Medical College of Virginia Hospitals		(804) 828-9000
Med Coll of VA Hosp		
1250 E Marshall St, Box 980510	Richmond, VA 23219	SOUTHEAST

Medical University of South Carolina Medical Center		(843) 792-2300
MUSC Med Ctr		
169 Ashley Ave	Charleston, SC 29425	SOUTHEAST

Memorial Health University Medical Center - Savannah		(912) 350-8000
Meml Hlth Univ Med Ctr - Savannah		
4700 Waters Ave	Savannah, GA 31404	SOUTHEAST

Memorial Hermann Hospital - Texas Medical Center		(713) 704-4000
Meml Hermann Hosp - Texas Med Ctr		
6411 Fannin	Houston, TX 77030	SOUTHWEST

Memorial Regional Hospital		(954) 987-2000
Meml Regl Hosp		
3501 Johnson Street	Hollywood, FL 33021	SOUTHEAST

Memorial Sloan-Kettering Cancer Center		(212) 639-2000
Meml Sloan-Kettering Cancer Ctr		
1275 York Avenue	New York, NY 10021	MID ATLANTIC

Methodist Hospital - Houston		(713) 790-3311
Methodist Hosp - Houston		
6565 Fannin St	Houston, TX 77030	SOUTHWEST

Methodist Hospital-Omaha		(402) 354-4000
Methodist Hosp - Omaha		
8303 Dodge St	Omaha, NE 68114	GREAT PLAINS AND MOUNTAINS

Methodist University Hospital - Memphis		(901) 516-7000
Methodist Univ Hosp - Memphis		
1265 Union Ave	Memphis, TN 38104	SOUTHEAST

MetroHealth Medical Center		(216) 778-7800
MetroHealth Med Ctr		
2500 MetroHealth Drive	Cleveland, OH 44109-1998	MIDWEST

Miami Children's Hospital		(305) 666-6511
Miami Children's Hosp		
3100 SW 62nd Ave	Miami, FL 33155	SOUTHEAST

Midwestern Regional Medical Center		(847) 872-4561
Midwest Reg Med Ctr		
2520 Elisha Ave	Zion, IL 60099	MIDWEST

Montefiore Medical Center - Henry and Lucy Moses Division		(718) 920-4321
Montefiore Med Ctr - Div. Moses		
111 East 210 Street	Bronx, NY 10467	MID ATLANTIC

Montefiore Medical Center - North Division		(718) 920-9000
Montefiore Med Ctr - Div. North		
600 E 233rd St	Bronx, NY 10466	MID ATLANTIC
Montgomery Rehabilitation Hospital		(215) 233-6200
Montgomery Rehab Hosp		
8601 Stenton Ave	Wyndmoor, PA 19038	MID ATLANTIC
Morristown Memorial Hospital		(973) 971-5000
Morristown Mem Hosp		
100 Madison Avenue	Morristown, NJ 07960	MID ATLANTIC
Mott Children's Hospital		(734) 936-4000
Mott Chldns Hosp		
1500 E Medical Center Dr	Ann Arbor, MI 48109	MIDWEST
Mount Clemens Regional Medical Center		(586) 493-8000
Mount Clemens Regional Med Ctr		
1000 Harrington Blvd	Mount Clemens, MI 48043	MIDWEST
Mount Sinai Medical Center		(212) 241-6500
Mount Sinai Med Ctr		
One Gustave L. Levy Pl	New York, NY 10029	MID ATLANTIC
Mount Sinai Medical Center - Miami		(305) 674-2121
Mount Sinai Med Ctr - Miami		
4300 Alton Rd	Miami Beach, FL 33140	SOUTHEAST
National Institutes of Health - Clinical Center		(301) 496-4000
Natl Inst of Hlth - Clin Ctr		
10 Center Drive	Bethesda, MD 20892-0001	MID ATLANTIC
Nationwide Children's Hospital		(614) 722-2000
Nationwide Chldn's Hosp		
700 Children's Drive	Columbus, OH 43205	MIDWEST
Nebraska Medical Center		(402) 559-2000
Nebraska Med Ctr		
42nd & Dewey St	Omaha, NE 68198	GREAT PLAINS AND MOUNTAINS
Nebraska Methodist Hospital		(402) 354-4000
Nebraska Meth Hosp		
8303 Dodge St	Omaha, NE 68114	GREAT PLAINS AND MOUNTAINS
New York Eye & Ear Infirmary		(212) 979-4000
New York Eye & Ear Infirm		
310 East 14th Street	New York, NY 10003	MID ATLANTIC

NewYork-Presbyterian Hospital/Columbia   (212) 305-2500
NY-Presby Hosp/Columbia
622 W 168th St   New York, NY 10032   MID ATLANTIC

NewYork-Presbyterian Hospital/Weill Cornell   (212) 746-5454
NY-Presby Hosp/Weill Cornell
525 E 68th St   New York, NY 10021   MID ATLANTIC

NewYork-Presbyterian/Morgan Stanley Children's Hospital   (212) 305-2500
NYPresby-Morgan Stanley Children's Hosp
622 W 168th St   New York, NY 10032   MID ATLANTIC

North Shore University Hospital   (516) 562-0100
N Shore Univ Hosp
300 Community Dr   Manhasset, NY 11030   MID ATLANTIC

Northern Memorial Health Care, Robbinsdale   (763) 520-5200
Northern Meml Hlth Care
3300 Oakdale Ave N   Robbinsdale, MN 55422   MIDWEST

NorthShore University HealthSystem   (847) 570-2000
NorthShore Univ HlthSys
1301 Central Ave   Evanston, IL 60201   MIDWEST

Northwest Hospital   (206) 364-0500
Northwest Hosp
1550 N 115th St   Seattle, WA 98133-0806   WEST COAST AND PACIFIC

Northwestern Memorial Hospital   (312) 926-2000
Northwestern Meml Hosp
251 E Huron St   Chicago, IL 60611   MIDWEST

Norton Hospital   (502) 629-8000
Norton Hosp
200 E Chestnut St   Louisville, KY 40202   SOUTHEAST

NYU Langone Medical Center   (212) 263-7300
NYU Langone Med Ctr
550 First Avenue   New York, NY 10016   MID ATLANTIC

Ochsner Baptist Medical Center   (504) 899-9311
Ochsner Baptist Med Ctr
2700 Napoleon Ave   New Orleans, LA 70115   SOUTHWEST

Ochsner Foundation Hospital   (504) 842-3000
Ochsner Fdn Hosp
1516 Jefferson Hwy   New Orleans, LA 70121   SOUTHWEST

Ohio State University Medical Center | (614) 293-8000
Ohio St Univ Med Ctr
410 W 10th Avenue | Columbus, OH 43210 | MIDWEST

Olathe Medical Center | (913) 791-4200
Olathe Med Ctr
20333 W 151st St | Olathe, KS 66061-5352 | GREAT PLAINS AND MOUNTAINS

Oregon Health & Science University | (503) 494-8311
OR Hlth & Sci Univ
3181 SW Sam Jackson Park Rd | Portland, OR 97239-3098 | WEST COAST AND PACIFIC

OU Medical Center | (405) 271-4700
OU Med Ctr
1200 Everett Dr | Oklahoma City, OK 73104-5098 | SOUTHWEST

Our Lady of the Lake Regional Medical Center | (225) 765-6565
Our Lady of the Lake Regl Med Ctr
5000 Hennessy Blvd | Baton Rouge, LA 70808-4398 | SOUTHWEST

Overland Park Regional Medical Center | (913) 541-5000
Overland Pk Regl Med Ctr
10500 Quivira Rd | Overland Park, KS 66215 | GREAT PLAINS AND MOUNTAINS

Palmetto Richland Memorial Hospital | (803) 434-7000
Palmetto Richland Mem Hosp
5 Richland Medical Park Drive | Columbia, SC 29203 | SOUTHEAST

Penn Presbyterian Medical Center - UPHS | (215) 662-8000
Penn Presby Med Ctr - UPHS
51 N 39th St | Philadelphia, PA 19104 | MID ATLANTIC

Penn State Milton S Hershey Medical Center | (717) 531-8521
Penn State Milton S Hershey Med Ctr
500 University Drive | Hershey, PA 17033-0850 | MID ATLANTIC

Pennsylvania Hospital | (215) 829-3000
Pennsylvania Hosp
800 Spruce St, Ste 240 | Philadelphia, PA 19107 | MID ATLANTIC

Phoenix Baptist Hospital & Medical Center | (602) 249-0212
Phoenix Baptist Hosp & Med Ctr
2000 West Bethany Home Rd | Phoenix, AZ 85015-2184 | SOUTHWEST

Physicians Regional Medical Center | (239) 348-4000
Physicians Regl Med Ctr
6101 Pine Ridge Rd | Naples, FL 34119 | SOUTHEAST

Presbyterian - St Luke's Medical Center   (303) 839-6000
Presby - St Luke's Med Ctr
1719 E 19th Ave   Denver, CO 80218   GREAT PLAINS AND MOUNTAINS

Presbyterian Hospital of Dallas   (214) 345-6789
Presby Hosp of Dallas
8200 Walnut Hill Ln   Dallas, TX 75231   SOUTHWEST

Primary Children's Medical Center   (801) 588-2000
Primary Children's Med Ctr
100 N Medical Drive   Salt Lake City, UT 84113-1100   GREAT PLAINS AND MOUNTAINS

Providence Hospital - Southfield   (248) 424-3000
Providence Hosp - Southfield
16001 W Nine Mile Rd   Southfield, MI 48075   MIDWEST

Providence Portland Medical Center   (503) 215-1111
Providence Portland Med Ctr
4805 NE Glisan   Portland, OR 97213-2967   WEST COAST AND PACIFIC

Providence Saint Joseph Medical Center   (818) 843-5111
Providence St Joseph Med Ctr
501 S Buena Vista St   Burbank, CA 91505   WEST COAST AND PACIFIC

Queen's Medical Center - Honolulu   (808) 538-9011
Queen's Med Ctr - Honolulu
1301 Punchbowl Street   Honolulu, HI 96813   WEST COAST AND PACIFIC

Rady Children's Hospital - San Diego   (858) 576-1700
Rady Children's Hosp - San Diego
3020 Children's Way   San Diego, CA 92123   WEST COAST AND PACIFIC

Rainbow Babies & Children's Hospital   (216) 844-1000
Rainbow Babies & Chldns Hosp
11100 Euclid Ave   Cleveland, OH 44106   MIDWEST

Rehabilitation Institute of Chicago   (312) 238-1000
Rehab Inst of Chicago
345 E. Superior Street   Chicago, IL 60611   MIDWEST

Rhode Island Hospital   (401) 444-4000
Rhode Island Hosp
593 Eddy Street   Providence, RI 02903-4923   NEW ENGLAND

Riley Hospital for Children   (317) 274-5000
Riley Hosp for Children
702 Barnhill Drive   Indianapolis, IN 46202   MIDWEST

Riverview Medical Center   (732) 741-2700
Riverview Med Ctr
1 Riverview Plaza   Red Bank, NJ 07701   MID ATLANTIC

Robert Wood Johnson University Hospital - New Brunswick   (732) 828-3000
Robert Wood Johnson Univ Hosp - New Brunswick
1 Robert Wood Johnson Pl   New Brunswick, NJ 08901   MID ATLANTIC

Rochester Methodist Hospital   (507) 284-2511
Rochester Methodist Hosp
201 W Center St   Rochester, MN 55905-3003   MIDWEST

Roper Hospital   (843) 724-2000
Roper Hosp
316 Calhoun St   Charleston, SC 29401   SOUTHEAST

Roswell Park Cancer Institute   (716) 845-5770
Roswell Park Cancer Inst
Elm and Carlton Streets   Buffalo, NY 14263   MID ATLANTIC

Rush University Medical Center   (312) 942-5000
Rush Univ Med Ctr
1653 W Congress Pkwy   Chicago, IL 60612-3833   MIDWEST

Sacred Heart Medical Center   (541) 686-7300
Sacred Heart Med Ctr
1255 Hilyard St   Eugene, OR 97440-3700   WEST COAST AND PACIFIC

Saint Francis Hospital - Memphis   (901) 765-1000
St Francis Hosp - Memphis
5959 Park Ave   Memphis, TN 38119   SOUTHEAST

Saint John's Health Center   (310) 829-5511
St John's Hlth Ctr, Santa Monica
1328 22nd St   Santa Monica, CA 90404   WEST COAST AND PACIFIC

Saint Vincent Catholic Medical Centers - St Vincent's Manhattan   (212) 604-7000
St Vincent Cath Med Ctrs - Manhattan
170 West 12th Street   New York, NY 10011   MID ATLANTIC

Salt Lake Regional Medical Center   (801) 350-4111
Salt Lake Regional Med Ctr
1050 E South Temple   Salt Lake City, UT 84102   GREAT PLAINS AND MOUNTAINS

San Diego Hospice   (619) 688-1600
San Diego Hospice
4311 3rd Ave0   San Diego, CA 92103-7499   WEST COAST AND PACIFIC

San Francisco General Hospital   (415) 206-8000
San Francisco Genl Hosp
1001 Potrero Avenue   San Francisco, CA 94110   WEST COAST AND PACIFIC

Santa Clara Valley Medical Center   (408) 885-5000
Santa Clara Vly Med Ctr
751 S Bascom Ave   San Jose, CA 95128   WEST COAST AND PACIFIC

Santa Monica - UCLA Medical Center and Orthopaedic Hospital   (310) 319-4000
Santa Monica - UCLA Med Ctr & Ortho Hosp
1250 16th St   Santa Monica, CA 90404   WEST COAST AND PACIFIC

Sarasota Memorial Hospital   (941) 917-9000
Sarasota Meml Hosp
1700 S Tamiami Trail   Sarasota, FL 34239   SOUTHEAST

Schneider Children's Hospital   (718) 470-3000
Schneider Chldn's Hosp
269-01 76th Ave   New Hyde Park, NY 11040   MID ATLANTIC

Scott & White Memorial Hospital   (254) 724-2111
Scott & White Mem Hosp
2401 S 31st St   Temple, TX 76508-0001   SOUTHWEST

Scottsdale Healthcare - Shea   (480) 860-3000
Scottsdale Hlthcare - Shea
9000 E Shea Blvd   Scottsdale, AZ 85258-4514   SOUTHWEST

Scripps Green Hospital   (858) 455-9100
Scripps Green Hosp
10666 N Torrey Pines Rd   La Jolla, CA 92037   WEST COAST AND PACIFIC

Scripps Memorial Hospital - La Jolla   (858) 457-4123
Scripps Meml Hosp - La Jolla
9888 Genesee Ave   La Jolla, CA 92037   WEST COAST AND PACIFIC

Sentara Norfolk General Hospital   (757) 668-3000
Sentara Norfolk Genl Hosp
600 Gresham Dr   Norfolk, VA 23507   SOUTHEAST

Shands at University of Florida   (352) 265-0111
Shands at Univ of FL
1600 SW Archer Rd   Gainesville, FL 32610   SOUTHEAST

Shands Jacksonville   (904) 244-0411
Shands Jacksonville
655 W 8th St   Jacksonville, FL 32209   SOUTHEAST

Sibley Memorial Hospital		(202) 537-4000
Sibley Mem Hosp		
5255 Loughboro Road NW	Washington, DC 20016	MID ATLANTIC

Sinai Hospital - Baltimore		(410) 601-9000
Sinai Hosp - Baltimore		
2401 W Belvedere Ave	Baltimore, MD 21215	MID ATLANTIC

Southern New Hampshire Medical Center		(603) 577-2000
Southern NH Med Ctr		
8 Prospect St	Nashua, NH 03061	NEW ENGLAND

Southwest Texas Methodist Hospital		(210) 575-4000
SW TX Meth Hosp		
7700 Floyd Curl Dr	San Antonio, TX 78229	SOUTHWEST

Spectrum Health - Blodgett Campus		(616) 774-7444
Spectrum Hlth Blodgett Campus		
1840 Wealthy St SE	Grand Rapids, MI 49506	MIDWEST

St Anthony Hospital - Oklahoma City		(405) 272-7000
St Anthony Hosp -Oklahoma City		
1000 N Lee St	Oklahoma City, OK 73102	SOUTHWEST

St Anthony's Hospital - St Petersburg		(727) 893-6814
St Anthony's Hosp - St Petersburg		
1200 7th Avenue North	St Petersburg, FL 33705	SOUTHEAST

St Barnabas Medical Center		(973) 322-5000
St Barnabas Med Ctr		
94 Old Short Hills Rd	Livingston, NJ 07039-5672	MID ATLANTIC

St Christopher's Hospital for Children		(215) 427-5000
St Christopher's Hosp for Chldn		
Erie Ave at Front St	Philadelphia, PA 19134	MID ATLANTIC

St Francis Hospital and Health Center		(317) 865-5000
St Francis Hosp		
8111 S Emerson Ave	Indianapolis, IN 46143	MIDWEST

St John's Hospital - Springfield		(217) 544-6464
St John's Hosp - Springfield		
800 E Carpenter St	Springfield, IL 62769	MIDWEST

St Joseph Hospital		(603) 882-3000
St Joseph Hosp		
172 Kinsley St	Nashua, NH 03060	NEW ENGLAND

St Joseph Hospital   (360) 734-5400
St Joseph Hosp - Bellingham
2901 Squalicum Pkwy   Bellingham, WA 98225-1898   WEST COAST AND PACIFIC

St Joseph Medical Center   (410) 337-1000
St Joseph Med Ctr
7601 Osler Drive   Baltimore, MD 21208   MID ATLANTIC

St Joseph's Children's Hospital   (813) 554-8500
St Josephs Chldns Hosp
3001 W Dr Martin Luther King Jr Blvd Tampa, FL 33607   SOUTHEAST

St Joseph's Hospital & Medical Center - Phoenix   (602) 406-3000
St Joseph's Hosp & Med Ctr - Phoenix
350 W Thomas Rd   Phoenix, AZ 85013-4496   SOUTHWEST

St Joseph's Hospital - Atlanta   (404) 851-7001
St Joseph's Hosp - Atlanta
5665 Peachtree Dunwoody Rd NE   Atlanta, GA 30342   SOUTHEAST

St Joseph's Hospital - Orange   (714) 633-9111
St Joseph's Hosp - Orange
1100 West Stewart Drive   Orange, CA 92868   WEST COAST AND PACIFIC

St Joseph's Hospital - Tucson   (520) 296-3211
St Joseph's Hosp - Tucson
350 N Wilmot Rd   Tucson, AZ 85711   SOUTHWEST

St Jude Children's Research Hospital   (901) 495-3300
St Jude Children's Research Hosp
262 Danny Thomas Pl   Memphis, TN 38105   SOUTHEAST

St Louis Children's Hospital   (314) 454-6000
St Louis Chldns Hosp
One Children's Pl   St Louis, MO 63110   MIDWEST

St Louis University Hospital   (314) 577-8000
St Louis Univ Hosp
3635 Vista at Grand Blvd   St Louis, MO 63110   MIDWEST

St Luke's - Roosevelt Hospital Center - Roosevelt Division   (212) 523-4000
St Luke's - Roosevelt Hosp Ctr - Roosevelt Div
1000 Tenth Avenue   New York, NY 10019   MID ATLANTIC

St Luke's - Roosevelt Hospital Center - St Luke's Hospital   (212) 523-4000
St Luke's - Roosevelt Hosp Ctr - St Luke's Hosp
1111 Amsterdam Ave   New York, NY 10025   MID ATLANTIC

St Luke's Episcopal Hospital-Houston (832) 355-1000
St Luke's Episcopal Hosp-Houston
6720 Bertner Avenue Houston, TX 77030 SOUTHWEST

St Luke's Hospital - Chesterfield, MO (314) 434-1500
St Luke's Hosp - Chesterfield, MO
232 S Woods Mill Rd Chesterfield, MO 63017 MIDWEST

St Mark's Hospital - Salt Lake City (801) 268-7111
St Mark's Hosp - Salt Lake City
1200 E. 3900 S Salt Lake City, UT 84124 GREAT PLAINS AND MOUNTAINS

St Mary's Hospital - Rochester, MN (Mayo Clinic) (507) 255-5123
St Mary's Hosp - Rochester
1216 2nd St SW Rochester, MN 55902 MIDWEST

St Mary's Medical Center - Huntington (304) 526-1234
St Mary's Med Ctr - Huntington
2900 First Ave Huntington, WV 25702-1272 MID ATLANTIC

St Mary's Medical Center - West Palm Beach (561) 844-6300
St Mary's Med Ctr - W Palm Bch
901 45th St West Palm Beach, FL 33407 SOUTHEAST

St Patrick Hospital & Health Sciences Center (406) 543-7271
St Patrick Hospital - Missoula
500 W Broadway Missoula, MT 59802 GREAT PLAINS AND MOUNTAINS

St Peter's University Hospital (732) 745-8600
St Peter's Univ Hosp
254 Easton Ave New Brunswick, NJ 08901-1780 MID ATLANTIC

St Vincent Carmel Hospital (317) 573-7000
St Vincent Carmel Hosp
13500 N Meridian St Carmel, IN 46032-1496 MIDWEST

St Vincent Hospital - Santa Fe (505) 983-3361
St Vincent Hosp - Santa Fe
455 St Michaels Dr Santa Fe, NM 87504-2107 SOUTHWEST

St Vincent Indianapolis Hospital (317) 338-2345
St Vincent Indianapolis Hosp
2001 W 86th St Indianapolis, IN 46260-1991 MIDWEST

St Vincent's Medical Center - Jacksonville (904) 308-7300
St Vincent's Med Ctr - Jacksonville
1800 Barrs St Jacksonville, FL 32204 SOUTHEAST

St. Luke's Regional Medical Center   (208) 381-2222
St. Luke's Reg Med Ctr - Boise
190 E Bannock St   Boise, ID 83712   GREAT PLAINS AND MOUNTAINS

Stanford University Medical Center   (650) 723-4000
Stanford Univ Med Ctr
300 Pasteur Dr   Stanford, CA 94305   WEST COAST AND PACIFIC

Stony Brook University Medical Center   (631) 689-8333
Stony Brook Univ Med Ctr
Nicolls Rd   Stony Brook, NY 11794-8410   MID ATLANTIC

SUNY Downstate Medical Center   (718) 270-1000
SUNY Downstate Med Ctr
450 Clarkson Ave   Brooklyn, NY 11203   MID ATLANTIC

Swedish Medical Center - Seattle   (206) 386-6000
Swedish Med Ctr - Seattle
747 Broadway   Seattle, WA 98122   WEST COAST AND PACIFIC

Tampa General Hospital   (813) 844-7000
Tampa Genl Hosp
PO BOX 1289   Tampa, FL 33601   SOUTHEAST

Temple University Hospital   (215) 707-2000
Temple Univ Hosp
3401 N Broad St   Philadelphia, PA 19140-5189   MID ATLANTIC

Texas Children's Hospital   (832) 824-1000
Texas Chldns Hosp
6621 Fannin St   Houston, TX 77030   SOUTHWEST

Thomas Jefferson University Hospital   (215) 955-6000
Thomas Jefferson Univ Hosp
111 S 11th St   Philadelphia, PA 19107   MID ATLANTIC

Tucson Medical Center   (520) 327-5461
Tucson Med Ctr
5301 E Grant Rd   Tucson, AZ 85712-2874   SOUTHWEST

Tufts Medical Center   (617) 636-5000
Tufts Med Ctr
800 Washington St   Boston, MA 02111   NEW ENGLAND

Tulane University Hospital & Clinic   (504) 588-5263
Tulane Univ Hosp & Clin
1415 Tulane Ave   New Orleans, LA 70112   SOUTHWEST

UCLA Ronald Reagan Medical Center		(310) 825-9111
UCLA Ronald Reagan Med Ctr		
757 Westwood Plaza	Los Angeles, CA 90095	WEST COAST AND PACIFIC
UCSD Medical Center		(619) 543-6222
UCSD Med Ctr		
200 W Arbor Dr	San Diego, CA 92103	WEST COAST AND PACIFIC
UCSF - Mount Zion Medical Center		(415) 567-6600
UCSF - Mt Zion Med Ctr		
1600 Divisadero St	San Francisco, CA 94115	WEST COAST AND PACIFIC
UCSF Medical Center		(415) 476-1000
UCSF Med Ctr		
500 Parnassus Ave	San Francisco, CA 94143	WEST COAST AND PACIFIC
UMass Memorial Medical Center		(508) 334-1000
UMass Memorial Med Ctr		
55 Lake Ave N	Worcester, MA 01655	NEW ENGLAND
UMDNJ-University Hospital-Newark		(973) 972-4300
UMDNJ-Univ Hosp-Newark		
150 Bergen St	Newark, NJ 07103-2406	MID ATLANTIC
Uniformed Services University of the Health Sciences		(301) 295-9390
Unif Serv Univ of the Hlth Sci		
4301 Jones Bridge Rd	Bethesda, MD 20814-4799	MID ATLANTIC
Union Memorial Hospital-Baltimore		(410) 554-2000
Union Meml Hosp-Baltimore		
201 E University Pkwy	Baltimore, MD 21218	MID ATLANTIC
University Health System-San Antonio		(210) 358-4000
Univ Hlth Syst-San Antonio		
4502 Medical Dr	San Antonio, TX 78229	SOUTHWEST
University Hospital - Cincinnati		(513) 584-1000
Univ Hosp - Cincinnati		
234 Goodman St	Cincinnati, OH 45219	MIDWEST
University Hospital - SUNY Upstate Medical University		(315) 464-5540
Univ Hosp - SUNY Upstate		
750 E Adams Street	Syracuse, NY 13210	MID ATLANTIC
University Hospitals Case Medical Center		(216) 844-1000
Univ Hosps Case Med Ctr		
11100 Euclid Ave	Cleveland, OH 44106	MIDWEST

University Medical Center of Southern Nevada - Las Vegas   (702) 383-2000
Univ Med Ctr - Las Vegas
1800 W Charleston Blvd   Las Vegas, NV 89102   WEST COAST AND PACIFIC

University Medical Center- Tucson   (520) 694-0111
Univ Med Ctr - Tucson
1501 N Campbell Ave   Tucson, AZ 85724-5128   SOUTHWEST

University Medical Center-Lubbock   (806) 775-8200
Univ Med Ctr-Lubbock
602 Indiana Ave   Lubbock, TX 79408   SOUTHWEST

University New Mexico Health & Science Center   (505) 272-2111
Univ NM Hlth & Sci Ctr
2211 Lomas Blvd NE   Albuquerque, NM 87106   SOUTHWEST

University of Alabama Hospital at Birmingham   (205) 934-4011
Univ of Ala Hosp at Birmingham
619 South 19th Street   Birmingham, AL 35249-6544   SOUTHEAST

University of Arkansas for Medical Sciences Medical Center   (501) 686-7000
UAMS Med Ctr
4301 W Markham St   Little Rock, AR 72205   SOUTHWEST

University of California - Davis Medical Center   (916) 734-2011
UC Davis Med Ctr
2315 Stockton Blvd   Sacramento, CA 95817   WEST COAST AND PACIFIC

University of California - Irvine Medical Center   (714) 456-6011
UC Irvine Med Ctr
101 The City Dr   Orange, CA 92868   WEST COAST AND PACIFIC

University of Chicago Medical Center   (773) 702-1000
Univ of Chicago Med Ctr
5841 S Maryland Ave   Chicago, IL 60637   MIDWEST

University of Colorado Hospital   (730) 848-4011
Univ Colorado Hosp
12605 E 16th Ave   Aurora, CO 80045   GREAT PLAINS AND MOUNTAINS

University of Connecticut Health Center, John Dempsey Hospital   (860) 679-2100
Univ of Conn Hlth Ctr, John Dempsey Hosp
263 Farmington Ave   Farmington, CT 06030   NEW ENGLAND

University of Illinois Medical Center at Chicago   (312) 996-7000
Univ of IL Med Ctr at Chicago
1740 W Taylor St   Chicago, IL 60612   MIDWEST

University of Iowa Hospitals and Clinics   (319) 356-1616
Univ Iowa Hosp & Clinics
200 Hawkins Drive   Iowa City, IA 52242   MIDWEST

University of Kansas Hospital   (913) 588-5000
Univ of Kansas Hosp
3901 Rainbow Blvd   Kansas City, KS 66160   GREAT PLAINS AND MOUNTAINS

University of Kentucky Chandler Hospital   (800) 333-8874
Univ of Kentucky Chandler Hosp
800 Rose Street   Lexington, KY 40536   SOUTHEAST

University of Louisville Hospital   (502) 562-3000
Univ of Louisville Hosp
530 S Jackson St   Louisville, KY 40202   SOUTHEAST

University of Maryland Medical Center   (410) 328-8667
Univ of MD Med Ctr
22 S Greene St   Baltimore, MD 21201   MID ATLANTIC

University of Miami Hosp & Clinics/Sylvester Comprehensive Cancer Cntr   (305) 243-1000
Univ of Miami Hosp & Clins/Sylvester Comp Canc Ctr
1475 NW 12th Ave   Miami, FL 33136   SOUTHEAST

University of Miami Hospital   (305) 325-5511
Univ of Miami Hosp
1400 NW 12 Ave   Miami, FL 33136   SOUTHEAST

University of Michigan Health System   (734) 936-4000
Univ Michigan Hlth Sys
1500 E Medical Center Dr   Ann Arbor, MI 48109   MIDWEST

University of Minnesota Medical Center, Fairview - University Campus   (612) 273-3000
Univ Minn Med Ctr, Fairview - Univ Campus
420 Delaware St SE   Minneapolis, MN 55455   MIDWEST

University of Mississippi Medical Center   (601) 984-1000
Univ Mississippi Med Ctr
2500 N State St   Jackson, MS 39216   SOUTHEAST

University of Missouri Hospitals & Clinics   (573) 882-4141
Univ of Missouri Hosp & Clins
1 Hospital Dr   Columbia, MO 65212   MIDWEST

University of North Carolina Hospitals   (919) 966-4131
Univ NC Hosps
101 Manning Drive, Box 7600   Chapel Hill, NC 27514   SOUTHEAST

University of Rochester Strong Memorial Hospital	(585) 275-2121
Univ of Rochester Strong Meml Hosp	
601 Elmwood Ave Rochester, NY 14642	MID ATLANTIC

University of South Alabama Medical Center	(251) 471-7000
Univ of S AL Med Ctr	
2451 Fillingim St Mobile, AL 36617	SOUTHEAST

University of South Florida - Tampa	(813) 974-2011
Univ of S FL - Tampa	
4202 E Fowler Ave Tampa, FL 33620	SOUTHEAST

University of Tennesee Memorial Hospital	(865) 544-9000
Univ of Tennesee Mem Hosp	
1924 Alcoa Hwy Knoxville, TN 37920	SOUTHEAST

University of Texas MD Anderson Cancer Center	(713) 792-2121
UT MD Anderson Cancer Ctr	
1515 Holcombe Blvd Houston, TX 77030-4095	SOUTHWEST

University of Toledo Medical Center	(419) 383-4000
Univ of Toledo Med Ctr	
3000 Arlington Ave Toledo, OH 43614	MIDWEST

University of Utah Hospitals and Clinics	(801) 581-2121
Univ Utah Hosps and Clins	
50 N Medical Dr Salt Lake City, UT 84132	GREAT PLAINS AND MOUNTAINS

University of Virginia Medical Center	(434) 924-0211
Univ Virginia Med Ctr	
1215 Lee Street Charlottesville, VA 22908-0001	SOUTHEAST

University of Washington Medical Center	(206) 598-3300
Univ Wash Med Ctr	
1959 NE Pacific St, Box 356355 Seattle, WA 98195	WEST COAST AND PACIFIC

University of Wisconsin Hospital & Clinics	(608) 263-6400
Univ WI Hosp & Clins	
600 Highland Avenue Madison, WI 53792	MIDWEST

UPMC Montefiore	(412) 647-2345
UPMC Montefiore	
200 Lothrop St Pittsburgh, PA 15213	MID ATLANTIC

UPMC Presbyterian	(412) 647-2345
UPMC Presby, Pittsburgh	
200 Lothrop St Pittsburgh, PA 15213	MID ATLANTIC

UPMC Shadyside		(412) 623-2121
UPMC Shadyside		
5230 Centre Ave	Pittsburgh, PA 15232	MID ATLANTIC

USC Norris Cancer Hospital		(323) 865-3000
USC Norris Cancer Hosp		
1441 Eastlake Ave	Los Angeles, CA 90033	WEST COAST AND PACIFIC

USC University Hospital		(323) 442-8444
USC Univ Hosp		
1500 San Pablo St	Los Angeles, CA 90033	WEST COAST AND PACIFIC

UT Southwestern Medical Center at Dallas		(214) 648-3111
UT Southwestern Med Ctr at Dallas		
5323 Harry Hines Blvd	Dallas, TX 75390	SOUTHWEST

VA Medical Center - Ann Arbor		(734) 769-7100
VA Med Ctr - Ann Arbor		
2215 Fuller Rd	Ann Arbor, MI 48105	MIDWEST

VA Medical Center - Atlanta		(404) 321-6111
VA Med Ctr - Atlanta		
1670 Clairmont Rd	Decatur, GA 30033	SOUTHEAST

VA Medical Center - Portland		(503) 220-8262
VA Medical Center - Portland		
3710 SW US Veteran Hospital Rd	Portland, OR 97239	WEST COAST AND PACIFIC

Vanderbilt Children's Hospital		(615) 936-1000
Vanderbilt Children's Hosp		
2200 Children's Way	Nashville, TN 37232	SOUTHEAST

Vanderbilt University Medical Center		(615) 322-5000
Vanderbilt Univ Med Ctr		
1313 21st Avenue South	Nashville, TN 37232	SOUTHEAST

Veterans Affairs Medical Center - Augusta		(706) 733-0188
VA Medical Ctr - Augusta		
One Freedom Way	Augusta, GA 30904	SOUTHEAST

Veterans Affairs Medical Center - Tucson		(520) 792-1450
VA Medical Center - Tucson		
3601 S 6th Avenue	Tucson, AZ 85723	SOUTHWEST

Virginia Mason Medical Center		(206) 223-6600
Virginia Mason Med Ctr		
1100 Ninth Ave, Box 900	Seattle, WA 98111	WEST COAST AND PACIFIC

Wake Forest University Baptist Medical Center　　　　　　(336) 716-2011
Wake Forest Univ Baptist Med Ctr
Medical Center Blvd　　　　　　　　Winston-Salem, NC 27157-1015　　　SOUTHEAST

WakeMed Cary Hospital　　　　　　　　　　　　　　　　(919) 350-2300
WakeMed Cary
1900 Kildaire Farm Rd　　　　　　　Cary, NC 27511-6616　　　　　SOUTHEAST

Washington Hospital Center　　　　　　　　　　　　　　(202) 877-7000
Washington Hosp Ctr
110 Irving St NW　　　　　　　　　Washington, DC 20010　　　MID ATLANTIC

Washington University Medical Center　　　　　　　　　　(314) 362-6828
Washington Univ Med Ctr
4444 Forest Park Ave　　　　　　　St Louis, MO 63108　　　　　MIDWEST

WellStar Windy Hill Hospital　　　　　　　　　　　　　　(770) 644-1000
WellStar Windy Hill Hosp
2540 Windy Hill Road　　　　　　　Marietta, GA 30067　　　　SOUTHEAST

West Virginia University Hospital - Ruby Memorial　　　　　(304) 598-4000
WV Univ Hosp - Ruby Memorial
1 Medical Center Drive　　　　　　Morgantown, WV 26506　　　MID ATLANTIC

Westchester Medical Center　　　　　　　　　　　　　　(914) 493-7000
Westchester Med Ctr
95 Grasslands Road　　　　　　　Valhalla, NY 10595　　　　MID ATLANTIC

William Beaumont Hospital　　　　　　　　　　　　　　(248) 551-5000
William Beaumont Hosp
3601 W 13 Mile Rd　　　　　　　Royal Oak, MI 48073　　　　MIDWEST

Wills Eye Hospital　　　　　　　　　　　　　　　　　(215) 928-3000
Wills Eye Hosp
840 Walnut St　　　　　　　　　Philadelphia, PA 19107-5598　　MID ATLANTIC

Winthrop - University Hospital　　　　　　　　　　　　　(516) 663-0333
Winthrop - Univ Hosp
259 1st St　　　　　　　　　　Mineola, NY 11501　　　　　MID ATLANTIC

Wolfson Children's Hospital　　　　　　　　　　　　　　(904) 202-8000
Wolfson Chldns Hosp
800 Prudential Dr　　　　　　　Jacksonville, FL 32207　　　　SOUTHEAST

Women & Infants Hospital of Rhode Island　　　　　　　(401) 274-1100
Women & Infants Hosp of RI
101 Dudley Street　　　　　　　Providence, RI 02905　　　　NEW ENGLAND

Women's and Children's Hospital of Buffalo, The   (716) 878-7000
Women's & Chldn's Hosp of Buffalo, The
219 Bryant St   Buffalo, NY 14222   MID ATLANTIC

Yakima Valley Memorial Hospital   (509) 575-8000
Yakima Valley Mem Hosp
2811 Tieton Dr   Yakima, WA 98902-3799   WEST COAST AND PACIFIC

Yale-New Haven Hospital   (203) 688-4242
Yale-New Haven Hosp
20 York St   New Haven, CT 06510   NEW ENGLAND

Yampa Valley Medical Center   (970) 879-1322
Yampa Valley Med Ctr
1024 Central Park Dr   Steamboat Springs, CO 80487GREAT PLAINS AND MOUNTAINS

Appendix C:
Selected Cancer Resources

AMERICAN CANCER SOCIETY
A site with many resources on types of cancer, treatments, coping, support, clinical research data, volunteering and current news articles. It also has a database which allows one to search by zip code to locate local resources, activities and news.

National Office
1599 Clifton Road, NE
Atlanta, GA 30329

800-ACS-2345
www.cancer.org

AMERICAN INSTITUTE FOR CANCER RESEARCH
Discusses current research findings on diet, nutrition and cancer prevention and provides an online Cancer Resource Book.

1759 R Street, NW
Washington, DC 20009-2552

800-843-8114
www.aicr.org

ANNIE APPLESEED PROJECT
Provides information, education, advocacy and awareness to those interested in complementary and alternative medical treatments.

7319 Serrano Terrace
Delray Beach, FL 33446-2215

www.annieappleseedproject.org
annfonfa@aol.com

ASSOCIATION OF CANCER ONLINE RESOURCES (ACOR)
Maintains many support groups and cancer-specific information, treatment options, clinical trial findings and a large collection of cancer-related online communities.

173 Duane Street
Suite 3A
New York, NY 10013-3334

212-226-5525
www.acor.org

CANCER CARE
Provides free resources and support to cancer patients, caregivers and families with all cancers through counseling, education, information, referrals and direct financial assistance.

National Office
275 7th Ave, Fl 22
New York, NY 10001

800-813-HOPE or 212-712-8400
www.cancercare.org

CANCER NEWS
News and information on cancer diagnosis, treatment and prevention.

www.cancernews.com

CANCER RESEARCH & PREVENTION FOUNDATION OF AMERICA

Scientific research and cancer education with a focus on cancers that can be prevented through lifestyle changes or early detection followed by prompt treatment. Includes breast, cervical, colorectal, lung, prostate, skin, oral and testicular cancers.

1600 Duke Street
Suite 500
Alexandria, VA 22314

800-227-2732
www.preventcancer.org

CANCER TRACK

Comprehensive source for links to news, research, medications, treatments, support groups, regulatory agencies and online references.

www.cancertrack.com

CANCERBACKUP

Europe-based organization with over 4,500 pages of online cancer information, practical advice and support for cancer patients and their families.

www.cancerbackup.org.uk

CANCEREDUCATION.COM

Provides cancer-specific information and educational programming for patients, their families and physicians.

750 Lexington Avenue
26th Floor
New York, NY 10022
NexCura, Inc.
1215 Fourth Age
Suite 1925
Seattle, WA 98161

212-531-5960
www.cancereducation.com
webmaster@cancereducation.com
206-270-0225
www.cancerfacts.com
answers@support.nextura.com

CANCERNETWORK.COM

Provides research findings and information on cancers, complications, therapies and insurance and payment issues.

CMP Heathcare Media
Oncology Publishing Group
600 Community Driv
Manhasset, NY 11050

516-734-2008
www.cancernetwork.com
info@cancernetwork.com

HEALTH FINDER

A service of the Department of Health and Human Services, Health Finder has many resources ranging from topics specifically related to cancer to broader health topics such as locating public clinics, nursing homes, health fraud advice, medical privacy and links to universities, medical dictionaries and journals. It also has a guide that presents information and resources to help patients and families get better quality healthcare.

P.O. Box 1133
Washington, DC 20013-1133

www.healthfinder.gov
healthfinder@nhic.org

NATIONAL CANCER INSTITUTE (NCI)

A branch of the US National Institutes of Health, NCI provides information about cancer, clinical trials, statistics, and research.

www.cancer.gov

The National Cancer Institute's (NCI's) Cancer Information Service (CIS) is a national information and education network. The CIS is a free public service of the NCI, the Nation's primary agency for cancer research. The CIS provides current cancer information to patients, their families, the public, and health professionals. The CIS provides personalized, confidential responses to specific questions about cancer.

NCI-Designated Cancer Centers
Cancer centers listed by state.

www.cancer.gov/cancercenters

NCI Dictionary of Cancer Terms
ww.cancer.gov/dictionary

NCI Public Inquiries Office
6116 Executive Blvd
Room 3056A
Bethesda, MD 20892-8322

1-800-4-CANCER (1-800-422-6237)
cis.nci.nih.gov

NATIONAL COMPREHENSIVE CANCER NETWORK (NCCN)

Outlines cancer treatment guidelines and offers cancer patients and their families information to help work with their physicians to make more informed decisions about care and treatments.

Treatment Guidelines for Patients

888.9009.NCCN

National Comprehensive Cancer Network
275 Commerce
Suite 300
Fort Washington, PA 19034

215-690-0300
www.nccn.org

ONCOLINK

Information on specific types of cancer, updates on cancer treatments and news about research advances

OncoLink
Abramson Cancer Center of the University of Pennsylvania
3400 Spruce Street - 2 Donner
Philadelphia, PA 19104

www.oncolink.com

215-349-8895

ONCOLOGY NURSING SOCIETY (ONS)

Resources on prevention, detection, diagnosis, treatment and survivorship.

Oncology Nursing Society
125 Enterprise Drive
Pittsburgh, PA 15275

866-257-4ONS
www.ons.org/patientEd
customer.service@ons.org

PEOPLE LIVING WITH CANCER

A website by the American Society of Clinical Oncology for patients that provides oncologist-approved information on more than 50 types of cancer and their treatments, side effects, coping, and clinical trials. It includes a "Find an Oncologist" database, live chats, message boards, a drug database and links to patient support organizations.

American Society of Clinical Oncology
2318 Mill Road
Suite 800
Alexandria, VA 22314

571-483-1780
www.cancer.net
contactus@cancer.net

YOUR DISEASE RISK

Provides education on cancers and focuses on prevention as the primary approach to controlling cancer and other chronic diseases.

Washington University in St. Louis
Siteman Cancer Center
660 S. Euclid Ave
Box 8100
St. Louis, MO 63110

314-747-7222
800-600-3606
www.yourdiseaserisk.wustl.edu

CHILDREN AND YOUNG ADULTS

BRAVE KIDS

Provides online resources for children with chronic, life-threatening illnesses and disabilities and their families. Local resources searchable by zip code.

800-568-1008
www.bravekids.org
info@bravekids.org

Brave Kids: East Coast
151 Sawgrass Corners Drive
Ste 204J
Ponte Verda Beach, FL 32082

904-827-9571
www.bravekids.org
info@bravekids.org

CANDLELIGHTERS CHILDHOOD CANCER FOUNDATION

Offers support, education and advocacy for families of children with cancer, survivors of childhood cancer and the professionals who care for them.

National Office
P.O. Box 498
Kensington, MD 20895-0498

800-366-CCCF or 301-962-3520
www.candlelighters.org
staff@candlelighters.org

CHILDREN'S ONCOLOGY GROUP

The Children's Oncology Group, in partnership with the National Childhood Cancer Foundation. Offers education and support resources.

Rush Operation Ctr
440 E. Hungton Dr., Ste 40
Arcadia, CA 91006

626-447-0064
www.childrensoncologygroup.org

CURESEARCH

Provides educational resources about cancer diagnoses, the different phases of treatment and support resources

CureSearch Headquarters
4600 East West Highway
Suite 600
Bethesda, MD

800-458-6223
www.curesearch.org

KIDSHEALTH.ORG

Site designed for parents, kids and teens that discusses many health topics including cancer.

www.kidshealth.org

LIVESTRONG™ YOUNG ADULT ALLIANCE (THE LANCE ARMSTRONG FOUNDATION).

The mission of the LIVESTRONG™ Young Adult Alliance is to improve survival rates and quality of life for young adults living with cancer by promoting relevant research and the delivery of patient care, generating awareness of the issue, being a voice for young adults with cancer and advancing helpful community-based programs and services.

Lanca Armstrong Foundation
PO Box 161150
Austin, TX 78716

512-238-8820
www.livestrong.org/yaa

NATIONAL CHILDHOOD CANCER FOUNDATION

National Childhood Cancer Foundation 800.458.NCCF

440 E Huntington Drive
Suite 300
Arcadia, CA 91066-0012

www.curesearch.org

PEDIATRIC ONCOLOGY RESOURCE CENTER

A site with resources, Internet links, and references for parents, friends and families of children who have or had childhood cancer.

www.acor.org/ped-onc

PLANET CANCER

A website for young adults with cancer that provides support and other resources, including an online forum.

www.planetcancer.org

TEENS LIVING WITH CANCER

A website for teenagers with cancer with information on treatments, combating fear, testimonials from other teens who have or had cancer and support chat rooms.

Melissa's Living Legacy Foundation
245 Citation Drive
Henrietta, NY 14467

585-334-0858
teenslivingwithcancer.org
info@teenslivingwithcancer.org

CLINICAL TRIALS

AMERICAN CANCER SOCIETY
Free clinical trial matching and referral service.

www.cancer.org

CENTERWATCH
Provides information and resources used by patients, pharmaceutical, biotechnology and medical device companies, CROs and research centers involved in clinical research around the world. The web site provides an extensive list of IRB approved clinical trials being conducted internationally and also lists promising therapies newly approved by the Food and Drug Administration. CenterWatch also offers reports on specific illnesses, clinical trial information and therapies that patients and advocates can buy.

100 N Washington Street
Ste 301
Boston, MA 02114

617-948-5100
www.centerwatch.com

COALITION OF NATIONAL CANCER COOPERATIVE GROUPS (CNCC)
A network of cancer clinical trials specialists including cooperative groups, cancer centers, academic medical centers, community hospitals, physician practices, and patient advocate groups, CNCC aims at improving the clinical trials experience for patients and physicians, and providing professional support services regulatory requirements, and providing professional support services. It offers a variety of programs and information for physicians, patient advocate groups, and patients designed to increase awareness of, and participation in cancer clinical trials.

1818 Market Street
#1100
Philadelphia, PA 19103

877-520-4457
www.cancertrialshelp.org

INTERNATIONAL FEDERATION OF PHARMACEUTICAL MANUFACTURERS & ASSOCIATIONS (IFPMA)
Provides a portal that allows one to search for comprehensive information on on-going clinical trials or results of completed trials conducted by the pharmaceutical industry.

www.ifpma.org/clinicaltrials

NATIONAL CANCER INSTITUTE (NCI)
A branch of the US National Institutes of Health, NCI provides information about cancer, clinical trials, statistics, and research.

www.cancer.gov/clinicaltrials

NATIONAL COMPREHENSIVE CANCER NETWORK (NCCN)
An alliance of 19 of the world's leading cancer centers, NCCN is a source of information to help patients and health professionals make informed decisions about cancer care. Through the collective expertise of its member institutions, the NCCN develops, updates, and disseminates a complete library of clinical practice guidelines.

275 Commerce Drive
Ste 200
Fort Washington PA,19034

Fax: 215-690-0280
888-909-NCCN
215.690.0300
www.nccn.org

SPECIFIC CANCERS

RARE CANCER ALLIANCE

Provides support and other resources for adults and children with rare cancers. Note: You are encouraged to explore the other websites listed in this appendix, as many also include information on rare cancers.

www.rare-cancer.org

SUPPORT

FERTILE HOPE

Provides reproductive information and support to cancer patients whose medical treatments present the risk of infertility.

Note: You are encouraged to explore the other websites listed in this appendix, as many also include resources for support including education materials, chat rooms, community groups and clinical advice.

www.fertilehope.org

SURVIVORS

CANCER SURVIVORS NETWORK

(American Cancer Society) Provides a forum for cancer survivors to share their stories, join chats, post messages on discussion boards and create their own webpage about their stories.

www.acscsn.org

CANCERVIVE

Provides support, public education and advocacy to those who have had cancer.

LANCE ARMSTRONG FOUNDATION (LAF)

LAF provides advocacy, education, support and research for both cancer survivors and people who currently have cancer.

PO Box 161150
Austin, TX 78716-1150

512-236-8820
www.livestrong.org

NATIONAL COALITION FOR CANCER SURVIVORSHIP (NCCS)

Provides education, advocacy and support to those affected by cancer and cancer survivors. Specifically addresses quality of care and minority issues.

1010 Wayne Avenue
Suite 770
Silver Spring, MD 20910

877.622.7937
www.canceradvocacy.org
info@canceradvocacy.org

Appendix C

TRAVEL ASSISTANCE

NATIONAL PATIENT AIR TRANSPORT HELPLINE (NPATH)
Provides information about and referrals to charitable medical air transportation programs that provide long-distance travel for medical, low income, and financially vulnerable patients. The information is provided at no cost and the HELPLINE is available 24 hours a day.

1-800-296-1217

TREATMENT

AMERICAN SOCIETY FOR THERAPEUTIC RADIOLOGY AND ONCOLOGY
Provides downloadable brochures and publications on treatment options for several specific cancers.

ASTRO Headquarters
8280 Willowoaks Corporate Drive
Suite 500
Fairfax, VA 22031

800-962-7876 703-502-1550
www.astro.org/patients

BLOOD AND MARROW TRANSPLANT INFORMATION NETWORK
Provides information about blood and marrow transplants, support groups, a list of transplant centers and testimonials from survivors.

BMI InfoNet
2310 Skokie Valley Road
Ste 104
Highland Park, IL 60035

1-847-433-3313
www.bmtinfonet.org

CANCERSYMPTOMS.ORG
(Oncology Nursing Society) Provides information and resources for learning about and managing symptoms often associated with cancer treatment.

www.cancersymptoms.org

WOMEN

BREASTCANCER.ORG
Offers information on breast cancer prevention, symptoms, treatment, research, recovery and support.

www.breastcancer.org

ENTRE MUJERES
Un guia sobre la recuperación física y emocional después de la mastectomía.

www.cancerlinks.com

LOOK GOOD. . . FEEL BETTER

Provides resources and links for women who are undergoing cancer treatment including cosmetic advice and support.

www.lookgoodfeelbetter.org

NATIONAL WOMEN'S HEALTH RESOURCE CENTER

Women's health site that includes information on various cancers.

NWHRC
157 Broad Street
Suite 106
Red Bank, NJ 07701

www.healthywomen.org (Note: Click on "Health Center" and select the appropriate topic.)
1-877-986-9472

NCI WOMEN OF COLOR

Provides basic data on how cancer affects women in minority populations.

WOMEN'S CANCER CENTER

Many resources for women with carious kinds of cancer.

www.womenscancercenter.com

YWCA

"ENCOREplus", a program available at some YWCA locations that focuses on cancer prevention, nutrition and rehabilitation.

YWCA USA
1015 18th Street, NW
Suite 1100
Washington, DC 20036

800-YWCA-US1 202-467-0801
www.ywca.org (Note: click on the "I need help" link.)

Appendix D:
NCI Designated Cancer Centers

National Cancer Institute (NCI) designated Cancer Centers are recognized for their scientific excellence and extensive resources focused on cancer and cancer-related problems.

The Cancer Centers are a major source of discovery of the nature of cancer and of the development of more effective approaches to cancer prevention, diagnosis, and therapy. They also deliver medical advances to patients and their families, educate health-care professionals and the public, and reach out to underserved populations. They may be freestanding organizations, a center within an academic institution, or part of a consortium of institutions.

NCI-designation is voluntary and is awarded via a grant using a peer-review process. All NCI-designated cancer centers receive substantial financial support from NCI grants and are reevaluated each time their cancer center support grant comes up for renewal (generally every 3 to 5 years). The NCI recognizes two types of centers: Cancer Centers and Comprehensive Cancer Centers, based on the type of grant received. In terms of patient care, there is no difference in the quality of care they each provide.

For more information on NCI-designated Cancer Centers, go to the Cancer Centers Program on the Internet at: http://cancercenters.cancer.gov.

Below is a list of states where a NCI-designated Cancer Center is located. There are two different types of cancer centers included in this appendix:

*Comprehensive Cancer Center:

Provides patient services; conducts basic, population sciences, and clinical research; and engages in outreach and education activities.

Cancer Center:

Provides patient services; and conducts basic, population sciences, and clinical research.

ALABAMA

*UNIVERSITY OF ALABAMA AT BIRMINGHAM COMPREHENSIVE CANCER CENTER (UAB)

Address:	North Pavilion 2500
	1802 Sixth Avenue South
	Birmingham, AL 35294
Telephone:	205-975-8222 (Cancer Answers) 205
	934-5077 (Administration)
	1-800-822-0933 (1-800-UAB-0933) (Cancer Answers)
	1-800-UAB-MIST (1-800-UAB-6478) (Referring Physicians)
Web site:	http://www3.ccc.uab.edu/

The University of Alabama at Birmingham Comprehensive Cancer Center is a National Cancer Institute (NCI)-designated Comprehensive Cancer Center that conducts research and provides services directly to cancer patients. Comprehensive Cancer Centers also conduct activities in outreach and education, and provide information on health care advances to both health care professionals and the public. An NCI-designated Cancer Center must meet a series of competitive requirements and demonstrate excellence in cancer research. For more general information about the Cancer Centers Program of NCI, please visit http://cancercenters.cancer.gov on the Internet

ARIZONA

*ARIZONA CANCER CENTER: UNIVERSITY OF ARIZONA

Address:	3838 North Campbell Avenue (clinic address)
	Tucson, AZ 85719
Telephone:	520-694-2873
	1-800-524-5928
Web site:	http://www.azcc.arizona.edu/

The Arizona Cancer Center is a National Cancer Institute (NCI)-designated Comprehensive Cancer Center that conducts research and provides services directly to cancer patients. Comprehensive Cancer Centers also conduct activities in outreach and education, and provide information on health care advances to both health care professionals and the public. An NCI-designated Cancer Center must meet a series of competitive requirements and demonstrate excellence in cancer research. For more general information about the Cancer Centers Program of NCI, please visit http://cancercenters.cancer.gov/ on the Internet.

---

*CHAO FAMILY COMPREHENSIVE CANCER CENTER: UNIVERSITY OF CALIFORNIA, IRVINE

Address:	101 The City Drive
	Building 23, Route 81
	Orange, CA 92868
Telephone:	714-456-8000 (Cancer Center)
	1-877-824-3627 (Physician Referral Service)
Web site:	http://www.ucihs.uci.edu/cancer/

The Chao Family Comprehensive Cancer Center is a National Cancer Institute (NCI)-designated Comprehensive Cancer Center that conducts research and provides services directly to cancer patients. Comprehensive Cancer Centers also conduct activities in outreach and education, and provide information on health care advances to both health care professionals and the public. An NCI-designated Cancer Center must meet a series of competitive requirements and demonstrate excellence in cancer research. For more general information about the Cancer Centers Program of NCI, please visit http://cancercenters.cancer.gov/ on the Internet.

*CITY OF HOPE
CITY OF HOPE NATIONAL MEDICAL CENTER AND BECKMAN RESEARCH INSTITUTE

Address:	1500 East Duarte Road
	Duarte, CA 91010
Telephone:	626-256-4673 (626-256-HOPE)
	1-800-826-4673 (New Patient Services)
	1-866-434-4673 (General Information)
E-mail:	becomingapatient@coh.org
Web site:	http://www.cityofhope.org

The City of Hope is a National Cancer Institute (NCI)-designated Comprehensive Cancer Center that conducts research and provides services directly to cancer patients. Comprehensive Cancer Centers also conduct activities in outreach and education, and provide information on health care advances to both health care professionals and the public. An NCI-designated Cancer Center must meet a series of competitive requirements and demonstrate excellence in cancer research. For more general information about the Cancer Centers Program of NCI, please visit http://cancercenters.cancer.gov/ on the Internet.

*MOORES UCSD CANCER CENTER
UNIVERSITY OF CALIFORNIA, SAN DIEGO

Address:	3855 Health Sciences Drive
	La Jolla, CA 92093
Telephone:	858-822-6100
	1-866-773-2703
Web site:	http://cancer.ucsd.edu/

The Rebecca and John Moores University of California, San Diego Comprehensive Cancer Center is a National Cancer Institute (NCI)-designated Comprehensive Cancer Center that conducts research and provides services directly to cancer patients. Comprehensive Cancer Centers also conduct activities in outreach and education, and provide information on health care advances to both health care professionals and the public. An NCI-designated Cancer Center must meet a series of competitive requirements and demonstrate excellence in cancer research. For more general information about the Cancer Centers Program of NCI, please visit http://cancercenters.cancer.gov/ on the Internet.

STANFORD CANCER CENTER (SCC)

Address: 875 Blake Wilbur Drive
             Stanford, CA 94305
Telephone: 650-498-6000 (Referral Center)
             1-877-668-7535 (Referral Center)
             1-877-487-0237 (International Medical Services)
E-mail: referral@stanfordmed.org
Web site: http://cancer.stanford.edu/

The Stanford Cancer Center is a National Cancer Institute (NCI)-designated Cancer Center that conducts research and provides services directly to cancer patients. An NCI-designated Cancer Center must meet a series of competitive requirements and demonstrate excellence in cancer research. For more general information about the Cancer Centers Program of NCI, please visit http://cancercenters.cancer.gov/ on the Internet.

UC DAVIS CANCER CENTER
UNIVERSITY OF CALIFORNIA, DAVIS

Address: Room 3003
             4501 X Street
             Sacramento, CA 95817
Telephone: 916-703-5210 (New Patient Referral Office)
             916-734-5959 (General Information)
             1-800-362-5566 (New Patient Referrals)
             1-800-282-3284 (General Information)
E-mail: cancer.center@ucdmc.ucdavis.edu
Web site: http://cancer.ucdmc.ucdavis.edu/

The UC Davis Cancer Center is a National Cancer Institute (NCI)-designated Cancer Center that conducts research and provides services directly to cancer patients. An NCI-designated Cancer Center must meet a series of competitive requirements and demonstrate excellence in cancer research. For more general information about the Cancer Centers Program of NCI, please visit http://cancercenters.cancer.gov/ on the Internet.

*UCLA'S JONSSON COMPREHENSIVE CANCER CENTER
UNIVERSITY OF CALIFORNIA, LOS ANGELES

Address: 8-684 Factor Building
             UCLA Box 951781
             Los Angeles, CA 90095
Telephone: 310-825-5268 (administrative office)
             1-888-662-8252 (UCLA Cancer Hotline)
             1-800-825-2631 (Cancer Screening or General Health Care)
E-mail: jcccinfo@mednet.ucla.edu
Web site: http://www.cancer.ucla.edu

UCLA's Jonsson Comprehensive Cancer Center is a National Cancer Institute (NCI)-designated Comprehensive Cancer Center that conducts research and provides services directly to cancer patients. Comprehensive Cancer Centers also conduct activities in outreach and education, and provide information on health care advances to both health care professionals and the public. An NCI-designated Cancer Center must meet a series of competitive requirements and demonstrate excellence in cancer research. For more general information about the Cancer Centers Program of NCI, please visit http://cancercenters.cancer.gov/ on the Internet.

*UCSF HELEN DILLER FAMILY COMPREHENSIVE CANCER CENTER
UNIVERSITY OF CALIFORNIA,
SAN FRANCISCO COMPREHENSIVE CANCER CENTER

Address:	Box 1297, UCSF
	1600 Divisadero Street
	San Francisco, CA 94143
Telephone:	415-353-8489 (International Inquiries)
	1-800-888-8664 (Cancer Referral Line)
	1-800-444-2559 (Physician Referral Service)
E-mail:	referral.center@ucsfmedctr.org
Web site:	http://cancer.ucsf.edu

The UCSF Helen Diller Family Comprehensive Cancer Center is a National Cancer Institute (NCI)-designated Comprehensive Cancer Center that conducts research and provides services directly to cancer patients. Comprehensive Cancer Centers also conduct activities in outreach and education, and provide information on health care advances to both health care professionals and the public. An NCI-designated Cancer Center must meet a series of competitive requirements and demonstrate excellence in cancer research. For more general information about the Cancer Centers Program of NCI, please visit http://cancercenters.cancer.gov/ on the Internet.

*USC/NORRIS COMPREHENSIVE CANCER CENTER

Address:	1441 Eastlake Avenue
	Los Angeles, CA 90033
Telephone:	323-865-3000 (general information)
	1-800-872-2273 (1-800-USC-CARE)
Web site:	http://ccnt.hsc.usc.edu/

The USC/Norris Comprehensive Cancer Center is a National Cancer Institute (NCI)-designated Comprehensive Cancer Center that conducts research and provides services directly to cancer patients. Comprehensive Cancer Centers also conduct activities in outreach and education, and provide information on health care advances to both health care professionals and the public. An NCI-designated Cancer Center must meet a series of competitive requirements and demonstrate excellence in cancer research. For more general information about the Cancer Centers Program of NCI, please visit http://cancercenters.cancer.gov/ on the Internet.

COLORADO

*UNIVERSITY OF COLORADO CANCER CENTER

Address: Box F-704
             1665 North Ursula Street
             Aurora, CO 80045
Telephone: 720-848-0300
             1-800-473-2288 (cancer referral line)
Web site: http://www.uccc.info

The University of Colorado Cancer Center is a National Cancer Institute (NCI)-designated Comprehensive Cancer Center that conducts research and provides services directly to cancer patients. Comprehensive Cancer Centers also conduct activities in outreach and education, and provide information on health care advances to both health care professionals and the public. An NCI-designated Cancer Center must meet a series of competitive requirements and demonstrate excellence in cancer research. For more general information about the Cancer Centers Program of NCI, please visit http://cancercenters.cancer.gov/ on the Internet.

CONNECTICUT

*YALE CANCER CENTER
YALE UNIVERSITY SCHOOL OF MEDICINE

Address: Post Office Box 208028 (mailing address)
             333 Cedar Street, WWW 205 (physical address)
             New Haven, CT 06520
Telephone: 203-785-4191
             1-866-925-3226 (1-866-YALECANCER)
Web site: http://yalecancercenter.org

The Yale Cancer Center is a National Cancer Institute (NCI)-designated Comprehensive Cancer Center that conducts research and provides services directly to cancer patients. Comprehensive Cancer Centers also conduct activities in outreach and education, and provide information on health care advances to both health care professionals and the public. An NCI-designated Cancer Center must meet a series of competitive requirements and demonstrate excellence in cancer research. For more general information about the Cancer Centers Program of NCI, please visit http://cancercenters.cancer.gov/ on the Internet.

DISTRICT OF COLUMBIA

*LOMBARDI COMPREHENSIVE CANCER CENTER
GEORGETOWN UNIVERSITY MEDICAL CENTER

Address: 3800 Reservoir Road, NW.
             Washington, DC 20007
Telephone: 202-444-2223 (Appointments)
             202-444-4000 (CancerLine)
Web site: http://lombardi.georgetown.edu/

The Lombardi Comprehensive Cancer Center, Georgetown University Medical Center is a National Cancer Institute (NCI)-designated Comprehensive Cancer Center that conducts research and provides services directly to cancer patients. Comprehensive Cancer Centers also conduct activities in outreach and education, and provide information on health care advances to both health care professionals and the public. An NCI-designated Cancer Center must meet a series of competitive requirements and demonstrate excellence in cancer research. For more general information about the Cancer Centers Program of NCI, please visit http://cancercenters.cancer.gov on the Internet.

FLORIDA

*H. LEE MOFFITT CANCER CENTER AND RESEARCH INSTITUTE AT THE
UNIVERSITY OF SOUTH FLORIDA

Address: 12902 Magnolia Drive
             Tampa, FL 33612
Telephone: 813-745-3980 (New Patient/Physician Referral)
             813-745-4673 (813-745-HOPE) (Main)
             1-888-860-2778 (New Patient/Physician Referral)
             1-800-456-7121 (Cancer Answers Line)
             1-888-663-3488 (1-888-MOFFITT) (Main)
Web site: http://www.moffitt.usf.edu/

The H. Lee Moffitt Cancer Center and Research Institute at the University of South Florida is a National Cancer Institute (NCI)-designated Comprehensive Cancer Center that conducts research and provides services directly to cancer patients. Comprehensive Cancer Centers also conduct activities in outreach and education, and provide information on healthcare advances to both healthcare professionals and the public. An NCI-designated Cancer Center must meet a series of competitive requirements and demonstrate excellence in cancer research. For more general information about the Cancer Centers Program of NCI please visit http://cancercenters.cancer.gov on the Internet.

Appendix D

WINSHIP CANCER INSTITUTE
EMORY UNIVERSITY

Address: 1365C Clifton Road
    Atlanta, GA 30322
Telephone: 404-778-5669 (Directors Office)
    404-778-1900 (Main)
    1-888-946-7447 (1-888-WINSHIP)
Web site: http://cancer.emory.edu/

The Winship Cancer Institute, Emory University, is a National Cancer Institute (NCI)-designated Cancer Center that conducts research and provides services directly to cancer patients. An NCI-designated Cancer Center must meet a series of competitive requirements and demonstrate excellence in cancer research. For more general information about the Cancer Centers Program of NCI, please visit http://cancercenters.cancer.gov/ on the Internet.

CANCER RESEARCH CENTER OF HAWAII (CRCH)
UNIVERSITY OF HAWAII

Address: Suite 510
    1236 Lauhala Street
    Honolulu, HI 96813
Telephone: 808-586-3010
Web site: http://www.crch.org

The Cancer Research Center of Hawaii (CRCH) is a National Cancer Institute (NCI)-designated Cancer Center that conducts research on the causes, prevention and treatment of cancer. Although CRCH does not treat patients at the facility, it can provide referrals to other facilities for medical care and second opinions and can refer patients to providers and institutions participating in clinical trials. An NCI-designated Cancer Center must meet a series of competitive requirements and demonstrate excellence in cancer research. For more general information about the Cancer Centers Program of NCI, please visit http://cancercenters.cancer.gov/ on the Internet.

ILLINOIS

*ROBERT H. LURIE COMPREHENSIVE CANCER CENTER
NORTHWESTERN UNIVERSITY

Address:	Galter Pavilion
	675 N. St. Clair, 21st Floor, Suite 100
	Chicago, IL 60611
Telephone:	312-908-5250
	1-866-587-4322 (1-866-LURIE-CC) appointment line
	1-800-543-7362 (1-800-KIDS-DOC) pediatric patients
E-mail:	cancer@northwestern.edu
Web site:	http://cancer.northwestern.edu/home/index.cfm

The Robert H. Lurie Comprehensive Cancer Center is a National Cancer Institute (NCI)-designated Comprehensive Cancer Center that conducts research and provides services directly to cancer patients. Comprehensive Cancer Centers also conduct activities in outreach and education, and provide information on health care advances to both health care professionals and the public. An NCI-designated Cancer Center must meet a series of competitive requirements and demonstrate excellence in cancer research. For more general information about the Cancer Centers Program of NCI, please visit http://cancercenters.cancer.gov/ on the Internet.

*UNIVERSITY OF CHICAGO CANCER RESEARCH CENTER

Address:	Mail Code 2115
	5841 South Maryland Avenue
	Chicago, IL 60637
Telephone:	773-702-6180
	1-888-824-0200 (new patients)
Web site:	http://www-uccrc.uchicago.edu/

The University of Chicago Cancer Research Center is a National Cancer Institute (NCI)-designated Comprehensive Cancer Center that conducts research and provides services directly to cancer patients. Comprehensive Cancer Centers also conduct activities in outreach and education, and provide information on health care advances to both health care professionals and the public. An NCI-designated Cancer Center must meet a series of competitive requirements and demonstrate excellence in cancer research. For more general information about the Cancer Centers Program of NCI, please visit http://cancercenters.cancer.gov/ on the Internet.

INDIANA

INDIANA UNIVERSITY MELVIN AND BREN SIMON CANCER CENTER
IU SIMON CANCER CENTER

Address:	535 Barnhill Drive
	Indianapolis, IN 46202
Telephone:	317-278-4822
	1-888-600-4822
Web site:	http://iucc.iu.edu

The Indiana University Melvin and Bren Simon Cancer Center is a National Cancer Institute (NCI)-designated Cancer Center that conducts research and provides services directly to cancer patients. An NCI-designated Cancer Center must meet a series of competitive requirements and demonstrate excellence in cancer research. For more general information about the Cancer Centers Program of NCI, please visit http://cancercenters.cancer.gov/ on the Internet.

IOWA

---

*HOLDEN COMPREHENSIVE CANCER CENTER
UNIVERSITY OF IOWA

Address:	4802 JPP
	200 Hawkins Drive
	Iowa City, IA 52242
Telephone:	319-356-4200 (Referrals & Appointments)
	319-356-3000 (General Information)
	1-800-777-8442 (Referrals & Appointments)
	1-800-237-1225 (General Information)
E-mail:	cancer-center@uiowa.edu
Web site:	http://www.uihealthcare.com/depts/cancercenter/

The Holden Comprehensive Cancer Center at the University of Iowa is a National Cancer Institute (NCI)-designated Comprehensive Cancer Center that conducts research and provides services directly to cancer patients. Comprehensive Cancer Centers also conduct activities in outreach and education, and provide information on health care advances to both health care professionals and the public. An NCI-designated Cancer Center must meet a series of competitive requirements and demonstrate excellence in cancer research. For more general information about the Cancer Centers Program of NCI, please visit http://cancercenters.cancer.gov/ on the Internet.

MARYLAND

GREENEBAUM CANCER CENTER (MARLENE AND STEWART) (UMGCC)
UNIVERSITY OF MARYLAND

Address:	22 South Greene Street
	Baltimore, MD 21201
Telephone:	410-328-7904 (Main and New Appointments)
	1-800-888-8823 (Main and New Appointments)
	1-800-373-4111 (Physician Referrals)
Web site:	http://www.umgcc.org/

The Greenebaum Cancer Center, University of Maryland, is a National Cancer Institute (NCI)-designated Cancer Center that conducts research and provides services directly to cancer patients. An NCI-designated Cancer Center must meet a series of competitive requirements and demonstrate excellence in cancer research. For more general information about the Cancer Centers Program of NCI please visit http://cancercenters.cancer.gov/ on the Internet.

*SIDNEY KIMMEL COMPREHENSIVE CANCER CENTER AT JOHNS HOPKINS UNIVERSITY

Address: The Harry and Jeanette Weinberg Building
Suite 1100, 401 North Broadway
Baltimore, MD 21231
Telephone: 410-955-8964 (Patient Referrals)
410-955-8804 (Clinical Trials)
410-955-5222 (Main# to SKCCC)
Web site: http://www.hopkinskimmelcancercenter.org/

The Sidney Kimmel Comprehensive Cancer Center at Johns Hopkins is a National Cancer Institute (NCI)-designated Comprehensive Cancer Center that conducts research and provides services directly to cancer patients. Comprehensive Cancer Centers also conduct activities in outreach and education, and provide information on health care advances to both health care professionals and the public. An NCI-designated Cancer Center must meet a series of competitive requirements and demonstrate excellence in cancer research. For more general information about the Cancer Centers Program of NCI, please visit http://cancercenters.cancer.gov/ on the Internet.

MASSACHUSETTS

*DANA FARBER/HARVARD CANCER CENTER

Address: 44 Binney Street
Boston, MA 02115
Telephone: 617-632-3673 (Spanish)
1-866-408-3324 (1-866-408-DFCI) (Adult/General)
Web site: http://www.dana-farber.org

The Dana Farber/Harvard Cancer Center is a National Cancer Institute (NCI)-designated Comprehensive Cancer Center that conducts research and provides services directly to cancer patients. Comprehensive Cancer Centers also conduct activities in outreach and education, and provide information on health care advances to both health care professionals and the public. An NCI-designated Cancer Center must meet a series of competitive requirements and demonstrate excellence in cancer research. For more general information about the Cancer Centers Program of NCI, please visit http://cancercenters.cancer.gov/ on the Internet.

Appendix D

*BARBARA ANN KARMANOS CANCER INSTITUTE
MEYER L. PRENTIS COMPREHENSIVE CANCER CENTER
OF METROPOLITAN DETROIT

Address: Wertz Clinical Cancer Center
              4100 John R Street
              Detroit, MI 48201
Telephone: 1-800-527-6266 (1-800-KARMANOS)
E-mail: info@karmanos.org
Web site: http://www.karmanos.org

The Barbara Ann Karmanos Cancer Institute is a National Cancer Institute (NCI)-designated Comprehensive Cancer Center that conducts research and provides services directly to cancer patients. Comprehensive Cancer Centers also conduct activities in outreach and education, and provide information on health care advances to both health care professionals and the public. An NCI-designated Cancer Center must meet a series of competitive requirements and demonstrate excellence in cancer research. For more general information about the Cancer Centers Program of NCI, please visit http://cancercenters.cancer.gov/ on the Internet.

*UNIVERSITY OF MICHIGAN COMPREHENSIVE CANCER CENTER
UNIVERSITY OF MICHIGAN HEALTH SYSTEM

Address: 1500 East Medical Center Drive
              Ann Arbor, MI 48109
Telephone: 734-763-5005
              1-800-865-1125 (Cancer Answer Line)
Web site: http://www.cancer.med.umich.edu/

The University of Michigan Comprehensive Cancer Center is a National Cancer Institute (NCI)-designated Comprehensive Cancer Center that conducts research and provides services directly to cancer patients. Comprehensive Cancer Centers also conduct activities in outreach and education, and provide information on health care advances to both health care professionals and the public. An NCI-designated Cancer Center must meet a series of competitive requirements and demonstrate excellence in cancer research. For more general information about the Cancer Centers Program of NCI, please visit http://cancercenters.cancer.gov/ on the Internet.

MINNESOTA

*MASONIC CANCER CENTER
UNIVERSITY OF MINNESOTA

Address:	Mayo Mail Code 806
	420 Delaware Street, SE.
	Minneapolis, MN 55455
Telephone:	612-624-8484 (administrative office)
	612-624-2620 (cancer information line)
	1-888-226-2376 (in IA, MN, ND, SD, WI)
E-mail:	ccinfo@cancer.umn.edu
Web site:	http://www.cancer.umn.edu

The Masonic Cancer Center is a National Cancer Institute (NCI)-designated Comprehensive Cancer Center that conducts research and provides services directly to cancer patients. Comprehensive Cancer Centers also conduct activities in outreach and education, and provide information on health care advances to both health care professionals and the public. An NCI-designated Cancer Center must meet a series of competitive requirements and demonstrate excellence in cancer research. For more general information about the Cancer Centers Program of NCI, please visit http://cancercenters.cancer.gov/ on the Internet.

*MAYO CLINIC CANCER CENTER

Address:	200 First Street SW.
	Rochester, MN 55905
Telephone:	507-284-4137 (Medical Oncology appt. office)
	507-284-8884 (international appointment services)
Web site:	http://cancercenter.mayo.edu/

The Mayo Clinic Cancer Center is a National Cancer Institute (NCI)-designated Comprehensive Cancer Center that conducts research and provides services directly to cancer patients. Comprehensive Cancer Centers also conduct activities in outreach and education, and provide information on health care advances to both health care professionals and the public. An NCI-designated Cancer Center must meet a series of competitive requirements and demonstrate excellence in cancer research. For more general information about the Cancer Centers Program of NCI, please visit http://cancercenters.cancer.gov/ on the Internet.

MISSOURI

*SITEMAN CANCER CENTER
BARNES-JEWISH HOSPITAL AND
WASHINGTON UNIVERSITY SCHOOL OF MEDICINE

Address:	Box 8100
	660 South Euclid Avenue
	Saint Louis, MO 63110
Telephone:	314-747-7222
	1-800-600-3606
E-mail:	info@ccadmin.wustl.edu
Web site:	http://www.siteman.wustl.edu/

The Siteman Cancer Center is a National Cancer Institute (NCI)-designated Comprehensive Cancer Center that conducts research and provides services directly to cancer patients. Comprehensive Cancer Centers also conduct activities in outreach and education, and provide information on health care advances to both health care professionals and the public. An NCI-designated Cancer Center must meet a series of competitive requirements and demonstrate excellence in cancer research. For more general information about the Cancer Centers Program of NCI, please visit http://cancercenters.cancer.gov/ on the Internet.

NEBRASKA

UNMC EPPLEY CANCER CENTER
UNIVERSITY OF NEBRASKA MEDICAL CENTER

Address:	The Peggy D. Cowdery Patient Care Center at UNMC
	43rd and Emilie Street
	Omaha, NE 68198
Telephone:	402-559-6500 (Peggy D. Cowdery Patient Care Center)
	1-800-922-0000 (Physician Referrals)
Web site:	http://www.unmc.edu/cancercenter/

The UNMC Eppley Cancer Center is a National Cancer Institute (NCI)-designated Cancer Center that conducts research and provides services directly to cancer patients. An NCI-designated Cancer Center must meet a series of competitive requirements and demonstrate excellence in cancer research. For more general information about the Cancer Centers Program of NCI, please visit http://cancercenters.cancer.gov/ on the Internet.

*NORRIS COTTON CANCER CENTER
DARTMOUTH-HITCHCOCK MEDICAL CENTER

Address:	One Medical Center Drive
	Lebanon, NH 03756
Telephone:	603-653-9000 (Administration)
	1-800-639-6918 (Cancer Help Line)
E-mail:	cancerhelp@dartmouth.edu
Web site:	http://www.cancer.dartmouth.edu/index.shtml

The Norris Cotton Cancer Center is a National Cancer Institute (NCI)-designated Comprehensive Cancer Center that conducts research and provides services directly to cancer patients. Comprehensive Cancer Centers also conduct activities in outreach and education, and provide information on health care advances to both health care professionals and the public. An NCI-designated Cancer Center must meet a series of competitive requirements and demonstrate excellence in cancer research. For more general information about the Cancer Centers Program of NCI, please visit http://cancercenters.cancer.gov/ on the Internet.

*CANCER INSTITUTE OF NEW JERSEY (CINJ)
ROBERT WOOD JOHNSON UNIVERSITY HOSPITAL

Address:	195 Little Albany Street
	New Brunswick, NJ 08903
Telephone:	732-235-2465 (CINJ)
	732-828-3000 (main RWJ number)
Web site:	http://www.cinj.org

The Cancer Institute of New Jersey, based at Robert Wood Johnson Medical School, is a National Cancer Institute (NCI)-designated Comprehensive Cancer Center that conducts research and provides services directly to cancer patients. Comprehensive Cancer Centers also conduct activities in outreach and education, and provide information on health care advances to both health care professionals and the public. An NCI-designated Cancer Center must meet a series of competitive requirements and demonstrate excellence in cancer research. For more general information about the Cancer Centers Program of NCI, please visit http://cancercenters.cancer.gov/ on the Internet.

NEW MEXICO

UNIVERSITY OF NEW MEXICO CANCER CENTER
UNM CANCER RESEARCH AND TREATMENT CENTER

Address: 900 Camino de Salud NE
1 University of New Mexico
Albuquerque, NM 87131
Telephone: 505-272-4946
1-800-432-6806 (in New Mexico)
Web site: http://cancer.unm.edu/

The UNM Cancer Center is a National Cancer Institute (NCI)-designated Cancer Center that conducts research and provides services directly to cancer patients. An NCI-designated Cancer Center must meet a series of competitive requirements and demonstrate excellence in cancer research. For more general information about the Cancer Centers Program of NCI, please visit http://cancercenters.cancer.gov/ on the Internet.

NEW YORK

ALBERT EINSTEIN CANCER CENTER (AECC)
ALBERT EINSTEIN COLLEGE OF MEDICINE OF YESHIVA UNIVERSITY

Address: 1300 Morris Park Avenue
Bronx, NY 10461
Telephone: 718-430-2302
E-mail: aecc@aecom.yu.edu
Web site: http://www.aecom.yu.edu/cancer/new/default.htm

The Albert Einstein Cancer Center is a National Cancer Institute (NCI)-designated Cancer Center that conducts research and provides services directly to cancer patients. An NCI-designated Cancer Center must meet a series of competitive requirements and demonstrate excellence in cancer research. For more general information about the Cancer Centers Program of NCI, please visit http://cancercenters.cancer.gov/ on the Internet.

*HERBERT IRVING COMPREHENSIVE CANCER CENTER
NEW YORK PRESBYTERIAN HOSPITAL,
COLUMBIA UNIVERSITY MEDICAL CENTER

Address: PH 18, Room 200
622 West 168th Street
New York, NY 10032
Telephone: 212-305-2500 (Main number for Columbia University Medical Center)
1-800-943-2782 (9 - 5) or 1-877-697-9355 (24 hours) (Physician Referrals)
Web site: http://hiccc.columbia.edu/

The Herbert Irving Comprehensive Cancer Center is a National Cancer Institute (NCI)-designated Comprehensive Cancer Center that conducts research and provides services directly to cancer patients. Comprehensive Cancer Centers also conduct activities in outreach and education, and provide information on health care advances to both health care professionals and the public. An NCI-designated Cancer Center must meet a series of competitive requirements and demonstrate excellence in cancer research. For more general information about the Cancer Centers Program of NCI, please visit http://cancercenters.cancer.gov/ on the Internet.

*MEMORIAL SLOAN-KETTERING CANCER CENTER

Address:	1275 York Avenue
	New York, NY 10065
Telephone:	212-639-2000 (General)
	1-800-525-2225 (Physician Referral)
Web site:	http://www.mskcc.org

The Memorial Sloan-Kettering Cancer Center is a National Cancer Institute (NCI)-designated Comprehensive Cancer Center that conducts research and provides services directly to cancer patients. Comprehensive Cancer Centers also conduct activities in outreach and education, and provide information on health care advances to both health care professionals and the public. An NCI-designated Cancer Center must meet a series of competitive requirements and demonstrate excellence in cancer research. For more general information about the Cancer Centers Program of NCI, please visit http://cancercenters.cancer.gov/ on the Internet.

NEW YORK UNIVERSITY CANCER INSTITUTE

Address:	550 First Avenue
	New York, NY 10016
Telephone:	212-731-5000 (Main)
	1-888-769-8633 (Physician Referral)
Web site:	http://ci.med.nyu.edu/

The New York University Cancer Institute is a National Cancer Institute (NCI)-designated Cancer Center that conducts research and provides services directly to cancer patients. An NCI-designated Cancer Center must meet a series of competitive requirements and demonstrate excellence in cancer research. For more general information about the Cancer Centers Program of NCI, please visit http://cancercenters.cancer.gov/ on the Internet.

*ROSWELL PARK CANCER INSTITUTE

Address:	Elm and Carlton Streets
	Buffalo, NY 14263
Telephone:	716-845-3516 (Physician Referral) or 716-845-2300 (Main)
	1-800-767-9355 (1-800-ROSWELL)
E-mail:	askrpci@roswellpark.org
Web site:	http://www.roswellpark.org/Home

The Roswell Park Cancer Institute is a National Cancer Institute (NCI)-designated Comprehensive Cancer Center that conducts research and provides services directly to cancer patients. Comprehensive Cancer Centers also conduct activities in outreach and education, and provide information on health care advances to both health care professionals and the public. An NCI-designated Cancer Center must meet a series of competitive requirements and demonstrate excellence in cancer research. For more general information about the Cancer Centers Program of NCI, please visit http://cancercenters.cancer.gov/ on the Internet.

NORTH CAROLINA

*DUKE COMPREHENSIVE CANCER CENTER
DUKE UNIVERSITY MEDICAL CENTER

Address:	Hock Plaza Suite 601
	2424 Erwin Road
	Durham, NC 27705
Telephone:	919-684-3377 (administrative offices)
	1-888-275-3853 (1-888-ASK-DUKE) (Consultation and Referral Service)
Web site:	http://www.cancer.duke.edu/

The Duke Comprehensive Cancer Center is a National Cancer Institute (NCI)-designated Comprehensive Cancer Center that conducts research and provides services directly to cancer patients. Comprehensive Cancer Centers also conduct activities in outreach and education, and provide information on health care advances to both health care professionals and the public. An NCI-designated Cancer Center must meet a series of competitive requirements and demonstrate excellence in cancer research. For more general information about the Cancer Centers Program of NCI, please visit http://cancercenters.cancer.gov/ on the Internet.

*UNC LINEBERGER COMPREHENSIVE CANCER CENTER
UNIVERSITY OF NORTH CAROLINA AT CHAPEL HILL

Address:	School of Medicine Campus Box #7295
	450 West Drive
	Chapel Hill, NC 27599
Telephone:	919-966-3036 (Main)
	1-866-828-0270 (Information or Appointments)
	1-877-668-0683 (Clinical Trials Information)
E-mail:	lccc@med.un.edu
Web site:	http://cancer.med.unc.edu/

The UNC Lineberger Comprehensive Cancer Center is a National Cancer Institute (NCI)-designated Comprehensive Cancer Center that conducts research and provides services directly to cancer patients. Comprehensive Cancer Centers also conduct activities in outreach and education, and provide information on health care advances to both health care professionals and the public. An NCI-designated Cancer Center must meet a series of competitive requirements and demonstrate excellence in cancer research. For more general information about the Cancer Centers Program of NCI, please visit http://cancercenters.cancer.gov/ on the Internet.

*WAKE FOREST UNIVERSITY COMPREHENSIVE CANCER CENTER
WAKE FOREST UNIVERSITY

Address:	Medical Center Boulevard
	Winston-Salem, NC 27157
Telephone:	336-716-4464
Web site:	http://www1.wfubmc.edu/cancer

The Wake Forest University Comprehensive Cancer Center is a National Cancer Institute (NCI)-designated Comprehensive Cancer Center that conducts research and provides services directly to cancer patients. Comprehensive Cancer Centers also conduct activities in outreach and education, and provide information on health care advances to both health care professionals and the public. An NCI-designated Cancer Center must meet a series of competitive requirements and demonstrate excellence in cancer research. For more general information about the Cancer Centers Program of NCI, please visit http://cancercenters.cancer.gov/ on the Internet.

OHIO

---

*CASE COMPREHENSIVE CANCER CENTER
CASE WESTERN RESERVE UNIVERSITY

Address:	11100 Euclid Avenue
	Cleveland, OH 44106
Telephone:	216-844-5432 (Phone greeting may say Ireland Cancer Center)
	1-800-641-2422 (Phone greeting may say Ireland Cancer Center)
E-mail:	cancer@case.edu
Web site:	http://cancer.case.edu/

Case Comprehensive Cancer Center of the Case Western Reserve University is a National Cancer Institute (NCI)-designated Comprehensive Cancer Center that conducts research and provides services directly to cancer patients. Comprehensive Cancer Centers also conduct activities in outreach and education, and provide information on health care advances to both health care professionals and the public. An NCI-designated Cancer Center must meet a series of competitive requirements and demonstrate excellence in cancer research. For more general information about the Cancer Centers Program of NCI, please visit http://cancercenters.cancer.gov/ on the Internet.

*THE OHIO STATE UNIVERSITY COMPREHENSIVE CANCER CENTER (OSUCCC - JAMES)
JAMES CANCER HOSPITAL AND SOLOVE RESEARCH INSTITUTE

Address:	Suite 519
	300 West 10th Avenue
	Columbus, OH 43210
Telephone:	614-293-5066
	1-800-293-5066
E-mail:	cancerinfo@jamesline.com
Web site:	http://www.jamesline.com/

The Ohio State University Comprehensive Cancer Center at the James Cancer Hospital and Solove Research Institute is a National Cancer Institute (NCI)-designated Comprehensive Cancer Center that conducts research and provides services directly to cancer patients. Comprehensive Cancer Centers also conduct activities in outreach and education, and provide information on health care advances to both health care professionals and the public. An NCI-designated Cancer Center must meet a series of competitive requirements and demonstrate excellence in cancer research. For more general information about the Cancer Centers Program of NCI, please visit http://cancercenters.cancer.gov/ on the Internet.

OREGON

OHSU KNIGHT CANCER INSTITUTE
OREGON HEALTH AND SCIENCE UNIVERSITY

Address:	Oregon Health and Science University
	3181 SW Sam Jackson Park Road, CR145
	Portland, OR 97239
Telephone:	503-494-1617 (Cancer Institute)
	503-494-8311 (Health Care Services and OHSU switchboard)
	1-888-222-6478 (Main operator at OHSU)
E-mail:	cancer@ohsu.edu
Web site:	http://ohsucancer.com

The OHSU Knight Cancer Institute is a National Cancer Institute (NCI)-designated Cancer Center that conducts research and provides services directly to cancer patients. An NCI-designated Cancer Center must meet a series of competitive requirements and demonstrate excellence in cancer research. For more general information about the Cancer Centers Program of NCI, please visit http://cancercenters.cancer.gov/ on the Internet. The OHSU Cancer Institute Web site offers a listing of staff doctors by cancer specialty.

PENNSYLVANIA

*ABRAMSON CANCER CENTER OF THE UNIVERSITY OF PENNSYLVANIA

Address:	Penn Tower, 15th Floor
	3400 Spruce Street
	Philadelphia, PA
Telephone:	215-662-4000 (main number)
	1-800-789-7366 (medical referrals)
Web site:	http://www.penncancer.org

The Abramson Cancer Center of the University of Pennsylvania is a National Cancer Institute (NCI)-designated Comprehensive Cancer Center that conducts research and provides services directly to cancer patients. Comprehensive Cancer Centers also conduct activities in outreach and education, and provide information on health care advances to both health care professionals and the public. An NCI-designated Cancer Center must meet a series of competitive requirements and demonstrate excellence in cancer research. For more general information about the Cancer Centers Program of NCI, please visit http://cancercenters.cancer.gov/ on the Internet.

*FOX CHASE CANCER CENTER

Address:	333 Cottman Avenue
	Philadelphia, PA 19111
Telephone:	215-728-2570 (Appointment scheduling)
	1-888-369-2427 (1-888-FOX-CHASE) (Cancer information)
Web site:	http://www.fccc.edu/

The Fox Chase Cancer Center is a National Cancer Institute (NCI)-designated Comprehensive Cancer Center that conducts research and provides services directly to cancer patients. Comprehensive Cancer Centers also conduct activities in outreach and education, and provide information on health care advances to both health care professionals and the public. An NCI-designated Cancer Center must meet a series of competitive requirements and demonstrate excellence in cancer research. For more general information about the Cancer Centers Program of NCI, please visit http://cancercenters.cancer.gov/ on the Internet.

KIMMEL CANCER CENTER
THOMAS JEFFERSON UNIVERSITY HOSPITAL

Address:	233 South 10th Street
	Philadelphia, PA 19107
Telephone:	215-503-4500 (Kimmel Cancer Center)
	1-800-533-3669 (1-800-JEFF-NOW) (Physician Referral)
Web site:	http://www.kimmelcancercenter.org/

The Kimmel Cancer Center, based at Thomas Jefferson University, is a National Cancer Institute (NCI)-designated Cancer Center that conducts research and provides services directly to cancer patients. Cancer Centers also conduct activities in outreach and education, and provide information on health care advances to both health care professionals and the public. An NCI-designated Cancer Center must meet a series of competitive requirements and demonstrate excellence in cancer research. For more general information about the Cancer Centers Program of NCI, please visit http://cancercenters.cancer.gov/ on the Internet.

*UNIVERSITY OF PITTSBURGH CANCER INSTITUTE
UNIVERSITY OF PITTSBURGH MEDICAL CENTER,
HILLMAN CANCER CENTER

Address:	5150 Centre Avenue
	Pittsburgh, PA 15232
Telephone:	412-647-2811
E-mail:	PCI-INFO@upmc.edu
Web site:	http://www.upci.upmc.edu/

The University of Pittsburgh Cancer Institute, based at the University of Pittsburgh Medical Center, is a National Cancer Institute (NCI)-designated Comprehensive Cancer Center that conducts research and provides services directly to cancer patients. Comprehensive Cancer Centers also conduct activities in outreach and education, and provide information on health care advances to both health care professionals and the public. An NCI-designated Cancer Center must meet a series of competitive requirements and demonstrate excellence in cancer research. For more general information about the Cancer Centers Program of NCI, please visit http://cancercenters.cancer.gov/ on the Internet.

Appendix D

HOLLINGS CANCER CENTER
MEDICAL UNIVERSITY OF SOUTH CAROLINA

Address: Post Office Box 250955
                86 Jonathan Lucas Street
                Charleston, SC 29425
Telephone: 843-792-9300 (Patient Care and Appointments)
                843-792-2200 (Physician Referral)
                1-800-424-6872 (1-800-424-MUSC) (Health Care Connection)
                1-800-922-5250 (Physician Referral)
Web site: http://hcc.musc.edu/

Hollings Cancer Center is a National Cancer Institute (NCI)-designated Cancer Center that conducts research and provides services directly to cancer patients. An NCI-designated Cancer Center must meet a series of competitive requirements and demonstrate excellence in cancer research. For more general information about the Cancer Centers Program of NCI please visit http://cancercenters.cancer.gov/ on the Internet.

*ST. JUDE CHILDREN'S RESEARCH HOSPITAL

Address: 332 North Lauderdale Street
                Memphis, TN 38105
Telephone: 901-595-3300 (General Information)
                1-866-278-5833 (Physician Referrals)
Web site: http://www.stjude.org

The St. Jude Children's Research Hospital is a National Cancer Institute (NCI)-designated Comprehensive Cancer Center that conducts research and provides services directly to cancer patients. Comprehensive Cancer Centers also conduct activities in outreach and education, and provide information on healthcare advances to both healthcare professionals and the public. An NCI-designated Cancer Center must meet a series of competitive requirements and demonstrate excellence in cancer research. For more general information about the Cancer Centers Program of NCI please visit http://cancercenters.cancer.gov/ on the Internet.

*THE VANDERBILT-INGRAM CANCER CENTER
VANDERBILT UNIVERSITY MEDICAL CENTER

Address: 691 Preston Research Building
                Nashville, TN 37232
Telephone: 615-936-5847 (Clinical Trials or Treatment Options)
                615-936-1782 (Admin.) 615-322-6053 (Main)
                1-800-811-8480 (Clinical Trials or Treatment Options)
                1-888-488-4089 (Admin.)
Web site: http://www.vicc.org/

The Vanderbilt-Ingram Cancer Center is a National Cancer Institute (NCI)-designated Comprehensive Cancer Center that conducts research and provides services directly to cancer patients. Comprehensive Cancer Centers also conduct activities in outreach and education, and provide information on health care advances to both health care professionals and the public. An NCI-designated Cancer Center must meet a series of competitive requirements and demonstrate excellence in cancer research. For more general information about the Cancer Centers Program of NCI, please visit http://cancercenters.cancer.gov/ on the Internet.

TEXAS

CANCER THERAPY & RESEARCH CENTER (CTRC)
UNIVERSITY OF TEXAS HEALTH SCIENCE AT SAN ANTONIO

Address:	7979 Wurzbach Road
	San Antonio, TX 78229
Telephone:	210-450-5798 (Clinical Trial Referral Office)
	210-450-1000 (Main Operator)
	1-800-340-2872 (Main Operator)
Web site:	http://www.ctrc.uthscsa.edu/

The Cancer Therapy & Research Center at the University of Texas Health Science Center at San Antonio is a National Cancer Institute (NCI)-designated Cancer Center that conducts research and provides services directly to cancer patients. An NCI-designated Cancer Center must meet a series of competitive requirements and demonstrate excellence in cancer research. For more general information about the Cancer Centers Program of NCI, please visit http://cancercenters.cancer.gov/ on the Internet.

THE DAN L. DUNCAN CANCER CENTER
BAYLOR COLLEGE OF MEDICINE

Address:	One Baylor Plaza
	Suite 450A
	Houston, TX 77030
Telephone:	713-798-1354
Web site:	http://www.bcm.edu/cancercenter/

The Dan L. Duncan Cancer Center at Baylor College of Medicine is a National Cancer Institute (NCI)-designated Cancer Center that conducts research and provides services directly to cancer patients. An NCI-designated Cancer Center must meet a series of competitive requirements and demonstrate excellence in cancer research. For more general information about the Cancer Centers Program of NCI, please visit http://cancercenters.cancer.gov/ on the Internet.

*THE UNIVERSITY OF TEXAS M.D. ANDERSON CANCER CENTER

Address:	1515 Holcombe Boulevard
	Houston, TX 77030
Telephone:	713-792-6161
	1-877-632-6789 (Patient Referral)
	1-800-392-1611 (Main)
	001-713-745-0450 (International)
Web site:	http://www.mdanderson.org/

Appendix D

The University of Texas M.D. Anderson Cancer Center is a National Cancer Institute (NCI)-designated Comprehensive Cancer Center that conducts research and provides services directly to cancer patients. Comprehensive Cancer Centers also conduct activities in outreach and education, and provide information on health care advances to both health care professionals and the public. An NCI-designated Cancer Center must meet a series of competitive requirements and demonstrate excellence in cancer research. For more general information about the Cancer Centers Program of NCI, please visit http://cancercenters.cancer.gov/ on the Internet.

UTAH

HUNTSMAN CANCER INSTITUTE
UNIVERSITY OF UTAH

Address:	2000 Circle of Hope
	Salt Lake City, UT 84112
Telephone:	801-585-0303
	1-877-585-0303 (Main)
	1-888-424-2100 (Cancer Information and Referrals)
E-mail:	patient.education@hci.utah.edu
Web site:	http://www.hci.utah.edu/

The Huntsman Cancer Institute is a National Cancer Institute (NCI)-designated Cancer Center that conducts research and provides services directly to cancer patients. An NCI-designated Cancer Center must meet a series of competitive requirements and demonstrate excellence in cancer research. For more general information about the Cancer Centers Program of NCI, please visit http://cancercenters.cancer.gov/ on the Internet.

VIRGINIA

MASSEY CANCER CENTER
VIRGINIA COMMONWEALTH UNIVERSITY

Address:	Post Office Box 980037
	401 College Street
	Richmond, VA 23298
Telephone:	804-828-0450 (General Information)
	804-828-5116 (New Patients)
	1-877-462-7739 (1-877-4-MASSEY)
E-mail:	massey@vcu.edu
Web site:	http://www.massey.vcu.edu/

The Massey Cancer Center is a National Cancer Institute (NCI)-designated Cancer Center that conducts research and provides services directly to cancer patients. An NCI-designated Cancer Center must meet a series of competitive requirements and demonstrate excellence in cancer research. For more general information about the Cancer Centers Program of NCI, please visit http://cancercenters.cancer.gov/ on the Internet.

UNIVERSITY OF VIRGINIA CANCER CENTER (UVA CANCER CENTER)
UNIVERSITY OF VIRGINIA HEALTH SCIENCE CENTER

Address:	Post Office Box 800334
	1300 Jefferson Park Avenue
	Charlottesville, VA 22908
Telephone:	434-924-9333
	1-800-223-9173
Web site:	http://www.uvacancer.com

The University of Virginia Cancer Center is a National Cancer Institute (NCI)-designated Cancer Center that conducts research and provides services directly to cancer patients. An NCI-designated Cancer Center must meet a series of competitive requirements and demonstrate excellence in cancer research. For more general information about the Cancer Centers Program of NCI, please visit http://cancercenters.cancer.gov/ on the Internet.

WASHINGTON

---

*FRED HUTCHINSON CANCER RESEARCH CENTER (FHCRC, SCCA)
SEATTLE CANCER CARE ALLIANCE

Address:	LA-205, Post Office Box 19024
	1100 Fairview Avenue North
	Seattle, WA 98109
Telephone:	206-288-1024 (SCCA)
	1-800-804-8824 (SCCA)
E-mail:	hutchdoc@seattlecca.org
Web site:	http://www.fhcrc.org/

The Fred Hutchinson Cancer Research Center is a National Cancer Institute (NCI)-designated Comprehensive Cancer Center that conducts research and provides services directly to cancer patients. Comprehensive Cancer Centers also conduct activities in outreach and education, and provide information on health care advances to both health care professionals and the public. An NCI-designated Cancer Center must meet a series of competitive requirements and demonstrate excellence in cancer research. For more general information about the Cancer Centers Program of NCI, please visit http://cancercenters.cancer.gov/ on the Internet.

Appendix D

*UNIVERSITY OF WISCONSIN
PAUL P. CARBONE COMPREHENSIVE CANCER CENTER

Address:	600 Highland Avenue
	K5/601
	Madison, WI 53792
Telephone:	608-263-8600 (General information)
	608-262-5223 (Cancer Connect)
	1-800-622-8922 (Cancer Connect)
E-mail:	uwccc@uwccc.wisc.edu
Web site:	http://www.cancer.wisc.edu

The University of Wisconsin Paul P. Carbone Comprehensive Cancer Center is a National Cancer Institute (NCI)-designated Comprehensive Cancer Center that conducts research and provides services directly to cancer patients. Comprehensive Cancer Centers also conduct activities in outreach and education, and provide information on health care advances to both health care professionals and the public. An NCI-designated Cancer Center must meet a series of competitive requirements and demonstrate excellence in cancer research. For more general information about the Cancer Centers Program of NCI, please visit http://cancercenters.cancer.gov/ on the Internet.

Section V
Indices

Subject Index

A

America's Top Doctors 11, 12, 15, 53

American Board of Medical Specialties (ABMS) 19, 57, 58, 64, 65

American Cancer Society 4

American Osteopathic Association (AOA) 19

Lance Armstrong 9

B

Board Certification 10, 19, 20, 21, 22, 53, 57, 65

Jane E. Brody 4

C

Centers for Disease Control and Prevention 4

CenterWatch 39

Clinical trials 37-45, 47-50

Consultation 31, 32, 33, 35

Continuing medical education 21

D

Directory of Graduate Medical Education Programs 18

F

Faculty Appointment 24, 53

Fellowship 19, 21, 22, 25, 26, 53

Food and Drug Administration 41

Foreign Medical Graduates 17

Friends of Cancer Research 15

J

Joint Commission on Accreditation of Healthcare Organizations 23

L

Liaison Committee for Medical Education (LCME) 16

M

Malpractice insurance 23

Managed care 7

Mark O. Hatfield Clinical Research Center 46

Medical College Admissions Tests 16

Medical records 32, 33, 35, 41, 46

N

National Cancer Institute (NCI) 4, 39, 43, 47, 48, 50

National Institutes of Health 3, 37, 39, 45

The New York Times 4

North American Association of Central Cancer Registries 4

Northwestern University 26

P

Partnership for Excellence Program 67

Primary care physician 7, 8, 16, 29

Professional Reputation 22

R

S

T

U

V

W

Special Expertise Index

This index lists the areas that the physicians listed in the Guide have identified as their "special expertise." These are not medical specialties. They are specific elements of disease, procedures, techniques and treatments for which these physicians are best known and are referred patients.

Spec	Name	St	Pg

A

Abdominal Imaging

Spec	Name	St	Pg
DR	Fishman, E	MD	391
DR	Levy, A	MD	391
DR	Weinreb, J	CT	390

Abdominal Wall Reconstruction

PlS	Stahl, R	CT	354

Adolescent/Young Adult Cancers

PHO	Fallon, R	IN	335

Adrenal Pathology

Path	Weiss, L	CA	317

Adrenal Tumors

S	Angelos, P	IL	424
S	Brunt, L	MO	424
S	Butler, J	CA	435
S	Duh, Q	CA	436
S	Grant, C	MN	426
S	Hanna, N	MD	415
S	Udelsman, R	CT	411
U	Donovan, J	OH	467
U	Libertino, J	MA	458
U	Vaughan, E	NY	463

Adrenal Tumors & Disorders

EDM	Waguespack, S	TX	114

Aerodigestive Tract Cancer

Onc	Fanucchi, M	NY	149

AIDS Related Cancers

Hem	Dezube, B	MA	126
Hem	Levine, A	CA	138
Inf	Palefsky, J	CA	485
Inf	Polsky, B	NY	485
Onc	Abrams, D	CA	189

Spec	Name	St	Pg
Onc	Ambinder, R	MD	145
Onc	Kaplan, L	CA	192
Onc	Mitsuyasu, R	CA	193
Onc	Remick, S	WV	156
Onc	Volberding, P	CA	197
Onc	Von Roenn, J	IL	179
Psyc	Breitbart, W	NY	360

Airway Reconstruction

Oto	Genden, E	NY	283

Anal Cancer

CRS	Fry, R	PA	89
CRS	Gorfine, S	NY	89
CRS	Nagle, D	MA	88
CRS	Welton, M	CA	95

Anal Disorders & Reconstruction

CRS	Rafferty, J	OH	93
CRS	Wong, W	NY	90

Anemia-Aplastic

Hem	Maciejewski, J	OH	134
PHO	Abella, E	AZ	339
PHO	Camitta, B	WI	334

Anemia-Cancer Related

Hem	Wisch, N	NY	129
Path	Rodgers, G	UT	313

Anemias & Red Cell Disorders

PHO	Finklestein, J	CA	341

Anorectal Disorders

CRS	Efron, J	AZ	94
CRS	Eisenstat, T	NJ	89
CRS	Fry, R	PA	89
CRS	Heppell, J	AZ	94
CRS	Senagore, A	MI	93
CRS	Shellito, P	MA	89
CRS	Stamos, M	CA	95
CRS	Stein, D	PA	90

Spec	Name	St	Pg

Appendix Cancer

S	Bartlett, D	PA	412
S	Mansfield, P	TX	433
S	Paty, P	NY	416
S	Sugarbaker, P	DC	418

Arteriovenous Malformations

RadRO	Isaacson, S	NY	373

Autoimmune Disease

D	Granstein, R	NY	102
Onc	Burt, R	IL	172
PHO	Bussel, J	NY	325

B

Barrett's Esophagus

Ge	Estores, D	FL	120
Ge	Fleischer, D	AZ	122
Ge	Gerdes, H	NY	118
Ge	Greenwald, B	MD	118
Ge	Lightdale, C	NY	119
Path	Montgomery, E	MD	307
S	Nava-Villarreal, H	NY	416
TS	Battafarano, R	MD	447
TS	Ferguson, M	IL	451

Bereavement/Traumatic Grief

Psyc	Roth, A	NY	361

Biliary Cancer

Onc	O'Reilly, E	NY	155
Onc	Patt, Y	NM	187
Onc	Posey, J	AL	167
Onc	Yen, Y	CA	197
S	Chari, R	TN	420
S	Drebin, J	PA	413
S	Ellison, E	OH	425
S	Heslin, M	AL	421
S	Yeo, C	PA	419

Special Expertise Index

America's Top Doctors® for Cancer 5th Edition

Special Expertise Index

Special Expertise Index

Special Expertise Index

Special Expertise Index

Special Expertise Index

America's Top Doctors® for Cancer 5th Edition

Special Expertise Index

H

Hand & Upper Extremity Tumors

Head & Neck Cancer

America's Top Doctors® for Cancer 5th Edition

Special Expertise Index

Spec	Name	St	Pg
Onc	Bashevkin, M	NY	145
Onc	Beatty, P	MT	180
Onc	Bergsagel, P	AZ	183
Onc	Bolwell, B	OH	172
Onc	Claxton, D	PA	147
Onc	Colon-Otero, G	FL	162
Onc	Deeg, H	WA	190
Onc	Erban, J	MA	141
Onc	Flinn, I	TN	163
Onc	Gabrilove, J	NY	150
Onc	Rosen, S	IL	178
Onc	Schilder, R	PA	157
Onc	Shields, P	DC	157
PHO	Hord, J	OH	336

Hematopathology

Path	Bagg, A	PA	305
Path	Banks, P	NC	309
Path	Behm, F	IL	311
Path	Braylan, R	FL	310
Path	Harris, N	MA	304
Path	Jaffe, E	MD	306
Path	Kinney, M	TX	314
Path	McCurley, T	TN	310
Path	Nathwani, B	CA	317
Path	Orazi, A	NY	307
Path	Rodgers, G	UT	313
Path	Swerdlow, S	PA	309
Path	Warnke, R	CA	317
Path	Weisenburger, D	NE	313
Path	Weiss, L	CA	317

Hemophilia

PHO	Tebbi, C	FL	334

Hepatobiliary Surgery

S	Adams, R	VA	419
S	Colquhoun, S	CA	436
S	Curley, S	TX	432
S	Emond, J	NY	414
S	Hemming, A	FL	421
S	Hoffman, J	PA	415
S	Jarnagin, W	NY	415
S	Moossa, A	CA	437
S	Nagorney, D	MN	427
S	Reich, D	PA	417
S	Vauthey, J	TX	434
S	Walsh, R	OH	430

Spec	Name	St	Pg

Hereditary Cancer

CG	Grody, W	CA	484
CG	Ostrer, H	NY	483
CG	Plon, S	TX	484
CG	Shapiro, L	NY	483
CG	Sutphen, R	FL	483
CG	Weitzel, J	CA	484
CG	Whelan, A	MO	484
Onc	Markowitz, S	OH	176
Onc	Nissenblatt, M	NJ	155
Onc	Olopade, O	IL	176
Onc	Toppmeyer, D	NJ	159

High Intensity Focused Ultrasound(HIFU)

U	Chang, S	TN	464

Hip & Knee Replacement in Bone Tumors

OrS	Healey, J	NY	273
OrS	Ready, J	MA	272

Histiocytoma

PHO	Arceci, R	MD	324

Hodgkin's Disease

Hem	Emanuel, P	AR	136
Hem	Gordon, L	IL	133
Hem	Habermann, T	MN	133
Hem	Slease, R	DE	129
Hem	Winter, J	IL	135
Onc	Ambinder, R	MD	145
Onc	Coleman, M	NY	147
Onc	Come, S	MA	141
Onc	Fisher, R	NY	149
Onc	Friedberg, J	NY	150
Onc	Glick, J	PA	150
Onc	Goy, A	NJ	151
Onc	Horning, S	CA	192
Onc	Lossos, I	FL	166
Onc	Moore, J	NC	167
Onc	Nichols, C	OR	194
Onc	Smith, M	PA	158
PHO	Brecher, M	NY	325
PHO	Chen, A	MD	325
PHO	Fallon, R	IN	335
PHO	Friedman, D	TN	331
PHO	Halpern, S	NJ	326
PHO	Hudson, M	TN	332
PHO	Hutchinson, R	MI	336

Spec	Name	St	Pg
PHO	Keller, F	GA	332
PHO	Nachman, J	IL	337
PHO	Schwartz, C	RI	324
PHO	Weiner, M	NY	330
RadRO	Donaldson, S	CA	387
RadRO	Hoppe, R	CA	387
RadRO	Mauch, P	MA	369
RadRO	Mendenhall, N	FL	378
RadRO	Nicolaou, N	PA	374
RadRO	Roberts, K	CT	370
RadRO	Yahalom, J	NY	375

Hodgkin's Disease Consultation

Onc	DeVita, V	CT	141

Hyperthermia Treatment of Cancer

RadRO	Myerson, R	MO	383
RadRO	Prosnitz, L	NC	378

I

Ileal Pouch Anal Anastomosis

CRS	Thorson, A	NE	93

Immune Deficiencies-Primary

Inf	Segal, B	NY	485

Immunopathology

Path	Bhan, A	MA	304
Path	Grogan, T	AZ	314
Path	McCurley, T	TN	310

Immunotherapy

GO	Giuntoli, R	MD	247
GO	Odunsi, A	NY	248
GO	Santin, A	CT	245
Hem	Maziarz, R	OR	139
Hem	Porcu, P	OH	135
Onc	Atkins, M	MA	140
Onc	Ball, E	CA	189
Onc	Borden, E	OH	172
Onc	Chapman, P	NY	147
Onc	Figlin, R	CA	191
Onc	Kirkwood, J	PA	153
Onc	Kwak, L	TX	185
Onc	Livingston, P	NY	154

Special Expertise Index

Spec	Name	St	Pg	Spec	Name	St	Pg	Spec	Name	St	Pg
Onc	Chachoua, A	NY	146	Onc	Ross, H	AZ	187	RadRO	Jose, B	KY	376
Onc	Chapman, R	MI	173	Onc	Ruckdeschel, J	MI	178	RadRO	Komaki, R	TX	385
Onc	Clamon, G	IA	173	Onc	Salgia, R	IL	178	RadRO	Le, Q	CA	388
Onc	Cohen, R	PA	147	Onc	Sandler, A	OR	195	RadRO	Lewin, A	FL	377
Onc	Cohen, S	NY	147	Onc	Schiller, J	TX	188	RadRO	Marks, L	NC	377
Onc	Conry, R	AL	163	Onc	Sherman, C	SC	168	RadRO	McGarry, R	KY	378
Onc	Crawford, J	NC	163	Onc	Simon, G	PA	158	RadRO	Mehta, M	WI	382
Onc	Dunphy, F	NC	163	Onc	Socinski, M	NC	169	RadRO	Movsas, B	MI	382
Onc	Edelman, M	MD	149	Onc	Stone, J	FL	169	RadRO	Roach, M	CA	388
Onc	Einhorn, L	IN	174	Onc	Stoopler, M	NY	158	RadRO	Rosenman, J	NC	379
Onc	Ettinger, D	MD	149	Onc	Thigpen, J	MS	169	RadRO	Schild, S	AZ	386
Onc	Fanucchi, M	NY	149	Onc	Vance, R	MS	170	RadRO	Seung, S	OR	389
Onc	Fossella, F	TX	184	Onc	Wierman, A	NV	197	RadRO	Streeter, O	DC	375
Onc	Gandara, D	CA	191	Path	Cagle, P	TX	314	RadRO	Videtic, G	OH	383
Onc	Garst, J	NC	163	Path	Hammar, S	WA	316	RadRO	Werner-Wasik, M	PA	375
Onc	Glisson, B	TX	184	Path	Katzenstein, A	NY	306	RadRO	Wilson, L	CT	370
Onc	Golomb, H	IL	175	Path	Koss, M	CA	316	TS	Altorki, N	NY	447
Onc	Greco, F	TN	164	Path	Leslie, K	AZ	314	TS	Bains, M	NY	447
Onc	Grunberg, S	VT	142	Path	Moran, C	TX	314	TS	Battafarano, R	MD	447
Onc	Herbst, R	TX	185	Path	Myers, J	MI	312	TS	Bueno, R	MA	446
Onc	Hoffman, P	IL	175	Path	Silverman, J	PA	308	TS	Cerfolio, R	AL	449
Onc	Holland, J	NY	152	Path	Suster, S	WI	313	TS	D'Amico, T	NC	449
Onc	Hong, W	TX	185	Path	Travis, W	NY	309	TS	De Meester, T	CA	453
Onc	Jahanzeb, M	FL	164	Path	Yousem, S	PA	309	TS	Demmy, T	NY	447
Onc	Johnson, B	MA	142	Pul	Alberts, W	FL	365	TS	Deschamps, C	MN	451
Onc	Johnson, D	TN	165	Pul	Garver, R	AL	365	TS	Ferguson, M	IL	451
Onc	Kalemkerian, G	MI	176	Pul	Goldman, A	FL	365	TS	Friedberg, J	PA	447
Onc	Karp, D	TX	185	Pul	Jett, J	MN	365	TS	Gaissert, H	MA	446
Onc	Kelly, K	KS	182	Pul	King, E	PA	364	TS	Gharagozloo, F	DC	447
Onc	Khuri, F	GA	165	Pul	Libby, D	NY	364	TS	Grannis, F	CA	454
Onc	Kies, M	TX	185	Pul	McLennan, G	IA	365	TS	Handy, J	OR	454
Onc	Koczywas, M	CA	192	Pul	Silver, M	IL	365	TS	Harpole, D	NC	450
Onc	Kris, M	NY	153	Pul	Steinberg, H	NY	364	TS	Heitmiller, R	MD	447
Onc	Langer, C	PA	153	Pul	Teirstein, A	NY	364	TS	Howington, J	IL	451
Onc	Lilenbaum, R	FL	165	Pul	Unger, M	PA	364	TS	Iannettoni, M	IA	451
Onc	Lippman, S	TX	186	Pul	White, D	NY	364	TS	Jablons, D	CA	454
Onc	Livingston, R	AZ	186	RadRO	Blackstock, A	NC	376	TS	Jones, D	VA	450
Onc	Lynch, J	FL	166	RadRO	Bogart, J	NY	370	TS	Karwande, S	UT	453
Onc	Martins, R	WA	193	RadRO	Bonner, J	AL	376	TS	Keenan, R	PA	448
Onc	Masters, G	DE	154	RadRO	Bradley, J	MO	380	TS	Keller, S	NY	448
Onc	Miller, A	NC	166	RadRO	Choi, N	MA	369	TS	Kernstine, K	CA	454
Onc	Miller, D	KY	167	RadRO	Choy, H	TX	385	TS	Kiernan, P	VA	450
Onc	Miller, V	NY	154	RadRO	Cox, J	TX	385	TS	Kiev, J	MD	448
Onc	Natale, R	CA	193	RadRO	Emami, B	IL	380	TS	Krasna, M	MD	448
Onc	Nemunaitis, J	TX	186	RadRO	Glatstein, E	PA	372	TS	Krellenstein, D	NY	448
Onc	Northfelt, D	AZ	186	RadRO	Greenberger, J	PA	372	TS	Lanza, L	AZ	453
Onc	Pasmantier, M	NY	156	RadRO	Haffty, B	NJ	372	TS	Maddaus, M	MN	452
Onc	Perry, D	DC	156	RadRO	Hahn, S	PA	373	TS	Marshall, M	DC	448
Onc	Perry, M	MO	177	RadRO	Halle, J	NC	376	TS	Mathisen, D	MA	446
Onc	Pisters, K	TX	187	RadRO	Haraf, D	IL	381	TS	Meyers, B	MO	452
Onc	Robert-Vizcarrondo, F	AL	168	RadRO	Hayman, J	MI	381	TS	Miller, D	GA	450

Lymphoma Consultation

Lymphoma, Cutaneous B Cell (CBCL)

Lymphoma, Cutaneous T Cell (CTCL)

Lymphoma, Non-Hodgkin's

Lymphoma-Ocular (eye)

Lymphoma-Primary CNS

M

Mammography

Mediastinal Tumors

Medulloblastoma

Melanoma

Special Expertise Index

Special Expertise Index

O

Special Expertise Index

Special Expertise Index

Special Expertise Index

Special Expertise Index

Special Expertise Index

Special Expertise Index

America's Top Doctors® for Cancer 5th Edition

Special Expertise Index

V

W

Alphabetical Listing of Doctors

Alphabetical Listing of Doctors

Name	Specialty	Pg	Name	Specialty	Pg
Arun, Banu (TX)	Onc	183	Bardot, Stephen (LA)	U	471
Asher, Anthony (NC)	NS	221	Barger, Geoffrey (MI)	N	237
Athanasian, Edward (NY)	HS	278	Barkin, Jamie (FL)	Ge	120
Atkins, Michael (MA)	Onc	140	Barlogie, Bart (AR)	Hem	136
Atlas, Scott (CA)	NRad	395	Barnes, Willard (DC)	GO	246
Attas, Lewis (NJ)	Onc	145	Barnett, Gene (OH)	NS	223
Audell, Laura (CA)	PM	300	Baron, Joseph (IL)	Hem	131
Augsburger, James (OH)	Oph	266	Barredo, Julio (FL)	PHO	330
August, David (NJ)	S	412	Barter, James (MD)	GO	246
Austin, John (NY)	DR	390	Bartlett, David (PA)	S	412
Averbook, Bruce (OH)	S	424	Basch, Samuel (NY)	Psyc	360
Axelrod, Deborah (NY)	S	412	Bashevkin, Michael (NY)	Onc	145
Axelrod, Rita (PA)	Onc	145	Basler, Joseph (TX)	U	471
Azodi, Masoud (CT)	GO	244	Bassett, Lawrence (CA)	DR	394
			Bastian, Boris (CA)	Path	315
			Battafarano, Richard (MD)	TS	447
			Beall, Michael (VA)	U	464
			Bear, Harry (VA)	S	419
B			Beart, Robert (CA)	CRS	94
Babiera, Gildy (TX)	S	431	Beatty, Patrick (MT)	Onc	180
Back, Anthony (WA)	Onc	189	Beauchamp, Robert (TN)	S	419
Badie, Behnam (CA)	NS	228	Beck, David (LA)	CRS	94
Baer, Maria (MD)	Hem	127	Becker, James (MA)	S	410
Bagg, Adam (PA)	Path	305	Bederson, Joshua (NY)	NS	217
Bagley, Demetrius (PA)	U	459	Beer, Tomasz (OR)	Onc	189
Bahn, Duke (CA)	RadRO	386	Behm, Frederick (IL)	Path	311
Bahnson, Robert (OH)	U	467	Behrns, Kevin (FL)	S	419
Baile, Walter (TX)	Psyc	361	Beitsch, Peter (TX)	S	431
Bailey, H Randolph (TX)	CRS	94	Belani, Chandra (PA)	Onc	146
Bailin, Philip (OH)	D	105	Belinson, Jerome (OH)	GO	252
Bains, Manjit (NY)	TS	447	Bell, Debra (MN)	Path	311
Bakay, Roy (IL)	NS	223	Belldegrun, Arie (CA)	U	472
Balch, Charles (MD)	S	412	Ben-Josef, Edgar (MI)	RadRO	380
Balducci, Lodovico (FL)	Onc	161	Benedetti, Costantino (OH)	PM	299
Bale, Allen (CT)	CG	483	Benedetto, Pasquale (FL)	Onc	161
Ball, Douglas (MD)	EDM	112	Benevenia, Joseph (NJ)	OrS	272
Ball, Edward (CA)	Onc	189	Benjamin, Robert (TX)	Onc	183
Balla, Andre (IL)	Path	311	Bennett, Richard (CA)	D	107
Ballantyne, Garth (NJ)	S	412	Bensinger, William (WA)	Onc	189
Banks, Peter (NC)	Path	309	Benson, Al (IL)	Onc	171
Bans, Larry (AZ)	U	470	Benson, Mitchell (NY)	U	459
Barakat, Richard (NY)	GO	246	Berchuck, Andrew (NC)	GO	249

America's Top Doctors® for Cancer 5th Edition

Name	Specialty	Pg	Name	Specialty	Pg
Berek, Jonathan (CA)	GO	256	Bonner, James (AL)	RadRO	376
Berg, Christine (MD)	RadRO	370	Bonomi, Philip (IL)	Onc	172
Berg, Daniel (WA)	D	107	Boop, Frederick (TN)	NS	221
Berg, Stacey (TX)	PHO	339	Borden, Ernest (OH)	Onc	172
Berg, Wendie (MD)	DR	390	Borgen, Patrick (NY)	S	412
Berger, Mitchel (CA)	NS	229	Borges, Lawrence (MA)	NS	216
Bergsagel, Peter Leif (AZ)	Onc	183	Bos, Gary (WA)	OrS	277
Berke, Gerald (CA)	Oto	293	Bosl, George (NY)	Onc	146
Berkowitz, Ross (MA)	GO	244	Boston, Barry (TN)	Onc	161
Berlin, Jordan (TN)	Onc	161	Bostwick, David (VA)	Path	309
Berman, Michael (CA)	GO	256	Bowen, Glen (UT)	D	106
Bernard, Stephen (NC)	Onc	161	Boxrud, Cynthia (CA)	Oph	268
Berrey, B Hudson (FL)	OrS	274	Boyd, Stuart (CA)	U	473
Bertolone, Salvatore (KY)	PHO	330	Bradford, Carol (MI)	Oto	289
Bhan, Atul (MA)	Path	304	Bradley, Jeffrey (MO)	RadRO	380
Bickers, David (NY)	D	101	Brandt, Keith (MO)	PlS	356
Bierman, Philip (NE)	Onc	181	Braun, Martin (DC)	D	101
Biermann, J Sybil (MI)	OrS	275	Braylan, Raul (FL)	Path	310
Bigelow, Carolyn (MS)	Hem	130	Brecher, Martin (NY)	PHO	325
Biggs, David (DE)	Onc	146	Breitbart, William (NY)	Psyc	360
Bilchik, Anton (CA)	S	435	Brem, Henry (MD)	NS	217
Billings, J Andrew (MA)	PM	298	Brem, Rachel (DC)	DR	390
Bilsky, Mark (NY)	NS	217	Brem, Steven (FL)	NS	221
Bitran, Jacob (IL)	Onc	171	Brems, John (IL)	S	424
Black, Keith (CA)	NS	229	Brendler, Charles (IL)	U	467
Black, Peter (MA)	NS	216	Brennan, Murray (NY)	S	412
Blackstock, Arthur William (NC)	RadRO	376	Brenner, Malcolm (TX)	Hem	136
Bland, Kirby (AL)	S	420	Bresalier, Robert (TX)	Ge	122
Blaney, Susan (TX)	PHO	339	Brescia, Frank (SC)	Onc	162
Blatt, Julie (NC)	PHO	330	Brewer, Molly (CT)	GO	244
Bleday, Ronald (MA)	CRS	88	Bricker, Leslie (MI)	Onc	172
Block, Susan (MA)	Psyc	360	Brien, Earl (CA)	OrS	277
Bockenstedt, Paula (MI)	Hem	131	Bristow, Robert (MD)	GO	246
Bogart, Jeffrey (NY)	RadRO	370	Brizel, David (NC)	RadRO	376
Boggan, James (CA)	NS	229	Brockstein, Bruce (IL)	Onc	172
Boice, Charles (MD)	GO	246	Brodland, David (PA)	D	101
Bojrab, Dennis (MI)	Oto	289	Brooks, Ari (PA)	S	413
Boland, C Richard (TX)	Ge	122	Brooks, John (PA)	Path	305
Bolger, Graeme (AL)	Onc	161	Brown, Kimberly (MI)	Ge	121
Bollen, Andrew (CA)	Path	315	Browne, J Dale (NC)	Oto	286
Bolton, John (LA)	S	431	Bruce, Jeffrey (NY)	NS	217
Bolwell, Brian (OH)	Onc	172	Bruera, Eduardo (TX)	Onc	184

Alphabetical Listing of Doctors

Alphabetical Listing of Doctors

Alphabetical Listing of Doctors

D

America's Top Doctors® for Cancer 5th Edition

Alphabetical Listing of Doctors

America's Top Doctors® for Cancer 5th Edition

Name	Specialty	Pg	Name	Specialty	Pg
Fleshman, James (MO)	CRS	92	Friedman, Debra (TN)	PHO	331
Fletcher, Christopher (MA)	Path	304	Friedman, Henry (NC)	PHO	331
Flickinger, John (PA)	RadRO	371	Frim, David (IL)	NS	224
Flinn, Ian (TN)	Onc	163	Fromm, Geri-Lynn (TX)	GO	255
Flomenberg, Neal (PA)	Onc	149	Fry, Robert (PA)	CRS	89
Flowers, Franklin (FL)	D	104	Fuchs, Charles (MA)	Onc	141
Flynn, Michael (KY)	S	420	Fung, John (OH)	S	426
Flynn, Patrick (MN)	Hem	132	Funk, Gerry (IA)	Oto	289
Fogt, Franz (PA)	Path	305	Furman, Wayne (TN)	PHO	331
Foley, Eugene (WI)	CRS	92	Futran, Neal (WA)	Oto	294
Follen, Michele (TX)	GO	255			
Fong, Yuman (NY)	S	414			
Fonseca, Rafael (AZ)	Hem	137			
Forastiere, Arlene (MD)	Onc	150	**G**		
Ford, James (CA)	Onc	191			
Forero, Andres (AL)	Onc	163	Gabram, Sheryl (GA)	S	420
Forman, Jeffrey (MI)	RadRO	381	Gabrilove, Janice (NY)	Onc	150
Forman, Stephen (CA)	Hem	138	Gaffney, David (UT)	RadRO	384
Formenti, Silvia (NY)	RadRO	372	Gaissert, Henning (MA)	TS	446
Forscher, Charles (CA)	Onc	191	Gajjar, Amar (TN)	PHO	331
Fossella, Frank (TX)	Onc	184	Galandiuk, Susan (KY)	CRS	90
Foster, Richard (IN)	U	468	Gamble, Gail (IL)	PMR	488
Foucar, M Kathryn (NM)	Path	314	Gandara, David (CA)	Onc	191
Fowble, Barbara (CA)	RadRO	387	Ganz, Patricia (CA)	Onc	191
Fowler, Jeffrey (OH)	GO	252	Garber, Judy (MA)	Onc	141
Fowler, Wesley (NC)	GO	250	Garnick, Marc (MA)	Onc	141
Fox, Kevin (PA)	Onc	150	Garrett, Algin (VA)	D	104
Fracasso, Paula (VA)	Onc	163	Garst, Jennifer (NC)	Onc	163
Fraker, Douglas (PA)	S	414	Garver, Robert (AL)	Pul	365
Francis, Kathleen (NJ)	PMR	487	Garvin, James (NY)	PHO	326
Frangoul, Haydar (TN)	PHO	331	Gaynor, Ellen (IL)	Hem	132
Frantz, Christopher (DE)	PHO	326	Gebhardt, Mark (MA)	OrS	272
Fraser, Lionel (MS)	U	464	Gejerman, Glen (NJ)	RadRO	372
Frassica, Frank (MD)	OrS	273	Geller, Kenneth (CA)	PO	345
Frazier, Thomas (PA)	S	414	Gelmann, Edward (NY)	Onc	150
Freedman, Gary (PA)	RadRO	372	Genden, Eric (NY)	Oto	283
Freifeld, Alison (NE)	Inf	485	Georgiade, Gregory (NC)	PlS	355
Friebert, Sarah (OH)	PHO	335	Gerdes, Hans (NY)	Ge	118
Friedberg, Jonathan (NY)	Onc	150	Geronemus, Roy (NY)	D	102
Friedberg, Joseph (PA)	TS	447	Gershenson, David (TX)	GO	255
Friedlaender, Gary (CT)	OrS	272	Gerson, Stanton (OH)	Onc	174
Friedman, Allan (NC)	NS	221	Gertz, Morie (MN)	Hem	132

Alphabetical Listing of Doctors

H

Alphabetical Listing of Doctors

Name	Specialty	Pg	Name	Specialty	Pg
Hartmann, Lynn (MN)	Onc	175	Hirsch, Barry (PA)	Oto	284
Harty, James (KY)	U	464	Hochster, Howard (NY)	Onc	152
Haskal, Ziv (MD)	VIR	395	Hoda, Syed (NY)	Path	306
Hatch, Kenneth (AZ)	GO	255	Hoffman, Andrew (CA)	EDM	115
Haughey, Bruce (MO)	Oto	289	Hoffman, Brenda (SC)	Ge	121
Hauke, Ralph (NE)	Onc	182	Hoffman, Henry (IA)	Oto	290
Haut, Paul (IN)	PHO	335	Hoffman, John (PA)	S	415
Hawkins, Douglas (WA)	PHO	341	Hoffman, Lloyd (NY)	PlS	354
Hayani, Ammar (IL)	PHO	336	Hoffman, Philip (IL)	Onc	175
Hayashi, Robert (MO)	PHO	336	Hogan, Thomas (WV)	Onc	152
Hayes, Daniel (MI)	Onc	175	Holden, Stuart (CA)	U	473
Hayman, James (MI)	RadRO	381	Holland, James (NY)	Onc	152
Healey, John (NY)	OrS	273	Holliday, Michael (MD)	Oto	284
Heber, David (CA)	EDM	114	Homans, Alan (VT)	PHO	323
Heimburger, Douglas (AL)	IM	486	Hong, Waun (TX)	Onc	185
Heinrich, Michael (OR)	Hem	138	Hoppe, Richard (CA)	RadRO	387
Heitmiller, Richard (MD)	TS	447	Hord, Jeffrey (OH)	PHO	336
Heller, Debra (NJ)	Path	306	Horn, Biljana (CA)	PHO	341
Helman, Lee (MD)	PHO	327	Hornicek, Francis (MA)	OrS	272
Helvie, Mark (MI)	DR	393	Horning, Sandra (CA)	Onc	192
Hemal, Ashok (NC)	U	465	Horowitz, Ira (GA)	GO	250
Hemming, Alan (FL)	S	421	Hortobagyi, Gabriel (TX)	Onc	185
Hendrickson, Michael (CA)	Path	316	Horwitz, Eric (PA)	RadRO	373
Heney, Niall (MA)	U	458	Horwitz, Steven (NY)	Onc	152
Henschke, Claudia (NY)	DR	391	Howe, James (IA)	S	426
Heppell, Jacques (AZ)	CRS	94	Howington, John (IL)	TS	451
Herbst, Roy (TX)	Onc	185	Hrebinko, Ronald (PA)	U	460
Herman, Terence (OK)	RadRO	385	Hricak, Hedvig (NY)	DR	391
Heros, Roberto (FL)	NS	221	Hruban, Ralph (MD)	Path	306
Herr, Harry (NY)	U	460	Hruza, George (MO)	D	105
Herrmann, Virginia (SC)	S	421	Huben, Robert (NY)	U	460
Herzog, Thomas (NY)	GO	247	Huber, Philip (TX)	CRS	94
Heslin, Martin (AL)	S	421	Hudes, Gary (PA)	Onc	152
Hester, T Roderick (GA)	PlS	356	Hudis, Clifford (NY)	Onc	152
Hetherington, Maxine (MO)	PHO	336	Hudson, Melissa (TN)	PHO	332
Hicks, Wesley (NY)	Oto	283	Hughes, Kevin (MA)	S	410
Hiesiger, Emile (NY)	N	236	Hunt, Kelly (TX)	S	432
Higano, Celestia (WA)	Onc	192	Huntoon, Marc (MN)	PM	299
Hilden, Joanne (IN)	PHO	336	Hurd, David (NC)	Onc	164
Himelstein, Andrew (DE)	Onc	151	Hussain, Maha (MI)	Onc	175
Hinkle, Andrea (NY)	PHO	327	Hutchins, Laura (AR)	Onc	185
Hinshaw, Daniel (MI)	S	426	Hutchinson, Raymond (MI)	PHO	336

Name	Specialty	Pg	Name	Specialty	Pg
Huynh, Phan Tuong (TX)	DR	393	Jhingran, Anuja (TX)	RadRO	385
Hyman, Neil (VT)	CRS	88	Jillella, Anand (GA)	Onc	164
			Johnson, Bruce (MA)	Onc	142
			Johnson, David (TN)	Onc	165
			Johnson, Denise (CA)	S	437
			Johnson, Jonas (PA)	Oto	284
I			Johnson, Ronald (PA)	S	415
Iannettoni, Mark (IA)	TS	451	Johnson, Stephen (CO)	NS	227
Iglehart, J Dirk (MA)	S	410	Johnson, Timothy (MI)	D	106
Iliff, Nicholas (MD)	Oph	264	Johnston, Carolyn (MI)	GO	252
Ilson, David (NY)	Onc	152	Johnston, J Martin (GA)	PHO	332
Ingle, James (MN)	Onc	175	Johr, Robert (FL)	D	104
Irwin, Ronald (MI)	OrS	275	Jones, David (VA)	TS	450
Isaacs, Claudine (DC)	Onc	152	Jones, Robert (DC)	Path	306
Isaacson, Steven (NY)	RadRO	373	Jordan, Gerald (VA)	U	465
Isik, Ferda (WA)	PlS	358	Jose, Baby (KY)	RadRO	376
Itzkowitz, Steven (NY)	Ge	119	Joyce, Michael J (OH)	OrS	276
			Juckett, Mark (WI)	Hem	133
			Judy, Kevin (PA)	NS	219
			Julian, Thomas (PA)	S	415
J			Jurcic, Joseph (NY)	Onc	153
Jablons, David (CA)	TS	454			
Jackler, Robert (CA)	Oto	294			
Jackman, Stephen (PA)	U	460	**K**		
Jackson, Gilchrist (TX)	S	433			
Jackson, Richard (TX)	PS	348	Kadmon, Dov (TX)	U	471
Jackson, Valerie (IN)	DR	393	Kadota, Richard (CA)	PHO	341
Jacobs, Charlotte (CA)	Onc	192	Kalaycio, Matt (OH)	Onc	176
Jaffe, Elaine (MD)	Path	306	Kalemkerian, Gregory (MI)	Onc	176
Jahanzeb, Mohammad (FL)	Onc	164	Kamani, Naynesh (DC)	PA&I	343
Jain, Subhash (NY)	PM	298	Kamen, Barton (NJ)	PHO	327
Jakacki, Regina (PA)	PHO	327	Kaminski, Mark (MI)	Onc	176
Jallo, George (MD)	NS	218	Kandeel, Fouad (CA)	EDM	115
Janeiro, John (NH)	U	458	Kane, Javier (TN)	PHO	332
Janss, Anna (GA)	N	237	Kane, Madeleine (CO)	Onc	182
Jarnagin, William (NY)	S	415	Kantarjian, Hagop (TX)	Hem	137
Jarow, Jonathan (MD)	U	460	Kantoff, Philip (MA)	Onc	142
Jayabose, Somasundaram (NY)	PHO	327	Kaouk, Jihad (OH)	U	468
Jenkins, Roger (MA)	S	410	Kaplan, Lawrence (CA)	Onc	192
Jett, James (MN)	Pul	365	Kaplan, Michael (CA)	Oto	294
Jewell, Mark (OR)	PlS	358	Kaplan, Steven (NY)	U	460

Alphabetical Listing of Doctors

America's Top Doctors® for Cancer 5th Edition

Alphabetical Listing of Doctors

Name	Specialty	Pg
Lydiatt, Daniel (NE)	Oto	292
Lydiatt, William (NE)	Oto	292
Lyerly, H Kim (NC)	S	422
Lyman, Gary (NC)	Onc	166
Lynch, James (FL)	Onc	166
Lyons, Roger (TX)	Hem	137

M

Name	Specialty	Pg
Machtay, Mitchell (PA)	RadRO	373
Maciejewski, Jaroslaw (OH)	Hem	134
Macklis, Roger (OH)	RadRO	382
Maddaus, Michael (MN)	TS	452
Maddox, Anne (AR)	Hem	137
Madoff, Robert (MN)	CRS	92
Magrina, Javier (AZ)	GO	256
Makhija, Sharmila (GA)	GO	251
Malawer, Martin (DC)	OrS	273
Malik, Ghaus (MI)	NS	225
Malkowicz, S Bruce (PA)	U	461
Maloney, David (WA)	Onc	193
Maloney, Mary (MA)	D	100
Mamelak, Adam (CA)	NS	230
Mamounas, Eleftherios (OH)	S	427
Mandelbaum, David (RI)	ChiN	239
Manera, Ricarchito (IL)	PHO	337
Mangan, Kenneth (PA)	Hem	128
Mansfield, Paul (TX)	S	433
Mantyh, Christopher (NC)	CRS	91
Mapstone, Timothy (OK)	NS	228
Marcet, Jorge (FL)	CRS	91
Marcom, Paul (NC)	Onc	166
Marcus, Robert (FL)	RadRO	377
Marentette, Lawrence (MI)	Oto	290
Margolin, Kim (WA)	Onc	193
Marina, Neyssa (CA)	PHO	342
Maris, John (PA)	PHO	328
Mark, Eugene (MA)	Path	304
Markert, James (AL)	NS	221
Markman, Maurie (TX)	Onc	186

Name	Specialty	Pg
Markoe, Arnold (FL)	RadRO	377
Markowitz, Sanford (OH)	Onc	176
Marks, Lawrence (NC)	RadRO	377
Marks, Stanley (PA)	Hem	128
Marsh, James (PA)	S	416
Marshall, Fray (GA)	U	465
Marshall, John (DC)	Onc	154
Marshall, Margaret Blair (DC)	TS	448
Martenson, James (MN)	RadRO	382
Martins, Renato G (WA)	Onc	193
Martuza, Robert (MA)	NS	217
Maslak, Peter (NY)	Onc	154
Mason, Joel (MA)	Ge	118
Masood, Shahla (FL)	Path	310
Masters, Gregory (DE)	Onc	154
Mathew, Paul (MA)	Onc	143
Mathisen, Douglas (MA)	TS	446
Matthay, Katherine (CA)	PHO	342
Matulonis, Ursula (MA)	Onc	143
Mauch, Peter (MA)	RadRO	369
Mauro, Matthew (NC)	VIR	396
Maxwell, G Patrick (TN)	PlS	356
May, James (MA)	PlS	354
Mayberg, Marc (WA)	NS	230
Maziarz, Richard (OR)	Hem	139
McCaffrey, Thomas (FL)	Oto	287
McCarthy, Shirley (CT)	DR	390
McConnell, John (NC)	U	465
McCormick, Beryl (NY)	RadRO	374
McCormick, Paul (NY)	NS	219
McCraw, John (MS)	PlS	356
McCurley, Thomas (TN)	Path	310
McDermott, Michael (CA)	NS	230
McDonald, Charles (RI)	D	100
McDonald, Douglas (MO)	OrS	276
McDougal, W Scott (MA)	U	458
McGahan, John (CA)	VIR	397
McGarry, Ronald (KY)	RadRO	378
McGill, Trevor (MA)	PO	344
McGlave, Philip (MN)	Hem	134
McGovern, Francis (MA)	U	458
McGrath, Patrick (KY)	S	422

Alphabetical Listing of Doctors

Name	Specialty	Pg	Name	Specialty	Pg
McGuire, William (MD)	Onc	154	Miller, Stanley (MD)	D	102
McLennan, Geoffrey (IA)	Pul	365	Miller, Thomas (AZ)	Onc	186
McMasters, Kelly (KY)	S	422	Miller, Timothy (CA)	PlS	358
McMenomey, Sean (OR)	Oto	295	Miller, Vincent (NY)	Onc	154
McVary, Kevin (IL)	U	469	Millis, J Michael (IL)	S	427
Meacham, Lillian (GA)	PEn	344	Mills, Stacey (VA)	Path	310
Mears, John Gregory (NY)	Hem	128	Milsom, Jeffrey (NY)	CRS	90
Medbery, Clinton (OK)	RadRO	386	Mintzer, David (PA)	Onc	154
Medich, David (PA)	CRS	90	Mischel, Paul (CA)	Path	317
Medina, Jesus (OK)	Oto	292	Mitchell, Beverly (CA)	Hem	139
Meehan, Kenneth (NH)	Hem	126	Mitnick, Julie (NY)	DR	391
Meek, Rita (DE)	PHO	328	Mitsuyasu, Ronald (CA)	Onc	193
Mehta, Minesh (WI)	RadRO	382	Mittal, Bharat (IL)	RadRO	382
Melamed, Jonathan (NY)	Path	307	Moley, Jeffrey (MO)	S	427
Melmed, Shlomo (CA)	EDM	115	Molo, Mary (IL)	RE	260
Melvin, W Scott (OH)	S	427	Monk, Bradley (CA)	GO	257
Mendenhall, Nancy (FL)	RadRO	378	Monsees, Barbara (MO)	DR	393
Mendenhall, William (FL)	RadRO	378	Montgomery, Elizabeth (MD)	Path	307
Menick, Frederick (AZ)	PlS	357	Montie, James (MI)	U	469
Menon, Mani (MI)	U	469	Moore, Anne (NY)	Onc	155
Merchant, Thomas (TN)	RadRO	378	Moore, David (IN)	GO	253
Meredith, Ruby (AL)	RadRO	378	Moore, Joseph (NC)	Onc	167
Merrick, Hollis (OH)	S	427	Moossa, AR (CA)	S	437
Meyer, William (OK)	PHO	340	Moran, Cesar (TX)	Path	314
Meyers, Bryan (MO)	TS	452	Morgan, Elaine (IL)	PHO	337
Meyers, Paul (NY)	PHO	328	Morgan, Linda (FL)	ObG	258
Meyers, Rebecka (UT)	PS	347	Morgan, Mark (PA)	GO	248
Meyskens, Frank (CA)	Onc	193	Morgan, Walter (TN)	PS	346
Michalski, Jeff M (MO)	RadRO	382	Morrison, Glenn (FL)	NS	222
Michelassi, Fabrizio (NY)	S	416	Morrow, Monica (NY)	S	416
Mickey, Bruce (TX)	NS	228	Mortimer, Joanne (CA)	Onc	193
Mieler, William (IL)	Oph	267	Moscow, Jeffrey (KY)	PHO	332
Mies, Carolyn (PA)	Path	307	Mostwin, Jacek (MD)	U	461
Mihm, Martin (MA)	D	101	Mott, Michael (MI)	OrS	276
Mikkelsen, Tommy (MI)	N	237	Motzer, Robert (NY)	Onc	155
Miles, Brian (TX)	U	471	Moul, Judd (NC)	U	465
Millenson, Michael (PA)	Hem	128	Movsas, Benjamin (MI)	RadRO	382
Miller, Antonius (NC)	Onc	166	Muggia, Franco (NY)	Onc	155
Miller, Daniel (GA)	TS	450	Mullett, Timothy (KY)	TS	450
Miller, Donald (KY)	Onc	167	Mulvihill, John (OK)	CG	484
Miller, Joseph (GA)	TS	450	Mulvihill, Sean (UT)	S	430
Miller, Kenneth (MA)	Hem	126	Mundt, Arno (CA)	RadRO	388

Name	Specialty	Pg
Munker, Reinhold (LA)	Hem	137
Muntz, Howard (WA)	GO	257
Murphree, A Linn (CA)	Oph	269
Murray, Timothy (FL)	Oph	265
Murtagh, F Reed (FL)	NRad	394
Muss, Hyman (NC)	Onc	167
Mutch, David (MO)	GO	253
Muto, Michael (MA)	GO	245
Myers, Jeffrey (TX)	Oto	293
Myers, Jeffrey (MI)	Path	312
Myers, Robert (MN)	U	469
Myerson, Robert (MO)	RadRO	383
Myseros, John (VA)	NS	222

N

Name	Specialty	Pg
Nabell, Lisle (AL)	Onc	167
Nabors, Louis (AL)	N	237
Nachman, James (IL)	PHO	337
Nademanee, Auayporn (CA)	Hem	139
Nadler, Lee (MA)	Onc	143
Nagle, Deborah (MA)	CRS	88
Nagorney, David (MN)	S	427
Nakakura, Eric (CA)	S	437
Nand, Sucha (IL)	Hem	135
Nascimento, Antonio (MN)	Path	312
Naslund, Michael (MD)	U	461
Natale, Ronald (CA)	Onc	193
Nathanson, S David (MI)	S	427
Nathwani, Bharat (CA)	Path	317
Naunheim, Keith (MO)	TS	452
Nava-Villarreal, Hector (NY)	S	416
Neel, Victor (MA)	D	101
Neglia, Joseph (MN)	PHO	337
Negrin, Robert (CA)	Hem	139
Neifeld, James (VA)	S	422
Nelson, Edward (UT)	S	431
Nelson, Heidi (MN)	CRS	92
Nelson, Joel (PA)	U	462
Nelson, Judith (NY)	Pul	364

Name	Specialty	Pg
Nemunaitis, John (TX)	Onc	186
Nerad, Jeffrey (OH)	Oph	267
Nesbitt, Jonathan (TN)	TS	450
Ness, John (MN)	PlS	356
Netterville, James (TN)	Oto	287
Neuberg, Ronnie (SC)	PHO	333
Neuburg, Marcelle (WI)	D	106
Neumann, Donald (OH)	NuM	398
Neuwelt, Edward (OR)	NS	230
Newman, Lisa (MI)	S	427
Newton, Herbert (OH)	N	238
Nichols, Craig (OR)	Onc	194
Nicholson, Henry (OR)	PHO	342
Nicolaou, Nicos (PA)	RadRO	374
Nicosia, Santo (FL)	Path	310
Nieder, Michael (FL)	PHO	333
Nigra, Thomas (DC)	D	102
Nimer, Stephen (NY)	Hem	128
Ninan, Mathews (TN)	TS	450
Nissen, Nicholas (CA)	S	437
Nissenblatt, Michael (NJ)	Onc	155
Nogueras, Juan (FL)	CRS	91
Noller, Kenneth (MA)	ObG	258
Noone, R Barrett (PA)	PlS	355
Nori, Dattatreyudu (NY)	RadRO	374
Northfelt, Donald (AZ)	Onc	186
Norton, Jeffrey (CA)	S	438
Norton, Larry (NY)	Onc	155
Nowak, Eugene (NY)	S	416
Noyes, Nicole (NY)	RE	260
Nuchtern, Jed (TX)	PS	348
Nugent, William (NH)	TS	446
Nuss, Daniel (LA)	Oto	293

O

Name	Specialty	Pg
O'Brien, Joan (CA)	Oph	269
O'Brien, Susan (TX)	Onc	186
O'Day, Steven (CA)	Onc	194
O'Donnell, Margaret (CA)	Hem	139

Alphabetical Listing of Doctors

Name	Specialty	Pg	Name	Specialty	Pg
Pensak, Myles (OH)	Oto	291	Polsky, Bruce (NY)	Inf	485
Penson, David (CA)	U	474	Pomeroy, Scott (MA)	ChiN	239
Perez, Edith (FL)	Onc	167	Ponn, Teresa (NH)	S	411
Perry, Arie (MO)	Path	312	Porayko, Michael (TN)	Ge	121
Perry, David (DC)	Onc	156	Porcu, Pierluigi (OH)	Hem	135
Perry, Michael (MO)	Onc	177	Porrazzo, Michael (DC)	RadRO	374
Persky, Mark (NY)	Oto	285	Portenoy, Russell (NY)	PM	299
Peschel, Richard (CT)	RadRO	369	Porter, David (PA)	Hem	128
Peters, Glenn (AL)	Oto	288	Posey, James (AL)	Onc	167
Petersdorf, Stephen (WA)	Onc	194	Posner, Jerome (NY)	N	236
Peterson, Bruce (MN)	Onc	177	Posner, Marshall (MA)	Onc	143
Peterson, Laura (HI)	S	438	Posner, Mitchell (IL)	S	428
Petrelli, Nicholas (DE)	S	417	Postier, Russell (OK)	S	434
Petruzzelli, Guy (IL)	Oto	291	Potkul, Ronald (IL)	GO	253
Petrylak, Daniel (NY)	Onc	156	Pow-Sang, Julio (FL)	U	466
Pezner, Richard (CA)	RadRO	388	Powell, Bayard (NC)	Hem	130
Pfister, David (NY)	Onc	156	Powell, Catherine (CA)	GO	257
Phillips, Peter (PA)	ChiN	239	Prados, Michael (CA)	Onc	194
Phuphanich, Surasak (CA)	N	239	Press, Oliver (WA)	Onc	194
Picozzi, Vincent (WA)	Onc	194	Presti, Joseph (CA)	U	474
Picus, Joel (MO)	Onc	177	Prieto, Victor (TX)	Path	314
Pienta, Kenneth (MI)	Onc	177	Prosnitz, Leonard (NC)	RadRO	378
Piepmeier, Joseph (CT)	NS	217	Provenzale, James (NC)	NRad	394
Pierce, Lori (MI)	RadRO	383	Puccetti, Diane (WI)	PHO	337
Pierson, Richard (MD)	TS	448	Pui, Ching-Hon (TN)	PHO	333
Pinson, C Wright (TN)	S	422	Pulido, Jose (MN)	Oph	267
Pinto, Harlan (CA)	Onc	194	Putnam, Joe (TN)	TS	450
Pisters, Katherine (TX)	Onc	187			
Pisters, Louis (TX)	U	472			
Pisters, Peter (TX)	S	434			
Pitman, Karen (MS)	Oto	288			
Plager, David (IN)	Oph	267	**Q**		
Plautz, Gregory (OH)	PHO	337	Quill, Timothy (NY)	IM	485
Plon, Sharon (TX)	CG	484	Quinn, David (CA)	Onc	194
Pochapin, Mark (NY)	Ge	119	Quivey, Jeanne (CA)	RadRO	388
Pockaj, Barbara (AZ)	S	434			
Podoloff, Donald (TX)	NuM	399			
Pohlman, Brad (OH)	Onc	177			
Poliakoff, Steven (FL)	GO	251			
Pollack, Alan (FL)	RadRO	378	**R**		
Pollack, Ian (PA)	NS	220	Rabinovitch, Rachel (CO)	RadRO	384
Pollock, Raphael (TX)	S	434	Rabow, Michael (CA)	IM	487

Alphabetical Listing of Doctors

Name	Specialty	Pg	Name	Specialty	Pg
Rader, Janet (MO)	GO	253	Rich, Keith (MO)	NS	226
Raffel, Corey (OH)	NS	225	Rich, Tyvin (VA)	RadRO	379
Rafferty, Janice (OH)	CRS	93	Richards, Jon (IL)	Onc	178
Raghavan, Derek (OH)	Onc	177	Richie, Jerome (MA)	U	458
Rai, Kanti (NY)	Hem	128	Ricketts, Richard (GA)	PS	347
Ramsay, David (NY)	D	103	Ridge, John Andrew (PA)	S	417
Randall, Marcus (KY)	RadRO	378	Ridgway, E (CO)	EDM	113
Randall, R Lor (UT)	OrS	277	Rigel, Darrell (NY)	D	103
Randall, Thomas (PA)	GO	248	Rikkers, Layton (WI)	S	428
Rao, Vijay (PA)	DR	392	Rilling, William (WI)	VIR	396
Raphael, Bruce (NY)	Hem	129	Ritchey, A Kim (PA)	PHO	329
Raptis, George (NY)	Onc	156	Rivlin, Richard (NY)	IM	486
Rashid, Asif (TX)	Path	315	Roach, Mack (CA)	RadRO	388
Rassekh, Christopher (WV)	Oto	285	Robb, Geoffrey (TX)	PlS	357
Ratain, Mark (IL)	Onc	177	Robbins, Richard (TX)	EDM	114
Rauch, Paula (MA)	Psyc	360	Robert, Nicholas (VA)	Onc	168
Rauck, Richard (NC)	PM	299	Robert-Vizcarrondo, Francisco (AL)	Onc	168
Rausen, Aaron (NY)	PHO	329	Roberts, Kenneth (CT)	RadRO	370
Razzouk, Bassem (IN)	PHO	338	Roberts, Patricia (MA)	CRS	88
Ready, John (MA)	OrS	272	Robertson, Cary (NC)	U	466
Ready, L Brian (WA)	PM	301	Robins, Perry (NY)	D	103
Reaman, Gregory (DC)	PHO	329	Robinson, Lary (FL)	TS	451
Reardon, Michael (TX)	TS	453	Rock, Jack (MI)	NS	226
Reber, Howard (CA)	S	438	Rodgers, George (UT)	Path	313
Recht, Abram (MA)	RadRO	369	Rogers, Lisa (MI)	N	238
Reed, Carolyn (SC)	TS	451	Roh, Mark (PA)	S	417
Regine, William (MD)	RadRO	374	Rohrich, Rod (TX)	PlS	357
Reich, David (PA)	S	417	Romaguera, Jorge (TX)	Onc	187
Reid, Tony (CA)	Onc	195	Rombeau, John (PA)	CRS	90
Reid, William (TN)	NS	222	Romond, Edward (KY)	Onc	168
Remick, Scot (WV)	Onc	156	Roodman, G David (PA)	Hem	129
Remmenga, Steven (NE)	GO	254	Rook, Alain (PA)	D	103
Rescorla, Frederick (IN)	PS	347	Rosato, Ernest (PA)	S	417
Reuter, Victor (NY)	Path	308	Rose, Christopher (CA)	RadRO	388
Rex, Douglas (IN)	Ge	121	Rose, Peter (OH)	GO	253
Reynolds, R Kevin (MI)	GO	253	Rosemurgy, Alexander (FL)	S	422
Rheingold, Susan (PA)	PHO	329	Rosen, Paul (NY)	Path	308
Riba, Michelle (MI)	Psyc	361	Rosen, Steven (IL)	Onc	178
Rice, Dale (CA)	Oto	295	Rosenberg, Steven (MD)	S	417
Rice, Henry (NC)	PS	346	Rosenblatt, Joseph (FL)	Hem	131
Rice, Laurel (WI)	GO	253	Rosenblum, Marc (NY)	Path	308
Rice, Thomas (OH)	TS	452	Rosenblum, Mark (MI)	NS	226

America's Top Doctors® for Cancer 5th Edition

Alphabetical Listing of Doctors

Name	Specialty	Pg	Name	Specialty	Pg
Scheithauer, Bernd (MN)	Path	312	Selvaggi, Kathy (PA)	Onc	157
Scher, Charles (LA)	PHO	340	Sen, Chandranath (NY)	NS	220
Scher, Howard (NY)	Onc	157	Senagore, Anthony (MI)	CRS	93
Scherr, Douglas (NY)	U	462	Sencer, Susan (MN)	PHO	338
Schiff, David (VA)	N	237	Sener, Stephen (IL)	S	428
Schiff, Peter (NY)	RadRO	374	Senzer, Neil (TX)	RadRO	386
Schiffer, Charles (MI)	Onc	178	Sepkowitz, Kent (NY)	Inf	485
Schiffman, Jade (TX)	Oph	268	Serletti, Joseph (PA)	PlS	355
Schild, Steven (AZ)	RadRO	386	Serody, Jonathan (NC)	Onc	168
Schilder, Russell (PA)	Onc	157	Seung, Steven (OR)	RadRO	389
Schiller, Alan (NY)	Path	308	Sewell, C Whitaker (GA)	Path	311
Schiller, Gary (CA)	Hem	139	Shaffrey, Mark (VA)	NS	222
Schiller, Joan (TX)	Onc	188	Shah, Jatin (NY)	S	418
Schilsky, Richard (IL)	Onc	178	Shamberger, Robert (MA)	PS	345
Schink, Julian (IL)	GO	254	Shapiro, Charles (OH)	Onc	178
Schlegel, Peter (NY)	U	462	Shapiro, Lawrence (NY)	CG	483
Schmidt, Richard (PA)	OrS	274	Shapiro, Scott (IN)	NS	226
Schnabel, Freya (NY)	S	417	Shapiro, William (AZ)	N	238
Schnipper, Lowell (MA)	Onc	143	Shapshay, Stanley (NY)	Oto	285
Schnitt, Stuart (MA)	Path	304	Shaw, Edward (NC)	RadRO	379
Schoenberg, Mark (MD)	U	462	Shea, Thomas (NC)	Onc	168
Schoetz, David (MA)	CRS	88	Shearer, Patricia (FL)	PHO	334
Schomberg, Paula (MN)	RadRO	383	Sheinfeld, Joel (NY)	U	463
Schraut, Wolfgang (PA)	S	417	Shellito, Paul (MA)	CRS	89
Schuchter, Lynn (PA)	Onc	157	Shen, Perry (NC)	S	423
Schuster, Michael (NY)	Hem	129	Shenk, Robert (OH)	S	429
Schusterman, Mark (TX)	PlS	357	Sherman, Carol (SC)	Onc	168
Schwartz, Burton (MN)	Onc	178	Sherman, Randolph (CA)	PlS	358
Schwartz, Cindy (RI)	PHO	324	Sherman, Steven (TX)	EDM	114
Schwartz, Herbert (TN)	OrS	274	Shibata, Stephen (CA)	Onc	195
Schwartz, L Matthew (PA)	PMR	487	Shields, Carol (PA)	Oph	265
Schwartz, Michael (FL)	Onc	168	Shields, Jerry (PA)	Oph	265
Schwartz, Peter (CT)	GO	245	Shields, Peter (DC)	Onc	157
Schwartzberg, Lee (TN)	Hem	131	Shike, Moshe (NY)	Ge	119
Schwartzentruber, Douglas (IN)	S	428	Shin, Dong Moon (GA)	Onc	169
Scott, Walter (PA)	TS	449	Shina, Donald (NM)	RadRO	386
Scott-Conner, Carol (IA)	S	428	Shindo, Maisie (OR)	Oto	295
Scully, Sean (FL)	OrS	274	Shipley, William (MA)	RadRO	370
See, William (WI)	U	469	Shochat, Stephen (TN)	PS	347
Segal, Brahm (NY)	Inf	485	Shrager, Joseph (CA)	TS	454
Seiff, Stuart (CA)	Oph	269	Shrieve, Dennis (UT)	RadRO	384
Sekhar, Laligam (WA)	NS	230	Shulman, Lawrence (MA)	Onc	143

Name	Specialty	Pg	Name	Specialty	Pg
Shulman, Lee (IL)	ObG	259	Slivka, Adam (PA)	Ge	120
Sibley, Richard (CA)	Path	317	Small, Eric (CA)	Onc	195
Sidransky, David (MD)	Onc	158	Small, William (IL)	RadRO	383
Siegel, Barry (MO)	NuM	398	Smalley, Stephen (KS)	RadRO	384
Siegel, Gordon (IL)	Oto	291	Smith, Barbara (MA)	S	411
Siegel, Herrick (AL)	OrS	274	Smith, David (FL)	PlS	356
Siegel, Stuart (CA)	PHO	343	Smith, Donna (IL)	GO	254
Sielaff, Timothy (MN)	S	429	Smith, Joseph (TN)	U	466
Sigurdson, Elin (PA)	S	418	Smith, Lloyd (CA)	GO	257
Sikic, Branimir (CA)	Onc	195	Smith, Matthew (MA)	Onc	143
Silbergeld, Daniel (WA)	NS	230	Smith, Mitchell (PA)	Onc	158
Sills, Allen (TN)	NS	223	Smith, Thomas (VA)	Onc	169
Silva, Elvio (TX)	Path	315	Smoot, Duane (DC)	Ge	120
Silver, Michael (IL)	Pul	365	Smythe, W Roy (TX)	TS	453
Silverberg, Steven (MD)	Path	308	Snyder, David (CA)	Hem	139
Silverman, Jan (PA)	Path	308	Snyder, Peter (PA)	EDM	112
Silverman, Lewis (NY)	Onc	158	Snyderman, Carl (PA)	Oto	285
Silverman, Paula (OH)	Onc	179	Sobel, Stuart (FL)	D	105
Silverstein, Melvin (CA)	S	438	Sober, Arthur (MA)	D	101
Sim, Franklin (MN)	OrS	276	Socinski, Mark (NC)	Onc	169
Simeone, Diane (MI)	S	429	Soiffer, Robert (MA)	Onc	144
Simon, George (PA)	Onc	158	Soisson, Andrew (UT)	GO	254
Sinanan, Mika (WA)	S	438	Sokol, Thomas (CA)	CRS	95
Singer, Daniel (HI)	OrS	278	Sokoloff, Daniel (FL)	D	105
Singer, Mark (CA)	Oto	295	Solberg, Lawrence (FL)	Hem	131
Singer, Samuel (NY)	S	418	Solin, Lawrence (PA)	RadRO	374
Singhal, Seema (IL)	Hem	135	Soloway, Mark (FL)	U	466
Singletary, S (TX)	S	434	Sondak, Vernon (FL)	S	423
Sinha, Uttam (CA)	Oto	295	Sondel, Paul (WI)	PHO	338
Siperstein, Allan (OH)	S	429	Sonett, Joshua (NY)	TS	449
Sisti, Michael (NY)	NS	220	Song, John (CO)	Oto	292
Skibber, John (TX)	S	434	Sood, Anil (TX)	GO	256
Skinner, Eila (CA)	U	474	Soparkar, Charles (TX)	Oph	268
Skinner, Kristin (NY)	S	418	Soper, John (NC)	GO	251
Skinner, Michael (TX)	PS	348	Sosman, Jeffrey (TN)	Onc	169
Sklar, Charles (NY)	PEn	344	Sotomayor, Eduardo (FL)	Onc	169
Slatkin, Neal (CA)	PM	301	Soulen, Michael (PA)	VIR	396
Slawin, Kevin (TX)	U	472	Spann, Cyril (GA)	GO	251
Slease, Robert (DE)	Hem	129	Spetzler, Robert (AZ)	NS	228
Sledge, George (IN)	Onc	179	Speyer, James (NY)	Onc	158
Slezak, Sheri (MD)	PlS	355	Spiegel, David (CA)	Psyc	362
Slingluff, Craig (VA)	S	423	Spirtos, Nicola (NV)	GO	258

Alphabetical Listing of Doctors

Name	Specialty	Pg	Name	Specialty	Pg
Spitzer, Thomas (MA)	Hem	126	Strome, Marshall (NY)	Oto	286
Spivak, Jerry (MD)	Hem	129	Strome, Scott (MD)	Oto	286
Spriggs, David (NY)	Onc	158	Strouse, Thomas (CA)	Psyc	362
Springfield, Dempsey (MA)	OrS	272	Strup, Stephen (KY)	U	466
Staats, Peter (NJ)	PM	299	Stryker, Steven (IL)	CRS	93
Stadelmann, Wayne (NH)	PlS	354	Stubblefield, Michael (NY)	PMR	487
Stadler, Walter (IL)	Onc	179	Suen, James (AR)	Oto	293
Stadtmauer, Edward (PA)	Onc	158	Sugarbaker, David (MA)	TS	446
Stahl, Donna (OH)	S	429	Sugarbaker, Paul (DC)	S	418
Stahl, Richard (CT)	PlS	354	Suh, John (OH)	RadRO	383
Stamos, Michael (CA)	CRS	95	Sultan, Mark (NY)	PlS	355
Staren, Edgar (IL)	S	429	Sun, Peter (CA)	NS	231
Stea, Baldassarre (AZ)	RadRO	386	Sun, Weijing (PA)	Onc	159
Stehman, Frederick (IN)	GO	254	Sundaram, Magesh (WV)	S	418
Stein, David (PA)	CRS	90	Suster, Saul (WI)	Path	313
Steinberg, Gary (IL)	U	469	Sutphen, Rebecca (FL)	CG	483
Steinberg, Harry (NY)	Pul	364	Sutton, John (NH)	S	411
Steingart, Richard (NY)	Cv	483	Sutton, Leslie (PA)	NS	220
Steinhagen, Randolph (NY)	CRS	90	Sutton, Linda (NC)	Onc	169
Steinherz, Laurel (NY)	PCd	343	Swain, Sandra (DC)	Onc	159
Steinherz, Peter (NY)	PHO	329	Swanson, David (TX)	U	472
Stern, Jeffrey (CA)	GO	258	Swanson, Neil (OR)	D	108
Sternberg, Paul (TN)	Oph	265	Swanson, Scott (MA)	TS	446
Stewart, Forrest (WA)	Onc	196	Swarm, Robert (MO)	PM	300
Stewart, Paula (AL)	PMR	487	Sweetenham, John (OH)	Hem	135
Stieg, Philip (NY)	NS	220	Swensen, Stephen (MN)	DR	393
Stiff, Patrick (IL)	Hem	135	Swerdlow, Steven (PA)	Path	309
Stock, Richard (NY)	RadRO	375	Swetter, Susan (CA)	D	108
Stockdale, Frank (CA)	Onc	196	Swisher, Stephen (TX)	TS	453
Stolar, Charles (NY)	PS	346	Swistel, Alexander (NY)	S	418
Stolier, Alan (LA)	S	434	Szabo, Robert (CA)	HS	278
Stone, Joel (FL)	Onc	169			
Stone, Richard (MA)	Hem	127			
Stoopler, Mark (NY)	Onc	158			
Stopeck, Alison (AZ)	Onc	188			
Stout, John (OR)	Oph	269	**T**		
Straus, David (NY)	Onc	159	Tafra, Lorraine (MD)	S	418
Strauss, Gary (MA)	Onc	144	Tagawa, Scott (NY)	Onc	159
Strauss, H William (NY)	NuM	397	Talamonti, Mark (IL)	S	429
Strauss, James (TX)	Hem	137	Tallman, Martin (IL)	Hem	135
Streeter, Oscar (DC)	RadRO	375	Tanabe, Kenneth (MA)	S	411
Stringer, Scott (MS)	Oto	288	Taneja, Samir (NY)	U	463

America's Top Doctors® for Cancer 5th Edition

Alphabetical Listing of Doctors

Alphabetical Listing of Doctors

Alphabetical Listing of Doctors

Acknowledgments

The publishers would like to thank the entire staff for their many hours and days of intense and precise work on this guide in order to further its goal of assisting consumers in making the best healthcare choices.

Castle Connolly Executive Management:

Chairman	John K. Castle
President & CEO	John J. Connolly, Ed.D.
Vice President, Chief Medical & Research Officer	Jean Morgan, M.D.
Vice President, Chief Strategy & Operations Officer	William Liss-Levinson, Ph.D.

Research Coordinators

Maryann Hynd, RN
Sara Belly
Mandy Guerrero
Terysia Herbert
Stephanie Sanchez

Book Layout, Database Management	Russell Hodgson
Office Manager, Book Coordination	Marcie Samartino
Corporate Services Manager	Jennifer Mojave

We also would like to extend our gratitude to the American Board of Medical Specialties (ABMS) for allowing us to use excerpts, especially the descriptions of medical specialties and subspecialties, from the text of their publication "Which Medical Specialist for You?"

Other Publications from Castle Connolly Medical Ltd.:
America's Top Doctors®; *Top Doctors: New York Metro Area*;
Top Doctors: Chicago Metro Area; *Cancer Made Easier: New York—Metro Area*, *Eldercare* and others...
Order online at http://www.castleconnolly.com/books

Doctor-Patient Advisor

Doctor-Patient Advisor is a Castle Connolly Medical Ltd. service providing one-on-one consultations with a physician or nurse to individuals who have serious or complex medical problems or to anyone who feels he/she needs assistance finding the right physician for any purpose. Each client will receive personalized assistance in identifying the appropriate specialists for his/her condition utilizing the Castle Connolly Medical Ltd. database of physicians and hospitals, as well as individual searches, to locate the best resources to meet the client's needs.

Fee: $375. For further information call (212) 367-8400 x 16.

Castle Connolly Corporate Membership

The Castle Connolly *Corporate Membership* provides an opportunity for employers to assist employees and their families to access the "Top Doctors" database as identified by Castle Connolly Medical Ltd. Through a Corporate Membership, the employer makes the Castle Connolly database of over 23,000 Top Doctors, in more than 70 medical specialties and sub-specialties, available to its employees through the company's website. Instead of asking a friend or neighbor for a recommendation of a doctor of simply choosing a name from a directory, employees can select from among doctorstop specialists and primary care physicians - who have been highly nominated by other physicians and thoroughly screened by our physician-led research team.

The result for employees is better health, reduced absence, less "fret and worry" about excellent healthcare and, overall, better morale. And that adds up to lower healthcare costs for employers. All of this can be achieved at a very low cost of a few dollars per employee a year; a remarkable return for a small investment, particularly at a time when most employers are reducing or freezing benefits. The Corporate Membership is suited for employers of varying sizes and can also be of great value to professional, social, civic, fraternal and religious associations. Castle Connolly may also be able to adapt and tailor the presentation of the database to meet the specific corporate client's needs.

For further information, contact:

Jennifer Mojave
Corporate Services Manager
212.367.8400, ext. 35
or
jmojave@castleconnolly.com

Strategic Partnerships

Castle Connolly Medical Ltd. has a number of strategic partnerships that may be of interest to consumers and physicians.

Access Medical LLC

Access Medical LLC is a diversified healthcare company that has partnered with Castle Connolly to help expand its top doctors database. Through its various resources and proprietary technologies, Access and Castle Connolly hope to build upon Castle Connolly's core nomination survey, research and selection process, thereby enabling Castle Connolly to identify 2-3 times more top doctors than it currently does.

Empowered Doctor

Empowered Doctor develops practice websites for physicians, all of whom must first be screened and vetted by Castle Connolly Medical Ltd.'s physician-led Research Department. Websites are designed for new patients to easily find the physician and request an appointment, as well as to serve as a resource for existing patients. Website features include: practice brochures; appointment and prescription refill request forms; patient intake forms; a patient education library; and a library of the latest news stories related to the physician's medical specialty.

For further information, call toll-free (866) 375-4007, or visit www.empowereddoctor.net.

Strategic Partnerships

DrScore.com

Founded by Steve Feldman, M.D., DrScore.com is an interactive online survey site where patients can rate their physicians, as well as find a physician based on their service level preference. DrScore's mission is to improve medical care by giving patients a forum for rating their physicians and by giving doctors an affordable, objective, non-intrusive means of documenting the quality of care that they provide. Visitors on Castle Connolly's website who are searching for "top doctors" have the option to also rate these and other physicians they have been to as patients, as well as to see if these physicians have been rated previously by other consumers on DrScore .com. Visitors to DrScore.com will be able to see if their doctors and/or other doctors are Castle Connolly "top doctors."

For more information, visit www.drscore.com.

America's Cosmetic Doctors Online
Castle Connolly has developed a website and database
www.AmericasCosmeticDoctors.com - to enable consumers to search and
find appropriately trained physicians for various cosmetic procedures and
treatments. The cosmetic doctors whose profiles are included on this site are
in one of only five medical specialties: Dermatology; Facial Plastic Surgery;
Ophthalmology; Otolaryngology; Plastic Surgery; or Surgery. They are
specially trained in cosmetic procedures and spend the majority of their time
in their medical practice doing cosmetic work. They are then included after a
careful review and screening by our physician-directed research team.

Valuable content on selecting the right cosmetic doctor for you, as well as
detailed information about some of the most common procedures is also
available on the site.

For more information visit www.AmericasCosmeticDoctors.com

Premium Membership at www.CastleConnolly.com
Reap the benefits of membership with Castle Connolly. Gain access to ALL
online top doctor listings and get discounts on book purchases from our
extensive catalog.

- Search among more than 23,000 Castle Connolly top doctor listings
- Search among select hospitals and centers of excellence
- Receive a 30% discount on all book purchases
- Read and print Healthcare Choice Guides
- Read and print Healthcare Advocate columns

Membership Levels:
- One year - $24.95
- Two years - $34.95

For more information, visit,
www.CastleConnolly.com/membership.index.cfm

Castle Connolly and Social Media

Castle Connolly has Facebook and Twitter accounts in an effort to keep consumers informed of the latest news at Castle Connolly Medical Ltd. Consumers who use our print guides, online database or refer to our regional magazine features can find up-to-date information about Castle Connolly by logging onto these social networking sites:

Become a Fan on Facebook (keyword: "Castle Connolly Medical ") or,

Follow us on Twitter (keyword: "CastleConnolly")

To find out more about our National Physician of the Year Award Honorees, distribution dates for our newest publications and news of Castle Connolly Top Doctors featured in local, regional and national media visit Facebook and Twitter.